Nurse's Pocket Guide

Problems, Diagnoses, Prioritized Solutions, and Rationales

SEVENTEENTH EDITION

Mary Frances Moorhouse, RN, MSN; CRRN-Retired
Nurse Consultant
TNT-RN Enterprises

Christina Baughn, DNP, RN, CNE
Assistant Professor, Adult Health Nursing
University of South Alabama College of Nursing
Fairhope, Alabama

Margaret Moore-Nadler, DNP, RN
Associate Professor Patient Education/Advocate, Community Mental Health
University of South Alabama College of Nursing-Retired
Mobile, Alabama

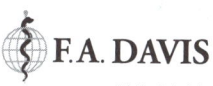

F. A. DAVIS
Philadelphia

F. A. Davis Company
1915 Arch Street
Philadelphia, PA 19103
www.fadavis.com

Copyright © 2026 by F. A. Davis Company

Copyright © 1985, 1988, 1991, 1993, 1996, 1998, 2000, 2002, 2004, 2006, 2008, 2010, 2013, 2016, 2019, 2022, 2026 by F. A. Davis Company. All rights reserved. This book is protected by copyright. No part of it may be reproduced, stored in a retrieval system, or transmitted in any form or by any means, electronic, mechanical, photocopying, recording, or otherwise, without written permission from the publisher.

Printed in the United States of America

10 9 8 7 6 5 4 3 2 1

Acquisitions Editor: Suzanne Czehut Toppy
Content Project Manager 2: Molly Shaffer
Design and Illustration Manager: Carolyn O'Brien

As new scientific information becomes available through basic and clinical research, recommended treatments and drug therapies undergo changes. The author(s) and publisher have done everything possible to make this book accurate, up to date, and in accordance with accepted standards at the time of publication. The author(s), editors, and publisher are not responsible for errors or omissions or for consequences from application of the book and make no warranty, expressed or implied, in regard to the contents of the book. Any practice described in this book should be applied by the reader in accordance with professional standards of care used in regard to the unique circumstances that may apply in each situation. The reader is advised always to check product information (package inserts) for changes and new information regarding dose and contraindications before administering any drug. Caution is especially urged when using new or infrequently ordered drugs.

Library of Congress Control Number: 2025942432

Authorization to photocopy items for internal or personal use, or the internal or personal use of specific clients, is granted by F. A. Davis Company for users registered with the Copyright Clearance Center (CCC) Transactional Reporting Service, provided that the fee of $.25 per copy is paid directly to CCC, 222 Rosewood Drive, Danvers, MA 01923. For those organizations that have been granted a photocopy license by CCC, a separate system of payment has been arranged. The fee code for users of the Transactional Reporting Service is: 978-1-7196-5036-6/26 0 + $.25.

DEDICATION

This book is dedicated to:

Our families, who helped with the mundane activities of daily living that allowed us to write this book and who provide us with love and encouragement in all our endeavors.

Our friends, who support us in our writing, put up with our memory lapses, and love us still.

Bob Martone, former Publisher, Nursing, who germinated the idea for this project so long ago.

Suzanne Toppy and Molly Shaffer, who have taken on the challenge of providing direct support and keeping us focused.

Robert Allen, who has guided us through the XML maze since the book went high tech and is a lifeline we greatly appreciate.

The F. A. Davis production staff, who coordinated and expedited the project through the editing and printing processes, meeting unreal deadlines, and sending pages to us with bated breath.

Robert H. Craven, Jr., and the F. A. Davis family, we could not have found a better company to work with.

And last and most important:

The nurses we are writing for, to those who have found the previous editions of the *Pocket Guide* helpful, and to other nurses who are looking for help to provide quality nursing care in a period of transition and change, we say, "Nursing Diagnosis is the way."

Tribute to Marilynn E. Doenges

It is an end of an era—a very long era. Marilynn Elizabeth Doenges died a few months short of her 102nd birthday. She was one of those special people who could honestly say, "Been there, done that, have the t-shirt!"

Marilynn was an Army nurse overseas at the end of WWII in Europe. While taking care of the troops, she used every free moment to travel the continent. After her return stateside, she worked in a number of nursing settings over the years while she raised a family and pursued her education, eventually becoming a psychiatric nurse specialist.

I first met Marilynn in the latter part of the 1970s, when we assisted on a project for another publisher. We had developed some material that was not used in the project, and a colleague, Mary Lisk-Jeffries, was committed to doing something with it. We received an offer from F. A. Davis, and the three of us signed our first contract on April 1, 1981—yes, April Fools'.

The project was a bigger challenge than expected. The initial attempt to use a transcriptionist was not successful, and in 1982, Marilynn became a pioneer and dived into the world of computers with an Osborne. This marvel was deemed portable, weighing only 24.5 lb, with 64K RAM, 5" monitor, and dual 5-1/4-inch floppy discs—yes really floppy! The care plans were constructed in two columns, so working on a 5" screen was a pain on multiple levels, and material lost was generally not retrievable.

Another new development was the beginning of Nursing Diagnosis. A list of titles (no definitions or guide as to how to use the labels) was obtained at a nursing conference, and the use of a standardized nursing language revolutionized the way the care plans were developed.

During the project, material was sent out for review. Two reviews were not complimentary, with one going so far as to say that "the project has merit but not with these ladies." A third review was eventually sent out, and as the partners were questioning whether to continue, the review was very favorable, and the die was cast. The combination of care plans and standardized nursing language was a huge success.

Marilynn and I were like oil and vinegar—both useful but better with a little agitation. As a critical care nurse, I tended to view the psych realm as "touchy, feely" versus my more hard science-based practice. Over time, we came to appreciate and value our different perspectives, which made our work more holistic and our care plans more inclusive, meeting the needs of the nurse and client alike.

In another pioneering moment, Marilynn opened a private counseling practice and demonstrated her commitment to standardized nursing language by using nursing diagnoses in documenting client visits and including it when billing for her services.

Receiving recognition as "Book of the Year" for several of the projects served to "doom" us to continue in this high-pressure endeavor. From a professional standpoint though, this was the highlight of Marilynn's career and brought her much joy and personal pride in sharing her work with students and professional nurses alike from around the world, including making two trips to China and holding a speaking engagement in Switzerland. In her last days, she continued to share her books with the hospice nurses caring for her—a dedicated nurse to the end.

Tribute to Alice C. Murr

How does one sum up 40 years in a few words? Forty years as a close friend, valued colleague, and indispensable writing partner.

As friends, we watched our kids grow up, and with my late husband Jan, we became the three amigos enjoying adventurous travels, great restaurants, and growing old together. We supported each other through losses and celebrated the many good times.

As colleagues, we both worked critical care, did travel nursing, and were legal nurse consultants before moving into different endeavors—Alice as a telehealth nurse and I as an adjunct nursing instructor. We had a broad range of experiences that enriched our writing. We did not always agree; however, our different perspectives allowed us a better grasp of the "big picture."

Alice and I worked well together. We needed each other to truly be successful. I stare at the blank piece of paper. Alice could throw thoughts, ideas, and research finds down and then pass them on for me to edit, rearrange, reimagine. She worked early (4 a.m.); I preferred the "evening" shift. She organized our contributors and kept an eye on the timeline. She kept it all together. Finishing this edition without her has been difficult. Fortunately, she participated in finding two talented nurses to mentor and help fill her shoes.

Alice, you were a hard worker all your life. I hope now you are peacefully enjoying a scone with your cup of tea and proud of your contribution to us all and to the profession of nursing.

Thank you to Mary F. Jeffries

Last, I'd like to take a moment to remember our first partner—Mary Frances Jeffries, who was the catalyst for beginning this incredible journey. She lived long enough to see how timely and successful that project was and how beneficial her idea of using standardized nursing language was. A heartfelt thank you to Mary for her vision.

ACKNOWLEDGMENTS

A special acknowledgment to Marilynn's friend, the late Diane Camillone, who provoked an awareness of the role of the patient and continues to influence our thoughts about the importance of quality nursing care, and to our late colleague, Mary Jeffries, who started us on this journey and introduced us to nursing diagnoses.

To our colleagues at NANDA International and the International Council of Nurses, who continue to formulate and refine nursing diagnoses to provide nursing with the tools to enhance and promote the growth of the profession.

Mary Frances Moorhouse
Christina Baughn
Margaret Moore-Nadler

CONTRIBUTORS

Our heartfelt thanks to our collaborators over the years. Your contributions made everything easier for us.

Christina Liebrecht, DNP, RN, CNE
Professor of Nursing, Chair of Health & Exercise Professions
Ohio Northern University
Ada, Ohio

CONTENTS

Health Conditions and Client Concerns appear on pages 1069–1196.

How to Use the Nurse's Pocket Guide xi

CHAPTER 1
The Nursing Process, Clinical Judgment, and Planning Client Care 1

CHAPTER 2
Nursing Diagnoses/Problems in Alphabetical Order 5
  For each nursing diagnosis, the following information is provided:
  Diagnostic Division
  Definition
  Recognizing Cues
    Related/Risk Factors
    Defining Characteristics: Subjective/Objective
    Clinical Connections
  Generate Solutions
    Plan Desired Outcomes
  Interventions/Take Action
    Nursing Priorities
  Documentation Focus
  Sample Nursing Outcomes & Nursing Interventions
    Classifications (NOC/NIC)

CHAPTER 3
Health Conditions and Client Concerns 1069

CHAPTER 4
Using Clinical Judgment to Create Client Plan of Care 1197
  Adult Medical/Surgical Assessment Tool 1198
    Diagnostic Divisions: Index of Nursing Diagnoses Included in This Text Organized According to a Nursing Focus 1205
  Using Tools and Engaging Clinical Judgment 1211
    Client Situation and Prototype Plan of Care 1212
    Plan of Care for Mr. R. S. with Diabetes Mellitus 1219
    Another Approach to Planning Client Care-Mind or Concept Mapping 1229

Bibliography (See FADavis.com)

Index 1231

HOW TO USE THE NURSE'S POCKET GUIDE

The American Nurses Association (ANA) *Social Policy Statement* of 1980 was the first to define nursing as the diagnosis and treatment of human responses to actual and potential health problems. This definition, when combined with the ANA *Standards of Practice*, provided impetus and support for the use of nursing diagnosis. Defining *nursing* and its effect on client care supports the growing awareness that nursing care is a key factor in client survival and in the maintenance, rehabilitative, and preventive aspects of healthcare. Changes and new developments in healthcare delivery in the past 40 years have given rise to the need for a common framework of communication to ensure continuity of care for the client moving between multiple healthcare settings and providers. Evaluation and documentation of care are important parts of this process.

This book is designed to aid the practitioner and student nurse in identifying interventions commonly associated with specific nursing diagnoses as proposed by NANDA International (NANDA-I) and the International Classification for Nursing Practice (ICNP). These interventions are the activities needed to implement and document care provided to the individual client and can be used in varied settings from acute to community/home care.

Chapter 1 presents a brief discussion of the nursing process, data collection, and care plan construction. Chapter 4 contains tools for choosing nursing diagnoses, an Adult Assessment Tool, and the Diagnostic Divisions list putting theory into practice with a sample assessment database and a corresponding plan of care. A mind or concept map is also provided. For more in-depth information and inclusive plans of care related to specific medical or psychiatric conditions, and maternal/newborn care (with rationale and the application of the diagnoses), the nurse is referred to the larger work, published by the F. A. Davis Company: *Nursing Care Plans: Guidelines for Individualizing Client Care Across the Life Span*, ed. 11 (Doenges, Moorhouse, Murr, Baughn, & Moore–Nadler, 2025). For nursing diagnoses and interventions with evidence-based citations, refer to the more in-depth work published by the F. A. Davis Company: *Nursing Diagnosis Manual: Identifying Problems and Individualizing Care*, ed. 8 (Moorhouse, Baughn, & Moore-Nadler, 2026).

Nursing diagnoses are listed alphabetically in Chapter 2 for ease of reference and include the diagnoses accepted for use by NANDA-I (2024–2026) and the International Council of Nurses (2019).* Each diagnosis includes a definition and cues to recognize, which include information divided into the categories of Risk/Related Factors and Defining Characteristics. Risk/Related Factors information reflects causative or contributing factors that can be useful for determining whether the diagnosis is applicable to a particular client. Defining Characteristics (signs and symptoms) are listed as subjective and/or objective and are used to confirm problem-focused diagnoses or readiness for enhanced diagnoses, aid in Generating Solutions to formulate outcomes, and provide additional data for choosing appropriate interventions. Clinical Connections have been included here to provide some suggested healthcare conditions/situations where the identified nursing diagnosis/problem could be used. The authors have not deleted or altered the nursing diagnosis information; however, on occasion, they have added to their definitions or suggested additional criteria to provide clarification and direction. These additions are denoted with brackets [ ].

The ANA, in conjunction with NANDA-I, proposed that specific nursing diagnoses currently approved and structured according to Taxonomy II Revised be included in the *International Classification of Diseases* (*ICD*) within the section "Family of Health-Related Classifications." Although the World Health Organization did not accept this initial proposal because of lack of documentation of the usefulness of nursing diagnoses at the international level, the NANDA-I list as well as the International Classification for Nursing Practice have been accepted by SNOMED (Systemized Nomenclature of Medicine) for inclusion in its international coding system and is included in the Unified Medical Language System of the National Library of Medicine. (Today, nurse researchers from around the world have submitted new nursing diagnoses and are validating current diagnoses in support for resubmission and acceptance of the NANDA-I list in future editions of the *ICD*.)

The authors have chosen to categorize the list of nursing diagnoses used in this text into Diagnostic Divisions, which is the framework for an assessment tool designed to assist the nurse to readily identify an appropriate nursing diagnosis from data collected and cues recognized during the assessment process. The Diagnostic Division label is listed under each nursing diagnosis heading.

Desired Outcomes are identified to assist the nurse in formulating individual client outcomes and to support the evaluation process.

Interventions/Actions in this pocket guide are primarily directed to adult care settings (although general age-span considerations are included) and are listed according to nursing priorities. Some solutions/actions require collaborative or interdependent orders (e.g., medical, psychiatric), and the nurse will need to determine when this is necessary and take appropriate action.

The inclusion of Documentation Focus suggestions is to remind the nurse of the importance and necessity of recording the steps of the nursing process.

Finally, in recognition of the ongoing work of numerous researchers over the past 35 years, the authors have referenced the Nursing Interventions and Outcomes labels developed by the Iowa Intervention Projects (Wagner et al.; Moorhead et al.). These groups have been classifying nursing interventions and outcomes to predict resource requirements and measure outcomes, thereby meeting the needs of a standardized language that can be coded for computer and reimbursement purposes. As an introduction to this work in progress, sample NIC and NOC labels have been included under the heading Sample Nursing Interventions & Outcomes Classifications at the conclusion of each nursing diagnosis section. The reader is referred to the various publications by Cheryl Wagner and Sue Moorhead for more in-depth information.

Chapter 3 presents more than 400 disorders/health conditions reflecting all specialty areas, with recognized cues that would likely be found in a specific Diagnostic Division of the assessment tool, and a corresponding nursing concept is suggested. After reviewing the Diagnostic Division and using the recognized cues to identify a nursing diagnosis label for the client problem, a client diagnostic statement can be written with the "related to" and "evidenced by" components, as appropriate. This section will facilitate and help validate the assessment and problem or needed identification steps of the nursing process.

We have chosen to use a variety of nursing languages and have incorporated the diagnoses and problems that we believe are most relevant to nursing education and clinical application. These languages include NANDA-I classification of nursing diagnoses, the Iowa Intervention and Outcome Projects: Nursing Interventions Classification (NIC), and the Nursing Outcomes Classification (NOC). We also include the International Classification for Nursing Practice (ICNP), which contains diagnoses, outcomes, and interventions. We believe that this approach will expose students to multiple standardized nursing languages that they may encounter during their career, thereby broadening their understanding of the nursing process, nursing diagnosis, and client problems.

As noted, with few exceptions, we presented NANDA-I's and the International Council of Nurses recommendations as formulated. In order to make safe and effective judgments using nursing diagnoses, it is essential that nurses refer to the definitions, related/risk factors, and defining characteristics of the diagnoses listed in this work. The authors have selected a portion of the nursing diagnoses from the current NANDA-I and ICNP terminology to use in the edition, which they believe are most relevant to nursing education. We support the belief that practicing nurses and researchers need to study, use, and evaluate the diagnoses as presented. Nurses can be creative as they use the standardized language, redefining and sharing information as the diagnoses are used with individual clients. Medical and nursing terminologies continue to evolve. As we developed this edition, we use the term chestfeeding in certain monographs, and breastfeeding in others reflecting the standardized nursing language provided. These terms are used throughout the text, and we encourage students and clinicians to use the term that their individual clients identify with. As new nursing diagnoses are developed, it is important that the data they encompass are added to assessment tools and current databases. As part of the process by clinicians, educators, and researchers across practice specialties and academic settings to define, test, and refine nursing diagnosis, nurses are encouraged to share insights and ideas with NANDA-I online (https://nanda.org/connect-engage/committees-task-forces/diagnosis-development/) or the International Council of Nurses at icnp@icn.ch.

---

*T. Heather Herdman/Shigemi Kamitsuru/Camila Takáo Lopes (Eds.), NANDA International, Inc.: Nursing Diagnoses: Definitions and Classification 2024–2026, Thirteenth Edition. © 2024 NANDA International, ISBN 978-1-68420-601-8. Used by arrangement with the Thieme Group, Stuttgart/New York.

International Council of Nurses International Classification for Nursing Practice. (2019). Version 2, Geneva, Switzerland.

CHAPTER 1

The Nursing Process, Clinical Judgment, and Planning Client Care

The Nursing Process

Nursing is both a science and an art concerned with the physical, psychological, sociological, cultural, and spiritual concerns of the individual receiving care. The science of nursing is based on a broad theoretical framework; its art depends on the caring skills and abilities of the individual nurse.

The nursing profession continues work to formally define what nurses do and what makes nursing unique, leading to a body of professional knowledge distinctive to nursing practice. A significant portion of defining the work of nursing has involved the establishment of a commonality of terminology or standardization of nursing language. Although several standardized nursing languages have been developed, the nursing diagnoses most commonly used today are the NANDA-I and International Classification for Nursing Practice (ICNP) nursing diagnoses (see Chapter 4 page 1197).*

In 1980, the American Nurses Association (ANA) defined nursing as "the diagnosis and treatment of human responses to actual or potential health problems." As the nursing profession has evolved, the definition of nursing has been expanded to reflect that growth—"nursing is the protection, promotion, and optimization of health and abilities, prevention of illness and injury, alleviation of suffering through the diagnosis and treatment of human responses, and advocacy in the care of individuals, families, communities, and populations" (ANA, 2003, p. 6).

Nursing process is patterned after the scientific method of observing, measuring, gathering data, and analyzing findings. This process incorporates an interactive and interpersonal approach with a problem-solving and decision-making

---

* As this edition was going to press, NANDA International announced that it would be undergoing a rebranding and renaming of the organization to The International Nursing Knowledge Association, but that nursing diagnoses and their definitions would still be known under the NANDA-I name.

process (King, 1971; Peplau, 1952; Yura & Walsh, 1988). Shore (1988) described the nursing process as "combining the most desirable elements of the art of nursing with the most relevant elements of systems theory, using the scientific method." It can be applied in any healthcare or educational setting, in any theoretical or conceptual framework, and within the context of any nursing theory. Therefore, because nursing process is the basis of all nursing action, we believe that it is the essence of nursing.

The five steps of the nursing process are (1) assessment—systematically gathering data, sorting and organizing the collected data, recognizing cues, and documenting the data in a retrievable format; (2) diagnosis—analyzing the recognized cues to identify the client's needs or problems; (3) planning/generating solutions—setting priorities, establishing goals, identifying desired client outcomes, and determining specific nursing interventions; (4) implementation/taking action—putting the plan of care into action and performing the planned interventions; and (5) evaluation—determining the client's progress toward attaining the identified outcomes and monitoring the client's response to and effectiveness of the selected nursing interventions. While the nursing process is the template for the work of nursing, clinical judgment is required to make it operational.

Using Clinical Judgment to Plan Care

The identification of client problems/needs is the cornerstone for the plan of care. We support that healthcare providers have a responsibility for planning care along with the client, with a goal toward the eventual outcome of an optimal state of wellness or a dignified death. Client-centered care engages the client in responsibility for their own care while helping to ensure that nursing interventions are timely and appropriate.

Creating a plan of care begins with the collection of data (assessment). The database consists of subjective and objective client information. Clinical judgment is used to determine what data needs to be collected and the analysis of the collected data leads to the identification of cues used to diagnose problems or areas of concern (including health promotion) specific to the client. These problems or needs are expressed as nursing diagnoses (NDs). To facilitate the diagnosis process, the authors have divided the NDs into Diagnostic Divisions (Chapter 4). A sample assessment tool is also provided, designed to assist the nurse to identify appropriate NDs as the data are collected.

When the needs are identified, nursing diagnoses are categorized as (1) *problem-focused* NDs; (2) *risk* NDs, which could develop due to specific vulnerabilities of the client; (3) *health promotion* NDs, which reflect a client's desire to improve their well-being; or (4) *syndrome* NDs, which reflect a specific cluster of NDs that occur together and are best addressed together and through similar interventions.

It is the belief of the authors that the majority of problem diagnoses can also be reframed and stated as a risk for or readiness for enhanced diagnosis.

Generating solutions by setting goals and choosing appropriate nursing interventions is also essential to the construction of a plan of care and the delivery of quality nursing care. Desired outcomes are the incremental steps formulated to give direction to and evaluate effectiveness of the care provided in achieving broader goals. Interventions, or actions are those activities that the nurse, client, and/or significant others perform to promote the client's movement toward achieving the desired outcomes. Clinical judgment is required to determine meaningful outcomes for the client and to choose appropriate actions to accomplish the outcomes.

An individualized client diagnostic statement can be formulated using the problem, etiology, and signs and symptoms (PES) format by combining the ND label (problem) with the individual's specific related factors (etiology) and defining characteristics (signs/symptoms) or risk factors when present. The resulting client diagnostic statement accurately represents the client's current situation, providing direction for nursing care.

Once the plan of care is put into action, changes in client needs must be continually monitored, because care is provided in a dynamic environment, and flexibility is required to allow changing circumstances. Periodic review of the client's responses to nursing interventions and progress toward attaining desired outcomes helps to determine the effectiveness of the plan of care. Based on findings, the plan may need to be modified, referrals to other resources may be required, or the client may be ready for discharge from the care setting.

Properly written and applied plans of care can save time by providing direction for continuity of care and by facilitating communication among nurses and other caregivers. The format for recording the plan of care is determined by agency policy; it may be handwritten or computer generated and may utilize standardized forms as with clinical pathways.

Ongoing changes in healthcare delivery and computerization of client records require a commonality of communication across clinical settings. By way of example, whereas a medical diagnosis of diabetes mellitus is the same label used for all individuals with this condition, the nursing diagnostic statement is individualized to reflect a specific client need or response.

We use the NANDA-I and the International Council of Nurses (ICNP) nursing diagnoses labels to define the client's responses to diabetes. For example, the diagnostic statement for a diabetic wound may read, "adult Pressure Injury related to surface friction, pressure over bony prominence as evidenced by tissue damage partial thickness loss of dermis, pain 4–5/10 at pressure point, draining wound left heel."

The plan of care not only is the end product of the nursing process, but it also documents client care in areas of accountability, quality assurance, and liability. It not only guides the nurse actively caring for the client (determining client's needs [NDs], goals/outcomes, and actions to be taken) but also substantiates the care provided for review by third-party payers, legal entities, and accreditation agencies. Therefore, the plan of care is a critical and permanent part of the client's healthcare record.

In Chapter 4, a sample scenario provides an opportunity to review a client assessment, the cues used to choose client problems/needs, and generate solutions. An alternate form of creating and documenting client care—a Mind Map is presented.

CHAPTER 2

Nursing Diagnoses/Problems in Alphabetical Order

ACTIVITY INTOLERANCE — ICNP

[Diagnostic Division: Activity/Rest]

Definition: Insufficient physical or mental energy to effectively perform the necessary or desired activities of daily living.

Recognizing Cues

Related/Risk Factors
Decreased muscle strength/muscle mass
Decreased physical endurance; physical deconditioning; sedentary lifestyle
Depressive symptoms
Pain
Imbalance between oxygen supply/demand
Malnutrition; overweight
Side effects of medication (e.g., beta blockers, antihistamines), substance misuse

Defining Characteristics

Subjective
Fatigue; generalized weakness
Exertional discomfort; dyspnea
Dizziness; headache; nausea

Objective
Abnormal heart rate or blood pressure in response to activity; orthostatic vital sign changes
Electrocardiogram change (e.g., arrhythmia, conduction abnormality, ischemia)

Clinical Connections
Neoplasms, neurodegenerative conditions, traumatic brain injury, myalgic encephalomyelitis/chronic fatigue syndrome (ME/CFS), respiratory disorders (e.g., pneumonia, chronic obstructive pulmonary disease), malnutrition, overweight,

cardiovascular disease (e.g., angina, aortic or mitral stenosis, heart failure, pericarditis, history of rheumatic fever), peripheral vascular disease, immunological dysfunction (e.g., HIV/AIDS, leukemias, thrombocytopenia), diabetes mellitus, anemia, failure to thrive, frailty

Functional Level Classification (Gordon, 2014):

Level I: Walk, regular pace, on level indefinitely; climb one flight or more but more short of breath than normal

Level II: Walk one city block [or] 500 ft on level; climb one flight slowly without stopping

Level III: Walk no more than 50 ft on level without stopping; unable to climb one flight of stairs without stopping

Level IV: Dyspnea and fatigue at rest

Generate Solutions

Plan Desired Outcomes

Client Will (Include Specific Time Frame)

- Identify negative factors affecting activity tolerance and eliminate or reduce their effects when possible.
- Use identified techniques to enhance activity tolerance.
- Participate willingly in necessary/desired activities.
- Report measurable increase in activity tolerance.
- Demonstrate a decrease in physiological signs of intolerance (e.g., pulse, respirations, and blood pressure remain within client's normal range).

Interventions/Take Action

Nursing Priority No. 1.

To identify causative/precipitating factors:

- Note presence of acute or chronic illness, such as heart failure, pulmonary disorders, hypothyroidism, diabetes mellitus, AIDS, malnutrition, anemias, stroke, cancers, moderate to severe brain injury, acute and chronic pain, early or delayed symptoms associated with recent viral diseases such as SARS and COVID-19 coronaviruses, hospital/facility-acquired deconditioning, ventilator-induced diaphragmatic dysfunction, and pregnancy-induced hypertension. **Many factors can cause or contribute to fatigue, having potential to interfere with client's ability to perform at a desired level of**

Information that appears in brackets has been added by the authors to clarify and enhance the use of nursing diagnoses.

 Acute Care 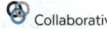 Collaborative 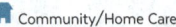 Community/Home Care Cultural activity. However, "activity intolerance" implies that the client cannot endure or adapt to increased energy or oxygen demands caused by an activity. (Refer to ND Fatigue.)

- Ask client/significant other (SO) about usual level of energy **to identify potential problems and/or client's/SO's perception of client's energy and ability to perform needed or desired activities.**
- Evaluate client's actual and perceived limitations and severity of deficit in light of usual status. **Provides a comparative baseline and information about needed education or interventions regarding quality of life (QOL).**
- Identify factors, such as age, functional decline, client resistive to efforts, painful conditions, breathing problems, vision or hearing impairments, climate or weather, unsafe areas to exercise, and need for mobility assistance, **that could block/affect the desired level of activity.**
- Note client reports of weakness, fatigue, pain, difficulty accomplishing tasks, and/or insomnia. **Symptoms may be a result of or contribute to intolerance of activity.**
- Assess cardiopulmonary response to physical activity, including vital signs, before, during, and after activity. Note accelerating fatigue. **Dramatic changes in heart rate and rhythm, changes in usual blood pressure, and progressively worsening fatigue result from an imbalance of oxygen supply and demand.**
- Assess for chest discomfort or tightness, dyspnea, severe cough, dizziness, headache, blurred vision, palpitations, excessive sweating, and instability. **These changes are potentially greater in the frail older adult population.**
- Ascertain the client's ability to stand and move about and the degree of assistance necessary or use of equipment **to determine current status and needs associated with participation in needed/desired activities.**
- Identify activity needs versus desires **to evaluate appropriateness (e.g., is barely able to walk upstairs but would like to play tennis).**
- Assess emotional and psychological factors affecting the current situation **(e.g., stress and/or depression may be increasing the effects of an illness, or depression might be the result of forced inactivity).**
- Note treatment-related factors, such as medication side effects and interactions. **For example, medications such as vasodilators, diuretics, or beta blockers can cause**

Information that appears in brackets has been added by the authors to clarify and enhance the use of nursing diagnoses.

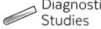 Diagnostic Studies   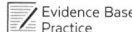 Evidence Based Practice   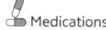 Medications   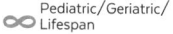 Pediatric/Geriatric/Lifespan

orthostatic hypotension with activity due to vasodilation, fluid shifts (diuresis), or compromised cardiac pumping function.

- Determine client's current activity level and physical condition with observation, exercise-capacity testing, or use of a functional-level classification system (e.g., Gordon's Functional Level Classification), as appropriate. **Provides a baseline for comparison, an opportunity to track changes, and enhanced care communication between the nurse, the client, and the care team.**

Nursing Priority No. 2.

To assist client to deal with contributing factors and manage activities within individual limits:

- Monitor vital and cognitive signs, watching for changes in blood pressure, heart rate, and respiratory rate; note skin pallor and/or cyanosis and presence of confusion with activity.
- Reduce intensity level or discontinue activities that cause undesired physiological changes **to prevent overexertion.**
- Provide and monitor response to supplemental oxygen, medications, and changes in treatment regimen.
- Increase exercise/activity levels gradually. **Current guidelines "recommend that adults (who do not have contraindications to exercise) should do at least 150 to 300 minutes per week of moderate-intensity aerobic physical activity, or at least 75 to 150 minutes per week of vigorous (higher)-intensity aerobic physical activity, or an equivalent combination of moderate- and vigorous-intensity aerobic activity." The use of step counters or digital fitness applications may be helpful in decreasing sedentary time and increasing lifestyle activities. Additionally, resistance training activities are recommended at least 2 days a week. Resistance training improves muscular strength, functional capacity, and QOL.**
- Teach methods to conserve energy and increase activity, such as stopping to rest for 3 min during a 10-min walk or sitting down to brush hair instead of standing. **Gradual increase in activity avoids excessive myocardial workload and associated oxygen demand and has been shown to exert positive health benefits, even in those with chronic diseases. In clients with chronic coronary disease, those who participate in cardiac rehabilitation have significantly better outcomes compared with those who do not participate,**

Information that appears in brackets has been added by the authors to clarify and enhance the use of nursing diagnoses.

 Acute Care   Collaborative 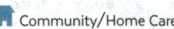 Community/Home Care   Cultural

including lower cardiovascular mortality rates, lower rehospitalization rates (total, cardiovascular, and non-cardiovascular), and improved QOL. Evidence suggests participation in cardiac rehabilitation may also improve symptom control, functional capacity, and QOL in patients with a variety of cardiac diseases or dysfunction.
- Plan care to balance rest periods with activities **to reduce fatigue.**
- Provide positive atmosphere while acknowledging the difficulty of the situation for the client. **Helps to minimize frustration and rechannel energy.**
- Encourage expression of feelings contributing to or resulting from the condition. **Acknowledging difficulty of situation can help reduce client's/SO's frustration and rechannel energy.**
- Involve client/SO(s) in planning activities as much as possible. **May give client opportunity to perform desired or essential activities during periods of peak energy.**
- Assist with activities and provide/monitor client's use of assistive devices (e.g., crutches, walker, wheelchair, oxygen tank) **to protect client from injury.**
- Administer supplemental oxygen, medications; prepare for surgery and other treatments, as indicated. **Type of therapy or medication is dependent on the underlying condition and might include medications (e.g., antiarrhythmics, short- and long-acting bronchodilators) or surgery (e.g., stents or coronary artery bypass graft) to improve breathing or myocardial perfusion and systemic circulation. Other treatments might include iron preparations or blood transfusion to treat severe anemia or use of oxygen during activities.**
- Promote comfort measures and provide for relief of pain **to enhance ability to participate in activities.** (Refer to NDs acute Pain; chronic Pain.)
- Provide referral to other disciplines, such as exercise physiologist, psychological counseling/therapy, occupational/physical therapists, and recreation/leisure specialists, as indicated, **to develop individually appropriate therapeutic program.**

Nursing Priority No. 3.

To promote maximum activity (Teaching/Discharge Considerations) and enhance well-being (long-term goals):

- Discuss with client/SO(s) the relationship between illness or debilitating condition and the ability to perform desired

---

Information that appears in brackets has been added by the authors to clarify and enhance the use of nursing diagnoses.

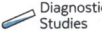 Diagnostic Studies 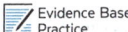 Evidence Based Practice 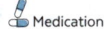 Medications 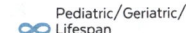 Pediatric/Geriatric/Lifespan

activities. **Understanding this relationship can help with acceptance of limitations or reveal opportunity for changes of practical value.**
- Assist client/SO(s) with planning for changes that may become necessary, such as use of supplemental oxygen, **to improve the client's ability to participate in desired activities.**
- Plan for maximal activity within the client's ability. **Promotes the idea of normalcy of progressive abilities in this area.**
- Review expectations of client/SO(s)/providers **to establish individual goals.** Explore conflicts and differences **to reach agreement for the most effective plan.**
- Instruct client/SO(s) in monitoring response to activity and in recognizing signs/symptoms that **indicate need to alter activity level.**
- Plan for progressive increase of activity level/participation in exercise training, as tolerated by client. **Both activity tolerance and health status may improve with progressive training.**
- Give client information that provides evidence of daily/weekly progress **to sustain motivation.**
- Assist client in learning and demonstrating appropriate safety measures **to prevent injuries.**
- Identify and discuss symptoms for which the client needs to seek medical assistance/evaluation, **providing for timely intervention.**
- Provide information about the effect of lifestyle on activity tolerance (e.g., nutrition, adequate fluid intake, getting sufficient rest and sleep, exercise, smoking cessation, and mental health status). **Many of these factors may be amenable to modification, thus reducing risk factors and promoting health.**
- Collaborate with dietician for information about proper nutrition to meet metabolic and energy needs, obtaining or maintaining normal body weight as indicated. **Energy is improved when nutrients are sufficient to meet metabolic demands. Unintentional weight loss may be a significant predictor of unfavorable client outcomes, including decline in activities of daily living, increased hospital complications, nursing home admission, poorer QOL, and overall functional decline.**
- Encourage client to maintain a positive attitude; suggest use of relaxation techniques, such as visualization or guided imagery, as appropriate, **to enhance sense of well-being.**

Information that appears in brackets has been added by the authors to clarify and enhance the use of nursing diagnoses.

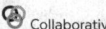
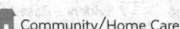

- Encourage participation in recreation, social activities, and hobbies appropriate for situation. (Refer to ND decreased Diversional Activity Engagement.)
- Refer to appropriate resources for assistance and/or equipment, as needed, **to sustain activity level.**
- Monitor laboratory values (such as for anemia) and pulse oximetry **to identify areas of concern that may require further assessment or intervention.**

Documentation Focus

Assessment/Reassessment
- Level of activity as noted in Functional Level Classification
- Causative, precipitating, or risk factors
- Client reports of fatigue or change in activity
- Vital signs before, during, and following activity

Planning
- Plan of care and who is involved in planning
- Treatment options, including physical therapy or exercise program; other assistive therapies and devices
- Lifestyle changes that are planned, who is to be responsible for each action, and monitoring methods

Implementation/Evaluation
- Response to interventions, teaching, and actions performed
- Implemented changes to plan of care based on assessment/reassessment findings
- Teaching plan and understanding of material presented
- Attainment of or progress toward desired outcome(s)

Discharge Planning
- Referrals to other resources
- Long-term needs and who is responsible for actions

Sample Nursing Outcomes & Interventions Classifications NOC/NIC

NOC—Activity Tolerance
NIC—Energy Management

ACUTE SUBSTANCE WITHDRAWAL SYNDROME **NANDA-I**

Definition: Serious, multifactorial sequelae following abrupt cessation of an addictive compound.

Information that appears in brackets has been added by the authors to clarify and enhance the use of nursing diagnoses.

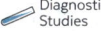 Diagnostic Studies   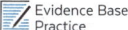 Evidence Based Practice   Medications   Pediatric/Geriatric/Lifespan

Recognizing Cues

Related/Risk Factors
Developed dependence to addictive substances
Inadequate knowledge of consequences of sudden cessation of addictive substance

Defining Characteristics

Subjective
Impaired physical comfort

Objective
Acute confusion
Excessive anxiety
Ineffective sleep pattern
Inadequate protein energy nutritional intake
Risk for physical injury

Clinical Connections
Alcohol intoxication, drug overdose

Generate Solutions

Plan Desired Outcomes

Client Will (Include Specific Time Frame)
- Be free of adverse reactions to withdrawal (e.g., stable vital signs, alert and oriented, with no cardiac dysrhythmias, electrolyte imbalance, hallucinations, or seizures).
- Commit to cessation of substance(s) used.
- Engage in behaviors/lifestyle changes to eliminate substance use.
- Use available personal, professional, and community resources.
- Manage own activities of daily living, including work/school schedule.
- Engage in appropriate social interactions.

Interventions/Take Action

Nursing Priority No. 1.
To determine degree or risk of impairment/compromise:
- Determine substance(s) taken, amount and time of last dosing, where possible. **Various drug classes have characteristic symptoms and withdrawal timelines. For example, opioids (e.g., heroin, certain prescription painkillers)**

Information that appears in brackets has been added by the authors to clarify and enhance the use of nursing diagnoses.

generally begin 8 to 24 hr after last use and last an average of 4 to 10 days; the first signs of alcohol withdrawal may appear within several hours after the last drink and peak over the course of 24 to 48 hr.

- Determine likelihood of withdrawal from two or more substances. Review toxicology results of urine and blood **to determine substances used, necessary interventions, and potential complications. Note: Symptoms and timing of occurrence depend on type of substance(s) used and last dose.**
- Identify comorbidities—medical conditions/psychiatric disorders and currently prescribed medications. **Underlying conditions are compounded by withdrawal, suggesting additional testing, monitoring, and potential treatment needs.**
- Determine if naloxone (Narcan) was administered, how many times, and time of last dose. **Used to reverse opioid overdose, but duration of action of some opioids may exceed that of Narcan, requiring repeat doses.**
- Assess level of consciousness, ability to speak, and response to commands. **Speech may be garbled, confused, or slurred. Response to commands may reveal inability to concentrate, impaired judgment, or muscle coordination deficits.**
- Determine stage of alcohol withdrawal syndrome (AWS) using Clinical Institute Withdrawal Assessment for Alcohol–Revised (CIWA-Ar) tool. **AWS usually begins 3 to 36 hr after last drink. Helps determine appropriate care setting and specific interventions. Note: The Prediction of Alcohol Withdrawal Severity Scale (PAWSS) has been found to have excellent predictive value helping clinicians identify those at risk for complicated AWS and allowing for prevention and timely treatment.**
- Observe for behavioral responses such as hyperactivity, disorientation, confusion, hallucinations, excitability, anger, sleeplessness. **Hyperactivity related to CNS disturbances may escalate rapidly. Sleep deprivation may aggravate disorientation or confusion. Progression of symptoms may indicate impending hallucinations or delirium tremens (DTs) in alcohol withdrawal.**
- Auscultate breath sounds, noting adventitious sounds such as rhonchi, wheezes, crackles. **Client is at risk for atelectasis related to hypoventilation and pneumonia.**

Information that appears in brackets has been added by the authors to clarify and enhance the use of nursing diagnoses.

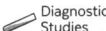 Diagnostic Studies 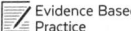 Evidence Based Practice 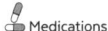 Medications Pediatric/Geriatric/Lifespan

- Review chest x-ray, arterial blood gas (ABG), or pulse oximetry. **Respiratory compromise (e.g., right lower lobe pneumonia) is common in alcohol-debilitated clients and is often due to chronic aspiration.**
- Measure weight and compare to usual weight and norms for age and body size. Note skin turgor, status of mucous membranes, muscle tone/wasting, presence of edema. **Substance abuse is often associated with malnutrition.**
- Review serum nutritional studies (e.g., albumin, transferrin, prealbumin, iron, liver function, electrolytes, hemoglobin, hematocrit). **Substance users are often malnourished, impacting organ function, energy/endurance level, immune status, general well-being.**

Nursing Priority No. 2.

To facilitate safe withdrawal from substance, when occurring:

- Consult with physician, medical toxicologist, or regional poison control center as needed. **Useful resources for diagnosis and management of acute/critically ill clients, especially those with multisubstance use.**
- Provide environmental safety (e.g., bed in low position, call device within reach, doors full open or closed position, padded side rails, family member or sitter at bedside), as indicated and appropriate.
- Monitor vital signs (VS) and level of consciousness (LOC) frequently during acute withdrawal. **VS and LOC can be labile based on specific substance(s) and length of time since last used.**
- Elevate head of bed. **Decreases potential for aspiration and lowers diaphragm, enhancing lung expansion.**
- Monitor respiratory rate, depth, and pattern. **Toxicity levels may change rapidly (e.g., hyperventilation common during acute alcohol withdrawal phase), or marked respiratory depression can occur because of CNS depressant effects of substance used.**
- Administer supplemental oxygen, as needed. **Hypoxia may occur with respiratory depression and chronic anemia.**
- Monitor body temperature. **Elevation may occur because of sympathetic stimulation, dehydration, and/or infection, causing vasodilation and compromising venous return and cardiac output.**
- Record intake/output, 24-hr fluid balance, skin turgor, status of mucous membranes. **Preexisting dehydration, nausea/vomiting, diuresis, and diaphoresis may compromise**

Information that appears in brackets has been added by the authors to clarify and enhance the use of nursing diagnoses.

 Acute Care 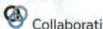 Collaborative 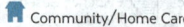 Community/Home Care Cultural

- cardiovascular function as well as renal perfusion, impacting drug clearance.
- Administer fluid/electrolytes as indicated. **Depending on substances used, client is susceptible to excessive fluid losses and electrolyte imbalances, especially losses of potassium and magnesium that can result in life-threatening dysrhythmias or seizures.**
- Reorient frequently to person, place, time, and surrounding environment. **May have calming effect and limit misinterpretation of external stimuli.**
- Encourage client to verbalize anxiety. Explain substance withdrawal increases anxiety and uneasiness. **Anxiety may be physiologically or environmentally caused, and client may be unable to identify and/or accept what is happening. Note: Individuals with alcohol use disorders often also have post-traumatic stress disorder (PTSD).**
- Monitor for suicidal tendencies. **May need to use emergency commitments or legal hold for client's safety once medically stable.**
- Provide symptom management as indicated. **Medications for nausea/vomiting, anxiety, trembling/"shakes," insomnia, seizure activity promote comfort and facilitate recovery.**
- Administer medications treating specific substance(s) used. **For example, for alcohol withdrawal, benzodiazepines, barbiturates, propofol, and ethanol may be used. Note: Beta-adrenergic blockers may speed up the alcohol withdrawal process but are not useful in preventing seizures or DTs. Acamprosate, disulfiram, and naltrexone can be used after the acute withdrawal phase to help avoid or limit alcohol use. Other drugs, such as methadone, buprenorphine, and naltrexone are used to assist opioid withdrawal. Note: There are no U.S. Food and Drug Administration–approved medications for treating cannabis, cocaine, or methamphetamine withdrawal, and medication-assisted treatments (MATs) are rarely used to treat adolescent alcohol use (Medications, Counseling, and Related Conditions, 2024).**
- Administer thiamine, vitamins C and B complex as indicated. **Vitamin deficiency, especially thiamine, is associated with ataxia, loss of eye movement and pupillary response, palpitations, postural hypotension, and exertional dyspnea.**

Information that appears in brackets has been added by the authors to clarify and enhance the use of nursing diagnoses.

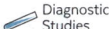 Diagnostic Studies   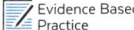 Evidence Based Practice   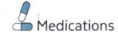 Medications   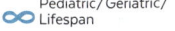 Pediatric/Geriatric/Lifespan

Nursing Priority No. 3.

To promote long-term sobriety:

- Develop trusting relationship; project an accepting attitude about substance use. **Provides client with a sense of humanness, helping to decrease paranoia and distrust. (Client will be able to detect biased or condescending attitude of caregivers, negatively impacting relationship.)**
- Determine understanding of current situation. **Provides information about degree of denial, acceptance of personal responsibility, and commitment to change.**
- Use motivational interviewing in controlled setting when client sufficiently recovered from withdrawal to address addiction issues. **Client is more likely to contract for treatment while still hurting from last substance use episode.**
- Identify use of defensive behaviors—denial, projection, and rationalization. **Helps client recognize the reality of the problems as they exist.**
- Identify individual triggers for substance use (e.g., exhaustion, loneliness/isolation, depression) and client's plans for living without drugs/alcohol. **Provides opportunity to discuss substance tension-reducing strategies and to develop and refine plan.**
- Use interventions based on client's stage of readiness for change to encourage desired behaviors. **Attempting interventions prior to readiness will be met with resistance.**
- Instruct in use of relaxation skills, guided imagery, and visualization techniques. **Helps client relax and develop new ways to deal with stress and to problem-solve.**
- Facilitate visit by a group member/possible sponsor as appropriate, such as Alcoholics Anonymous (AA), Narcotics Anonymous (NA), Crystal Methamphetamine Anonymous (CMA), Smart Recovery. **Puts client in direct contact with support system necessary for managing sobriety and drug-free life.**
- Administer antipsychotic medications as necessary. **May be indicated for prolonged or profound psychosis following lysergic acid diethylamide (LSD) or phencyclidine (PCP) intoxication.**
- Engage entire family in multidimensional family therapy as indicated. **Program developed for adolescents with substance use disorder and their families to address the various influences on client's substance use by improving family functioning and collaboration with other systems such as school and juvenile justice.**

Information that appears in brackets has been added by the authors to clarify and enhance the use of nursing diagnoses.

 Acute Care   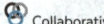 Collaborative   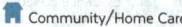 Community/Home Care   Cultural

Nursing Priority No. 4.

To support/sustain sobriety (Teaching/Discharge Considerations) and enhance well-being (long-term goals):

- Review effects of substance(s) used—physical, psychological, social. **Information needed for client to make informed decisions and commit to therapeutic regimen.**
- Discuss potential for reemergence of withdrawal symptoms in stimulant abuse as early as 3 months or as late as 9 to 12 months after discontinuing use. **Early recognition of recurrence of withdrawal symptoms provides for timely intervention.**
- Review specific aftercare needs (e.g., alcohol abuser with liver damage should refrain from medications, anesthetics, or use of household cleaning products that are detoxified in the liver). **Promotes individualized care related to specific situation.**
- Encourage balanced diet, adequate rest, exercise such as walking, biofeedback, deep meditative techniques. **These activities help restore natural biochemical balance, aid detoxification, and manage stress and anxiety.**
- Review long-term therapeutic regimen/MAT. **Medications such as methadone (for opioid use) or acamprosate (for alcohol use) may be prescribed to help maintain sobriety and reduce risk of relapse.**
- Identify community/social assistance resources (e.g., housing, food pantry, senior center/feeding station, transportation, medical care). **Provides for basic human needs, enhances coping abilities, reduces sense of isolation, and decreases risk of relapse.**
- Refer for vocational counseling/alternative schooling program as appropriate. **Provides opportunity to learn skills and obtain employment to promote independence and enhance self-esteem.**
- Encourage continued involvement in peer group therapy, individual/family counseling, drug recovery education programs. **Provides follow-up support to maintain sobriety.**
- Monitor results of periodic drug screening as appropriate. **Important to identify return to substance use or change to another drug.**

Documentation Focus

Assessment/Reassessment

- Individual findings including general health status, comorbidities, signs/stages of withdrawal

---

Information that appears in brackets has been added by the authors to clarify and enhance the use of nursing diagnoses.

 Diagnostic Studies 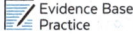 Evidence Based Practice 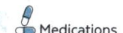 Medications 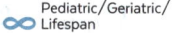 Pediatric/Geriatric/Lifespan

- Substance(s) used, dose, frequency, last dose
- Results of laboratory tests/diagnostic studies
- Effects of substance use on life and relationships

Planning
- Plan of care and who is involved in planning
- Teaching plan
- Plan for sobriety

Implementation/Evaluation
- Response to interventions, teaching, and actions performed
- Attainment of or progress toward desired outcomes
- Modifications to plan

Discharge Planning
- Long-term needs and who is responsible for actions to be taken
- Specific referrals made
- Plan for monitoring sobriety

Sample Nursing Outcomes & Interventions Classifications NOC/NIC

NOC—Alcohol [or] Drug Abuse Cessation Behavior
NIC—Substance Use Treatment: Alcohol [or] Drug Withdrawal

---

impaired AIRWAY CLEARANCE ICNP

[Diagnostic Division: Respiration]

Definition: Decreased ability to expectorate secretions or potential obstructions that may lead to occlusion or narrowing of the respiratory tract.

Recognizing Cues

Related/Risk Factors
Inadequate hydration; NPO status, poor fluid intake
Copious secretions; tenacious, sticky mucus
Exposure to airway irritants; smoking/vaping
Ineffective/weak cough
Pain; respiratory muscle fatigue
Decreased level of consciousness (LOC), postanesthetic

Information that appears in brackets has been added by the authors to clarify and enhance the use of nursing diagnoses.

 Acute Care 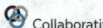 Collaborative 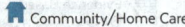 Community/Home Care 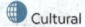 Cultural

Defining Characteristics

Objective
Copious sputum; ineffective sputum elimination
Adventitious breath sounds, decreased breath sounds
Irregular respiratory rhythm; increased, decreased respiratory rate
Intercostal/subcostal retraction; accessory muscle use; nasal flaring
Unable to clear airways; inability to speak
Cyanosis; hypoxemia
Changes in mentation
Postoperative thoracic/abdominal surgery

Clinical Connections
Chronic obstructive pulmonary disease (COPD), asthma, pneumonia, influenza, acute respiratory distress syndrome (ARDS), cancer of the lung, cancer of head and neck, congestive heart failure (CHF), neuromuscular diseases such as cerebral palsy, inhalation injuries, spinal cord injury (SCI), Guillain-Barré syndrome, traumatic brain injury, cystic fibrosis, drug or alcohol toxicity, malnutrition/failure to thrive (FTT) postanesthesia

Generate Solutions

Plan Desired Outcomes

Client Will (Include Specific Time Frame)
- Maintain airway patency.
- Expectorate/clear secretions readily.
- Demonstrate absence/reduction of congestion with breath sounds clearing, noiseless respirations, and improved oxygen exchange (e.g., absence of cyanosis and arterial blood gas [ABG]/pulse oximetry results within client norms).
- Verbalize understanding of cause(s) and therapeutic management regimen.
- Demonstrate behaviors to improve or maintain clear airway.
- Identify potential complications and how to initiate appropriate preventive or corrective actions.

Interventions/Take Action

Nursing Priority No. 1.
To maintain adequate, patent airway:
- Identify client populations at risk. **Persons with impaired ciliary function (e.g., cystic fibrosis or lung transplant);**

Information that appears in brackets has been added by the authors to clarify and enhance the use of nursing diagnoses.

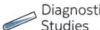 Diagnostic Studies   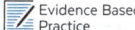 Evidence Based Practice   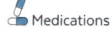 Medications   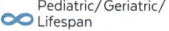 Pediatric/Geriatric/Lifespan

those with excessive or abnormal mucus production (e.g., asthma, COPD, pneumonia, dehydration, bronchiectasis, or mechanical ventilation); those with impaired cough function (e.g., neuromuscular diseases, such as muscular dystrophy; multiple sclerosis neuromotor conditions, such as cerebral palsy; or spinal cord injury); those with swallowing abnormalities (e.g., poststroke, seizures, head/neck cancer, coma/sedation, tracheostomy, or facial burns/trauma/surgery); those who are immobile (e.g., sedated individual, frail elderly, developmentally delayed, institutionalized client with multiple high-risk conditions); infant/child (e.g., feeding intolerance, abdominal distention, and emotional stressors that may compromise airway) are all at risk for problems with the maintenance of open airways.

- Assess behaviors indicating respiratory distress (e.g., wide-eyed, irritable, restless) as well as level of consciousness/cognition and ability to protect own airway. **This information is essential for identifying potential for airway problems, providing baseline level of care needed, and influencing choice of interventions.**
- Monitor respirations and breath sounds, noting rate and sounds (e.g., tachypnea, stridor, crackles, or wheezes) **indicative of respiratory distress and/or accumulation of secretions.**
- Assess for a sawtooth pattern on the ventilator flow waveform in clients receiving mechanical ventilation. Assess for visible secretions in the artificial airway (i.e., endotracheal tube, tracheostomy tube).
- Evaluate client's cough/gag reflex, amount and type of secretions, and swallowing ability **to determine ability to protect own airway.**
- ∞ Position head appropriately for age and condition **to open or maintain open airway in an at-rest or compromised individual.**
- ∞ Suction nose, mouth, and trachea prn using correct-size catheter and suction timing for child or adult **to clear airway when excessive or viscous secretions are blocking airway or client is unable to swallow or cough effectively.**
- ∞ Insert an airway adjunct (using correct size for adult or child) when needed **to maintain anatomical position of tongue and natural airway, especially when tongue/laryngeal edema or thick secretions may block airway.**
- Elevate head of bed, encourage early ambulation, and change client's position every 2 hr **to take advantage**

Information that appears in brackets has been added by the authors to clarify and enhance the use of nursing diagnoses.

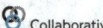 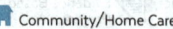

of gravity decreasing pressure on the diaphragm and enhancing drainage of/ventilation to different lung segments.
- Exercise diligence in providing oral hygiene and keeping oral mucosa hydrated. **Airways can be obstructed by substances such as blood or thickened secretions. These can be managed by strict attention to good oral hygiene, especially in the client who is unable to provide that for self.**
- Monitor infant/child for feeding intolerance, abdominal distention, and emotional stressors **that may compromise airway.**
- Prepare for/assist with appropriate testing (e.g., pulmonary function or sleep studies) **to identify causative/precipitating factors.**
- Instruct in/review postoperative breathing exercises, effective coughing, and use of adjunct devices (e.g., active cycle of breathing technique [ACBT], chest physiotherapy [CPT], forced exhalation technique [FET], intrapulmonary percussive ventilation [IPV], positive expiratory pressure [PEP], mechanical insufflation-exsufflation [MIE], oscillating PEP therapy [OPEP], incentive spirometer) in preoperative teaching.
- Assist with procedures (e.g., bronchoscopy or tracheostomy) **to clear/maintain open airway.**
- Keep environment allergen free (e.g., dust, feather pillows, or smoke) according to individual situation.

Nursing Priority No. 2.
To mobilize secretions:

- Mobilize client as soon as possible. **Reduces risk or effects of atelectasis, enhancing lung expansion and drainage of different lung segments.**
- Encourage deep-breathing and coughing exercises or splint chest/incision **to maximize effort.**
- Administer analgesics **to improve cough when pain is inhibiting effort. (Caution: Overmedication can depress respirations and cough effort.)**
- Administer medications (e.g., expectorants, anti-inflammatory agents, bronchodilators, and mucolytic agents), as indicated, **to relax smooth respiratory musculature, reduce airway edema, and mobilize secretions.**
- Increase fluid intake to at least 2,000 mL/day within cardiac tolerance (may require IV in acutely ill, hospitalized client). Encourage/provide warm versus cold liquids as appropriate.

Information that appears in brackets has been added by the authors to clarify and enhance the use of nursing diagnoses.

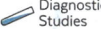 Diagnostic Studies   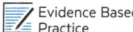 Evidence Based Practice   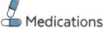 Medications   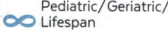 Pediatric/Geriatric/Lifespan

Provide supplemental humidification if needed (ultrasonic nebulizer or room humidifier). **Hydration can help prevent the accumulation of viscous secretions and improve secretion clearance.** Monitor for signs/symptoms of congestive heart failure (crackles, edema, or weight gain) when the client is at risk.

- Perform or assist client in learning airway clearance techniques such as ACBT, CPT, FET, IPV, PEP, MIE, and OPEP (e.g., flutter devices and high-frequency chest compression with an inflatable vest). **Various therapies/modalities may be required to acquire and maintain adequate airways and improve respiratory function and gas exchange.** (Refer to NDs ineffective Breathing Pattern; impaired Gas Exchange; impaired spontaneous Ventilation.)
- Support reduction/cessation of smoking **to improve lung function.**
- Position appropriately (e.g., head of bed elevated, side lying) and discourage use of oil-based products around nose **to prevent vomiting with aspiration into lungs.** (Refer to NDs risk for Aspiration; impaired Swallowing.)

Nursing Priority No. 3.
To assess changes, note complications:

- Auscultate breath sounds and assess air movement **to ascertain current status and note effects of treatment in clearing airways.**
- Monitor vital signs, noting respiratory rate, oxygen saturation, blood pressure, and heart rate.
- Observe for signs of respiratory distress (increased rate, restlessness/anxiety, or use of accessory muscles for breathing).
- Evaluate changes in sleep pattern, noting insomnia or daytime somnolence, **which may be evidence of nighttime airway incompetence or sleep apnea.** (Refer to NDs Insomnia, Sleep Deprivation.)
- Document response to drug therapy and/or development of adverse side effects or interactions with antimicrobials, steroids, expectorants, and bronchodilators. **Pharmacological therapy is used to prevent and control symptoms, reduce severity of exacerbations, and improve health status.**
- Observe for signs/symptoms of infection (e.g., increased respiratory rate, dyspnea, onset of fever, change in sputum color, amount, or character) **to identify the infectious process and promote timely intervention.**

Information that appears in brackets has been added by the authors to clarify and enhance the use of nursing diagnoses.

 Acute Care 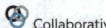 Collaborative 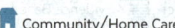 Community/Home Care   Cultural

- Obtain sputum specimen, preferably before antimicrobial therapy is initiated, **to point to effective antimicrobial agent.**
- Monitor/document serial chest x-rays, arterial blood gases, and pulse oximetry readings.

Nursing Priority No. 4.

To maintain patent airways (Teaching/Discharge Considerations) and enhance well-being (long-term goals):

- Assess client's/significant other's (SO) knowledge of contributing causes, treatment plan, specific medications, and therapeutic procedures **to determine educational and support needs.**
- Provide information about the necessity of raising and expectorating secretions versus swallowing them **to report changes in color and amount in the event that medical intervention may be needed to prevent or treat infection.**
- Demonstrate/assist client/SO in performing specific airway clearance techniques (e.g., forced expiratory breathing [also called *huffing*] or respiratory muscle strength training, chest percussion, or use of a vest), as indicated.
- Instruct client/SO/caregiver in use of inhalers and other respiratory drugs. Include expected effects and information regarding possible side effects and interactions of respiratory drugs with other medications, over-the-counter medications, and herbals. Discuss symptoms requiring medical follow-up. **Client is often taking multiple medications that have similar side effects and potential for interactions. It is important to understand the difference between nuisance side effects (e.g., fast heartbeat after albuterol inhaler) and adverse effects (e.g., chest pain, hallucinations, or uncontrolled cardiac arrhythmia).**
- Encourage/provide opportunities for rest; limit activities to level of respiratory tolerance. **Prevents/reduces fatigue.**
- Urge reduction or cessation of smoking. **Smoking is known to increase production of mucus and to paralyze (or cause loss of) cilia needed to move secretions to clear airway and improve lung function.**
- Refer to appropriate support groups (e.g., stop smoking clinic, COPD exercise group, weight reduction, American Lung Association, Cystic Fibrosis Foundation, or Muscular Dystrophy Association).
- Determine that the client has equipment and is informed in the use of nocturnal continuous positive airway pressure (CPAP) **for the treatment of obstructive sleep apnea, when indicated.** (Refer to ND ineffective Sleep Pattern.)

Information that appears in brackets has been added by the authors to clarify and enhance the use of nursing diagnoses.

 Diagnostic Studies   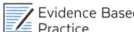 Evidence Based Practice   Medications   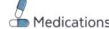 Pediatric/Geriatric/Lifespan

Documentation Focus

Assessment/Reassessment
- Related factors for individual clients
- Breath sounds, presence and character of secretions, use of accessory muscles for breathing
- Level of consciousness; skin color
- Character of cough and sputum
- Respiratory rate, pulse oximetry/O_2 saturation, vital signs

Planning
- Plan of care and who is involved in planning
- Teaching plan

Implementation/Evaluation
- Client's response to interventions, teaching, and actions performed
- Use of respiratory devices/airway adjuncts
- Response to medications administered
- Attainment of or progress toward desired outcome(s)
- Modifications to plan of care

Discharge Planning
- Long-term needs and who is responsible for actions to be taken
- Education on symptoms to report to providers
- Specific referrals made, such as pulmonary rehabilitation

Sample Nursing Outcomes & Interventions Classifications NOC/NIC

NOC—Respiratory Function: Airway Patency
NIC—Airway Management

---

risk for **ALLERGY REACTION** NANDA-I

[Diagnostic Division: Safety]

Definition: Susceptible to an excessive immune response to allergens.

Recognizing Cues

Risk Factors
Inadequate knowledge of avoidance of relevant allergens
Inattentive to potential allergen exposure

Information that appears in brackets has been added by the authors to clarify and enhance the use of nursing diagnoses.

 Acute Care   Collaborative 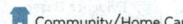 Community/Home Care   Cultural

Inadequate knowledge of, or management of factors contributing to allergic reaction severity

Risk-taking behavior

Clinical Connections

Asthma, conjunctivitis; eczema and other allergic skin rashes; food allergies and intolerances; hay fever; hives; insect stings

Generate Solutions

Plan Desired Outcomes

Client Will (Include Specific Time Frame)

- Be free of signs of hypersensitive response.
- Verbalize understanding of individual risks and responsibilities in avoiding exposure.
- Identify signs/symptoms requiring prompt response.

Interventions/Take Action

Nursing Priority No. 1.

To identify causative/precipitating factors related to risk:

- Question the client regarding known allergies upon admission to healthcare facility. **Basic safety information will help healthcare providers prepare a safe environment for the client while providing care.**
- Ascertain the type of allergy and usual symptoms if the client reports a history of allergies (e.g., seasonal rhinitis ["hay fever"], allergic dermatitis, conjunctivitis, environmental asthma, environmental substances [e.g., mold, dust, pet dander or water/air pollution], insect sting reactions, food intolerance, immunodeficiency such as Addison disease, or drug or transfusion reaction). **Allergies can manifest as local reactions (as may occur in skin rashes) or may be systemic. The client/caregiver may be aware of some, but not all, allergies. It is also possible that client is having a first-time allergic reaction to a substance and does not know what caused the reaction.**
- Obtain a written list of drug allergies upon first contact with the client and document it in appropriate place(s) in client records. **Helps prevent adverse drug events while the client is in facility care and aids in differentiating side effects from allergic responses. May also help improve client's understanding of reportable symptoms.**

Information that appears in brackets has been added by the authors to clarify and enhance the use of nursing diagnoses.

 Diagnostic Studies 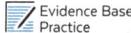 Evidence Based Practice 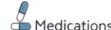 Medications 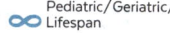 Pediatric/Geriatric/Lifespan

- Discuss the possibility of a latex allergy when entering facility care, especially when procedures are anticipated (e.g., laboratory, emergency department, operating room, wound care management, one-day surgery, or dental) **so that proper precautions can be taken by healthcare providers.** (Refer to ND risk for Latex Allergy for related interventions.)
- Note the client's age. **Although allergies can occur at any time in a client's life span, there are some that can start early in life. These include food allergies (e.g., peanuts) and respiratory ailments (e.g., asthma).**
- Perform challenge or patch test, if appropriate, **to identify specific allergens in a client with known type IV hypersensitivity.**
- Note response to allergen-specific IgE antibody tests, where available. **Performed to measure the quantity of IgE antibodies in serum after exposure to specific antigens and have generally replaced skin tests and provocation tests. Note: These tests are useful in nonemergent evaluations.**

Nursing Priority No. 2.

To take measures to avoid exposure and reduce/limit allergic response:

- Discuss the client's current symptoms, noting reports of rash, hives, itching; teary eyes; localized swelling (e.g., of lips) or diarrhea; nausea; or a feeling of faintness. Ascertain if client/care provider associates these symptoms with certain food, substances, or environmental factors (triggers). **May help isolate the cause of a reaction. Provides a baseline for determining where the client is along a continuum of symptoms so that appropriate treatments can be initiated.**
- Provide an allergen-free environment (e.g., clean, dust-free room or use air filters to reduce mold and pollens in the air) **to reduce client exposure to allergens.**
- Collaborate with all healthcare providers to administer medications and perform procedures with client's allergies in mind.
- Encourage the client to wear a medical ID bracelet/necklace **to alert providers to condition if the client is unresponsive or unable to relay information for any reason.**
- Refer to physician/allergy specialists as indicated **for interventions related to specific allergy conditions.**

Information that appears in brackets has been added by the authors to clarify and enhance the use of nursing diagnoses.

Nursing Priority No. 3.

To promote safety (Teaching/Discharge Criteria) and enhance well-being (long-term goals):

- Instruct/review with client and care provider(s) ways to prevent or limit client exposures. **They may need or desire information regarding ways to reduce allergens at home, school, or work; may desire information regarding potential exposures when traveling or how to manage food allergies when eating in restaurants.**
- Instruct in signs of reaction and emergency treatment needs. **Allergic reactions range from skin irritation to anaphylaxis. Reaction may be gradual but progressive, affecting multiple body systems, or may be sudden, requiring life-saving treatment.**
- Emphasize the critical importance of taking immediate action for moderate to severe hypersensitivity reactions **to limit life-threatening symptoms.**
- Demonstrate equipment and injection procedure and recommend that the client carry auto-injectable epinephrine **to provide timely emergency treatment, as needed.**
- Emphasize the necessity of informing all new care providers of allergies **to reduce preventable exposures.**
- Provide educational resources and assistance numbers for emergencies. **When allergy is suspected or the potential for allergy exists, protection must begin with identification and removal of possible sources.**

Documentation Focus

Assessment/Reassessment
- Individual risk factors identified
- Client concerns or difficulty making and following through with plans

Planning
- Plan of care and who is involved in planning
- Teaching plan

Implementation/Evaluation
- Response to interventions, teaching, and actions performed
- Attainment of or progress toward outcomes

Discharge Planning
- Referrals to other resources
- Long-term need and who is responsible for actions

Information that appears in brackets has been added by the authors to clarify and enhance the use of nursing diagnoses.

Sample Nursing Outcomes & Interventions Classifications NOC/NIC

NOC—Allergy Response: Systemic
NIC—Allergy Management

[mild, moderate, severe, panic] ANXIETY　　　iCNP

[Diagnostic Division: Stress Management]

Definition: Persistent thoughts fearing the unknown and intense worry of impending disaster or catastrophe not based on reality and impairing function and well-being.

Recognizing Cues

Related/Risk Factors
Chronic medical or life-threatening health conditions; pain
Traumatic life experience; stressful environments (home, work, school); unfamiliar situations
Expected performance (e.g., stage fright, test anxiety)
Substance abuse/misuse; some pharmaceuticals
Insecurity; low self-esteem; transference of feelings from/to others
Family history of anxiety

Defining Characteristics

Subjective

Mild: Expresses fear or worry, difficulty concentrating; nausea; insomnia; shortness of breath
Moderate: Inability to relax/jittery most days of the week; preoccupation with fear or worry; dry mouth; able to attend to activities of daily living most days of the week
Severe: Feels detached; dizziness; tingling sensations; headache; nausea; diarrhea; urinary frequency/urgency; chest pain; sense of impending doom
Panic: Sense of terror; unrealistic perception of situation; heart palpitations; chest pain; intense fear of repeat panic attacks

Objective

Mild: Muscle tension; restlessness; irritable mood; flight of ideas; rumination

---

Information that appears in brackets has been added by the authors to clarify and enhance the use of nursing diagnoses.

Acute Care　　Collaborative　　Community/Home Care　　Cultural

Moderate: Narrowed focus; scanning behavior; hypervigilance; reduced eye contact; voice quivers; rapid speech; crying; trembling; tachycardia

Severe: Scattered thoughts; decreased productivity; difficulty meeting personal care needs; erratic behavior; indecision; cold extremities; shaking/trembling; facial flushing; sweating; vomiting; hyperventilation; pupil dilation; psychomotor agitation

Panic: Rapid onset of signs/symptoms; increased pulse and blood pressure; confusion; hyperventilation; unable to speak/move (paralyzed with fear); potential loss of consciousness or fainting

Clinical Connections

Major life changes or events; hospital admissions; surgery; cancer; hyperthyroidism; drug intoxication or abuse; mental health disorders (e.g., anxiety, post-traumatic stress, personality disorders)

Generate Solutions

Plan Desired Outcomes

Client Will (Include Specific Time Frame)

- Verbalize awareness of thoughts and feelings regarding fear or worry causing anxiety.
- Appear relaxed and report that anxiety is reduced to a manageable level.
- Identify healthy ways to cope with and express anxiety.
- Demonstrate problem-solving skills.
- Use resources/support systems effectively.

Interventions/Take Action

Nursing Priority No. 1.

To assess level of anxiety:

- Review familial and physiological factors (e.g., genetic depressive factors), psychiatric condition, active medical conditions (e.g., thyroid problems, metabolic imbalances, cardiopulmonary disease, anemia, or dysrhythmias), and recent/ongoing stressors (e.g., family member illness or death, spousal conflict/abuse, or loss of job). **These factors can cause/exacerbate anxiety and anxiety disorders.**
- Determine current prescribed medications and recent drug history of prescribed or over-the-counter (OTC) medications (e.g., steroids, thyroid preparations, weight loss pills,

---

Information that appears in brackets has been added by the authors to clarify and enhance the use of nursing diagnoses.

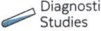 Diagnostic Studies   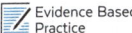 Evidence Based Practice   Medications   Pediatric/Geriatric/Lifespan

or caffeine) and substance use. **These medications can heighten feelings and sense of anxiety or may be used to self-treat anxiety disorders, which are frequently underdiagnosed and undertreated in primary care.**

- Identify the client's perception of the threat represented by the situation. **Distorted perceptions of the situation may magnify feelings. Understanding client's point of view promotes a more accurate plan of care.**

- Note cultural and spiritual factors that may influence anxiety. **Individual responses are influenced by cultural values and beliefs and culturally learned patterns of their family of origin. In addition, cultural or spiritual abandonment can occur when client has odd or different behaviors from the norm within the family, community, or society.**

- Monitor physical responses (e.g., rapid or irregular pulse, rapid breathing/hyperventilation, changes in blood pressure, diaphoresis, tremors, irritability, or restlessness) **to identify signs/symptoms associated with both medical and emotional conditions.**

- Observe behaviors symptomatic of anxiety. **Symptomatic behaviors can be a clue to the client's level of anxiety:**

Mild

Alert, more aware of environment, attention focused on environment and immediate events

Restless, irritable, wakeful; reports of insomnia

Motivated to deal with existing problems in this state

Moderate

Narrowed perception, concentration increased on fear or worry, able to ignore distractions in dealing with problem(s)

Voice quivers or changes pitch

Trembling, increased pulse/respirations

Severe

Range of perception is reduced; anxiety interferes with effective functioning

Preoccupied with feelings of discomfort; gastric distress, chest pain, sense of impending doom

Increased pulse/respirations with reports of dizziness, tingling sensations, headaches, and so forth

Panic

Inability to concentrate, behavior is disintegrated, and the client distorts the situation and does not have realistic perceptions of what is happening

---

Information that appears in brackets has been added by the authors to clarify and enhance the use of nursing diagnoses.

 Acute Care 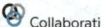 Collaborative 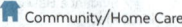 Community/Home Care   Cultural

May be experiencing terror or confusion or be unable to speak or move (paralyzed with fear)

- Note use of drugs (including alcohol or other drugs), insomnia or excessive sleeping, and limited or avoidance of interactions with others. **May be behavioral indicators used to withdraw from others to cope with problems.**
- Review results of diagnostic tests (e.g., drug screens, cardiac testing, complete blood count, and chemistry panel), **which may point to physiological sources of anxiety.**
- Determine ability to manage life responsibilities and meet self-care needs. **Anxiety disorders that interfere with activities of daily living may indicate a need for medications and nonpharmacological interventions to help client regain control.**

Nursing Priority No. 2.

To assist client with identifying feelings and beginning to deal with problems:

- Establish a therapeutic relationship, conveying empathy and unconditional positive regard. **When client is treated with dignity and respect, it promotes client comfort and allows them to begin looking at feelings and coping with the situation.**
- Ask permission to provide age-appropriate touch/contact as client desires (e.g., touching arm/holding adult's hand or rocking child). **Touching clients without permission may increase the level of anxiety. For clients who accept therapeutic touch, it can help soothe fear and provide assurance for client. Note: Clients, especially children, need to recognize that their feelings are not different from those of others.**
- Acknowledge client's anxiety as worry or fear. Respond truthfully with facts related to reality. Avoid denying or reassuring client that everything will be all right. **Clients need honest and respectful feedback to help them recognize unrealistic thinking. False reassurances may be interpreted as lack of understanding or dishonesty, further isolating client.**
- Active-listen client's feelings and observe nonverbal communication (e.g., crying, laughing, restlessness, or trembling). **Provides opportunity to clarify and understand the client's thoughts, feelings, and beliefs regarding the current event while discussing the reality of the present situation.**

Information that appears in brackets has been added by the authors to clarify and enhance the use of nursing diagnoses.

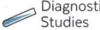 Diagnostic Studies 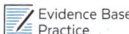 Evidence Based Practice 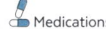 Medications 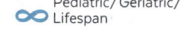 Pediatric/Geriatric/Lifespan

- Encourage client to identify meaning of behaviors and feelings, such as crying (sadness), laughing (fear or denial), or swearing (fear or anger). **Self-awareness aids client in controlling actions and beginning to deal with issues that are causing anxiety.**
- Determine use of defense mechanisms (e.g., denial, regression, or transference) and ineffective coping skills (e.g., anger, avoidance, eating, smoking, substance use). **Defense mechanisms may be useful for the moment but may eventually interfere with resolution of current situation and divert the energy that the client needs for healing, thus delaying the client from focusing on and coping with the actual problem.**

Nursing Priority No. 3.

To provide measures to comfort and aid client to handle problematic situations:

- Manage environmental factors, such as harsh lighting, high traffic flow, and excessive noise, guiding client to calmness and intellectual engagement. **May be especially confusing or stressful to older individuals. Milieu management promotes learning to live at home or in community setting as independently as client is capable. These factors can lessen anxiety, especially when client is in strange and unusual circumstances.**
- Limit/modify procedures as necessary (e.g., substitute oral for intramuscular medications, combine blood draws or use finger-stick method). **Limits degree of stress and avoids overwhelming child or anxious adult.**
- Teach, provide calming measures/relaxation techniques (e.g., soft music, deep breathing, meditation, yoga, warm bath, or therapeutic touch) if approved by client. **Aids in meeting basic human need, decreasing sense of isolation, encouraging client to select interventions that work best for them. Note: Therapeutic touch requires the nurse to have specific knowledge of and experience in using the hands to correct energy field disturbances by redirecting human energies to help or heal.**
- Accept client as is. **The client may need to be where they are at this point in time, such as in denial after receiving the diagnosis of a terminal illness.**
- Recognize client owns their behaviors while treating client with respect and dignity without responding personally. **Allows client to take responsibility and work on**

Information that appears in brackets has been added by the authors to clarify and enhance the use of nursing diagnoses.

 Acute Care 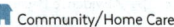 Collaborative Community/Home Care Cultural

self-improvement. **Limits manipulation of staff and staff stress. Responding personally to the client's behavior can escalate the situation, promoting a nontherapeutic situation and increasing anxiety.**
- Permit client to use anxiety for coping with the situation if helpful. **Moderate anxiety heightens awareness and can help client to focus on coping with problems. However, constant daily worry/fear creates fatigue, gastrointestinal distress, restlessness, and sleep disorders.**
- Encourage awareness of negative self-talk and encourage replacing with positive statements, such as using "can" instead of "can't." **Negative self-talk promotes feelings of anxiety and self-doubt. Becoming aware of and replacing negative thoughts can provide a starting point for enhancing sense of self-worth and helping control anxiety.**

Panic

- Stay with client, maintaining a calm, confident manner. **Presence communicates caring and helps client to regain control and sense of calm.**
- Communicate using simple language and brief statements. **Client is not able to comprehend complex information at this time.**
- Provide for nonthreatening, consistent environment or atmosphere, moving client to quiet area/room as indicated. **Minimizes stimuli and interactions with others, lessening effect of transmission of anxious feelings.**
- Allow client to pace if needed, setting limits on behaviors that are harmful to self or others.
- Administer antianxiety medications, as ordered. **Appropriate medication can be helpful in enabling client to regain control.**
- Use therapeutic communication/cognitive therapy **to refocus on reality opposed to catastrophic interpretations of physical symptoms or the environment. For example, thoughts of dying increase anxiety and feelings of panic. Refocusing/controlling these thoughts allows client to look at situation more realistically and begin to cope more calmly with what is happening.**
- Monitor response to medication and gradually increase activities and involvement with others as tolerated. **Promotes sense of normalcy, helps control feelings of anxiety.**

Information that appears in brackets has been added by the authors to clarify and enhance the use of nursing diagnoses.

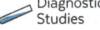 Diagnostic Studies   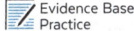 Evidence Based Practice   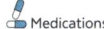 Medications   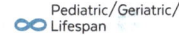 Pediatric/Geriatric/Lifespan

Nursing Priority No. 4.

To promote ongoing sense of safety (Teaching/Discharge Considerations) and enhance well-being (long-term goals):

- Assist client to identify precipitating factors, thoughts, and feelings preceding anxiety. **Awareness provides opportunity to prevent/lessen possibility of repeat episodes.**
- Review actions and activities the client has previously used to cope successfully when feeling nervous/anxious. **Realizing that the individual already has some coping skills that can be applied in current and future situations can empower client.**
- Review coping strategies such as role-playing, use of visualizations to practice anticipated events, mindfulness, and prayer or meditation. **These activities can help the client practice behaviors in a safe and supportive environment, enabling individual to manage anxiety-provoking situations.**
- Identify resources/referrals for contact person/crisis manager, available hotline, individual/group therapy, and community support group. **Anxiety disorders can be a lifelong struggle requiring ongoing/timely support to aid client in controlling anxiety.**
- Encourage client to develop an exercise/activity program. **May be helpful in relieving tension and has been shown to raise endorphin levels to enhance sense of well-being.**
- Review medication regimen, benefits, side effects, and possible interactions with over-the-counter drugs, other prescription drugs, alcohol, and herbal products. **Enhances understanding of reason for medication and can help client avoid untoward or harmful reactions from incompatible drugs. Important for client to understand benzodiazepines are for short-term use due to tolerance/dependence and that possible use of selective serotonin reuptake inhibitors (SSRIs) may be indicated for long-term management.**
- Discuss appropriate drug substitutions or changes in dosage or time of dose. **Ensures proper dosage and avoids untoward side effects. This is especially important in older adults, who are particularly susceptible to multidrug complications.**
- Refer to the physician for drug management alteration of the prescription regimen. **Drugs that often cause symptoms of anxiety include aminophylline/theophylline, anticholinergics, dopamine, levodopa, salicylates, and steroids.**

Information that appears in brackets has been added by the authors to clarify and enhance the use of nursing diagnoses.

Monitoring provides opportunity to correct possible undesirable effects of these drugs.

Documentation Focus

Assessment/Reassessment
- Level of anxiety and precipitating/aggravating factors
- Description of feelings (expressed and displayed)
- Awareness and ability to recognize and express feelings
- Related substance use, if present

Planning
- Treatment plan and individual responsibility for specific activities
- Teaching plan

Implementation/Evaluation
- Client involvement and response to interventions, teaching, and actions performed
- Attainment of or progress toward desired outcome(s)
- Modifications to plan of care

Discharge Planning
- Referrals and follow-up plan
- Specific referrals made

Sample Nursing Outcomes & Interventions Classifications NOC/NIC

NOC—Anxiety Level
NIC—Anxiety Reduction

---

risk for ASPIRATION NANDA-I

[Diagnostic Division: Respiration]

Definition: Susceptible to entry of gastrointestinal secretions, oropharyngeal secretions, solids or fluids to the tracheobronchial passages.

Recognizing Cues

Risk Factors
Barrier to elevating upper body
Decreased gastrointestinal (GI) motility
Difficulty swallowing; difficulty clearing airway

Information that appears in brackets has been added by the authors to clarify and enhance the use of nursing diagnoses.

 Diagnostic Studies 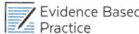 Evidence Based Practice 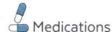 Medications Pediatric/Geriatric/Lifespan

Enteral nutrition tube displacement
Increased gastric residual
Inadequate knowledge of modifiable factors

Clinical Connections

Facial, jaw, oral, neck injury/surgery; vomiting, bulimia nervosa, presence of nasogastric tube, enteral feedings; stroke/brain injury; Parkinson disease; spinal cord injury

Generate Solutions

Plan Desired Outcomes

Client Will (Include Specific Time Frame)

- Experience no aspiration as evidenced by noiseless respirations; clear breath sounds; and clear, odorless secretions.
- Identify causative/risk factors.
- Demonstrate techniques to prevent and/or correct aspiration.

Interventions/Take Action

Nursing Priority No. 1.

To assess causative/contributing factors:

- Identify at-risk clients according to condition or disease process, as listed in Risk Factors/Clinical Connections, **to determine when observation and/or interventions may be required.**
- Assess for age-related risk factors potentiating risk of aspiration (e.g., premature infant, elderly infirm). **Aspiration pneumonia is more common in extremely young or old patients and commonly occurs in individuals with chronically impaired airway defense mechanisms.**
- Note client's level of consciousness, awareness of surroundings, and cognitive function, **as impairments in these areas increase the client's risk of aspiration owing to the inability to cough or swallow well and/or the presence of an artificial airway, mechanical ventilation, and/or tube feedings.**
- Determine the presence of neuromuscular disorders, noting muscle groups involved, degree of impairment, and whether they are of an acute or progressive nature (e.g., stroke, Parkinson disease, progressive supranuclear palsy, and similar disabling brain diseases; Guillain-Barré syndrome, or amyotrophic lateral sclerosis). **May result in temporary or chronic, progressive impairment of protective muscle functions.**

Information that appears in brackets has been added by the authors to clarify and enhance the use of nursing diagnoses.

- Assess the client's ability to swallow and cough; note quality of voice. **Sudden respiratory symptoms (e.g., severe coughing and cyanosis; wet, phlegmy voice quality) are indicative of potential aspiration. Also, individuals with impaired or absent cough reflexes (such as may occur after a stroke, in Parkinson disease, or during sedation) are at high risk for "silent" aspiration.**
- Observe for neck and facial edema. **A client with a head/neck surgery or a tracheal/bronchial injury (e.g., upper torso burns or inhalation/chemical injury) is at particular risk for airway obstruction and an inability to handle secretions.**
- Assess for coughing and note amount and consistency of respiratory secretions. **Helps differentiate the potential cause for risk of aspiration.**
- Auscultate lung sounds periodically (especially in a client who is coughing frequently or not coughing at all; a client with artificial airways, endotracheal and tracheostomy tubes; or a ventilator client being tube-fed, immediately following extubation), **to determine decreased breath sounds, rales, or dullness to percussion that could indicate the presence of aspirated secretions and "silent aspiration" leading to aspiration pneumonia.** Also observe chest radiographs.
- Evaluate for/note presence of GI pathology and motility disorders. **Nausea with vomiting (associated with metabolic disorders, or following surgery, and with certain medications) and gastroesophageal reflux disease (GERD) can cause inhalation of gastric contents.**
- Note the administration of enteral feedings, which may be initiated when oral nutrition is not possible. **The potential exists for regurgitation and aspiration with the use of feeding tubes, the risk is increased with nasogastric feeding tubes, even with proper tube placement.**
- Ascertain lifestyle habits (e.g., chronic use of alcohol and drugs, alcohol intoxication, tobacco, and other central nervous system [CNS] suppressant drugs). **Can affect awareness as well as impair gag and swallow mechanisms.**
- Assist with/review diagnostic studies (e.g., videofluoroscopy or fiberoptic endoscopy), **which may be done to assess for presence/degree of swallowing impairment.**

Nursing Priority No. 2.
To assist in correcting factors that can lead to aspiration:
- Elevate the client to the highest or best possible position (e.g., sitting upright in chair) for eating and drinking and

---

Information that appears in brackets has been added by the authors to clarify and enhance the use of nursing diagnoses.

during tube feedings. **Adults and children should be upright for meals to decrease the likelihood of drainage into the trachea and to reduce reflux and improve gastric emptying.**

- Encourage the client to cough, as able, to clear secretions. **The client may simply need to be reminded or encouraged to cough (such as might occur in an elderly person with delayed gag reflex or in a postoperative, sedated client).**
- Monitor the use of oxygen masks in clients at risk for vomiting. Refrain from using oxygen masks for comatose individuals.
- Keep wire cutters/scissors with the client at all times when jaws are wired/banded **to facilitate clearing the airway in emergency situations.**
- Assist with oral care, postural drainage, and other respiratory therapies **to remove or mobilize thickened secretions that may interfere with swallowing and block airway.**
- **In client requiring suctioning to manage secretions:**
  Maintain operational suction equipment at bedside/chairside.
  Suction (oral cavity, nose, and endotracheal/tracheostomy tube), as needed, and avoid triggering the gag mechanism when performing suction or mouth care **to clear secretions while reducing the potential for aspiration of secretions.**
  Avoid keeping the client supine/flat when on mechanical ventilation (especially when also receiving enteral feedings). **Supine positioning and enteral feedings have been shown to be independent risk factors for the development of aspiration pneumonia.**
  Perform scrupulous oral care **to prevent the accumulation of thickened secretions in the oral pharynx and to remove secretions that may interfere with the movement of air.**
- **For a verified swallowing problem:**
  Provide a rest period prior to feeding time. **The rested client may have less difficulty with swallowing.**
  Feed slowly, using small bites, instructing the client to chew slowly and thoroughly.
  Vary the placement of food in the client's mouth according to type of swallowing deficit (e.g., place food in right side of mouth if facial weakness is present on the left side).
  Provide soft foods that stick together/form a bolus (e.g., casseroles, puddings, or stews) **to aid the swallowing effort.**

Information that appears in brackets has been added by the authors to clarify and enhance the use of nursing diagnoses.

 Acute Care 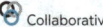 Collaborative 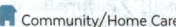 Community/Home Care Cultural

Determine liquid viscosity best tolerated by client. Add thickening agent to liquids, as appropriate. **Some individuals may swallow thickened liquids more easily than thin liquids.**

Offer very warm or very cold liquids. **Activates temperature receptors in the mouth that help to stimulate swallowing.**

Avoid washing solids down with liquids **to prevent bolus of food pushing down too rapidly, increasing risk of aspiration.**

- **When feeding tube is in place:**

Ascertain that the feeding tube (when used) is in the correct position. **Placement may be done under fluoroscopy and/or measurement of aspirate pH following placement of feeding tube may be indicated.** Ask the client about feeling of fullness and/or measure residuals (just prior to feeding and several hours after feeding), when appropriate, **to reduce risk of aspiration.**

Elevate head of bed 30 degrees during and for at least 30 min after bolus feedings. Note: Head of bed should remain at 30 degrees or higher at all times during continuous feedings.

Determine the best resting position for infant/child (e.g., with the head of the bed elevated 30 degrees and the infant propped on the right side after feeding). An elevated, right, side-lying position uses gravity to prevent esophageal (and potential tracheal) reflux while promoting gastric emptying.

Provide oral medications in elixir form or crush, if appropriate.

Minimize the use of sedatives/hypnotics whenever possible. **These agents can impair coughing and swallowing.**

Refer to physician and/or speech-language therapist for medical or surgical interventions and/or exercises **to strengthen muscles and learn specific techniques to enhance swallowing/reduce potential aspiration.**

Nursing Priority No. 3.

To promote safety (Teaching/Discharge Considerations) and enhance well-being (long-term goals):

- Review with client/significant other individual risk or potentiating factors.
- Provide information about the signs and effects of aspiration on the lungs. **Severe coughing and cyanosis (associated with eating or drinking) or changes in vocal quality**

Information that appears in brackets has been added by the authors to clarify and enhance the use of nursing diagnoses.

after swallowing indicate onset of respiratory symptoms associated with aspiration and require immediate intervention.
- Instruct in safety concerns regarding oral or tube feeding. (Refer to ND impaired Swallowing.)
- Train the client how to self-suction or train family members in suction techniques (especially if the client has constant or copious oral secretions) **to enhance safety/self-sufficiency.**
- Instruct the individual/family member to avoid or limit activities after eating that increase intra-abdominal pressure (straining, strenuous exercise, or tight/constrictive clothing), **which may slow digestion/increase risk of regurgitation.**

Documentation Focus

Assessment/Reassessment
- Assessment of findings, conditions that could lead to problems of aspiration
- Verification of tube placement, observations of physical findings

Planning
- Interventions to prevent aspiration or reduce risk factors and who is involved in the planning
- Teaching plan

Implementation/Evaluation
- Client's responses to interventions, teaching, and actions performed
- Foods/fluids client handles with ease or difficulty
- Amount and frequency of intake
- Attainment of or progress toward desired outcome(s)
- Modifications to plan of care

Discharge Planning
- Long-term needs and who is responsible for actions to be taken

Sample Nursing Outcomes & Interventions Classifications NOC/NIC

NOC—Risk Control: Aspiration
NIC—Aspiration Precautions

Information that appears in brackets has been added by the authors to clarify and enhance the use of nursing diagnoses.

risk for AUTONOMIC DYSREFLEXIA   ICNP

[Diagnostic Division: Circulation]

Definition: At risk for an uncoordinated, autonomic response as a consequence of a stimulus below the level of injury in clients with a spinal cord injury (SCI)/lesion at, or above, thoracic vertebra 6 (T6) and if left untreated may result in a life-threatening emergency.

Recognizing Cues

Risk Factors

Gastrointestinal Stimuli
Bowel distention; constipation; fecal impaction
Hemorrhoids; anal fissures
Digital stimulation; enemas, suppositories
Gastroesophageal reflux; gastric ulcers

Integumentary Stimuli
Cutaneous stimulation; skin irritation; sunburn
Wounds, wound care, ingrown toenails

Musculoskeletal-Neurological Stimuli
Irritating, painful stimuli below level of injury
Pressure over bony prominence
Range-of-motion exercises; muscle spasm

Regulatory-Situational Stimuli
Constricting clothing
Environmental temperature fluctuations
Venous thromboembolism

Reproductive-Urological Stimuli
Urinary tract infection (UTI); bladder spasm or distention; urolithiasis
Sexual intercourse excitation; genital pressure
Pregnancy/labor/delivery
Instrumentation (e.g., catheter insertion, obstruction, irrigation)

Other
Inadequate knowledge of physiological triggers
Failure to take adequate precautions

Clinical Connections

High-level SCI (level of T6 or above) with bone fractures, heterotopic bone, constipation, gastric ulcer, UTI, epididymitis; ovarian cyst, dysmenorrhea, surgery, venous thromboembolism

---

Information that appears in brackets has been added by the authors to clarify and enhance the use of nursing diagnoses.

 Diagnostic Studies 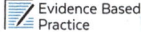 Evidence Based Practice 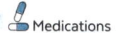 Medications ∞ Pediatric/Geriatric/Lifespan

Generate Solutions

Plan Desired Outcomes

Client/Caregiver Will (Include Specific Time Frame)
- Identify risk factors present.
- Demonstrate preventive of corrective techniques.

Client Will (Include Specific Time Frame)
- Be free of episodes of dysreflexia.

Interventions/Take Action

Nursing Priority No. 1.
To assess for **risk** or precipitating factors:

- Note client's level and degree of SCI to identify potential risk for Autonomic Dysreflexia (AD). **The higher the level of SCI and the more complete the cord injury, the higher is the risk for increased frequency and severity of AD episodes. Clients with a complete SCI are greater than three times more likely to experience AD than clients with incomplete SCI.**
- Determine the client's SCI timeline **to identify the client's current risk for AD and accurately interpret clinical manifestations; spinal shock, neurogenic shock, and AD all may occur after SCI; however, all occur at different times and have different symptoms. Note: The risk for AD increases as the client moves away from their initial injury and spinal shock.**
- Monitor for potential precipitating factors, including urological (e.g., bladder distention, UTI, urolithiasis, etc.), gastrointestinal (e.g., constipation, hemorrhoids, digital stimulation), cutaneous (e.g., pressure injury, temperature fluctuation, dressing changes, etc.), reproductive (e.g., sexual activity, menstruation, pregnancy/delivery, etc.), and miscellaneous (e.g., venous thromboembolism, drug reaction, etc.).

Nursing Priority No. 2.
To prevent occurrence:

- Monitor vital signs regularly, noting changes in blood pressure, heart rate, and temperature, especially during times of physical stress, **to identify trends and intervene promptly. Note: Baseline blood pressure in spinal cord–injured clients (adults and children) is lower than in the general**

Information that appears in brackets has been added by the authors to clarify and enhance the use of nursing diagnoses.

population; therefore, an elevation of 20 to 40 mm Hg above baseline may be indicative of AD.

- Instruct client and all caregivers in regularly timed elimination and safe bowel, bladder, and catheter care **to reduce risk of AD episode. Note: The two most common inciting stimuli are bladder and bowel distention, respectively; commonly a blocked urinary catheter.**
- Instruct client and all caregivers in interventions for long-term prevention of skin stress or breakdown (e.g., prevent pressure injury, appropriate padding for skin and tissues, proper positioning, routine foot and toenail care) **to reduce risk of AD episode. (Refer to NDs impaired Skin Integrity and adult, child, and neonatal Pressure Injury for related assessments and interventions.)**
- Instruct client/caregivers in additional preventive interventions (e.g., temperature control; checking frequently for tight clothes or leg straps; sunburn and other burn prevention).
- Administer antihypertensive medications, as ordered **to reduce the severity and duration of AD episodes. Clients at an increased risk for AD may be prescribed a regularly scheduled medication (e.g., α1-adrenergic antagonists [prazosin, terazosin]) when noxious stimuli cannot be removed (e.g., presence of chronic sacral pressure injury, fracture, acute postoperative pain).**

Nursing Priority No. 3.

To promote autonomic stability (Teaching/Discharge Considerations) and enhance well-being (long-term goals):

- Determine client/caregiver's understanding regarding AD prevention. Provide education and periodically reinforce teaching regarding the following **to avoid an episode of AD and/or initiate prompt interventions as needed:**
  Keep indwelling catheter free of kinks, keep the urinary drainage bag empty and situated below bladder level, and check daily for deposits (bladder grit) inside catheter
  Catheterize as often as necessary **to prevent bladder distention**
  Monitor voiding patterns for adequate frequency and amount
  Perform regular bowel evacuation program
  Perform regular skin assessments
  Monitor all organ systems for signs/symptoms of infection and report promptly to the provider **for prompt medical treatment**
- Review warning signs of AD with client/caregiver (i.e., sudden, severe pounding headache; flushed face; increased

---

Information that appears in brackets has been added by the authors to clarify and enhance the use of nursing diagnoses.

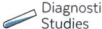 Diagnostic Studies
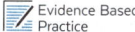 Evidence Based Practice
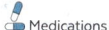 Medications
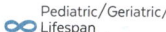 Pediatric/Geriatric/Lifespan

blood pressure/acute hypertension; nasal congestion; anxiety; blurred vision; metallic taste in mouth; diaphoresis and/or flushing above the level of SCI; piloerection; bradycardia; cardiac irregularities). **AD can develop rapidly (in minutes) and thus requires prompt intervention.**

- Consider client's communication abilities and monitor nonverbal behaviors. **AD can occur at any age, from infant to very old, and the individual may not be able to verbalize AD symptoms, such as a pounding headache, which is often the first symptom during onset of AD.**
- Instruct family member/caregiver in blood pressure monitoring, including return demonstration **to ensure competency of skill performance.**
- Review proper use/administration of medication, as ordered. **Some clients take medications routinely, and if so, they should receive instructions for routine administration, as well as symptoms to report for immediate or emergent care, when blood pressure is not responsive. Note: Additional education should be provided to client using phosphodiesterase inhibitors (e.g., sildenafil, tadalafil, etc.) for erectile dysfunction to avoid drug interaction with nitrate antihypertensives.**
- Emphasize the importance of regularly scheduled medical evaluations **to monitor status and to identify developing problems.**
- Recommend wearing a medical alert bracelet or necklace with information card about signs/symptoms of AD and methods of treatment **to provide vital information in emergencies. Note: The Reeves Foundation provides online printable wallet cards in many languages to inform client/caregivers/emergency healthcare providers about AD's most common causes and treatments.**
- Assist the client/family in identifying emergency referrals (e.g., physician, rehabilitation nurse, home care supervisor, etc.). Place phone number(s) in a prominent place or program into the client's/caregiver's cell phone **to ensure rapid access in case of an emergency.**

Documentation Focus

Assessment/Reassessment

- Individual risk factors or findings (e.g., episodic bladder distention, severe headache, spike in blood pressure), noting number and severity of previous episodes, precipitating factors when known, and individual's typical signs/symptom

---

Information that appears in brackets has been added by the authors to clarify and enhance the use of nursing diagnoses.

Planning
- Plan of care and who is involved in planning
- Teaching plan

Implementation/Evaluation
- Client's responses to interventions and actions performed, understanding of teaching
- Attainment of or progress toward desired outcome(s)
- Modifications to plan of care

Discharge Planning
- Long-term needs and who is responsible for actions to be taken

Sample Nursing Outcomes & Interventions Classifications NOC/NIC

NOC—Risk Control
NOC—Neurological Function: Autonomic
NIC—Dysreflexia Management

---

risk for excessive BLEEDING NANDA-I

[Diagnostic Division: Circulation]

Definition: Susceptible to significant blood loss.

Recognizing Cues

Risk Factors
Inadequate knowledge of bleeding precautions, or management strategies
Ineffective medication self-management
Inadequate follow-through with bleeding precautions, or management strategies
Inattentive to early warning signs of complications
Inadequate vitamin intake
Psychomotor agitation

Clinical Connections
Aortic aneurysm; gastrointestinal ulcer, varices; cirrhosis; pancreatitis; sickle cell anemia; surgical procedures; femur/pelvic fractures; disseminated intravascular coagulopathy (DIC); use of anticoagulants; pregnancy or postpartum complications; circumcision

---

Information that appears in brackets has been added by the authors to clarify and enhance the use of nursing diagnoses.

 Diagnostic Studies 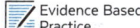 Evidence Based Practice Medications 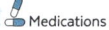 Pediatric/Geriatric/Lifespan

Generate Solutions

Plan Desired Outcomes

Client Will (Include Specific Time Frame)
- Be free of signs of active bleeding, such as hemoptysis, hematuria, hematemesis, or excessive blood loss, as evidenced by stable vital signs, skin and mucous membranes free of pallor, and usual mentation and urinary output.
- Display laboratory results for clotting times and factors within normal range for individual.
- Identify individual risks and engage in appropriate behaviors or lifestyle changes to prevent or reduce the frequency of bleeding episodes.

Interventions/Take Action

Nursing Priority No. 1.
To assess risk factors:

- Assess client risk, noting possible medical diagnoses or disease processes that may lead to bleeding.
- Note the type of injury/injuries when the client presents with trauma. **The pattern and extent of injury and bleeding may or may not be readily determined. For example, unbroken skin can hide a significant injury where a large amount of blood is lost within soft tissues; or a crush injury resulting in interruption of the integrity of the pelvic ring can cause life-threatening bleeding from three sources: arterial, venous, and bone edge bleeding.**
- Determine the presence of hereditary factors, obtain a detailed history if a familial bleeding disorder is suspected, such as hereditary hemorrhagic telangiectasia (HHT), hemophilia, other factor deficiencies, or thrombocytopenia. **Hereditary bleeding or clotting disorders predispose the client to bleeding complications, necessitating specialized testing and/or referral to a hematologist.**
- Note the client's gender. **While bleeding disorders are common in both men and women, women are affected more owing to the increased risk of blood loss related to menstrual cycle and pregnancy complications/delivery procedures.**
- Identify pregnancy-related factors, as indicated. **Many factors can occur, including overdistention of the uterus, pregnancy with multiples, prolonged or rapid labor, lacerations occurring during vaginal delivery, or retained**

Information that appears in brackets has been added by the authors to clarify and enhance the use of nursing diagnoses.

 Acute Care 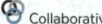 Collaborative 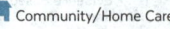 Community/Home Care 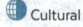 Cultural

placenta, which can place the mother at risk for postpartum bleeding.
- Evaluate the client's medication regimen. **The use of medications, such as nonsteroidal anti-inflammatories (NSAIDs), anticoagulants, and antiplatelet agents; a variety of drugs that can decrease or destroy platelets (e.g., antidepressants, antineoplastic agents, iodinated contrast agents, certain cardiac medications and diuretics); corticosteroids; and certain herbals (e.g., garlic, ginseng, Ginkgo biloba, fish oil), predispose client to bleeding.**

Nursing Priority No. 2.
To evaluate for potential bleeding:

- Recognition of the components of the "triad of death," e.g., hypothermia, acidosis, and coagulopathy, as a potential cause for excessive bleeding. Monitor perineum and fundal height in a postpartum client, and wounds, dressings, or tubes in a client with trauma, surgery, or other invasive procedures **to identify active blood loss. Note: Hemorrhage may occur because of the inability to achieve hemostasis in the setting of injury or may result from the development of a coagulopathy.**
- Evaluate and mark boundaries of soft tissues in enclosed structures, such as a leg or abdomen, **to document expanding bruises or hematomas.**
- Assess vital signs, including blood pressure, pulse, and respirations. Measure blood pressure lying/sitting/standing as indicated to evaluate for orthostatic hypotension; monitor invasive hemodynamic parameters when present **to determine if an intravascular fluid deficit exists. Note: Fit, young people may lose 40% of their blood volume before the systolic blood pressure drops below 100 mm Hg, whereas the elderly may become hypotensive with volume loss of as little as 10%.**
- Send stool for occult blood **to determine possible sources of bleeding.**
- Note client report of pain in specific areas, and whether pain is increasing, diffuse, or localized. **Can help to identify bleeding into tissues, organs, or body cavities.**
- Assess skin color and moisture, urinary output, level of consciousness, or mentation. **Changes in these signs may be indicative of blood loss affecting systemic circulation or local organ function, such as kidneys or brain.**

Information that appears in brackets has been added by the authors to clarify and enhance the use of nursing diagnoses.

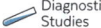 Diagnostic Studies 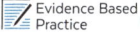 Evidence Based Practice 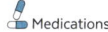 Medications 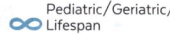 Pediatric/Geriatric/Lifespan

- Review laboratory data (e.g., complete blood count [CBC], platelet numbers and function, reticulocyte count, and other coagulation factors such as Factor I, Factor II, international normalized ratio [INR], prothrombin time [PT], partial thromboplastin time [PTT], activated clotting time [aPTT], fibrinogen) **to evaluate bleeding risk. The common problem in life-threatening anemia is a sudden reduction in the oxygen-carrying capacity of the blood. Depending on the etiology, this may occur with or without reduction in the intravascular volume. It is generally accepted that an acute drop in hemoglobin to a level of 7 to 8 g/dL is symptomatic.**
- Prepare the client for or assist with diagnostic studies such as x-rays, computed tomography (CT), or magnetic resonance imaging (MRI) scans, ultrasound, or colonoscopy **to determine the presence of injuries or disorders that could cause internal bleeding.**

Nursing Priority No. 3.

To prevent bleeding/correct potential causes of excessive blood loss:

- Apply direct pressure and cold pack to bleeding site, utilize compression devices, insert nasal packing, or perform fundal massage as appropriate for site and cause of bleeding.
- Restrict activity and encourage bedrest or chair rest until bleeding abates.
- Maintain the patency of vascular access **for fluid administration or blood replacement as indicated.**
- Administer isotonic IV fluids, as indicated. **Supports intravascular volume until (and in addition to) blood products can be administered. Current evidence supports a less aggressive administration of isotonic IV fluids with concomitant administration of blood products (e.g., plasma, platelets, and red blood cells) as appropriate to prevent a dilutional coagulopathy and worsen bleeding. Likewise, bleeding patients should be covered with heated blankets, IV and blood products should be warmed prior to administration.**
- Assist with the treatment of underlying conditions causing or contributing to blood loss, such as medical treatment of systemic infections or balloon tamponade of esophageal varices prior to sclerotherapy; use of proton pump inhibitor medications or antibiotics for gastric ulcer; or surgery for internal abdominal trauma or retained placenta. **Treatment of underlying conditions may prevent or halt bleeding complication.**

Information that appears in brackets has been added by the authors to clarify and enhance the use of nursing diagnoses.

 Acute Care 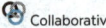 Collaborative 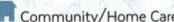 Community/Home Care 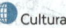 Cultural

- Provide special intervention for the at-risk client, such as an individual with bone marrow suppression, chemotherapy, or uremia, **to prevent bleeding associated with tissue injury:** Monitor closely for overt bleeding.

  Observe for petechiae and diffuse oozing from tubes, wounds, or orifices with no observable clotting **to identify excessive bleeding and/or possible coagulopathy.**

  Maintain direct pressure or pressure dressings as indicated for a longer period of time over arterial puncture sites **to prevent oozing or active bleeding.**

  Protect the client from trauma such as falls, accidental or intentional blows, or lacerations.

  Use soft toothbrush or Toothettes for oral care **to reduce risk of injury to the oral mucosa.**

- Collaborate in evaluating the need for replacing blood loss or specific components and be prepared for emergency interventions. **Institution or physician may have specific guidelines for transfusion, such as platelet count less than 20,000/mcL or Hg less than 7 g/dL, in addition to the client's clinical status.**

- Be prepared to administer hemostatic agents, if needed, **to promote clotting and diminish bleeding by increasing coagulation factors,** or medications such as proton pump inhibitors **to reduce risk of gastrointestinal bleeding.**

Nursing Priority No. 4.

To maintain normal hemostasis (Teaching/Discharge Considerations) and enhance well-being (long-term goals):

- Provide information to the client/family about hereditary or familial problems that predispose to bleeding complications.
- Instruct at-risk client and family regarding:

  Specific signs of bleeding requiring healthcare provider notification, such as active bright bleeding anywhere, prolonged epistaxis or trauma in a client with known factor bleeding tendencies, black tarry stools, weakness, vertigo, syncope, and so forth.

  Need to inform healthcare providers when on (1) antiplatelet agents (e.g., aspirin, Plavix, Brilinta, Xarelto) and (2) anticoagulants (e.g., Pradaxa, Eliquis, Lovenox, Coumadin), especially when elective surgery or other invasive procedure is planned. **These agents will most likely be withheld for a period of time prior to elective procedures to reduce potential for excessive blood loss.**

  Importance of periodic review of client's medication regimen **to identify medications (prescriptions,**

Information that appears in brackets has been added by the authors to clarify and enhance the use of nursing diagnoses.

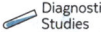 Diagnostic Studies   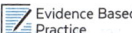 Evidence Based Practice   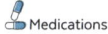 Medications   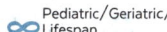 Pediatric/Geriatric/Lifespan

over-the-counter, and herbals) that might cause or exacerbate bleeding problems.

Necessity of regular medical and laboratory follow-up when on warfarin (Coumadin) **to determine needed dosage changes or client management issues requiring monitoring and/or modification.**

Dietary measures to improve blood clotting, such as foods rich in vitamin K.

Need to avoid alcohol in diagnosed liver disorders or seek treatment for alcoholism in the presence of alcoholic varices.

Techniques for postpartum client to check her own fundus and perform fundal massage as indicated and to contact physician for postdischarge bleeding that is bright red or dark red with large clots **(may prevent blood loss complications, especially if client is discharged early from hospital).**

Documentation Focus

Assessment/Reassessment
- Individual factors that may potentiate blood loss—type of injuries, surgical, trauma, obstetrical complications, and so on
- Baseline vital signs and trends, mentation, urinary output, and subsequent assessments
- Results of laboratory tests or diagnostic procedures

Planning
- Plan of care and who is involved in the planning
- Teaching plan

Implementation/Evaluation
- Responses to interventions, teaching, and actions performed
- Attainment of or progress toward desired outcome(s)
- Modifications to plan of care

Discharge Planning
- Long-term needs, identifying who is responsible for actions to be taken
- Community resources or support for chronic problems
- Specific referrals made

Sample Nursing Outcomes & Interventions Classifications NOC/NIC

NOC—Blood Loss Severity
NIC—Bleeding Precautions

Information that appears in brackets has been added by the authors to clarify and enhance the use of nursing diagnoses.

BLOOD GLUCOSE WITHIN NORMAL LIMITS ICNP

[Diagnostic Division: Food/Fluid]

Definition: Promotion of euglycemia to enhance short- and long-term health outcomes.

Recognizing Cues

Related/Risk Factors
Excessive stressors; changes in activity level
Excessive weight gain or loss; inadequate/inappropriate dietary intake; food insecurity
Ineffective adherence to treatment regimen; ineffective medication management
Lack of/incorrect blood glucose or diabetes monitoring; lack of knowledge of disease management, modifiable factors
Sedentary lifestyle; alcohol abuse

Defining Characteristics

Subjective
Headache, blurred vision
Irritability; anxiety
Dizziness; light-headedness; fatigue
Thirst; hunger

Objective
Pale
Diaphoresis, shaking
Irregular or fast heartbeat
Increased/frequent urination
Hyperglycemia, hypoglycemia
Changes in mentation; confusion; impaired concentration

Clinical Connections
Diabetes mellitus, diabetic ketoacidosis, hyperosmolar hyperglycemic state (HHS), hypoglycemia, surgical procedures, hepatitis, cirrhosis, gestational diabetes, corticosteroid use, total parenteral nutrition (TPN), infection, sepsis, Cushing syndrome, Addisonian crisis

---

Information that appears in brackets has been added by the authors to clarify and enhance the use of nursing diagnoses.

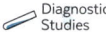 Diagnostic Studies 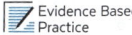 Evidence Based Practice 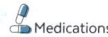 Medications 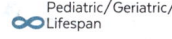 Pediatric/Geriatric/Lifespan

Generate Solutions

Plan Desired Outcomes

Client Will (Include Specific Time Frame)
- Acknowledge factors that may lead to unstable glucose.
- Verbalize understanding of body and energy needs.
- Verbalize plan for modifying factors to prevent or minimize shifts in glucose level.
- Maintain glucose within satisfactory range.

Interventions/Take Action

Nursing Priority No. 1.
To assess cause/contributing factors:
- Identify/investigate client factors (as suggested in Related/Risk Factors and Clinical Connections) that increase the probability of serum glucose fluctuations (e.g., client or family history of diabetes, poor glucose control, eating disorders, poor exercise habits, failure to recognize changes in glucose needs, or serum glucose lability [e.g., thyrotoxicosis, renal failure, Cushing syndrome, steroid use/dependence, pheochromocytoma, sepsis, insulin, or food insecurity, etc.]) **to understand the etiology of client's issue and assist in developing an appropriate treatment plan.**
- Determine client's/significant other's (SO's) knowledge and understanding of the client's condition and treatment needs.
- Identify individual perceptions and expectations of treatment regimen.
- Interview client and discuss relevant cultural, spiritual, and socioeconomic influences that may impact diabetes recognition and care, including family and community perceptions of a diabetes diagnosis; healthcare management plan (e.g., dietary practices, weight, blood pressure, and exercise); and expectations of outcomes. **These factors influence client's ability to manage their condition and must be considered when planning care. Racial and ethnic minorities (i.e., American Indians, Alaska Natives, African Americans, Hispanics, Asian Americans, Native Hawaiians, and other Pacific Islanders) have a higher prevalence of diabetes compared to White people, and often higher rates of complications. Some studies show differences in individuals receiving treatment for hyperlipidemia or albuminuria, control of glucose and hypertension, and preventive self-care. Among some minority groups,**

Information that appears in brackets has been added by the authors to clarify and enhance the use of nursing diagnoses.

a diagnosis of diabetes has a particularly negative connotation; the presence of these cultural perceptions adds to the burden of disease. Access to care and disease management may seem overwhelming. Some people/groups use folk medicine (e.g., bitter food and herbs to reduce blood sugar or practice fasting or prayer) as well as popular remedies. Full knowledge of alternative treatment strategies is important for optimal client outcomes.

- Consider client's age, developmental factors, and ability to care for self. Impacts the client's ability **to assess a problem as well as the ability to prevent harm. Children with type 1 diabetes and their care provider should receive culturally sensitive and age-appropriate care starting at diagnosis and routinely thereafter. Client management should include a plan to ensure continuity of care throughout the client's transition into adult care.**
- Assess family/SO(s) support of the client. **The client may need assistance with lifestyle changes (e.g., food preparation or consumption, exercise, administration of medications) to achieve treatment goals, including serum glucose within the normal range. Children with type 1 diabetes and their care provider should receive education regarding diabetes self-management, medical nutrition therapy, and psychosocial support at diagnosis and regularly thereafter. Treatment plans for the client with diabetes may include devices to monitor blood glucose and/or administer insulin. For the client whose diabetes is partially or wholly managed by someone else (e.g., child, physically impaired, cognitively unable, etc.), caregiver support will be integral for optimal client outcomes.**
- Evaluate client's health status in general terms. **Many clients diagnosed with diabetes or prediabetes have concomitant health concerns (e.g., depression, hypertension, atherosclerosis, renal disease, etc.) that contribute to blood sugar levels.**
- Review client's medication regimen to identify potential causes for unstable blood glucose. **Certain medications have been identified to increase the risk for hyperglycemia (e.g., glucocorticoids, antipsychotic medications, thiazide diuretics, etc.) or hypoglycemia (e.g., quinidine, indomethacin, SGLT2 inhibitors, sulfonylureas, levofloxacin, etc.).**
- Determine client's nutritional status and the effect of dietary patterns on blood glucose.**Overnutrition and undernutrition may have significant implications for blood glucose**

Information that appears in brackets has been added by the authors to clarify and enhance the use of nursing diagnoses.

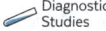 Diagnostic Studies   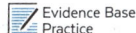 Evidence Based Practice   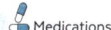 Medications   Pediatric/Geriatric/Lifespan

levels and, subsequently, the action of insulin (endogenous or exogenous). **Note: Dietary/food patterns are often learned in a family context and may have highly symbolic associations; food choices and preparation may be some of the most difficult aspects of diabetes management.**

- Evaluate client's body mass index (BMI), waist-to-hip ratio (WHR), waist circumference, and waist-to-height ratio (WHtR). **Although no single anthropometric measurement may be used conclusively, the trending of several measurements provides greater evidence of client risk and the need for intervention.**
- Review laboratory results (e.g., fasting plasma glucose [FPG], hemoglobin A_{1c} [$HgbA_{1C}$], random plasma glucose test, oral glucose tolerance test [OGTT], and lipid studies [as needed]) **to evaluate indicators and causative factors of glucose intolerance/insulin dysfunction.**
- Note the availability and use of resources.

Nursing Priority No. 2.

To assist client to develop preventive strategies to avoid glucose instability:

- Provide client/family/caregiver with age/education-appropriate, culturally sensitive education regarding the client's specific pathophysiology and treatment needs **to facilitate client support and promote continuity of care.**
- Review client's dietary patterns and provide education on the impact of macronutrients on glucose levels, especially carbohydrate intake. **Glucose balance is primarily determined by the amount of carbohydrates consumed, the client's age, weight, and activity level. Recommendations for the client's diet will be based on medications and the etiology of the problem (i.e., hypo- or hyperglycemia). However, avoidance of spikes in blood glucose associated with diet is recommended.**
- Demonstrate to client and SO(s) how to read food labels and choose foods with carbohydrates described as having a low glycemic index (GI), adequate protein, higher fiber, and low fat content. **These foods produce a slower rise in blood glucose and a more stable release of insulin. Note: For most people with diabetes, the first tool for managing blood glucose is some form of carbohydrate counting. Not all carbohydrates work the same in the body. Some trigger a quick spike in blood sugar, while others work more slowly, keeping blood sugar more stable. The**

Information that appears in brackets has been added by the authors to clarify and enhance the use of nursing diagnoses.

54 Acute Care 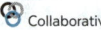 Collaborative 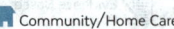 Community/Home Care Cultural

GI addresses these differences by assigning a number to foods that reflects how quickly they increase blood glucose compared to pure glucose. Using the GI may be helpful in "fine-tuning" blood glucose management.
- Assist client and SO(s) to determine a plan for blood glucose monitoring (i.e., intermittent blood glucose monitoring [BGM] or continuous glucose monitoring [CGM]) as appropriate. **Technological advances in the care of diabetic clients offer additional options beyond traditional finger sticks for blood glucose readings. Continuous blood glucose monitoring may be integrated with automatic insulin administration. However, the selection of monitoring should be individualized to the client's needs.**
- Demonstrate the use of approved blood glucose monitoring device (i.e., BGM, CGM) with a return demonstration by the client and/or SO(s) **to ensure competency and accuracy of the device results.**
- Discuss with client and SO(s) common situations that could contribute to client's daily glucose instability **such as missing meals, dehydration, acute infection, level of activity, or stress.**
- Administer antidiabetic medications as prescribed **to facilitate normal blood glucose levels. Early initiation of pharmacological therapy is associated with improved glycemic control and reduced long-term complications in type 1 and 2 diabetes. Drugs and combinations of drugs work in varying ways to achieve blood glucose control.**
- Provide education to client and SO(s) on the client's antidiabetic medication(s) regimen and each medication's mechanism of action (MOA). **The many classes of antidiabetic agents for treatment of type 2 diabetes have varied MOA. Treatment of type 1 diabetes includes a variety of insulins; safe and efficacious glucose control requires a clear understanding of the MOA of how each medication lowers blood glucose and how the actions of medications may overlap to adversely affect the client. This knowledge can help the client avoid or reduce the risk of potential hypoglycemic reactions.**
- Discuss the importance of exercise as part of the diabetes management plan. **Physical exercise is a relevant component of dealing with diabetes; exercise reduces insulin resistance, lowers serum blood glucose levels, and may decrease medication requirements.**
- Provide education to client and SO(s) on balancing food intake, antidiabetic agents, and energy expenditure.

Information that appears in brackets has been added by the authors to clarify and enhance the use of nursing diagnoses.

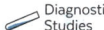 Diagnostic Studies 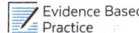 Evidence Based Practice 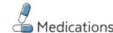 Medications 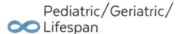 Pediatric/Geriatric/Lifespan

- Review and trend laboratory screening and monitoring tests for diabetes. **Screening tests may include FPG, HgbA$_{1C}$, random plasma glucose test, OGTT, and lipid studies. HgbA$_{1C}$ and estimated average glucose may help determine glucose control over time (few months). Some guidelines suggest that an HgbA$_{1C}$ ≥ 6.5% is suggestive for diabetes, while others indicate that a level of less than 7% is a reasonable goal for most clients; however, evaluation of the client's risk for complications should be considered when establishing therapeutic goals.**

For Client Receiving Insulin

- Include client and SO(s) in determining a plan for insulin administration (i.e., insulin administered by syringe, pen, patch devices, or pump [continuous subcutaneous insulin via automated insulin delivery (AID) systems]). **For most clients, injecting insulin with a syringe or pen is safe and effective in achieving therapeutic goals; however, current research supports the use of AID systems to achieve therapeutic goals and reduce the risk of long-term complications associated with diabetes.**
- Stress the importance of checking expiration dates of insulin, inspecting for cloudiness if it is normally clear, and monitoring proper storage and preparation (when mixing required). **Improper storage affects insulin absorbability and effectiveness.**
- Provide education to client and SO(s) on the type(s) of insulin used (e.g., rapid, short, intermediate, long-acting, combinations, premixed). Discuss timing of administration based on type of insulin prescribed. Remind client that only short-acting insulin (e.g., lispro, aspart, glulisine) is used in a pump. **The type of insulin and the timing of its effects on client's blood glucose level provide valuable information on diet, activity, and potential timing of glucose instability.**
- Recommend keeping a log of injections and sites used. **Verifies that all medication injections are being given. Children, teenagers, and elderly clients may forget injections or be unable to self-inject; the client may need reminders or supervision.**
- Check injection sites periodically **to assess for the development of lipohypertrophy. Insulin administration into lipohypertrophic tissue can cause variable insulin absorption resulting in both hypo- and hyperglycemia.**

Information that appears in brackets has been added by the authors to clarify and enhance the use of nursing diagnoses.

Nursing Priority No. 3.

To promote euglycemia (Teaching/Discharge Considerations) and enhance well-being (long-term goals):

- Review individual risk factors and provide information to assist client in efforts to avoid complications, such as those caused by chronic hyperglycemia and acute hypoglycemia. **Note: Alterations in blood glucose are commonly caused by alterations in nutrition needs, changes in activity levels, or incorrect use of antidiabetic medications or administration devices.**
- Discuss the effects of lifestyle and treatment choices—both immediate and long term—**to help promote informed and effective decision making. Prevention and/or management of high blood pressure and blood lipids can go a long way toward reducing complications associated with diabetes. Research suggests that close control of glucose levels over time may delay onset and reduce severity of complications, enhancing quality of life.**
- Engage client/family/caregiver in formulating a plan **to manage blood glucose level incorporating lifestyle, age and developmental level, and physical and psychological ability to manage the client's condition.**
- Encourage client to develop a system for self-monitoring **to provide a sense of control and enable the client to follow their progress and assist with making choices.**
- Consult with the dietitian about specific dietary needs based on the client's needs (e.g., growth spurt, pregnancy, or change in activity level, comorbidities, etc.).
- Refer to appropriate community resources, such as diabetic educator, medical management, support for insulin pump or glucose monitoring equipment, financial assistance for supplies, support groups, as needed, **for lifestyle modification, etc.**

Documentation Focus

Assessment/Reassessment

- Findings related to individual situation, risk factors, current caloric intake, and dietary pattern; prescription medication use; monitoring of condition
- Client's/caregiver's understanding of individual risks and potential complications
- Results of laboratory tests and finger-stick testing

Information that appears in brackets has been added by the authors to clarify and enhance the use of nursing diagnoses.

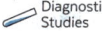 Diagnostic Studies 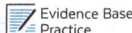 Evidence Based Practice 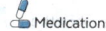 Medications 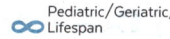 Pediatric/Geriatric/Lifespan

Planning
- Plan of care and who is involved in planning
- Teaching plan

Implementation/Evaluation
- Individual responses to interventions, teaching, and actions performed
- Specific actions and changes that are made
- Attainment of or progress toward desired outcomes
- Modifications to plan of care

Discharge Planning
- Long-term plans for ongoing needs, monitoring and management of condition, and who is responsible for actions to be taken
- Sources for equipment/supplies
- Specific referrals made

Sample Nursing Outcomes & Interventions Classifications NOC/NIC

NOC—Blood Glucose Control
NIC—Hyperglycemia/Hypoglycemia Management

risk for imbalanced BLOOD PRESSURE   NANDA-I

[Diagnostic Division: Circulation]

Definition: Susceptible to recurrent elevation or decrease in the force exerted by blood flow on the arterial wall, above or below desired individual levels.

Recognizing Cues

Risk Factors
Anxiety; excessive stress
Inadequate fluid volume; excessive bleeding
Excessive fluid volume; edema
Inappropriate dietary habits; ineffective overweight self-management
Inadequate knowledge of risk factors; inadequate self-management of orthostasis
Sedentary behavior occurring for ≥2 hr/day; ineffective sleep pattern

---

Information that appears in brackets has been added by the authors to clarify and enhance the use of nursing diagnoses.

 Acute Care 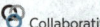 Collaborative 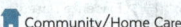 Community/Home Care 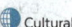 Cultural

Inadequate follow-through with treatment regimen
Tobacco use; substance misuse

Clinical Connections

Fluid retention or fluid shifts; hypertension; cardiac disease/
dysrhythmia; stroke/brain injury; spinal cord injury; surgery; trauma; burns; eating disorders (anorexia/bulimia); sepsis; hemorrhagic conditions; diabetes ketoacidosis; Cushing syndrome; hyperparathyroidism; hyperthyroidism or hypothyroidism; pregnancy complications; medication effect/drug use

[This nursing diagnosis encompasses assessments and nursing interventions found in many other nursing diagnoses. For specific related information, refer to NDs risk for ineffective cerebral Tissue Perfusion; risk for Allergy Reaction; risk for Autonomic Dysreflexia; risk for excessive Bleeding; impaired Cardiac Output; inadequate Health Knowledge; risk for impaired Water-Electrolyte Balance; inadequate Fluid Volume; excessive Fluid Volume; Hyperthermia; risk for Infection; risk for Shock.]

Generate Solutions

Plan Desired Outcomes

Client Will (Include Specific Time Frame)

- Maintain blood pressure within acceptable limits.
- Experience no cardiovascular or systemic complications.
- Verbalize understanding of condition, therapeutic regimen, and preventive measures.
- Initiate necessary lifestyle/behavioral changes.

Interventions/Take Action

Nursing Priority No. 1.

To identify contributing risk factors:

- Identify presence of associated conditions, for example, (1) cardiac dysfunction (including myocardial infarction, dysrhythmias, heart failure, cardiomyopathy); (2) brain injury (including traumatic injury, stroke); (3) fluid imbalances (either deficit or excess) and electrolyte imbalances; (4) endocrine disorders (e.g., primary aldosteronism, adrenal gland tumors, thyroid issues); (5) acute or chronic renal disease; (6) trauma (causing damage to central and autonomic systems, including radiation for head and neck cancers,

---

Information that appears in brackets has been added by the authors to clarify and enhance the use of nursing diagnoses.

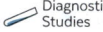 Diagnostic Studies 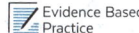 Evidence Based Practice 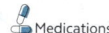 Medications 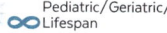 Pediatric/Geriatric/Lifespan

spinal cord injury); (7) fever (such as accompanies infections/sepsis); (8) substance use/abuse/overdose/withdrawal (e.g., caffeine, cocaine, alcohol/other drugs of abuse); (9) great physical/emotional stress (e.g., traumas causing anxiety, fear/panic); (10) pregnancy; and (11) allergic reactions, **which can cause or exacerbate blood pressure instability.**

- Review current medication regimen. **Use of certain medications, such as dysrhythmia agents, vasodilators, antihypertensives, diuretics, tricyclic antidepressants, medications for Parkinson disease, can have direct effects on blood pressure.**

- Determine how client takes medications, whether assistance is provided and by whom. **Blood pressure fluctuations can occur (1) in client who is not taking blood pressure medications as prescribed (e.g., older client living alone who doesn't understand or chooses not to follow directions and takes less or more than prescribed dose); (2) in client who is taking medications as prescribed but failing to report adverse side effects (e.g., blood pressure too low on current dose of amlodipine); (3) when caregiver is not involved with client medications, does not understand dosing instructions, inadvertently gives incorrect doses, or makes decisions for client (e.g., "My husband doesn't like the way that medication makes him feel, so we stopped the blood pressure medication"); or (4) if client/caregiver receives inadequate teaching.**

- Note client age, general health, developmental and cognitive status. Determine how client takes medications, whether assistance is provided and by whom. **These factors affect client's abilities to manage own symptoms or respond to emergent conditions affecting blood pressure.**

- Ascertain client's current and ongoing blood pressure measurements, noting trends and sudden changes.

- Measure blood pressure to determine risk for hypertension or hypotension, using the appropriate size and type of equipment, proper position (e.g., seated, legs uncrossed, feet flat on floor), and free of contributing factors (e.g., recent consumption of caffeine, recent administration of influential medications, agitation). Be aware of numbers that are currently used to identify normal ranges of blood pressure. **Incorrect readings may result in inappropriate or lack of needed treatment.**

- Note client reports of headaches, blurred vision, chest pain, weakness or numbness in arms, legs, or face, **which may**

Information that appears in brackets has been added by the authors to clarify and enhance the use of nursing diagnoses.

indicate that blood pressure is elevated (although high blood pressure often fails to produce any noticeable symptoms until damage to the blood vessels results in serious conditions or blood pressure rise is sudden).

- Observe for (or assess client/significant [SO] reports of) sudden high blood pressure. **This condition usually occurs in a small percentage of people with high blood pressure. It can occur in young adults. The at-risk population includes a high number of African American men and individuals experiencing collagen vascular disorders, kidney issues, or pregnancy.**
- Note client reports of dizziness or fainting, blurred vision, nausea, shortness of breath, and thirst, **which may indicate that blood pressure is fluctuating downward.**
- Note whether client has potential causes for low blood pressure, or hypotension. **The reason (1) may not be pathological (e.g., client reports typical blood pressure lower depending on time of day or with medication effect; chronic kidney disease); or (2) may be indicative of pathological-associated conditions (e.g., heart attack, blood loss, allergic response).**

Nursing Priority No. 2.
To assist client/caregiver to reduce risk:

- Refer for and collaborate in treatment/management of underlying condition(s) **that can restore hemodynamic stability or reduce risk of blood pressure fluctuations.**
- Monitor blood pressure as indicated and evaluate trends. Correlate client's symptoms with potential or identified cause for blood pressure instability.
- Address personal factors (e.g., age and developmental level, social and cultural influences, life experiences, cognitive/emotional/psychological impairment) **that require modifications in healthcare management, teaching, and follow-up.**
- Discuss with client/SO those risk factors that are modifiable (e.g., dietary modifications such as reduced sodium and weight loss where indicated, taking medications as prescribed, avoiding substance misuse/[abuse]).
- Recommend changing position from supine to standing slowly and in stages, avoiding standing motionless or for long periods of time, or sitting with legs crossed **to enhance safety and reduce gravitational blood pooling in the lower extremities.**

Information that appears in brackets has been added by the authors to clarify and enhance the use of nursing diagnoses.

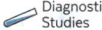 Diagnostic Studies 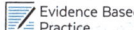 Evidence Based Practice 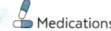 Medications 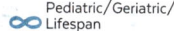 Pediatric/Geriatric/Lifespan

- Identify available support systems, as needed. **Client or caregiver may need community resources (e.g., home healthcare services, assistance with medication setup/administration, supervision or day care for frail elderly or child).**
- Emphasize importance of regular and long-term medical follow-up appointments **for monitoring blood pressure and disease/condition trends and to provide for early intervention to reduce risk of complications.**

Nursing Priority No. 3.

To promote stable blood pressure (Teaching/Discharge Considerations) and enhance well-being (long-term goals):

- Determine most urgent need from client's/caregiver's and healthcare provider's viewpoints, **which may differ and require adjustments in teaching plan.**
- Teach home monitoring of blood pressure, where indicated, and obtain return demonstration of ability to take blood pressure (and medications) accurately.
- Recommend client keep diary of pressure readings taken at different times of the day and note any associated symptoms. **Provides opportunity to follow trends and identify contributing factors, such as medication effects.**
- Instruct client/SO in healthy eating and adequate fluid intake. **For example, obesity is a risk factor for hypertension, and dehydration is a risk for hypotension. Furthermore, sodium intake can influence blood pressure in hyper- and hypotension.**
- Instruct client/SO in lifestyle modifications based on identified risks. **Exercise program, smoking cessation, stress management techniques, and substance use programs not only reduce risk of blood pressure issues but also enhance general well-being.**
- Elicit client's knowledge of reportable blood pressure measurements and symptoms and to whom to report. **Provides opportunity for timely intervention.**
- Review specifics and rationale for components of treatment plan. Ask client/SO if they have questions and/or if they are willing to adhere to plan. **Helps to identify areas of concern and need for further instruction/interventions.**
- Refer to specific underlying condition for related teaching/discharge considerations.

Documentation Focus

Assessment/Reassessment
- Baseline and subsequent blood pressure measurements

Information that appears in brackets has been added by the authors to clarify and enhance the use of nursing diagnoses.

 Acute Care 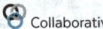 Collaborative 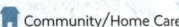 Community/Home Care Cultural

- Medications (correct use, understanding of expected and reportable side effects)
- Individual risk factors

Planning
- Plan of care and who is involved in planning
- Teaching plan, such as dietary modification, consistent exercise, safety issues, consistent fluid volume status

Implementation/Evaluation
- Client's response to interventions, teaching, and actions performed
- Status and disposition at discharge
- Attainment of or progress toward desired outcome(s)
- Modifications to plan of care

Discharge Planning
- Discharge considerations and who will be responsible for carrying out individual actions
- Long-term needs and available resources
- Specific referrals made

Sample Nursing Outcomes & Interventions Classifications NOC/NIC

NOC—Cardiac Pump Effectiveness
NIC—Hypertension [or] Hypotension Management

---

disturbed BODY IMAGE ICNP

[Diagnostic Division: Self-Perception/Concept]

Definition: Individual's negative perceptions, thoughts, and feelings of how they view their body, or fear others view their body.

Recognizing Cues

Related/Risk Factors
Presence of visible physical disabilities (e.g., use prosthesis, crutches/wheelchair); chronic health conditions, pain
Perceived conflict with social medias' presentations of an ideal body; cultural differences in ideal body type/beauty
Eating disorders; substance misuse/abuse to control weight
Depression
Gender dysphoria

Information that appears in brackets has been added by the authors to clarify and enhance the use of nursing diagnoses.

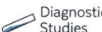 Diagnostic Studies 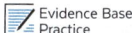 Evidence Based Practice 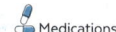 Medications Pediatric/Geriatric/Lifespan

Defining Characteristics

Subjective
Highly critical of appearance/function

Repeatedly compares past and present appearance/function (e.g., weight loss, sexual attractiveness, change in body-functions, physical strength)

Concerns of not meeting cultural expectations related to appearance or sexuality

Fears response of others to appearance or disability

Names or uses impersonal pronouns to describe impaired body part/missing body part

Self-deprecating statements

Objective
Routinely monitors changes in body (e.g., repeated weighing); compares body structure and functioning with others

Attempts to cover/hide perceived negative body part; prevents contact with the deformed/malfunctioning body part

Lacks proprioception (sense of self-movement or body position); body part(s) not moving as expected, involuntary body movements (e.g., tremors, tics, repetitious muscle contractions, tardive dyskinesia, cerebral palsy)

Anxious (e.g., restlessness, fidgeting, inability to concentrate); social anxiety; decreased social interactions; loss of self-confidence, self-esteem

Compulsive eating; excessive exercise; fasting; purging; laxative or diuretic use

Refuses to acknowledge change

Depressive symptoms (e.g., lack of eye contact, fatigue, sadness); substance misuse

Clinical Connections
Anorexia/bulimia nervosa, traumatic injuries/burns, cerebrovascular accident, spinal cord injury, surgical procedures (e.g., ostomy, amputation, mastectomy, hysterectomy), chronic conditions (e.g., arthritis, psoriasis), renal dialysis, sexually transmitted diseases (e.g., human immunodeficiency virus [HIV] infections, genital herpes), depression, anxiety, borderline personality disorder

Generate Solutions

Plan Desired Outcomes

Client Will (Include Specific Time Frame)
- Recognize and discuss their body change while maintaining positive self-esteem and self-concept.

Information that appears in brackets has been added by the authors to clarify and enhance the use of nursing diagnoses.

 Acute Care 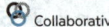 Collaborative 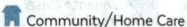 Community/Home Care Cultural

- Actively seek information to improve health status/function.
- Recognize and verbalize they are a valuable human being with responsibilities for self and others.
- Verbalize importance and demonstrate appropriate use of adaptive devices/prosthetics.

Interventions/Take Action

Nursing Priority No. 1.

To assess causative/contributing factors:

- Identify client's thoughts and feelings related to the current situation. **Helps to understand the client's perceptions of what they are thinking about their body image, which may indicate acceptance or nonacceptance of the situation.**
- Discuss present pathophysiology and/or situation affecting the individual (e.g., neurological deficit; cerebrovascular accident [CVA]; severe, ongoing pain; amputee; disfigurement; or inadequate sexual function). **Understanding the client's perception of their condition can suggest additional NDs such as chronic Pain, impaired Sexual Functioning, ineffective adolescent or child Eating Dynamics, Body Weight Problem for focused interventions.**
- Determine whether the condition is permanent with no expectation for resolution. **Identifies appropriate interventions based on reality of situation and need to plan for long- or short-term prognosis. Note: There is always something that can be done to enhance acceptance, and it is important to hold out the possibility of living a good life with the disability/situation.** (Refer to other NDs situational, or chronic inadequate Self-Esteem; inadequate Self-Compassion for additional interventions as appropriate.)
- Assess mental and physical illnesses or conditions influencing client's emotional state (e.g., diseases of the endocrine system or use of steroid therapy, schizophrenia, depression, or anxiety). **Some diseases or conditions can have a profound effect on one's emotions and need to be considered in the evaluation and treatment of the individual's behavior and reaction to the current situation. May interfere with ability to engage in therapy and indicate need to provide interventions to deal with concern before beginning therapy.**
- Have the client describe self, noting what is positive and what is negative. Be aware of how the client believes others see self. **Identifies self-image and whether there is a discrepancy between own view and how client's view is**

Information that appears in brackets has been added by the authors to clarify and enhance the use of nursing diagnoses.

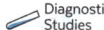 Diagnostic Studies 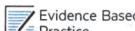 Evidence Based Practice 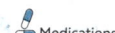 Medications 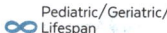 Pediatric/Geriatric/Lifespan

affected by social media or how client believes others see self, which may have an effect on how client perceives changes that have occurred.
- Discuss the meaning of loss/change to client. **A small (seemingly trivial) loss may have a big impact (e.g., the use of a urinary catheter or enema for continence). A change in function (e.g., immobility in elderly) may be more difficult for some to deal with than a change in appearance. The change could be devastating (e.g., permanent facial scarring of child).**
- Use developmentally appropriate communication techniques for determining exact expression of body image in a child (e.g., puppet play or constructive dialogue for toddler). **Developmental capacity must guide interaction to gain accurate information.**
- Note signs of grieving or indicators of severe or prolonged depression **to evaluate need for counseling and/or medications.**
- Determine ethnic background and cultural and religious perceptions or considerations. **Understanding how these factors affect the individual in this situation and how they may influence how individual deals with what has happened is necessary to develop appropriate intervention.**
- Identify social aspects of illness or condition (e.g., sexually transmitted diseases, sterility, vitiligo, multiple sclerosis, or chronic conditions). **May affect how client views self and functions in social settings as well as how others view the client.**
- Observe interaction of client with significant other (SO). **Distortions in body image may be unconsciously reinforced by family members, and/or secondary gain issues may interfere with progress.**

Nursing Priority No. 2.
To determine coping abilities and skills:

- Assess the client's current level of adaptation and progress. **Client may have already adapted somewhat, and information provides starting point for developing plan of care.**
- Active-listen client's comments and responses to the situation. **Different situations are upsetting to different people, depending on individual coping skills and past experiences.**
- Identify use of defense mechanisms (e.g., denial, displacement). **May be a normal response to a situation or may**

Information that appears in brackets has been added by the authors to clarify and enhance the use of nursing diagnoses.

 Acute Care  Collaborative 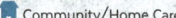 Community/Home Care   Cultural

be indicative of mental illness (e.g., schizophrenia). (Refer to ND difficulty Coping.)
- Identify dependence on prescription medications or use of addictive substances, such as alcohol or other drugs. **May reflect defensive coping opposed to healthy coping strategies.**
- Identify previously used coping strategies and effectiveness. **Familiar coping strategies can be used to begin adaptation to current situation.**
- Determine individual/family/community resources available to client. **Can provide efficient assistance and support to enable client to adapt to changing circumstances.**

Nursing Priority No. 3.

To assist client and SO(s) to deal with/accept issues of self-concept related to body image:

- Establish a therapeutic nurse-client/SO relationship, conveying an attitude of caring and developing a sense of trust. **Conveys an attitude of caring and develops a sense of trust in which client can discuss concerns and find answers to issues confronting the client in new situation.**
- Assess and monitor client frequently while acknowledging the individual as someone who is worthwhile. **Provides opportunities for listening to concerns and answering questions to promote dealing positively with individual situation and change in body image.**
- Identify and assist in correcting underlying fears or concerns when possible. **Promote optimal healing and adaptation to individual situation (i.e., amputation, presence of colostomy, mastectomy, impotence).**
- Provide assistance with self-care needs as necessary while promoting individual abilities and independence. **Client may need support to achieve the goal of independence and positive return to managing own life.**
- Work with the client's self-concept, avoiding moral judgments regarding client's efforts or progress (e.g., "You should be progressing faster"; "You're weak or not trying hard enough"). **Such statements diminish self-esteem and are counterproductive to progress. Positive reinforcement encourages the client to continue efforts and strive for improvement.**
- Discuss concerns about fear of mutilation, prognosis, or rejection when the client is facing surgery or a potentially poor outcome of procedure/illness, **to address realities and provide emotional support to enable client to be ready to deal with whatever the outcome may be.**

Information that appears in brackets has been added by the authors to clarify and enhance the use of nursing diagnoses.

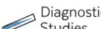 Diagnostic Studies   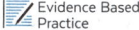 Evidence Based Practice   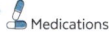 Medications   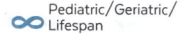 Pediatric/Geriatric/Lifespan

- Acknowledge and accept feelings of dependency, grief, and hostility. **Conveys a message of understanding.**
- Encourage verbalization of and role-play anticipated conflicts **to enhance the handling of potential situations.**
- Encourage client and SO(s) to communicate feelings to each other and discuss situation openly. **Helps to enhance handling of potential situations. Provides an opportunity to imagine and practice how different situations can be dealt with, thus promoting confidence.**
- Alert staff to monitor their own facial expressions and other nonverbal behaviors. **Important to convey acceptance and not revulsion when the client's appearance is affected. Clients are very sensitive to reactions of those around them, and negative reactions will affect self-esteem and may retard adaptation to situation.**
- Encourage family members to treat client normally and not as an invalid. **Helps client return to own routine and begin to gain confidence in ability to manage own life.**
- Encourage client to look at/touch affected body part. **Helps to incorporate changes into body image. Acceptance will enhance self-esteem and enable client to move forward in a positive manner.**
- Allow client to use denial without participating (e.g., client may at first refuse to look at a colostomy; the nurse says, "I am going to change your colostomy now," and proceeds with the task). **Provides the individual with time to adapt to the situation.**
- Set limits on maladaptive behavior and assist client to identify positive behaviors. **Self-esteem will be damaged if client is allowed to continue behaviors that are destructive or are not helpful, and adaptation to new image will be delayed.**
- Provide accurate information as desired/requested. Reinforce previously given information. **Accurate knowledge helps client make better decisions for the future.**
- Discuss the availability of prosthetics, reconstructive surgery, and physical/occupational therapy or other referrals as dictated by the individual situation. **Provides hope that situation is not impossible, and the future does not look so bleak.**
- Assist client to select and use clothing or makeup appropriately. **Helps to minimize body changes and enhance appearance.**
- Discuss the reasons for infectious isolation and treatment procedures when used, and make time to sit down and

---

Information that appears in brackets has been added by the authors to clarify and enhance the use of nursing diagnoses.

 Acute Care 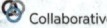 Collaborative 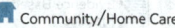 Community/Home Care   Cultural

talk/listen to client while in the room. **Promotes understanding and decreases sense of isolation/loneliness.**

Nursing Priority No. 4.

To promote ongoing self acceptance (Teaching/Discharge Considerations) and enhance well-being (long-term goals):

- Begin counseling/other therapies (e.g., biofeedback, relaxation) as soon as possible. **Provides early/ongoing sources of support to promote rehabilitation in a timely manner.**
- Provide information at the client's level of acceptance and in small segments. **Allows for easier assimilation.**
- Clarify misconceptions and reinforce explanations given by other health team members. **Ensures client is hearing factual information to make the best decisions for own situation.**
- Include client in the decision-making process and problem-solving activities. **Promotes adherence to decisions and plans that are made.**
- Assist client in incorporating the therapeutic regimen into activities of daily living (e.g., including specific exercises and housework activities). **Promotes continuation of a program by helping client see that progress can be made within own daily activities.**
- Identify/plan for alterations to home and work environment/activities. **Accommodates individual needs and supports independence.**
- Assist client in learning strategies for dealing with feelings and venting emotions. **Helps individual move toward healing and optimal recuperation.**
- Offer positive reinforcement for efforts made (e.g., wearing makeup or using a prosthetic device). **Client needs to hear that what they are doing is helping.**
- Refer to appropriate support groups. **May need additional help/positive role models to adjust to new situation and life changes.**

Documentation Focus

Assessment/Reassessment

- Observations, presence of maladaptive behaviors, emotional changes, stage of grieving, level of independence
- Physical wounds, dressings; use of life support–type machine (e.g., ventilator, dialysis machine)
- Meaning of loss or change to client
- Support systems available (e.g., SOs, friends, and groups)

Information that appears in brackets has been added by the authors to clarify and enhance the use of nursing diagnoses.

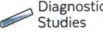 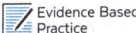 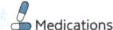 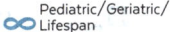

Planning
- Plan of care and who is involved in planning
- Teaching plan

Implementation/Evaluation
- Client's response to interventions, teaching, and actions performed
- Attainment of or progress toward desired outcome(s)
- Modifications of plan of care

Discharge Planning
- Long-term needs and who is responsible for actions
- Specific referrals made (e.g., rehabilitation center and community resources)

Sample Nursing Outcomes & Interventions Classifications NOC/NIC

NOC—Body Image
NIC—Body Image Enhancement

---

decreased BODY TEMPERATURE   NANDA-I

[Diagnostic Division: Safety]

Definition: Unintended drop in the internal thermal state below the normal diurnal range in individuals >28 days of life.

Recognizing Cues

Related/Risk Factors
Alcohol intoxication; malnutrition
Excessive conductive, convective, evaporative, or radiative heat transfer
Low environmental temperature; inactivity
Inadequate caregiver knowledge of importance of body temperature management, or of hypothermia prevention
Inappropriate clothing for environmental temperature; wet clothing in low temperature environment

Defining Characteristics

Objective
Hypothermia I—mild
Core temperature 32°C–35°C (89.6°F–95°F)

Information that appears in brackets has been added by the authors to clarify and enhance the use of nursing diagnoses.

 Acute Care   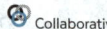 Collaborative   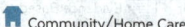 Community/Home Care   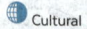 Cultural

Piloerection
Skin cool to touch; shivering
Hypothermia II—moderate
Core temperature 28°C to less than 32°C (82.4°F–89.6°F); skin cool to touch; slow capillary refill
Increased blood pressure; hypertension
Tachycardia; increased cardiac output
Peripheral vasoconstriction; slow capillary refill
Increased respiratory rate, oxygen consumption
Cyanotic nailbeds; acrocyanosis
Decreased blood glucose level; hypoglycemia
Impaired consciousness
Hypothermia III—severe
Core temperature less than 28°C (82.4°F)
Hypotension; bradycardia; ventricular arrhythmias
Bradypnea; hypoxia
Unconsciousness

Clinical Connections

Dementia, malnutrition, anorexia nervosa, brain trauma, stroke, endocrine disorders, infection, traumatic injury, alcohol intoxication, radiotherapy, abuse or neglect, prematurity, near drowning

Generate Solutions

Plan Desired Outcomes

Client Will (Include Specific Time Frame)
- Display core temperature within normal range.
- Be free of complications, such as cardiac failure, respiratory infection or failure, and thromboembolic phenomena.
- Identify underlying cause or contributing factors that are within client control.
- Verbalize understanding of specific interventions to prevent hypothermia.
- Demonstrate behaviors to monitor and promote normothermia.

Caregiver Will (Include Specific Time Frame)
- Maintain a safe environment.
- Identify underlying cause or contributing factors that are within caregiver control.
- Verbalize an understanding of specific interventions to prevent hypothermia.
- Demonstrate behaviors to monitor and promote normothermia.

Information that appears in brackets has been added by the authors to clarify and enhance the use of nursing diagnoses.

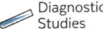 Diagnostic Studies   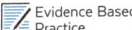 Evidence Based Practice   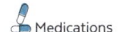 Medications   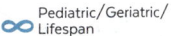 Pediatric/Geriatric/Lifespan

Interventions/Take Action

Nursing Priority No. 1.
To assess causative/contributing factors:

- Note underlying cause, for example, (1) *decreased heat production,* such as occurs with hypopituitary, hypoadrenal, and hypothyroid conditions; hypoglycemia; and neuromuscular inefficiencies seen in extremes of age; (2) *increased heat loss,* such as occurs with exposure to cold weather, winter outdoor activities; cold water drenching or immersion; improper clothing, shelter, or food for conditions; vasodilation from medications, drugs, or poisons; skin-surface problems such as burns or psoriasis; fluid losses, dehydration; surgery, open wounds, exposed skin or viscera; multiple rapid infusions of cold solutions or transfusions of banked blood; overtreatment of hyperthermia; or (3) *impaired thermoregulation.* Hypothalamus failure might occur with central nervous system (CNS) trauma or tumor, intracranial bleeding or stroke, toxicological and metabolic disorders, Parkinson disease, or multiple sclerosis (MS).
- Note contributing or risk factors, such as age of client (e.g., premature infant, child, elderly person); concurrent or coexisting medical problems (e.g., brainstem injury, CNS trauma, near drowning, sepsis, hypothyroidism); other factors (e.g., alcohol or other drug use or abuse; homelessness); living conditions; or relationship status (e.g., age of cognitive impaired client living alone).

Nursing Priority No. 2.
To prevent a further decrease in body temperature

Mild to moderate hypothermia:
Remove wet clothing and bedding.
Add layers of clothing and wrap in warm blankets.
Increase physical activity if possible.
Provide warm liquids after shivering stops if client is alert and can swallow.
Provide warm, nutrient-dense food (carbohydrates, proteins, and fats) and fluids (hot sweet liquids are easily digestible and absorbable).
Avoid alcohol, caffeine, and tobacco **to prevent vasodilation, diuresis, or vasoconstriction, respectively.**
Place in warm ambient temperature environment and protect from drafts; safely provide external heat sources.

Information that appears in brackets has been added by the authors to clarify and enhance the use of nursing diagnoses.

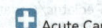 Acute Care 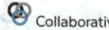 Collaborative 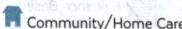 Community/Home Care   Cultural

- Provide barriers to heat loss, monitoring temperature closely. **Measures might include the use of protective hats and/or heating blanket.**

Severe hypothermia:

- Remove the client from causative or contributing factors.
  Remove tight-fitting clothing or jewelry. Let affected skin dry passively, cover with blankets, and provide shelter with warm ambient temperature; use radiant lights.
  Provide heat to trunk, not to extremities, initially. Avoid the use of heat lamps or hot water bottles. **Surface rewarming can result in rewarming shock due to surface vasodilation.**
  Elevate affected body parts and separate affected fingers/toes with a loose bulky dressing. Avoid rubbing or massaging the injured skin **to prevent soft tissue injury.**
  Immerse affected extremity in warmed water (37°C–39°C). **The preferred method for rewarming and prevention of further tissue damage.**
  Keep the individual lying down. Avoid jarring (**can trigger an abnormal heart rhythm**).

Nursing Priority No. 3.
To evaluate effects of hypothermia:

- Measure the core temperature with a low-register thermometer (measuring below 94°F [34.4°C]).
- Assess respiratory effort (**rate and tidal volume are reduced when metabolic rate decreases and respiratory acidosis occurs**).
- Auscultate lungs, noting adventitious sounds. **Pulmonary edema, respiratory infection, and pulmonary embolus are possible complications of hypothermia.**
- Monitor heart rate and rhythm. **Cold stress reduces pacemaker function, and bradycardia (unresponsive to atropine), atrial fibrillation, atrioventricular blocks, and ventricular tachycardia can occur. Ventricular fibrillation occurs most frequently when core temperature is 82°F (27.7°C) or below.**
- Monitor blood pressure, noting hypotension. **Can occur due to vasoconstriction and shunting of fluids as a result of cold injury effect on capillary permeability.**
- Measure urine output. **Oliguria and renal failure can occur due to low flow state and/or following hypothermic osmotic diuresis.**
- Note CNS effects (e.g., mood changes, sluggish thinking, amnesia, complete obtundation) and peripheral CNS effects

---

Information that appears in brackets has been added by the authors to clarify and enhance the use of nursing diagnoses.

 Diagnostic Studies   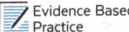 Evidence Based Practice   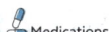 Medications   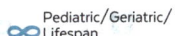 Pediatric/Geriatric/Lifespan

(e.g., paralysis—87.7°F [30.9°C]; dilated pupils—below 86°F [30°C]; flat electroencephalogram [EEG]—68°F [20°C]).

- Monitor laboratory studies, such as arterial blood gas (ABGs) **(respiratory and metabolic acidosis);** electrolytes; complete blood count (CBC) **(increased hematocrit, decreased white blood cell count);** cardiac enzymes **(myocardial infarct may occur owing to electrolyte imbalance, cold-stress catecholamine release, hypoxia, or acidosis);** coagulation profile; glucose; and pharmacological profile **(for possible cumulative drug effects).**

Nursing Priority No. 4.

To restore normal body temperature/organ function/organ function:

- Assist with measures to normalize core temperature, such as warmed IV solutions and warm solution lavage of body cavities (gastric, peritoneal, bladder) or cardiopulmonary bypass, if indicated.
- Rewarm no faster than 1 to 2 degrees per hour **to avoid sudden vasodilation, increased metabolic demands on heart, and hypotension (rewarming shock).**
- Assist with surface warming by means of heated blankets, warm environment or radiant heater, electronic heating/cooling devices. Cover head, neck, and thorax. Leave extremities uncovered, as appropriate, **to maintain peripheral vasoconstriction.** Refrain from instituting surface rewarming prior to core rewarming in severe hypothermia, **as it may cause after-drop of temperature by shunting cold blood back to the heart in addition to rewarming shock as a result of surface vasodilation.**
- Protect the skin and tissues by repositioning, applying lotion or lubricants, and avoiding direct contact with heating appliance or blanket. **Impaired circulation can result in severe tissue damage.**
- Keep client quiet; handle gently **to reduce the potential for fibrillation in a cold heart.**
- Provide CPR, as necessary, with compressions initially at one-half the normal heart rate **(severe hypothermia causes slowed conduction, and a cold heart may be unresponsive to medications, pacing, and defibrillation).**
- Maintain patent airway. Assist with intubation and mechanical ventilation, if indicated.
- Provide heated, humidified oxygen when used.
- Turn off warming blanket when temperature is within 1 to 3 degrees of desired temperature **to allow for drift and avoid hyperthermia situation.**

Information that appears in brackets has been added by the authors to clarify and enhance the use of nursing diagnoses.

 Acute Care 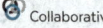 Collaborative 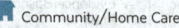 Community/Home Care 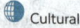 Cultural

- Administer IV fluids with caution **to prevent overload as the vascular bed expands (a cold heart is slow to compensate for increased volume).**
- Avoid vigorous drug therapy. **As rewarming occurs, organ function returns, correcting endocrine abnormalities, and tissues become more receptive to the effects of drugs previously administered.**
- Perform range-of-motion exercises, provide sequential compression devices (SCDs), reposition, encourage coughing and deep-breathing exercises, avoid restrictive clothing or restraints **to reduce effects of circulatory stasis.**
- Provide well-balanced, high-calorie diet or feedings **to replenish glycogen stores and nutritional balance.**

Nursing Priority No. 5.

To maintain normothermia (Teaching/Discharge Considerations) and enhance well-being (long-term goals):

- Review specific risk factors or causes of hypothermia. Note that hypothermia can be *accidental* or *intentional* (such as occurs when induced-hypothermia therapy is used after cardiac arrest or brain injury), requiring interventions to protect client from adverse effects.
- Maintain a warm ambient environment, especially in facility settings (e.g., operating room, bath areas).
- Heed severe cold weather warnings, staying inside when possible, and storing blankets, emergency gear, and extra batteries for cell phones in car in event of winter storms.
- Recommend appropriate warm clothing (layers plus appropriate outwear, hats, gloves, shoes, socks, and boots) in cold weather, with children and frail elderly well wrapped up when outdoors, and limit time exposures.
- Suggest eating and drinking warm fluids regularly when outside during cold weather and avoiding alcohol.
- Remove wet clothing and bedding promptly. Add extra clothing and warmed blankets.
- Discuss signs/symptoms of early hypothermia (e.g., changes in mentation, poor judgment, somnolence, impaired coordination, slurred speech) **to facilitate recognition of problem and timely intervention.**
- Identify assistive community resources, as indicated (e.g., social services, emergency shelters, clothing suppliers, food bank, public service company, financial resources). **Individual/significant other may be in need of numerous resources if hypothermia was associated with inadequate housing, homelessness, or malnutrition.**

Information that appears in brackets has been added by the authors to clarify and enhance the use of nursing diagnoses.

 Diagnostic Studies 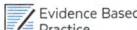 Evidence Based Practice 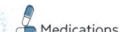 Medications 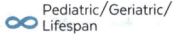 Pediatric/Geriatric/Lifespan

Documentation Focus

Assessment/Reassessment
- Findings, noting degree of system involvement, respiratory rate, ECG pattern, capillary refill, and level of mentation
- Graph temperature

Planning
- Plan of care and who is involved in planning
- Teaching plan

Implementation/Evaluation
- Responses to interventions, teaching, and actions performed
- Attainment of or progress toward desired outcome(s)
- Modifications to plan of care

Discharge Planning
- Long-term needs, identifying who is responsible for each action

Sample Nursing Outcomes & Interventions Classifications NOC/NIC

NOC—Thermoregulation
NIC—Hypothermia Treatment

---

decreased neonatal BODY TEMPERATURE NANDA-I

[Diagnostic Division: Safety]

Definition: Unintended drop in the thermal state below the normal diurnal range in individuals up to 28 days of life.

Recognizing Cues

Related/Risk Factors
Delivery room with temperatures below 25°C (77°F); low environmental temperature
Inadequate skin-to-skin contact immediately after birth
Immature stratum corneum
Delayed chestfeeding; malnutrition
Early bathing of newborn; weighing of newborn less than 6 h of age
Inadequate clothing; inappropriate clothing for environmental temperature; wet clothing in low-temperature environment
Excessive conductive, convective, evaporative, or radiative heat transfer

---

Information that appears in brackets has been added by the authors to clarify and enhance the use of nursing diagnoses.

 Acute Care 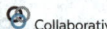 Collaborative 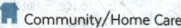 Community/Home Care   Cultural

Inadequate caregiver knowledge of hypothermia prevention, or importance of body temperature management

Defining Characteristics

Objective

Hypothermia I—mild
Axillary temperature 36°C to 36.4°C (96.8°F–97.5°F)
Pallor; decreased peripheral perfusion
Increased oxygen demand; tachypnea; tachycardia
Decreased blood glucose level; weight gain less than 30 g/day
Hypothermia II—moderate
Axillary temperature 32°C to 35.9°C (89.6°F–96.6°F); skin cool to touch; slow capillary refill
Dyspnea; grunting; acrocyanosis
Inadequate energy to maintain sucking; unaddressed hypoglycemia; metabolic acidosis
Bradycardia; hypertension
Irritable crying; lethargy
Hypothermia III—severe
Axillary temperature less than 32°C (89.6°F)
Peripheral vasoconstriction
Respiratory distress; hypoxia

Clinical Connections

Newborn infant, low-birth-weight neonate, premature neonate, hypoglycemia, adolescent pregnancy, cesarean delivery, out-of-hospital birth, sepsis

Generate Solutions

Plan Desired Outcomes

Client Will (Include Specific Time Frame)

- Display core temperature within normal range.
- Be free of signs/symptoms of hypothermia such as pale, cool skin; bradycardia, tachypnea, restlessness, hypoglycemia.
- Be free of complications such as cardiac failure, respiratory infection or failure, and thromboembolic phenomena.

Caregiver Will (Include Specific Time Frame)

- Maintain safe environment.
  Identify underlying cause or contributing factors that are within caregiver control.
  Verbalize understanding of specific interventions to prevent hypothermia.

Information that appears in brackets has been added by the authors to clarify and enhance the use of nursing diagnoses.

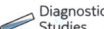 Diagnostic Studies   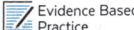 Evidence Based Practice   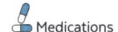 Medications   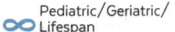 Pediatric/Geriatric/Lifespan

- Demonstrate behaviors to monitor and promote normothermia.

Interventions/Take Action

Nursing Priority No. 1.

To assess contributing or risk factors:

- Note potential cause for cold stress; for example, (1) *Radiant heat loss:* **Bare skin is exposed to an environment containing objects of cooler temperature.** (2) *Evaporative heat loss:* **Neonate wet with amniotic fluid.** (3) *Conductive heat loss:* **Neonate placed in contact with a cool surface or object.** (4) *Convective heat loss:* **A flow of cooler ambient air carries heat away from neonate.**
- Note contributing factors: *age* (e.g., preterm or full-term neonate); *concurrent or coexisting medical disorders that impair thermoregulation* (e.g., sepsis, intracranial hemorrhage, drug withdrawal); *environmental factors* (inadequate housing, homelessness); or a *combination.* Prolonged, unrecognized cold stress can produce an unwanted metabolically induced thermogenisis. This reaction increases metabolic rate and oxygen consumption and can result in tissue hypoxia and neurological damage.
- Monitor temperature regularly, measuring core body temperature. Exercise care in selecting appropriate thermometer for neonate's age and clinical condition. **Normal newborn temperature usually refers to the rectal temperature (true reflection of core temperature); however, temporal readings are useful for trending and safer than rectal. On average, neonate's body temperature often hovers around 98.6°F (37°C). However, it can fluctuate anywhere in the range of 96.8°F to 100.3°F (36°C–37.9°C). Abdominal (skin probe) temperature monitoring is preferred method for the premature neonate.**

Nursing Priority No. 2.

To maintain body temperature or prevent further decrease in body temperature:

- Maintain optimal ambient temperature in delivery room and newborn care areas. **The optimal ambient temperature for neonates to maintain body temperature is typically 74°F to 77°F (23°C–25°C).**
- Place newborn under radiant warmer, cover infant's head with cap, and use layers of lightweight blankets. Warm

---

Information that appears in brackets has been added by the authors to clarify and enhance the use of nursing diagnoses.

neonate in incubator or under a radiant warmer. Place premature infant in a polyethylene bag, according to facility policy. **Heat loss is greatest through the head and by evaporation and convection. Studies have shown that use of polyethylene bag prevents heat loss at delivery in preterm infant less than 32 wks' gestation.**
- Dry and swaddle full-term neonates at delivery and after bathing.
- Remove wet clothing and bedding immediately.
- Add layers of clothing and wrap in warm blankets.
- Provide skin-to-skin care where possible. **Skin-to-skin care was shown to be effective in reducing the risk of hypothermia when compared to conventional incubator care for infants and can rewarm newborn experiencing mild to moderate hypothermia.**
- Encourage/promote early breastfeeding, preferably within first hour of life. **Provides calories for neonate to produce body heat.**
- Postpone bathing until vital signs stable, preferably following transition period (6–8 hr), as indicated. **Bathing newborn soon after birth causes drop in body temperature, increasing risk of hypothermia and hypoglycemia.**
- Limit time neonate is uncovered, and place infant on warmed surface or under appropriate heat source/radiant warmer during assessment/interventions.

Nursing Priority No. 3.

To promote normothermia (Teaching/Discharge Considerations) and enhance well-being (long-term goals):

- Review specific risk factors or causes of hypothermia.
- Identify factors that parent can control (if any), such as protection from environment, adequate heat in home, layering of clothing and blankets, minimizing heat loss from head with hat or blanket, appropriate cold weather clothing.
- Discuss signs/symptoms of early hypothermia (e.g., cool, pale skin; slowed breathing; unwillingness to feed; somnolence) **to facilitate recognition of problem and promote timely intervention.**
- Identify assistive community resources, as indicated (e.g., social services, emergency shelters, clothing suppliers, food bank, public service company, financial resources). **Parent may be in need of numerous resources if hypothermia was associated with inadequate housing, homelessness, or malnutrition.**

Information that appears in brackets has been added by the authors to clarify and enhance the use of nursing diagnoses.

Documentation Focus

Assessment/Reassessment
- Individual findings, including fluctuations in temperature
- Specific causative/contributing or risk factors
- Graph temperature

Planning
- Plan of care and who is involved in planning
- Parent/care provider teaching plan

Implementation/Evaluation
- Responses to interventions and actions performed
- Attainment of or progress toward desired outcome(s)
- Modifications to plan of care
- Parent/caregiver response to teaching

Discharge Planning
- Long-term needs, identifying who is responsible for each action
- Specific referrals made

Sample Nursing Outcomes & Interventions Classifications NOC/NIC

NOC—Thermoregulation: Newborn
NIC—Hypothermia Treatment

---

risk for decreased perioperative BODY TEMPERATURE — NANDA-I

[Diagnostic Division: Safety]

Definition: Susceptible to an inadvertent drop in core body temperature below 36°C/96.8°F occurring 1 hr before to 24 hr after surgery.

Recognizing Cues

Risk Factors
Anxiety
Underweight for age and gender
Environmental temperature less than 21°C/69.8°F
Inadequate availability of appropriate warming equipment
Wound area uncovered

Information that appears in brackets has been added by the authors to clarify and enhance the use of nursing diagnoses.

 Acute Care 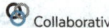 Collaborative 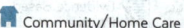 Community/Home Care Cultural

Clinical Connections

Surgical procedures/anesthesia greater than 2 hr, combined regional and general anesthesia, open surgical procedures

Generate Solutions

Plan Desired Outcomes

Client Will (Include Specific Time Frame)
- Display core temperature within normal range.
- Be free of complications such as cardiac failure, respiratory infection or failure, thromboembolic phenomena, and delayed healing.

Caregiver Will (Include Specific Time Frame)
- Identify client condition/situations that may lead to problems with temperature regulation.
- Engage in protective actions to control body temperature.

Interventions/Take Action

Nursing Priority No. 1.
To identify risk factors affecting current situation:

- Ascertain the type of surgical procedure the client is having. **Helps in identifying elements of risk. For example, some procedures carry a higher risk of hypothermia (e.g., laparoscopic abdominal procedure with carbon dioxide insufflation; extensive surgical procedure of any sort with prolonged exposure of body surfaces and long period of anesthesia).**
- Assess client conditions/comorbidities (e.g., diabetes, impaired skin and tissue integrity, respiratory, cardiac, vascular, or neurological disorders, hypothyroidism) **that may place the client at a higher risk for perioperative complications, including hypothermia.**
- Note the client's body type and age. **Very thin, malnourished, or dehydrated individuals, as well as the very young or elderly, are more susceptible to perioperative hypothermia.**
- Review client's medication regimen. **Medications, including some vasodilators, antipsychotics, and sedatives, can impair the body's ability to regulate its temperature.**

Information that appears in brackets has been added by the authors to clarify and enhance the use of nursing diagnoses.

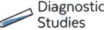 Diagnostic Studies 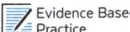 Evidence Based Practice 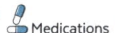 Medications 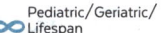 Pediatric/Geriatric/Lifespan

Nursing Priority No. 2.

To maintain appropriate body temperature/prevent hypothermia complications:

- Measure client's temperature preoperatively and report temperature below ideal range to surgical team/anesthesiologist. Confirm that continuous monitoring of temperature is occurring during the procedure. **Method of measuring temperature should reflect core temperature or a direct estimate of core temperature.**
- Implement preventive warming techniques using single strategies such as forced-air warming, which are more effective than passive warming (e.g., blankets from a warmer); however, combined strategies, including preoperative commencement, use of warmed fluids plus forced-air warming, and other active strategies, were more effective in vulnerable groups. **In the preoperative phase, identification of the client at risk for hypothermia will allow for initiation of prewarming interventions to normalize client body temperature before surgery and prevent hypothermia intraoperatively. Evidence suggests preoperative prewarming results in higher postoperative temperatures, higher core body temperatures intraoperatively, and lower rates of hypothermia.**
- Provide passive warming. **Increase operating room temperature, as indicated. It is currently thought that optimal operating room temperatures for the client should be no less than 69.8°F (21°C) to reduce risk of hypothermia complications while still providing a comfortable environment for scrubbed personnel under surgical lights. Recovery room temperatures of 68°F (20°C) to 75°F (24°C) may be ideal for rewarming client.**
- Use conductive warming devices such as heated blankets from a warming cabinet or warming pad. **Note: While easy to use and effective, blankets on top of client can limit access to surgical site. A warming pad is an electrical resistive/conductive device that warms underneath the client's body allowing for greater surgical access.**
- Consider convective warming devices. **Warm air is pumped through a hose into a disposable blanket that covers the client. Heat transfer results from the movement of warm air across the surface of the patient's skin, which allows forced-air blankets to transfer more heat at a lower temperature. Current evidence suggests forced air systems are the most effective and frequently used systems to reduce the burden of perioperative hypothermia.**

Information that appears in brackets has been added by the authors to clarify and enhance the use of nursing diagnoses.

 Acute Care Collaborative 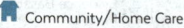 Community/Home Care Cultural

• Warm IV fluids and blood products to 37°C using a warming device as appropriate. Additionally, all irrigation fluids used intraoperatively should be warmed to a temperature of 38°C to 40°C. **Heated fluids can increase core temperature by approximately half a degree versus use of room-temperature fluids.**

Documentation Focus

Assessment/Reassessment
- Findings, noting degree of system involvement
- Graph temperature

Planning
- Plan of care

Implementation/Evaluation
- Responses to interventions and actions performed
- Attainment of desired outcome(s)
- Modifications to plan of care

Sample Nursing Outcomes & Interventions Classifications NOC/NIC

NOC—Thermoregulation
NIC—Temperature Regulation: Perioperative

BODY WEIGHT PROBLEM · ICNP

[Diagnostic Division: Food/Fluid]

Definition: Susceptible to health risks and chronic illness associated with abnormal or excessive adiposity (body fat accumulation).

Related/Risk Factors

Excessive eating behavior; frequent snacking; frequent intake of high-calorie food and beverages; large portion sizes
Inadequate daily physical activity (i.e., less than recommended for age and gender); energy expenditure below energy intake based on standard assessment; sedentary behavior occurring for ≥2 hr/day
Impaired sleep patterns, insomnia; nocturnal eating
Alcohol/substance misuse
Food insecurity

Information that appears in brackets has been added by the authors to clarify and enhance the use of nursing diagnoses.

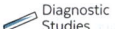 Diagnostic Studies   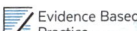 Evidence Based Practice   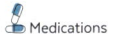 Medications   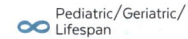 Pediatric/Geriatric/Lifespan

Solid foods as a major food source for children less than 5 months of age

Defining Characteristics

Subjective
Reports lack of balanced diet regarding appropriate intake of fruits/vegetables, starches, proteins, and fats

Objective
ADULT: Body mass index (BMI) of greater than 30 kg/m^2; waist circumference male greater than 102 cm (40 in.), female greater than 88 cm (36 in.)

CHILD younger than 2 years: BMI-for-age percentile is graphed for males/females greater than 95th percentile considered obese

CHILD 2 to 18 years: BMI greater than 95th percentile or greater than 30 kg/m^2 for age and gender

Clinical Connections
Familial obesity, premature pubarche, morbid obesity, diseases requiring long-term steroid use (e.g., chronic obstructive pulmonary disease [COPD]), conditions associated with immobility (e.g., stroke/paralysis, multiple sclerosis [MS], amputation), Alzheimer disease, depression, developmental delay

Generate Solutions

Plan Desired Outcomes

Client Will (Include Specific Time Frame)
- Verbalize a realistic self-concept or body image (congruent mental and physical picture of self).
- Participate in development of, and commit to, a personal weight loss program.
- Demonstrate appropriate changes in lifestyle and behaviors, including eating patterns, food quantity/quality, and exercise program.
- Show progress toward/attain desirable body weight with optimal maintenance of health.

Interventions/Take Action

Nursing Priority No. 1.
To identify contributing factors/health status:

 • Obtain weight history, noting if client has weight gain out of character for self or family, is or was obese as a child,

---

Information that appears in brackets has been added by the authors to clarify and enhance the use of nursing diagnoses.

or used to be much more physically active than now **to identify trends. Note: According to Centers for Disease Control and Prevention (CDC) 2018 statistics: (1) About 40% of young adults between 20 and 39 years old are obese; (2) 42.8% of those aged 60 years and older are obese; 18.4% of children between the ages of 6 and 11 years are obese, and 20.6% of those between 12 and 19 years are obese. Being overweight during older childhood is highly predictive of adult obesity, especially if a parent is also obese.**

- Assess risk and presence of factors or conditions associated with obesity (e.g., familial pattern of obesity; genetic disorders in children [e.g., Prader-Willi syndrome, Laurence-Moon-Biedl syndrome]; hypothyroidism; type 2 diabetes; reproductive dysfunction; menopause; chronic disorders, such as heart disease, kidney disease, chronic pain; food or other substance addictions; dyssomnia/insomnia, nocturnal eating; stressful or sedentary lifestyle; depression; use of certain medications such as steroids, birth control pills; physical disabilities or limitations; lack of socioeconomic resources for obtaining or preparing healthy foods) **to determine treatments and interventions that may be indicated in addition to weight management. Note: Studies have shown that the strongest correlate of weight gain over 20 years was susceptibility to overeating in response to everyday cues within the environment (habitual disinhibition); and susceptibility to overeating in response to emotional states such as depression (emotional disinhibition).**

- Investigate client's current and previous dieting history. **Client may report normal or excessive food intake, but calories and intake of certain food groups (e.g., sweets and fats) are often underestimated. Client may report experimentation with numerous types of diets, repeated dieting efforts ("yo-yo" dieting) with varying results, or may never have attempted a weight-management program.**

- Assess client's knowledge of own body weight, nutritional needs, and cultural expectations regarding body size. **Although nutritional needs are not always understood, being overweight or having a large body size may not be viewed negatively by client because it aligns with family eating patterns and peer and cultural influences. Ethnicity factors may influence the age of onset and the rapidity of weight gain. Race and ethnicity are associated with increased rates of obesity in children and adolescents.**

Information that appears in brackets has been added by the authors to clarify and enhance the use of nursing diagnoses.

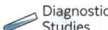 Diagnostic Studies
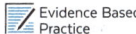 Evidence Based Practice
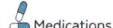 Medications
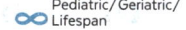 Pediatric/Geriatric/Lifespan

Puerto Rican, Cuban American, and Native American preschoolers have an increased incidence of obesity; Black, Native American, Puerto Rican, Mexican, and native Hawaiian school-aged children have the highest rates of obesity in this age group. Adolescent obesity is predictive of adult obesity, with 80% of teenagers who are obese continuing to be obese as adults. Note: In 2017, a CDC report noted that in the United States (in most states examined), almost half (48.4%) of non-Hispanic Black adults were considered to be obese, and about 12.4% were considered to have extreme obesity. Among Hispanic adults, 42.6% were considered to have obesity, and about 7% were considered to have extreme obesity.

- Investigate familial and cultural influences regarding food. **People of many cultures place high importance on food and food-related events, while some cultures routinely observe fasting days (e.g., Muslim, Greek, Irish, Jewish) that may be done for health or religious purposes.**
- Ascertain how client perceives food and the act of eating. **Individual beliefs, values, and the types of foods available influence what people eat, avoid, or alter. Client may be eating to satisfy an emotional need rather than physiological hunger, not only because food plays a significant role in socialization but also because food can offer comfort, a sense of security, and acceptance.**
- Evaluate client's routine medications. **Some medications can contribute to weight gain (e.g., cortisol and other glucocorticoids; sulfonylureas, tricyclic antidepressants, monoamine oxidase inhibitors; oral contraceptives; insulin [in excessive doses]; risperidone).**
- Assess dietary practices through collection of a client food diary—recalling 3 to 7 days. **Recall of foods and fluids ingested; times, patterns, and place of eating; whether alone or with other(s); and feelings before, during, and after eating can increase client's understanding of eating behavior and serve as the basis for dietary modifications.**
- Identify problems with client energy balance. **Studies indicate that few people can accurately estimate the number of calories they should consume daily for a person their age, height, weight, and physical activity. Note: Eating and physical activity patterns focused on consuming fewer calories, making informed food choices, and being physically active can help people attain and maintain a healthy weight, reduce their risk of chronic disease, and promote overall health. Clients who are overweight**

Information that appears in brackets has been added by the authors to clarify and enhance the use of nursing diagnoses.

 Acute Care 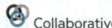 Collaborative 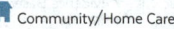 Community/Home Care Cultural

or obese will need to consume fewer calories from both foods and beverages.

- Review client's daily activity and assess for a regular exercise program **for a comparative baseline and to identify areas for activity modification. Note: According to 2020 state maps of adult physical inactivity, all states and territories had more than 15% of adults who were physically inactive. Inactivity levels vary among adults by race/ethnicity and location.**
- Obtain client's anthropometric measurements **to determine the presence and severity of obesity:**
  Calculate BMI **to estimate the degree of client fatness. Note: The CDC has standardized BMI calculations, removing age and sex differences for adults with obesity being defined as 30 and above. Note: Obesity is also divided into classes. Class 3 obesity is sometimes categorized as "extreme" or "severe" obesity (may replace term *morbid obesity*) and is defined as BMI equal to or greater than 40. The CDC has recommended that children (over age 2 years) and adolescents be considered obese if their BMI exceeds the 95th percentile on growth curves or exceeds 30 kg/m at any age. Note: Normal BMI in children changes with age and as growth occurs and is also different between the sexes.**
  Refer to ND ineffective Overweight Self-Management and readiness for enhanced Weight Self-Management for additional diagnostic studies information.
- Collaborate in assessment and interventions for client with disordered eating habits or eating perceptions:
  Obtain a comparative body drawing, having client draw self on a wall with chalk, then standing against it have actual body outline drawn to demonstrate the difference between the two. **Determines whether client's view of self-body image is congruent with reality.**
  Investigate the occurrence of negative feedback from significant others (SOs). **May reveal control issues and impact motivation for change.**
  Identify unhelpful eating behaviors (e.g., eating over the sink; "gobbling, nibbling, or grazing") and address kinds of activities associated with eating (e.g., watching television or reading, being unmindful of eating or food) **that result in taking in too many calories as well as eliminating the joy of food because of failure to notice flavors or sensation of fullness or satiety.**

Information that appears in brackets has been added by the authors to clarify and enhance the use of nursing diagnoses.

Nursing Priority No. 2.

To establish a weight-reduction program:

- Refer to ND ineffective Overweight Self-Management and readiness for enhanced Weight Self-Management, Nursing Priority No. 2 for interventions common to weight-loss programs.
- Use motivational interviewing to determine client's stage of readiness for change. **Assists in choice of interventions reducing client's resistance.**
- Collaborate with dietician in addressing/implementing client's specific needs (e.g., what foods to incorporate or limit, how to identify nutrient-dense foods and beverages). **A healthy eating pattern limits intake of sodium, saturated fats, added sugars, and refined grains and emphasizes nutrient-dense foods and beverages (e.g., vegetables, fruits, whole grains, fat-free or low-fat milk and dairy products), seafood, lean meats, poultry, eggs, beans and peas, and nuts and seeds.**
- Assist client and family in using technology to manage food choices. **Technology offers applications that can assist in monitoring dietary intake and food choices. Some calculate calories, providing immediate feedback and generating individualized reminders. The best applications include (1) a large database of foods with nutritional information for various serving sizes, (2) a bar scanner that allows users to add information about prepared foods to their database, (3) a calorie tracker that is easy to use, and (4) the ability to track other nutrients (e.g., carbohydrates, protein, calcium).**
- Engage client and family in structured weight loss programs, as indicated. **Approaches to the treatment of severely obese individuals may include lifestyle modifications, physical activity, very controlled diets, and intensive psychiatric interventions, including individual, group, and family therapy. Note: DeBar et al. reported that an intensive, group therapy approach was superior to standard, family-based therapy in achieving lifestyle changes (e.g., less consumption of fast foods) and in reducing the BMI of overweight adolescents.**
- Administer medication(s), as indicated. **The Food and Drug Administration (FDA) has approved medications (e.g., glucagon-like peptide-1 [GLP-1] agonist) for the treatment of weight management concerns.**

Information that appears in brackets has been added by the authors to clarify and enhance the use of nursing diagnoses.

- Refer to bariatric physician/surgeon, as indicated. **Evaluation for special measures (e.g., supervised fasting or bariatric surgery) may be needed for obese persons with comorbidities and for morbidly obese persons with BMI greater than 40. Currently, there are several bariatric surgical procedures (e.g., gastric bypass [Roux-en-Y], biliopancreatic diversion [rare], vertical gastric sleeve).**

Nursing Priority No. 3.

To promote a healthy weight and weight loss (Teaching/Discharge Considerations) and enhance well-being (long-term goals):
- Refer to ND ineffective Overweight Self-Management, and readiness for enhanced Weight Self-Management for related interventions.

Documentation Focus

Assessment/Reassessment
- Individual findings, including current weight, dietary pattern; perceptions of self, food, and eating; motivation for loss, support, or feedback from SO(s).
- Results of laboratory and diagnostic testing.

Planning
- Plan of care, specific interventions, and who is involved in planning.
- Teaching plan.

Implementation/Evaluation
- Responses to interventions and actions performed.
- Attainment or progress toward desired outcome(s).
- Modifications to plan of care.

Discharge Planning
- Long-term needs and who is responsible for actions to be taken.
- Specific referrals made.

Sample Nursing Outcomes & Interventions Classifications (NOC/NIC)

NOC—Eating Disorder Self-Control
NIC—Weight Reduction Assistance

Information that appears in brackets has been added by the authors to clarify and enhance the use of nursing diagnoses.

difficulty performing BREASTFEEDING — ICNP

[Diagnostic Division: Food/Fluid]

Definition: Perceived or actual problems incurred by the breastfeeding dyad associated with the process of delivering human milk from the breast to a neonate, infant, or child.

Recognizing Cues

Related/Risk Factors

Mother
Lack of knowledge/instruction of effective breastfeeding techniques
Inadequate fluid intake; alcohol/tobacco use; malnutrition; overweight
Multiple stressors/responsibilities; inadequate partner/family support
History of unsatisfactory breastfeeding (self, others); previous early cessation of breastfeeding
Fatigue; anxiety; ambivalence; depression
Use of supplemental bottle feedings; pacifier use
Breast anomaly (e.g., flat/inverted nipples)

Infant or Child
Uncoordinated suck-swallow and breathing reflex during feeding
Resists latching on to breast; refusal to breastfeed
Prematurity
Oral anomaly (e.g., tongue-tied, cleft lip/pallet)

Defining Characteristics

Subjective

Mother
Sore nipples; nipple pain (beyond first few minutes of breastfeeding)
Breast tenderness; persistent pain
Expresses dissatisfaction with feeding process; concern about adequacy of milk supply

Objective

Mother
Cracked, bleeding nipples
Breast swelling, engorgement, erythema; lump in breast
Incomplete emptying of breast(s) following feedings

Information that appears in brackets has been added by the authors to clarify and enhance the use of nursing diagnoses.

 Acute Care   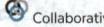 Collaborative   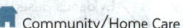 Community/Home Care   Cultural

Improper positioning of infant during feeding

Infant or Child

Poor latch on to breast; weak suck-swallow; clicking sounds during feedings

Feeding less than 8 times/24 hr

Inadequate number of wet diapers/day (less than 6 after first 5 days)

Bowel movements less than 3/day initially, (frequency may decline after first 6 wk)

Fussy/crying after feeding; displays cues of hunger

Regurgitation, or vomiting following feeding

Prolonged feeding time greater than 30 min; repeatedly detaching from breast during feeding

Falls asleep, not alert when feeding

Inadequate weight gain for age; weight loss; failure to thrive

Clinical Connections

Prematurity, cleft lip/palate, ankyloglossia (tongue-tie), Down syndrome, child abuse or neglect, failure to thrive, diseases/infections of the breast

Generate Solutions

Plan Desired Outcomes

Client Will (Include Specific Time Frame)

- Verbalize understanding of causative or contributing factors.
- Demonstrate techniques to enhance breastfeeding experience.
- Assume responsibility for effective breastfeeding.
- Achieve mutually satisfactory breastfeeding regimen with infant content after feedings, gaining weight appropriately, and output within normal range.

Interventions/Take Action

Nursing Priority No. 1.

To identify maternal causative or contributing factors:

- Assess client knowledge about breastfeeding and extent of instruction that has been given.
- Identify cultural expectations and conflicts about breastfeeding and beliefs or practices regarding lactation, letdown techniques, and maternal food preferences. **Understanding impact of culture and idiosyncrasies of specific feeding practices is important to determine the effect on infant feeding. For example, in many cultures, such as Mexican American, Navajo, and Vietnamese, colostrum is not**

Information that appears in brackets has been added by the authors to clarify and enhance the use of nursing diagnoses.

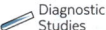 Diagnostic Studies   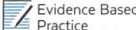 Evidence Based Practice   Medications   Pediatric/Geriatric/Lifespan

offered to the newborn. Intervention is necessary only if the practice/belief is harmful to the infant.

- ∞ Note myths/misunderstandings, especially in teenage clients, **who are more likely to have limited knowledge and more concerns about body image issues.**
- Encourage discussion of current and previous breastfeeding experience(s).
- Note previous unsatisfactory experience (including self or others), **because it may lead to negative expectations.**
- Perform physical assessment, noting appearance of breasts and nipples, marked asymmetry of breasts, obvious inverted or flat nipples, or minimal or no breast enlargement during pregnancy. **Identifies existing problems that may interfere with successful breastfeeding experience and provides opportunity to correct them when possible.**
- Determine whether lactation failure is primary (**i.e., maternal prolactin deficiency/serum prolactin levels, inadequate mammary gland tissue, breast surgery that has damaged the nipple, areola enervation [irremediable], and pituitary disorders**) or secondary (**i.e., sore nipples, severe engorgement, plugged milk ducts, mastitis, inhibition of letdown reflex, and maternal/infant separation with disruption of feedings [treatable]**).
- Review history of pregnancy, labor, and delivery (vaginal or cesarean section); other recent or current surgery; preexisting medical problems (e.g., diabetes, seizure disorder, cardiac diseases, or presence of disabilities); or adoptive parent. **While some conditions may preclude breastfeeding, and alternate plans need to be made, others will need specific plans for monitoring and treatment to ensure successful breastfeeding.**
- 🏠 Identify client's support systems or presence and response of significant others (SOs), extended family, and friends. **The infant's father and maternal grandmother (in addition to caring healthcare providers) are important factors that contribute to successful breastfeeding.**
- Ascertain client's age, number of children at home, and need to return to work. **These factors may have a detrimental effect on desire to breastfeed. Immaturity may influence mother to avoid breastfeeding, believing that it will be inconvenient, or may cause her to be insensitive to the infant's needs. The stress of the responsibility of other children or the need to return to work can affect the ability to manage effective breastfeeding; mother will need support and information to be successful.**

Information that appears in brackets has been added by the authors to clarify and enhance the use of nursing diagnoses.

 Acute Care 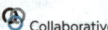 Collaborative 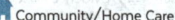 Community/Home Care 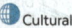 Cultural

- Determine client's feelings (e.g., fear/anxiety, ambivalence, or depression), **which are indicators of underlying emotional state that may suggest need for intervention and referral.**
- Note myths or misunderstandings, especially in teenage clients **who are more likely to have limited knowledge and more concerns about body image issues.**

Nursing Priority No. 2.

To assess infant causative/contributing factors:

- Determine suckling problems, as noted in Recognizing Cues.
- Note prematurity and/or infant anomaly (e.g., cleft lip/palate) **to determine special equipment/feeding needs.**
- Review feeding schedule to note increased demand for feeding (at least eight times a day, taking both breasts at each feeding for more than 15 min on each side) or use of supplements with artificial nipple.
- Evaluate observable signs of inadequate infant intake (e.g., baby latches onto nipples with sustained suckling but minimal audible swallowing or gulping noted, infant arching and crying at the breasts with resistance to latching on, decreased urinary output and frequency of stools, or inadequate weight gain).
- Determine whether the baby is content after feeding or exhibits fussiness and crying within the first hour after breastfeeding, **suggesting unsatisfactory breastfeeding process.**
- Note any correlation between client's ingestion of certain foods and "colicky" response of infant. **Some foods may seem to result in reaction by the infant, and identification and elimination from mother's diet may correct the problem.**

Nursing Priority No. 3.

To assist mother to develop skills of successful breastfeeding:

- Provide emotional support to the client. Use one-to-one instruction with each feeding during hospital stay and clinic or home visit. Refer adoptive clients choosing to breastfeed to a lactation consultant **to assist with induced lactation techniques.**
- Discuss early infant feeding cues (e.g., rooting, lip smacking, and sucking fingers/hand) versus late cue of crying. **Early recognition of infant hunger promotes timely/more rewarding feeding experience for infant and client.**

Information that appears in brackets has been added by the authors to clarify and enhance the use of nursing diagnoses.

 Diagnostic Studies   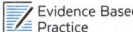 Evidence Based Practice   Medications   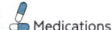 Pediatric/Geriatric/Lifespan

- Inform client how to assess and correct a latch if needed. Demonstrate asymmetric latch aiming infant's lower lip as far from base of the nipple as possible, then bringing infant's chin and lower jaw in contact with breast while mouth is wide open and before upper lip touches breast. **This position allows infant to use both tongue and jaw more effectively to obtain milk from the breast.**
- Recommend avoidance or overuse of supplemental feedings and pacifiers (unless specifically indicated), **which can lessen the infant's desire to breastfeed/increase risk of early weaning. Note: Adoptive clients may not develop a full breast milk supply, necessitating supplemental feedings.**
- Restrict the use of nipple shields (i.e., only temporarily to help draw the nipple out, deal with sore nipples) and then place the baby directly on the nipple. **Conflicting research findings provide support for their use or suggest a number of possible negatives, including decreased release of prolactin (promoting milk production) affecting adequate milk supply. However, temporary use of shield may be beneficial in the presence of severe nipple cracking.**
- Demonstrate the use of hand expression, hand pump, and piston-type electric breast pump with bilateral collection chamber when necessary **to maintain or increase the milk supply.**
- Discuss/demonstrate breastfeeding aids (e.g., infant sling, nursing pillows, or footstool) **to find the most comfortable ones for mother and infant.**
- Suggest using a variety of nursing positions. **Positions particularly helpful for plus-sized women or those with large breasts include the "football" hold with the infant's head to the client's breast and body curved around behind client or lying down to nurse.**
- Encourage frequent rest periods, sharing household/childcare duties **to limit fatigue and facilitate relaxation at feeding times.**
- Recommend abstinence/restriction of tobacco, caffeine, alcohol, drugs, and excess sugar, as appropriate, **because they may affect milk production and the letdown reflex or be passed on to the infant.**
- Promote early management of breastfeeding problems. For example:
  Engorgement: Wear a supportive bra, apply heat and/or cool applications to the breasts, and massage from chest

---

Information that appears in brackets has been added by the authors to clarify and enhance the use of nursing diagnoses.

wall down to nipple **to enhance letdown reflex;** soothe a "fussy baby" before latching on the breast; properly position the baby on the breast/nipple; alternate the side baby starts nursing on; nurse around the clock and/or pump with piston-type electric breast pump with bilateral collection chambers at least 8 to 12 times a day; and avoid using bottle, pacifier, or supplements.

Sore nipples: Wear 100% cotton fabrics; do not use soap or alcohol/other drying agents on nipples; avoid the use of nipple shields or nursing pads that contain plastic; cleanse and then pat dry with a clean cloth; apply a thin layer of USP-modified lanolin on the nipple, and administer a mild pain reliever as appropriate. **Note:** The infant should latch on to the least sore side, or the client should begin with hand expression **to establish the letdown reflex.** Properly position the infant on the breast/nipple and use a variety of nursing positions. Gently break suction after breastfeeding is complete.

Clogged ducts: Use a larger bra or extender to avoid pressure on the site; use moist or dry heat; gently massage from above the plug down to the nipple; nurse the infant, hand express, or pump after massage; nurse more often on the affected side.

Inhibited letdown: Use relaxation techniques before nursing (e.g., maintain quiet atmosphere, massage the breast, apply heat to breasts, have beverage available, assume a position of comfort, place the infant on the client's chest skin-to-skin). Develop a routine for nursing, and encourage client to enjoy her baby.

Mastitis: Promote bedrest (with infant) for several days; administer antibiotics; provide warm, moist heat before and during nursing; and empty breasts completely. Continue to nurse the baby at least 8 to 12 times a day or pump breasts for 24 hr and then resume breastfeeding as appropriate.

- Demonstrate use of hand expression, hand pump, and electric piston-type breast pump with bilateral collection chamber when necessary to maintain or increase milk supply. **Note: Studies indicate that teaching hands-on pumping increased the mean daily volume of milk by 48%. The need to use a pump in order to store milk for feedings while the client is away (i.e., going back to work or simply to allow time away from the infant) demands some degree of proficiency in the use of the pump.**

Information that appears in brackets has been added by the authors to clarify and enhance the use of nursing diagnoses.

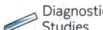 Diagnostic Studies 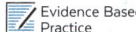 Evidence Based Practice 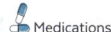 Medications 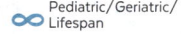 Pediatric/Geriatric/Lifespan

Nursing Priority No. 4.
To condition the infant to breastfeed:
- Scent breast pad with breast milk and leave in bed with infant along with client's photograph when separated for medical purposes (e.g., prematurity).
- Increase skin-to-skin contact (kangaroo care).
- Provide practice times at breast for infant to "lick and learn."
- Express small amounts of milk into the baby's mouth.
- Have client pump breast after feeding to enhance milk production.
- Use supplemental nutrition system cautiously when necessary.
- Identify special interventions for feeding in the presence of cleft lip/palate. **These measures promote optimal interaction between client and infant and provide adequate nourishment for the infant, enhancing successful breastfeeding.**

Nursing Priority No. 5.
To promote optimal success (Teaching/Discharge Considerations) and enhance well-being (long-term goals):
- Schedule a follow-up visit with the healthcare provider 48 hr after hospital discharge and 2 wk after birth **for evaluation of milk intake/breastfeeding process and to answer the client's questions.**
- Recommend monitoring the number of infant's wet/soiled diapers. **Stools should be yellow in color, and the infant should have at least six wet diapers a day to determine that the infant is receiving sufficient intake.**
- Weigh the infant at least every third day initially, as indicated, and record **to verify adequacy of nutritional intake.**
- Educate partner/SO about benefits of breastfeeding and how to manage common lactation challenges. **Enlisting the support of the partner/SO is associated with a higher ratio of successful breastfeeding at 6 mo.**
- Instruct in use of relaxation techniques. **Facilitates release of oxytocin improving milk removal.**
- Promote peer and cultural group counseling for teen clients. **Provides a positive role model that the teen can relate to and feel comfortable with when discussing concerns/feelings.**
- Discuss with partner/SO the client's need for rest, relaxation, and time with other children as appropriate. **Promotes**

Information that appears in brackets has been added by the authors to clarify and enhance the use of nursing diagnoses.

understanding of client's needs and cooperation with incorporation of new member into family.
- Discuss the importance of adequate nutrition and fluid intake, prenatal vitamins, or other vitamin/mineral supplements, such as vitamin C, as indicated. **During lactation, there is an increased need for energy, and supplementation of protein, minerals, and vitamins is necessary to provide nourishment for the infant and to protect client's stores, along with extra fluid intake.**
- Address specific problems (e.g., suckling problems or prematurity, facial anomalies).
- Discuss the timing of the introduction of solid foods and the importance of delaying until the infant is at least 4 mo, preferably 6 mo old. If supplementation is necessary, the infant can be finger fed, spoon fed, cup fed, or syringe fed.
- Inform the client that return of menses while nursing varies and usually averages 3 to 36 wk with ovulation returning in 17 to 28 wk. **Return of menstruation does not affect breastfeeding, and breastfeeding is not a reliable method of birth control.**
- Refer to certified lactation counselor or support groups (e.g., La Leche League, parenting support groups, stress reduction, or other community resources, as indicated).
- Provide bibliotherapy/appropriate websites for further information.

Documentation Focus

Assessment/Reassessment
- Identified assessment factors, for client and infant (e.g., engorgement present, is infant demonstrating adequate weight gain without supplementation)

Planning
- Plan of care, specific interventions, and who is involved in planning
- Teaching plan

Implementation/Evaluation
- Client's/infant's responses to interventions, teaching, and actions performed
- Changes in infant's weight and output
- Attainment of or progress toward desired outcome(s)
- Modifications to plan of care

Information that appears in brackets has been added by the authors to clarify and enhance the use of nursing diagnoses.

 Diagnostic Studies 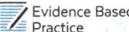 Evidence Based Practice 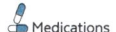 Medications 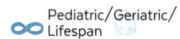 Pediatric/Geriatric/Lifespan

Discharge Planning
- Referrals that have been made and mother's choice of participation

Sample Nursing Outcomes & Interventions Classifications NOC/NIC

NOC—Breastfeeding Establishment: Maternal [or] Infant
NIC—Lactation Counseling

---

interrupted BREASTFEEDING ICNP

[Diagnostic Division: Food/Fluid]

Definition: Unplanned or undesired break in the process of delivering human milk from the breast to a neonate, infant, or child.

Recognizing Cues

Related/Risk Factors
Lack of knowledge/instruction of effective breastfeeding techniques
Multiple stressors/responsibilities; inadequate family/employer support
Fatigue; ambivalence; depression
Inadequate fluid intake; alcohol/tobacco use; malnutrition
Pain
History of unsatisfactory breastfeeding (self, others); previous early cessation of breastfeeding
Use of supplemental feedings; early introduction of solid foods
Illness; prescribed medication use; treatment regimen; substance misuse

Defining Characteristics

Subjective
Mother
Sore, cracked nipples
Breast tenderness; persistent pain
Difficulty meeting needs of infant, self, family
Expresses concern about adequacy of milk supply, infant nutrition
Mother
Cracked, bleeding nipples
Breast swelling, engorgement, erythema; lump in breast

Information that appears in brackets has been added by the authors to clarify and enhance the use of nursing diagnoses.

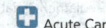 Acute Care 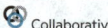 Collaborative 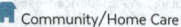 Community/Home Care Cultural

Improper positioning of infant during feeding
Use of formula feedings in place of human breast milk
Infant or Child
Poor latch; weak suck-swallow; clicking sounds during feedings
Feeding less than eight times/24 hr, less than six times/24 hr at 3 mo of age
Prolonged feeding time greater than 30 min; repeatedly detaching from breast during feeding
Falls asleep, not alert when feeding
Inadequate weight gain for age

Clinical Connections
Prematurity, postpartum depression, client illness, client substance misuse, hospitalization of infant or client

Generate Solutions

Plan Desired Outcomes

Client Will (Include Specific Time Frame)
- Identify and demonstrate techniques to sustain lactation until breastfeeding is reinitiated.
- Achieve mutually satisfactory feeding regimen, with infant content after feedings and gaining weight appropriately.
- Achieve weaning and cessation of lactation if desired or necessary.

Interventions/Take Action

Nursing Priority No. 1.
To identify causative/contributing factors:

- Assess client knowledge and perceptions about breastfeeding and extent of instruction that has been given.
- Note myths/misunderstandings, especially in some cultures and in teenage mothers, **who are more likely to have limited knowledge and more concerns about body image issues.**
- Ascertain cultural expectations/conflicts. **Breastfeeding influences one's relationship with body and identity. When breasts are perceived as sexual, appearance influences breastfeeding decisions, and people may have a concern with embarrassment, discomfort in public, and potential sexual implications of breastfeeding. In the United States, breastfeeding rates vary not only by race and ethnicity but also by geographic location.**

Information that appears in brackets has been added by the authors to clarify and enhance the use of nursing diagnoses.

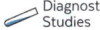 Diagnostic Studies   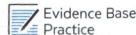 Evidence Based Practice   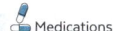 Medications   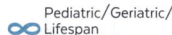 Pediatric/Geriatric/Lifespan

- Encourage discussion of current/previous breastfeeding experience(s). Note previous unsatisfactory experience (including self or others). **Useful for determining efforts needed to continue breastfeeding, if desired, while circumstances interrupting process are resolved, if possible. Often unsolved problems and stories told by others may cause doubt about chance for success.**
- Identify client's feelings (e.g., fear, anxiety, ambivalence, depression). **Indicators of underlying emotional state that may impact commitment to breastfeeding and suggest need for intervention and referral.**
- Determine client's responsibilities, routines, and scheduled activities. **Caretaking of siblings, employment in or out of the home, and work or school schedules of family members may affect ability to visit hospitalized infant when this is the reason for mother-infant separation.**
- Identify factors necessitating interruption, or occasionally cessation, of breastfeeding (e.g., maternal illness, drug use) and desire or need to wean infant. **In general, infants with chronic diseases benefit from breastfeeding. Only a few maternal infections (e.g., HIV, active/untreated tuberculosis for initial 2 wk of multidrug therapy, active herpes simplex of the breasts, and development of chickenpox within 5 days prior to delivery or 2 days after delivery) are hazardous to breastfeeding infants. Also, the use of antiretroviral medications/chemotherapy agents or client's substance abuse may require weaning of the infant. (Refer to Drugs and Lactation Database [LactMed] for specific information.) Exposure to radiation therapy requires interruption of breastfeeding for the length of time radioactivity is known to be present in breast milk and is therefore dependent on the agent used. Note: Client can "pump and dump" her breast milk to maintain supply and continue to breastfeed after her condition has resolved (e.g., chickenpox).**
- Determine support systems available to the client/family. **The infant's father and maternal grandmother, in addition to caring healthcare providers, are important factors that contribute to successful breastfeeding.**

Nursing Priority No. 2.
To assist the mother to maintain breastfeeding if desired:

- Provide information as needed regarding the need/decision to interrupt breastfeeding.
- Give emotional support to client and support her decision regarding cessation or continuation of breastfeeding.

Information that appears in brackets has been added by the authors to clarify and enhance the use of nursing diagnoses.

Many women are ambivalent about breastfeeding, and providing information about the pros and cons of both breastfeeding and bottle feeding, along with support for the mother's/couple's decision, will promote a positive experience.

- Promote peer counseling for teen clients. **This provides a positive role model that the teen can relate to and feel comfortable with discussing concerns/feelings.**
- Educate the partner/significant other (SO) about the benefits of breastfeeding and how to manage common lactation challenges. **Enlisting the support of the partner/SO is associated with a higher ratio of successful breastfeeding at 6 mo.**
- Discuss/demonstrate breastfeeding aids (e.g., infant sling, nursing footstool/pillows, hand expression, manual and/or piston-type electric breast pumps). **Enhances comfort and relaxation for breastfeeding. When circumstances dictate that the client and infant are separated for a time, whether by illness, prematurity, or returning to work or school, the milk supply can be maintained by use of the pump. Storing the milk for future use enables the infant to continue to receive the value of breast milk. Learning the correct technique is important for successful use of the pump.**
- Suggest abstinence/restriction of tobacco, caffeine, excess sugar, alcohol, certain medications, all illicit drugs, as appropriate, when breastfeeding is reinitiated, **because they may affect milk production/letdown reflex or be passed on to the infant.**
- Review techniques for expression and storage of breast milk **to provide optimal nutrition and promote continuation of breastfeeding process.**
- Problem-solve return-to-work (or school) issues or periodic infant care requiring bottle/supplemental feeding.
- Provide privacy/calm surroundings when the mother breastfeeds in a hospital/work setting. **Note: Federal Law 2010 requires an employer to provide a place and reasonable break time for an employee to express her breast milk for her baby for 1 yr after birth.**
- Determine if a routine visiting schedule or advance warning can be provided **so that the infant will be hungry/ready to feed.**
- Recommend using expressed breast milk instead of formula or at least partial breastfeeding for as long as client and child are satisfied. **Prevents permanent interruption in breastfeeding, decreasing the risk of premature weaning.**

Information that appears in brackets has been added by the authors to clarify and enhance the use of nursing diagnoses.

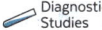 Diagnostic Studies
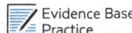 Evidence Based Practice
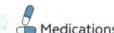 Medications
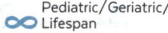 Pediatric/Geriatric/Lifespan

- Encourage client to obtain adequate rest, maintain fluid and nutritional intake, continue her prenatal vitamins, and schedule breast pumping every 3 hr while awake, as indicated, **to sustain adequate milk production and breastfeeding process.**
- Refer to NDs difficulty performing Breastfeeding; inadequate Human Milk Production as indicated for additional interventions.

Nursing Priority No. 3.
To promote successful infant feeding:

- Determine suckling problems or infant oral anomaly (e.g., cleft lip/palate), signs of hunger post feeding. **These factors can negatively impact both infant and client's satisfactions with feedings, resulting in concern about adequacy of client's milk supply and infant's nutrition necessitating interventions directed at correcting individual situation. Note: Conditions such as cleft palate need evaluation for correction and individualized instruction in holding infant upright and using special nipple or feeding device, such as a Haberman Feeder.**
- Recommend/provide for infant sucking on a regular basis, especially if gavage feedings are part of the therapeutic regimen. **Reinforces that feeding time is pleasurable and enhances digestion.**
- Explain anticipated changes in feeding needs and frequency. **Growth spurts require increased intake or more feedings by infant.**
- Discuss the proper use and choice of supplemental nutrition and alternate feeding methods (e.g., bottle/syringe) if desired. **If infant is not receiving sufficient nourishment, whether by client's choice to reduce number of feedings (e.g., returning to work) or necessity (e.g., specific client illness, medication use), other means for supplementing intake must be taken, and client needs to be given information regarding method chosen.**
- Review safety precautions (e.g., proper flow of formula from nipple, frequency of burping, holding bottle instead of propping, formula preparation, and sterilization techniques). **Identifying importance of proper flow of formula from nipple, frequency of burping, holding bottle instead of propping, techniques of formula preparation, and sterilization techniques are necessary for successful bottle feeding.**

Information that appears in brackets has been added by the authors to clarify and enhance the use of nursing diagnoses.

Nursing Priority No. 4.

To promote continued success (Teaching/Discharge Considerations) and enhance well-being (long-term goals):

- Encourage client to obtain adequate rest, maintain fluid and nutritional intake, continue to take her prenatal vitamins, and schedule breast pumping every 3 hr while awake, as indicated. **Sustains adequate milk production and enhances breastfeeding process when mother and infant are separated for any reason. Note: Research suggests a correlation between psychological stress and development of breast disease (e.g., breast pain, milk stasis, mastitis) leading to early weaning.**
- Suggest abstinence or restriction of tobacco, caffeine, alcohol, drugs, and excess sugar, as appropriate, when breastfeeding is reinitiated. **These substances may affect milk production/letdown reflex and can be passed on to the infant.**
- Recommend avoidance or overuse of supplemental bottle feedings and pacifiers (unless specifically indicated). **These can lessen infant's desire to breastfeed. The shape of the mouth and lips and the sucking mechanism are different for breast and bottle, and the infant may be confused by the difference, causing interference in the breastfeeding process and increasing risk of early weaning.**
- Identify other means (other than breastfeeding) of nurturing and strengthening infant attachment (e.g., comforting, consoling, or play activities).
- Refer to support groups (e.g., La Leche League or Lact-Aid), community resources (e.g., a public health nurse; a lactation specialist; Women, Infants, and Children program; and electric pump rental programs).
- Promote the use of bibliotherapy/appropriate websites for further information.
- Discuss the timing of the introduction of solid foods and the importance of delaying until the infant is at least 4 mo, preferably 6 mo old, if possible. **The American Academy of Pediatrics and the World Health Organization (WHO) recommend delaying solids until at least 6 mo. If supplementation is necessary, the infant can be finger fed, spoon fed, cup fed, or syringe fed.**

Nursing Priority No. 5.

To assist the client in the weaning process when desired:

- Provide emotional support to client and accept decision regarding cessation of breastfeeding. **Feelings of sadness are common, even if weaning is the client's choice.**

Information that appears in brackets has been added by the authors to clarify and enhance the use of nursing diagnoses.

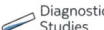 Diagnostic Studies 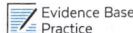 Evidence Based Practice 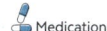 Medications 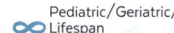 Pediatric/Geriatric/Lifespan

- Discuss reducing the frequency of daily feedings and breast pumping by one session every 2 to 3 days. **This is the preferred method of weaning, if circumstance permits, to reduce problems associated with engorgement.**
- Encourage wearing a snug, well-fitting bra, but refrain from binding breasts **because of increased risk of clogged milk ducts and inflammation.**
- Recommend expressing some milk from breasts regularly each day over a period of 1 to 3 wk, if necessary, **to reduce discomfort associated with engorgement until milk production decreases.**
- Suggest holding the infant differently during bottle feeding/interactions or having another family member give the infant's bottle feeding **to prevent infant rooting for breast and to prevent stimulation of nipples.**
- Discuss the use of ibuprofen/acetaminophen **for discomfort during the weaning process.**
- Suggest the use of ice packs to breast tissue (not nipples) for 15 to 20 min at least four times a day **to help reduce swelling during sudden weaning.**

Documentation Focus

Assessment/Reassessment
- Baseline findings of maternal and infant factors, including mother's milk supply and infant nourishment
- Reason for interruption or cessation of breastfeeding
- Number of wet/soiled diapers daily, log of intake and output, as appropriate; periodic measurement of weight

Planning
- Method of feeding chosen
- Plan of care and who is involved in planning
- Teaching plan

Implementation/Evaluation
- Maternal response to interventions, teaching, and actions performed
- Infant's response to feeding and method
- Whether infant appears satisfied or still seems to be hungry
- Attainment of or progress toward desired outcome(s)
- Modifications to plan of care

Discharge Planning
- Plan for follow-up and who is responsible
- Specific referrals made

Information that appears in brackets has been added by the authors to clarify and enhance the use of nursing diagnoses.

Sample Nursing Outcomes & Interventions Classifications NOC/NIC

NOC—Breastfeeding Maintenance
NIC—Lactation Counseling

ineffective BREATHING PATTERN NANDA-I

[Diagnostic Division: Respiration]

Definition: Difficulty maintaining adequate ventilation through inspiration and/or expiration.

Recognizing Cues

Related/Risk Factors
Anxiety; [panic attacks]
Excessive airway secretions; ineffective cough
Body position that inhibits lung expansion; respiratory muscle fatigue
Ineffective overweight self-management
Excessive fatigue burden; increased physical exertion
Pain

Defining Characteristics

Subjective
Dsypnea

Objective
Abdominal paradoxical respiratory pattern; altered chest excursion; increased anterior-posterior chest diameter
Altered respiratory depth; altered respiratory rhythm
Altered tidal volume; decreased minute ventilation or vital capacity; decreased expiratory or inspiratory pressures; prolonged expiration phase
Bradypnea; tachypnea; hyperventilation; hypoventilation
Adventitious respiratory sounds
Cyanosis
Hypercapnia; hypoxemia; hypoxia
Nasal flaring; orthopnea; uses three-point position; pursed-lip breathing; subcostal retraction; excessive use of accessory respiratory muscles

Clinical Connections
Chronic obstructive pulmonary disease (COPD), emphysema, asthma, pneumonia, sleep apnea syndromes, chest trauma

---

Information that appears in brackets has been added by the authors to clarify and enhance the use of nursing diagnoses.

 Diagnostic Studies 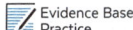 Evidence Based Practice 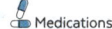 Medications ∞ Pediatric/Geriatric/Lifespan

105

or surgery, scoliosis, spinal cord injury, Guillain-Barré syndrome, traumatic brain injury, cystic fibrosis, drug or alcohol toxicity

Generate Solutions

Plan Desired Outcomes

Client Will (Include Specific Time Frame)
- Establish a normal, effective respiratory pattern as evidenced by absence of cyanosis and other signs/symptoms of hypoxia, with arterial blood gasses (ABGs) within client's normal or acceptable range.
- Verbalize awareness of causative factors.
- Initiate needed lifestyle changes.
- Demonstrate appropriate coping behaviors.

Interventions/Take Action

Nursing Priority No. 1.
To identify etiology/precipitating factors:
- Determine the presence of factors/conditions as noted in Defining Characteristics **that would demonstrate breathing impairments.**
- Identify age of client who may be at increased risk. **Respiratory ailments in general are increased in infants, children with neuromuscular disorders, the smoking and vaping population (tobacco and other products), the frail elderly, and persons living or working in highly polluted environments. People most at risk for infectious pneumonia include the very young and frail elderly and those with compromised immune systems.**
- Ascertain if client has history of underlying respiratory disorder or if this is a new condition with potential for breathing problems or exacerbation of preexisting problems (e.g., asthma, other acute upper respiratory infection, lung cancer, neuromuscular disorders, heart disease, sepsis, burns, acute chest or brain trauma). **Respiratory ailments in general are increased in infants, children with neuromuscular disorders, the smoking and vaping population (tobacco and other products), the frail elderly, and persons living or working in highly polluted environments.**
- Note current symptoms and how they relate to past history.

Information that appears in brackets has been added by the authors to clarify and enhance the use of nursing diagnoses.

 Acute Care 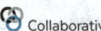 Collaborative 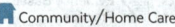 Community/Home Care 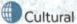 Cultural

- Assess for pregnancy, other abdominal distention, and muscle guarding. **Distended abdomen and muscle tension can impede diaphragmatic excursion and reduce lung expansion.**
- Note emotional state. **Emotional changes can accompany a condition or precipitate or aggravate ineffective breathing patterns.**
- Assess client's awareness and cognition. **Affects ability to manage own airway and cooperate with interventions such as controlling breathing and managing secretions.**
- Assess for concomitant pain/discomfort **that may restrict respiratory effort.**
- ∞ Evaluate client's respiratory status:

    Note rate and depth of respirations, counting for 1 full minute, if rate is irregular. **Rate may be faster or slower than usual. In infants and younger children, rate increases dramatically relative to anxiety, crying, fever, or disease. Depth may be difficult to evaluate but is usually described as shallow, normal, or deep.**

    Note client's reports and perceptions of breathing ease. **Client may report a range of symptoms (e.g., air hunger, shortness of breath with speaking, activity, or at rest) and demonstrate a wide range of signs (e.g., tachypnea, gasping, wheezing, coughing).**

    Observe characteristics of breathing pattern. **May see use of accessory muscles for breathing, sternal retractions (infants and young children), nasal flaring, or pursed-lip breathing. Irregular patterns (e.g., prolonged expiration, periods of apnea, obvious agonal breathing) may be pathological.**

    Auscultate and percuss chest, describing presence, absence, and character of breath sounds. **Abnormal breath sounds are indicative of numerous problems and must be evaluated further.**

    Observe chest size, shape, and symmetry of movement. **Changes in movement of chest wall (such as might occur with chest trauma, chest wall deformities) can impair breathing patterns.**

    Note color of skin and mucous membranes. **If pallor, duskiness, and/or cyanosis are present, supplemental oxygen and/or other interventions may be required.** (Refer to ND impaired Gas Exchange.)

- ∞ Note presence and character of cough. **Cough function may be weak or ineffective in conditions such as extremes in age (e.g., premature infant or elderly) or**

Information that appears in brackets has been added by the authors to clarify and enhance the use of nursing diagnoses.

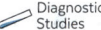 Diagnostic Studies   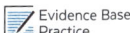 Evidence Based Practice   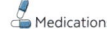 Medications   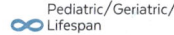 Pediatric/Geriatric/Lifespan

in diseases (e.g., cerebral palsy, muscular dystrophy, spinal cord injury, brain injury). Cough that is persistent and constant (such as can occur with asthma, acute bronchitis, cystic fibrosis, croup, whooping cough) can interfere with breathing. (Refer to ND impaired Airway Clearance.)
- Assist with/review results of necessary testing (e.g., chest x-rays, lung volumes/flow studies, and pulmonary function [determines vital capacity/tidal volume]/sleep studies) **to diagnose the presence/severity of lung diseases.**
- Review laboratory data, such as ABGs **(determines degree of oxygenation and carbon dioxide [CO_2] retention),** drug screens, and pulmonary function studies.

Nursing Priority No. 2.
To provide for relief of causative factors:

- Assist in treatment of underlying conditions, administering medications and therapies as ordered.
- Administer oxygen at the lowest concentration indicated and prescribed respiratory medications **for management of underlying pulmonary condition, respiratory distress, or cyanosis.**
- Suction airway, as needed, **to clear secretions.**
- Assist with bronchoscopy or chest tube insertion as indicated.
- Elevate the head of the bed and/or have the client sit up in a chair, as appropriate, **to promote physiological and psychological ease of maximal inspiration.**
- Direct client in breathing efforts as needed. Encourage slower and deeper respirations and use of the pursed-lip technique **to assist client in "taking control" of the situation, especially when condition is associated with anxiety and air hunger.**
- Monitor pulse oximetry, as indicated, **to verify maintenance/improvement in O_2 saturation.**
- Maintain a calm attitude while dealing with the client and significant other(s) **to limit the level of anxiety.**
- Assist the client in the use of relaxation techniques.
- Deal with fear/anxiety that may be present. (Refer to NDs Fear; Anxiety.)
- Encourage a position of comfort. Reposition the client frequently if immobility is a factor.
- Coach client in effective coughing techniques. Place in appropriate position for clearing airways. Splint the rib cage during deep-breathing exercises/cough, if indicated.

Information that appears in brackets has been added by the authors to clarify and enhance the use of nursing diagnoses.

Acute Care   Collaborative   Community/Home Care   Cultural

Promotes more effective breathing and airway management, especially when client is guarding, as might occur with chest, rib cage, or abdominal injuries or surgeries.

- Medicate with analgesics, as appropriate, **to promote deeper respiration and cough.** (Refer to NDs acute Pain; chronic Pain.)
- Encourage ambulation/exercise, as individually indicated, **to prevent onset or reduce severity of respiratory complications and to improve respiratory muscle strength.**
- Avoid overfeeding, such as might occur with young infant or client on tube feedings. **Abdominal distention can interfere with breathing as well as increase the risk of aspiration.**
- Provide/encourage use of adjuncts, such as incentive spirometer, **to facilitate deeper respiratory effort.**
- Supervise the use of respirator/diaphragmatic stimulator, rocking bed, apnea monitor, and so forth, **when neuromuscular impairment is present.**
- Ascertain that the client possesses and properly operates continuous positive airway pressure (CPAP) machine **when obstructive sleep apnea is causing breathing problems.**
- Maintain emergency equipment in readily accessible location and include age-/size-appropriate endotracheal/trach tubes (e.g., infant, child, adolescent, or adult) **when ventilatory support might be needed.**

Nursing Priority No. 3.

To promote optimal ventilation (Teaching/Discharge Considerations) and enhance well-being (long-term goals):

- Review the etiology of respiratory distress, treatment options, and possible coping behaviors.
- Emphasize the importance of good posture and effective use of accessory muscles **to maximize respiratory effort.**
- Instruct and reinforce breathing retraining. **Education may include many measures, such as conscious control of breathing rate, breathing exercises (diaphragmatic, abdominal breathing, inspiratory resistive, pursed-lip), and assistive devices such as rocking bed.**
- Recommend energy conservation techniques and pacing of activities.
- Refer for general exercise program (e.g., upper and lower extremity endurance and strength training), as indicated, **to maximize the client's level of functioning.**
- Encourage adequate rest periods between activities **to limit fatigue.**

Information that appears in brackets has been added by the authors to clarify and enhance the use of nursing diagnoses.

 Diagnostic Studies 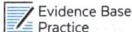 Evidence Based Practice Medications 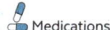 Pediatric/Geriatric/Lifespan

- Encourage the client/significant other(s) to develop a plan **for smoking cessation.** Provide appropriate referrals.
- Review environmental factors (e.g., exposure to dust, high pollen counts, severe weather, perfumes, animal dander, household chemicals, fumes, secondhand smoke; insufficient home support for safe care) **that may require avoidance of triggers or modification of lifestyle or environment to limit the impact on the client's breathing.**
- Encourage self-assessment and symptom management:
  Use of equipment to identify respiratory decompensation, such as a peak flow meter
  Appropriate use of oxygen (dosage, route, and safety factors)
  Medication regimen, including actions, side effects, and potential interactions of medications, over-the-counter (OTC) drugs, vitamins, and herbal supplements
  Adherence to home treatments such as metered-dose inhalers (MDIs), compressors, nebulizers, and chest physiotherapy
  Dietary patterns and needs; access to foods and nutrients supportive of health and breathing
  Management of personal environment, including stress reduction, rest and sleep, social events, travel, and recreation issues
  Avoidance of known irritants, allergens, and sick persons
  Immunizations against influenza and pneumonia
  Early intervention when respiratory symptoms occur, knowing what symptoms require reporting to medical providers, and seeking emergency care
- Provide referrals as appropriate. **May include a wide variety of services and providers, including support groups, a comprehensive rehabilitation program, occupational nurse, oxygen and durable medical equipment companies for supplies, home health services, occupational and physical therapy, transportation, assisted or alternate living facilities, local and national Lung Association chapters, and websites for educational materials.**

Documentation Focus

Assessment/Reassessment
- Relevant history of problem
- Respiratory pattern, breath sounds, use of accessory muscles
- Laboratory values
- Use of respiratory aids or supports, ventilator settings, and so forth

---

Information that appears in brackets has been added by the authors to clarify and enhance the use of nursing diagnoses.

Planning
- Plan of care, specific interventions, and who is involved in the planning
- Teaching plan

Implementation/Evaluation
- Response to interventions, teaching, actions performed, and treatment regimen
- Mastery of skills; level of independence
- Attainment of or progress toward desired outcome(s)
- Modifications to plan of care

Discharge Planning
- Long-term needs, including appropriate referrals and action taken, available resources
- Specific referrals provided

Sample Nursing Outcomes & Interventions Classifications NOC/NIC

NOC—Respiratory Function: Ventilation
NIC—Ventilation Assistance

---

impaired CARDIAC OUTPUT — ICNP

[Diagnostic Division: Circulation]

Definition: Failure of the heart to pump blood at a rate and rhythm that meets systemic metabolic requirements.

Recognizing Cues

Related/Risk Factors
Dysrhythmia (bradycardia/tachycardia)
Reduced stroke volume
Systemic loss of vascular tone, reduced mean arterial pressure (MAP)
Hypertension; coronary disease; myocardial injury
Fluid/electrolyte imbalance

Defining Characteristics (Decreased Cardiac Output)

Subjective
Fatigue; syncope; nausea/vomiting; anorexia
Dyspnea, progressive/activity intolerance
Anxiety

Information that appears in brackets has been added by the authors to clarify and enhance the use of nursing diagnoses.

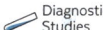 Diagnostic Studies   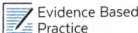 Evidence Based Practice   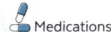 Medications   ∞ Pediatric/Geriatric/Lifespan

Objective
Adventitious breath sounds; persistent cough
Edema; decreased peripheral pulses
Altered blood pressure; narrowed pulse pressure
Paroxysmal nocturnal dyspnea (PND); orthopnea
Neck vein distention; pulmonary edema; visceral congestion
Presence of S_3 or S_4 sounds (gallop rhythm)
Electrocardiogram (ECG) changes; decreased pulse oximetry
Skin color changes; clammy skin
Decreased urinary output
 Cognitive/behavioral changes; decreased mentation

Clinical Connections
Myocardial infarction (MI), congestive heart failure, valvular heart disease, dysrhythmias, cardiomyopathy, cardiac contusions/trauma, pericarditis, ventricular aneurysm, spinal cord injury, kidney failure

American College of Cardiology/American Heart Association (ACC/AHA) Heart Failure guidelines.[1]

Stage A patients are at high risk for heart failure but have no structural heart disease or symptoms of heart failure.
Stage B patients have structural heart disease but have no symptoms of heart failure.
Stage C patients have structural heart disease and have symptoms of heart failure.
Stage D patients have refractory heart failure requiring specialized interventions.

Generate Solutions

Plan Desired Outcomes

Client Will (Include Specific Time Frame)
- Display hemodynamic stability (e.g., blood pressure, cardiac output, renal perfusion/urinary output, peripheral pulses).
- Report/demonstrate decreased episodes of dyspnea, angina, and dysrhythmias.
- Demonstrate an increase in activity tolerance.
- Verbalize knowledge of the disease process, individual risk factors, and treatment plan.
- Participate in activities that reduce the workload of the heart (e.g., stress management or therapeutic medication regimen

---

Information that appears in brackets has been added by the authors to clarify and enhance the use of nursing diagnoses.

 Acute Care 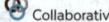 Collaborative 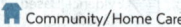 Community/Home Care 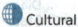 Cultural

program, weight reduction, balanced activity/rest plan, proper use of supplemental oxygen, cessation of smoking).
- Identify signs of cardiac decompensation, alter activities, and seek help appropriately.

Interventions/Take Action

Nursing Priority No. 1.
To identify causative/contributing factors:

- Identify clients exhibiting symptoms as noted in Related/Risk Factors. **Current evidence continues to show a strong correlation for the risk of heart failure in clients with type 2 diabetes, cardiovascular disease, hypertension, sedentary lifestyle, overweight/obesity, and smoking history.[1,7] In addition to individuals obviously at risk with known cardiac problems, there is a potential for cardiac output problems in persons with trauma; hemorrhage, substance abuse/overdose or withdrawal; pregnant/postpartum women with cardiovascular history; individuals with chronic renal disease; individuals with brainstem trauma or spinal cord injury at T8 or above.**
- Note age- and ethnic-related cardiovascular considerations. **In infants, failure to thrive with poor ability to suck and feed can be indications of heart problems. When in the supine position, pregnant women incur decreased vascular return during the second and third trimesters, potentially compromising cardiac output. Contractile force is naturally decreased in the elderly with reduced ability to increase cardiac output in response to increased demand. Also, arteries are stiffer, veins are more dilated, and heart valves are less competent, often resulting in systemic hypertension and blood pooling. Generally, higher-risk populations for decreased cardiac output due to heart failure include African Americans, Hispanics, Native Americans, and recent immigrants from developing nations, directly related to the higher incidence and prevalence of hypertension and diabetes. According to a report from the ACC and AHA Joint Committee on Clinical Practice Guidelines, African American and Hispanic clients with established heart failure experienced higher rates of heart failure–associated hospitalization compared with White clients. Asian and Pacific Islander clients with heart failure had a similar rate of hospitalization as White clients but lower rates of death.**

Information that appears in brackets has been added by the authors to clarify and enhance the use of nursing diagnoses.

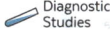 Diagnostic Studies 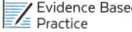 Evidence Based Practice 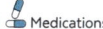 Medications 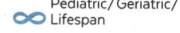 Pediatric/Geriatric/Lifespan

- Review diagnostic studies, including, but not limited to, chest radiograph, cardiac stress testing, ECG, echocardiogram, cardiac output and ventricular ejection studies, and heart scan or catheterization. **For example, ECG may show previous or evolving MI, left ventricular hypertrophy. Doppler flow echocardiogram showing an ejection fraction (EF) less than 40% is indicative of systolic dysfunction, but many clients with clinical diagnosis of heart failure have a normal EF. Although cardiac output can be normal in certain types of heart failure, a client with severe left-sided heart failure will have decreased cardiac output (less than 4 L/min) owing either to an increased hemodynamic burden or to a reduction in oxygen delivery to the myocardium, resulting in impaired contraction. Additional cardiac studies (e.g., radionuclide scans or catheterization) may be indicated to assess left ventricular function, valvular function, and coronary circulation. Chest radiography may show enlarged heart, pleural effusions.**
- Review laboratory data, including but not limited to complete blood count (CBC), electrolytes (e.g., serial sodium [Na] and potassium [K] levels), arterial blood gases (ABGs), cardiac biomarkers (e.g., creatine kinase and its subclasses, troponins, myoglobin, and LDH); lactate; brain natriuretic peptide (BNP); kidney, thyroid, and liver function studies; cultures (e.g., blood, wound, or secretions); and bleeding and coagulation studies **to identify imbalances, disease processes, and desired or adverse effects of treatments.**
- Assess the potential for/type of developing shock states: hypovolemic, distributive, cardiogenic, obstructive, and psychogenic.

Nursing Priority No. 2.
To assess degree of debilitation:

- Assess for signs of poor ventricular function or impending cardiac failure and shock using clinical staging/classification (e.g., New York Heart Association [NYHA] classification, American Heart Association Heart Failure guidelines, Framingham Diagnostic Criteria for Heart Failure, etc.) **for assessment of heart failure and evaluating degree of debilitation:**
  Reports of extreme fatigue, intolerance for activity, sudden or progressive weight gain, swelling of extremities, and progressive shortness of breath.
  Chest pain. **May indicate evolving heart attack; can also accompany congestive heart failure. Chest pain may be atypical in women experiencing an MI and**

Information that appears in brackets has been added by the authors to clarify and enhance the use of nursing diagnoses.

is often atypical in the elderly owing to altered pain perception.

Mental status changes. **Confusion, agitation, decreased cognition, and coma may occur due to decreased brain perfusion.**

Changes in heart rate or rhythm (e.g., tachycardia at rest, bradycardia, atrial fibrillation, or varied dysrhythmias). **Heart irritability is common, reflecting conduction defects and/or ischemia.**

Heart sounds distant, with irregular rhythms; murmurs—systolic (**valvular stenosis and shunting**) and diastolic (**aortic or pulmonary insufficiency**) or gallop rhythm (S_3, S_4) noted **when heart failure is present and ventricles are stiff.**

Peripheral pulses weak and thready, **reflecting hypotension, vasoconstriction, shunting.**

∞ Changes in skin color, moisture, temperature, and capillary refill time. **Pallor or cyanosis; cool, moist skin; and slow capillary refill time may be present because of peripheral vasoconstriction (i.e., shunting of blood to vital organs) and decreased oxygen saturation.**

Blood pressure changes. **Hypertension may be chronic or blood pressure elevated initially in client with impending cardiogenic, hypovolemic, or septic shock (i.e., distributive shock). Later, as cardiac output decreases, profound hypotension can be present, often with narrowed pulse pressure.**

Breath sounds distant, muffled, or diminished *associated with pleural fluid accumulation*, **or reveal bilateral crackles and wheezing associated with congestion.**

Edema with neck vein distention; pitting edema in extremities and dependent portions of body **because of impaired venous return.**

∞ Urinary output decreased or absent, **reflecting poor perfusion of kidneys and activation of the renin-angiotensin-aldosterone system (RAAS). Note: Output less than 0.5 to 1.5 mL/kg/hr for adults and children indicates inadequate renal perfusion.**

Nursing Priority No. 3.

To minimize/correct causative factors, maximize cardiac output:

Acute/Severe Phase

Care focus for the critically ill and hospitalized client

- Wash hands before and after client contact, maintain aseptic technique during invasive procedures, and provide

---

Information that appears in brackets has been added by the authors to clarify and enhance the use of nursing diagnoses.

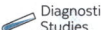 Diagnostic Studies 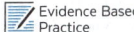 Evidence Based Practice 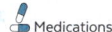 Medications 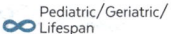 Pediatric/Geriatric/Lifespan

site care, as indicated, **to prevent hospital-acquired infection.** (Refer to ND risk for Infection for additional interventions.)

- Provide antipyretics and fever control actions as indicated. Adjust ambient environmental temperature **to maintain body temperature in near-normal range, reducing metabolic oxygen demands.**
- Minimize activities that can elicit Valsalva response (e.g., rectal straining, vomiting, spasmodic coughing with suctioning, prolonged breath-holding during pushing stage of labor) and encourage client to breathe deeply in and out during activities that increase risk of Valsalva effect. **Valsalva response to breath-holding causes increased intrathoracic pressure, reducing cardiac output and blood pressure.**
- Maintain patency of invasive intravascular monitoring and infusion lines and tape connections **to prevent exsanguination or air embolus.**
- Promote rest in bed or chair with upper body elevated as comfortable. **Decreases oxygen consumption and demand and catecholamine-induced stress response, thus reducing myocardial workload and risk of decompensation.**
- Promote energy conservation:
  Decrease stimuli, providing quiet environment.
  Schedule activities and assessments to maximize sleep periods.
  Assist with or perform self-care activities for client.
  Avoid use of restraints whenever possible, especially if client is confused.
  Use sedation and analgesics, as indicated, with caution **to achieve desired rest state without compromising hemodynamic responses.**
- Administer supplemental oxygen, as indicated (by cannula, mask, or endotracheal/tracheostomy tube with mechanical ventilation), **to improve cardiac function by increasing available oxygen and reducing work of breathing.**
- Elevate legs when in sitting position (if heart failure present or extremities are edematous). **Note: During an acute heart failure exacerbation, use caution elevating severely edematous extremities to prevent rapid intravascular volume expansion.**
- Apply antiembolic hose or sequential compression devices when indicated, being sure they are individually fitted

---

Information that appears in brackets has been added by the authors to clarify and enhance the use of nursing diagnoses.

 Acute Care 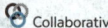 Collaborative 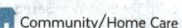 Community/Home Care Cultural

and appropriately applied. **Improves venous return and reduces the risk of thrombophlebitis.**
- Monitor vital signs frequently **to evaluate response to treatments and activities.**
- Perform periodic hemodynamic measurements, as indicated. **Perform periodic hemodynamic measurements, as indicated (e.g., arterial, central venous pressure [CVP], pulmonary artery wedge pressure [PAWP], pulmonary artery pressure; cardiac output and cardiac index, saturation of venous oxygen [Svo_2]).**
- Monitor cardiac rhythm continuously **to note changes and evaluate effectiveness of medications and devices (e.g., implanted pacemaker/defibrillator).**
- Be aware of waveforms natural to client's particular device, and be prepared to take appropriate action if device is not functioning correctly.
- Administer or restrict fluids, provide electrolytes as indicated **to maximize cardiac output, improve tissue perfusion, and prevent dysrhythmias. Note: Replacement of blood and large amounts of IV fluids may be needed if low output state is due to hypovolemia.**
- Use infusion pumps **to monitor IV rates closely to prevent bolus or exacerbation of fluid overload.**
- Assess hourly or periodic urinary output and daily weight, noting 24-hr total fluid balance and presence of edema **to evaluate kidney function and effects of interventions as well as to allow for timely alterations in therapeutic regimen.**
- Administer medications as indicated. **For clients in ACC/AHA stage C and D, guideline-directed medical therapy (GDMT) suggests the use of the angiotensin-converting enzyme inhibitors/angiotensin receptor blockers (ACEI/ARB), beta blockers, or angiotensin receptor–neprilysin inhibitors (ARNIs), in conjunction with loop diuretics for fluid retention, aldosterone receptor blockers, hydralazine and nitrates, with consideration of ivabradine, a sinoatrial node modulator.** Additional therapies may include inotropic drugs **to enhance myocardial contractility and improve stroke volume;** antiarrhythmics **to reduce myocardial irritability and improve cardiac output;** vasopressors and/or dilators, as indicated, **to manage systemic effects of vasoconstriction and low cardiac output;** pain medications **to reduce cardiac pain and muscle tension;** antidiabetic

---

Information that appears in brackets has been added by the authors to clarify and enhance the use of nursing diagnoses.

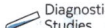 Diagnostic Studies   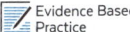 Evidence Based Practice   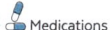 Medications   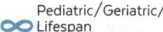 Pediatric/Geriatric/Lifespan

agents **to maintain tight glycemic control in client with diabetes during acute phase of cardiovascular care or to reduce risk of heart failure;** anti-anxiety agents **to reduce oxygen demand and myocardial workload;** and anticoagulants **to prevent thromboemboli.**

- Investigate reports of anorexia or nausea and limit or withhold oral intake as indicated. **Symptoms may be a systemic reaction to low cardiac output, visceral congestion, or a reaction to medications or pain.**
- Assist with preparations for and monitor response to support procedures or devices as indicated (e.g., cardioversion, pacemaker/implantable cardioverter-defibrillator (ICD), angioplasty/stent placement, coronary artery bypass graft [CABG] or valve replacement, intra-aortic balloon pump [IABP], left ventricular assist device [LVAD], total artificial heart [TAH], transplantation). **Any number of interventions may be required to correct a condition causing heart failure or to support a failing heart during recovery from myocardial infarction, while awaiting transplantation, or for long-term management of chronic heart failure.**
- Provide for nutritional needs/diet restrictions (**e.g., IV nutrition or total parenteral nutrition, low-sodium, bland, soft, carbohydrate restriction, low-cholesterol/low-fat diet, with frequent small feedings**) as indicated.
- Collaborate with nutritionist/dietitian **to determine/adjust individually appropriate diet plan.**
- Provide skin-protective measures (e.g., frequent position changes, early ambulation, monitoring of bony prominences, sheepskin or special flotation mattress) **to avoid the development of pressure injury in the setting of impaired circulation and generalized weakness or debilitation.**
- Provide information about testing procedures and client participation.
- Explain limitations imposed by condition and dietary and fluid restrictions.
- Share information about positive signs of improvement.
- Promote visits from family/significant others to provide positive social interaction.
- Provide psychological support to reduce anxiety and its adverse effects on cardiac function:
  Maintain calm attitude and limit stressful stimuli.
  Provide and encourage use of relaxation techniques, such as massage therapy, soothing music, or quiet activities.

Information that appears in brackets has been added by the authors to clarify and enhance the use of nursing diagnoses.

 Acute Care 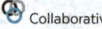 Collaborative 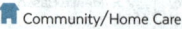 Community/Home Care Cultural

Nursing Priority No. 4.
To support cardiac output, minimize risk factors:

Postacute/Chronic Phase
Care focus for the chronically ill client

- Provide for adequate rest, positioning client for maximum comfort.
- Provide skin care, a special bed or mattress (e.g., air, water, gel, foam), and assist with frequent position changes **to avoid the development of pressure injury in the setting of impaired circulation and generalized weakness or debilitation.**
- Encourage changing positions slowly, dangling legs before standing to reduce risk of orthostatic hypotension.
- Avoid a prolonged sitting position for all clients, and supine position for sleep or exercise for gravid clients (second and third trimesters) **to maximize venous return.**
- Elevate legs when in a sitting position if extremities are edematous.
- Increase activity levels gradually, as permitted by individual condition, noting vital sign response to activity.
- Monitor weight changes and swelling as well as intake/output, calculating 24-hr fluid balance. Increase or restrict fluids, as indicated, **to maximize cardiac output and improve tissue perfusion.**
- Educate client/caregivers about drug regimen, including indications, dose and dosing schedules, potential adverse side effects, or drug/drug interactions. **Client is often on multiple medications, which can be difficult to manage, thus increasing potential that medications can be missed or incorrectly used.**
- Emphasize reporting of adverse and nuisance side effects of medications **so that adjustments can be made in dosing or another class of medication considered.**
- Discuss significant signs/symptoms that need to be reported to healthcare provider, **such as unrelieved or increased chest pain, dyspnea, fever, swelling of ankles, especially when accompanied by weight gain; and sudden unexplained cough; these are all "danger signs" that require immediate evaluation and possible change of usual therapies.**
- Encourage relaxation techniques such as soothing music or quiet activities **to reduce anxiety, muscle tension.**
- Refer for nutritional needs assessment and management **to provide for supportive nutrition while meeting dietary restrictions (e.g., sodium-restricted, carbohydrate restriction, low-cholesterol/low-fat diet, or other**

Information that appears in brackets has been added by the authors to clarify and enhance the use of nursing diagnoses.

 Diagnostic Studies 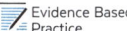 Evidence Based Practice 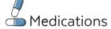 Medications 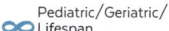 Pediatric/Geriatric/Lifespan

types of diet). **Current data suggest whole grain, plant-based dietary plans (e.g., Mediterranean diet, Dietary Approaches to Stop Hypertension [DASH]) may offer protection from heart failure exacerbation and improve patient outcomes.**
- Monitor weight changes and swelling as well as intake/output, calculating 24-hr fluid balance. Increase or restrict fluids, as indicated, **to maximize cardiac output and improve tissue perfusion.**

Nursing Priority No. 5.

To maintain optimal cardiac function (Teaching/Discharge Considerations) and enhance well-being (long-term goals):

- Emphasize importance of regular medical follow-up care.
- Review "danger" signs requiring immediate physician notification (e.g., unrelieved or increased chest pain, functional decline, dyspnea, or edema) **which may indicate deteriorating cardiac function, heart failure.**
- Recommend annual flu shot, pneumonia and other vaccinations as needed.
- Provide information to clients/caregivers on individual condition, treatment plan, and expected outcomes using various forms of teaching according to client needs, desires, and learning style. **Treatment plan is usually complex and can be overwhelming to client/caregiver. Providing information in multiple formats increases learning and likelihood of retention to achieve goals of treatment.**
- Provide instruction for home monitoring of weight, pulse, and blood pressure, as appropriate, **to detect change and allow for timely intervention.**
- Encourage participation in regular exercise and cardiac rehabilitation (CR) program as appropriate. **Current evidence from multiple random controlled trials indicates CR improves client quality of life, functional status, and activity tolerance; CR is recommended in ACC/AHA-guideline-directed medical therapy (GDMT).**
- Review individual's particular risk factors (e.g., smoking, stress, elevated blood glucose/diabetes; obesity, recent MI). **Providing printed information sheets and direction to helpful websites for client/caregiver to refer to postdischarge enhances retention of learning and self-management of health.**
- Refer to classes/programs to address specific risk factors such as smoking cessation, nutrition, energy conservation, and stress management techniques **to achieve long-term goals and improve general well-being.**

Information that appears in brackets has been added by the authors to clarify and enhance the use of nursing diagnoses.

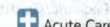 Acute Care 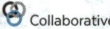 Collaborative 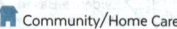 Community/Home Care 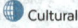 Cultural

- Direct client and/or caregivers to community resources as indicated. **Clients with impaired functional capabilities may require home/respite care, meal prep/delivery, financial assistance, psychosocial support, and resources for durable medical supplies and equipment, e.g., 24-hr oxygen, LVAD support.**
- Refer to NDs Activity Intolerance, decreased Diversional Activity Engagement, difficulty Coping, ineffective Breathing Pattern, impaired family Coping, inadequate/excessive Fluid Volume, inadequate Nutritional Intake, Body Weight Problem, acute/chronic Pain, risk for impaired Cardiovascular Function, ineffective peripheral Tissue Perfusion, impaired Sexual Functioning, as indicated.

Documentation Focus

Assessment/Reassessment
- Baseline and subsequent findings and individual hemodynamic parameters, heart and breath sounds, chest x-ray results, ECG pattern, presence/strength of peripheral pulses, skin/tissue status, renal output, and mentation.

Planning
- Plan of care and who is involved in planning
- Teaching plan

Implementation/Evaluation
- Client's responses to interventions, teaching, and actions performed
- Status and disposition at discharge
- Attainment of or progress toward desired outcome(s)
- Modifications to plan of care

Discharge Planning
- Discharge considerations and who will be responsible for carrying out individual actions
- Long-term needs and available resources
- Specific referrals made

Sample Nursing Outcomes & Interventions Classifications NOC/NIC

NOC—Cardiac Pump Effectiveness
NIC—Hemodynamic Regulation
NIC—Cardiac Care

Information that appears in brackets has been added by the authors to clarify and enhance the use of nursing diagnoses.

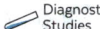 Diagnostic Studies 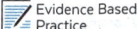 Evidence Based Practice 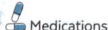 Medications 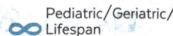 Pediatric/Geriatric/Lifespan

risk for impaired CARDIOVASCULAR FUNCTION

NANDA-I

[Diagnostic Division: Circulation]

Definition: Susceptible to changes in the normal process of substance transport, body homeostasis, tissue metabolic residue removal, and organ function.

Recognizing Cues

Risk Factors
Excessive anxiety; excessive stress
Average daily physical activity is less than recommended for age and gender
Ineffective overweight self-management; excessive accumulation of fat for age and gender
Excessive alcohol consumption; inappropriate dietary habits; inattentive to secondhand smoke; tobacco use; substance misuse
Inadequate knowledge of modifiable factors
Ineffective blood glucose level management; inadequate blood pressure self-management; ineffective lipid balance management

Clinical Connections
Angina, coronary artery disease, hypertension, diabetes mellitus, cardiac surgery, bariatric surgery, substance abuse

Generate Solutions

Plan Desired Outcomes

Client Will (Include Specific Time Frame)
- Be free of cardiovascular symptoms, such as hypertension, chest pain, activity intolerance, altered mental status, changes in heart rate or rhythm, syncope, decreased skin temperature, or diminished peripheral pulses.
- Verbalize knowledge of the disease process, individual risk factors, and treatment plan.
- Participate in activities that promote cardiovascular health (e.g., stress management, therapeutic medication regimen program, weight reduction, balanced activity/rest plan, and cessation of smoking).

Information that appears in brackets has been added by the authors to clarify and enhance the use of nursing diagnoses.

 Acute Care 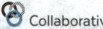 Collaborative 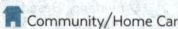 Community/Home Care 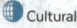 Cultural

Interventions/Take Action

Nursing Priority No. 1.
To identify client at risk:

- Note the client's age and gender and family history when assessing risk for cardiovascular disease (CVD). **Risks that cannot be controlled include advancing age, gender, and heredity. The American College of Cardiology Foundation and American Heart Association Task Force reported in 2019 that "risk for heart disorders increases with age, and men are still considered at higher risk for myocardial infarction and experience them earlier in life" (Arnett et al., 2019).**
- Review with the client their past history of conditions associated with cardiovascular impairment, such as heart attack, stroke, diabetes, and peripheral vascular conditions **to help assess current risk for recurrence.**
- Determine if the client has condition known as "metabolic syndrome" (i.e., large waistline, high triglyceride level, low high-density lipoprotein [HDL], [or is on medications to lower triglycerides or cholesterol]); is hypertensive, and has high fasting blood glucose or hemoglobin A_{1C}. **Metabolic risk factors are strongly associated with increased risk for heart disease and stroke, especially when combined with other risk factors such as smoking, sedentary lifestyle, and obesity.**
- Inquire about the client's current and past history of smoking. **Smoking is associated with vasoconstriction, which causes decreased blood flow and reduced oxygenation of organs, which can impair cardiovascular function.**
- Note the client's weight and dietary habits **to determine if obesity or poor nutrition are risk factors. Note: Studies have shown that being overweight/obesity predispose and are associated with coronary heart disease, heart failure, and sudden death because of their impact on the cardiovascular system.**
- Inquire about client's use of alcohol, opioids, stimulants, sedatives, and cannabis. *The abuse of alcohol, opioids, stimulants (i.e., methamphetamine, cocaine), sedatives, and cannabis are associated with an increased risk of CVD (i.e., coronary artery disease, heart failure, and arrhythmias).*

Information that appears in brackets has been added by the authors to clarify and enhance the use of nursing diagnoses.

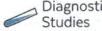 Diagnostic Studies 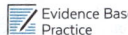 Evidence Based Practice 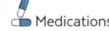 Medications 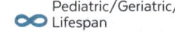 Pediatric/Geriatric/Lifespan

Nursing Priority No. 2.
To determine changes in cardiovascular status:
- Investigate reports of chest pain, headache, or pain in the extremities **to identify potential problem with cardiovascular perfusion.**
- Measure the client's blood pressure at each medical provider visit **to identify the client with high blood pressure (risk factor) or unknown or uncontrolled hypertension. Encourage client to monitor blood pressure at home, keep a daily log, and bring the log to follow-up appointments.**
- Review diagnostic studies, including but not limited to electrocardiogram (ECG), echocardiogram, body mass scan or other nutrition screen, or coronary calcium scan/calcium scoring **to determine if cardiovascular concerns are developing.**
- Review laboratory data, including but not limited to lipid studies (e.g., cholesterol, triglycerides), electrolytes, fasting blood glucose, glucose tolerance, insulin resistance, and hemoglobin A_{1C}; cardiac biomarkers; kidney, thyroid, and liver function studies **to identify imbalances or disease processes and to take preventive measures when needed. Note: Familial hypercholesterolemia (FH) is an inherited disorder that is thought to lead to aggressive and premature-onset cardiovascular disease. Also, it has long been known that an association exists between diabetes mellitus and increased cardiovasular risk.**
- Assess for restlessness, fatigue, changes in level of consciousness, increased capillary refill time, diminished peripheral pulses, and pale, cool skin. **These are signs and symptoms of inadequate systemic perfusion, which can cause or affect cardiovascular function.**
- Assess heart sounds and pulses. **Helps identify conditions associated with inadequate myocardial or systemic tissue perfusion, dehydration, immobility, electrolyte or acid-base imbalances.**
- Investigate reports of difficulty breathing; note respiratory rate outside of acceptable parameters, **which can be indicative of oxygen exchange problems with potential for cardiopulmonary dysfunction.**
- Assess for extremity discoloration; changes in pulses, temperature, or color; and client report of discomfort/pain. **These signs and symptoms are associated with systemic or peripheral vascular conditions.**

Information that appears in brackets has been added by the authors to clarify and enhance the use of nursing diagnoses.

Nursing Priority No. 3.

To promote cardiovascular health (Teaching/Discharge Considerations) and enhance well-being (long-term goals):

- Discuss the risk factors (e.g., family history, obesity, age, smoking, hypertension, diabetes, and clotting disorders) and potential outcomes of atherosclerosis (e.g., systemic and cardiac disease conditions). **This information is necessary for the client to make informed decisions concerning risk factors and to commit to lifestyle changes necessary to prevent onset of complications or manage symptoms when condition present.**
- Review difference between modifiable and nonmodifiable risk factors **to assist client/significant other (SO) in understanding those areas in which they can take action or make healthy choices.**
- Recommend maintenance of normal weight or weight loss if client is an unhealthy weight **to decrease risk associated with overweight and obesity.**
- Encourage smoking cessation, when indicated, offering information about stop-smoking aids and programs. **Smoking cessation is important in the medical management of many contributors to heart attack and stroke. These include atherosclerosis (fatty buildups in arteries), thrombosis (blood clots), artery spasm (e.g., coronary, carotid, or cerebral), and cardiac dysrhythmias.**
- Encourage the client to engage in regular exercise **to enhance circulation and promote healthy blood pressure and general well-being.**
- Review medications on a regular basis **to manage those that affect cardiac function or those given to prevent blood pressure or thromboembolic problems.**
- Discuss drug use, as indicated, alcohol, opioids, stimulants (i.e., cocaine, methamphetamine), sedatives, and cannabis, **to educate client regarding effect of drug on cardiovascular system.**
- Encourage the client in high-risk categories (e.g., strong family history, diabetic, or prior history of cardiac event) to have regular medical examinations **to provide timely intervention when needed.**
- Refer to educational or community resources, as indicated. **The client/SO may benefit from instruction and support provided by agencies to engage in healthier heart activities (e.g., weight loss, smoking cessation, or exercise) and**

Information that appears in brackets has been added by the authors to clarify and enhance the use of nursing diagnoses.

promote healthier diet through meal planning, cooking classes, and addressing food insecurity.

- Instruct in blood pressure monitoring at home if indicated; advise purchase of home monitoring equipment; refer to community resources as indicated. **Facilitates management of hypertension, which is a major risk factor for damage to blood vessels or organ function.**

Documentation Focus

Assessment/Reassessment
- Individual findings, noting specific risk factors including diet, exercise, smoking
- Vital signs, pulse oximetry, cardiac rhythm, presence of dysrhythmias, capillary refill
- Status of organ function (e.g., mentation, breath sounds, or renal output)

Planning
- Plan of care and who is involved in planning
- Teaching plan

Implementation/Evaluation
- Response to interventions, teaching, and actions performed
- Attainment of or progress toward desired outcome(s)
- Modifications to plan of care

Discharge Planning
- Long-term needs and who is responsible for actions to be taken
- Available resources, specific referrals made

Sample Nursing Outcomes & Interventions Classifications NOC/NIC

NOC—Circulation Status
NIC—Cardiac Risk Management

---

impaired, CAREGIVER CHILD ATTACHMENT ICNP

[Diagnostic Division: Roles/Relationships]

Definition: Lacking reliable and nurturing response of primary caregiver(s) to child, or response of child to caregiver, that limits reciprocal relationship and psychosocial development.

Information that appears in brackets has been added by the authors to clarify and enhance the use of nursing diagnoses.

 Acute Care   Collaborative 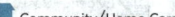 Community/Home Care   Cultural

Recognizing Cues

Related/Risk Factors
Parents lack ability to meet personal needs of child
 Parent/child separation due to illness, physical barriers (e.g., infant in isolette, pediatric/adult ICU); a lack of sufficient privacy preventing effective initiation/continuation of bonding process
Anxiety; stressors; financial concerns; unwanted pregnancy; unwanted gender
Parent lacks understanding/knowledge of child's disorganized neurobehavioral manifestations resulting in a relational conflict disorganized behavior
Parental substance abuse

Defining Characteristics

Subjective
Reports difficulty for infant to latch, pain/discomfort with breastfeeding; concerned milk supply is inadequate
Avoids clingy, touchy, or needy people or relationships
Feels insecure, lacks confidence; expresses poor self-image or self-loathing

Objective
Difficulty expressing love, nurturing, comforting, touching, or is avoidant of child
Decreased sensitivity; does not recognize or honor personal space or boundaries
Reacts negatively to criticism
Depressive symptoms; frequent emotional outbursts or erratic behaviors

Clinical Connections
Prematurity, genetic or congenital conditions, autism, attention deficit disorder, developmental delay (parent or child), oppositional defiant, conduct disorders. Parent disorders: substance abuse, depression, anxiety, schizophrenia, bipolar disorder, antisocial or borderline personality disorders

Generate Solutions

Plan Desired Outcomes

Parent Will (Include Specific Time Frame)
- Verbalize family strengths and needs.
- Demonstrate nurturing, supportive, and protective behaviors toward child.

Information that appears in brackets has been added by the authors to clarify and enhance the use of nursing diagnoses.

 Diagnostic Studies   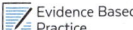 Evidence Based Practice   Medications   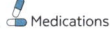 Pediatric/Geriatric/Lifespan

- Demonstrate newly learned skills to modify behavioral disorganization of the child.
- Commit to family counseling/therapy and follow-up as indicated.
- Access available community resources appropriately.

Child Will (Include Specific Time Frame)
- Be receptive of parents' loving attention.
- Verbalize/demonstrate affection towards parents.
- Demonstrate ability to hug/hold parents hands within level of comfort.
- Accept and follow parents' guidance and instructions.
- Verbalize positive self affirmations.

Interventions/Take Action

Nursing Priority No. 1.
To identify causative/contributing factors:

- Assess parents' perception of situation, understanding of attachment process, and individual concerns. **Attachment is a powerful predictor of a child's later social and emotional outcome. Identifying problem areas and strengths is important to formulate appropriate plans to promote positive outcome.**
- Monitor parent/child interactions. **Identifies relationships, communication skills, and feelings about one another. The way in which a parent responds to a child and how the child responds to the parent largely determines how the child develops. Identifying the way in which the family responds to one another is crucial in determining the need for and type of interventions required.**
- Determine parenting skill level, considering intellectual, emotional, and physical strengths and limitations. **Identifies areas of need for further education, skill training, and factors that might interfere with ability to assimilate new information.**
- Determine availability and use of resources to include extended family, parenting classes, support groups, and financial resources. **Lack of support from or presence of extended family, lack of involvement in groups (e.g., church, school, cultural, or social organizations) or specific resources (e.g., La Leche League), and financial stresses can affect family negatively, interfering with ability to deal effectively with parenting responsibilities.**
- Determine emotional and behavioral challenges of the child/parent. **Attachment-disordered children are unable to**

Information that appears in brackets has been added by the authors to clarify and enhance the use of nursing diagnoses.

 Acute Care 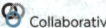 Collaborative 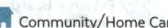 Community/Home Care 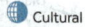 Cultural

give and receive love and affection. They defy parental rules and authority, creating ongoing stress and turmoil in the family. Adults with an attachment disorder may have challenges responding to child.

- Evaluate parents' ability to provide a protective environment and participate in a reciprocal relationship. **Parents may be immature, may be substance abusers, or may be mentally ill and unable or unwilling to assume the task of parenting. The ways in which parents respond to the child are critical to the child's development, and interventions need to be directed at helping the parents to deal with their own issues and learn positive parenting skills.**
- Observe attachment behaviors between parent and child(ren) for biological, adopted, or blended families, recognizing cultural background. **For example, lack of eye-to-eye contact, use of en face (facing to face) position, and talking to the infant in a high-pitched voice are indicative of attachment behaviors in American culture but may not be practiced in another culture. Failure to bond effectively is thought to affect subsequent parent-child interaction.**

Nursing Priority No. 2.

To enhance behavioral organization of the child:

- Identify the infant's/child's strengths and vulnerabilities. **Each person is born with their own temperament that affects interactions with caregivers, and when these are known, actions can be taken to assist parents/caregivers to parent or care for family members appropriately.**
- Educate parents regarding child growth and development and the perceptions of parenting styles. **Parents often have misconceptions about the abilities of their child, and providing correct information clarifies expectations and is more realistic.**
- Assist parents in modifying the environment. **The environment can be changed to provide appropriate stimulation (e.g., to diminish stimulation before bedtime, to simplify when the environment is too complex to handle, to provide life space where the child can play unrestricted, resulting in freedom for the child to meet their needs).** (Refer to ND impaired infant Neurodevelopmental Organization.)
- Model caregiving techniques that best support neurobehavioral organization. **Recognizing that the child deserves to**

Information that appears in brackets has been added by the authors to clarify and enhance the use of nursing diagnoses.

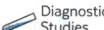 Diagnostic Studies   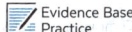 Evidence Based Practice   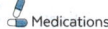 Medications   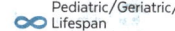 Pediatric/Geriatric/Lifespan

have their needs taken seriously and responding to those needs in a loving fashion promotes trust, and children learn to model their behavior after what they have seen the parents do.
- Respond consistently with nurturing to infant/child. **Babies signal their needs by crying; when parents respond to these signals, they develop a sensitivity that in turn develops parental intuition, providing infants with gratification of their needs and trust in their environment.**

Nursing Priority No. 3.

To enhance best functioning of parents:
- Develop a therapeutic nurse-client relationship. Provide a consistently caring, nurturing, and nonjudgmental environment and consistent point of contact. **Parents are often surprised to find that a tiny infant can cause so many changes in their lives and need help to adjust to this new experience. The caring/supportive relationship of the nurse can help with this adjustment and provide the information and empathy they need at this time.**
- Assist parents in identifying and prioritizing family strengths and needs. **Promotes a positive attitude by looking at what they already do well and using those skills to address needs.**
- Support and guide parents in the process of assessing resources. **Outside support is important at this time, and making sure that parents receive the help they need will help them in this adjustment period.**
- Involve parents in activities with the child that they can accomplish successfully. **Parent participation (mentoring and modeling) in activities recommended such as for infant the Gymboree Play and Music creative play, or baby yoga can enable the parents to get to know their child and themselves, enhancing their confidence and self-concept.**
- Recognize and provide positive feedback for nurturing and protective parenting behaviors. **Reinforces the continuation of desired behaviors.**

Nursing Priority No. 4.

To support parent/child attachment during separation:
- Advise parent to use telephone/electronic device contact, as appropriate. **Knowing there is someone or a client electronic health record they can contact if they have problems provides a sense of security.**

Information that appears in brackets has been added by the authors to clarify and enhance the use of nursing diagnoses.

- Establish a routine time for daily calls/initiate calls, as indicated when child or parent is hospitalized. **Provides a sense of consistency and control and allows for the planning of other activities.**
- Minimize the number of professionals on the team with whom parents must have contact. **Family begin to know the individuals they are dealing with on a regular basis. Fosters trust in these relationships, providing opportunities for modeling and learning.**
- Determine if family is able to use resources such as the Ronald McDonald House or provide them with a list of a variety of local accommodations and restaurants. **When a family member is hospitalized out of town, families need to have a place to stay so they can have ready access to the hospital and be able to rest and refresh from time to time.**
- Arrange for the family to receive progress reports. **Provides information and comfort as the client progresses, allowing the family to continue to have hope for a positive resolution.**
- Suggest that parents keep a journal of child progress. **Serves as a reminder of the progress that is being made, especially when they become discouraged and believe the infant/child is "never" going to be better.**
- Provide a comfortable and quiet environment for situations requiring supervision of visits. **Supports the family as they work toward resolving conflicts and promotes a sense of hopefulness, enabling them to experience success when the family is involved with a legal situation.**

Nursing Priority No. 5.

To strengthen attachment process (Teaching/Discharge Considerations) and enhance well-being (long-term goals):

- Identify and coordinate services for transportation, financial resources, housing, and other needs identified by family. **Coordination with parents and social services helps families (e.g., limited education, financial, or community resources) focus on therapeutic regimen and on issues of parenting or supporting the family to improve their relationships/dynamics.**
- Develop support systems appropriate to the situation (e.g., extended family, friends, or social worker). **Depending on individual situation, support from extended family, friends, social worker, or therapist can assist the family to deal with attachment disorders.**

Information that appears in brackets has been added by the authors to clarify and enhance the use of nursing diagnoses.

- 🕲 Explore community resources (e.g., support groups, religious affiliations, or day/respite care). **Can help parents who are overwhelmed with the care of a loved one with special needs. Support groups provide opportunity for parents to learn from others with similar issues/concerns.**
- 🕲 Refer to addiction counseling, individual counseling, family therapies, or treatment as indicated. **May need additional assistance when a situation is complicated by drug abuse (including alcohol), mental illness, disruptions in caregiving, parents who are burned out with caring for child with attachment or other difficulties.**

Documentation Focus

Assessment/Reassessment
- Identified behaviors of both parents and child, separation anxiety
- Specific risk factors, parent conflict/infant behaviors, individual perceptions and concerns
- Understanding of attachment process
- Interactions between parent and child

Planning
- Plan of care and who is involved in planning
- Teaching plan

Implementation/Evaluation
- Parents'/child's responses to interventions, teaching, and actions performed
- Attainment of or progress toward desired outcomes
- Modifications to plan of care

Discharge Planning
- Long-term needs and who is responsible
- Plan for home visits to support parents and to ensure infant/child safety and well-being
- Specific referrals made

Sample Nursing Outcomes & Interventions Classifications NOC/NIC

NOC—Parent-Infant Attachment
NIC—Attachment Promotion

Information that appears in brackets has been added by the authors to clarify and enhance the use of nursing diagnoses.

excessive CAREGIVING BURDEN NANDA-I

[Diagnostic Division: Roles/Relationships]

Definition: Overwhelming multidimensional strain when caring for a significant other.

Recognizing Cues

Related/Risk Factors
Difficulty prioritizing competing role commitments
Inadequate equipment, or physical environment for providing care; inadequate privacy
Inadequate knowledge about community resources; difficulty accessing support, or community resources
Difficulty navigating complex healthcare systems
Impaired resilience; ineffective use of coping strategies; impaired family process
Inadequate use of prescribed medication
Unaddressed abuse from care receiver

Defining Characteristics

Subjective
Behavioral
Difficulty performing required tasks
Difficulty meeting own personal or healthcare needs
Difficulty enjoying leisure activities
Physiological
Fatigue; altered sleep-wake cycle
Gastrointestinal discomfort; inadequate appetite
Headache
Psychological
Anxiety; frustration; feels lonely
Overwhelming responsibility

Objective
Behavioral
Substance misuse; somatoform disorder
Physiological
Muscle tension; rash
Hypertension; weight change
Frequent illness
Psychological
Anger behaviors; emotional lability; impatience
Depressive symptoms
Helplessness; suicidal ideation

Information that appears in brackets has been added by the authors to clarify and enhance the use of nursing diagnoses.

 Diagnostic Studies 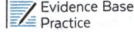 Evidence Based Practice 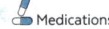 Medications 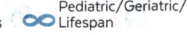 Pediatric/Geriatric/Lifespan

Clinical Connections

Chronic conditions (e.g., severe brain injury, spinal cord injury [SCI], severe developmental delay), progressive debilitating conditions (e.g., muscular dystrophy, multiple sclerosis [MS], Parkinson disease, dementia or Alzheimer disease, end-stage chronic obstructive pulmonary disease [COPD], renal failure, renal dialysis), substance abuse, end-of-life care, psychiatric conditions (e.g., schizophrenia, personality disorders).

NOTE: The presence of this problem may encompass other numerous problems/high-risk concerns, such as deficient Diversional Activity Engagement; ineffective Sleep Pattern; Fatigue; Anxiety; difficulty Coping; impaired family Coping; Grief; lack of Resilience; impaired Spiritual Well-Being; ineffective Health Self-Management; ineffective Home Maintenance Behaviors; impaired Sexual Functioning; impaired Family Process; and inadequate Social Connectedness. Careful attention to data gathering will identify and clarify the client's specific needs, which can then be coordinated under this single diagnostic label.

Generate Solutions

Plan Desired Outcomes

Client Will (Include Specific Time Frame)
- Identify resources to help cope with situation.
- Provide opportunity for care receiver to deal with situation in own way.
- Express more realistic understanding and expectations of the care receiver.
- Demonstrate behavior or lifestyle changes to cope with or resolve problematic factors.
- Report improved general well-being, ability to cope with situation.

Interventions/Take Action

Nursing Priority No. 1
To assess degree of impaired function:
- Verify role acceptance by caregiver. **Caregiver's reluctance or apathy to the role will hinder the well-being of the care receiver and the caregiver.**

Information that appears in brackets has been added by the authors to clarify and enhance the use of nursing diagnoses.

 Acute Care 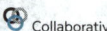 Collaborative 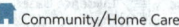 Community/Home Care  Cultural

- Identify relationship and proximity of caregiver to care receiver (e.g., spouse/lover, parent/child, sibling, friend). **There is added stress in maintaining own life and responsibilities when caregiver has to travel some distance to provide care. Close relationships may make it more difficult to manage feelings of guilt, loneliness, anger, and resentment or create problems of codependency and identification that can be counterproductive to caregiving. Note: The number of family caregivers grew to 53 million in 2020 with many individuals providing care for longer periods of time (i.e., 5 years or more).**
- Identify caregiver's level of knowledge and abilities/inabilities to provide specific care. **Caregiver's knowledge, level of required skills (e.g., chair to bed, bed to chair, chair to walking), or performance of specific activities related to personal hygiene (e.g., bathing or cleaning/changing adult briefs) may require assistance or training.**
- Assess caregiver's current state of physical/mental health (e.g., caregiver has multiple medical issues; is unable to get enough sleep, developmental level, physical abilities, has poor nutritional intake, employed, raising family, personal appearance and demeanor are indicating stress). **Provides basis for determining needs that indicate caregiver is having difficulty coping with role. Younger-aged family caregivers are at increased risk for lower levels of hope and higher levels of caregiver strain. Note: Today's caregivers and their needs are diverse, cross-generational, cross-gender, and cross-cultural.**
- Determine caregiver's use of medications/drugs (e.g., prescription, over-the-counter, or illicit drugs and/or alcohol). **Caregiver may turn to using these substances to deal with situation.**
- Identify safety issues concerning caregiver and receiver. **The stress and anxiety of caregiving situations can lead to inattention. Identifying these issues provides an opportunity to correct problems before injury occurs.**
- Assess current actions of caregiver and how they are received by care receiver. **Caregiver may be trying to be helpful but is not perceived as helpful; may be too protective or may have unrealistic expectations of care receiver's abilities, which can lead to misunderstanding and conflict.**
- Identify choice and frequency of social involvement and recreational activities. **Caregiver needs to take time away**

Information that appears in brackets has been added by the authors to clarify and enhance the use of nursing diagnoses.

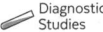 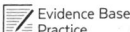 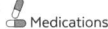

from situation to maintain own sense of self and ability to continue in role.
- Determine use and effectiveness of resources and support systems. **May not be aware of what is available or may need help in using them to the best advantage.**
- Inquire about physical/mental health condition of care receiver and surroundings to identify needs. **Important to determine factors that may indicate problems that can interfere with ability to continue caregiving.**

Nursing Priority No. 2
To identify the causative/contributing factors relating to current difficulties:

- Identify presence of high-risk situations (e.g., elderly client with total care dependence on spouse; or caregiver with several small children, with one child requiring extensive assistance due to physical condition or developmental delays). **Such situations result in daily added and ever-changing stressors (e.g., imposing unwanted role reversal, placing excessive demands on parenting skills).**
- Determine current knowledge of the situation, noting misconceptions and lack of information. **May interfere with caregiver/care receiver's response to situation.**
- Determine quality of couple's relationship/presence of intimacy issues. **Disease/condition, caregiving activities, and possible change in role responsibilities may strain relationship, adding to sense of loss and unmet needs.**
- Determine proximity of caregiver to care receiver. **Caregiver could be living in the home of care receiver (e.g., spouse or parent of disabled child) or could be adult child stopping by to check on elderly parent each day, providing support, food preparation, shopping, and assistance in emergencies. Note: There is added stress in maintaining own life and responsibilities when caregiver has to travel some distance to provide care.**
- Determine caregiver's level of involvement in and preparedness for the responsibilities of caring for the client and anticipated length of care. **Information needed to develop plan of care that takes into consideration who will provide basic care needs, technical or skilled care, scheduling/timing of activities/appointments, and other specific activities to maintain coverage for situation.**
- Identify caregiver's use of coping skills or defense mechanisms used to contend with caregiver burden. Use tools such as Zarit Burden Interview, Caregiver Reaction Scale,

---

Information that appears in brackets has been added by the authors to clarify and enhance the use of nursing diagnoses.

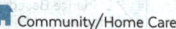

Perceived or Benefits of Caregiving (not a comprehensive list). **Caregiver's unidentified stressors and coping skills can lead to burnout resulting in neglect of the care receiver.**

- Identify individual cultural factors and impact on caregiver. **Helps clarify expectations of caregiver and receiver, family, and community. Many cultures believe strongly in keeping care receivers in the home and caring for them.**
- Identify presence and degree of conflict between caregiver/care receiver/family. **Stressful situations can exacerbate underlying feelings of anger and resentment, resulting in difficulty managing caregiving needs**
- Determine pre-illness and current behaviors that may be interfering with the care or recovery of the care receiver. **Underlying personality of care receiver may create situation in which old conflicts interfere with current treatment regimen.**
- Note codependency needs and enabling behaviors of caregiver. **These behaviors can interfere with competent caregiving and contribute to caregiver burnout.**

Nursing Priority No. 3.

To assist caregiver in identifying feelings and look toward the future.

- Establish a therapeutic relationship, conveying empathy and unconditional positive regard. **A compassionate approach, blending the nurse's expertise in healthcare with the caregiver's firsthand knowledge of the care receiver can provide encouragement, especially in a long-term difficult situation.**
- Acknowledge difficulty of the situation for the caregiver/family. **Research shows that the two greatest predictors of caregiver strain are poor health and the feeling that there is no choice but to take on additional responsibilities.**
- Discuss caregiver's view of and concerns about situation, including quality of couple's relationship/presence of intimacy issues. **Important to identify issues so planning and solutions can be developed.**
- Encourage caregiver to acknowledge and express feelings. Discuss normalcy of the reactions without using false reassurance. **Individual needs to understand that all feelings are acceptable to be expressed and dealt with, but not acted on in the situation.**

Information that appears in brackets has been added by the authors to clarify and enhance the use of nursing diagnoses.

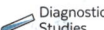 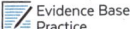 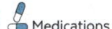 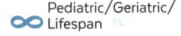

- Discuss caregiver's and family members' life goals, perceptions, and expectations of self. **Clarifies unrealistic thinking and identifies potential areas of flexibility or compromise.**
- Discuss caregiver's perception of impact of and ability to handle role changes necessitated by situation. **People initially do not realize changes that will be encountered as situation develops, and it helps to identify and plan for changes before they arise.**

Nursing Priority No. 4.

To enhance caregiver's ability to manage current situation:

- Identify strengths of caregiver and care receiver. **Bringing them to the individual's awareness promotes positive thinking and helps with problem-solving to deal more effectively with circumstances.**
- Discuss strategies to coordinate caregiving tasks and other responsibilities (e.g., employment, care of children/dependents, or housekeeping activities).
- Facilitate family conference, as appropriate, **to share information and develop plan for involvement in care activities.**
- Identify classes for caregiver (e.g., first aid and cardiopulmonary resuscitation [CPR] classes) or needed specialists (e.g., enterostomal specialist, physical therapist, home health assistance). **Provides information needed to manage tasks of caregiving more effectively, giving individuals more sense of control.**
- Determine need for, and sources of, additional resources (e.g., financial, legal, resources available to military personnel and families, respite care, social, and spiritual). **Can help to resolve problems that arise in the course of caregiving that are out of the knowledge or abilities of the individual. Solving these issues can relieve caregiver of anxiety and concern.**
- Provide information or demonstrate techniques for handling acting out, violent, or disoriented behavior. **Presence of dementia necessitates learning these techniques or skills to enhance safety of caregiver and receiver.**
- Identify equipment needs or adaptive aids and resources **to enhance the independence and safety of the care receiver.**
- Provide contact person/case manager to partner with in-home care provider(s) in coordinating care, providing physical and social support, assist with problem solving as

---

Information that appears in brackets has been added by the authors to clarify and enhance the use of nursing diagnoses.

needed or desired, or discuss/consider long-term care facilities. **As care receiver's condition declines or caregiving activities are prolonged/intensify, caregiver strain may escalate, and psychological well-being of caregiver may decline. Ongoing support by health and social services promotes more effective caregiving and thereby lessens strain on caregiver.**

Nursing Priority No. 5.

To promote continued growth and improve coping abilities (Teaching/Discharge Considerations) and enhance well-being (long-term goals):

- Advocate for and assist caregiver to plan for and implement changes that may be necessary (e.g., home-care providers, adult day care, eventual placement in long-term care facility). **As caregiving tasks become more difficult, other options need to be considered, and planning ahead can promote acceptance of necessary changes.**
- Encourage attention to own needs (e.g., eating and sleeping regularly, setting realistic goals, talking with trusted friend, periodic respite from caregiving), accepting own feelings, acknowledging frustrations and limitations, and being realistic about loved one's condition. **Supports and enhances caregiver's general well-being and coping ability.**
- Discuss with caregiver(s) signs of burnout (e.g., emotional or physical exhaustion, changes in appetite and sleep, withdrawal from friends/family or life interests). **Recognition of developing problem allows for timely intervention.**
- Review stress management techniques and importance of self-nurturing (e.g., pursuing self-development interests, hobbies, social activities, spiritual enrichment). **Being involved in activities such as these can prevent caregiver burnout.**
- Encourage involvement in caregiver support group. **Having others to share concerns and fears is therapeutic and provides ideas for different ways to manage problems, helping caregivers deal more effectively with the situation.**
- Refer to recreational, hobbies, or exercise classes that are therapeutic. **Provides additional information as needed.**
- Encourage involvement in caregiver/other specific support group(s). **Having others with whom to share concerns and fears is therapeutic and provides ideas for different ways to manage problems, helping caregivers deal more effectively with the situation.**

Information that appears in brackets has been added by the authors to clarify and enhance the use of nursing diagnoses.

- Refer to classes/other therapies, as indicated.
- Identify available 12-step/other recovery or support program, when indicated. **Support groups help caregiver to cope with enabling or codependent behaviors that impair level of function and healthy relationships.**
- 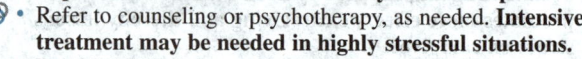 Refer to counseling or psychotherapy, as needed. **Intensive treatment may be needed in highly stressful situations.**
- Provide bibliotherapy using professional references and websites for self-paced learning and updated information, and contact with other caregivers. **Further information can help individuals understand what is happening and manage more effectively.**

Documentation Focus

Assessment/Reassessment
- Assessment findings, functional level or degree of impairment, caregiver's understanding and perception of situation
- Reactions of care receiver and family
- Involvement of family members and others
- Identification of inner resources, and lifestyle changes to be made

Planning
- Plan of care and individual responsibility for specific activities
- Teaching plan

Implementation/Evaluation
- Caregiver/receiver response to interventions, teaching, and actions performed
- Attainment of or progress toward desired outcome(s)
- Modifications to plan of care

Discharge Planning
- Needed resources, including type and source of assistive devices and durable equipment
- Plan for continuation and follow-through of needed changes
- Referrals for assistance and reevaluation

Sample Nursing Outcomes & Interventions Classifications NOC/NIC

NOC—Caregiver Role Endurance
NOC—Caregiver Stressors
NIC—Caregiver Support

Information that appears in brackets has been added by the authors to clarify and enhance the use of nursing diagnoses.

ineffective CHILDBEARING PROCESS NANDA-I

[Diagnostic Division: Sexuality/Reproduction]

Definition: Inability to prepare for and/or maintain a healthy pregnancy, childbirth process, and care of the newborn for ensuring well-being.

Recognizing Cues

Related/Risk Factors

Birth parent malnutrition; inconsistent prenatal health visits; inadequate prenatal care

Inadequate knowledge of childbearing process; unrealistic birth plan, inadequate mental preparation for pregnancy

Inadequate confidence in chestfeeding parent

Inadequate mental preparation for parenting; inadequate parental role model; inadequate social support

Birth parent powerlessness; birth parent psychological distress

Unaddressed domestic violence; unsafe environment; substance misuse

Defining Characteristics

Subjective

Throughout Pregnancy
Failure to use social support
Inadequate attachment behavior

During Pregnancy
Inadequate prenatal lifestyle
Inadequate management of unpleasant symptoms in pregnancy
Unrealistic expectations about labor and delivery

During Labor and Delivery Period
Inadequate lifestyle for stage of labor

After Birth
Inappropriate lifestyle

Objective

During Pregnancy
Inadequate respect for unborn baby; inadequate preparation of newborn care items, or home environment

During Labor and Delivery Period
Inappropriate response to onset of labor; decreased proactivity during labor and delivery

---

Information that appears in brackets has been added by the authors to clarify and enhance the use of nursing diagnoses.

 Diagnostic Studies 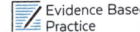 Evidence Based Practice 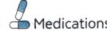 Medications 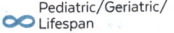 Pediatric/Geriatric/Lifespan

After Birth
Inadequate baby care techniques
Inappropriate baby feeding techniques; inappropriate breast care
Inadequate infant clothing; unsafe environment for an infant

Clinical Connections
First, second, and third trimesters of pregnancy; adolescent pregnancy, unplanned or unwanted pregnancy, labor and delivery, postpartum, newborn

Generate Solutions

Plan Desired Outcomes

Client Will (Include Specific Time Frame)
- Acknowledge and address individual related/risk factors.
- Demonstrate healthy pregnancy free of preventable complications.
- Engage in activities to prepare for birth process and care of newborn.
- Experience complication-free labor and childbirth.
- Verbalize understanding of care requirements to promote health of self and infant.

Interventions/Take Action

Nursing Priority No. 1.
To determine causative factors and individual needs:

During Pregnancy
- Determine maternal health/nutritional status, usual pregravid weight, and dietary pattern. **Research studies have found a positive correlation between pregravid maternal obesity and increased perinatal morbidity rates (e.g., hypertension and gestational diabetes) associated with preterm births and macrosomia.**
- Note use of alcohol/other drugs and nicotine. **Maternal pregnancy complications and negative effects on the developing fetus are increased with the use of tobacco, alcohol, and illicit drugs. Note: Prescription medications may also be dangerous to the fetus, requiring a risk/benefit analysis for therapeutic choices and appropriate dosage.**
- Evaluate current knowledge regarding physiological and psychological changes associated with pregnancy. **Provides information to assist in identifying needs and creating an individual plan of care.**

Information that appears in brackets has been added by the authors to clarify and enhance the use of nursing diagnoses.

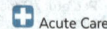 Acute Care 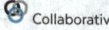 Collaborative 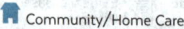 Community/Home Care   Cultural

- Identify involvement/response of child's father to pregnancy. **Helps clarify whether the father is likely to be supportive or has the potential of posing a threat to the safety and well-being of mother/fetus.**
- Determine individual family stressors, economic situation/financial needs, and availability/use of resources **to identify necessary referrals. Impact of pregnancy on family with limited resources can create added stress and result in limited prenatal care and preparation for newborn.**
- Verify environmental well-being and safety of client/family. **Women experiencing intimate partner violence before and/or during pregnancy are at higher risk for multiple poor maternal and infant health outcomes.**
- Determine cultural expectations/beliefs about childbearing, self-care, and so on. Identify who provides support/instruction within the client's culture (e.g., grandmother/other family member, cuerandero/doula, or other cultural healer). Work with support person(s) as desired by the client, using an interpreter as needed. **Helps ensure quality and continuity of care because support person(s) can reinforce information provided.**
- Ascertain the client's commitments to work, family, and self; roles/responsibilities within family unit; and use of supportive resources. **Helps in setting realistic priorities to assist the client in making adjustments, such as changing work hours, shifting household chores, curtailing some outside commitments.**
- Determine the client's/couple's perception of the fetus as a separate entity and extent of preparations being made for this infant. **The absence of activities such as choosing a name or nicknaming the baby in utero and home preparations indicate lack of completion of psychological tasks of pregnancy. Note: Cultural or familial beliefs may limit visible preparations out of concern that a bad outcome might result.**

During Labor and Delivery Period

- Ascertain the client's understanding and expectations of the labor process and who will participate/provide support. **The client's/couple's coping skills are more challenged during the active and transitional phases as contractions become increasingly intense. Lack of knowledge, misconceptions, or unrealistic expectations can have a negative impact on coping abilities.**

Information that appears in brackets has been added by the authors to clarify and enhance the use of nursing diagnoses.

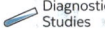 Diagnostic Studies 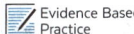 Evidence Based Practice 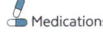 Medications 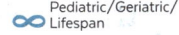 Pediatric/Geriatric/Lifespan

- Determine the presence/appropriateness of the birth plan developed by the client/couple and any associated cultural expectations/preferences. **Identifies areas to address to ensure that choices made are amenable to the specific care setting, reflect reality of client/fetal status, and accommodate individual wishes.**

After Birth

- Determine the plan for discharge after delivery and home care support/needs. **Important for facilitating discharge and ensuring client/infant needs will be met.**
- Appraise the level of the parent's understanding of physiological needs and adaptation to extrauterine life associated with maintenance of body temperature, nutrition, respiratory needs, and bowel and bladder functioning. **Identifies areas of concern/need requiring development of a teaching plan and/or demonstration of care activities.**
- Assess the mother's strengths and needs, noting age, relationship status, and reactions of family members. **Identifies potential risk factors that may influence the client's/couple's ability to assume the role of parenthood. For example, an adolescent still formulating goals and identity may have difficulty accepting the infant as a person. The single parent who lacks support systems may have difficulty assuming sole responsibility for parenting.**
- Ascertain the nature of emotional and physical parenting that the client/couple received during their childhood. **The parenting role is learned, and individuals use their own parents as role models. Those who experienced a negative upbringing or poor parenting may require additional support to meet the challenges of effective parenting.**

Nursing Priority No. 2.
To promote optimal maternal well-being:

During Pregnancy

- Emphasize the importance of maternal well-being, including discussion of nutrition, regular moderate exercise, comfort measures, rest, breast care, and sexual activity. **Fetal well-being is directly related to maternal health, especially during the first trimester, when developing organ systems are most vulnerable to injury from environmental or hereditary factors:**

   Review nutrition requirements and optimal prenatal weight gain to support maternal-fetal needs. **Inadequate**

Information that appears in brackets has been added by the authors to clarify and enhance the use of nursing diagnoses.

 Acute Care 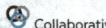 Collaborative 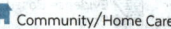 Community/Home Care Cultural

prenatal weight gain and/or below normal prepregnancy weight increases the risk of intrauterine growth retardation (IUGR) in the fetus and delivery of a low-birth-weight (LBW) infant.

Encourage moderate exercise such as walking or non-weight-bearing activities (e.g., swimming, bicycling) in accordance with the client's physical condition and cultural beliefs. **Exercise tends to shorten labor, increases likelihood of a spontaneous vaginal delivery, and decreases need for oxytocin augmentation.**

Recommend a consistent sleep and rest schedule (e.g., 1- to 2-hr daytime nap and 8 hr of sleep each night) in a dark, comfortable room. **Provides rest to meet metabolic needs associated with growth of maternal and fetal tissues.**

- Provide necessary referrals (e.g., dietitian, social services, supplemental nutrition assistance programs) as indicated. **Federal/state food programs promote optimal maternal, fetal, and infant nutrition.**
- Encourage participation in smoking cessation program, alcohol/drug abstinence, as appropriate. **Reduces the risk of premature birth, stillbirth, low birth weight, congenital defects, drug withdrawal of newborn, and fetal alcohol syndrome.**
- Explain psychological reactions including ambivalence, introspection, stress reactions, and emotional lability as characteristic of pregnancy. **Helps client/couple understand mood swings and may provide opportunity for partner to offer support and affection at these times. Note: The stressors associated with pregnancy can lead to abuse or exacerbate existing abusive behavior.**
- Discuss personal situation and options, providing information about resources available to client. **The partner may be upset about an unplanned pregnancy, have financial concerns regarding supporting the child, or may even be jealous that attention is shifting to the unborn child, creating safety issues for client/family.**
- Identify reportable potential danger signals of pregnancy, such as bleeding, cramping, acute abdominal pain, backache, edema, visual disturbances, headaches, and pelvic pressure. **Helps the client distinguish normal from abnormal findings, thus assisting her in seeking timely, appropriate healthcare.** (Refer to ND risk for impaired Maternal-Fetal Dyad for additional interventions.)

Information that appears in brackets has been added by the authors to clarify and enhance the use of nursing diagnoses.

During Labor and Delivery Period

- Monitor labor progress and maternal and fetal well-being per protocol. Provide continuous intrapartal professional support/doula. **Fear of abandonment can intensify as labor progresses, and client may experience increased anxiety and/or loss of control when left unattended.**
- Identify the client's support person/coach and ascertain that the individual is providing support the client requires. **The coach may be the client's husband/significant other (SO) or doula and needs to provide physical and emotional support for the mother and aid in initiation of bonding with the neonate.**

After Birth

- Promote sleep and rest. **Reduces the metabolic rate and allows energy and oxygen to be used for the healing process.**
- Ascertain the client's perception of labor and delivery, length of labor, and fatigue level. **There is a correlation between length of labor and the ability of some clients to assume responsibility for self-care/infant-care tasks and activities.**
- Assess the client's readiness for learning. Assist the client in identifying needs. **The postpartum period provides an opportunity to foster maternal growth, maturation, and competence.**
- Provide information about self-care, including perineal care and hygiene; physiological changes, including normal progression of lochial flow; need for sleep and rest; importance of progressive postpartum exercise program; and role changes. **Helps prevent infection, fosters healing and recuperation, and contributes to positive adaptation to physical and emotional changes, enhancing feelings of general well-being.**
- Review nipple and breast care, special dietary needs for lactating mother, factors that facilitate or interfere with successful breastfeeding, use of breast pump and appropriate suppliers, proper storage of expressed milk or preparation/storage of formula, as indicated. **Prevents nipple cracking and soreness, enhancing comfort; facilitates role of breastfeeding mother; and helps ensure an adequate milk supply.**
- Discuss normal psychological changes and needs associated with the postpartal period. **The client's emotional state may be somewhat labile at this time and often is**

Information that appears in brackets has been added by the authors to clarify and enhance the use of nursing diagnoses.

influenced by physical well-being. Anticipating such changes may reduce the stress associated with this transition period that necessitates learning new roles and taking on new responsibilities.
- Discuss sexuality needs and plans for contraception. Provide information about available methods, including advantages/disadvantages. **Client/couple may need clarification regarding available contraception methods and the fact that pregnancy could occur even prior to the 4- to 6-wk postpartum visit.**
- Reinforce the importance of postpartum examination by a healthcare provider and interim follow-up as appropriate. **A follow-up visit is necessary to evaluate recovery of reproductive organs, healing of episiotomy/laceration repair, general well-being, and adaptation to life changes.**

Nursing Priority No. 3.

To promote appropriate participation in childbearing process:

During Pregnancy

- Develop nurse-client relationship and maintain an open attitude toward beliefs of the client/couple. **Acceptance is important to developing and maintaining a relationship and supporting independence.**
- Explain office visit routine and rationale for ongoing screening and close monitoring (e.g., urine testing, blood pressure monitoring, weight, fetal growth). Emphasize the importance of keeping regular appointments. **Reinforces the relationship between health assessment and positive outcomes for mother and baby.**
- Suggest father/siblings attend office visits and listen to fetal heart tones (FHTs) as appropriate. **Promotes a sense of involvement and helps make baby a reality for family members.**
- Provide anticipatory guidance regarding health habits/lifestyle and employment concerns:
  Review physical changes to be expected during each trimester. **Prepares client/couple for managing common discomforts associated with pregnancy.**
  Discuss signs/symptoms requiring evaluation by primary provider during prenatal period (e.g., excessive vomiting, fever, unresolved illness of any kind, and decreased fetal movement). **Allows for timely intervention.**
  Identify anticipatory adaptations for SO/family necessitated by pregnancy. **Family members will need to be flexible**

Information that appears in brackets has been added by the authors to clarify and enhance the use of nursing diagnoses.

 Diagnostic Studies 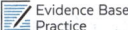 Evidence Based Practice 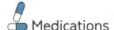 Medications 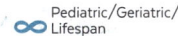 Pediatric/Geriatric/Lifespan in adjusting own roles and responsibilities in order to assist client to meet her needs related to the demands of pregnancy.

- Provide information about potential teratogens, such as alcohol, nicotine, illicit drugs, the STORCH group of viruses (syphilis, toxoplasmosis, other, rubella, cytomegalovirus [CMV], herpes simplex), and HIV. **Helps the client make informed decisions/choices about behaviors and environment that can promote healthy offspring. Note: Research supports the attribution of a wide range of negative effects in the neonate to alcohol, recreational drug use, and smoking.**
- Provide information about the need for additional laboratory studies, diagnostic tests, or procedure(s). Review risks and potential side effects **to facilitate the decision-making process.**
- Discuss signs of labor onset; how to distinguish between false and true labor; when to notify healthcare provider; when to leave for birth center/hospital as appropriate; and stages of labor and delivery. **Helps ensure timely arrival and enhances coping with the labor/delivery process.**
- Determine anticipated infant feeding plan. Discuss physiology and benefits of breastfeeding. **Breastfeeding provides a protective effect against respiratory illnesses, ear infections, gastrointestinal diseases, and allergies, including asthma, eczema, and atopic dermatitis.**
- Encourage attendance at prenatal and childbirth classes. Provide information about father/sibling or grandparent participation in classes and delivery if client desires. **Knowledge gained helps reduce fear of the unknown and increases confidence that client/couple can manage the preparation for the birth of their child. Helps family members to realize they are an integral part of the pregnancy and delivery.**

During Labor and Delivery Period

- Support use of positive coping mechanisms. **Enhances feelings of competence and fosters self-esteem.**
- Demonstrate behaviors and techniques (e.g., breathing, focused imagery, music, other distractions; aromatherapy; abdominal effleurage, back or leg rubs, sacral pressure, repositioning, back rest; oral care, linen changes, shower/tub use) that a partner can use **to assist with pain control and relaxation.**

Information that appears in brackets has been added by the authors to clarify and enhance the use of nursing diagnoses.

 Acute Care 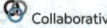 Collaborative 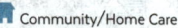 Community/Home Care Cultural

- Discuss available analgesics, appropriate timing, usual responses and side effects (client and fetal), and duration of analgesia effect in light of the current situation. **Allows the client to make informed choices about means of pain control and can allay the client's fears and anxieties about medication use.**
- Honor the client's decision about the use or nonuse of medication in a nonjudgmental manner. Continue encouragement for efforts and use of relaxation techniques. **Enhances the client's sense of control and may prevent or reduce the need for medication.**

After Birth

- Monitor and document the client's/couple's interactions with the infant. **The presence of bonding acquaintance behaviors (e.g., making eye contact, using a high-pitched voice and en face [face-to-face] position as culturally appropriate, calling infant by name, and holding infant closely) are indicators of beginning attachment process.**
- Initiate early breastfeeding or oral feeding according to facility protocol and client preference. **Initiating feeding for breastfed infants usually occurs in the delivery room. Otherwise, 5 to 15 mL of sterile water may be offered in the nursery to assess effectiveness of sucking, swallowing, gag reflexes, and patency of esophagus.**
- Provide for unlimited participation of father and siblings. Ascertain whether siblings attended orientation program. **Facilitates family development and ongoing process of acquaintance.**

Nursing Priority No. 4.

To facilitate newborn transition (Teaching/Discharge Considerations) and enhance well-being of family (long-term goals):

- Provide information about newborn interactional capabilities, states of consciousness, and means of stimulating cognitive development. **Helps parents recognize and respond to infant cues during interactional process and fosters optimal interaction, attachment behaviors, and cognitive development in the infant.**
- Note the father's/partner's response to birth and to the parenting role. **The client's ability to adapt positively to parenting may be strongly influenced by the partner's reaction.**

Information that appears in brackets has been added by the authors to clarify and enhance the use of nursing diagnoses.

- Discuss normal variations and characteristics of the infant, such as caput succedaneum, cephalohematoma, pseudomenstruation, breast enlargement, physiological jaundice, and milia. **Helps parents recognize normal variations and may reduce anxiety.**
- Demonstrate/supervise infant care activities related to feeding and holding; bathing, diapering, and clothing; care of umbilical cord stump; and care of circumcised male infant. **Promotes an understanding of the principles and techniques of newborn care, fosters parents' skills as caregivers, and enhances self-confidence.**
- Note the frequency, amount, and length of feedings. Encourage demand feedings instead of scheduled feedings. Note frequency, amount, and appearance of regurgitation. **Hunger and length of time between feedings vary from feeding to feeding, and excessive regurgitation increases replacement needs.**
- Evaluate neonate and maternal satisfaction following feedings. **Provides an opportunity to answer client questions, offer encouragement for efforts, identify needs, and problem-solve situations.**
- Appraise the level of parent's understanding of physiological needs and adaptation to extrauterine life associated with maintenance of body temperature, nutrition, respiratory needs, and bowel and bladder functioning.
- Emphasize the newborn's need for follow-up laboratory tests, regular evaluations by the healthcare provider, and timely immunizations.
- Identify manifestations of illness and infection and when to contact healthcare provider. Demonstrate proper technique for taking temperature, administering oral medication, or providing other care activities for the infant as required. **Early recognition of illness and prompt use of healthcare facilitate timely treatment and positive outcomes.**
- Provide oral and written/pictorial information and reliable websites about infant care and development, feeding, and safety issues. Offer appropriate resources in client's dominant language and reflecting cultural beliefs. **Maximizes learning, providing the opportunity to review information as needed.**
- Refer the breastfeeding client to a lactation consultant/support group (e.g., La Leche League, Lact-Aid) **to promote a successful breastfeeding outcome.**
- Discuss available community support groups/parenting class, as indicated. **Increases the parents' knowledge of**

Information that appears in brackets has been added by the authors to clarify and enhance the use of nursing diagnoses.

child rearing and child development and provides a supportive atmosphere while parents incorporate new roles.

Documentation Focus

Assessment/Reassessment
- Assessment findings, general health, previous pregnancy experience, any risks or safety concerns
- Knowledge of pre-/postpartum needs and newborn care
- Cultural beliefs and expectations
- Specific birth plan and individuals to be involved in delivery
- Arrangement for postpartum period and preparation for newborn

Planning
- Plan of care and who is involved in planning
- Individual teaching plans for pregnancy, labor/delivery, postpartum self-care, and infant care

Implementation/Evaluation
- Response to interventions, teaching, and actions performed
- Attainment of or progress toward desired outcomes
- Modifications to plan of care

Discharge Planning
- Long-term needs and who is responsible for actions to be taken
- Available resources, specific referrals made

Sample Nursing Outcomes & Interventions Classifications NOC/NIC

NOC—Prenatal Health Behavior
NIC—Prenatal/Intrapartal/Postpartal Care

---

impaired verbal COMMUNICATION   NANDA-I

[Diagnostic Division: Roles/Relationships]

Definition: Limitation or absence of ability to use spoken or written words that are used to convey a message to other people.

Information that appears in brackets has been added by the authors to clarify and enhance the use of nursing diagnoses.

 Diagnostic Studies   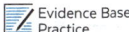 Evidence Based Practice   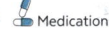 Medications   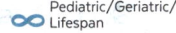 Pediatric/Geriatric/Lifespan

Recognizing Cues
Related/Risk Factors
Inadequate self-concept or self-esteem; perceived vulnerability
Dyspnea
Emotional lability; psychological barriers
Unaddressed environmental constraints
Inadequate stimulation
Inability to speak language of caregiver
Values incongruent with cultural normals; substance misuse

Defining Characteristics
Objective
Appears shy, withdrawn; does not engage in social situations
Difficulty responding to others; does not engage in conversation; obstinate refusal to speak
Decreased speech productivity; impaired ability to adjust communication rate; slurred speech; impaired ability to speak; conversation becomes tiresome
Difficulty following conversational rules; difficulty understanding humor; difficulty adjusting speech to different social contexts
Difficulty following directions, understanding nonexplicit information; misunderstanding what is asked; inappropriately responds to questions
Inappropriate verbalization
Agraphia [loss of ability to communicate through writing]; anarthria [inability to control or coordinate muscles needed for speech]; aphasia [impairment of language, speech, comprehension, and the ability to read and write]; dysarthria [difficult or unclear articulation of speech]; dysgraphia [inability to write]; dyslalia [inability to articulate comprehensible speech or pronounce certain sounds properly]; dysphonia [disorder of the voice, often caused by abnormalities that affect vocal cord vibration]
Difficulty using alternative or augmentative communication

Clinical Connections
Brain injury or stroke, facial trauma, head or neck cancer, radical neck surgery, laryngectomy, cleft lip/palate, spinal cord injury, ventilator dependent, dementia, Tourette syndrome, autism, schizophrenia, developmental disabilities

---

Information that appears in brackets has been added by the authors to clarify and enhance the use of nursing diagnoses.

 Acute Care 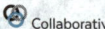 Collaborative 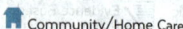 Community/Home Care   Cultural

Generate Solutions

Plan Desired Outcomes

Client Will (Include Specific Time Frame)

- Verbalize or indicate an understanding of the communication difficulty and plans for ways of handling.
- Establish method of communication in which needs can be expressed.
- Participate in therapeutic communication (e.g., using silence, acceptance, restating, reflecting, active-listening, and I-messages).
- Demonstrate congruent verbal and nonverbal communication.
- Use resources appropriately.

Interventions/Take Action

Nursing Priority No. 1.

To assess causative/contributing factors:

- Identify physiological or neurological conditions impacting speech. **Numerous underlying causes and diagnoses can lead to communication difficulties (e.g., severe shortness of breath, cleft palate, facial trauma, neuromuscular and certain psychiatric disorders, stroke, brain trauma, tumors or infections, dementia, deafness/impaired hearing, developmental and learning disorders).**
- Obtain history surrounding hearing- and speech-related pathophysiology or trauma (e.g., cleft lip/palate, traumatic brain injury, shaken baby syndrome, frequent ear infections affecting hearing, sensorineural changes associated with aging).
- Note new onset or diagnosis of deficits that will progress or permanently affect speech.
- Note results of neurological tests (e.g., electroencephalogram [EEG]; or computed tomography/magnetic resonance imaging [CT/MRI] scans; language/speech tests [e.g., Boston Diagnostic Aphasia Examination, the Action Naming Test]) **to assess and delineate underlying conditions affecting verbal communication.**
- Interview parent to determine the child's developmental level of speech and language comprehension.
- Note parental speech patterns and the manner of communicating with the child, including gestures.

Information that appears in brackets has been added by the authors to clarify and enhance the use of nursing diagnoses.

 Diagnostic Studies   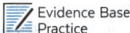 Evidence Based Practice   Medications   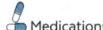 Pediatric/Geriatric/Lifespan

- ∞ Consider age and developmental considerations when performing verbal examination, noting: (1) child too young for language or has developmental delays affecting speech and language skills or comprehension; (2) autism or other mental impairments; (3) older client does not or is not able to speak, verbalizes with difficulty, or has difficulty hearing or comprehending language or concepts. (The verbal examination should be adapted to the client's communication skills and should use clear and concrete language, structure, reassurance, and support.)
- Note presence of physical barriers, including tracheostomy/intubation, wired jaws, or condition resulting in failure of voice production or "problem voice" (**pitch, loudness, or quality calls attention to voice rather than what speaker is saying, as might occur with electronic voice box or "talking valves" when tracheostomy in place**).
- Determine the presence of psychological or emotional barriers, history or presence of psychiatric conditions (e.g., bipolar disorder, schizoid or affective behavior); high level of anxiety, frustration, or fear; presence of angry, hostile behavior. Note the effects on speech and communication. Assess psychological response to communication impairment and willingness to find an alternate means of communication.
- Determine if client with communication impairment has a speech or language problem or both. **With a speech problem, words might be garbled, client may stutter, or there may be a problem with voice. Language is a code made up of rules (e.g., what words mean, how to make new words, how to combine words, what combinations work in what situations). Inability to understand the code creates a reception problem. Language and speech problems can exist individually or together.**
- Assess the style of speech (as outlined in Defining Characteristics).
- Note whether aphasia is temporary, permanent, or progressive, and type—motor (**expressive: loss of images for articulated speech**), sensory (**receptive: unable to understand words and does not recognize the defect**), conduction (**slow comprehension: uses words inappropriately but knows the error**), and/or global (**total loss of ability to comprehend and speak**). Evaluate the degree of impairment.

Information that appears in brackets has been added by the authors to clarify and enhance the use of nursing diagnoses.

- Note diagnosis of apraxia, **which causes impairment in carrying out purposeful movements affecting rhythm and timing of speech**; dysarthria, **when language code can be correct but the right body parts do not move at the right time to produce the right message**; or dementia, **where defect is part of a decline in mental functions, including memory, attention, intellect, and personality.**
- Determine dominant language spoken. **Knowing the client's primary language and fluency in other languages is important to communication. For example, while some individuals may seem to be fluent in conversational English, they may still have limited understanding, especially the language of health professionals, and have difficulty answering questions, describing symptoms, or following directions.**
- Determine cultural factors affecting communication, such as beliefs concerning touch and eye contact, gestures, and verbal communications. **Certain cultures may prohibit client from speaking directly to healthcare provider; some cultures (e.g., Native Americans, Appalachians, or young African Americans) may interpret direct eye contact as disrespectful, impolite, an invasion of privacy, or aggressive; and other cultures (e.g., Latinos, Arabs, and Asians) may shout and gesture when excited.**
- Identify information barriers, such as lack of knowledge or misunderstanding of terms related to client's medical conditions, procedures, treatments, and equipment.
- Assess level of understanding in a sensitive manner. **Client may be reluctant to say they do not understand or may be embarrassed to ask for help. Head nodding and smiles do not always mean comprehension.**
- Investigate client reports of problems such as constantly raising voice to be heard, cannot hear someone 2 ft away, conversation in the room sounds muffled or dull, too much energy required to listen, or pain or ringing in ears after exposure to noise.
- Identify environmental barriers, such as recent or chronic exposure to hazardous noise in home, job, recreation, or healthcare setting (e.g., rock music, jackhammer, snowmobile, lawn mower, truck traffic or busy highway, heavy equipment, medical equipment). **Noise not only affects hearing but also can have negative cardiovascular**

Information that appears in brackets has been added by the authors to clarify and enhance the use of nursing diagnoses.

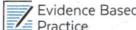 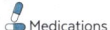

effects, increases fatigue, causes irritability, and reduces attention to tasks.
- Note results of neurological tests (e.g., electroencephalogram [EEG]; computed tomography/magnetic resonance imaging scans; language/speech tests [e.g., Boston Diagnostic Aphasia Examination, the Action Naming Test]) **to assess and delineate underlying conditions affecting verbal communication.**

Nursing Priority No. 2.

To assist client to establish a means of communication to express needs, wants, ideas, and questions:

- Determine that you have the client's attention before communicating. **Sitting down and maintaining eye contact (as appropriate), preferably at client's level, and spending time with client conveys that the nurse has time and interest in communicating.**
- Establish rapport with client, initiate eye contact or shake hands (depending on their culture), address by preferred name, and meet the family members present; ask simple questions, smile, and engage in brief social conversation if appropriate. **Helps establish a trusting relationship with client/family, demonstrating caring about the client as a person.**
- Maintain a calm, unhurried manner. Active-listen and provide sufficient time for client to respond/share information. **Active-listening communicates acceptance, respect, and that client is a capable and competent person creating an atmosphere in which client feels free to speak without fear of criticism and to explore issues involved in making decisions to improve communication skills.**
- Determine the ability to read and write. Evaluate neuromuscular status, including manual dexterity (e.g., ability to hold a pen and write) and the need or desire for pictures or written communications and instructions as part of treatment plan.
- Advise other healthcare providers of client's communication deficits (e.g., deafness, aphasia, intubation/presence of mechanical ventilation) and needed means of communication (e.g., writing pad, signing, yes/no responses, gestures, or picture board) **to minimize the client's frustration and promote understanding.**
- Obtain a professional interpreter with language or signing abilities and preferably with medical knowledge when

---

Information that appears in brackets has been added by the authors to clarify and enhance the use of nursing diagnoses.

needed. **Federal law mandates that interpretation services be made available. A trained, professional interpreter who translates precisely and possesses a basic understanding of medical terminology and healthcare ethics is preferred (over a family member) to enhance client and provider interactions and ensure client understanding of words and language concepts to ascertain that interpretation of communication is accurate.**

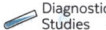

- Facilitate hearing and vision examinations **to obtain necessary aids, when indicated.**
- Check that hearing aid(s) are in place and batteries are charged and/or glasses are clean and worn when needed **to facilitate and improve communication.** Assist the client to learn to use and adjust to aids.
- Reduce environmental distractions and background noise (e.g., close the door, turn down the radio or television). Provide adequate lighting, especially if the client is reading lips or attempting to write. **A distracting environment can interfere with communication, limiting attention to tasks, and making speech and communication more difficult.**
- Identify family member who can speak for client and who is the family decision maker regarding healthcare decisions.
- Note significant other's (SO's)/parents'/caregiver's speech patterns and interactive manner of communicating with client, including gestures.
- Keep communication simple, speaking in short sentences, using appropriate words, and using all modes for accessing information: visual, auditory, and kinesthetic.
- Refrain from shouting when directing speech to confused, deaf, or hearing-impaired client. Speak slowly and clearly, pitching voice low **to increase the likelihood of being understood.**
- Determine the meaning of words used by the client and congruency of communication and nonverbal messages.
- Evaluate the meaning of words that are used/needed to describe aspects of healthcare (e.g., pain), and ascertain how to communicate important concepts.
- Validate the meaning of verbal and nonverbal communication; refrain from making assumptions, and seek assistance from others as appropriate. **Assumptions may be incorrect leading to misunderstandings. Family members, or other care providers, may better understand client's intention, preventing confusion and frustration for all parties.**

Information that appears in brackets has been added by the authors to clarify and enhance the use of nursing diagnoses.

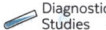 Diagnostic Studies   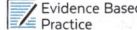 Evidence Based Practice   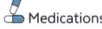 Medications   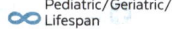 Pediatric/Geriatric/Lifespan

- Be honest and let the speaker know when you have difficulty understanding. Repeat part of the message that you do understand **so client does not have to repeat the entire message.**
- Individualize techniques using breathing for relaxation of the vocal cords, rote tasks (e.g., counting), and singing or melodic intonation **to assist aphasic clients in relearning speech.**
- Answer call light promptly. Anticipate client needs and avoid leaving client alone with no way to summon assistance. **Reduces fear, conveys caring to client, and prevents problems associated with failure to provide due care.**
- Plan for and provide alternative methods of communication, incorporating information about type of disability present:
  Provide pad and pencil, slate board, or computer/tablet **when the client is able to write but cannot speak.**
  Use letter or picture board **when the client cannot write and picture concepts are understandable to both parties.**
  Establish hand or eye signals **when the client can understand language but cannot speak or has physical barrier to writing.**
  Remove isolation mask where possible or use special mask with plastic insert over mouth area **when the client is deaf and reads lips.**
  Obtain or provide access to voice-enabled computer **if communication impairment is long-standing or the client is used to this method.**
- Identify and use previous successful communication solutions used if the situation is chronic or recurrent.
- Respectfully set limits with behaviors or speech that are unacceptable. **Sets the tone for a professional nurse-client relationship and helps client to maintain self-esteem.**
- Refer for appropriate therapies and support services (e.g., speech therapist, individual/family or psychiatric counseling). **Client and family may have multiple needs (e.g., sources for further examinations and rehabilitation services, obtaining necessary aids for improving communication).**

Nursing Priority No. 3.

To maintain communication (Teaching/Discharge Considerations) and enhance general well-being (long-term goals):

- Encourage family engagement in client's plan of care. **Involving client and family members in planning care**

Information that appears in brackets has been added by the authors to clarify and enhance the use of nursing diagnoses.

enhances participation and commitment to the plan and assists in normalizing family role patterns.
- Review information about client's condition, prognosis, and treatment with client/SO, reinforcing that loss of speech does not imply loss of intelligence.
- Teach client and family the needed techniques for communication, whether it be speech or language techniques or alternative modes of communicating. Encourage the family to involve the client in family activities using enhanced communication techniques. **Reduces the stress of a difficult situation and promotes earlier return to more normal life patterns.**
- Discuss individual methods of dealing with impairment, capitalizing on client's and caregiver's strengths.
- Discuss ways to provide/adjust environmental stimuli as appropriate **to maintain contact with reality or reduce environmental stimuli or noise. Displeasing sound affects physical health, increases fatigue, reduces attention to tasks, and makes speech communication more difficult.**
- Recommend that care providers notify the local police, fire, and first responders that deaf or communication-impaired persons live at the address. **Plan can be established for dealing with emergency assistance.**
- Use and assist client/SO(s) to learn therapeutic communication skills of acknowledgment, active-listening, and I-messages. **This improves general communication skills and may be especially useful in clients with emotional/psychological conditions affecting communication.**
- Involve family/SO(s) in plan of care as much as possible. **Enhances participation and commitment to communication with a loved one.**
- Refer to additional resources (e.g., language classes, local or national support groups such as stroke club, services for disabled, financial assistance).
- Refer to NDs difficulty Coping, impaired family Coping, Anxiety, Fear for additional interventions.

Documentation Focus

Assessment/Reassessment
- Assessment findings, pertinent history information (i.e., physical, psychological, cultural concerns)
- Meaning of nonverbal cues, level of anxiety client exhibits

---

Information that appears in brackets has been added by the authors to clarify and enhance the use of nursing diagnoses.

 Diagnostic Studies 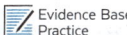 Evidence Based Practice 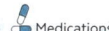 Medications 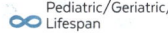 Pediatric/Geriatric/Lifespan

Planning
- Plan of care and interventions (e.g., type of alternative communication/translator)
- Teaching plan

Implementation/Evaluation
- Response to interventions, teaching, and actions performed
- Attainment of or progress toward desired outcome(s)
- Modifications to plan of care

Discharge Planning
- Discharge needs, referrals made; additional resources available

Sample Nursing Outcomes & Interventions Classifications NOC/NIC

NOC—Communication
NIC—Communication Enhancement: Speech Deficit

---

acute CONFUSION   NANDA-I

[Diagnostic Division: Neurosensory]

Definition: Reversible disturbances of consciousness, attention, cognition, and perception that develop over a short period of time, and which last less than 3 months.

Recognizing Cues

Related/Risk Factors
Unaddressed sleep deprivation; severe pain
Inadequate fluid volume; protein-energy malnutrition; unaddressed vitamin B_{12} deficiency
Sedentary behaviors; inappropriate use of physical restraint; environmental sensory deprivation, or overestimation
Hyperthermia
Substance misuse
Urinary retention

Defining Characteristics (acute Confusion)

Subjective
Disorientation to person, place, time
Hallucinations (visual or auditory); illusions, [delusions]

Information that appears in brackets has been added by the authors to clarify and enhance the use of nursing diagnoses.

 Acute Care   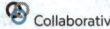 Collaborative   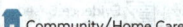 Community/Home Care   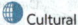 Cultural

Objective
Irritable mood, hypersensitivity
Impaired attention, concentration, memory; disorganized thinking
Fluctuating levels of consciousness
Fluctuations in psychomotor activity; psychomotor slowing, or agitation; restlessness; repetitive movements

Clinical Connections
Brain injury or stroke, respiratory conditions with hypoxia, medication adverse reactions, drug or alcohol intoxication or withdrawal, hyperthermia, infectious processes, malnutrition, eating disorders, fluid and electrolyte imbalances, chemical exposure

Generate Solutions

Plan Desired Outcomes

Client Will (Include Specific Time Frame)
- Regain and maintain usual reality orientation and level of consciousness.
- Verbalize understanding of causative or risk factors when known.
- Initiate lifestyle or behavior changes to prevent or reduce risk of problem.

Interventions/Take Action

Nursing Priority No. 1.
To assess causative/contributing **or risk** factors:

- Identify factors present, such as recent surgery or trauma; use of large numbers of medications (polypharmacy); intoxication with/withdrawal from a substance (e.g., prescription and over-the-counter [OTC] drugs; alcohol or illicit drugs); history or current seizure activity; episodes of fever or pain, or presence of acute infection (especially occult urinary tract infection [UTI] in elderly clients); traumatic events; or person with dementia experiencing sudden change in environment, unfamiliar surroundings, or people. **Acute confusion is a symptom associated with numerous causes (e.g., hypoxia; metabolic/endocrine/neurological conditions, toxins; electrolyte abnormalities; systemic or central nervous system [CNS] infections; nutritional deficiencies; or acute psychiatric disorders).**
- Assess mental status. **Typical symptoms of delirium include anxiety, disorientation, tremors, hallucinations,**

Information that appears in brackets has been added by the authors to clarify and enhance the use of nursing diagnoses.

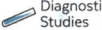 Diagnostic Studies   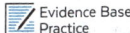 Evidence Based Practice   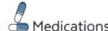 Medications   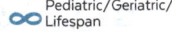 Pediatric/Geriatric/Lifespan

delusions, and incoherence. **Onset is usually sudden, developing over a few hours or days, and resolving over varying periods of time.**
- Evaluate vital signs **for indicators of poor tissue perfusion (i.e., hypotension, tachycardia, or tachypnea) or stress response (tachycardia, tachypnea).**
- Determine the client's functional level, including the ability to provide self-care and move about at will. **Conditions and situations that limit a client's mobility and independence (e.g., acute or chronic physical or psychiatric illnesses and their therapies, trauma or extensive immobility, confinement in unfamiliar surroundings, and sensory deprivation) potentiate the prospect of acute confusional state.**
- Determine current medications/drug use—especially antianxiety agents, barbiturates, certain antipsychotic agents, methyldopa, disulfiram, cocaine, alcohol, amphetamines, hallucinogens, or opiates **associated with a high risk of confusion and delirium**—and schedule of use, such as cimetidine + antacid or digoxin + diuretics **(combinations can increase the risk of adverse reactions and interactions).**
- Evaluate for exacerbation of psychiatric conditions (e.g., mood or dissociative disorders or dementia). **Identification of the presence of mental illness provides opportunity for correct treatment and medication.**
- Investigate the possibility of alcohol or other drug intoxication or withdrawal or prescription or OTC medication toxicity, side effects, or interactions.
- Ascertain life events (e.g., death of spouse/other family member, absence of known care provider, move from lifelong home, catastrophic natural disaster) **that can affect client's perceptions, attention, and concentration.**
- Assess diet and nutritional status **to identify possible deficiencies of essential nutrients and vitamins (e.g., thiamine) that could affect mental status.**
- Evaluate sleep and rest status, noting insomnia, sleep deprivation, or oversleeping. **Discomfort, worry, and lack of sleep and rest can cause or exacerbate confusion.** (Refer to ND ineffective Sleep Pattern, as appropriate.)
- Monitor laboratory values (e.g., complete blood count [CBC], blood cultures; oxygen saturation, and in some cases, arterial blood gases [ABGs]; blood urea nitrogen [BUN] and creatinine [Cr] levels; electrolytes; thyroid

---

Information that appears in brackets has been added by the authors to clarify and enhance the use of nursing diagnoses.

function studies; liver function studies, ammonia levels; serum glucose; urinalysis for infection and drug analysis; specific drug toxicologies and drug levels [including peak and trough, as appropriate]) **to identify imbalances that have potential for causing confusion.**

Nursing Priority No. 2.
To determine degree of impairment:

- Talk with SO(s) to determine historic baseline, observed changes, and onset or recurrence of changes **to understand and clarify current situation.**
- Collaborate with medical and psychiatric providers. Review results of diagnostic studies (e.g., delirium assessment tools, such as the Confusion Assessment Method [CAM], delirium index [DI], Mini-Mental State Examination [MMSE]; **to evaluate the extent of impairment in orientation, attention span, ability to follow directions, send and receive communication, and appropriateness of response.**
- Note occurrence and timing of agitation, hallucinations, and violent behaviors. **("Sundown syndrome" may occur, with client oriented during daylight hours but confused during nighttime.)**
- Determine threat to safety of client/others. **Delirium can cause the client to become verbally and physically aggressive, resulting in behavior threatening the safety of self and others.**

Nursing Priority No. 3.
To maximize level of function, prevent further deterioration, and correct existing risk factors:

- Assist with treatment of the underlying problem (e.g., drug intoxication/substance abuse, infectious process, hypoxemia, biochemical imbalances, nutritional deficits, or pain management).
- Monitor/adjust medication regimen and note response. Determine medications that can be changed or eliminated **when polypharmacy, side effects, or adverse reactions are determined to be associated with current condition.**
- Orient client to surroundings, staff, necessary activities, as needed. Present reality concisely and briefly. Avoid challenging illogical thinking—**defensive reactions may result.**
- Encourage family/significant others (SO[s]) to participate in reorientation as well as provide ongoing input (e.g., current

---

Information that appears in brackets has been added by the authors to clarify and enhance the use of nursing diagnoses.

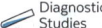 Diagnostic Studies   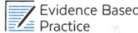 Evidence Based Practice   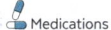 Medications   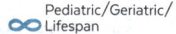 Pediatric/Geriatric/Lifespan

news and family happenings). **The client may respond positively to a well-known person and familiar items.**
- Maintain a calm environment and eliminate extraneous noise or other stimuli **to prevent overstimulation.** Provide normal levels of essential sensory and tactile stimulation—include personal items, pictures, and so forth.
- Mobilize an elderly client (especially after orthopedic injury) as soon as possible. **An older person with low level of activity prior to crisis is at particular risk for acute confusion and may fare better when out of bed.**
- Provide adequate supervision: remove harmful objects from environment, provide siderails and seizure precautions, place call bell and position needed items within reach, clear traffic paths, and ambulate with devices **to meet client's safety needs and reduce risk of falls.**
- Avoid or limit use of restraints. **Can cause agitation and increase likelihood of untoward complications.**
- Encourage client to use vision or hearing aids when needed **to assist client in interpretation of environment and communication.**
- Give simple directions. Allow sufficient time for the client to respond, communicate, and make decisions.
- Establish and maintain elimination patterns. **Disruption of elimination may be a cause for confusion, or changes in elimination may also be a symptom of acute confusion.**
- Note behavior that may be indicative of a potential for violence and take appropriate actions. (Refer to ND risk for other-directed Violence.)
- Assist with treatment of alcohol or drug intoxication and/or withdrawal, as indicated.
- Administer psychotropics cautiously **to control restlessness, agitation, and hallucinations.**
- Provide undisturbed rest periods.
- Refer to NDs impaired Memory; impaired verbal Communication for additional interventions.

Nursing Priority No. 4.
To promote ongoing recovery (Teaching/Discharge Considerations) and enhance well-being (long-term goals):

- Explain reason(s) for confusion, if known. **Although acute confusion usually subsides over time as the client recovers from the underlying cause and/or adjusts to a situation, it can initially be frightening to a client/SO. Therefore, information about the cause and appropriate**

Information that appears in brackets has been added by the authors to clarify and enhance the use of nursing diagnoses.

treatment to improve the condition may be helpful in managing a sense of fear and powerlessness.
- Discuss the need for ongoing medical review of the client's medications **to limit the possibility of misuse or potential for adverse actions or reactions.**
- Assist in identifying ongoing treatment needs and emphasize the necessity of periodic evaluation **to support early intervention.**
- Educate SO/caregivers to monitor client at home for sudden change in cognition and behavior. **An acute change is a classic presentation of delirium and should be considered a medical emergency. Early intervention can often prevent long-term complications.**
- Emphasize the importance of keeping vision/hearing aids in good repair **to improve the client's interpretation of environmental stimuli and communication.**
- Review ways to maximize the sleep environment (e.g., preferred bedtime rituals, comfortable room temperature, bedding and pillows, and elimination or reduction of extraneous noise or stimuli and interruptions) **to prevent confusional state caused by sleep deprivation.**
- Provide appropriate referrals (e.g., cognitive retraining, substance abuse treatment and support groups, medication monitoring program, Meals on Wheels, home health, or adult day care).

Documentation Focus

Assessment/Reassessment
- Existing conditions, risk factors for individual
- Nature, duration, frequency of problem
- Current and previous level of function and effect on independence and lifestyle (including safety concerns)

Planning
- Plan of care and who is involved in planning
- Teaching plan

Implementation/Evaluation
- Response to interventions and actions performed
- Attainment of or progress toward desired outcomes
- Modifications to plan of care

Discharge Planning
- Long-term needs and who is responsible for actions to be taken
- Available resources and specific referrals

Information that appears in brackets has been added by the authors to clarify and enhance the use of nursing diagnoses.

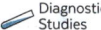 Diagnostic Studies 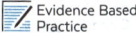 Evidence Based Practice 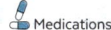 Medications 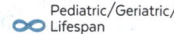 Pediatric/Geriatric/Lifespan

Sample Nursing Outcomes & Interventions Classifications NOC/NIC

NOC—Delirium Level
NIC—Delirium Management

chronic CONFUSION NANDA-I

[Diagnostic Division: Neurosensory]

Definition: Irreversible, progressive, insidious disturbances of consciousness, attention, cognition, and perception, which last more than 3 months.

Recognizing Cues

Related/Risk Factors
Chronic sorrow
Sedentary behaviors
Inadequate environmental stimulation
Excessive alcohol consumption; substance misuse

Defining Characteristics

Objective
Altered personality; impaired psychosocial functioning; behavioral change; repetition of behaviors
Difficulty retrieving information when speaking; tangential speech; neologisms; poverty of speech; incoherent speech
Difficulty with decision-making; impaired executive functioning skills; long-term or short-term memory loss
Loosening of associations; rumination; blocking of thoughts
Inability to perform at least one daily activity

Clinical Connections
Brain injury or stroke, dementia/Alzheimer disease, human immunodeficiency virus infections, medication adverse reactions, drug or alcohol abuse, malnutrition, eating disorders, chemical exposure

Generate Solutions

Plan Desired Outcomes

Client Will (Include Specific Time Frame)
- Remain safe and free from harm.
- Maintain usual level of orientation.

Information that appears in brackets has been added by the authors to clarify and enhance the use of nursing diagnoses.

 Acute Care   Collaborative 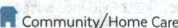 Community/Home Care 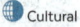 Cultural

Family/Significant Other Will (Include Specific Time Frame)
- Verbalize an understanding of the disease process, prognosis, and client's needs.
- Identify and participate in interventions to deal effectively with the situation.
- Provide for maximal independence while meeting the safety needs of the client.

Interventions/Take Action

Nursing Priority No. 1.
To assess degree of impairment:

- Evaluate responses on diagnostic examinations (e.g., memory impairments, reality orientation, attention span, calculations, and quality of life). **A combination of tests (e.g., Confusion Assessment Method [CAM], the Mini-Mental State Examination [MMSE], the Alzheimer's Disease Assessment Scale [ADAS-cog], the Brief Dementia Severity Rating Scale [BDSRS], or the Neuropsychiatric Inventory [NPI]) is often needed to complete an evaluation of the client's overall condition relating to a chronic/irreversible condition.**
- Test the client's ability to receive and send effective communication. **The client may be nonverbal or require assistance with/interpretation of verbalizations.**
- Talk with significant others (SO[s]) regarding baseline behaviors, length of time since onset and progression of problem, their perception of prognosis, and other pertinent information and concerns for client. **If the history reveals an insidious decline over months to years, and if abnormal perceptions, inattention, and memory problems are concurrent with confusion, a diagnosis of dementia is likely.**
- Obtain information regarding recent changes or disruptions in client's health or routine. **Decline in physical health or disruption in daily living situation (e.g., hospitalization, change in medications, or moving to new home) can exacerbate agitation or bring on acute confusion.** (Refer to ND acute Confusion.)
- Ascertain interventions previously used or tried.
- Evaluate response to care providers and receptiveness to interventions **to determine areas of concern to be addressed.**
- Determine anxiety level in relation to situation and problem behaviors **that may be indicative of potential for violence.**

Information that appears in brackets has been added by the authors to clarify and enhance the use of nursing diagnoses.

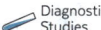 Diagnostic Studies   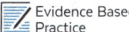 Evidence Based Practice   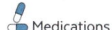 Medications   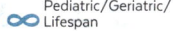 Pediatric/Geriatric/Lifespan

Nursing Priority No. 2.
To limit effects of deterioration/maximize level of function:

- Assist in treating conditions (e.g., infections, malnutrition, electrolyte imbalances, and adverse medication reactions) **that may contribute to/exacerbate confusion, discomfort, and agitation.**
- Provide a calm environment, minimize relocations, and eliminate extraneous noise/stimuli **that may increase the client's level of agitation/confusion.**
- Be open and honest in discussing the client's disease, abilities, and prognosis.
- Use touch judiciously. Tell the client what is being done before initiating contact **to reduce sense of surprise and negative reaction.**
- Avoid challenging illogical thinking **because defensive reactions may result.**
- Use positive statements; offer guided choices between two options. Simplify the client's tasks and routines **to accommodate fluctuating abilities and to reduce agitation associated with multiple options or demands.**
- Be supportive when the client is attempting to communicate, and be sensitive to increasing frustration, fears, and misperceived threats.
- Encourage family/SO(s) to provide ongoing orientation and input to include current news and family happenings.
- Maintain reality-oriented relationship and environment (e.g., clocks, calendars, personal items, and seasonal decorations). Encourage participation in resocialization groups.
- Allow the client to reminisce or exist in own reality if not detrimental to well-being.
- Provide safety measures (e.g., close supervision, identification bracelet, alarm on unlocked exits; medication lockup, removal of car or car keys; and lower temperature on hot water tank).
- Set limits on unsafe and/or inappropriate behavior, being alert to potential for violence.
- Avoid use of restraints as much as possible. Use vest (instead of wrist) restraints, or investigate the use of alternatives (such as bed nets, electronic bed pads, laptop trays) when required. **Although restraints may prevent falls, they can increase client's agitation and distress and are a safety risk.**
- Administer medications, as ordered (e.g., antidepressants or antipsychotics). Monitor for therapeutic action, as well

---

Information that appears in brackets has been added by the authors to clarify and enhance the use of nursing diagnoses.

as adverse reactions, side effects, and interactions. **Medications may be used judiciously to manage symptoms of psychosis, depression, or aggressive behavior.**
- Implement complementary therapies (e.g., music or dance therapy, animal-assisted therapy, massage, Therapeutic Touch [if touch is tolerated], aromatherapy, bright light treatment) as ordered or desired. Monitor client's response to each modality and modify as indicated. **Use of alternative therapies tailored to the client's preferences, skills, and abilities can be calming and provide relaxation and can be carried out by a wide range of health and social care providers and volunteers.**
- Refer to NDs acute Confusion; impaired Memory; impaired verbal Communication for additional interventions.

Nursing Priority No. 3.
To assist SO(s) to develop coping strategies:

- Determine family dynamics, cultural values, resources, availability, and willingness to participate in meeting client's needs. Evaluate SO's attention to own needs, including health status, grieving process, and respite. **Primary caregiver and other members of family will suffer from the stress that accompanies caregiving and will require ongoing support.**
- Involve family/SO(s) in planning and care activities as needed/desired. Maintain frequent interactions with SO(s) **to relay information, change care strategies, try different responses, or implement other problem-solving solutions.**
- Discuss caregiver burden and signs of burnout, when appropriate. (Refer to ND excessive Caregiving Burden.)
- Provide educational materials, bibliographies, list of available local resources, help lines, websites, and so on, as desired, **to assist SO(s) in dealing and coping with long-term care issues.**
- Identify appropriate community resources (e.g., Alzheimer's Association [AA], stroke or brain injury support groups, senior support groups, specialist day services, home care, and respite care; adult placement and short-term residential care; clergy, social services, occupational and physical therapists; assistive technology and telehealth services; attorney services for advance directives and durable power of attorney) **to provide client/SO with support and assist with problem-solving.**

Information that appears in brackets has been added by the authors to clarify and enhance the use of nursing diagnoses.

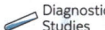 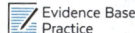 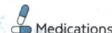 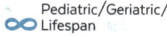

Nursing Priority No. 4.

To promote optimal functioning and safety (Teaching/Discharge Considerations) and enhance well-being (long-term goals):

- Discuss the nature of the client's condition (e.g., chronic stable, progressive, or degenerative), treatment concerns, and follow-up needed **to promote maintaining client at highest possible level of functioning.**
- Determine age-appropriate ongoing treatment and socialization needs and appropriate resources.
- Review medications with SO/caregiver(s), including dosage, route, action, expected and reportable side effects, and potential drug interactions **to prevent or limit complications associated with multiple psychiatric and central nervous system medications.**
- Develop plan of care with family **to meet client's and SO's individual needs.**
- Provide appropriate referrals (e.g., Meals on Wheels, adult day care, home care agency, or respite care). **May need additional assistance to maintain the client in the home setting or make arrangements for placement, if necessary.**

Documentation Focus

Assessment/Reassessment
- Individual findings, including current level of function and rate of anticipated changes
- Safety issues

Planning
- Plan of care and who is involved in planning

Implementation/Evaluation
- Response to interventions and actions performed
- Attainment of or progress toward desired outcomes
- Modifications to plan of care

Discharge Planning
- Long-term needs, referrals made, and who is responsible for actions to be taken
- Available resources, specific referrals made

Sample Nursing Outcomes & Interventions Classifications NOC/NIC

NOC—Cognitive Orientation
NIC—Dementia Management

Information that appears in brackets has been added by the authors to clarify and enhance the use of nursing diagnoses.

chronic functional CONSTIPATION   NANDA-I

[Diagnostic Division: Elimination]

Definition: chronic functional Constipation: Infrequent or difficult evacuation of feces, which has been present for a prolonged period of time.

Recognizing Cues

Related/Risk Factors
Decreased food intake; inadequate nutritional intake; inadequate caloric intake

Inadequate fluid intake, or fluid volume

Diet disproportionately high in fat, or protein; inadequate fiber intake

Elder frailty syndrome; impaired physical mobility; sedentary behaviors

Habitually suppresses urge to defecate

Inadequate knowledge of modifiable factors

Defining Characteristics (chronic functional Constipation)
General

Subjective
Pain with defecation
Prolonged straining

Objective
Distended abdomen; palpable abdominal mass

Fecal impaction

Leakage of feces with digital stimulation

Positive fecal occult blood

Type 1 or 2 Bristol Stool Chart

Two or more of the following symptoms on Rome IV classification system:

Symptoms present for greater than 25% of defecations at least 3 of the prior 12 months, in individuals older than 18 years old

Lumpy feces; straining; sensation of incomplete evacuation; sensation of anorectal obstruction/blockage; manual maneuvers to facilitate defecations (digital manipulation, pelvic floor support)

Bristol Stool Form Scale of 1–2

Information that appears in brackets has been added by the authors to clarify and enhance the use of nursing diagnoses.

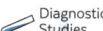 Diagnostic Studies   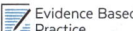 Evidence Based Practice   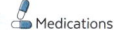 Medications   ∞ Pediatric/Geriatric/Lifespan

Two or more criteria on Rome IV Pediatric classification system

[Symptoms present] in 4- to 18-year-old children for greater than 2 months; in children up to 4 years for ≥1 month

Large-diameter stools that may obstruct the toilet

Recurrent painful bowel movements; hard feces

Presence of large fecal mass in the rectum

Retentive posturing

Two or less defecations per week; one or more episodes of fecal incontinence per week in toilet-trained children

Clinical Connections

Abdominal surgeries, hemorrhoids, anal lesions/strictures, perineal injury, irritable bowel syndrome, diverticulitis, spinal cord injury (SCI), multiple sclerosis (MS), degenerative neurological diseases, hypothyroidism, iron deficiency, scleroderma, Alzheimer disease/dementia; depressive disorders

Generate Solutions

Plan Desired Outcomes

Client Will (Include Specific Time Frame)

- Establish or regain a normal pattern of bowel functioning.
- Document that bowel function has improved through the use of a bowel function diary noting an increase in the frequency of stools, and/or decrease in straining at stool.
- Verbalize an understanding of etiology and appropriate interventions or solutions for the individual situation.

Interventions/Take Action

Nursing Priority No. 1.

To identify causative/contributing or risk factors:

- **Review medical/surgical history to identify conditions commonly associated with functional constipation. Primary causes are related to problems inherent to the intestine, subdivided into normal-transit constipation, slow-transit constipation, and anorectal dysfunction. Secondary causes include (1) gastrointestinal (GI) disorders (e.g., intestinal tumors; idiopathic megacolon; rectal prolapse, anal fissure; and irritable bowel syndrome); (2) metabolic and endocrine disorders (e.g., diabetes, chronic renal insufficiency); (3) neurological conditions (e.g., stroke, dementia syndromes, MS, SCIs);**

Information that appears in brackets has been added by the authors to clarify and enhance the use of nursing diagnoses.

 Acute Care  Collaborative 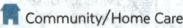 Community/Home Care Cultural

(4) psychogenic disorders (e.g., anxiety, depression); (5) dehydration; and (6) use of a variety of medications.

- Note the client's age, gender, and general health status. **Constipation is more likely to occur in individuals older than 65 years of age but may occur in a client of any age with chronic, debilitating conditions. Approximately 95% of childhood constipation is functional in nature without any obvious cause. Prevalence estimates by gender support a female-to-male ratio of 3:1.**
- Evaluate current medications or drug usage **for agents that could slow the passage of stool and cause or exacerbate constipation (e.g., opioids, anti-inflammatories, calcium channel blockers, calcium and iron supplements, anticholinergics, antidepressants, antipsychotics, antihistamines, anticonvulsants, diuretics, chemotherapy, contrast media, and steroids).**
- Note interventions the client has tried **to relieve the current situation (e.g., fiber pills, laxatives, suppositories, or enemas),** and document success or lack of effectiveness.
- Assist with medical workup (e.g., lower GI series x-rays, abdominal imaging [e.g., defecography], colonoscopy, or sigmoidoscopy; anorectal function tests [e.g., anal manometry, balloon expulsion tests]; and colonic transit studies) **for identification of possible causative factors and to show how well food moves through the colon.**

Nursing Priority No. 2.
To assess current pattern of elimination:

- Note color, odor, consistency, amount, and frequency of stool following each bowel movement during assessment phase. **Provides a baseline for comparison, promoting recognition of changes.**
- Auscultate abdomen for presence, location, and characteristics of bowel sounds **reflecting bowel activity.**
- Palpate abdomen for hardness, distention, and masses, **indicating possible obstruction or retention of stool.**
- Perform digital rectal examination, as indicated, **to evaluate rectal tone and detect tenderness, blood, or fecal impaction.**

Nursing Priority No. 3.
To reduce actual unacceptable pattern of elimination:

- Collaborate in the treatment of underlying medical cause when appropriate (e.g., surgery to repair rectal prolapse, biofeedback to retrain anorectal or pelvic floor dysfunction, medications, and combinations of therapies as indicated) **to**

Information that appears in brackets has been added by the authors to clarify and enhance the use of nursing diagnoses.

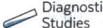 Diagnostic Studies   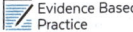 Evidence Based Practice   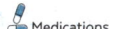 Medications   Pediatric/Geriatric/Lifespan

improve body and bowel function. **Note: Treatment is highly individual. For example, clients with slow-transit constipation tend to benefit from fiber, osmotic laxatives, and stimulant laxatives (e.g., bisacodyl), whereas those with evacuation disorders usually do not need medication other than fiber supplementation following pelvic floor retraining.**

- Review the client's current medication regimen with the provider **to determine if drugs contributing to constipation can be discontinued or changed.**
- Administer medications as indicated by the client's particular bowel dysfunction, such as stool softeners (e.g., docusate sodium [Colace, Surfak]) **to provide moisture to stool,** mild stimulants (e.g., bisacodyl [Dulcolax, Bisco-Lax]) **to cause rhythmic muscle contractions and improve transit time,** osmotic agents (e.g., polyethylene glycol [PEG; MiraLAX]) **to absorb water in intestine,** and opioid antagonist (e.g., methylnaltrexone [Relistor]) **to treat constipation in client with advanced/terminal illness necessitating long-term opioid analgesia.**
- Remove impacted stool digitally, when necessary, after applying lubricant and anesthetic ointment to anus **to soften impaction and decrease rectal pain.**
- Administer enemas (e.g., hyperosmolar agents [e.g., Fleet enema] or suppositories), as indicated.
- Promote lifestyle changes:
  Instruct in and encourage a personalized dietary program that involves adjustment of dietary fiber and bulk in diet (e.g., fruits, vegetables, and whole grains) and fiber supplements (e.g., wheat bran, psyllium) **to improve consistency of stool and increase transit time through colon, if slow transit through colon is causing symptoms.**
  Promote adequate fluid intake, including water, high-fiber fruit, and vegetable juices, fruit/vegetable smoothies, popsicles. Suggest drinking warm, stimulating fluids (e.g., decaffeinated coffee, hot water, or tea) **to avoid dehydration; promote moist, soft feces; and facilitate passage of stool.**
- Instruct in/assist with other means of triggering defecation (e.g., abdominal massage, digital stimulation, placement of rectal stimulant suppositories) **to provide predictable and effective elimination and reduce evacuation problems when long-term or permanent bowel dysfunction is present.**

Information that appears in brackets has been added by the authors to clarify and enhance the use of nursing diagnoses.

 Acute Care   Collaborative 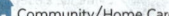 Community/Home Care   Cultural

- Refer to physical therapy or other medical/surgical practitioners for additional interventions as indicated. **Physical therapy may be useful in improving mobility, pelvic floor retraining, and activity levels. Biofeedback treatment can result in a cure for constipation associated with certain evacuation disorders. Surgical interventions may be used in some instances to treat long-term, intractable constipation due to neurogenic bowel.**

Nursing Priority No. 4.

To promote regular, comfortable defecation (Teaching/Discharge Considerations) and enhance well-being (long-term goals):

- Discuss the client's particular anatomy and physiology of bowel and acceptable variations in elimination.
- Provide information and resources to client/significant other about relationship of diet, exercise, fluid, and appropriate use of laxatives, as indicated.
- Provide social and emotional support **to help client manage actual or potential disabilities associated with long-term bowel management.** Discuss rationale for and encourage continuation of successful interventions.
- Encourage the client to maintain an elimination diary, if appropriate, **to facilitate management of long-term condition and reveal the most helpful interventions.**
- Educate client/significant other about safe and risky practices for managing constipation. **Information can assist client to make beneficial choices when need arises.**
- Collaborate with medical providers and client/caregiver in designing bowel management program to be easily replicated in home and community settings.
- Identify specific actions to be taken if the problem does not resolve (e.g., return to physician for additional testing and interventions) **to promote timely intervention, thereby enhancing the client's independence.**

Documentation Focus

Assessment/Reassessment

- Usual and current bowel pattern, duration of the problem, and interventions used
- Characteristics of stool
- Individual contributing factors

Information that appears in brackets has been added by the authors to clarify and enhance the use of nursing diagnoses.

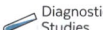 Diagnostic Studies   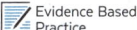 Evidence Based Practice   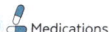 Medications   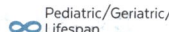 Pediatric/Geriatric/Lifespan

Planning
- Plan of care, specific interventions or changes in lifestyle necessary to correct individual situation, and who is involved in planning
- Teaching plan

Implementation/Evaluation
- Responses to interventions, teaching, and actions performed
- Change in bowel pattern, character of stool
- Attainment of or progress toward desired outcomes
- Modifications to plan of care

Discharge Planning
- Individual long-term needs, noting who is responsible for actions to be taken
- Recommendations for follow-up care
- Specific referrals made

Sample Nursing Outcomes & Interventions Classifications NOC/NIC

NOC—Bowel Elimination
NIC—Bowel Management

CONTAMINATION EXPOSURE ICNP

[Diagnostic Division: Safety]

Definition: Significant exposure to environmental contaminants resulting in negative health effects

Recognizing Cues

Related/Risk Factors

Exposure to:

Toxins via ingestion/topical exposure to chemicals (e.g., household/industrial cleaners, insecticides, paint, lead, waste/sewage, etc.)

Toxins via food (i.e., mercury [fish], salmonella, *Escherichia coli*, nitrates, etc.)

Toxins via inhalation (e.g., air pollution, mold, volatile organic compounds [VOCs], carbon monoxide, pet dander, radon, etc.)

Information that appears in brackets has been added by the authors to clarify and enhance the use of nursing diagnoses.

 Acute Care Collaborative 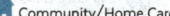 Community/Home Care Cultural

Toxins via injury (i.e., jellyfish, stingray, scorpion, insect bite/stings, venomous snakes, etc.)

Toxins via infectious agents (i.e., bacteria, viruses, fungi, parasites, etc.)

Radiation exposure (e.g., nuclear accidents, medical procedures using radioactive materials, naturally occurring radioactive elements in the environment, etc.)

Defining Characteristics

AUTHOR NOTE: Defining characteristics are dependent on the causative agent. Agents cause a variety of individual organ responses as well as systemic responses.

Subjective/Objective

Integumentary: Dermatitis, generalized skin irritation, burns, premature aging, acne flare-ups, exacerbation of eczema or psoriasis, skin dryness, increased sensitivity to sunlight

Pulmonary: Coughing, wheezing, shortness of breath, chest tightness, airway irritation, inflammation in the lungs, asthma symptoms, reduced lung function, susceptibility to respiratory infections

Gastrointestinal: Diarrhea, nausea, vomiting, stomach cramps, abdominal pain, bloody stools

Neurological: Memory problems, cognitive impairment, headaches, mood changes, difficulty concentrating, motor coordination issues, numbness/tingling

Renal: Reduced kidney function, proteinuria (albuminuria), proximal tubular dysfunction, acute kidney injury (AKI), chronic kidney disease (CKD), hypertension, and in severe cases, kidney failure (e.g., accumulation of heavy metals like lead, mercury, and arsenic in the kidneys with damage to the tubules)

Hepatic: Inflammation (hepatitis), fatty liver, fibrosis, altered liver function

Immunological: Hematologic suppression and or dysfunction

Clinical Connections

E coli infection, plague, hantavirus, asthma, botulism, cholera, lead or other heavy metal poisoning, renal failure, chemical burns, asbestosis, carbon monoxide poisoning, radiotherapy, radiation sickness

---

Information that appears in brackets has been added by the authors to clarify and enhance the use of nursing diagnoses.

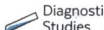 Diagnostic Studies 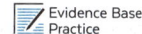 Evidence Based Practice 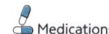 Medications 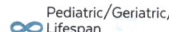 Pediatric/Geriatric/Lifespan

Generate Solutions

Plan Desired Outcomes

Client Will (Include Specific Time Frame)
- Be free of injury/adverse health effects.
- Verbalize an understanding of individual factors that contributed to injury and take steps to correct situation(s).
- Demonstrate behaviors or lifestyle changes to reduce risk factors and protect self from injury.
- Modify environment, as indicated, to enhance safety.

Client/Community Will (Include Specific Time Frame)
- Identify hazards that lead to exposure or contamination.
- Correct environmental hazards, as identified.
- Demonstrate necessary actions to promote community safety.
- Support community activities for disaster preparedness.

Interventions/Take Action

In reviewing this ND, it is apparent there is overlap with other diagnoses. We have chosen to present generalized interventions. Although there are commonalities to contamination situations, we suggest that the reader refer to other primary diagnoses as indicated, such as ineffective Airway Clearance; ineffective Breathing Pattern; impaired Gas Exchange; ineffective Home Maintenance Behaviors; risk for Infection; risk for physical Injury; risk for Poisoning; impaired Skin Integrity; risk for Suffocation; ineffective Tissue Perfusion [specify].

Nursing Priority No. 1.
To evaluate degree/source of exposure inherent in the home, community, and work site:

- Ascertain the type of contaminant(s) (e.g., chemical, biological, or air pollutant) **that has exposed (or is posing a potential hazard to) client and/or community.**
- Determine manner of exposure when contamination has occurred (e.g., inhalation, ingestion, topical, or physical injury), whether exposure was accidental or intentional, and immediate/delayed reactions. **Determines the course of action to be taken by all emergency/other care providers. Note: Typically, law enforcement and public health workers will participate in the joint threat assessment**

Information that appears in brackets has been added by the authors to clarify and enhance the use of nursing diagnoses.

 Acute Care   Collaborative 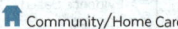 Community/Home Care   Cultural

of a suspicious exposure, illness, or outbreak involving a biological or toxic agent.

- Note age and gender: **Children less than 5 years are at greater risk for adverse effects from exposure to contaminants because (1) smaller body size causes them to receive a more concentrated "dose" than adults; (2) they spend more time outside than most adults, increasing exposure to air and soil pollutants; (3) they spend more time on the floor, increasing exposure to toxins in carpets and low cupboards; (4) they consume more water and food per pound than adults, increasing their bodyweight-to-toxin ratio; and (5) fetus's/infant's and young children's developing organ systems can be disrupted. Older adults have a normal decline in function of immune, integumentary, cardiac, renal, hepatic, and pulmonary systems; an increase in adipose tissue mass; and a decline in lean body mass. Females, in general, have a greater proportion of body fat, increasing the chance of accumulating more lipid-soluble toxins than males.**
- Ascertain client's geographical location for home and work (e.g., lives where crop spraying is routine; works in a nuclear plant; contract worker or soldier returning from combat area) where exposure occurred. **Individual and/or community intervention may be needed to modify or correct problem.**
- Note socioeconomic status and availability and use of resources. **Living in poverty increases potential for multiple exposures, delayed/lack of access to healthcare, and poor general health, potentially increasing the severity of adverse effects of exposure.**
- Determine client's/significant other's understanding of potential risk and appropriate protective measures.
- Determine factors associated with particular contaminant:
  Pesticides: Ingestion of contaminated foods (e.g., fruits, vegetables, or commercially raised meats) or inhaled agent (e.g., aerosol bug sprays, in vicinity of crop spraying).
  Chemicals: Use of environmental contaminants in the home or at work (e.g., pesticides, chemicals, chlorine household cleaners) and fails to use/inappropriately uses protective clothing.
  Biologics: Exposure to biological agents (bacteria, viruses, fungi, other microorganisms and their associated toxins) or bacterial toxins (e.g., *botulinum, anthrax, ricin,*

Information that appears in brackets has been added by the authors to clarify and enhance the use of nursing diagnoses.

diphtheria, Staphylococcal enterotoxin B [SEB]). **Exposure occurring as a result of an act of terrorism would be rare; however, individuals may be exposed to bacterial agents or toxins through contaminated or poorly prepared foods.**

Pollution air/water: Exposure/is sensitive to atmospheric pollutants (e.g., radon, benzene [from gasoline], carbon monoxide, automobile emissions [numerous chemicals], chlorofluorocarbons [refrigerants, solvents], ozone or smog particles [acids, organic chemicals; particles in smoke; commercial plants, such as pulp and paper mills]).

Home-based exposure to air pollution. **Toxins may include carbon monoxide; automobile exhaust; many consumer products, including paint, hairspray, charcoal starter fluid, chemical solvents, plastic popcorn packaging; factories/commercial plants (e.g., power plants, pulp and paper mills).**

Home-based exposure to water pollution. **Water pollutants come from many sources, including and not limited to oil, grease, chemical toxins from paint thinners, cleaning products, pharmaceuticals, personal care products; pesticides and nutrients from lawns/gardens, heavy metals, viruses, bacteria and nutrients from animal waste; failing septic systems or improper sewage disposal; dirt/groundwater runoff.**

Injury: Exposure to venomous or toxic exposure through injury (i.e., bite, sting, scratch, infestation, etc.). **Client exposure risk is directly associated with the client's immediate environment and will vary greatly depending on client-specific situation and geographic location.**

Waste: Living in an area where trash or garbage accumulates or is exposed to raw sewage or industrial wastes that **can contaminate soil and water.**

Radiation: Client/household member experienced accidental exposure (e.g., occupation in radiography; living near, or working in, nuclear industries or electrical generation plants; radon gas seeping from soil into home).

- Observe for signs and symptoms of infective agent and sepsis, such as fatigue, malaise, headache, fever, chills, diaphoresis, skin rash, and altered level of consciousness. **Initial symptoms of some diseases that mimic influenza may be misdiagnosed if healthcare providers do not maintain an index of suspicion.**

Information that appears in brackets has been added by the authors to clarify and enhance the use of nursing diagnoses.

- Note the presence and degree of chemical burns and initial treatment provided.
- Obtain/assist with diagnostic studies, as indicated. **Provides information about the type and degree of exposure/organ involvement or damage.**
- Identify psychological responses (e.g., anger, shock, acute anxiety, confusion, or denial) to accidental or mass exposure incident. **Although these are normal responses, they may be recycled repeatedly and result in post-trauma syndrome if not dealt with adequately.**
- Alert the proper authorities to the presence of or exposure to contamination, as appropriate. **Depending on the agent involved, there may be reporting requirements to local, state, or national agencies, such as the local health department, local/other law enforcement agencies, the Environmental Protection Agency (EPA), and the Centers for Disease Control and Prevention (CDC).**

Nursing Priority No. 2.

To assist in treating the effects of exposure and reduce/correct individual risk factors:

- Implement a coordinated decontamination plan (e.g., removal of clothing, showering with soap and water), when indicated, following consultation with medical toxicologist, hazardous materials team, and industrial hygiene and safety officer **to prevent further harm to client and to protect healthcare providers.**
- Ensure availability of and educate client in use of personal protective equipment (PPE) (e.g., high-efficiency particulate air [HEPA] filter masks, special garments, and barrier materials including gloves/face shield) **to protect from exposure to biological, chemical, and radioactive hazards.**
- Provide for isolation or group individuals with same diagnosis or exposure, as resources require. **Limited resources may dictate open ward–like environment; however, the need to control the spread of infection still exists. A number of bioterrorism precautions require more than standard infection control measures. Some of these include pneumonic plague, smallpox, and viral hemorrhagic fevers; coronaviruses such as severe acute respiratory syndrome coronavirus 2 (SARS-CoV-2); and the present outbreak of a coronavirus-associated acute respiratory disease labeled** *coronavirus disease 19 (COVID-19).*
- Provide/assist with therapeutic interventions, as individually appropriate. **Specific needs of the client and the level**

Information that appears in brackets has been added by the authors to clarify and enhance the use of nursing diagnoses.

 Diagnostic Studies 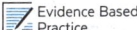 Evidence Based Practice Medications 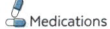 Pediatric/Geriatric/Lifespan of care available at a given time/location determine response.

- Refer pregnant client for individually appropriate diagnostic procedures or screenings. **This helps to determine effects of teratogenic exposure on fetus, allowing for informed choices/preparations.**
- Emphasize importance of pregnant or lactating women following fish or wildlife consumption guidelines provided by state, U.S. territorial, or Native American tribes. Ingestion of noncommercial fish or wildlife **can be a significant source of pollutants.**
- Screen breast milk in lactating client following radiation exposure or if mother is herself ill because of toxin exposure (e.g., lead, mercury). **Depending on type and amount of exposure, breastfeeding may need to be briefly interrupted or, occasionally, terminated.**
- Cooperate with and refer to appropriate agencies (e.g., CDC; U.S. Army Medical Research Institute of Infectious Diseases [USAMRIID]; Federal Emergency Management Agency [FEMA]; U.S. Department of Health and Human Services [DHHS]; Office of Emergency Preparedness [OEP]; EPA, U.S. National Park Service) **to prepare for/manage mass casualty incidents.**

Nursing Priority No. 3.

To assist client to reduce or correct individual factors:

- Assist client to develop a plan to address individual safety needs and injury/illness prevention in home, community, and work settings.
- Repair or replace unsafe household items and situations (e.g., flaking/peeling paint or plaster; filter for unsafe tap water).
- Review effects of secondhand smoke and importance of refraining from smoking in home/car **where others are likely to be exposed.**
- Encourage the removal or proper cleaning of carpeted floors, especially for small children and persons with respiratory conditions. **Carpets may trap pollutants like dust mites, pet dander, cockroach allergens, particle pollution, lead, mold spores, pesticides, dirt, and dust.**
- Encourage timely cleaning and replacement of air filters on furnace and/or air-conditioning unit. **Good ventilation cuts down on indoor air pollution from carpets, machines, paints, solvents, cleaning materials, and pesticides.**

Information that appears in brackets has been added by the authors to clarify and enhance the use of nursing diagnoses.

- Recommend periodic inspection of well water or tap water **to identify possible contaminants.**
- Encourage client to install carbon monoxide monitors and other air pollutant detectors in the home, as appropriate.
- Recommend placing a dehumidifier in damp areas **to retard growth of molds.**
- Review proper handling of household chemicals:
  Read chemical labels. Know primary hazards (especially in commonly used household cleaning and gardening products).
  Follow directions printed on product label (e.g., avoid use of certain chemicals on food preparation surfaces, refrain from spraying garden chemicals on windy days).
  Use products labeled "nontoxic" wherever possible. Choose the least hazardous products for the job, preferably multi-use products, **to reduce number of different chemicals used and stored.**
  Use a form of chemical that most reduces risk of exposure (e.g., cream instead of liquid or aerosol).
  Wear protective clothing, gloves, and safety glasses when using chemicals. Avoid mixing chemicals at all times, and use in well-ventilated areas.
  Store chemicals in locked cabinets. Keep chemicals in original labeled containers and do not pour into other containers.
  ∞ Place safety stickers on chemicals **to warn children of harmful contents.**
- Review proper food handling, storage, and cooking techniques.
- Encourage client/caregiver to participate in recommended travel vaccinations.
- Encourage client/caregiver to utilize insect repellant and protective attire **to prevent injury (e.g., insect stings/bites, snake bite, ticks, etc.).**

Nursing Priority No. 4.

To promote a contaminant-free environment (Teaching/Discharge Considerations) and enhance well-being (long-term goals):

Client/Caregiver

- Discuss individual nutritional needs, appropriate exercise program, and need for rest. **These are essentials for well-being and recovery.**

Information that appears in brackets has been added by the authors to clarify and enhance the use of nursing diagnoses.

 Diagnostic Studies   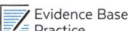 Evidence Based Practice   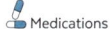 Medications   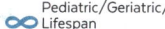 Pediatric/Geriatric/Lifespan

- ∞ Emphasize the importance of supervising infant/child or individuals with cognitive limitations **to protect those who are unable to protect themselves.**
- Discuss protective actions for specific "bad air days" (e.g., limiting or avoiding outdoor activities).
- 🔄 Refer to smoking-cessation program, as needed.
- Emphasize the importance of posting emergency and poison control numbers in a visible location.
- Encourage learning CPR and first aid.
- Encourage the client/caregiver to develop a personal/family disaster plan, to gather needed supplies to provide for self and family during a community emergency, and to learn how specific public health threats might affect client and actions **to reduce the risk to health and safety.**
- 🔄 Refer to counselor/support groups **for ongoing assistance in dealing with traumatic incident/aftereffects of exposure.**
- Provide bibliotherapy including written resources and appropriate websites **for review and self-paced learning.**
- 🏠 Discuss general safety concerns with client/significant other **to ensure that people are educated about potential risks and ways to manage risks.**
- Discuss protective actions for specific "bad air" days (e.g., limiting or avoiding outdoor activities). **Measures may include limiting or avoiding outdoor activities, especially in sensitive groups (e.g., children who are active outdoors, adults involved in moderate or strenuous outdoor activities, and persons with respiratory diseases).**
- Identify commercial cleaning resources, if appropriate, **for safe cleaning of contaminated articles/surfaces.**

Community

- Promote community education programs in different modalities, languages, cultures, and educational levels geared **to increasing awareness of safety measures and resources available to individuals/community.**
- Encourage community members/groups to engage in problem-solving activities.
- Review pertinent job-related health department and Occupational Safety and Health Administration (OSHA) regulations. Emphasize necessity of wearing appropriate protective equipment.
- 🔄 Ascertain that there is a comprehensive disaster plan for the community that includes a chain of command, equipment, communication, training, decontamination area(s), and

---

Information that appears in brackets has been added by the authors to clarify and enhance the use of nursing diagnoses.

 Acute Care 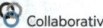 Collaborative 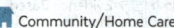 Community/Home Care   Cultural

safety and security plans **to ensure an effective response to any emergency (e.g., flood, toxic spill, infectious disease outbreak, radiation release).**

- Refer to appropriate agencies (e.g., CDC; USAMRIID; FEMA; DHHS; OEP; EPA) **to prepare for and manage mass casualty incidents.**

Documentation Focus

Assessment/Reassessment
- Details of specific exposure including location and circumstances
- Client's/caregiver's understanding of individual risks and safety concerns

Planning
- Plan of care and who is involved in planning
- Teaching plan

Implementation/Evaluation
- Individual responses to interventions, teaching, and actions performed
- Specific actions and changes that are made
- Attainment of or progress toward desired outcome(s)
- Modifications to plan of care

Discharge Planning
- Long-range plans for discharge needs, lifestyle and community changes, and who is responsible for actions to be taken
- Specific referrals made

Sample Nursing Outcomes & Interventions Classifications NOC/NIC

NOC—Symptom Severity
NOC—Risk Control: Environmental Hazards
NIC—Environmental Risk Protection

---

impaired fecal CONTINENCE   NANDA-I

[Diagnostic Division: Elimination]

Definition: Inability to control anal sphincters, with involuntary passage of feces and flatus.

Information that appears in brackets has been added by the authors to clarify and enhance the use of nursing diagnoses.

Recognizing Cues

Related/Risk Factors

Avoidance of nonhygienic toilet use; embarrassment regarding toilet use in social situations

Constipation; diarrhea; incomplete emptying of bowel; laxative misuse

Decreased toileting ability; difficulty finding a toilet; difficulty obtaining timely assistance to toilet

Unaddressed environmental constraints

Sedentary behaviors; muscle hypotonia; impaired physical mobility or postural balance

Inappropriate dietary habits

Excessive stress; inattentive to urge to defecate; inadequate bowel retraining

Defining Characteristics

Subjective

Abdominal discomfort; fecal urgency; inability to delay defecation; inability to hold flatus

Impaired ability to expel formed feces despite recognition of rectal fullness

Inability to reach toilet in time

Objective

Fecal staining; leakage of feces during activities

Clinical Connections

Hemorrhoids, rectal prolapse, anal/gynecological surgery, childbirth injuries/uterine prolapse, spinal cord injury (SCI), stroke, multiple sclerosis (MS), degenerative neurological diseases, ulcerative colitis, enlarged prostate, dementia

Generate Solutions

Plan Desired Outcomes

Client Will (Include Specific Time Frame)

- Verbalize understanding of causative and controlling factors.
- Identify individually appropriate interventions.
- Participate in therapeutic regimen to control incontinence.
- Establish/maintain as regular a pattern of bowel functioning as possible.

Information that appears in brackets has been added by the authors to clarify and enhance the use of nursing diagnoses.

 Acute Care 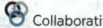 Collaborative 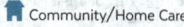 Community/Home Care Cultural

Interventions/Take Action

Nursing Priority No. 1.
To assess causative/contributing factors:

- Determine the type of bowel incontinence present, as possible: **(1) loss of anal sphincter control (such as might occur with sphincter trauma); (2) stool seepage (as may result from fistulas or prolapse); or (3) poor bowel control (as might occur with inflammatory bowel disease, following intestinal surgery, chronic constipation with weakening musculature, laxative abuse, parasitic infection, and toxins).**
- Determine historical aspects of incontinence with preceding/precipitating events. **Common factors include (1) structural changes in the sphincter muscle (e.g., hemorrhoids; rectal prolapse; prostate, anal, or gynecological surgery; vaginal delivery; inadequate repair of obstetric injury); (2) injuries to sensory nerves (e.g., spinal cord injury, multiple sclerosis), major trauma, stroke, tumor, or radiation therapy; (3) strong-urge or severe prolonged diarrhea (e.g., ulcerative colitis, Crohn disease, infectious diarrhea); (4) dementia (e.g., acute or chronic cognitive impairment, not necessarily related to sphincter control); (5) result of toxins. Note: Acute diarrhea may be caused by viral (e.g., Norwalk virus, rotavirus), bacterial (e.g., *Staphylococcus aureus*, *Escherichia coli*, salmonella, shigella), or parasitic infections (e.g., giardia, amebiasis); (6) aging, particularly in menopausal women; and (7) effects of improper diet or type and rate of enteral feedings.**
- Note client's age and gender. **Bowel incontinence is more common in children, women of childbearing age, and elderly adults (difficulty responding to urge in a timely manner, problems walking or undoing zippers, decrease of maximum squeeze pressure); more common in boys than girls, but more common in elderly women than elderly men.**
- Auscultate abdomen **for presence, location, and characteristics of bowel sounds reflecting bowel activity.**
- Palpate abdomen for hardness, distension, and masses **indicating possible obstruction or retention of stool.**
- Review medication regimen, including over-the-counter drugs (e.g., sedatives/hypnotics, narcotics, muscle relaxants, antacids [constipation risk]). **Laxative abuse and**

Information that appears in brackets has been added by the authors to clarify and enhance the use of nursing diagnoses.

 Diagnostic Studies 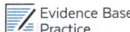 Evidence Based Practice 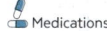 Medications 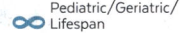 Pediatric/Geriatric/Lifespan drugs with a side effect of diarrhea (such as antibiotics [e.g., cephalosporins, erythromycin, penicillins, quinolones, tetracyclines]: cardiovascular drugs [e.g., digitalis, angiotensin-converting enzyme inhibitors]; antidiabetic agents [e.g., metformin]; NSAIDs; chemotherapy agents [e.g., 5-fluorouracil, ipilimumab]; psychotropics [e.g., lithium]; and cholesterol-lowering drugs [e.g., atorvastatin] can cause or exacerbate diarrhea, particularly in the elderly and in those who have had surgery on the intestinal tract) or constipation (e.g., sedatives, hypnotics, opioids, muscle relaxants) may impact bowel control.

- Review results of diagnostic studies (e.g., sonography, abdominal x-rays, colon endoscopy/other imaging, nerve studies, complete blood count, serum chemistries, stool for blood), as appropriate. **Pelvic and/or anal ultrasound may be used to identify structural abnormalities; endoanal ultrasonography is a primary imaging modality; endoscopy may be used to visualize lower gastrointestinal tract; manometry may be used to measure pressure and strength of anal muscles; and nerve studies may be used to check for nerve damage. Blood tests and stool cultures may be done to identify presence of bacteria and toxins.**

Nursing Priority No. 2.

To determine current pattern of elimination:

- Ascertain timing and characteristic aspects of incontinent occurrence, noting preceding or precipitating events, and what client is experiencing at the time. **Changes in usual routines, dietary patterns, surrounding environment, general health condition, and the addition of emotional stressors can cause or exacerbate incontinence behaviors. Interventions are different for sudden acute accidents than for chronic long-term incontinence problems.**
- Note stool characteristics, including **consistency** (e.g., soft to watery stools, bloody, greasy, liquid, hard formed, or hard at first and then soft), **amount** (e.g., may be a small amount of liquid or entire solid bowel movement), **frequency** (e.g., more than normal number of stools/day), **duration** (e.g., discern from a long-standing condition that the client has "lived with" and an acute incontinence), **and associated signs/symptoms** (e.g., fever/chills, abdominal cramping,

---

Information that appears in brackets has been added by the authors to clarify and enhance the use of nursing diagnoses.

emotional upset, weight loss). **Provides information that can help differentiate the type of incontinence present and provide comparative baseline for response to interventions.**
- Encourage client/significant other (SO) to record times at which incontinence occurs **to note relationship to meals, activity, medications, or client's behavior.**

Nursing Priority No. 3.
To promote control/management of incontinence:
- Assist in the treatment of causative/contributing factors. **Although incontinence is a symptom and not a disease, appropriate treatment can often correct the problem or at least improve the client's quality of life.**
- Establish bowel program in client requiring constant bowel care, with predictable time for defecation efforts; use suppositories and/or digital stimulation when indicated. Maintain daily program initially. Progress to alternate days dependent on usual pattern or amount of stool. **A toileting program within a consistent environment may promote predictable and effective elimination and reduce evacuation problems when long-term or permanent bowel dysfunction is present.**
- Establish a toileting program where possible:
  Take client to the bathroom or place on commode or bedpan at specified intervals, taking into consideration individual needs and incontinence patterns.
  Use the same type of facility for toileting as much as possible.
  Make sure bathroom is safe for impaired person (good lighting, support rails, good height for getting onto and up from stool).
  Provide time and privacy for elimination.
  Remove stool promptly and use room deodorizers to reduce noxious odors and limit embarrassment.
  For sources of fecal incontinence associated with **constipation, encopresis, or overflow constipation,** demonstrate techniques and assist client/caregiver to practice contracting abdominal muscles, leaning forward on commode **to increase intra-abdominal pressure during defecation,** and left to right abdominal massage **to stimulate peristalsis.**
  Encourage and instruct client/caregiver in providing diet high in bulk/fiber and adequate fluids (minimum of

---

Information that appears in brackets has been added by the authors to clarify and enhance the use of nursing diagnoses.

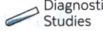 Diagnostic Studies 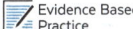 Evidence Based Practice 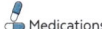 Medications 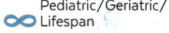 Pediatric/Geriatric/Lifespan

2,000 mL/day if cardiac or renal conditions allow) **to help manage constipation.** Encourage warm fluids after meals **to promote intestinal motility and avoid constipation, dry hard stools, or fecal impaction.**

Identify and eliminate problem foods such as alcohol, caffeine, dairy products (in lactose-intolerant clients), spicy foods, cured or smoked meats, artificial sweeteners (e.g., fructose, mannitol, sorbitol, and xylitol) **to avoid diarrhea, constipation, and gas formation.**

- Administer medications, as indicated. Stool softeners, laxatives, or bulk formers may be used **when the cause of incontinence is related to constipation, encopresis, or overflow constipation.** Antidiarrheals, including cholinergics, anti-infectives, bulk formers, or antispasmodics may be used **to decrease bowel motility if diarrhea is cause for incontinence.**
- Adjust enteral feedings and/or change formula, as indicated, **to reduce diarrhea effect.**
- Recommend walking and a regular exercise program, pelvic floor exercises, and biofeedback, as individually indicated, **to improve abdominal and pelvic muscles and strengthen rectal sphincter tone.**
- Provide incontinence aids/pads until control is obtained. **Note: Incontinence pads should be changed frequently to reduce incidence of skin rashes/breakdown.**
- Encourage or provide perineal care with frequent gentle cleansing and use of emollients after incontinent stools. Discourage excessive rubbing with toilet paper, encourage cleaning with warm water, pat dry, and apply barrier cream to maintain skin integrity **to reduce excoriation of skin. Protection and hygiene of the perianal skin are important to prevent pruritis ani. Excessive rubbing with tissue paper causes secondary injury to the skin and may lead to scratching, further worsening bowel seepage.**
- Refer to ND chronic functional Constipation if incontinence is due to impaction.

Nursing Priority No. 4.

To promote ongoing bowel continence (Teaching/Discharge Considerations) and enhance well-being (long-term goals):

- Review and encourage continuation of successful interventions as individually identified.
- Instruct in use of suppositories or stool softeners, if indicated, **to stimulate timed defecation.**

Information that appears in brackets has been added by the authors to clarify and enhance the use of nursing diagnoses.

- Identify foods (e.g., daily bran muffins, prunes) **that promote soft stool consistency and bowel regularity.**
- Recommend avoidance of problem foods **such as caffeine and high-fat (e.g., butter, fried foods) or high-protein (e.g., meats) foods known to cause or aggravate diarrhea (e.g., extremely hot or cold foods, chili), milk, and fruits or fruit juices** dependent on individual reactions.
- Provide emotional support to client and significant other(s), especially when condition is long term or chronic. **Fecal incontinence can be a source of great embarrassment and can lead to social isolation and feeling of powerlessness. Intimate relationship and sexual activity may be affected and need specific interventions to resolve.**
- Encourage scheduling of social activities within time frame of bowel program, as indicated (e.g., avoid a 4-hr excursion if bowel program requires toileting every 3 hr and facilities will not be available), **to maximize social functioning and success of bowel program.**
- Refer client/caregivers to outside resources when condition is long term or chronic **to obtain care assistance and respite, or psychological support to enhance coping with difficult situation.**

Documentation Focus

Assessment/Reassessment
- Current and previous pattern of elimination, physical findings, character of stool, actions tried

Planning
- Plan of care and who is involved in planning
- Teaching plan

Implementation/Evaluation
- Client's/caregiver's responses to interventions, teaching, and actions performed
- Changes in pattern of elimination, characteristics of stool
- Attainment of or progress toward desired outcome(s)
- Modifications to plan of care

Discharge Planning
- Identified long-term needs, noting who is responsible for each action
- Specific bowel program at time of discharge

Information that appears in brackets has been added by the authors to clarify and enhance the use of nursing diagnoses.

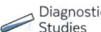 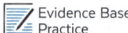 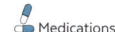 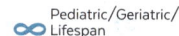

Sample Nursing Outcomes & Interventions Classifications NOC/NIC

NOC—Bowel Continence
NIC—Bowel Incontinence Care

difficulty COPING ICNP

[Diagnostic Division: Stress Management]

Definition: Pattern of using ineffective strategies to solve problems resulting in psychological distress and conflict when managing, responding to, or making decisions when confronted with a stressful situation.

Recognizing Cues

Related/Risk Factors

Significant loss—personal, professional, economic; health status change

Fear of the unknown, or the future, humiliations, repercussions, economics, health status

Inability to analyze interpersonal communication and emotions

Decreased self-confidence or confidence in others or lacks resilience; lacks sense of self-control, unrealistic expectations

Lack of knowledge, or access to resources; lack of, or ineffective support system

Defining Characteristics

Subjective

Anxiety; concern for future; headaches; depressive symptoms

Lack of knowledge, or access to resources; lack of or ineffective support system

Inability to handle change or a new situation; excessive use of defense mechanisms (e.g., denial, displacement); strategies used fail to resolve problems

Sense of guilt, or shame

Fatigue; does not feel rested on awakening

Inability to attend to daily responsibilities, or meet role expectations

---

Information that appears in brackets has been added by the authors to clarify and enhance the use of nursing diagnoses.

 Acute Care   Collaborative 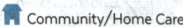 Community/Home Care 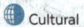 Cultural

Objective
Increased irritability; difficulty concentrating
Increased blood pressure, gastrointestinal distress (heartburn, nausea, change in bowel habits)
Disorganization of thoughts, activities, or goal obtainment
Frequent infections, or illness
Suicidal thoughts, attempts or harms others
Loss of sexual desire
Suicidal thoughts, attempts or harm to others

Clinical Connections
Eating disorders, chronic medical conditions, substance misuse, depression; anxiety, bipolar, adjustment, personality disorders; schizophrenia, post-traumatic stress disorders

Generate Solutions

Plan Desired Outcomes

Client Will (Include Specific Time Frame)
- Verbalize acceptance of, and responsibility for own actions with success or failures.
- Verbalize self-awareness of own coping abilities.
- Recognize other's emotions during interpersonal communications.
- Identify how a lack of handling stress can affect health status.
- Meet psychological needs as evidenced by appropriate expression of feelings, identification of options, and use of resources.

Interventions/Take Action

Nursing Priority No. 1.
To determine degree of impairment:
- Develop a therapeutic relationship conversing at the client's developmental level, and using client-centered open-ended questions. **Clients treated with respect and dignity feel regard as a worthy person that encourages them to share their thoughts, feelings, and behaviors associated with current stressors and life's concerns.**
- Active-listen client's responses in respectful, nonjudgmental manner. **Client's sharing is crucial to understanding their perception of the situation and desire to change.**
- Evaluate client's ability (while telling their story) to realistically comprehend current situation based on their

---

Information that appears in brackets has been added by the authors to clarify and enhance the use of nursing diagnoses.

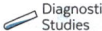 Diagnostic Studies 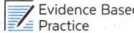 Evidence Based Practice Medications 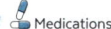 Pediatric/Geriatric/Lifespan

psychosocial developmental level. **Tendency for individuals to regress to a lower developmental stage during crisis can impact ability to recognize effect of situation and resulting unhealthy lifestyle.**
- Observe and note congruent/incongruent verbal and nonverbal behaviors. **Verbal and nonverbal communication is a process of conveying thoughts and beliefs during interpersonal communication. Nonverbal communication often expresses more salient points of client's thoughts and beliefs requiring clarification.**
- Identify current situation, crisis, or problem and the impact on daily living and personal relationships. **Attentively listening to client's concerns demonstrates an interest in the client's distress and caring about the client's well-being.**
- Determine cultural background and how family beliefs, speech, and communication patterns, including nonverbal behavior, possibly influence or contribute to coping with stressors in daily living. **Family of origin can have a positive or negative effect on the individual's ability to contend with stressful situations.**
- Identify use of defense mechanisms (e.g., projections, denial, rationalization). *Use of defense mechanisms is a protective approach that negatively impacts client's self-esteem, self-expectations, resulting in a fear of failure influencing decision-making and ability to resolve issues.*
- Perform and review results of testing, such as nine-time Emotional Reactivity Scale, and physiological evaluations, as indicated. **Tools help with assessing a client's thoughts and beliefs while reflecting on the situation.**
- Directly ask client if they have thoughts of harming self or others. **Impaired thinking and poor decision-making can negatively influence the client's ability to see a positive resolution to the crisis and may lead to thoughts of harming self or others.**
- Determine client's level of readiness to change from unproductive behaviors to a healthier lifestyle. **Attempting to implement interventions prior to client's readiness will be met with resistance.**

Nursing Priority No. 2.
To assist client to cope with current situation:
- Encourage verbalization of fears, anxieties, and issues related to grief. **Free expression allows client to contend**

Information that appears in brackets has been added by the authors to clarify and enhance the use of nursing diagnoses.

with emotions instead of repressing them to a point of sudden outburst. Helping the client to recognize the use of defense mechanisms (e.g., denial, repression, projection, or displacement) limits coping with stress as well as how they receive and respond to others during social interaction that helps build positive/negative relationships. Note: Concerns of sexual nature require sensitive questioning, allowing client to respond when ready to cope with situation. (Refer to ND dysfunctional Grief for additional interventions.)

- Explain client-centered care and shared decision making. **Client-centered care promotes empowerment and autonomy when acting as the expert of their mind and body while working with the treatment team to develop a plan of care. Depression or anxiety, psychosocial level of development, or use of defense mechanisms may hinder client's ability to determine or select a path leading to personal growth.**

- Provide an explanation of the rules for the treatment program and consequences for actions. **Clients must understand the structure of the milieu/program policy and procedures for the program to be effective and facilitate client achieving identified goals.**

- Assist client to recognize use of maladaptive behaviors. **Clients overwhelmed with stress or fear learn to self-protect at early ages with a constellation of defense mechanisms and may delay psychosocial development. Setting limits on manipulative behaviors helps the client to develop self-awareness.**

- Engage in Motivational Interviewing using empathy and open-ended questions. **Empowers client to express their desire, reason, ability, and need for change in their lifestyle.**

- Identify successful coping strategies used in the past. **Provides opportunity for positive reinforcement increasing likelihood of repeating desired behaviors rather than trying to manipulate staff/therapist or environment.**

- Incorporate past strengths with new coping techniques such as relaxation skills, appropriate exercise, mindfulness/self-awareness, respectful communication, accepting reality, and what can and cannot be changed. **Enhances sense of self-worth and provides opportunity for positive reinforcement increasing the likelihood of repeating desired behaviors.**

Information that appears in brackets has been added by the authors to clarify and enhance the use of nursing diagnoses.

- 🤝 Coordinate mental and medical treatments for illnesses as indicated. **Taking care of physical concerns will enable client to contend with emotional and physical issues more effectively.**

Nursing Priority No. 3.

To provide for meeting psychological needs:

- Ask client how they prefer to be addressed. **Honors and respects the client as a human being who is valued.**
- Ask permission to touch the client as appropriate. **Prevents misinterpretation of touch with clients who have experienced trauma/abuse. Note all clients are not receptive to therapeutic touch.**
- Active-listen to client's perception of current stressors. **Reflecting client's statements and thoughts provides a forum for understanding client's perceptions in relation to reality and helps to provide interventions based on client's psychosocial developmental level.**
- Review verbalization of fears and anxieties and expression of feelings of denial, depression, or anger. Let the client know these are common reactions. **Encourages client to contend with these feelings and respond with open and honest communication opposed to use of defense mechanisms. Learning to recognize stress and applying emotional intelligence/self-awareness helps build positive relationships.**
- Continue motivational interviewing/communication when interacting with client. **Understanding the client's stage of readiness to change (e.g., precontemplation, contemplation, preparation, action, and maintenance) helps to coordinate the correct stage of intervention and empowers client to change behavior.**
- Discuss the level of stress and anxiety felt when using defense mechanisms (e.g., denial, repression, alcohol, drugs, or smoking). **Brings self-awareness of distress that results in poor decision making (e.g., substance misuse, blaming others, angry outbursts, or aggression).**
- Assist client to learn how to substitute positive thoughts for negative ones (i.e., "I can do this; I am in charge of myself"). **Applying positive thinking when contending with stress and anxiety will increase self-awareness and the opportunity to choose new ways to cope with life stressors. Positivity can enhance one's response to stressors, while negative thoughts can actually increase the impact of the stressor.**

Information that appears in brackets has been added by the authors to clarify and enhance the use of nursing diagnoses.

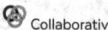 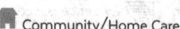

- Help client to set limits on acting-out behaviors and learn ways to cope with emotions in an acceptable manner. **Enables client to gain sense of self-esteem, promoting internal locus of control. Mindfulness, Emotional Intelligence (recognizing others' responses), and other coping strategies are designed to prevent acting-out behaviors, enhancing safety for self/others.**

Nursing Priority No. 4.

To assist client to develop enhanced coping skills:

- Active-listen and clarify client's perception of new coping skills taught. **Reflecting client's statements and thoughts provides a forum for understanding client's perceptions in relation to reality and helps to provide interventions based on client's psychosocial developmental level.**
- Listen for client's words of desire, ability, reason, or need (DARN words) to improve or change behaviors. **Helps empower client's readiness to change unhealthy behaviors for self-sufficiency and identifies areas of concern for client.**
- Identify client's current stage of readiness to change (e.g., precontemplation, contemplation, preparation, action, and maintenance). **Knowing client's stage of change guides a specific choice of interventions helping client progress to a healthy lifestyle and higher level/stage of change that requires applying appropriate interventions for the new level/stage.**
- Role-play while engaging in newly learned coping strategies. **Provides a safe environment to practice managing stressful situations using new skills.**

Nursing Priority No. 5.

To promote ongoing success (Teaching/Discharge considerations) and enhance general well-being (long-term goals):

- Review progress to date, reinforcing client's ability to change thoughts, feelings, beliefs regarding stressors. **Encourages an atmosphere of realistic hope. An optimistic outlook energizes the client. Empowered individuals develop self-respect and confidence to continue their emotional growth. Learning may need to be repeated over time due to defensive coping, psychosocial level of development, or self-defeating thinking and beliefs.**

Information that appears in brackets has been added by the authors to clarify and enhance the use of nursing diagnoses.

Improving client's health literacy, healthy lifestyle, and how to defend self with affective coping skills empowers client to manage their life.

- Discuss how to apply newly learned coping strategies to future stressors, including potential for future losses (e.g., personal, professional, economic, grief, health status change). **Knowledge helps reduce anxiety and allows client to cope with reality. Improving client's health literacy, healthy lifestyle, and how to defend self with affective coping skills empowers client to manage their future.**

- Discuss potential for, or reoccurrence of harmful self-depreciating thoughts or thoughts of harming self or others. **Relapse, encountering multiple stressors, and/or medication side-effects may influence negative thinking necessitating immediate evaluation/emergent care. Promoting other strategies can help client handle anger, sadness, or hostile thoughts and feelings. Important to support and refer client to emergent care to resolve human emotions, as opposed to hurting self or others, thus fostering a healthy outcome.**

- Provide updated or additional information needed about mental/medical condition, treatment, medications, and prognosis. **Knowledge helps reduce anxiety/fear and allows the client to deal with reality. Learning may need to be repeated over time due to defensive coping, psychosocial level of development, or self-defeating thinking and beliefs.**

- Encourage and support client in evaluating current lifestyle, occupation, and leisure activities. **Client's review/evaluation of conflicted/congenial communication at home, work/school, or social gatherings alters or brings self-awareness of using defense mechanism or positive coping skills that demonstrates the need for further help, as well as improving relationships.**

- Emphasize the importance of follow-up care by healthcare professionals. **Personal growth and lifestyle changes require periodic review of progress and appropriateness of plan of care as client progresses. Changing one's thoughts, feelings, and behaviors is a process that will progress, relapse, and can advance to higher levels of coping even with setbacks. Client needs to realize this is a part of growth and development.**

Information that appears in brackets has been added by the authors to clarify and enhance the use of nursing diagnoses.

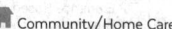

- Refer to community resources, spiritual/religious counselors, self-help groups (e.g., Alcohol/Narcotics Anonymous, grief and loss, sexual abuse survivors), as indicated or ordered. **Resources are needed for clients and families to continue the emotional growth.**
- Provide information and/or refer for consultation, as indicated, for sexual concerns. Provide privacy when the client is not in their own home. **Sexual needs are an integral part of being human, and determining and meeting individual preferences help client deal with concerns and desires for discussion or assistance in this area.**

Documentation Focus

Assessment/Reassessment
- Baseline findings, specific stressors, degree of impairment, and client's perceptions of situation
- Coping abilities and previous ways of dealing with life problems

Planning
- Plan of care, specific interventions, and who is involved in planning
- Teaching plan

Implementation/Evaluation
- Client's responses to interventions, teaching, and actions performed
- Medication dose, time, and client's response
- Attainment of or progress toward desired outcome(s)
- Modifications to plan of care

Discharge Planning
- Long-term needs and actions to be taken
- Support systems available, specific referrals made, and who is responsible for actions to be taken

Sample Nursing Outcomes & Interventions Classifications NOC/NIC

NOC—Coping
NIC—Coping Enhancement

Information that appears in brackets has been added by the authors to clarify and enhance the use of nursing diagnoses.

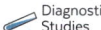 Diagnostic Studies 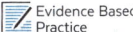 Evidence Based Practice 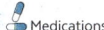 Medications 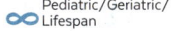 Pediatric/Geriatric/Lifespan

impaired community COPING ICNP

[Diagnostic Division: Social Interaction]

Definition: Lacking communication and teamwork necessary to meet the needs and demands of the community.

Recognizing Cues

Related/Risk Factors
Lack of resources for interprofessional collaboration that promotes a united approach to solve problems
Conflict between agencies; limited/lack of financial resources
Lack of, or outdated plan for community needs

Defining Characteristics

Subjective
Community members' needs not adequately addressed
Vulnerable communities' perception of hopelessness, powerlessness
Community members/groups report feeling stress/distress

Objective
Lack of willingness to engage in community projects/events
Higher rates of community illness
Neighborhood/community communications leading to conflict
Increased crime rate (e.g., homicides, vandalism, robbery, terrorism, abuse, unemployment, poverty, militancy, mental illness)

Generate Solutions

Plan Desired Outcomes

Community Will (Include Specific Time Frame)
- Recognize negative and positive factors affecting community's ability to meet its own demands or needs.
- Identify alternatives to inappropriate activities for adaptation/problem-solving.
- Report a measurable increase in necessary/desired activities to improve community functioning.

Information that appears in brackets has been added by the authors to clarify and enhance the use of nursing diagnoses.

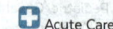 Acute Care 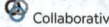 Collaborative 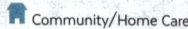 Community/Home Care   Cultural

Interventions/Take Action

Nursing Priority No. 1.

To identify causative or precipitating factors:

- Perform community needs assessment to evaluate social determinants of health. **A needs assessment is an in-depth and complex view of the community to determine what activities are currently available and what needs are not being met, either by the local or county/state entities. Provides information on which to base the steps needed to begin planning for desired changes.**
- Identify if a community needs assessment has been completed in the recent past. **Community nongovernment and government agencies are responsible for identifying needed changes for improvement. Compare and contrast the past needs assessment with present concerns since it will reflect past improvements or failures.**
- Identify unmet demands or needs of the community. **Determining deficiencies is a crucial step to developing an accurate plan for correction. Elected bodies may see problems differently from the general population, and conflict can arise.**
- Identify effects of Related Factors on community activities limiting/preventing the development of community collaboration. Note immediate needs (e.g., healthcare, food, shelter, transportation, funding). **Once immediate needs are known, community collaboration is required to begin the problem-solving process.**
- Determine the availability and use of resources. **Promoting agency cooperation requires clearly identifying roles, boundaries, and expectations of the outcomes. While resources may be available, they may not be appropriately used, requiring further evaluation.**

Nursing Priority No. 2.

To assist the community to reactivate/develop skills to deal with needs:

- Encourage community members/groups/agencies/government to engage in problem-solving activities. **Individuals who are involved in the problem-solving process and make a commitment to the solutions have an investment and are more apt to follow through on their commitments.**

Information that appears in brackets has been added by the authors to clarify and enhance the use of nursing diagnoses.

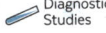 Diagnostic Studies 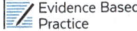 Evidence Based Practice 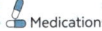 Medications 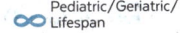 Pediatric/Geriatric/Lifespan

- Determine community strengths. **Promotes understanding of ways in which community is already meeting identified needs, and once identified, they can be built on to develop plan to improve community.**
- Identify and prioritize community goals. **Goals enable the identification of actions to direct the changes that are needed to improve the community. Prioritizing enables actions to be taken in order of importance.**
- Develop a plan jointly with community members to correct community deficits. **Working together will enhance efforts and help to meet identified goals.**

Nursing Priority No. 3.

To promote wellness as related to future needs for community health and well-being:

- Assist the community to form partnerships including nongovernmental and governmental agencies. **Promotes long-term development of the community to cope with current and future challenges.**
- Create and update plans addressing community goals based on prioritized needs. **Ongoing diverse partnerships are required to meet the needs of all community members or groups.**
- Engage community members, governmental agencies, and nonprofit organizations in formulating a comprehensive disaster plan. **This is vital for mounting an effective response to local emergencies (e.g., flood, tornado, wildfire, toxic spill, infectious disease outbreak).**
- Provide channels for dissemination of information to the community as a whole (e.g., print media; radio/television reports and community bulletin boards; speakers' bureau; and reports to committees, councils, and advisory boards), keeping material on file and accessible to the public. **Having information readily available for everyone provides opportunity for all members of the community to know what is being planned and have input into the planning. Keeping community informed promotes understanding of needs and plans and probability of follow-through to successful outcomes.**
- Make information available in different modalities and geared to differing educational levels and cultural and ethnic populations of the community.
- Seek out and evaluate underserved populations, including the homeless. **These members of the community often need**

Information that appears in brackets has been added by the authors to clarify and enhance the use of nursing diagnoses.

help to become productive citizens and to be involved in changes that are occurring.
- Work with community members to identify lifestyle changes that can be made to meet the goals identified to improve community deficits. **Changing lifestyles can promote a sense of power and encourage members to become involved in improving their community.**

Documentation Focus

Assessment/Reassessment
- Assessment findings, including perception of community members regarding problems
- Availability and use of resources

Planning
- Plan of care and who is involved in planning
- Teaching plan

Implementation/Evaluation
- Response of community entities to plan, interventions, and actions performed
- Attainment of or progress toward desired outcome(s)
- Modifications to plan of care

Discharge Planning
- Long-term plans and who is responsible for actions to be taken

Sample Nursing Outcomes & Interventions Classifications NOC/NIC

NOC—Community Competence
NIC—Environmental Management: Community

---

impaired family COPING ICNP

[Diagnostic Division: Roles/Relationships]

Definition: An emotionally connected family (e.g., parent[s], child or significant other) where a member disrupts cohesiveness preventing family support for emotional and physical well-being.

Information that appears in brackets has been added by the authors to clarify and enhance the use of nursing diagnoses.

 Diagnostic Studies 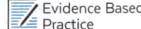 Evidence Based Practice 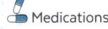 Medications 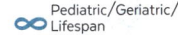 Pediatric/Geriatric/Lifespan

Recognizing Cues

Related/Risk Factors
Physical or emotional conditions affecting primary support person; illness of one or more family members

Controlling behaviors of support person requiring others to yield to their demands

Emotional distancing/isolating/abandonment from family; marital conflict; difficulty structuring activities of daily living

Conflict resulting from different parenting/coping styles

Defining Characteristics

Subjective
Lack of concern or response by primary support person for others' physical or emotional health

Family feels controlled, lacks autonomy by support person

Family member/client reports feeling isolated

Denies problems; criticizes others, manipulation, mistrust of others

Objective
Limited interaction and support between primary support person and client or family members

Communication controlled, incongruent, abusive, and/or aggressive by primary support person or others

Physical and emotional aggression toward family members

Refuses to seek help

At-Risk Population: Families with member in altered family role

Families with support person experiencing depleted capacity due to prolonged disease

Families with support person experiencing developmental or situational crisis

Clinical Connections
Chronic conditions (e.g., chronic obstructive pulmonary disease [COPD], heart failure, AIDS, Alzheimer disease, pain, renal failure), substance abuse, cancer, depression, anxiety, schizophrenia, borderline personality, antisocial, narcissistic personality disorders, hypochondriasis

---

Information that appears in brackets has been added by the authors to clarify and enhance the use of nursing diagnoses.

Generate Solutions

Plan Desired Outcomes

Family Will (Include Specific Time Frame)
- Identify effective problem-solving and decision-making skills with the family.
- Describe basic communication patterns that promote supportive relationships.
- Acknowledge importance of each family member's ability to express their thoughts and feelings openly and honestly.
- Verbalize acceptance of differences in family roles, knowledge and understanding of illness, disability, or condition.
- Identify need for continued individual and family support.

Interventions/Take Action

Nursing Priority No. 1.
To assess causative/contributing factors:

- Identify who client is in the family and how family members describe the individual. **Family members may present client (e.g., child, adolescent, or geriatric member) as challenging, disruptive, angry, aggressive, violent, or physically/mentally ill. For example, triangulation is a three-party relationship with two emotionally attached members blaming the third member for all problems, scapegoating. The scapegoated client may have developed depression, anxiety, or a physical illness resulting in a focus by family to fix what is wrong with the client rather than recognizing their emotional abuse.**
- Identify underlying circumstance(s) occurring prior to current situation that may contribute to the inability to provide support and assistance to the client. **Conflicts may have preceded the illness and now have a significant effect on the family (e.g., client is/was a substance abuser; client has acute/chronic physical or mental health condition).**
- Identify family members' relationships and roles. **Illness affects how a client performs usual functions in the family and affects how others in the family take over those responsibilities. These changes may result in dysfunctional behaviors, anger, hostility, and hopelessness. Family roles are diverse; however, general roles include**

Information that appears in brackets has been added by the authors to clarify and enhance the use of nursing diagnoses.

 Diagnostic Studies 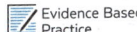 Evidence Based Practice 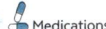 Medications 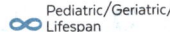 Pediatric/Geriatric/Lifespan parent/caregiver, leader/decision-maker, hero/high achiever, scapegoat, and lost child (withdrawn/isolated). **The roles identified in a family significantly influence relationships and contribute to the family/individual identity. Expectations are defined to the members who impact self-perception and relationships within the family unit.**

- Note factors (besides the client's condition) that are affecting abilities of family members to provide needed support. **Additionally, caregivers may incur decreased or lost income or risk losing own health insurance if they alter their work hours to care for client.**

- Note cultural factors related to family relationships that may be involved in problems of caring for member who is ill. **Cultural families view family composition, structure, methods of decision making, gender issues, and expectations with their own point of view related to an illness or a negative prognosis. Depending on the role of the ill client, absent parent/caregiver, or migration status, other members may have difficulty assuming an assertive role and managing the family.**

- Note prognosis, length of illness or condition (e.g., heart failure, cancer, multiple sclerosis), and/or other long-term situations that are present. **Chronic or unresolved illness, accompanied by changes in role performance or responsibility, often exhausts supportive capacity and coping abilities of significant other (SO)/family.**

- Assess knowledge regarding illness/condition available to and understood by the family/SO. **Understanding information regarding the specific situation, treatment, and prognosis are essential to family cooperation and care of the client.**

- Discuss family perceptions and expectations of the situation/crisis. **Expectations of client and family members may/may not be realistic and may interfere with ability to cope with situation.**

Nursing Priority No. 2.

To determine family's readiness to change:

- Active-listen client's/SO's comments, remarks, and expression of concern(s). Note nonverbal behaviors with responses and congruency. **Provides information and promotes understanding of client's/family's view of the illness and needs related to current situation.**

Information that appears in brackets has been added by the authors to clarify and enhance the use of nursing diagnoses.

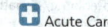 Acute Care 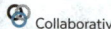 Collaborative 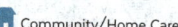 Community/Home Care Cultural

- Encourage family members to verbalize feelings openly and clearly. **Promotes understanding of feelings in relationship to current events and helps them to hear what other person is saying, leading to more appropriate interactions.**
- Identify client/family members' readiness to change (e.g., precontemplation, contemplation, preparation, action, maintenance), family communication pattern and relationships. **Attempting to implement interventions that are beyond the family's level of readiness to change will be met with resistance.**
- Develop a plan of care based on the client's/family's readiness to change. **Collaborating with the family to meet their needs helps to improve support, trust, and relationships within the family.**

Nursing Priority No. 3.
To assist family to cope with current situation:

- Discuss client's behaviors and their influence on family members. **Helps family/SO recognize client behaviors that may be triggered by emotional or physical effects of situation.**
- Assist the family and client to understand "who owns the problem" and who is responsible for resolution. **Avoids blaming or placing guilt on others. When these boundaries are defined, each individual can begin to take care of own self and stop taking care of others in inappropriate ways.**
- Encourage client and family to develop problem-solving skills to cope with the situation. **Use of these skills enables each member of the family to identify what is seen as the problem to be dealt with and contribute ideas for solutions that are acceptable to each member, promoting more effective interactions among the family members.**
- Recommend family develop regular family meetings to plan for work, socialization, problem-solving and decision making. **Regular democratic family meetings help with role development, setting boundaries, building trust, respect, and relationships.**

Nursing Priority No. 4.
To promote continued family growth (Teaching/Discharge Considerations) and enhance well-being (long-term goals):

- Provide information for family/SO(s) about specific illness or condition. **Promotes better understanding of need**

Information that appears in brackets has been added by the authors to clarify and enhance the use of nursing diagnoses.

for following therapeutic regimen to provide maximum benefit.
- Encourage family to continue providing client care, as appropriate. **Identifies ways of demonstrating support while maintaining client's independence (e.g., providing favorite foods, engaging in diversional activities).**
- Review with client and family the progress achieved and the need for continuation of planning for the future. **Helps family recognize improvement achieved. When family members are knowledgeable and understand needs, commitment to plan is enhanced.**
- Promote the assistance of family in providing client care, as appropriate (e.g., counseling, psychotherapy, financial, spiritual). **May need additional help, and getting to the appropriate resource provides accurate help for individual situation (e.g., family counseling, financial planning).**
- Refer to community resources for assistance, as indicated (e.g., counseling, psychotherapy, financial, and spiritual). **May need additional help, and getting to the appropriate resource provides accurate help for individual situation.**
- Refer to NDs Anxiety, difficulty Coping, Death Anxiety, impaired Family Process, Fear, dysfunctional Grief, as appropriate.

Documentation Focus

Assessment/Reassessment
- Assessment findings, including current and past coping behaviors, emotional response to situation and stressors, and support systems available

Planning
- Plan of care, who is involved in planning, and areas of responsibility
- Teaching plan

Implementation/Evaluation
- Responses of family members/client to interventions, teaching, and actions performed
- Attainment of or progress toward desired outcome(s)
- Modifications to plan of care

Discharge Planning
- Long-term plan and who is responsible for actions
- Specific referrals made

Information that appears in brackets has been added by the authors to clarify and enhance the use of nursing diagnoses.

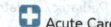 Acute Care 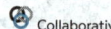 Collaborative 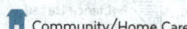 Community/Home Care   Cultural

Sample Nursing Outcomes & Interventions Classifications NOC/NIC

NOC—Family Coping
NIC—Family Involvement Promotion

DEATH ANXIETY ICNP

[Diagnostic Division: Stress Management]

Definition: Fear and worry due to thoughts of own death or the death of a loved.

Recognizing Cues

Related/Risk Factors

Phobias (lasting 6 months or more)
Obsessive-compulsive disorder (OCD) with unexpected changes in routine; fear of undiagnosed illness
Depression; separation anxiety (leaving loved ones); past traumatic/near-death experiences
Prognosis undecided; terminal illness; expectation of pain
Religious/spiritual distress doubting the existence of a higher power or what happens after death

Defining Characteristics

Subjective

Expresses:
- Unrealistic beliefs (e.g., death is unfair, fear for family after death, separation from family and friends)
- Powerlessness; helplessness; loneliness; isolated
- Anxiety; fear of the unknown (e.g., pain/suffering, the future, negative thoughts related to premature death, or prolonged dying process, and afterlife)
- Feeling weak, tired; short of breath; nausea
- Depressive symptoms; suicidal ideation

Objective

Alteration in vital signs
Irritability; trembling, sweating; somatic complaints
Inability to manage activities of daily living
Decreased social interactions
Substance misuse/abuse

Information that appears in brackets has been added by the authors to clarify and enhance the use of nursing diagnoses.

 Diagnostic Studies 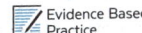 Evidence Based Practice 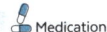 Medications ∞ Pediatric/Geriatric/Lifespan

Clinical Connections
Chronic health conditions (e.g., cardiovascular and respiratory conditions, cancer), accidents, or assaults, terminal illness, hospitalization, impending surgery, depression

Generate Solutions

Plan Desired Outcomes

Client Will (Include Specific Time Frame)
- Discuss how thoughts, feelings, and behaviors interfere with activities of daily living and relationships.
- Participate in developing a plan of care or goal setting for the future while working on goal achievement one day at a time.
- Identify effective ways to cope with social and physical concerns as well as the eventualities of dying/death.

Interventions/Take Action

Nursing Priority No. 1.
To assess causative/contributing factors:
- Determine how client sees self in usual lifestyle, role, daily functioning; determine perception and meaning of anticipated death of client/significant other (SO) and influence on family. **Provides information that can help understand the client's perceptions in contrast to the reality of the present situation. Understanding these factors are helpful for planning. Note one recent study stated that "over the years, research has shown two separate but connected constructs of death anxiety: fear of death or fear of the dying process. Many variables influence death anxiety, amongst them religiosity, gender, psychological state and age."**
- Identify client's current knowledge of the situation. **Identifies misconceptions, lack of information, and other pertinent issues.**
- Determine the client's role in the family constellation. Observe patterns of communication in family and response of family/SOs to client's situation and concerns. **Identifies areas of need/concern and reveals strengths useful in addressing the current concerns.**
- Assess the impact of client reports of subjective experiences and past experience with death (or exposure to death), for

---

Information that appears in brackets has been added by the authors to clarify and enhance the use of nursing diagnoses.

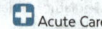 Acute Care 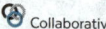 Collaborative 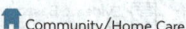 Community/Home Care   Cultural

example, witnessed violent death, viewed body in casket as a child, and so on. **Identifies possible feelings that may be affecting current situation, thus promoting accurate planning.**

- Identify cultural factors/expectations and impact on current situation and feelings. **These factors affect client attitude toward events and impending loss. Note: Culture is the mix of beliefs, values, behaviors, traditions, and rituals that members of a cultural group share. Culture influences how people care for people as they approach death (e.g., who is present and what ceremonies are performed at the moments before and after death). Culture can dictate whether grief is expressed quietly and privately or loudly and publicly. However, people often adapt the beliefs and values of their culture to meet their own unique needs and circumstances. As a result, grief responses within a culture vary from person to person. Many cultures prefer to keep the client at home instead of in a long-term care facility or hospital. In the United States, hospice is often used to provide palliative care and comfort during the client's final days in any setting.**
- Note client's age, physical and mental condition, and complexity of therapeutic regimen. **May affect ability to cope with current situation.**
- Determine the ability to manage self-care, end-of-life and other affairs, and awareness/use of available resources. **Information will be necessary for determining needs and planning care.**
- Observe behavior indicative of the level of anxiety present (mild to panic). **The level of anxiety affects client's/SO's ability to process information and participate in activities.**
- Identify coping skills currently used and degree of effectiveness. **Note, defense mechanisms are protective strategies used by the client to protect self-esteem. Over time, they may result in a lack of coping and resolving of current issues/problems.**
- Note the use of alcohol or other drugs of abuse, reports of insomnia, excessive sleeping, and avoidance of interactions with others. **May be behavioral indicators of withdrawal symptoms and need for intervention to cope with symptoms or help client deal realistically with diagnosis or illness. Note: In a recent study comparing death anxiety in**

Information that appears in brackets has been added by the authors to clarify and enhance the use of nursing diagnoses.

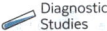 Diagnostic Studies 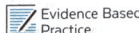 Evidence Based Practice 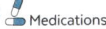 Medications 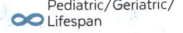 Pediatric/Geriatric/Lifespan

addicted and nonaddicted individuals, findings indicated that death anxiety in the addicted group was significantly more than in the nonaddicted group.

- Note client's religious and spiritual orientation and involvement in religious activities; note presence of conflicts regarding spiritual beliefs. **Helps to understand their values and beliefs of death.**
- Active-listen client's/SOs' reports/expressions of anger and concern, alienation from God/higher power, or belief that impending death is a punishment for wrongdoing. **Indicates the stage of grief client is experiencing.**
- Determine sense of futility; feelings of hopelessness or helplessness; lack of motivation to help self. **May indicate the presence of depression and need for intervention.**
- Listen for expressions of inability to find meaning in life or suicidal ideation. **Signs of depression indicate need for referral to therapist/psychiatrist and possible pharmacological treatment to help client deal with terminal illness or situation.**

Nursing Priority No. 2.

To assist client to cope with situation:

- Provide an open and trusting relationship. **Promotes opportunity to explore feelings about impending death.**
- Use therapeutic communication skills of active-listening, silence, and acknowledgment. Respect the client's desire or request not to talk. Provide hope within parameters of the individual situation.
- Encourage expressions of feelings (anger, fear, sadness, etc.). Acknowledge anxiety/fear. Do not deny or reassure client that everything will be all right. Be honest when answering questions/providing information. **This enhances trust and therapeutic relationship.**
- Provide information about the normalcy of feelings and individual grief reaction. **Most individuals question their reactions and whether they are normal, and information can provide reassurance.**
- Make time for nonjudgmental discussion of philosophical issues and questions about the spiritual impact of the illness and provide hope within parameters of the individual situation.
- Review life experiences of loss and previous use of coping skills, noting the client's strengths and successes. **Provides a starting point to plan care and assists client to**

Information that appears in brackets has been added by the authors to clarify and enhance the use of nursing diagnoses.

acknowledge reality and deal more effectively with what is happening.
- Provide a calm, peaceful setting and privacy as appropriate. **Promotes relaxation and the ability to deal with a situation.**
- Respect client's desire or request not to talk. **Promotes open environment that encourages client to talk freely about thoughts and feelings. Client may not be ready to talk about situation or concerns about death, or client may be denying the reality of what is happening.**
- Provide information about normalcy of feelings and individual grief reaction. **Most individuals question their reactions and whether they are normal, and information can provide reassurance.**
- Note client's religious or spiritual orientation, involvement in religious or church activities, and presence of conflicts regarding spiritual beliefs. **May benefit from referral to appropriate resource to help client resolve issues, if desired.**
- Assist the client to engage in spiritual growth activities, if desired, and experience prayer/meditation and forgiveness to heal past hurts. Provide information that anger with God is a normal part of the grieving process. **Reduces feelings of guilt/conflict, allowing the client to move forward toward resolution.**
- Refer to therapists, spiritual advisors, and counselors **to facilitate grief work.**
- Refer to community agencies/resources **to assist client/SO(s) in planning for eventualities (legal issues, funeral plans, etc.).**

Nursing Priority No. 3.
To promote independence:
- Support the client's efforts to develop realistic steps to put plans into action. **Provides sense of control over situation in which client does not have much control.**
- Direct the client's thoughts beyond the present state to enjoyment of each day and the future when appropriate. **Being in the moment can help client enjoy this time rather than dwelling on what is ahead.**
- Provide opportunities for the client to make simple decisions. **Enhances sense of control.**
- Develop an individual plan using the client's locus of control. **Incorporating locus of control (internal or external)**

Information that appears in brackets has been added by the authors to clarify and enhance the use of nursing diagnoses.

enhances success of plan by enabling client/family to manage situation.
- Treat expressed decisions and desires with respect and convey to others as appropriate. **Expresses regard for the individual and enhances sense of control in situation that is not controllable.**
- Assist with completion of advance directives, CPR instructions, and durable medical power of attorney.
- Refer to palliative, hospice, or end-of-life care resources, as appropriate. **Provides support and assistance to client and SO/family through potentially complex and difficult process.**

Documentation Focus

Assessment/Reassessment
- Assessment findings, including client's fears, anticipation of pain, reality of terminal disease, and signs/symptoms being exhibited
- Responses and actions of family/SO(s)
- Client's concern about caregiver
- Availability and use of resources

Planning
- Plan of care and who is involved in planning

Implementation/Evaluation
- Client's response to interventions, teaching, and actions performed
- Attainment of or progress toward desired outcome(s)
- Modifications to plan of care

Discharge Planning
- Identified needs and who is responsible for actions to be taken
- Specific referrals made, including palliative/hospice care

Sample Nursing Outcomes & Interventions Classifications NOC/NIC

NOC—Dignified Life Closure
NIC—Dying Care

Information that appears in brackets has been added by the authors to clarify and enhance the use of nursing diagnoses.

impaired DECISION-MAKING   NANDA-I

[Diagnostic Division: Values/Beliefs]

Definition: Inability to make appropriate choices, which may have negative impact on health related goals, well-being and quality of life.

Recognizing Cues

Related Factors

Inexperience with decision making; interference in decision making

Inadequate information; conflicting information sources

Inadequate social support

Unclear personal beliefs, values

Perceived danger to value system

Conflict with moral obligation; moral principle, rule, or value supports mutually inconsistent actions

Defining Characteristics

Subjective

Uncertainty about choices

Recognizes undesired consequences of potential actions

Questions personal beliefs or values while attempting decision

Questions moral principle, rule, or values while attempting decision

Objective

Delayed decision making; vacillating among choices

Self-focused attention

Distressed during decision making; physical sign of tension, distress

Clinical Connections

Any condition/situation requiring healthcare decisions: Parkinson disease, depression, schizophrenia, substance abuse, traumatic brain injury, therapeutic options with undesired side effects (e.g., amputation, visible scarring) or conflicting with belief system (e.g., blood transfusion, termination of pregnancy); chronic disease states, dementia, Alzheimer disease, terminal or end-of-life situations

---

Information that appears in brackets has been added by the authors to clarify and enhance the use of nursing diagnoses.

 Diagnostic Studies 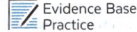 Evidence Based Practice 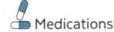 Medications 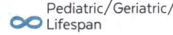 Pediatric/Geriatric/Lifespan

Generate Solutions

Plan Desired Outcomes

Client Will (Include Specific Time Frame)

- Verbalize awareness of positive and negative aspects of choices and alternative actions.
- Identify personal values and beliefs concerning issues.
- Make decision(s) and express satisfaction with choices.
- Meet psychological needs as evidenced by appropriate expression of feelings, identification of options, and use of resources.
- Display relaxed manner and calm demeanor, and be free of physical signs of distress.

Interventions/Take Action

Nursing Priority No. 1.

To assess causative/contributing factors:

- Begin developing the nurse-client relationship during the initial assessment. **Initial nurse communication skills with client begins developing trust that allows equal distribution of power, fostering patient-centered care and good decision making by the client.**
- Determine client's capacity and cognition as key factors to make a decision (e.g., capacity to understand, express a choice, appreciate the situation, reason treatment options; cognition is brain function) to manage own affairs. Assessment tools such as the Mini-Mental State Examination (MMSE) does not assess for capacity; however, lower scores (e.g., 16 or lower out of 30 points) are noted in clients with dementia. Clarify who has legal right to intervene on behalf of child/adolescent/adult (e.g., parent, other relative, or court-appointed guardian/advocate). **Family disruption or conflicts can complicate decision-making process. All adults have the right to make their own decisions unless a legal court has ruled the individual is incompetent and a guardian is appointed.**
- Observe/note expressions of indecision, dependence on others, availability, and involvement of support persons (e.g., lack of or conflicting advice). **Care providers need to be sensitive to the physical, cognitive, and emotional effects of illness on decision-making capabilities and whether the individual wants to be involved in making the decision.**
- Determine dependency of other(s) on client and/or issues of codependency. **Influence of others may lead client to**

Information that appears in brackets has been added by the authors to clarify and enhance the use of nursing diagnoses.

make decision that is not what is really wanted or in client's best interest.
- Active-listen and identify reason for indecisiveness. **Helps client to clarify problem and begin looking for resolution. May talk about uncertainty—and alternative choices that can lead to risky, uncertain outcomes—and the need to make value judgments about losses versus gains.**
- Identify cultural values and beliefs or moral obligations and principles that may be creating conflict for client and complicating decision-making process. **These issues must be addressed before client can be at peace with the decision that is made.**
- Determine effectiveness of current problem-solving techniques. **Provides information about client's ability to make decisions that are needed or desired.**
- Note presence and intensity of physical signs of anxiety (e.g., increased heart rate, muscle tension). **Client may be conflicted about the decision that is required and may need help to deal with anxiety to begin to deal with reality of situation. Different treatment decisions may have more uncertainty and generate more conflict in client.**
- Listen for expressions of inability to find meaning in life or reason for living, feelings of futility, or alienation from God or others. (Refer to ND impaired Spiritual Well-Being as indicated.) **May need to talk about reasons for feelings of alienation to resolve concerns and may engage in questioning about own values.**
- Review information client has to support the decision to be made. **Inaccurate or incomplete information and misinterpretations complicate the process and may result in a poor outcome.**

Nursing Priority No. 2.

To assist client to develop/effectively use problem-solving skills:

- Promote safe and hopeful environment, as needed. **Client needs to be protected and supported while regaining inner control.**
- Encourage verbalization of conflicts and concerns. **Helps client to clarify these issues so client can come to a resolution of the situation.**
- Accept verbal expressions of anger or guilt. Set limits on maladaptive behavior. **Verbalization of feelings enables client to sift through feelings and begin to deal with**

Information that appears in brackets has been added by the authors to clarify and enhance the use of nursing diagnoses.

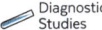 Diagnostic Studies 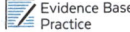 Evidence Based Practice 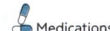 Medications 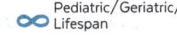 Pediatric/Geriatric/Lifespan

situation. **Behavior that is inappropriate is not helpful for dealing with the situation and will lead to feelings of guilt and low self-worth.**
- Clarify and prioritize individual goals, noting where the subject of the "conflict" falls on this scale. **Helps to identify importance of problems client is addressing, enabling realistic problem-solving.**
- Identify strengths and use of positive coping skills (e.g., use of relaxation techniques, willingness to express feelings). **Helpful for developing solutions to current situation.**
- Identify positive aspects of this experience and assist client to view it as a learning opportunity. **Reframing the situation can help the client see things in a different light, enabling client to develop new and creative solutions.**
- Correct misperceptions client may have and provide factual information, as needed. **Promotes understanding and enables client to make better decisions for own situation.**
- Provide opportunities for client to make simple decisions regarding self-care and other daily activities. Accept choice not to do so. Advance complexity of choices, as tolerated. **Acceptance of what client wants to do, with gentle encouragement to progress, enhances self-esteem and ability to try more. Providing individualized decision support can help the client move to more difficult decisions.**
- Encourage child to make developmentally appropriate decisions concerning own care. **Fosters child's sense of self-worth and enhances ability to learn and exercise coping skills.**
- Discuss time considerations, setting time line for small steps and considering consequences related to not making or postponing specific decisions to facilitate resolution of conflict. **When time is a factor in making a decision, these strategies can promote movement toward solution.**
- Have client list some alternatives to present situation or decisions, using a brainstorming process. Include family in this activity, as indicated (e.g., placement of parent in long-term care facility, use of intervention process with addicted member). **Involving family and looking at different options can promote successful resolution of decision to be made.** Refer to NDs impaired Family Process, impaired family Coping, Moral Distress.
- Practice use of problem-solving process with current situation and decision. **Promotes identification of different possibilities that may not have been thought of otherwise.**

Information that appears in brackets has been added by the authors to clarify and enhance the use of nursing diagnoses.

 Acute Care 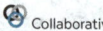 Collaborative 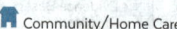 Community/Home Care 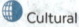 Cultural

- Discuss and clarify spiritual concerns, accepting client's values in a nonjudgmental manner. **Client will be willing to consider own situation when accepted as an individual of worth.**

Nursing Priority No. 3.

To promote personal success (Teaching/Discharge Considerations) and enhanced well-being:

- Promote opportunities for using conflict-resolution skills, identifying steps as client does each one. **Emphasizing each step as it is used will help with learning these skills. Allows client to practice communication of desires to others.**
- Provide positive feedback for efforts and progress noted. **Promotes a continuation of efforts.**
- Encourage involvement of family/SO(s), as desired/available. **Can provide support for client and encourages family members to work together.**
- Support the client for decisions made, especially if consequences are unexpected and/or difficult to cope with.
- Encourage attendance at stress reduction or assertiveness classes. **Using these skills can strengthen decision-making process.**
- Refer to other resources, as necessary (e.g., clergy, psychiatric clinical nurse specialist/psychiatrist, family/marital therapist, or addiction support groups). **Client/SO(s) may need this additional help to deal with complicated problems and facilitate problem-solving and decision making.**

Documentation Focus

Assessment/Reassessment
- Assessment findings, behavioral responses, degree of impairment in lifestyle functioning.
- Individuals involved in the conflict.
- Personal values and beliefs.

Planning
- Plan of care, specific interventions, and who is involved in the planning process.
- Teaching plan.

Implementation/Evaluation
- Client's and involved individuals' responses to interventions, teaching, and actions performed.
- Ability to express feelings and identify options.
- Use of resources.
- Attainment or progress toward desired outcome(s).
- Modifications to plan of care.

Information that appears in brackets has been added by the authors to clarify and enhance the use of nursing diagnoses.

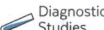 Diagnostic Studies 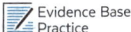 Evidence Based Practice 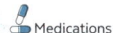 Medications 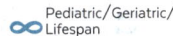 Pediatric/Geriatric/Lifespan

Discharge Planning
- Long-term needs, actions to be taken, and who is responsible for doing.
- Specific referrals made.

Sample Nursing Outcomes & Interventions Classifications NOC/NIC

NOC—Decision-Making
NIC—Decision-Making Support

---

delayed child DEVELOPMENT — NANDA-I

[Diagnostic Division: Health Management]

Definition: Consistent failure to achieve developmental milestones within the expected time frame, in individuals 1–9 years of age.

Recognizing Cues

Related/Risk Factors
Infant or Child Factors:
Inadequate access to health personnel
Inadequate attachment behavior; inadequate stimulation
Unaddressed abuse or psychological neglect
Caregiver Factors:
Excessive anxiety; inadequate emotional support; depressive symptoms
Excessive stress
Unaddressed domestic violence

Defining Characteristics

Objective
Consistent difficulty performing cognitive, or language, or motor, or psychosocial skills typical of age group

Clinical Connections
Congenital or genetic disorders, Down syndrome, prematurity, low birth weight, delayed growth, infection, nutritional problems (malnutrition, anorexia, failure to thrive), toxic exposures (e.g., lead), substance abuse, endocrine disorders, abuse or neglect, developmental delay

---

Information that appears in brackets has been added by the authors to clarify and enhance the use of nursing diagnoses.

 Acute Care 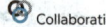 Collaborative 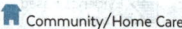 Community/Home Care   Cultural

Generate Solutions

Plan Desired Outcomes

Client Will (Include Specific Time Frame)
- Perform self-regulatory behavior and motor, social, cognitive, and language skills appropriate for age within scope of present capabilities.

Parent/Caregiver Will (Include Specific Time Frame)
- Verbalize an understanding of age-appropriate development and expectations.
- Identify individual developmental delay or deviation.
- Formulate plan(s) for management of developmental deviation.
- Initiate interventions and lifestyle changes promoting appropriate development.

Interventions/Take Action

Nursing Priority No. 1.
To assess for causative/contributing or **risk** factors:

- Identify condition(s) that could contribute to developmental deviations. **This list is extensive and widely variable. Potential for developmental issues might be apparent at birth (e.g., neonatal brain injury occurring before or at time of birth; prematurity; extremes of maternal age; unwanted or complicated pregnancy; known prenatal substance abuse, etc.). However, risks are not confined to the child's birth events but also encompass parent/family issues and environment (e.g., family history of developmental disorders; mother with mental illness or intellectual limitations, child with acute or chronic severe illness and lengthy hospitalizations; family poverty with inadequate living quarters, nutrition, nurturing, or supervision; family instability or violence; shaken baby syndrome and other maltreatment or child abuse; institutional home or foster system during early life or prior to adoption).**
- Participate in screening child's development level by means of observation and history related by concerned parents/significant others. **Developmental delay occurs when a child fails to achieve one or more developmental milestones (e.g., cognitive, social and emotional, speech and**

Information that appears in brackets has been added by the authors to clarify and enhance the use of nursing diagnoses.

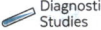 Diagnostic Studies 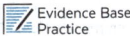 Evidence Based Practice 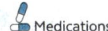 Medications 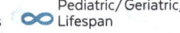 Pediatric/Geriatric/Lifespan

language, fine motor skills or gross motor skills) and may be the result of one or multiple factors.
- Obtain information from variety of sources. **Parents are often the first ones to think that there is a problem with their baby's development and should be encouraged to have routine well-baby checkups and screening for developmental delays. Teachers, family members, daycare or foster care providers, physicians, and others interacting with a client (older than infant) may have valuable input regarding behaviors that may indicate problems or developmental issues.**
- Identify cultural beliefs, norms, and values, as they may impact parent/caregiver view of situation. **Culture shapes parenting practices, family roles and goals, understanding of health and illness, perceptions related to development, school readiness, and beliefs about individuals affected by developmental disorders.**
- Ascertain nature of required parent/caregiver activities, and evaluate caregiver's abilities to perform needed activities.
- Note severity and pervasiveness of situation (e.g., potential for long-term stress leading to abuse or neglect versus situational disruption during period of crisis or transition that may eventually level out). **Situations require different interventions in terms of the intensity and length of time that assistance and support may be critical to the parent/caregiver. A crisis can produce great change within a family, some of which can be detrimental to the individual or family unit.**
- Evaluate environment in which long-term care will be provided. **The physical, emotional, financial, and social needs of a family are impacted by and intertwined with the needs of the client. Changes may be needed in the physical structure of the home, or family roles, resulting in disruption and stress, placing everyone at risk.**
- Refer for and assist with evaluation, when indicated, using screening tools or an authoritative text. **Provides guide for comparative measurement as child/individual progresses. A diagnosis is often determined over months or years. Note: Often, there is no single diagnostic test for a specific developmental delay. Pediatrician may screen with the Ages and Stages Questionnaire (ASQ) and Modified Checklist for Autism in Toddlers (M-CHAT) (commonly used screening tools for developmental delay and autism, respectively).**

Information that appears in brackets has been added by the authors to clarify and enhance the use of nursing diagnoses.

Nursing Priority No. 2.

To assist in managing child with developmental delays:

- Note chronological age and review with parents the expectations for "normal development" in infancy and early childhood at clinic visits **to help determine developmental expectations (e.g., when child should walk, climb stairs, speak three-word sentences, engage in storytelling, follow three-part commands, dress and feed self, use crayons/pencil to draw pictures/letters, cooperate with other children, etc.) and how the expectations may be altered by child's condition. Note: For high-risk individuals, including children affected by biological (e.g., low birth weight) and psychosocial (e.g., foster care, homelessness) risk factors, earlier and more frequent formal developmental screening may be warranted.**
- Describe realistic, age-appropriate patterns of development to parent/caregiver, and promote activities and interactions that support developmental tasks where client is at this time. **Important in planning interventions in keeping with the individual's current status and potential. Each child will have own unique strengths and challenges.**
- Collaborate with related professional resources, as indicated (e.g., physical, occupational, rehabilitation, speech therapists; home health agencies; social services, nutritionist; special education teacher, family therapists; technological and adaptive equipment specialists; vocational counselor). **Multidisciplinary team care increases the likelihood of developing a well-rounded plan of care that meets client/family's specialized and varied needs, minimizing identified risks.**
- Engage parents/caregivers in carrying out home plan of care that considers child's behavioral style and temperament patterns such as:
- Discuss developmentally appropriate toys and activities, items available in the home that can be used
- Encourage healthy hobbies/activities that promote fitness and large/fine motor skill development including time outdoors
- Read stories and encourage child to read aloud as able, engage in storytelling
- Provide opportunity for interaction/play with children of similar age or developmental level
- Role-model interaction skills/behaviors, facilitate role-playing or imaginative play
- Reinforce child sharing and taking turns

Information that appears in brackets has been added by the authors to clarify and enhance the use of nursing diagnoses.

 Diagnostic Studies   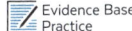 Evidence Based Practice   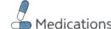 Medications   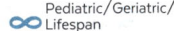 Pediatric/Geriatric/Lifespan

- Assist child to express emotions in safe manner; protect from overstimulation
- Limit rules, but consistently enforce them
- Provide positive reinforcement for efforts and desired behaviors
- Encourage/assist with self-care skills (e.g., feeding, toileting, washing hands, dressing, brushing teeth)
- Promote positive body image and self-esteem

Nursing Priority No. 3.

To promote maximum development (Teaching/Discharge Considerations) and enhance well-being (long-term goals):

- Engage parents/caregivers in harm-prevention strategies (e.g., referral for treatment programs; referral for violence prevention counseling; anticipatory guidance for potential handicaps [vision, hearing, failure to thrive]). **Promoting child wellness starts with preventing complications and acting early to limit severity of anticipated problems.**
- Evaluate client's progress on continual basis. Identify target symptoms requiring intervention **to make referrals in a timely manner and/or to make adjustments in plan of care, as indicated.**
- Emphasize importance of follow-up appointments as indicated **to promote ongoing evaluation, support, or management of situation.**
- Discuss proactive wellness actions to take (e.g., periodic laboratory studies to monitor nutritional status, getting immunizations on schedule to prevent serious infections) **to avoid preventable complications.**
- Maintain a positive, hopeful attitude. Encourage setting of short-term realistic goals for achieving developmental potential. **Small, incremental steps are often easier to deal with, and successes enhance hopefulness and well-being.**
- Provide information as appropriate, including pertinent reference materials and reliable internet sites, being sensitive to parent's/caregiver's health literacy, cultural and socioeconomic concerns.
- Encourage attendance at educational programs (e.g., parenting classes, infant stimulation sessions; food buying, cooking, and nutrition; home and family safety, anger management, seminars on life stresses, aging process) **to address specific learning need or desires and interact with others with similar life challenges.**

Information that appears in brackets has been added by the authors to clarify and enhance the use of nursing diagnoses.

 Acute Care 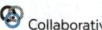 Collaborative 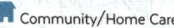 Community/Home Care Cultural

• Refer to available community and national resources if appropriate (e.g., early intervention programs, gifted and talented programs, sheltered workshop, disabled children's services, medical equipment and supplier, caregiver support, and respite services).

Documentation Focus

Assessment/Reassessment
- Assessment findings, individual needs, including developmental level
- Caregiver's understanding of situation and individual role

Planning
- Plan of care and who is involved in the planning
- Teaching plan

Implementation/Evaluation
- Client's response to interventions, teaching, and actions performed
- Caregiver response to teaching
- Attainment of or progress toward desired outcome(s)
- Modifications to plan of care

Discharge Planning
- Identified long-term needs and who is responsible for actions to be taken
- Specific referrals made; sources for assistive devices, educational tools

Sample Nursing Outcomes & Interventions Classifications NOC/NIC

NOC—Child Development: [specify age]
NIC—Teaching: Early Childhood Development 1–5 years [or] 6–12 years

---

risk for compromised DIGNITY NANDA-I

[Diagnostic Division: Self-Perception/Self-Concept]

Definition: Susceptible to sense of lack of respect, absence of compassion; feeling humiliation that can negatively impact self-image and self-worth, creating sense of alienation.

Information that appears in brackets has been added by the authors to clarify and enhance the use of nursing diagnoses.

Recognizing Cues

Related/Risk Factors
Lack of privacy; open doors, curtains; entering room before knocking

Not speaking upon entry; rushing client to speak, not listening to the response

Violating personal space; fails to seek consent or ask client's preferences or desires prior to any task, exposing body/body parts; contempt or distress at client's appearance, loss of control of body functions

Values or actions not congruent with spiritual and cultural customs of client

Referring to or treating client as an object or condition (e.g., client 18, frequent flyer, drug seeker, TB client, the obsessive-compulsive); not protecting personal information

Clinical Connections
Chronic conditions (e.g., multiple sclerosis [MS], stroke, quadriplegia, amyotrophic lateral sclerosis [ALS]), overweight, personality disorders, substance abuse

Generate Solutions

Plan Desired Outcomes

Client Will (Include Specific Time Frame)
- Acknowledge not all people recognize the value of differences.
- Identify respectful strategies to respond to rude and disrespectful people.
- Demonstrate assertiveness skills.
- Demonstrate ability to participate in decision making.
- Verbalize self-worth.

Interventions/Take Action

Nursing Priority No. 1.
To determine individual situation as perceived by client:
- Determine the client's perceptions and specific factors that could lead to a sense of loss of dignity. **Human dignity is a totality of the individual's uniqueness: totality of mind, body, and spirt.**
- Note and discuss labels, terms, lack of privacy used by staff or friends/family that stigmatize the client. **All people are worthy of being treated with honor, respect, and**

Information that appears in brackets has been added by the authors to clarify and enhance the use of nursing diagnoses.

 Acute Care  Collaborative 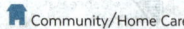 Community/Home Care 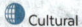 Cultural

dignity in all settings, and human dignity is threatened by insensitive as well as inadequate healthcare. **Identifies opportunities to educate staff and others in advocating for client's physical and emotional well-being.**

- Identify cultural beliefs, values, and degree of importance to client. **Individuals cling to their basic culture, especially during times of stress, and recognizing these factors facilitates choosing interventions that build the value of being human while dealing with illness, disability, aging, or other life events, especially when grave injustices have occurred.**
- Assess family/SO's response to clients reported lack of respect and dignity. **Physical/emotional responses are dependent on perceptions of moral justice. Supportive family/friends may need help verbalizing concerns while a lack of support or conflict may require the client to consider separating self from those with negative influences.**
- Identify client's/significant other's healthcare goals and expectations. **Shared decision making empowers client and the family while restoring self-worth to set goals and beginning the healing process to becoming a resilient human being able to overcome injustices.**
- Note the availability of family/friends for support and encouragement. **Vulnerable clients unable to defend themselves against cruelty require others to protect their dignity.**

Nursing Priority No. 2.

To assist client to deal with situation in positive ways:

- Ask the client how they wish to be addressed. **Client-centered care begins with respectful communication, and use of desired name supports a person's identity and recognizes their individuality.**
- Develop nurse-client therapeutic relationship. **Communicates respect for client and allows individual to express self freely.**
- Active-listen client's thoughts, feelings, and beliefs while encouraging verbalization of concerns. **Can help client discover underlying reasons for feelings. Observing both verbal and body language will alert listener to possible incongruences in client's story/unexpressed conflicts.**
- Honor client's wishes for quiet/silence and for privacy during care, procedures, or when discussing sensitive or

---

Information that appears in brackets has been added by the authors to clarify and enhance the use of nursing diagnoses.

personal issues. **Demonstrates respect for client, promoting a sense of safe environment, and helps client feel honored and respected.**

- ∞ Use understandable/age-appropriate terms and communication aids, as appropriate, when interacting with client/family regarding medical condition, procedures, and treatments (component of informed consent). **Enhances client/family understanding of what is/will be taking place.**
- ∞ Educate client/family/SO(s) in how to effectively and respectfully communicate when attempting to understand what is being reported, especially when the client may be irritable, angry, have conflicted relationships, or lack ability to comprehend the situation. **Teaching Emotional Intelligence, Mindfulness, respectful and assertive communication helps empower client/family/SO's to protect self regardless of age or individual abilities or frailty. Promotes personal growth and development of self-worth.**
- ᗧ Include client and family (if client desires) in decision making, especially regarding end-of-life issues. **Helps individuals feel respected and valued, and allows interprofessional team to provide client-centered care respecting client's needs and desires.**
- ᗧ Involve the facility/local ethics committee to facilitate mediation or resolution of conflicts between client/family, or staff/client/family members related to healthcare treatments or other issues, as appropriate. **Moral courage and support are required to effectively advocate and speak for vulnerable clients who are afraid or unable to speak up for themselves.**

Nursing Priority No. 3.

To maintain dignity/self-worth (Teaching/Discharge Considerations) and enhance well-being (long-term goals):

- 🏠 Discuss the client's human and civil rights as an individual. **Although hospitals and other care settings have a client's bill of rights, a broader view of human dignity is enshrined in laws of most countries and the United Nations.**
- ᗧ Use a shared decision-making model incorporating identified familial, spiritual, and cultural factors that have meaning for the client when planning for future. **Collaboration between healthcare team members and client, honoring client's desires and needs, increases feelings of inclusion for the client and likelihood of success of plan.**
- Stress importance of continuing use of new skills such as mindfulness and assertive communication. **Learning and**

Information that appears in brackets has been added by the authors to clarify and enhance the use of nursing diagnoses.

➕ Acute Care   ᗧ Collaborative   🏠 Community/Home Care   🌐 Cultural

using skills such as mindfulness and assertive communication is an ongoing process for growth and development of self-worth.
- Refer to community resources/services (e.g., pastoral care, counseling, organized support groups, classes), as appropriate. **May need additional assistance to access supports that promote diversity and inclusion for everyone in dealing with illness/disability or life situation.**

Documentation Focus

Assessment/Reassessment
- Assessment findings, including individual risk factors, client's perceptions, and concerns about involvement in care
- Individual cultural and spiritual beliefs, values, healthcare goals
- Responses and involvement of family/SO(s)

Planning
- Plan of care and who is involved in planning
- Teaching plan

Implementation/Evaluation
- Client's response to interventions, teaching, and actions performed
- Attainment or progress toward desired outcome(s)
- Modifications to plan of care

Discharge Planning
- Long-term needs and who is responsible for actions to be taken
- Specific referrals made

Sample Nursing Outcomes & Interventions Classifications NOC/NIC

NOC—Client Satisfaction: Protection of Rights
NIC—Cultural Care Negotiation

DISCOMFORT ICNP

[Diagnostic Division: Comfort]

Definition: Physical or mental uneasiness, unpleasant feelings, personal suffering negatively affecting individual's sense of well-being.

Information that appears in brackets has been added by the authors to clarify and enhance the use of nursing diagnoses.

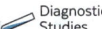 Diagnostic Studies   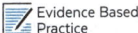 Evidence Based Practice   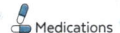 Medications   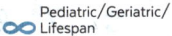 Pediatric/Geriatric/Lifespan

Recognizing Cues

Related/Risk Factors
Unmet/unrelieved physical symptoms, pain
Psychological distress
Unpleasant environmental stimuli
Lack of control of situation
Inadequate health knowledge, resources, support

Defining Characteristics

Subjective
Lack of physical comfort
Feeling sadness, annoyance, anxious
Depressive symptoms
Unable to relax; impaired sleep pattern; fatigue

Objective
Distorted facial expressions, frowning, grimacing
Moaning; crying
Restless; irritable mood; agitated
Sighing; withdrawn; avoids social contact
Impaired concentration

Clinical Connections
Presence of chronic physical or psychological conditions

Generate Solutions

Plan Desired Outcomes

Client Will (Include Specific Time Frame)
- Engage in behaviors or lifestyle changes to increase level of ease.
- Verbalize sense of comfort or contentment.
- Participate in desirable and realistic health-seeking/wellness behaviors.

Interventions/Take Action

Nursing Priority No. 1.
To assess etiology/precipitating contributory factors:
- Determine the type of discomfort the client is experiencing, such as physical pain; feeling of discontent; lack of

---

Information that appears in brackets has been added by the authors to clarify and enhance the use of nursing diagnoses.

 Acute Care Collaborative 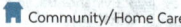 Community/Home Care Cultural

ease with self, environment, or sociocultural settings; or inability to rise above one's problems or pain (lack of transcendence). Have the client rate total comfort, using a scale of 0 to 10, with 10 being as comfortable as possible, or a "general comfort" questionnaire using a Likert-type scale. **A comfort scale is similar to a pain rating scale and can help the client identify the focus of discomfort (e.g., physical, emotional, or social).**

- Note cultural or religious beliefs and values that impact perceptions and expectations of comfort. **Client does not think, feel, or believe the same ideas.**
- Ascertain locus of control. **The presence of an external locus of control may hamper efforts to achieve a sense of peace or contentment.**
- Discuss concerns with the client and active-listen to identify underlying issues (e.g., physical and emotional stressors or external factors such as environmental surroundings; social interactions) that could impact the client's ability to control own well-being. **Helps to determine the client's specific needs and ability to change own situation.**
- Establish context(s) in which lack of comfort is realized: *physical* (pertaining to bodily sensations), *psychospiritual* (pertaining to internal awareness of self and meaning in one's life, relationship to a higher order or being), *environmental* (pertaining to external surroundings, conditions, and influences), or *sociocultural* (pertaining to interpersonal, family, and societal relationships). **Note: A recent integrative review study showed that "Comfort is multidimensional, experienced by patients as a sense of positivity and strength characterized not only by the relief of physical discomfort but an integration of positive emotions that include feeling confident, competent, having a sense of personal control, feeling cared for, valued, safe (able to trust) and at ease."**

Physical

- Determine how the client is managing pain and pain components. **Lack of comfort may be exacerbated by other issues or emotions such as fear, loneliness, anxiety, noxious stimuli, or anger.**
- Identify client's environmental needs such as privacy, room temperature, natural lighting, windows to view outdoors,

---

Information that appears in brackets has been added by the authors to clarify and enhance the use of nursing diagnoses.

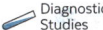 Diagnostic Studies 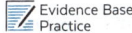 Evidence Based Practice 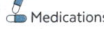 Medications 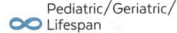 Pediatric/Geriatric/Lifespan

loud noises, pollution, and allergies. **Enhancing comfort includes manipulating the environment for clients as appropriate.**
- Ascertain what has been tried or is required for comfort or rest (e.g., head of bed up or down, music on or off, white noise, rocking motion, certain person or thing; ability to express and/or manage conflicts).

Psychological
- Determine how psychological, social, and spiritual indicators overlap (e.g., meaningfulness, faith, identity, and self-esteem) for the client. **Clients experiencing grief/loss of family or cultural support, social isolation, or feelings of spiritual abandonment may find prayer helpful. Research reports prayer and spirituality can improve distress and health outcomes.**
- Identify meaning of comfort in context of interpersonal, family, and cultural values and societal relationships. **Clients experiencing ordinary discomforts of life feel uneasy because they cannot control changes such as birth or death. Or change is not accepted when having to accept doing or giving up something important to the client. A conditional state of discomfort is a client whose thoughts, judgments, or self-commentary result in butterflies, or nervousness. In general, a client's lack of confidence, thoughts, and feelings regarding interactions with others may cause an uneasiness/nervousness/stress. Culture has a significant impact on both diagnoses and treatment options, primarily because of different social beliefs but also because of biological factors. Many studies have shown that people from different cultures see and perceive things differently, probably due to how their culture shaped the way they view the world. However, culture shapes a person's thoughts in a unique way for each individual.**
- Identify length of time client has had nervous or unpleasant feelings. **Lengthy periods of discord can lead to mental health disorders such as depression or anxiety.**
- Identify the client's ideas of comfort/discomfort with family/friends during interactions or with relationships. **Clients experiencing ordinary discomforts of life feel uneasy because they cannot control changes such as birth or death. Or change is not accepted when having to accept doing or giving up something important to the client. Last, a conditional state of discomfort is a client whose**

Information that appears in brackets has been added by the authors to clarify and enhance the use of nursing diagnoses.

 Acute Care Collaborative 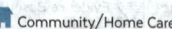 Community/Home Care  Cultural

thoughts, judgments, or self-commentary result in butterflies, or nervousness. In general, a client's lack of confidence, thoughts, and feelings regarding interactions with others may cause an uneasiness/nervousness/stress to participate.

- Determine if the client/significant other (SO) desires support regarding spiritual enrichment, including prayer, meditation, or access to a spiritual counselor of choice. **A recent review study reported statistical correlations between religiosity, spirituality, and health outcomes, including cardiovascular conditions common among older persons (e.g., heart disease, blood pressure, cholesterol, myocardial infarction, and stroke). Beneficial effects were seen with respect to disability and functional limitation, kidney function, cirrhosis, emphysema, chronic pain, cancer, and self-rated overall health.**

Nursing Priority No. 2.

To assist client to alleviate discomfort:

- Interact with the client in a therapeutic manner. **The nurse could be the most important comfort intervention for meeting clients' needs. For example, assuring the client that nausea can be treated successfully with both pharmacological and nonpharmacological methods may be more effective than simply administering an antiemetic without reassurance and a comforting presence.**
- Encourage verbalization of feelings and be available for listening/interacting. **Promotes self-esteem and guides interactions and interventions with the client.**
- Review knowledge base and note coping skills that have been used previously to change behavior/promote well-being. **Brings these to client's awareness and promotes use in the current situation.**
- Acknowledge the client's strengths in the present situation and build on these strengths in planning for the future.

Physical

- 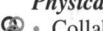 Collaborate in treating or managing medical conditions involving oxygenation, elimination, mobility, cognitive abilities, electrolyte balance, thermoregulation, and hydration **to promote physical stability.**
- Work with the client to prevent pain, nausea, itching, and thirst/other physical discomforts.
- Review medications or treatment regimen **to determine possible changes or options to reduce side effects.**

Information that appears in brackets has been added by the authors to clarify and enhance the use of nursing diagnoses.

- ∞ • Suggest that the parent be present during procedures **to comfort child.**
- ∞ • Provide age-appropriate comfort measures (e.g., presence, gentle touch, change of position, cuddling, and use of heat/cold) **to provide nonpharmacological pain management.**
- 💊 • Discuss interventions/activities such as Therapeutic Touch, massage, healing touch, biofeedback, self-hypnosis, guided imagery, and breathing exercises; play therapy; and humor **to promote ease and relaxation and to refocus attention.**
- 💊 • Assist the client to use and modify medication regimen **to make the best use of pharmacological pain or symptom management.**
- Assist the client/SO(s) to develop a plan for activity and exercise within individual ability, emphasizing the necessity of allowing sufficient time to finish activities.
- Maintain open and flexible visitation as client desires.
- Provide for periodic changes in the personal surroundings when client is confined. Use the individual's input in creating the changes (e.g., seasonal bulletin boards, color changes, rearranging furniture, pictures).
- Encourage/plan care to allow individually adequate rest periods **to prevent fatigue. Schedule activities for periods when the client has the most energy to maximize participation.**
- Discuss routines to promote restful sleep and modifications to environment to enhance comfort.

Psychological

- Encourage client to make use of beneficial coping behaviors and to develop assertiveness skills, prioritizing goals and activities. **Promotes sense of control and improves self-esteem.**
- Establish realistic activity goals with the client. **Enhances self-esteem, independence, and a sense of wellness. Note: Wellness can exist in the presence of disease as individuals live the experience of striving to function at maximum ability with minimal symptoms and suffering. Many people are functioning with a diagnosed disease—diabetes, asthma, arthritis, advanced heart or kidney disease, cancer, hypertension, to name but a few.**
- Involve the client/SO(s) in schedule planning and decisions about timing and spacing of treatments **to promote relaxation/reduce sense of boredom.**

Information that appears in brackets has been added by the authors to clarify and enhance the use of nursing diagnoses.

- Encourage the client to do whatever possible (e.g., self-care, sit up in chair, or walk). **Enhances self-esteem, independence, and a sense of wellness. For the most part, individuals say of themselves that they are "well" when they are functioning at their perceived highest level.**
- Avoid overstimulation or understimulation (cognitive and sensory). **Maintaining a balance with a daily schedule of activities of daily living, socialization, activities/interest/hobbies, and rest promotes comfort and enjoyment.**
- Encourage age-appropriate diversional activities (e.g., TV, radio, music, computer/video games, playtime, chatting, texting with family/friends, socialization/outings with others, volunteering). **Limits dwelling on negatives and helps to transcend unpleasant sensations and situations. Facilitates activities with others, develops relationships, and prevents isolation. Note: Avoid activities such as computer games unless others are included.**
- Support cultural interests and activities (e.g., festivals, art, language, music, foods, or dance). **Participating in own and other cultural activities (cultural exchange) develops an appreciation, and awareness of self and others.**
- Identify ways to achieve connectedness or harmony with self, others, nature, or a higher power. **Encouraging meditation, mindfulness, yoga, walks in nature, and showing gratitude foster spiritual wellness.**
- Assist client/family/SO to identify and provide a stress-free or a pleasant environment. **Reducing loud noises, comfortable room temperatures, adequate lighting, windows allowing client to view outdoors, moving furniture or changing wall decorations promote relaxation and sense of well-being.**

Nursing Priority No. 3.

To promote sense of physical/psychological comfort (Teaching/Discharge Considerations) and enhance well-being (long-term goals):

- Provide information about conditions/health risk factors or concerns in desired format (e.g., pictures, TV programs, articles, handouts, or audio/visual materials; classes, group discussions, internet websites, and other databases), as appropriate. **The use of multiple modalities enhances acquisition/retention of information and gives the client choices for accessing and applying information.**

Information that appears in brackets has been added by the authors to clarify and enhance the use of nursing diagnoses.

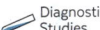 Diagnostic Studies 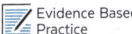 Evidence Based Practice 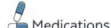 Medications 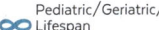 Pediatric/Geriatric/Lifespan

- Discuss potential complications and the possible need for medical follow-up or alternative therapies. **Timely recognition and intervention can promote wellness.**
- Promote overall health measures (e.g., nutrition, adequate fluid intake, appropriate vitamin or iron supplementation).
- Assist the client/SO(s) to identify and acquire necessary equipment (e.g., lifts, commode chair, safety grab bars, or personal hygiene supplies) to meet individual needs. Refer to appropriate suppliers.
- Collaborate with others when the client expresses interest in lessons, counseling, coaching, and/or mentoring. **Enhance emotional growth and development supporting issues of comfort.**
- Encourage client's contributions toward meeting realistic goals. **Encouraging sensible and obtainable goals builds confidence in life.**
- Advocate for growth-promoting environment in conflict situations and consider issues from client/family and cultural perspective. **Developing awareness of others' emotions and responses while communicating can be a starting point to resolving conflict.**
- Recommend client take time to be introspective in the search for contentment or transcendence. **Client's discovering ways to practice gratitude, volunteering for acts of kindness, employing spiritual practices (e.g., meditation, reading books on philosophy and personal growth to expand new ideas or worldviews, or joining a spiritual group) keep client aware of their inner self that is centered and connected to the world surrounding the client.**
- Recommend participation in diverse cultural activities. **Facilitates developing a diverse appreciation of others and self-awareness of own identity.**
- Encourage creation of a compassionate supportive and therapeutic environment incorporating client's cultural, age, and developmental factors. **Stimulates a sense of well-being and a caring atmosphere where individuals function at their highest level of potential.**
- Discuss long-term plan for taking care of environmental needs.
- Identify resources or referrals (e.g., knowledge and skills, financial resources or assistance, personal or psychological support group, social activities). **External support promotes knowledge and skills that promote growth and development with self-sufficiency.**

Information that appears in brackets has been added by the authors to clarify and enhance the use of nursing diagnoses.

Documentation Focus

Assessment/Reassessment
- Individual findings including client's description of current status/situation and factors impacting sense of comfort
- Pertinent cultural and religious beliefs and values
- Medication use and nonpharmacological measures

Planning
- Plan of care, specific interventions, and who is involved in planning
- Teaching plan

Implementation/Evaluation
- Responses to interventions, teaching, and actions performed
- Attainment of or progress toward desired outcome(s)
- Modifications to plan of care

Discharge Planning
- Long-term needs and who is responsible for actions to be taken
- Specific referrals made

Sample Nursing Outcomes & Interventions Classifications NOC/NIC

NOC—Comfort Status
NIC—Environmental Management

---

decreased DIVERSIONAL ACTIVITY ENGAGEMENT NANDA-I

[Diagnostic Division: Activity/Rest]

Definition: Reduced stimulation, interest, or participation in recreational or leisure activities.

Recognizing Cues

Related/Risk Factors
Current setting does not allow engagement in activities; inadequate available activities
Unaddressed environmental distractions
Impaired physical mobility; prolonged inactivity; inadequate physical endurance
Inadequate motivation; psychological distress

Information that appears in brackets has been added by the authors to clarify and enhance the use of nursing diagnoses.

 Diagnostic Studies 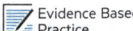 Evidence Based Practice 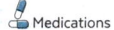 Medications ∞ Pediatric/Geriatric/Lifespan

Defining Characteristics

Subjective
Lacks motivation; discontentment with environment or situation

Objective
Altered mood; flat affect
Physical deconditioning; frequent naps

Clinical Connections
Traumatic injuries, chronic pain, prolonged recovery (e.g., postoperative, complicated fractures), cancer therapy, chronic/debilitating conditions (e.g., congestive heart failure, chronic obstructive pulmonary disease, renal failure, multiple sclerosis), awaiting organ transplantation, depression, phobias, or anxiety

Generate Solutions

Plan Desired Outcomes

Client Will (Include Specific Time Frame)
- Recognize own psychological response (e.g., hopelessness and helplessness, anger, depression) and initiate appropriate coping actions.
- Engage in satisfying activities within personal limitations.

Interventions/Take Action

Nursing Priority No. 1.
To assess precipitating/etiological factors:
- Assess client's physical, cognitive, emotional, and environmental status limiting recreational activities. **Validates the reality of environmental deprivation (Social Determinants of Health) where it exists and considers potential for loss of desired diversional activities in order to plan for prevention or early interventions. Note: Studies show that key problems faced by clients who are hospitalized (or immobilized) for extended periods of time include dull, tedious repetition, stress, and depression. These negative states can impede recovery and lead clients to report symptoms more frequently.**
- Observe for restlessness, flat facial expression, withdrawal, hostility, yawning, or statements of boredom as noted earlier, especially in individual likely to be confined either

---

Information that appears in brackets has been added by the authors to clarify and enhance the use of nursing diagnoses.

 Acute Care 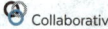 Collaborative 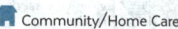 Community/Home Care 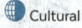 Cultural

temporarily or long term. **May be indicative of need for diversional interventions.**

- Note potential impact of disability or illness on lifestyle (e.g., young child with leukemia, elderly person with fractured hip, individual with severe depression). **A lack of activities to stimulate interest in visual, auditory, olfactory, or tactile senses limits client's ability to enjoy or relax to the quality of the surrounding environment. For example, bird watching, smelling the fresh air, flowers, or watching the sunrise/sunset, listening to music, working with clay for pottery, finger painting, or other arts of interest to the client are easy to engage in and require few resources.**
- Be aware of age and developmental level, gender, cultural factors, and the importance of a given activity in the client's life. **Cultural issues include gender roles, communication styles, privacy and personal space, expectations and views regarding time and activities, control of the immediate environment, family traditions, and social patterns. When illness interferes with an individual's ability to engage in usual activities, the person may have difficulty engaging in meaningful substitute activities.**
- Determine client's ability to participate and interest in available activities, noting attention span, physical limitations and tolerance, level of interest or desire, and safety needs. **The presence of acute illness, depression, problems of mobility, protective isolation, or sensory deprivation may interfere with desired activity. However, lack of involvement may not reflect client's abilities but may rather be a matter of misperception of their abilities.**

Nursing Priority No. 2.

To motivate and stimulate client involvement in solutions:

- Establish nurse/client therapeutic relationship, acknowledging reality of situation and client's feelings. **Client may be feeling sense of loss when unable to participate in usual activities or to interact socially as desired.**
- Include new activities or continue activities that help client cope with conditions such as anxiety, depression, grief, dementia, physical injury, isolation and immobility, malnutrition, acute or chronic pain, etc. **Health conditions may interfere with the individual's ability to engage in meaningful diversional activities. Creative approaches may be required to engage client.**

Information that appears in brackets has been added by the authors to clarify and enhance the use of nursing diagnoses.

- Introduce activities at client's current level of functioning, progressing to more complex activities, as tolerated. **Provides opportunity for client to experience successes, reaffirming capabilities and enhancing self-esteem.**
- Show interest in client's stated activities, hobbies, or desire to develop a new hobby. **Encourages continuation of desired arts, recreation, or crafts. Also, demonstrates support and enhances the therapeutic relationship.**
- Accept hostile expressions while limiting aggressive acting-out behavior. **Permission to express feelings of anger and hopelessness allows for beginning resolution. However, destructive behavior is counterproductive to self-esteem and problem-solving.**
- Involve client and parent/significant other/caregiver in determining client's needs, desires, and available resources. **Client-centered care (client/provider collaboration) helps ensure that plan is attentive to client's interests and resources, increasing likelihood of client participation**
- Encourage parent/caregiver of young child to engage in play with confined child. **Play is essential to young child's development, can help redirect child's attention from pain of condition, and reduce child's boredom and stress.**
- Review history of lifelong activities and hobbies client has enjoyed. Discuss reasons client is not doing these activities now and whether client can or would like to resume these activities. **Diversional activities can provide positive and productive avenues into which client can channel thoughts and feelings.**
- Assist client/caregiver to set realistic goals for diversional activities, communicating hope and patience. **Can help client realize that this situation is not hopeless, that there are choices for improving the current situation, and that the future can hold the promise for improvement.**
- Provide instruction in relaxation techniques (e.g., meditation, yoga, deep breathing exercises, soft music, guided visualization). **Enhances coping skills.**
- Participate in decisions about timing and spacing of visitors, leisure, and care activities. **Scheduling time for relaxation and activities can reduce sense of dissatisfaction or restlessness, as well as prevent overstimulation and exhaustion.**
- Encourage client to assist in scheduling required and optional activity choices. **For example, client may want to watch favorite television show at bath time; if bath**

Information that appears in brackets has been added by the authors to clarify and enhance the use of nursing diagnoses.

 Acute Care Collaborative 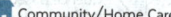 Community/Home Care Cultural

can be rescheduled later, client's sense of control is enhanced.
- Encourage a mix of desired activities and stimuli (e.g., music, news, educational presentations—TV/videos/podcasts, movies, computer or internet access, books and other reading materials, visitors, games, arts and crafts, sensory enrichment [e.g., massage, aromatherapy], grooming and beauty care, cooking, social outings, gardening, or discussion groups, as appropriate). **Activities need to be personally meaningful and not physically or emotionally overwhelming for the client to derive the most benefit.**
- Refrain from making changes in the schedule without discussing with the client. **It is important for staff to be responsible in making and following through on commitments to client.**
- Provide a change of scenery (indoors and outdoors where possible) to **provide positive sensory stimulation, reduce sense of boredom, and improve sense of normalcy and control.**
- Identify requirements for mobility (wheelchair, walker, van, volunteers, etc.). **Makes it possible for the individual to participate safely in desired activities.**
- Suggest activities, such as bird feeders or baths for bird watching, a garden in a window box or terrarium, or a fish bowl or aquarium **to stimulate observation as well as involvement and participation in activity, such as identification of birds, choice of seeds, and so forth.**
- Identify and involve recreational, occupational, play, music, and/or movement therapist as appropriate. **Activities should be enjoyable for client, and collaborating with therapist helps in procuring assistive devices or modifying activities for individual situation. Assists client to express needs and feelings, share experiences, escape healthcare routines, and participate in self-healing.**

Nursing Priority No. 3.

To promote continued involvement (Teaching/Discharge Considerations) and enhance general well-being (long-term goals):

- Explore options for useful activities using the person's strengths and abilities. **Finding hands-on or observational activities keeps the client engaged with others or the environment, thus, preventing distress and boredom.**
- Make referrals to available professional resources (e.g., exercise groups, senior activities, hobby clubs, volunteering, companion and service organizations) **to provide new**

Information that appears in brackets has been added by the authors to clarify and enhance the use of nursing diagnoses.

contacts/support to continue diversional activities in community/home settings enhancing self-worth.
- Refer to NDs difficulty Coping; lack of Resilience, inadequate Social Connectedness for additional interventions.

Documentation Focus

Assessment/Reassessment
- Specific assessment findings, including blocks to desired activities
- Individual choices for activities

Planning
- Plan of care, specific interventions, and who is involved in planning
- Teaching plan

Implementation/Evaluation
- Client's responses to interventions, teaching, and actions performed
- Attainment of or progress toward desired outcome(s)
- Modifications to plan of care

Discharge Planning
- Long-term needs and who is responsible for actions to be taken
- Referrals and community resources

Sample Nursing Outcomes & Interventions Classifications NOC/NIC

NOC—Leisure Participation
NIC—Recreation Therapy

---

risk for **DRY EYE**   NANDA-I

[Diagnostic Division: Comfort]

Definition: Susceptible to persistently unstable and/or deficient tear film causing discomfort and/or visual impairment.

Recognizing Cues

Risk Factors
Decreased blinking frequency; inappropriate use of contact lenses; inadequate fluid intake

---

Information that appears in brackets has been added by the authors to clarify and enhance the use of nursing diagnoses.

Air pollution; excessive wind; low air humidity; prolonged sunlight exposure

Caffeine consumption; unaddressed vitamin A deficiency; omega-3 fatty acids deficiency

Inadequate knowledge of modifiable factors; excessive screen time; tobacco use; inattentive to secondhand smoke

Inappropriate use of fans, or hair dryer; prolonged air-conditioning exposure

Use of products with benzalkonium chloride preservatives

Clinical Connections

Any condition where client is unable to protect self from drying of eye tissues, including facial or general trauma or surgery; mechanical ventilation; brain injury, cerebrovascular accident; neurological conditions such as Parkinson disease, Bell palsy; diabetic retinopathy; lupus; rheumatoid arthritis; allergies, chemotherapy, radiotherapy

Generate Solutions

Plan Desired Outcomes

Client Will (Include Specific Time Frame)
- Be free of discomfort or damage to eye related to dryness.
- Verbalize understanding of risk factors and ways to prevent dry eye.

Interventions/Take Action

Nursing Priority No. 1.
To identify causative/precipitating factors related to risk:

- Obtain a history of eye conditions when assessing client concerns overall. Note reports of dry sensation, burning, itching, pain, foreign body sensation, light sensitivity (photophobia), and blurred vision. **These symptoms can be associated with dry eye syndrome and, if present, require further evaluation and possible treatment.**
- Note the presence of conditions listed in risk factors/Clinical Connections leading to **dry eye syndrome. It is caused by increased tear evaporation or insufficient aqueous tear production and can occur because of damage to the eye surface (e.g., chemical burn) or may be associated with disease conditions, neurological disorders, environmental factors, and electronic device use.**

Information that appears in brackets has been added by the authors to clarify and enhance the use of nursing diagnoses.

- Note the client's gender and age. **Studies show a higher prevalence of dry eye syndrome in females than in males, especially aged over 50.**
- Determine the client's current situation (e.g., admitted to facility for procedures/surgery, recent neurological event, mechanical ventilation, facial or eye trauma; eye infections, lower eyelid malposition) **that places the client at high risk for dry eye associated with low or absent blink reflex and/or decreased tear production.**
- Determine the client's history/presence of seasonal or environmental allergies, **which may cause or exacerbate conjunctivitis.**
- Review living and work environments to identify factors (e.g., exposure to smoke, wind, or chemicals; poor lighting; long periods of computer use or eye-straining work).
- Assess the client's medications, noting the use of certain drugs (e.g., antihistamines, beta blockers, antidepressants, and oral contraceptives) **known to decrease tear production.**
- Refer for diagnostic evaluation and interventions as indicated.

Nursing Priority No. 2.
To promote eye health/comfort:

- Assist in/refer for treatment of underlying cause of dry eyes. **Interventions could range from changing a medication that is causing decreased tear production to surgery to correcting an anatomical abnormality of the eyelid that interferes with blinking. Referral may be needed (e.g., to rheumatologist or endocrinologist for treatment of autoimmune condition or diabetes).**
- Administer artificial tears, lubricating eyedrops, or ointments as indicated, **when the client is unable to blink or otherwise protect eyes while in healthcare facility.**

Nursing Priority No. 3.
To promote safety (Teaching/Discharge Considerations) and enhance well-being (long-term goals):

- Instruct high-risk client in self-management interventions **to prevent or limit symptoms of dry eye:**
- Avoid air blowing in eyes **such as might occur with hair dryers, car heaters, air conditioners, or fans directed toward eyes.**
- Wear eyeglasses or safety shield glasses on windy days **to reduce effects of the wind** and goggles while swimming **to protect eyes from chemicals in the water.**

Information that appears in brackets has been added by the authors to clarify and enhance the use of nursing diagnoses.

- Take proper care of contact lenses and adhere to prescribed wearing time.
- Add moisture to indoor air, especially in winter.
- Take eye breaks during long reading and computer tasks or when watching TV for long periods of time.
- Blink repeatedly for a few seconds **to help spread tears evenly over eye.**
- Position computer screen below eye level. **May help slow the evaporation of tears between eye blinks.**
- Recommend cessation of smoking and avoidance of smoking environments. **Smoke can worsen dry eye symptoms.**
- Discuss dietary changes if indicated. **Some physicians and nutritionists recommend a diet high in vitamin A and/or a diet high in omega-3 fatty acids to prevent dry eye associated with vitamin A deficiency.**

Documentation Focus

Assessment/Reassessment
- Individual risk factors identified
- Client concerns or difficulty making and following through with plan

Planning
- Plan of care and who is involved in planning
- Teaching plan

Implementation/Evaluation
- Response to interventions, teaching, and actions performed
- Attainment of or progress toward outcomes

Discharge Planning
- Referrals to other resources
- Long-term need and who is responsible for actions

Sample Nursing Outcomes & Interventions Classifications NOC/NIC

NOC—Dry Eye Severity
NIC—Dry Eye Prevention

Information that appears in brackets has been added by the authors to clarify and enhance the use of nursing diagnoses.

 Diagnostic Studies   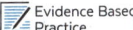 Evidence Based Practice   Medications   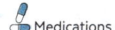 Pediatric/Geriatric/Lifespan

ineffective DRY MOUTH SELF-MANAGEMENT NANDA-I

[Diagnostic Division: Comfort]

Definition: Unsatisfactory handling of treatment regimen, consequences, and lifestyle changes associated with reduced salivary secretion.

Recognizing Cues

Related Factors

Inadequate knowledge of modifiable factors; inadequate action to address modifiable factors
Inadequate knowledge of substance that increases mouth dryness
Inadequate knowledge of oral hygiene; inadequate access to dental care
Inadequate knowledge of treatment regimen; inadequate commitment to plan of care
Competing demands; competing lifestyle preferences; conflict between health behaviors and social norms
Inadequate health literacy; inadequate self-efficacy; inadequate social support
Excessive stress; depressive symptoms
Difficulty managing complex treatment regimen
Nonacceptance of condition; unaware of seriousness of condition; unaware of susceptibility to sequelae
Negative feelings toward treatment regimen; perceived barrier to treatment regimen
Unrealistic expectation of treatment benefits
Inadequate caregiver knowledge of modifiable factors

Defining Characteristics

Subjective

Dry mouth symptoms
Mouth dryness; oral discomfort; burning sensation; halitosis
Decreased taste perception; difficulty chewing, swallowing
Exacerbation of dry mouth symptoms
Difficulty speaking
Behaviors
Inadequate oral hygiene practices

Objective

Dry mouth signs
Dry mucous membranes; pale, lusterless mucous membranes

Information that appears in brackets has been added by the authors to clarify and enhance the use of nursing diagnoses.

 Acute Care   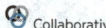 Collaborative   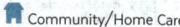 Community/Home Care   Cultural

Atrophic mucous membranes; ruptured mucous membranes
Oral fissure; lip fissure
Excessive dental plaque
Exacerbation of dry mouth signs
Dry mouth complications
Dental caries; marginal periodontitis; gingivitis; oral ulcer
Glossitis; oral infections
Behaviors
Mouth breathing
Inadequate oral hygiene practices
Inadequate use of dry mouth guard, oral lubricant, saliva stimulant or substitute
Eats foods that increase mouth dryness; frequent consumption of fluids during meals
Uses substances, nonprescription drugs that increase mouth dryness
Inadequate fluid intake; inadequate maintenance of air humidity

Clinical Connections
Chemotherapy; radiotherapy to the head and neck; radical oral/neck surgery; conditions restricting oral intake; renal dialysis; thyroid disease; oxygen therapy

Generate Solutions

Plan Desired Outcomes

Client Will (Include Specific Time Frame)
- Be free of discomfort or damage to mouth related to dryness.
- Verbalize understanding of risk factors and ways to prevent dry mouth.
  Note: Many of the assessments and interventions in this ND are the same as or similar to those in ND: impaired oral Mucous Membrane.

Interventions/Take Action

Nursing Priority No. 1.
To identify causative/contributing factors:

- Perform oral screening or comprehensive assessment upon admission to facility using tool (e.g., Oral Health Assessment Tool for Long-Term Care), as indicated. **Use of standardized tool is beneficial in evaluating health of entire mouth, including lips, tongue, gums, and other soft tissues.**

Information that appears in brackets has been added by the authors to clarify and enhance the use of nursing diagnoses.

 Diagnostic Studies 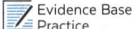 Evidence Based Practice Medications Pediatric/Geriatric/Lifespan

- Note presence of diseases/conditions (e.g., Sjögren syndrome, dementias, diabetes, anemia, cystic fibrosis, rheumatoid arthritis, hypertension, Parkinson disease, stroke; dehydration [as might occur with fever, vomiting, diarrhea, blood loss, burns]) and treatments (e.g., nerve damage to the head and neck from injury or surgery; damage to the salivary glands as might occur from radiation to the head and neck, or chemotherapy for various cancers). **These factors/conditions are often associated with dry mouth.**
- Review client's medications. **Dry mouth is a common side effect of many prescription and nonprescription drugs, including (but not limited to) muscle relaxants, sedatives, antidepressants, psychotropics, anti-anxiety agents; analgesics, antihistamines/decongestants; antiepileptics, antihypertensives, diuretics; antidiarrheals, antiemetics, bronchodilators.**
- Perform regular oral examinations (periodically, such as when seen in clinic) or daily (in acute care). Pay attention to client reports of thirst, burning in mouth or tongue; dry throat; problems swallowing or speaking. Observe for dried, flaky, whitish saliva in and around the mouth, thick saliva that sticks to lip, bits of food or other matter on the teeth, tongue, and gums; cracked lips, raw-appearing red tongue, sores in corners of mouth; bad breath. **These signs and symptoms are associated with severely dry mouth, reduced saliva, and possible systemic dehydration. Note: If client is receiving radiation therapy for cancer, the symptoms can greatly increase client's discomfort.**
- Determine status of oral hygiene. Observe for chipped, sharp-edged, or malpositioned teeth. Note fit of dentures or other prosthetic appliances when used. **Healthy teeth or well-fitting dentures have a strong effect on oral health and comfort of the oral mucosa, as well as the ability to eat (chewing, swallowing). Conversely, dry mouth can contribute to dental cavities and mouth infections.**
- Determine problems with food and fluid intake (e.g., avoiding eating, reports change in taste, chews painstakingly, swallows numerous times for even small bites; insufficient fluid intake/dehydration; unexplained weight loss). **Malnutrition and dehydration are associated with problems with oral mucous membranes.**
- Evaluate lifestyle concerns (e.g., smoking, chewing tobacco, breathing or sleeping with open mouth) **that may be contributing to dryness.**

Information that appears in brackets has been added by the authors to clarify and enhance the use of nursing diagnoses.

Nursing Priority No. 2.
- To correct identified/developing problems:
- Collaborate in treatment of underlying conditions. **May correct or reduce problem with dry mouth.**
- Adjust medication regimen, if indicated, **to reduce use of drugs with potential for causing or exacerbating painful dry mouth.**
- Provide or encourage regular oral care (e.g., after meals and at bedtime) using soft-bristle brush to cleanse teeth and oral tissues.
- Provide mouth care (e.g., water, sodium bicarbonate solutions, mucosal coating agents, topical anesthetic gargles). Use petroleum jelly, cocoa butter, or a mild lip balm to keep lips moist. **May improve client comfort by hydration of mucous membrane surfaces.**
- Avoid mouthwashes containing alcohol **(drying effect)** or hydrogen peroxide **(drying and foul tasting).**
- Use lemon/glycerin swabs with caution. **The use of glycerin swabs appears to be controversial, with some stating that glycerin should not be used, as it absorbs water and actually dries the oral cavity.**
- Encourage use of sugar-free chewing gum or sucking on hard candy **to stimulate flow of saliva to neutralize acids and limit bacterial growth.**
- Avoid dry foods, such as crackers, cookies, and toast, or soften them with liquids before eating. Sip liquids with meals to moisten foods and help with swallowing.
- Encourage adequate fluids **to prevent dehydration and oral dryness and limit bacterial overgrowth.**
- Suggest use of vaporizer or room humidifier **to increase humidity if client is mouth breather or ambient humidity is low.**
- Discuss and instruct caregiver(s) in special mouth care required during end-of-life care/hospice **to promote optimal comfort in client who has stopped eating or drinking, has dry mouth, and may not have sensation of thirst.**

Nursing Priority No. 3.
To promote appropriate salivation and subsequent oral health (Teaching/Discharge Considerations) and enhance well-being (long-term goals):
- Recommend regular dental checkups and care, as well as episodic evaluation of oral health prior to certain medical treatments (e.g., chemotherapy, radiation), **to maintain oral health and reduce risks associated with impaired tissues.**

Information that appears in brackets has been added by the authors to clarify and enhance the use of nursing diagnoses.

- Review current oral hygiene practices and concerns. Provide informational resources, including reliable websites about oral health **to reinforce learning and encourage proper care.**
- Provide nutritional information **to correct deficiencies, reduce mucosal inflammation or gum disease, and prevent dental caries.**
- Emphasize benefit of avoiding alcohol and smoking or chewing tobacco, **which can contribute to mucosal inflammation and gum disease.**
- Discuss need for and demonstrate use of special appliances (e.g., power toothbrushes, dental water jets, flossing instruments, applicators) if indicated.
- Identify community resources (e.g., low-cost dental clinics, smoking-cessation resources, cancer information services or support group, Meals on Wheels, supplemental nutrition program, home-care aide).

Documentation Focus

Assessment/Reassessment
- Condition of oral mucous membranes, routine oral care habits and interferences
- Availability of oral care equipment and products
- Knowledge of proper oral hygiene and care
- Availability and use of resources

Planning
- Plan of care and who is involved in planning
- Teaching plan

Implementation/Evaluation
- Responses to interventions, teaching, and actions performed
- Attainment of or progress toward desired outcome(s)
- Modifications to plan of care

Discharge Planning
- Long-term needs and who is responsible for actions to be taken
- Specific referrals made, resources for special appliances

Sample Nursing Outcomes & Interventions Classifications NOC/NIC

NOC—Oral Health
NIC—Oral Health Restoration

Information that appears in brackets has been added by the authors to clarify and enhance the use of nursing diagnoses.

ineffective adolescent EATING DYNAMICS   NANDA-I

[Diagnostic Division: Food/Fluid]

Definition: Altered attitudes and behaviors resulting in over or undereating patterns that compromise nutritional health in individual 11 to 19 years of age.

Recognizing Cues

Related/Risk Factors
Altered family relations; negative parental influences on eating behaviors

Anxiety; excessive stress; food insecurity

Changes to self-esteem upon entering puberty; inappropriate peer pressure

Eating disorder; eating in isolation; inappropriate dietary habits

Excessive family mealtime control; intrusive parenting behaviors; irregular mealtime; stressful mealtimes

Media influence on knowledge of, or eating behaviors of high-caloric unhealthy foods

Psychological neglect; unaddressed abuse

Defining Characteristics

Subjective
Complains of hunger between meals; inadequate appetite; food refusal

Objective
Frequent snacking; frequently consumes fast food or low-quality food; diet high in processed foods

Avoids participation in regular mealtimes

Overeating, undereating

Shifting toward less-nutritious, lower-cost, or nonperishable foods

Depressive symptoms

Clinical Connections
Anorexia, bulimia nervosa, obesity, bariatric surgery, substance abuse, depression, anxiety disorder, parental psychiatric disorder

---

Information that appears in brackets has been added by the authors to clarify and enhance the use of nursing diagnoses.

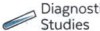 Diagnostic Studies 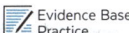 Evidence Based Practice Medications 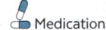 Pediatric/Geriatric/Lifespan

Generate Solutions

Plan Desired Outcomes

Client Will (Include Specific Time Frame)
- Make nutritionally adequate choices of food/fluids.
- Assume control over mealtime.
- Identify feelings and underlying dynamics of low self-esteem/ changes of puberty.
- Display normalization of laboratory values reflecting appropriate nutrient intake.

Parent/Caregiver Will (Include Specific Time Frame)
- Verbalize understanding of under-/overinvolved parenting style.
- Identify specific actions that affect eating habits.
- Demonstrate willingness to work together as a family to resolve presenting problems.

Refer to NDs Nutritional Intake, inadequate; Body Weight Problem; Overweight Self-Management, ineffective; Weight Self-Management, readiness for enhanced, as indicated, for additional interventions specific to client's situation.

Interventions/Take Action

Nursing Priority No. 1.
To assess causative/contributing factors:
- Begin developing the nurse/client relationship during the initial assessment. **Initial nurse communication skills with clients begin developing trust that allows equal distribution of power, fostering client-centered care and good decision making by the client.**
- Note age and developmental level of client and place in family order. **The adolescent period of development is a period of vulnerability for the development of problems with eating.**
- Discuss client's perception of the current situation and motivation for change. **Understanding client's belief and whether current situation is viewed as a problem directly impacts likelihood of successful outcome.**
- Assess eating habits and nutritional intake using a food log/journal. **Helps determine behaviors to be addressed and provides basis for planning care.**
- Identify family cultural/spiritual factors and finances. **Personal beliefs and finances affect choices when developing meal plans.**

Information that appears in brackets has been added by the authors to clarify and enhance the use of nursing diagnoses.

- Determine dynamics of family system. **How the family deals with the adolescent is critical to the outcome of the situation.**
- Perform a complete physical examination. **Provides a baseline for comparison as client progresses through treatment.**
- Assess current weight and recent changes **to identify deviations from the norm and establish baseline parameters.**
- Evaluate possibility of attention deficit-hyperactivity disorder (ADHD). **Although research has lagged in this area, there are reasons to believe that girls with this disorder may be at increased risk for eating disorders, such as body dissatisfaction, showing distress through eating disorders, under- or overweight.**
- Note issues of self-esteem client may express. **Adolescents often struggle with concerns about their body in relation to others and often believe they are not as worthwhile as their peers.**
- Note gender of the client, male or female. **Although females outnumber males by a significant number, males make up an important aspect of this problem, are more reluctant to seek help, and may need special accommodations, such as an all-male treatment team.**
- Discuss client's/family's eating patterns and attitudes toward food. Note variance from family diet (e.g., teen choosing vegan diet). **Helpful in identifying possible conflicts and may reveal problems of other family members needing to be addressed.**
- Review laboratory studies reflecting nutritional status. **Helpful in identifying deficiencies and therapeutic needs.**

Nursing Priority No. 2.

To assist client to develop skills to manage adequate nutritional needs:

- Advance the therapeutic nurse/client/family relationship while making plans for improved health/weight outcomes. **During the working phase of the relationship, the nurse/client/family collaborate, allowing the client to freely share their ideas for improving health.**
- Assist client to make achievable goals to maintain healthy eating habits. **Increases likelihood of successful change.**
- Include nutritionist in the planning of care. **Provides information and guidance in determining individual nutritional needs incorporating child's likes and being mindful of dislikes.**

Information that appears in brackets has been added by the authors to clarify and enhance the use of nursing diagnoses.

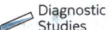 Diagnostic Studies   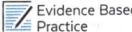 Evidence Based Practice   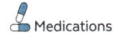 Medications   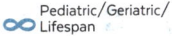 Pediatric/Geriatric/Lifespan

- Talk about frequent use of processed or fast food sources for meals. **Although such foods may expedite meals for the busy family, they do not provide the nutrition needed for growing children as well as for general health of other family members and are not cost effective.**
- Assist client in developing own/family meal plans, healthy snacks, and food preparation, as appropriate. **Involvement in the process supports teen's growth and increases chances for success.**
- Encourage client to read nutritional labels on food packaging or on menus when eating out. **Helps teen to make informed food choices.**
- Emphasize need to avoid comparing self with others, encouraging client to look at positive aspects of self. **Adolescents tend to look at friends, TV, fashion models, sports figures, and others to model themselves after rather than accepting their body as all right as is.**
- Note perceptions client may express and discuss versus realities. **Correcting misperceptions helps the adolescent adjust choices of food and activities for more positive results.**
- Address physical/safety issues client presents. **Physical changes in body that are occurring with client's current eating habits affect how client views self-esteem and contributes to lack of attention to safety issues.**
- Remind family/friends that teasing client about body/eating habits is not to be done. **Teasing can be damaging, regardless of whether client is obese or thin, and is counterproductive.**
- Refer for family therapy, as indicated. **May help resolve parent and adolescent issues interfering with relationship and manifested in unhealthy eating behaviors.**
- Encourage client to become involved in enjoyable physical activities. **Participation in these activities can enhance self-esteem, promote self-reliance and confidence, and lead to improved weight management.**
- Refer to ND Self-Esteem, chronic inadequate for additional interventions.

Nursing Priority No. 3.

To promote continued dietary success (Teaching/Discharge Considerations) and enhanced well-being:

- Involve client in school and social activities. **Continuing studies will improve sense of accomplishment, and involvement in social groups provides opportunities to**

Information that appears in brackets has been added by the authors to clarify and enhance the use of nursing diagnoses.

make friends and enjoy activities that may involve eating in accepted manner.
- Talk with adolescent about involvement with social media. **Social media is found to have a negative effect on self-esteem for adolescents, and sharing this information can help the individual change their attitude.**
- Identify appropriate online reference sites. **Can provide information and recipes to help with meal planning over time to achieve long-term goals.**
- Identify age-appropriate community support programs and resources as needed. **Provides opportunity to interact with peers facing similar issues and useful in sustaining efforts for change.**
- Assist client/family to access available nutritional assistance program, community food banks, budget counseling, and so on. **Assists family in providing nutritional meals.**
- Refer parents to parenting classes, such as Parent Effectiveness Training, group therapy, and so on. **Will help parents learn how to interact with their growing adolescent as both develop positive relationships.**

Documentation Focus

Assessment/Reassessment
- Individual findings, including eating habits, attitude toward them, food choices, likes and dislikes
- Current weight, recent changes
- Interactions with others, peers, and family
- Motivation for change

Planning
- Plan of care and who is involved in planning
- Teaching plan

Implementation/Evaluation
- Responses to interventions, teaching, and changes
- Attainment of or progress toward desired outcome(s)
- Modification to plan of care

Discharge Planning
- Long-term needs and who is responsible for actions
- Specific referrals made

Sample Nursing Outcomes & Interventions Classifications NOC/NIC

NOC—Eating Disorder: Self-Control
NIC—Nutritional Counseling

Information that appears in brackets has been added by the authors to clarify and enhance the use of nursing diagnoses.

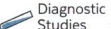 Diagnostic Studies 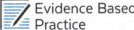 Evidence Based Practice 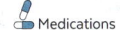 Medications 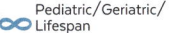 Pediatric/Geriatric/Lifespan

ineffective child EATING DYNAMICS — NANDA-I

[Diagnostic Division: Food/Fluid]

Definition: Altered attitudes, behaviors, and influences on child eating patterns resulting in compromised nutritional health, in individuals 1 to 10 years of age.

Recognizing Cues

Related/Risk Factors

Eating Habit:

Bribing or forcing child to eat; excessive parental control over child's eating experience; limiting child's diet; rewarding child to eat

Consumption of large volumes of food in a short period of time; inappropriate dietary habits

Eating in isolation; abnormal or unpredictable eating patterns

Excessive parental control over family mealtime; absence of regular mealtimes; stressful mealtimes

Unstructured eating of snacks between meals

Family Processes:

Abusive interpersonal relationships

Anxious, hostile, insecure, or tense parent-child relations

Disengaged, intrusive, or uninvolved parenting

Parent:

Inadequate appetite; inability to support healthy eating patterns

Ineffective use of coping strategies; substance misuse

Inability to divide eating or feeding responsibility between parent and child

Inadequate confidence in child to develop healthy eating habits, or grow appropriately

Environmental Factors:

Media influence on knowledge of or eating behaviors of high-caloric unhealthy foods

Defining Characteristics

Subjective

Complains of hunger between meals

Objective

Frequent snacking; frequently consumes fast food; frequently eats low-quality food

Diet high in processed foods

Information that appears in brackets has been added by the authors to clarify and enhance the use of nursing diagnoses.

 Acute Care   Collaborative 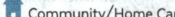 Community/Home Care 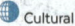 Cultural

Avoids participation in regular mealtimes; food refusal
Overeating, undereating

Clinical Connections
Obesity, anorexia, depression, substance abuse

Generate Solutions

Plan Desired Outcomes

Client Will (Include Specific Time Frame)
- Ingest appropriate amount of calories/nutrients to meet metabolic needs.
- Achieve/maintain body weight appropriate for height.

Parent/Caregiver Will (Include Specific Time Frame)
- Acknowledge that child is having problems with eating.
- Verbalize understanding of under-/overinvolved parenting style.
- Identify specific actions that affect eating habits.
- Demonstrate willingness to work together as a family to resolve presenting problems.

Refer to NDs Nutritional Intake, inadequate; Body Weight Problem; Overweight Self-Management, ineffective; Weight Self-Management, readiness for enhanced, as indicated, for additional interventions specific to client's situation.

Interventions/Take Action

Nursing Priority No. 1.
To assess causative/contributing factors:
- Begin developing the nurse/client relationship during the initial assessment. **Initial nurse communication skills with clients begin developing trust that allows for equal distribution of power, fostering patient-centered care and good decision making by the client.**
- Determine individual dynamics (e.g., bribing or forcing child to eat, excessive parental control over child's eating experience, stressful mealtimes, inappropriate choice of foods). **Identify issues to be addressed in plan of care.**
- Identify family's eating patterns and attitudes toward food. **Helpful in identifying possible conflicts and may reveal problems of other family members needing to be addressed. Parental food habits and feeding strategies**

Information that appears in brackets has been added by the authors to clarify and enhance the use of nursing diagnoses.

are the most dominant determinants of a child's eating behavior and food choices.
- Assess child's health status, weight, age, stage of growth, and development. **Information needed to determine nutritional needs and desired change in weight goal.**
- Determine family functioning and relationships that may affect child's eating disorder. **How family members interact with one another, arguments, or disagreements can affect child's eating behaviors.**
- Note child's eating habits, eating in isolation, unpredictable eating patterns, eating snacks between meals. **These factors can lead to weight gain as child grows.**
- Determine family habits of watching TV and other social media, especially while eating. **The influence of media (especially food commercials) on family and child's eating of high-calorie unhealthy foods is well documented.**
- Evaluate physical activities of all family members. **Inactivity can contribute to increased risk of obesity. A significant number of children are obese or overweight at an earlier age than in the past.**
- Note environmental factors, including family functioning and parenting style, mother's eating disorder or mental status, relationships between mother and child. **Self-report interviews reveal problem areas for mothers and children to determine needs for intervention. Note: Although the primary focus has been directed toward mothers, either or both parents may have issues to be addressed.**
- Identify family cultural/spiritual beliefs and finances. **Personal beliefs and financial resources affect how family views food and impacts meal planning.**

Nursing Priority No. 2.

To assist family/child to develop new habits/patterns of family functioning and eating behaviors:

- Advance the therapeutic nurse/client/family relationship to the working phase of the relationship. Listen for client/family ideas on improving healthy eating patterns, patient-centered care, while developing the plan of care. Be attentive, provide encouragement for efforts, use skills of active-listening and I-messages to maintain open communication. **Promotes trusting situation in which client is able to express self and be honest and open with self and nurse.**
- Discuss eating behaviors with family/child, identifying areas for improvement. **Realizing how eating patterns**

Information that appears in brackets has been added by the authors to clarify and enhance the use of nursing diagnoses.

affect children can enable parents to be willing to make changes for better nutrition and overall health.
- Help parents learn new methods of planning and cooking foods. **Learning healthy ways of eating can help parents and children establish nutritionally sound habits of eating.**
- Discuss parental involvement with child's eating behaviors. **Parents may not trust child to make healthy choices for eating, resulting in overinvolvement or anxious behaviors affecting child's eating.**

Nursing Priority No. 3.

To establish nutritionally adequate plan that meets needs of family members:

- Involve parents and child in developing achievable short- and long-term goals. **Increases likelihood of success if all parties agree on the goals.**
- Include dietitian in care planning. **Provides information and guidance in determining individual nutritional needs incorporating child's likes and being mindful of dislikes.**
- Develop plan taking into account previously identified problems of family's eating behaviors. **Sitting down as a family at regularly scheduled times in a "media-free zone" that encourages open family communication can reduce stress levels and enhance food intake.**
- Encourage parents to relax and allow child to make own decisions among foods offered for meal. **Children will eat what they need when given the opportunity to make own choices.**
- Talk about frequent use of processed or fast food sources for meals. **Although such foods may expedite meals for the busy family, they do not provide the nutrition needed for growing children as well as for general health of other family members and are not cost effective.**

Nursing Priority No. 4.

To promote continued dietary success (Teaching/Discharge Considerations) and enhanced well-being:

- Emphasize importance of well-balanced nutrition intake within financial concerns. **Individuals may never have learned how to shop for and prepare affordable quality foods.**
- Assist client/family to access available nutritional assistance program, community food banks, budget counseling, and

---

Information that appears in brackets has been added by the authors to clarify and enhance the use of nursing diagnoses.

 Diagnostic Studies 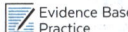 Evidence Based Practice 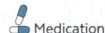 Medications 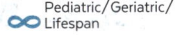 Pediatric/Geriatric/Lifespan

so on. **Enhances family's ability to provide nutritional meals/snacks, especially in presence of food insecurity.**
- Identify appropriate online reference sites. **Can provide information and recipes to help with meal planning over time to achieve long-term goals.**
- Assist in developing regular exercise and stress reduction programs. **Helps family members learn ways to manage weight and stress levels, improving general well-being.**
- 🐊 Refer parents to classes in parenting, nutritional food preparation, or therapeutic needs. **Can be helpful when needed to assist family to learn new ways of dealing with issues/problems.**
- 🐊 Identify community support programs and resources as needed. **Useful in sustaining efforts for change.**

Documentation Focus

Assessment/Reassessment
- Health status and weight of child and parents
- Parent-child interactions/relationship
- Eating habits, food choices
- Parents' understanding of or perception of problems

Planning
- Plan of care and who is involved in planning
- Teaching plan

Implementation/Evaluation
- Parent/child responses to interventions, teaching, and actions performed
- Attainment or progress toward desired outcomes
- Modifications to plan of care

Discharge Planning
- Long-term needs and who is responsible for actions
- Specific referrals made

Sample Nursing Outcomes & Interventions Classifications NOC/NIC

NOC—Knowledge: Eating Disorder Management
NIC—Nutritional Counseling

Information that appears in brackets has been added by the authors to clarify and enhance the use of nursing diagnoses.

ELDER FRAILTY SYNDROME NANDA-I

[Diagnostic Division: Health Management]

Definition: Dynamic state of disequilibrium that includes deterioration of functions and reserves across physiological systems.

Recognizing Cues

Related/Risk Factors
Anxiety; fear of falling; sadness
Decreased energy; exhaustion; sedentary behaviors; muscle weakness; impaired postural balance
Inadequate knowledge of modifiable factors; inadequate social support
Malnutrition; anorexia of aging; ineffective overweight self-management
Confusion
Inadequate caregiver knowledge of modifiable factors

Defining Characteristics

AUTHOR NOTE: NANDA-I has defined a syndrome as "a clinical judgment concerning a specific cluster of nursing diagnoses [NDs] that occur together and are best addressed together and through similar interventions" (Herdman, Kamitsuru, and Lopes 2024). Defining Characteristics contain these ND titles:

Subjective
Decreased activity tolerance
Excessive fatigue burden

Objective
Decreased bathing, dressing, grooming, feeding, or toileting abilities
Disability-associated urinary incontinence
Inadequate nutritional intake; less than body requirements
Impaired memory
Impaired physical mobility; impaired walking ability; risk for adult falls
Inadequate social connectedness

Clinical Connections
Chronic debilitating conditions (e.g., chronic obstructive pulmonary disease (COPD), diabetes, AIDS, Alzheimer

---

Information that appears in brackets has been added by the authors to clarify and enhance the use of nursing diagnoses.

disease, multiple sclerosis [MS]), cancer, terminal illnesses, major depression, long-term care residents

Generate Solutions

Plan Desired Outcomes

Client Will (Include Specific Time Frame)
- Acknowledge the presence of factors affecting well-being.
- Identify corrective/adaptive measures for individual situation.
- Demonstrate behaviors/lifestyle changes necessary to enhance functional status.
- Look to the future, expressing a sense of control.

Interventions/Take Action

Refer to NDs Activity Intolerance; chronic Confusion; difficulty Coping; risk for Fall; dysfunctional Grief; excessive Loneliness; inadequate Nutritional Intake; risk for Relocation Stress; Self-Care Deficit [specify]; chronic inadequate Self-Esteem; impaired Spiritual Well-Being; ineffective Self-Health Management, as appropriate, for additional relevant interventions.

Nursing Priority No. 1.
To identify causative/contributing **or risk** factors:
- Identify the presence of "frailty syndrome (FS)." **Demonstrated in an elderly person by three or more symptoms together: unintentional weight loss (5% or more of body weight within the past year [also called "shrinking"]), weakness marked by grip strength, a feeling of exhaustion, slow walking speed (more than 6 sec to walk 15 ft), and low levels of physical activity. Note: The presence of FS is a predictor for hospitalization, disability, decreasing mobility, falls, and even death.**
- Note the individual's age, gender, ethnicity, and socioeconomic status. **Higher prevalence of frailty has been observed among older persons, women and racial/ethnic minorities, persons in residential care, and persons with lower incomes.**
- Note individual's age, gender, ethnicity, and socioeconomic status. **Geriatric persons, women, racial/ethnic minorities, persons with lower incomes, and long-term care clients have a higher prevalence than White persons with higher incomes.**

Information that appears in brackets has been added by the authors to clarify and enhance the use of nursing diagnoses.

- Identify presence of physical complaints (e.g., fatigue/exhaustion, unintentional weight loss, muscle weakness, slow walking, inability to participate in usual physical activities) and the presence of conditions (e.g., heart disease, undetected diabetes mellitus, dementia, stroke, renal failure, long-term period of being bedridden, or terminal conditions). **Note: These factors associated with frailty may or may not be recognized by the client but may be reported or documented by others. Clients with serious heart disease and FS may not be able to provide adequate self-care.**
- Determine nutritional status (i.e., nutritional assessment, observation, physical examination, and if available, review of medical records). **Review anthropometric measurements, laboratory abnormalities, and factors contributing to failure to eat (e.g., chronic nausea, loss of appetite, no access to food or cooking, poorly fitting dentures, no one with whom to share meals, depression, financial problems) that greatly impact health status and quality of life, especially for the elderly individual. Evidence indicates that when obesity and muscle impairment coexist, they act synergistically on the risk of developing multiple health-related outcomes.**
- Evaluate the medication regimen. **Polypharmacy (e.g., use of four or more prescribed medications) and use of over-the-counter drugs can contribute to side effects, adverse reactions, and risk of falling. Medications that cause electrolyte imbalances (e.g., diuretics) can exacerbate weakness. Drugs that slow reaction time (e.g., sedatives and antidepressants) can interfere with balance and coordination, as can alcohol.**
- Note the client's living situation (e.g., lives alone or lives in a facility). **Helps identify environmental risk factors such as risk for falls, problem with food shopping or preparation, depression, or other contributing factors.**
- Evaluate the client's level of adaptive behavior and client/caregiver knowledge and skills about health maintenance, environment, and safety. **Caring for the frail client is complex due to a multitude of physical and psychological contributions to the condition. FS can be preventable or reversible with an interprofessional approach (e.g., nursing, geriatrician, occupational and physical therapists).**
- Discuss with the client/significant other (SO) previous and current life situations, including role changes, multiple losses (e.g., death of loved ones, change in living

---

Information that appears in brackets has been added by the authors to clarify and enhance the use of nursing diagnoses.

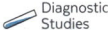 Diagnostic Studies   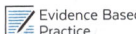 Evidence Based Practice   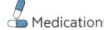 Medications   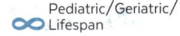 Pediatric/Geriatric/Lifespan

arrangements, finances, and independence), social isolation, and grieving. **Psychological stressors may affect or complicate the current situation.**

- Determine safety of the home environment and persons providing care. **The potential for/presence of neglectful or abusive situations and/or need for referrals may be indicated to keep the client safe and free from harm.**

Nursing Priority No. 2.
To assess degree of impairment:

- Collaborate with client/family/SO and with multidisciplinary team to determine the severity of the client's limitations. **A complete geriatric assessment helps to identify risk factors and symptoms; however, a starting point is routine blood test, urine analysis, chest x-rays, and an ECG. Presently, recommendations or treatment guidelines for routine screening are not available. Some evidence suggests considering screening for diabetes, COPD, stroke, dementia, multiple sclerosis, connective tissue disease, osteoarthritis, or chronic fatigue syndrome.**

- Encourage client and family/SO to express their goals. Provide information about the benefits or harms of extensive testing. **Evaluation and management are individualized for each client based on medical history, degree of frailty, healthcare goals, and life expectancy. Depending on expressed goals, extensive testing may not be beneficial.**

- Identify client's level of ability to attend to activities of daily living (ADLs), need for assistive devices and/or care assistance. **Information necessary for developing plan of care to meet client's needs and provide for safe environment.**

Nursing Priority No. 3.
To assist client to achieve general well-being:

- Assist with treatment of underlying comorbid medical, functional, cognitive, or psychiatric conditions. **Resolving underlying medical issues can positively influence current health status (e.g., resolution of infection, treating anemia and malnutrition, addressing diabetes, cardiovascular conditions, delirium, social isolation, depression).**

Information that appears in brackets has been added by the authors to clarify and enhance the use of nursing diagnoses.

- Develop a plan of action with the client/caregiver. **Collaborative (e.g., nurse, dietitian/nutritionist, social worker, occupational and physical therapy) care plans developed with client/caregiver are more likely to meet the immediate needs for nutrition, safety, self-care, and home health services, and facilitate implementation of actions.**
- Assess client's cognitive status using the Mini-Mental State Examination (MMSE). **Geriatric clients' cognitive functions decline. Use stimulating activities (e.g., memory training, exercises, and place calendars and clocks available for clients to see). Mood may decline with cognitive changes.**
- Administer medications as appropriate. **Clients and caregivers who understand the importance of medication administration in a timely manner reflect optimized management of congestive heart failure, chronic pulmonary disease, or improved glycemic control of diabetes, resulting in improved health status, fewer hospitalizations, and reductions in the physical declines associated with the frailty syndrome.**
- Discuss individual concerns about feelings of loss/loneliness and the relationship between these feelings and a current decline in well-being. Note desire or willingness to change situation. **Motivation or lack thereof can impede—or facilitate—achieving desired outcomes.**
- Explore mental strengths and successful coping skills the individual has previously used and apply to current situation. Refine or develop new strategies, as appropriate. **Incorporating these into problem-solving builds on past successes.**
- Recommend client/SO develop routine schedule to engage in physical activities. **Exercises/activities (e.g., chair/water aerobics, stretching, resistance training, walking, tai chi) can improve balance, muscle and core strength, as well as physical endurance.**
- Encourage stimulating activities (e.g., memory training, exercises, and place calendars and clocks available for clients to see). **Facilitates persevering and maintaining orientation and memory.**
- Assist the client to develop goals for dealing with life or illness situation. Involve the SO in long-range planning. **Promotes commitment to goals and plan, thereby maximizing outcomes.**

Information that appears in brackets has been added by the authors to clarify and enhance the use of nursing diagnoses.

Nursing Priority No. 4.

To promote optimal function (Teaching/Discharge Considerations) and enhance well-being (long-term goals):

- Review client/family/SO concerns/needs. Discuss how to intervene in dangerous situations and who to contact for help. **Enhances sense of safety and support for providing care, and promotes independence in daily living for client.**
- Assist client/SO(s) to identify and/or access useful community resources (e.g., support groups, Meals on Wheels, social worker, housekeeping/handyman services, home care, day care programs, or placement services). **Enhances coping, assists with problem-solving, and may reduce risks to client and caregiver.**
- Encourage client to talk about positive aspects of life and to keep as physically active as possible. **Social interactions with family/friends/SOs prevent a feeling of being disconnected, loneliness, feeling isolated, or feeling devalued. Including afternoon walks and conversations with others improves emotions and physical strength.**
- Offer opportunities to discuss life goals and support the client/SO in setting/attaining new goals for this time in their life. **Enhances present enjoyment in life and offers hope for the future.**
- Help client explore reasons for living or begin to cope with end-of-life issues and provide support for grieving. **Enhances hope and sense of control, providing opportunity for client to take charge of their own future.**
- Assist client/SO/family to understand that frailty commonly occurs near the end of life and cannot always be reversed. **Discussions help client/family/SOs to consider addressing issues and reality, as appropriate.**
- Discuss appropriateness of and refer to palliative services or hospice care, as indicated. **Helps client/family to understand the differences in palliative services and hospice care and make informed decision about options.**
- Refer to pastoral care, counseling, or psychotherapy. **Grief work or other issues may arise during the early stages of frailty, and client and/or others may need support to deal with situation.**

Documentation Focus

Assessment/Reassessment

- Individual findings, including current weight, dietary pattern, food and eating, perceptions of self, motivation for loss, support and feedback from SOs

---

Information that appears in brackets has been added by the authors to clarify and enhance the use of nursing diagnoses.

- Perception of losses or life changes
- Ability to perform ADLs, participate in care, meet own needs
- Motivation for change, support and feedback from SO(s)

Planning
- Plan of care, specific interventions, and who is involved in planning
- Teaching plan

Implementation/Evaluation
- Responses to interventions and actions performed, general well-being, weekly weight
- Attainment of or progress toward desired outcome(s)
- Modifications to plan of care

Discharge Planning
- Long-term needs and who is responsible for actions to be taken
- Community resources and support groups
- Specific referrals made

Sample Nursing Outcomes & Interventions Classifications NOC/NIC

NOC—Personal Health Status
NIC—Resilience Promotion

---

impaired intestinal ELIMINATION   NANDA-I

[Diagnostic Division: Elimination]

Definition: Change in the normal process of defecation from the rectum or ostomy.

Recognizing Cues

Related/Risk Factors
Altered regular routine; inadequate privacy; habitually suppresses urge to defecate
Exposure to toxins
Impaired physical mobility; impaired postural balance
Average daily physical activity is less than recommended for age and gender

---

Information that appears in brackets has been added by the authors to clarify and enhance the use of nursing diagnoses.

 Diagnostic Studies   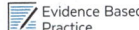 Evidence Based Practice   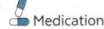 Medications   ∞ Pediatric/Geriatric/Lifespan

Inadequate fluid, or fiber intake; inadequate access to safe food or safe drinking water; malnutrition; early formula feeding

Inadequate knowledge about sanitary food preparation, or storage

Inadequate personal hygiene practices

Anxiety; excessive stress; communication barriers

Laxative misuse; substance misuse

Inadequate knowledge about rotavirus vaccine

Defining Characteristics

Subjective

Abdominal cramping, pain

Fecal urgency

Sensation of incomplete evacuation; sensation of anorectal obstruction

Evidence of symptoms in standardized diagnostic criteria

Objective

Constipation; diarrhea

Hyperactive bowel sounds

Straining with defecation

Need for manual maneuvers to facilitate defecation

Clinical Connections

Abdominal or pelvic surgeries; hemorrhoids, anal lesions, irritable bowel syndrome, diverticulitis, inflammatory bowel disease, gastritis; spinal cord injury (SCI), multiple sclerosis (MS); hypothyroidism, iron-deficiency anemia; uremia, kidney dialysis; dementia; AIDS; food allergies or contamination; infection, parasites; enteral feedings; alcohol/substance abuse; radiation

Generate Solutions

Plan Desired Outcomes

Client Will (Include Specific Time Frame)

- Reestablish and maintain normal pattern of bowel functioning.
- Verbalize understanding of etiology and appropriate interventions or solutions for individual situation.
- Demonstrate appropriate behaviors or lifestyle changes to resolve problem/prevent recurrence.
- Participate in bowel program, as indicated.

Information that appears in brackets has been added by the authors to clarify and enhance the use of nursing diagnoses.

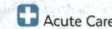 Acute Care 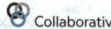 Collaborative 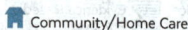 Community/Home Care   Cultural

Interventions/Take Action

Nursing Priority No. 1.
To assess causative factors/etiology:

- Review medical/surgical history as indicated in Related Factors **to identify conditions commonly associated with constipation or diarrhea.** (Refer to ND chronic functional Constipation).
- Note client's age and evaluate client's/caregiver's perception of the severity of symptoms:
- Diarrhea: **Acute diarrhea is usually caused by an infection, while chronic diarrhea is usually related to a functional disorder or intestinal disease. Viral diarrhea is most common among young children. Adults tend to average one bout of acute diarrhea each year. Chronic (persistent) diarrhea may be a symptom of a chronic disease and often affects adults more than children. People perceive having diarrhea in many different ways, but generally, if client is having loose, watery stools occurring more than three times a day for 3 days or more, the diagnosis of diarrhea can be made. The condition can affect people of all ages, although its effect is more dangerous for infants and frail elders (due to risk of dehydration).**
- Constipation: **Constipation is more likely to occur in individuals older than 65 years of age but can occur in any age from infant to elderly. A bottle-fed infant is more prone to constipation than a breastfed infant, especially when formula contains iron. Toddlers are at risk because of developmental factors (e.g., too young, too interested in other things, rigid schedule during potty training), and children and adolescents are at risk because of unwillingness to take breaks from play, poor eating and fluid intake habits, and withholding because of perceived lack of privacy. Many older adults experience constipation because of duller nerve sensations, immobility, dehydration, and electrolyte imbalances; incomplete emptying of the bowel; or failing to attend to signals to defecate.**
- Obtain a comprehensive history of symptoms **to identify conditions commonly associated with constipation or diarrhea.**
- Observe and investigate client reports of stool characteristics (e.g., soft to watery stools, bloody, greasy; hard, dry), frequency (e.g., more than normal number of stools/day for client),

---

Information that appears in brackets has been added by the authors to clarify and enhance the use of nursing diagnoses.

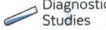 Diagnostic Studies   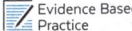 Evidence Based Practice   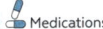 Medications   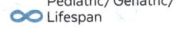 Pediatric/Geriatric/Lifespan

time of day (e.g., after meals), and volume **to provide a baseline for comparison, promoting recognition of changes.**

- Determine if incontinence is present. **May indicate the presence of fecal impaction, particularly in the elderly, where impaction may be accompanied by diarrhea.** (Refer to ND impaired fecal Continence.)
- Identify any associated signs/symptoms (e.g., fever/chills, abdominal cramping, emotional upset, weight loss), aggravating factors (e.g., stress, foods), or mitigating factors (e.g., changes in diet, poor oral/dental health, use of prescription or over-the-counter [OTC] medications).
- Observe and investigate client reports of onset and pattern of defecation changes (i.e., constipation or diarrhea), noting whether it is acute or chronic. **Acute diarrhea is caused by (1) viral, bacterial, or parasitic infections (e.g., Norwalk virus, rotavirus; salmonella, shigella; giardia, amebiasis, respectively); (2) bacterial food-borne toxins (e.g., *Staphylococcus aureus, Escherichia coli*); (3) medications (e.g., antibiotics, chemotherapy agents, colchicine, laxatives); and (4) enteral tube feedings. It may last a few days up to a week. Chronic diarrhea is caused by irritable bowel syndrome, infectious diseases, inflammatory bowel disease, colon cancer and treatments, severe constipation, malabsorption disorders, laxative abuse, and certain endocrine disorders (e.g., hyperthyroidism, Addison disease). It often lasts for more than 3 weeks.**
- Auscultate client's abdomen for the presence, location, and characteristics of bowel sounds. **High-pitched, rapidly occurring, and loud or tinkling bowel sounds often accompany diarrhea. Hypoactive or absent bowel sounds may indicate slowed or impaired gastrointestinal (GI) motility.**
- Palpate client's abdomen **to assess for hardness, distension, and masses indicating possible obstruction or retention of stool.**
- Assess client reports of pain (e.g., abdominal or rectal pain, pain with defecation). **Pain is often present with inflammatory bowel disease, irritable bowel syndrome, and mesenteric ischemia. Hemorrhoids, rectal fissures or prolapse, skin breakdown, etc., may hinder the passage of stool or cause client to hold stool.**
- Perform digital rectal examination, as indicated, **to evaluate client's rectal tone and detect tenderness, the presence of blood, or fecal impaction.**

Information that appears in brackets has been added by the authors to clarify and enhance the use of nursing diagnoses.

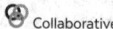 Acute Care 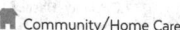 Collaborative Community/Home Care   Cultural

- Assess client for personal **strategies to stimulate bowel activity or personal preferences that affect bowel patterns (e.g., not wanting to use a particular facility or not wanting to interrupt play or an activity). Client may describe having to sit in a particular position, needing to apply perineal pressure or digital stimulation to start stool.**
- Evaluate diet history, noting food allergies or intolerances, food and water safety issues, amount of dietary fiber (i.e., dietary fiber influences the amount and consistency of feces), and general nutritional, fluid, and electrolyte status (i.e., that may be causing or exacerbating diarrhea) **to evaluate potential impact on client condition.**
- Determine fluid intake to note deficits **that may contribute to hard, dry stool.**
- Evaluate and investigate client's activity level and exercise pattern. **Lack of physical activity or regular exercise is often a factor in constipation.**
- Evaluate and investigate client's access to bathroom, privacy, and ability to perform self-care activities **to evaluate potential impact on client condition.**
- Review client's drug regimen. **Medications such as laxatives, antibiotics, cardiovascular drugs, antidiabetic agents, anticholesterol agents, opiates, sedatives, and iron preparations may cause or exacerbate intestinal issues. Note reports of laxative abuse or overuse of stimulant laxatives; this is most common among older adults preoccupied with having daily bowel movement.**
- Note lifestyle issues that can affect GI function (e.g., travel to developing countries or foreign environments, change in drinking water or food intake, consumption of unsafe food, swimming in untreated surface water, or similar illness of family members/significant others [SOs] close to client) **to identify causative environmental factors.**
- Assess client for life changes or stressors. **Factors such as pregnancy, traumas, changes in personal relationships, occupational factors, or financial concerns can cause or exacerbate defecation habits.**
- Assist client with and evaluate results of diagnostic/laboratory evaluation (e.g., x-rays, abdominal imaging, colonoscopy, proctosigmoidoscopy, anorectal function tests; colonic transit studies, stool sample tests, etc.) **for identification of possible causative factors.** Refer to ND: chronic functional Constipation for further assessments and interventions.

Information that appears in brackets has been added by the authors to clarify and enhance the use of nursing diagnoses.

 Diagnostic Studies 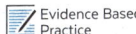 Evidence Based Practice 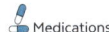 Medications 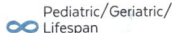 Pediatric/Geriatric/Lifespan

Nursing Priority No. 2.

To minimize/correct causative factors:

- Assist with treatment of underlying conditions (e.g., infections, malabsorption syndrome, cancer) and complications associated with constipation or diarrhea. **Treatments are varied and may be as simple as allowing time for recovery from self-limiting gastroenteritis or may require complex treatments, including antimicrobials, dietary intervention, rehydration, or community health interventions for contaminated food or water sources.**
- Promote client activity as indicated for intestinal dysfunction:

    Client with diarrhea: Encourage bedrest during an acute episode, especially if fever is present and/or client is dehydrated and weak. **Rest reduces intestinal motility and metabolic rate when infection or hemorrhage is a complication.**

    Client with constipation: Encourage daily activity and exercise within limits of individual ability **to stimulate contractions of the intestines.**

- Promote and provide client nutrition as indicated for intestinal dysfunction:

    Recommend products such as natural fiber, plain natural yogurt, and Lactinex, as indicated **to restore normal bowel flora.**

    Client with diarrhea: Restrict solid food intake, if indicated. **May help in the short term to allow for bowel rest and reduced intestinal workload, especially if cause of diarrhea is under investigation or vomiting is present. Caffeine, high-fat (e.g., butter, fried foods), or high-protein (e.g., meats) foods may cause or aggravate diarrhea. Note: A child's preferred or usual diet may be continued to prevent or limit dehydration, with the possible limitation of fruit, fruit juices, or milk, if these factors are exacerbating the diarrhea. Infants may require a change in infant formula. Diarrhea may be the result of or aggravated by intolerance to a specific formula.**

    Client with constipation: Limit foods with little or no fiber or diet high in fats (e.g., ice cream, cheese, meats, fast foods, processed foods). **Note: Clients with descending or sigmoid colostomy must avoid constipation. Some may find it helpful to create their own dietary bulk laxative by combining unprocessed miller's bran, applesauce, and prune juice.**

Information that appears in brackets has been added by the authors to clarify and enhance the use of nursing diagnoses.

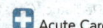 Acute Care 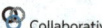 Collaborative 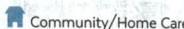 Community/Home Care Cultural

- Promote and provide client hydration and electrolytes, as indicated for intestinal dysfunction. **Offer and encourage water, oral beverages (e.g., Gatorade, Pedialyte, Infalyte, Smartwater, etc.) plus broth or soups that contain sodium, or soft fruits or vegetables that contain potassium to replace water and electrolytes. Commercial rehydration solutions containing electrolytes may prevent or correct imbalances:**

  Client with diarrhea: Adjust strength and/or rate of enteral feedings, or change formula as indicated **when diarrhea is associated with enteral feedings.**

  Client with constipation: Offer water, high-fiber fruit and vegetable juices, fruit/vegetable smoothies, and Popsicles. Suggest drinking warm, stimulating fluids (e.g., decaffeinated coffee, hot water, tea) **to avoid dehydration; promote moist, soft feces; and facilitate passage of stool.**

- Administer IV fluids, electrolytes, and enteral or parenteral feedings, as indicated. **IV fluids may be needed either in the short term to restore hydration status (e.g., acute gastroenteritis) or long term (severe osmotic diarrhea). Enteral or parenteral nutrition is reserved for clients unable to maintain adequate nutritional status because of long-term diarrhea (e.g., wasting syndrome, malnutrition states).**

- Review client's current medication regime with physician **to determine if drugs contributing to client problem can be discontinued or changed.**

- Administer medications as indicated, depending on the cause of client condition (e.g., antidiarrheals, anti-infectives, antispasmodics, stool softeners, laxatives [i.e., mild stimulants, hyperosmolar laxatives, or bulk-forming agents], or lubricants).

- Provide sitz bath before stools **to relax sphincter and after stools for cleansing and soothing effect to rectal area.**

- Encourage client to not ignore the defecation urge. **Persistent delay in response to the defecation urge may ultimately suppress the gastrocolic reflex, potentially worsening intestinal complaints.**

- Provide client privacy and time for defecation **to promote psychological readiness and comfort. Prompt removal of stool and use of room deodorizers may reduce noxious odors and limit client embarrassment.**

- Initiate a bowel program, including predictable interval timing for colostomy irrigation or toileting, use of particular position for defecation, abdominal massage, biofeedback

---

Information that appears in brackets has been added by the authors to clarify and enhance the use of nursing diagnoses.

for pelvic floor dysfunction, etc., **to provide predictable and effective elimination and reduce evacuation problems when long-term or permanent bowel dysfunction is present.**
- Assist client to manage elimination needs:
  Respond to call for assistance promptly.
  Place bedpan or bedside commode near bed **to provide quick access and reduce the need to wait for assistance from others.**
  Offer client incontinence pads/briefs, depending on the severity of the problem.
- Promote the use of relaxation techniques (e.g., progressive relaxation exercises, visualization techniques) **to decrease client stress and anxiety.**

Nursing Priority No. 3.

To promote normal bowel function (Teaching/Discharge Considerations) and enhance well-being (long-term goals):

- Review individual's causative factors and appropriate interventions **to prevent recurrence.**
- Provide information and resources to client/SO about relationship of diet, fluid, exercise, and healthy elimination.
- Discuss medication regimen, including prescription and over-the-counter (OTC) drugs, **especially when client has multiple medications with the potential for side effects or interaction.**
- Encourage client to maintain elimination diary, if appropriate, **to facilitate monitoring of long-term problem and choice of interventions.**
- Instruct clients planning to travel outside the United States about traveler's diarrhea and ways to prevent or limit food- and waterborne illness **(e.g., do not drink tap water, use tap water ice cubes, or brush your teeth with tap water; avoid raw fruits and vegetables unless they can be peeled; avoid raw or rare meat or fish; discuss destination with local health department for particular recommendations, such as advisability of use of protective antibiotics).**
- Encourage/refer for vaccines, as indicated. **Vaccines could include those recommended for travelers to susceptible areas of the world (e.g., cholera or typhoid vaccines) and/or could be preventative therapies for infants.**
- Identify specific actions to be taken if the problem does not resolve **to promote timely intervention, thereby enhancing client's independence.**

Information that appears in brackets has been added by the authors to clarify and enhance the use of nursing diagnoses.

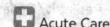 Acute Care 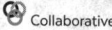 Collaborative 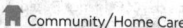 Community/Home Care 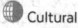 Cultural

- Instruct parent/caregiver in signs of dehydration and importance of fluid and electrolyte replacement, as well as simple food and fluids **to provide rehydration.**
- Educate client/SO/caregiver on clinical manifestations that require provider follow-up (e.g., dehydration, obstruction, indications of electrolyte abnormalities, etc.) **to ensure client safety and timely intervention.**
- Provide social and emotional support **to help client manage actual or potential disabilities associated with long-term bowel management concerns. Discuss rationale for and encourage continuation of successful interventions.**

Documentation Focus

Assessment/Reassessment
- Assessment findings, including characteristics and pattern of elimination.
- Characteristics of stool.
- Individual contributing factors.

Planning
- Plan of care, specific interventions or changes in lifestyle necessary to correct individual situation, and who is involved in planning.
- Teaching plan.

Implementation/Evaluation
- Client's response to treatment, teaching, and actions performed.
- Change in bowel pattern, character of stool.
- Attainment or progress toward desired outcome(s).
- Modifications to plan of care.

Discharge Planning
- Individual long-term needs, noting who is responsible for actions to be taken.
- Recommendations for follow-up care.
- Specific referrals made.

Sample Nursing Outcomes & Interventions Classifications NOC/NIC

NOC—Bowel Elimination
NIC—Bowel Management

Information that appears in brackets has been added by the authors to clarify and enhance the use of nursing diagnoses.

 Diagnostic Studies 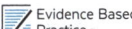 Evidence Based Practice 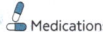 Medications 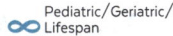 Pediatric/Geriatric/Lifespan

impaired urinary ELIMINATION

NANDA-I

[Diagnostic Division: Elimination]

Definition: Inability to effectively excrete fluids and wastes stored in the bladder through the urethra.

Recognizing Cues

Related/Risk Factors
Alcohol or caffeine consumption; use of aspartame
Unaddressed environmental constraints; inadequate privacy
Fecal impaction; involuntary sphincter relaxation
Improper toileting posture; ineffective toileting habits
Pelvic organ prolapse; weakened bladder muscle; weakened pelvic floor
Ineffective overweight self-management
Tobacco use

Defining Characteristics

Subjective
Increased urinary frequency; urinary hesitancy, incontinence, or urgency
Dysuria
Nocturia; [enuresis]

Objective
Urinary retention

Clinical Connections
Urinary tract infection (UTI), benign prostatic disease (BPH), bladder cancer, interstitial cystitis, spinal cord injury (SCI), multiple sclerosis (MS), pregnancy, childbirth, pelvic trauma, abdominal surgery, dementia, Alzheimer disease

Generate Solutions

Plan Desired Outcomes

Client Will (Include Specific Time Frame)
- Verbalize understanding of condition.
- Identify specific causative factors.
- Achieve normal elimination pattern or participate in measures to correct or compensate for defects.

Information that appears in brackets has been added by the authors to clarify and enhance the use of nursing diagnoses.

- Demonstrate behaviors and techniques to prevent urinary infection.
- Manage care of urinary catheter, or stoma, and appliance following urinary diversion.

Interventions/Take Action

Nursing Priority No. 1.

To assess causative/contributing factors:

- Note the presence of physical diagnoses that may be involved, such as UTI, fecal incontinence or constipation; dehydration; surgery (including urinary diversion); neurological involvement (e.g., MS, stroke, Parkinson disease, paraplegia/tetraplegia); mental or emotional dysfunction (e.g., impaired cognition, delirium or confusion, depression, Alzheimer disease); prostate disorders; overweight; postmenopausal hormonal factors; recent or multiple pregnancies; and pelvic trauma.
- Determine pathology of bladder dysfunction relative to the medical diagnosis identified. **While urinary incontinence (UI) is the most common elimination problem (categorized as stress, urge, mixed, or disability associated), other issues may need further evaluation such as in neurological or demyelinating diseases (e.g., MS), the problem may be related to the inability to store urine, empty the bladder, or both.**
- Assist with physical examination (e.g., cough test for incontinence, palpation for bladder retention or masses, prostate size, and observation for urethral stricture).
- Note age and gender of client. **Incontinence is twice as common in women as in men and affects at least one in three older women. While increasing age increases the risk for UI in both men and women, risk factors specific to women include parity, obesity, and history of hysterectomy. Evidence suggests UI is more common in men with the following risk factors: immobility, UTIs, diabetes, cognitive impairment, prostate disease/dysfunction, and neurological disease.**
- Investigate reports of pain, noting location, duration, intensity; presence of bladder spasms; or back or flank pain **to assist in differentiating between bladder and kidney as cause of dysfunction. Note: Bladder pain located suprapubically, vaginally, in the perineum, low back, or medial aspects of the thighs that is relieved by voiding and often recurs with bladder filling suggests the**

Information that appears in brackets has been added by the authors to clarify and enhance the use of nursing diagnoses.

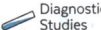 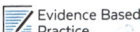 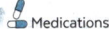 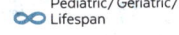

presence of painful bladder syndrome (PBS)/interstitial cystitis (IC).

- Observe current voiding pattern and time, color, and amount voided, as indicated. Note client's ability to recognize urge to void. **Helps determine type of problem present and assists in finding likely cause. Utilization of validated screening tools (e.g., The 3 Incontinence Questions, the International Consultation on Incontinence Questionnaire Urinary Incontinence Short Form, the Revised Urinary Incontinence Scale) can easily be completed to screen for UI symptoms and discern the effect that UI has on quality of life (QOL).**
- Measure postvoid urinary residual using bladder scanner, if available. **Determines adequacy of bladder emptying and urinary retention.**
- Have client complete standardized self-report tool, such as the Pelvic Pain and Urgency/Frequency client symptom survey, as indicated. **Helpful in evaluating the presence and severity of symptoms.**
- Note reports of exacerbations and spontaneous remissions of symptoms of urgency and frequency, which may or may not be accompanied by pain, pressure, or spasm.
- Determine the client's usual daily fluid intake (both amount and beverage choices, use of caffeine). Note the condition of skin and mucous membranes and the color of urine **to help determine level of hydration.**
- Review medication regimen **for drugs that can alter bladder or kidney function (e.g., antihypertensive agents such as angiotensin-converting enzyme [ACE] inhibitors, beta-adrenergic blockers; diuretics, anticholinergics, antihistamines; antiparkinsonian drugs; antidepressants or antipsychotics; sedatives, hypnotics, narcotics/opioids; caffeine and alcohol).**
- Obtain urine specimen (midstream clean-voided or catheterized) for culture and sensitivities in the presence of signs of UTI—cloudy, foul odor; bloody urine.
- Review laboratory tests for hyperglycemia, hyperparathyroidism, or other metabolic conditions; changes in renal function; culture for presence of infection or sexually transmitted infections (STIs); urine cytology for cancer.
- Prepare for/review results of cystoscopy and bladder distention test as appropriate. **May be done to diagnose painful bladder syndrome/interstitial cystitis (PBS/IC). Note: Bladder distention test can also be used as initial therapy.**

Information that appears in brackets has been added by the authors to clarify and enhance the use of nursing diagnoses.

- Review results of diagnostic studies (e.g., uroflowmetry; cystometrogram; postvoid residual ultrasound (bladder scan); pressure flow and leak point pressure measurement; videourodynamics; electromyography; kidney, ureter, and bladder [KUB] imaging) **to identify presence and type of elimination problem.**
- Refer to NDs disability-associated urinary Incontinence; mixed urinary Incontinence; stress urinary Incontinence; urge urinary Incontinence; urinary Retention for related assessments and interventions.

Nursing Priority No. 2.
To assess degree of interference/disability:

- Compare client's previous pattern of elimination with current situation. Note reports of problems (e.g., frequency, urgency, painful urination; leaking or incontinence; changes in size and force of urinary stream; problems emptying bladder completely; nocturia or enuresis) **to assist in identification and treatment of particular dysfunction.**
- Ascertain the client's/significant other's (SO's) perception of problem and degree of disability (e.g., client is restricting social, employment, or travel activities; having sexual or relationship difficulties; incurring sleep deprivation; experiencing depression).
- Note influence of culture/ethnicity or gender on client's view of problems of incontinence. **Limited evidence exists to understand and help people cope with the physical and psychosocial consequences of this chronic, socially isolating, and potentially devastating disorder.**
- Have the client keep a voiding diary for a prescribed number of days to record fluid intake, voiding times, precise urine output, and dietary intake. **Helps determine baseline symptoms, severity of frequency or urgency, and whether diet is a factor (if symptoms worsen).**

Nursing Priority No. 3.
To assist in treating/preventing urinary alteration:

- Encourage fluid intake up to 1,500 to 2,000 mL/day (within cardiac tolerance), including cranberry juice. **Adequate fluid intake supports optimal renal function, prevents infection and formation of urinary stones, and may reduce crust formation around indwelling catheter. Some studies suggest a clear correlation between cranberry juice and the prevention and treatment of UTIs.**

Information that appears in brackets has been added by the authors to clarify and enhance the use of nursing diagnoses.

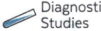 Diagnostic Studies
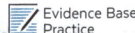 Evidence Based Practice
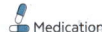 Medications
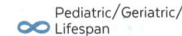 Pediatric/Geriatric/Lifespan

- Discuss possible dietary restrictions (e.g., especially coffee, alcohol, carbonated drinks, citrus, tomatoes, and chocolate) based on individual symptoms.
- Assist with developing toileting routines (e.g., timed voiding, bladder training, prompted voiding, habit retraining), as appropriate. **For adults who are cognitively intact and physically capable of self-toileting, bladder training, timed voiding, and habit retraining may be beneficial.**
- Encourage the client to verbalize fears and concerns (e.g., disruption in sexual activity or inability to work). **Open expression allows the client to deal with feelings and begin problem-solving.**
- Modify medication regimens as appropriate. For example, administer prescribed diuretics in the morning **to lessen nighttime voiding,** and reduce or eliminate use of hypnotics, if possible, **as client may be too sedated to recognize or respond to urge to void.**
- Implement and monitor interventions for specific elimination problem (e.g., pelvic floor exercises or other bladder retraining modalities; medication regimen, including antimicrobials [single dose is frequently being used for UTI], sulfonamides, antispasmodics); and evaluate client's response **to modify treatment, as needed.**
- Refer to appropriate resources (e.g., medical supply company, ostomy nurse, rehabilitation team) **for assistance, as desired or needed, to promote self-care.**
- Discuss possible surgical procedures and medical regimen, as indicated (e.g., client with benign prostatic hypertrophy bladder or prostatic cancer, PBS/IC). **For example, cystoscopy with bladder hydrodistention may be used for PBS/IC, or an electrical stimulator may be implanted to treat chronic urinary urge incontinence, nonobstructive urinary retention, and symptoms of urgency and frequency.**

Nursing Priority No. 4.
To assist in management of long-term urinary alterations:

- Instruct client/SO/caregivers in cues (e.g., voiding on routine schedule; showing client location of the bathroom; providing adequate room lighting, signs, color coding of door) that client needs **to assist in continued continence, especially when in unfamiliar surroundings.**
- Keep bladder deflated by use of an indwelling catheter connected to closed drainage. Investigate alternatives when possible. **Measures such as intermittent catheterization,**

Information that appears in brackets has been added by the authors to clarify and enhance the use of nursing diagnoses.

surgical interventions, urinary drugs, voiding maneuvers may be preferable to the indwelling catheter to provide more effective control and prevent the possibility of recurrent infections.
- Educate client/SO in use of/or assist with urinary devices or adjuncts (e.g., urethral closure devices [FemAssist, CapSure Shield, Reliance Urinary Control Insert, etc.], pads/absorbency devices [Purewick, condom cath]). **Adjuncts may be helpful to improve client skin integrity, improve sense of control, reduce fall risk, and improve QOL.**
- Provide latex-free catheter and care supplies, if indicated. **Reduces the risk of developing sensitivity to latex, which can develop in individuals requiring frequent catheterization or who have long-term indwelling catheters.**
- Check frequently for bladder distention and observe for overflow **to reduce the risk of infection and/or autonomic hyperreflexia (risk for clients with SCI).**
- Adhere to a regular bladder or diversion appliance emptying schedule. **Avoids reflux of urine (i.e., risk of infection) and accidents (i.e., prevents embarrassment to the individual).**
- Provide for routine diversion appliance care and assist the client to recognize and deal with problems, such as alkaline salt encrustation, ill-fitting appliance, malodorous urine, and infection. **Provides information and promotes competence in care, increasing self-confidence in dealing with appliance on a regular basis.**
- Refer to NDs disability-associated urinary Incontinence; mixed urinary Incontinence; stress urinary Incontinence; urge urinary Incontinence; urinary Retention for additional interventions.

Nursing Priority No. 5.
To promote maximum elimination management (Teaching/Discharge Considerations) and enhance well-being (long-term goals):

- Review expectations and prognosis of underlying condition (e.g., MS, prostate disease). **Provides information to assist client/SO to make informed decisions and plan for possible changes.**
- Emphasize the importance of keeping the perineal area clean and dry **to reduce the risk of infection and/or skin breakdown.**
- Instruct female clients with UTI to drink large amounts of fluid, wipe from front to back, promptly treat vaginal

---

Information that appears in brackets has been added by the authors to clarify and enhance the use of nursing diagnoses.

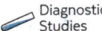 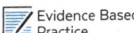 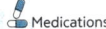 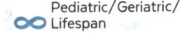

infections, and take showers rather than tub baths **to limit risk or avoid reinfection.**

- Recommend smoking cessation program, as appropriate. **Cigarette smoking can be a source of bladder irritation.**
- Encourage SO(s) who participate in routine care to recognize complications (including latex allergy) necessitating medical evaluation or intervention.
- Instruct in proper application and care of appliance for urinary diversion. Encourage liberal fluid intake, avoidance of foods or medications that produce strong odor, use of white vinegar or deodorizer in pouch. **These measures help to ensure patency of device and prevent embarrassing situations for client.**
- Identify sources for supplies and programs or agencies providing financial assistance. **Lack of access to necessities can be a barrier to management of incontinence, and having help to obtain needed equipment can assist with daily care.**
- Recommend avoidance of gas-forming foods in the presence of ureterosigmoidostomy, **as flatus can cause urinary incontinence.**
- Recommend use of silicone catheter. **Although these catheters are more expensive than rubber catheters, they are more comfortable and generally cause fewer problems with infection when permanent or long-term catheterization is required.**
- Demonstrate proper positioning of catheter drainage tubing and bag below level of the bladder **to facilitate drainage, prevent reflux, and complications of infection.**
- Refer client/SO(s) to appropriate community resources, such as ostomy specialist, support group, sex therapist, or psychiatric clinical nurse specialist, **to deal with changes in body image and function, when indicated.**

Documentation Focus

Assessment/Reassessment
- Individual findings, including previous and current pattern of voiding, nature of problem, and effect on desired lifestyle
- Cultural factors or concerns

Planning
- Plan of care and who is involved in planning
- Teaching plan

Information that appears in brackets has been added by the authors to clarify and enhance the use of nursing diagnoses.

 Acute Care 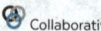 Collaborative 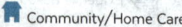 Community/Home Care  Cultural

Implementation/Evaluation
- Response to interventions, teaching, and actions performed
- Attainment of or progress toward desired outcome(s)
- Modifications to plan of care

Discharge Planning
- Long-term needs and who is responsible for actions to be taken
- Available resources and specific referrals made
- Individual equipment needs and sources

Sample Nursing Outcomes & Interventions Classifications NOC/NIC

NOC—Urinary Elimination
NIC—Urinary Elimination Management

---

risk for ELOPEMENT ICNP

[Diagnostic Division: Safety]

Definition: Susceptible to individual in supervised setting seeking to leave or wandering away without knowledge or permission.

Recognizing Cues

Risk Factors
Disorientation; confusion; persistent seeking of exit doors; aimless wandering

Unfamiliar environment; concern for personal safety

Limited, ineffective caregiver supervision; lack of social support

Irritability; frustration with perceived "confinement" or restriction of movement; fear of losing autonomy

Concern for unfulfilled obligations to family/friends, financial consequences

Dissatisfied with treatment plan or care provided

Intention of harm to self or others; substance misuse

Clinical Connections
Mental health conditions (e.g., Autism Spectrum Disorder, dementia, depression, manic phase of bipolar disorder, schizophrenia), traumatic brain injury, developmental delays, substance abuse

---

Information that appears in brackets has been added by the authors to clarify and enhance the use of nursing diagnoses.

 Diagnostic Studies 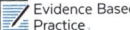 Evidence Based Practice 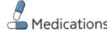 Medications ∞ Pediatric/Geriatric/Lifespan

Generate Solutions

Plan Desired Outcomes

Caregiver Will (Include Specific Time Frame)
- Recognize signs and symptoms of a client who is at risk of elopement.
- Alleviate environmental risks for elopement.

Client Will (Include Specific Time Frame)
- Remain in facility/designated area.

Interventions/Take Action

Nursing Priority No. 1.
To determine degree of risk:

- Determine presence of psychiatric behavioral health issues, noting history of prior attempts to leave without permission. **Elopement has been defined as "a patient that is aware that he/she is not permitted to leave, but does so with intent" (DeRosier & Taylor, 2005), which distinguishes it from wandering. In many cases of elopement, client may have diminished mental capacity related to developmental disorders, dementia, or acute substance intoxication, disease, or traumatic injury.**

- Evaluate at-risk client and note presence/severity of individual factors (using an elopement assessment tool), as indicated. At-risk clients may include:

  Those who have a court-appointed legal guardian or have been legally committed to care.

  Those with physical, developmental, or mental impairments that increase the risk of being a danger to self or others.

  Those who lack cognitive, intellectual, or developmental abilities to make relevant decisions.

  Those with history of elopement.

  Why and where did the client want to go.

  Review behavioral areas of concern:

  Mobility: **Client might be fully ambulatory or be able to propel self in some manner, or may enlist assistance from others unaware of elopement risk.**

  Mental stability: **Client's mental status may be acutely or chronically impaired if diagnoses include related conditions (e.g., intellectual disabilities, brain injuries, short-term delirium; mental illness or dementia). Note: Psychiatric diagnoses, such as delusions, hallucinations, and schizophrenia, also place residents at**

Information that appears in brackets has been added by the authors to clarify and enhance the use of nursing diagnoses.

high risk for elopement. Depression is known to mimic symptoms associated with dementia, and akathisia (motor restlessness characterized by pacing, standing and sitting, or rocking back and forth) may be caused by psychotropic and antidepressant medications.

Emotional status: Client may have many emotional reactions (e.g., be agitated, angry, or expressing desire to leave) or could be calm but delusional, believing they need to go to another location (such as work).

History of elopement attempts: One recent legal article noted that 80% of current cases were known to be chronic wanderers with prior elopements.

Behaviors: Client may attempt to communicate strong emotion or a need, such as wandering near the bathroom or getting away from an undesired activity or person; a client in a new and unfamiliar setting may be trying to return to known environment or people but be unable to communicate.

Medications: Medications that cause confusion and restlessness and addictive substances (alcohol and other drugs) can impair thinking and cause harm. Akathisia may be caused by psychotropic and antidepressant medications.

- Note client's age and developmental level. **Although elopement is a risk at any age, individuals at extremes of age who cannot protect themselves, individuals with ASD, teenagers (rebelling or asserting independence), and younger individuals with dementia may be more prone to elopement attempts than others. Note: Research shows that one in three young children with ASD has tried to wander off. This behavior may continue to happen into adulthood. It is concerning because many people with ASD may not be able to share their name, address, or phone number if they get lost.**

- Gather information about the behavior from multiple sources (e.g., observe individual engaging in elopement and record what happens immediately and after the behavior). **Information may need to be obtained from numerous persons involved in client's life (e.g., babysitter, treatment care staff, school staff) to obtain a comprehensive picture when client is frequently attempting to leave.**

- Evaluate client's activity/lifestyle (e.g., individual typically hyperactive, or reacts to stress with physical activity

---

Information that appears in brackets has been added by the authors to clarify and enhance the use of nursing diagnoses.

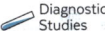 Diagnostic Studies 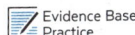 Evidence Based Practice 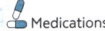 Medications 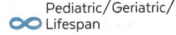 Pediatric/Geriatric/Lifespan

rather than emotional reactions) to help identify likelihood of wanting to leave. **For example, client may enjoy running or exploring, or wants to get out of a situation that causes stress (e.g., being asked to do something at school or getting away from noisy environments or crowds). Note: One study showed that a history of prior elopement is a high predictor (72%) of further incidents.**

- Document timing and pattern of wandering behavior, which could result in elopement. **For example, client may attempt to leave at 5 p.m. every day, believing he is going home from work or school. Client may be goal-directed (e.g., searching for person or object, escaping from something) or non–goal directed (wandering aimlessly). Knowledge of patterns can prompt caregivers to anticipate need for personal attention. Note: Studies have shown that many elopements (in clients with dementia) occur in the late afternoon and evening hours (often due to sundowning syndrome).**

Nursing Priority No. 2.

To promote client safety:

- Practice client safety at all times. **Elopement can place the client in immediate jeopardy (loss of life or major injury); upset/undermine family unit; result in negligence or malpractice litigation, monetary penalties, lack of reimbursement by payers, and loss of public confidence. Understand the potential costs of negligent behaviors and how to prevent client injury as well as practice/civil liability.**
- Provide for 24-hr supervision, as indicated. Institute "whereabouts" checks so that staff/caregivers can account for all individuals at regular intervals on each shift. Communicate client's history and supervision needs with ancillary team members, as appropriate. **Some clients may require documentation every 15 min, while others may need to be on one-to-one supervision (within arm's length at all times). Client safety is the responsibility of all staff. Legally, elopement is considered unacceptable and can result in litigation. Failure to monitor, whether as a result of neglect or understaffing, is not acceptable.**
- Establish that environmental safety measures are in place and operating (e.g., video observation of client areas; exits equipped with alarms and pressure-sensitive doormats, safety locks on doors and windows; complex and inaccessible door latches). **Technology is vital for helping to**

Information that appears in brackets has been added by the authors to clarify and enhance the use of nursing diagnoses.

prevent elopement, and it is critical for staff/caregivers to monitor equipment, monitor the client, and document the client's presence.
- Provide client safety measures (e.g., picture of client, physical description, identification necklace/dog tags, ankle/wrist sensors/monitors, dead bolt and door locks/safety locks that are secured at all times and out of reach of toddlers. **Important to have availability to share a picture and description with first responders; necklace such as military-style dog tags may help with identification. Ankle/wrist sensors/monitors help locate the individual.**
- Schedule maintenance to update, repair, or replace faulty equipment. **Routine inspection is required for equipment to operate properly.**
- Recommend that family work with behavior analyst, especially if child elopes often or elopes in dangerous situations (e.g., high-traffic areas or after dark). **Helps family to understand safety measures in any health setting.**

Nursing Priority No. 3.

To promote continued safety (Teaching/Discharge Considerations) and enhance well-being (long-term goals):

- Identify problems that are remediable and assist client/significant other (SO) to seek appropriate assistance and access resources. **Encourages problem-solving to improve client's condition and seek help from community resources, family, and friends.**
- Provide structured activities dependent upon age, intellectual, educational, and psychosocial development level (e.g., engaging client with dementia in simple repetitive actions such as folding towels/napkins; music, art projects, exercise program, or games). **Providing a variety of activities keeps the client involved and interested in present environment.**
- Refer to community resources, such as day-care programs, support groups. **Caregiver(s) will require access to multiple kinds of assistance and opportunities to promote problem-solving, enhance coping, and obtain necessary respite.**
- Notify neighbors about client's condition and request that they contact client's family or local police if they see client outside alone; request community signage about client's condition (if appropriate). **Community awareness can prevent or reduce risk of client being lost or injured.**

Information that appears in brackets has been added by the authors to clarify and enhance the use of nursing diagnoses.

- Help client/SO and family members develop plan of care when problem is progressive. **Client may initially need part-time assistance at home, progressing to enrollment in day-care program, and then full-time home care or placement in care facility. Include respite care for family, making a weekly schedule (e.g., eating out, visiting friends, or social activities.)**
- Refer to community resources, such as day-care programs, support groups, respite care. **Caregiver(s) will require access to multiple kinds of assistance and opportunities to promote problem-solving, enhance coping.**
- Refer to NDs acute/chronic Confusion, risk for physical Injury, or Sensory Deficit for additional interventions as indicated.

Documentation Focus

Assessment/Reassessment
- Assessment findings, including individual concerns, family involvement, and support factors
- Availability and use of resources

Planning
- Plan of care and who is involved in planning
- Teaching plan

Implementation/Evaluation
- Responses of client/SO(s) to plan interventions and actions performed
- Attainment of or progress toward desired outcome(s)
- Modifications to plan of care

Discharge Planning
- Long-term needs and who is responsible for actions to be taken
- Specific referrals made

Sample Nursing Outcomes & Interventions Classifications NOC/NIC

NOC—Elopement Propensity Risk
NIC—Elopement Precautions

Information that appears in brackets has been added by the authors to clarify and enhance the use of nursing diagnoses.

impaired EMANCIPATED DECISION-MAKING   NANDA-I

[Diagnostic Division: Health Management]

Definition: A process of choosing a healthcare decision that does not include personal knowledge and/or consideration of social norms, or does not occur in a flexible environment, resulting in decisional dissatisfaction.

Recognizing Cues

Related/Risk Factors
Decreased understanding of available healthcare options; inadequate information regarding healthcare options

Inadequately verbalizes beliefs about healthcare options; inadequate confidence to openly discuss healthcare options; inadequate self-confidence in decision making

Inadequate privacy to openly discuss healthcare options; inadequate time to discuss healthcare options

Defining Characteristics

Subjective

Difficulty choosing a healthcare option that best fits current lifestyle; impaired ability to describe how option will fit into current lifestyle

Uses constraint in describing own option; excessive concern about others' opinions; excessive fear of what others think about a decision

Objective

Delayed enactment of healthcare option

Limited verbalization about healthcare option in other's presence; discomfort with other's opinion

Clinical Connections
Any condition/situation requiring healthcare decisions

Generate Solutions

Plan Desired Outcomes

Client Will (Include Specific Time Frame)
- Verbalize concern about healthcare decision making.
- Express understanding of available healthcare options.

Information that appears in brackets has been added by the authors to clarify and enhance the use of nursing diagnoses.

 Diagnostic Studies   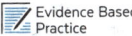 Evidence Based Practice   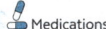 Medications   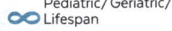 Pediatric/Geriatric/Lifespan

- Discuss healthcare options openly and with confidence.
- Participate in decision making freely and openly.

Interventions/Take Action

Nursing Priority No. 1.

To assess causative/contributing factors (e.g., dementia, delirium, intellectual disability, substance abuse, lack of confidence):

- Determine usual ability to make decisions and factors that are currently interfering with making a personal choice. **The individual may not have sufficient knowledge or may be influenced by family pressures, which may prevent making an independent decision.**
- Note expressions of indecision, dependence on others, availability and involvement of support persons. **Healthcare providers need to be sensitive to the physical, emotional, and cognitive effects of the situation on decision-making capabilities and client's desire for family/friend support.**
- Discuss if client feels comfortable, confident, or wants to be involved in decision making. **External influences may pressure the person to give up their own responsibility for the decision.**
- Identify previous decisions the individual has made and the environment in which those and current decisions were/are made. **Provides information about the client's ability and circumstances surrounding decision making.**
- Active-listen and identify reasons for indecisiveness. **Helps the client to clarify the problem and begin to look at alternatives for the situation.**
- Identify cultural values, beliefs, moral obligations, or ethical concerns that may be creating conflict in the current situation. **These issues need to be resolved before the client will be comfortable with the decision.**
- Review information the client has to support the decision to be made. **Provides an opportunity to clarify and correct misinformation or inaccurate perceptions that can affect the outcome.**

Nursing Priority No. 2.

To determine readiness to improve/effectively use problem-solving skills:

- Determine the client's level of readiness to change (e.g., precontemplation, contemplation, preparation, action,

---

Information that appears in brackets has been added by the authors to clarify and enhance the use of nursing diagnoses.

maintenance, termination). **Recognizing state of readiness to change guides choice of interventions. Attempting to take action prior to client readiness will be met with resistance and lack of improvement.**
- Use Motivational Interviewing skills to help establish a therapeutic relationship. **The interviewing style lets the client know you are interested in them, want to understand their life and help with improving their circumstances.**
- Listen and observe for verbal and nonverbal communication patterns. **Responses from Motivational Interviewing help to determine the client's desires, abilities, reasons, and needs for change. Nonverbal communication reflects the congruency of the client's verbal expressions.**
- Identify cultural and spiritual health beliefs and expectations. **Different cultures and spiritual health beliefs expect family members to respond to family/tribe's/clan's lifestyle of choice. Awareness of the diversity and differences in decision making helps to guide the client/family to accept or reject change. Motivational Interviewing is a respectful approach to help clients who reject change to begin thinking about making changes.**

Nursing Priority No. 3.

To assist client to become empowered and able to make effective decisions:

- Promote safe and hopeful environment as needed. **The client needs to feel safe and supported to be comfortable in own ability to make satisfactory decisions.**
- Encourage verbalization of conflicts and concerns. **Helps to identify and clarify these issues so the individual can reach a satisfying solution.**
- Discuss importance of open and honest communication and not holding on to secrets. **Functional communication is clear, direct, and honest, with congruence between verbal and nonverbal expressions. Dysfunctional communication is indirect, vague, and controlled, with many double-binded (conflicting) messages. Awareness of this information can enhance relationships among family members.**
- Demonstrate techniques such as active-listening, "I" messages, and problem-solving. **Learning these skills can promote effective communication and improve interactions among the family.**

Information that appears in brackets has been added by the authors to clarify and enhance the use of nursing diagnoses.

 Diagnostic Studies 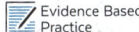 Evidence Based Practice 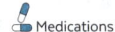 Medications 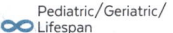 Pediatric/Geriatric/Lifespan

- Provide time to talk with family to discuss their views of the situation. **Provides an opportunity to clarify family's understanding and determine how realistic their ideas are for planning how they are going to cope with the current situation in the most positive manner.**
- Clarify and prioritize individual goals. **Enables the client to look at the importance of the issues of the conflict and reach realistic problem-solving.**
- Identify strengths and use of positive coping skills, relaxation techniques, and willingness to express feelings. **Encourages the individual to view self as a capable person who can make a desired decision.**
- Discuss time constraints related to the decision to be made. **Healthcare decisions (i.e., breastfeeding) may need to be made quickly depending on the circumstances.**
- Help client to understand, value, and learn the problem-solving process. **Provides a structure for the individual to look at alternatives for making a decision in the current situation and for other decisions that need to be made in the future.**
- Discuss and clarify spiritual concerns, accepting the client's values in a nonjudgmental manner. **The client will be willing to consider own situation when accepted as an individual of worth.**

Nursing Priority No. 4.

To promote independence (Teaching/Discharge Considerations) and enhance well-being (long-term goals):

- Provide opportunities for role-playing and practicing problem-solving skills. **Helps the client to become more confident and solve current and future situations.**
- Encourage the family to become involved as desired by client. **Facilitates an understanding of the individual's needs and abilities, promoting support and acceptance of the ability of the family member.**
- Recommend client attendance at assertiveness and stress-reduction classes. **Learning these skills helps the client to become able to make decisions in a more decisive manner.**
- Refer to other resources as indicated (e.g., public health, healthcare providers, support group, clergy, psychiatrist/psychiatric clinical nurse specialist). **The client may need**

Information that appears in brackets has been added by the authors to clarify and enhance the use of nursing diagnoses.

additional support to manage difficult decision making and/or support for long-term needs.

Documentation Focus

Assessment/Reassessment
- Assessment findings, behavioral responses and degree of impairment in lifestyle functioning
- Individual involved in the conflict
- Personal values and beliefs, moral or ethical concerns

Planning
- Plan of care, specific interventions, and who is involved in the planning process
- Teaching plan

Implementation/Evaluation
- Client's and involved individual's responses to interventions, teaching, and actions performed
- Ability to express feelings and identify options
- Use of resources
- Attainment of or progress toward desired outcome(s)
- Modifications to plan of care

Discharge Planning
- Long-term needs, actions to be taken, and who is responsible for actions
- Specific referrals made

Sample Nursing Outcomes & Interventions Classifications NOC/NIC

NOC—Decision-Making
NIC—Decision-Making Support

---

ineffective EMOTION REGULATION — NANDA-I

[Diagnostic Division: Stress Management]

Definition: Inability to control feelings, thoughts, behaviors and interactions, leading to mismatched responses and expressions in social situations.

Information that appears in brackets has been added by the authors to clarify and enhance the use of nursing diagnoses.

 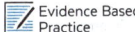 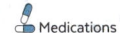

Recognizing Cues

Related/Risk Factors
Depression, inadequate self-esteem
Limited coping strategies; excessive use of defense mechanisms
Fatigue; muscle weakness
Inadequate knowledge of disease process, or about symptom control
Social distress
Substance misuse

Defining Characteristics

Subjective
Excessive crying without feeling sadness, or laughing without feeling happiness
Embarrassment regarding emotional expression
Incongruent expression of emotion with social interactions

Objective
Absence of eye contact; impaired nonverbal communication
Blunted affect (showing lack of emotions); restricted affect (limited range of expressions); flat affect (showing no emotion); labile affect (shows rapid changes with emotions)
Emotions incongruent with triggering factor; phobias; panic attacks
Crying; involuntary or uncontrollable crying or laughing
Withdrawal from occupational situations; social alienation

Clinical Connections
Traumatic brain injury, autism, stroke, multiple sclerosis, depression, anxiety, post-traumatic stress disorder, schizophrenia, schizoaffective disorder, bipolar disorder, schizoid and borderline personality disorders, substance abuse

Generate Solutions

Plan Desired Outcomes

Client Will (Include Specific Time Frame)
- Acknowledge problem with emotional control.
- Identify feelings that occur with episodes of uncontrollable emotions.
- Follow medication regimen.
- Participate in recommended activities/rehabilitation.

Information that appears in brackets has been added by the authors to clarify and enhance the use of nursing diagnoses.

 Acute Care 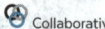 Collaborative 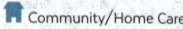 Community/Home Care Cultural

Interventions/Take Action

Nursing Priority No. 1.
To assess causative/contributing factors:

- Identify medical and psychiatric history influencing emotional dysregulation (e.g., traumatic brain injury, schizophrenia, depression, narcissism/borderline personality disorders) in client in the current situation. **Many different physiological/psychological factors may be involved in the loss of emotional control for a given person. Identifying these factors will help to develop a plan of care that is specific to this individual.**
- Note when episodes of loss of control occur. **Helps in determining the frequency of incidents and factors associated with the condition (e.g., outcomes of first stroke), or inability to manage emotions during social interactions.**
- Identify client's awareness and perception of emotional dysregulation. **Most people are embarrassed by these outbursts and may consider suicide, while others believe they can control their outbursts. Individuals with multiple sclerosis are prone to pseudobulbar affect (PBA) resulting in emotional outbursts. PBA needs to be recognized as different, as treatments are different for this condition.**
- Evaluate for depression and suicidal ideation. **Clients may experience social isolation due to emotional outbursts, resulting in depression and suicidal ideation.**

Nursing Priority No. 2.
To determine effective control of labile episodes:

- Develop plan of care to meet needs of individual's medical or mental diagnosis/situation. **Assists in providing effective care for specific problems the person is experiencing.**
- Establish a therapeutic nurse–client relationship. **Promotes trust and willingness to share concerns about problems that arise.**
- Identify feelings of emotional exhaustion and social isolation. **The individual may not recognize that PBA is a medical condition and may tend to remove self from situations that trigger the episodes.**
- Assure client with multiple sclerosis and PBA that symptoms are real and need to be treated. **Client may not recognize that these are symptoms and neglect reporting problems of emotional outbursts to all their healthcare providers.**

Information that appears in brackets has been added by the authors to clarify and enhance the use of nursing diagnoses.

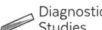 Diagnostic Studies 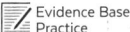 Evidence Based Practice 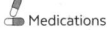 Medications ∞ Pediatric/Geriatric/Lifespan

- Correct misperceptions and provide accurate information. **Promotes understanding and helps the client to be proactive in care.**

Nursing Priority No. 3.
To stabilize emotions and interactions (Teaching/Discharge Considerations) and enhance well-being (long-term goals):

- Involve the family in the treatment plan. **Provides support for the client and promotes understanding of the uncontrollable episodes.**
- Discuss the use of medication. **Antidepressants (e.g., selective serotonin reuptake inhibitors [SSRIs], selective norepinephrine reuptake inhibitors [SNRIs]), antipsychotics (e.g., Thorazine, Serentil), mood stabilizers (e.g., lithium or anticonvulsants, Depakote) are used in clinical practice; a PBA-specific treatment, Nuedexta, is a fixed-dose combination of dextromethorphan hydrobromide/quinidine sulfate (DHQ).**
- Encourage involvement in social activities. **Enhances the ability to participate with others, reducing sense of social isolation.**
- Refer for physical therapy and rehabilitation. **The client may benefit from these activities, enhancing sense of well-being.**
- Refer to other resources as necessary: group therapy, psychiatric therapy, assertiveness training. **This additional help will enable the client to develop a more positive lifestyle.**

Documentation Focus

Assessment/Reassessment
- Assessment findings, characteristics/frequency of episodes, other pertinent information

Planning
- Plan of care, specific interventions, and who is involved in the planning process
- Teaching plan

Implementation/Evaluation
- Response to intervention, teaching, and actions performed
- Ability to express feelings, control emotions
- Use of resources
- Attainment of or progress toward desired outcome(s)
- Modifications to plan of care

Information that appears in brackets has been added by the authors to clarify and enhance the use of nursing diagnoses.

Discharge Planning
- Long-term needs, who is responsible for actions to be taken
- Specific referrals made

Sample Nursing Outcomes & Interventions Classifications NOC/NIC

NOC—Mood Equilibrium
NIC—Mood Management

---

impaired END-OF-LIFE COMFORT SYNDROME NANDA-I

[Diagnostic Division: Comfort]

Definition: Deterioration in a set of physical, psychological, social, and spiritual manifestations due to the imminence of the death process.

Recognizing Cues

Related/Risk Factors
Anxiety; excessive stress; fear
Depressive symptoms; suffering; despair
Decreased activity tolerance; feeling bad for depending on others
Feeling threatened by current condition, or by death
Dry mouth; indigestion; unaddressed vomiting
Impaired skin or tissue integrity
Urinary retention
Increased oxygen demand

Defining Characteristics

Subjective
Acute pain; chronic pain; impaired physical or psychological comfort
Excessive fatigue burden; ineffective sleep pattern
Excessive death anxiety; impaired spiritual well-being

Objective
Acute or chronic confusion
Impaired physical mobility
Excessive fluid volume; inadequate nutritional intake
Impaired urinary or intestinal elimination
Ineffective breathing pattern

Information that appears in brackets has been added by the authors to clarify and enhance the use of nursing diagnoses.

 Diagnostic Studies 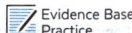 Evidence Based Practice 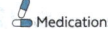 Medications 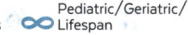 Pediatric/Geriatric/Lifespan

Ineffective thermoregulation
Maladaptive grieving; inadequate social support

Clinical Connections
Chronic conditions, elder individuals

Generate Solutions

Plan Desired Outcomes

Client Will (Include Specific Time Frame)
- Be free of pain/discomfort, relaxing in a comfortable position.
- Discuss physical changes and be able to express own desires.
- Express fears and concerns freely.
- Verbalize acceptance of outcome regarding efforts to resolve conflicts/make amends with others.

Interventions/Take Action

Nursing Priority No. 1.
To assess comfort needs at end of life:
- Identify physical concerns such as discomfort/pain, breathing problems, skin irritation, digestive concerns, too warm/too cold, or being fatigued. Note an increase in wakefulness, restlessness, crying, or agitation. **Managing a dying person's comfort/pain can be difficult. Not all clients experience pain at the end of life. Provide as much pain medication as prescribed by the doctor.**
- Assess for bed sores/pressure ulcers every 2 hr while repositioning client. **Poor circulation at end of life allows for bed sores to develop quickly.**
- Identify mental and emotional concerns (e.g., fear of being alone, unresolved conflicts, anger/resentment toward others, feelings of guilt). **Allows client to express their thoughts and feelings and what they would like to happen in their final hours.**
- Identify spiritual needs (e.g., visitation by spiritual leader, conflict resolution, accepting conditions of life/death). **Understanding client's needs helps with planning nursing actions.**
- Determine end-of-life desires noting cultural preferences. **Client may want to finalize or re-write living will or will, make plans for pet care, organ donation, burial/cremation, or determine what happens with personal items.**

Information that appears in brackets has been added by the authors to clarify and enhance the use of nursing diagnoses.

Nursing Priority No. 2.
To maximize client comfort:

- Explain palliative care versus hospice care. **Client/family/SO may not understand the differences in care issues between palliative and hospice care.**
- Encourage client to express thoughts about past, present, death, and settling affairs. Listen for comments about pain, agitation, fear of death, or auditory/visual hallucinations. **Relating memories and experiences may be calming to client or disruptive depending on their life experiences. Client may also want to settle business/financial affairs. Last, client may want to amend relationships with family/friends.** Refrain from challenging client regarding hallucinations, **which distresses client leading to agitation and possible mistrust of provider.**
- Speak to client in soft and calming voice, being sensitive to cultural and spiritual background and keeping conversation focused on positive memories, as appropriate. **Reinforcing your presence can be calming to client.**
- Monitor environment making adjustments based on client desires (e.g., temperature, smells, level of lighting, noise level, privacy or presence). **Allowing client to select environmental comfort measures provides a sense of calm and relaxation while entering their final hours.**
- Encourage family to provide small amounts of food/fluids if desired by client. **Small feedings/tastes can be pleasurable to client while preventing gastrointestinal distress as organ function declines at end of life.**
- Provide ice chips, lip balm as indicated to maintain oral comfort, especially if client is mouth breathing. **Dry mouth and lips are uncomfortable for people.**
- Arrange visitation of family/friends based on client wishes. Provide support of counselor/spiritual leader if desired to address past conflicts, grievances, reconciliation. **While client may enjoy reminiscing and sharing fond memories, resolving emotional conflict helps in limiting distress for the client and others.**

Nursing Priority No. 3.
To assist client/family/SO to cope with end of life:

- Identify resources (e.g., home health, palliative care, hospice agencies, nursing facilities, healthcare clinic, and other resources the family may need or request). **Hospitalized client's family/SO may desire transfer to home for**

Information that appears in brackets has been added by the authors to clarify and enhance the use of nursing diagnoses.

end-of-life care. **Family/SO caregivers will need help with identifying resources.**
- Include client and family/SO, as appropriate, in developing plan of care. **Maintains sense of control and provides opportunity to clarify and meet wishes, including how much care is to be provided (e.g., medications, use of oxygen).**
- Administer pain medications, anxiolytic, sedatives, antinausea, antipyretic drugs as indicated. **Provides relief of distressing symptoms based on client's plan of care.**
- Monitor for cold extremities, changes in skin color (e.g., pale, bluish), sleepiness, and unresponsiveness. **Client changes that often take place 24 hr prior to death can be very distressing to family and signal need for presence so client does not die alone.**

Documentation Focus

Assessment/Reassessment
- Identification of risk factors related to skin care, behavioral/emotional responses of client/family/SO
- Client's perception of the situation
- Cultural/spiritual beliefs and expectations
- Availability and use of resources

Planning
- Plan of care and who will be included
- Teaching plan

Implementation/Evaluation
- Response to interventions, teaching, and actions performed
- Attainment or progress toward desired outcome(s)

Discharge Planning
- Long-term needs and who is responsible for actions to be taken
- Referrals made

Sample Nursing Outcomes & Interventions Classifications NOC/NIC

NOC—Comfort Status
NIC—Dying Care

Information that appears in brackets has been added by the authors to clarify and enhance the use of nursing diagnoses.

 Acute Care Collaborative 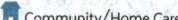 Community/Home Care Cultural

disrupted ENERGY FIELD ICNP

[Diagnostic Division: Stress Management]

Definition: Disturbance or deficiency in the flow, rhythm, symmetry, or gentle vibration characterizing the luminous field of energy extending beyond one's physical body.

Recognizing Cues

Related/Risk Factors
Stress; anxiety; situational crisis
Acute illness; chronic conditions; injury
Physical pain
Psychological distress

Defining Characteristics

Subjective
Sense of disharmony, disconnectedness, depletion
Fatigue; malaise; discomfort
Difficulty concentrating

Objective
Change in rate or strength of energy flow
Uneven distribution, congestion, blockage, or breaks in energy flow
Temperature changes in energy field
Change in color, vibrational frequency of aura; tingling sensation
Crisis; individuals experiencing personal crisis/life transition

Clinical Connections
Illness, trauma, cancer, chronic pain, impaired immune system, fatigue, surgical procedures, depression, post-traumatic stress disorder (PTSD), high-risk pregnancy, labor and delivery, end of life

Generate Solutions

Plan Desired Outcomes

Client Will (Include Specific Time Frame)
- Acknowledge feelings of anxiety and distress.
- Verbalize sense of relaxation and well-being.
- Display reduction in severity or frequency of symptoms.

Information that appears in brackets has been added by the authors to clarify and enhance the use of nursing diagnoses.

 Diagnostic Studies
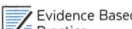 Evidence Based Practice
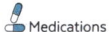 Medications
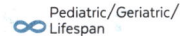 Pediatric/Geriatric/Lifespan

Interventions/Take Action

Nursing Priority No. 1.
To determine causative/contributing factors:

- Review current situation and concerns of client. Provide opportunity for client to talk about condition, past history, emotional state, or other relevant information. Note body gestures, tone of voice, and words chosen to express feelings or issues. **Research suggests biofield, or energy field, therapies (Healing Touch, Therapeutic Touch [TT]) may be beneficial in reducing levels of anxiety and pain perception, improving sense of well-being. Therapy may be effective in reducing PTSD symptoms, and TT may also be beneficial in reducing behavioral symptoms of dementia (e.g., manual manipulation/restlessness, vocalization, pacing).**
- Explain therapeutic process and expected results, and determine client's motivation or desire for treatment. **This therapy is the knowledgeable and purposeful patterning of client's environmental energy field to relieve discomfort and anxiety. Providing information that the fundamental focus is on healing and wholeness, not curing signs/symptoms of disease, helps client understand the process and can clarify any unrealistic expectations.**
- Note use of medications, other drug use (e.g., alcohol). **May affect client's ability to relax and take full advantage of the therapy process. Therapy may be helpful in reducing anxiety level in individuals undergoing alcohol withdrawal.**
- Perform/review results of testing, as indicated, such as the State-Trait Anxiety Inventory (STAI) or the Affect Balance Scale (ABS), **to provide measures of the client's anxiety.**

Nursing Priority No. 2.
To evaluate energy field:

- Develop therapeutic nurse–client relationship, initially accepting role of healer/guide as client desires. **This relationship is one in which both participants recognize each other as unique and important human beings and in which mutual learning occurs. The role of the nurse and the use of self as a therapeutic tool are recognized.**
- Place client in sitting or supine position with legs and arms uncrossed. Place pillows or other supports to enhance comfort and relaxation. **Promotes relaxation and feelings of**

Information that appears in brackets has been added by the authors to clarify and enhance the use of nursing diagnoses.

 Acute Care 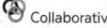 Collaborative 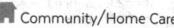 Community/Home Care Cultural

peace, calm, and security, preparing the client to derive the most benefit from the procedure.
- Center self physically and psychologically **to quiet mind and turn attention to the healing intent.**
- Move hands slowly over the client at level of 2 to 6 in. above skin to assess state of energy field and flow of energy within the system. **Assesses state of energy field and flow of energy within the system. The feelings that may be noted are tingling, warmth, coolness, comfort, relaxation, emotional release, and security.**
- Identify areas of imbalance or obstruction in the field (i.e., areas of asymmetry; feelings of heat or cold, tingling, congestion, or pressure).

Nursing Priority No. 3.
To provide therapeutic intervention:
- Discuss findings of evaluation with client and proposed intervention. **Including the client in the process by sharing the findings of the nurse combined with sensations the client experienced provides the best opportunity to derive benefit from the procedure.**
- Assist client with exercises (e.g., deep breathing, guided imagery) to promote "centering" and increase potential to self-heal, enhance comfort, and reduce anxiety.
- Perform unruffling process, keeping hands 2 to 6 in. from client's body **to dissipate impediments to free flow of energy within the system and between nurse and client.**
- Focus on areas of disturbance identified, holding hands over or on skin, and/or place one hand in back of body with other hand in front while concentrating on the intent to help the client heal. **Allows client's body to pull or repattern energy as needed.**
- ∞ Shorten duration of treatment to 2 to 3 min, as appropriate. **Children, elderly individuals, those with head injuries, and others who are severely debilitated are generally more sensitive to overloading energy fields.**
- Make coaching suggestions (e.g., pleasant images or other visualizations, deep breathing) in a soft voice **for enhancing feelings of relaxation.**
- Use hands-on massage/apply pressure to acupressure points, as appropriate, during process.
- Note changes in energy sensations as session progresses, stopping when the energy field is symmetric and there is a change to feelings of peaceful calm.

Information that appears in brackets has been added by the authors to clarify and enhance the use of nursing diagnoses.

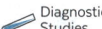 Diagnostic Studies 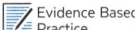 Evidence Based Practice 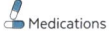 Medications 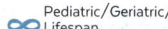 Pediatric/Geriatric/Lifespan

- Hold client's feet for a few minutes at end of session **to assist in "grounding" the body energy.**
- Provide client time following procedure **for a period of peaceful rest.**

Nursing Priority No. 4.

To promote ongoing harmony (Teaching/Discharge Considerations) and enhance well-being (long-term goals):

- Allow period of client dependency, as appropriate, **for client to strengthen own inner resources.**
- Encourage ongoing practice of the therapeutic process.
- Instruct in use of activities (e.g., energy-focusing or centering/meditation techniques, stretching exercises, stress reduction and relaxation exercises) **to promote mind-body-spirit harmony.**
- Discuss importance of integrating techniques into daily activity plan, **helping to keep energy fields open and sustaining/enhancing sense of well-being.**
- Have client practice each step and demonstrate the complete process following the session as client displays readiness to assume responsibilities for self-healing.
- Promote attendance at a support group **where members can help each other practice and learn the techniques of TT.**
- Reinforce that biofield therapies are complementary interventions, and stress importance of seeking timely evaluation and continuing other prescribed treatment modalities, as appropriate.
- Refer to other resources, as identified (e.g., psychotherapy, clergy, medical treatment of disease processes, hospice), **for the individual to address maximal well-being or facilitate peaceful death.**

Documentation Focus

Assessment/Reassessment
- Assessment findings, including characteristics and differences in the energy field
- Client's perception of problem or motivation for treatment

Planning
- Plan of care and who is involved in planning
- Teaching plan

Implementation/Evaluation
- Characteristics of energy work performed
- Changes in energy field

Information that appears in brackets has been added by the authors to clarify and enhance the use of nursing diagnoses.

- Client's response to interventions (physical, mental, emotional), teaching, and actions performed
- Attainment of or progress toward desired outcomes
- Modifications to plan of care

Discharge Planning
- Long-term needs and who is responsible for actions to be taken
- Specific referrals, if made

Sample Nursing Outcomes & Interventions Classifications NOC/NIC

NOC—Personal Well-Being
NIC—Therapeutic Touch; Healing Touch

---

readiness for ENHANCED EXERCISE ENGAGEMENT   NANDA-I

[Diagnostic Division: Health Management]

Definition: Pattern of attention to physical activity characterized by planned, structured, repetitive body movements, which can be strengthened.

Recognizing Cues

Defining Characteristics

Subjective
Expresses desire to enhance:
  Autonomy for activities of daily living
  Competence to interact with physical or social environment
  Knowledge about environmental conditions, group opportunities, or physical settings for participation in physical activity; or about need for physical activity
  Physical abilities, or appearance, or condition

Desires to:
  Maintain motivation to participate in physical activity plan
  Maintain physical abilities; maintain physical well-being through physical activities
  Meet other's expectations about physical activity plans

Information that appears in brackets has been added by the authors to clarify and enhance the use of nursing diagnoses.

 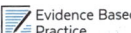 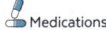

Clinical Connections
As a health-seeking behavior, the client may be healthy or this diagnosis can occur in any clinical condition or life process

Generate Solutions

Plan Desired Outcomes

Client Will (Include Specific Time Frame)
- Identify/reduce negative factors affecting exercise performance.
- Use identified techniques to enhance exercise tolerance.
- Report measurable increase in exercise engagement.

Interventions/Take Action

Nursing Priority No. 1.
To assess client's readiness and motivation:
- Determine client's current exercise lifestyle, as well as physical and psychological readiness for increased exercise. **Determinants of readiness may have to do with desire to eliminate risk factors, or to manage medical conditions with exercise, or to continue with a lifetime of physical activity.**
- Note client reports of difficulty accomplishing tasks or desired activities. Evaluate current limitations or degree of deficit in light of usual health status and what the client perceives causes, exacerbates, and helps the problem. **Provides comparative baseline; influences choice of interventions; and may reveal causes affecting energy (of which client might be unaware), such as sleep deprivation, smoking, poor diet, depression, or lack of support.**
- Identify activity needs versus desires (e.g., client barely able to walk up stairs but states would like to play racquetball). **Assists caregiver in dealing with reality and feasibility of goals client wants to achieve when developing activity plan.**

Nursing Priority No. 2.
To assist client to deal with potentially inhibiting factors and enhance exercise:
- Note client's age and developmental level when developing exercise plan(s). **The benefits of physical activity and exercise have been demonstrated across the life span. For example, studies show that moderate to vigorous physical activity and exercise during the day**

Information that appears in brackets has been added by the authors to clarify and enhance the use of nursing diagnoses.

are associated with elevation in self-esteem, improved concentration, reduction in depressive symptoms, and improvement in sleep.

- Discuss and implement client's choice of exercise where possible. **Recent studies note that granting people choice increases the perception of autonomy and motivation to perform and that choice provision can also enhance physical performance.**
- Emphasize small incremental changes instead of exercising at a level that is overly stressful at the beginning. **Increasing exercise levels gradually but steadily promotes continuation of activity as well as builds stamina and strength.**
- Involve client/significant others (SOs) in planning the timing and progression of exercise. **Gives client opportunity to perform desired or essential activities during periods of peak energy and promotes support from others.**
- Encourage expression of feelings contributing to or resulting from challenges in meeting goals. Provide encouragement based on objective measurements. **Helps to minimize frustration and rechannel energy.**
- Promote comfort measures and provide for relief of pain, when needed, **to enhance client's ability and desire to participate in activities.**
- Implement graded exercise or rehabilitation program under direct medical supervision if appropriate. **Gradual increase in activity has been shown to exert positive health benefits even in those with chronic diseases.**
- Provide referral to collaborative disciplines, such as an exercise physiologist, occupational/physical therapist, and recreation/leisure specialist. **Client may want to participate in particular type of exercise program or may need assistance in developing individually appropriate therapeutic regimens.**

Nursing Priority No. 3.

To promote continued activity (Teaching/Discharge Considerations) and enhance well-being (long-term goals):

- Review expectations of client/SOs/providers and explore conflicts or differences. **Helps to establish goals and to reach agreement for the most effective plan.**
- Assist or direct client/SOs to plan for progressive increase of activity level, aiming for maximal activity within the client's ability. **Promotes improved or more normal activity level, stamina, and conditioning.**

Information that appears in brackets has been added by the authors to clarify and enhance the use of nursing diagnoses.

 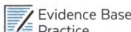 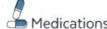

- Instruct client/SOs in monitoring response to activity and in recognizing signs and symptoms that indicate need to alter activity level. **Assists in self-management of condition and in understanding of reportable problems.**
- Suggest an exercise journal that provides evidence of daily or weekly progress **to sustain motivation.**
- Assist client to learn and demonstrate appropriate safety measures, such as using assistive devices correctly, wearing glasses, and having a companion when walking, where appropriate, **to prevent injuries.**
- Provide information about proper nutrition to meet metabolic and energy needs, obtaining or maintaining normal body weight. **Energy is improved when nutrients are sufficient to meet metabolic demands.**
- Encourage participation in self-care, recreation, or social activities and hobbies appropriate for situation. **Client may report these as desired goals for increasing exercise but may need encouragement to pursue the increased social involvement.**

Documentation Focus

Assessment/Reassessment
- Current level of exercise tolerance and performance
- Client motivation for increasing activity

Planning
- Plan of care and who is involved in planning
- Teaching plan

Implementation/Evaluation
- Response to interventions and teaching
- Modifications to plan of care
- Attainment of or progress toward desired outcome(s)

Discharge Planning
- Referrals to other resources
- Long-term needs and who is responsible for actions

Sample Nursing Outcomes & Interventions Classifications NOC/NIC

NOC—Exercise Participation
NIC—Exercise Promotion

Information that appears in brackets has been added by the authors to clarify and enhance the use of nursing diagnoses.

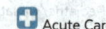 Acute Care 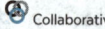 Collaborative 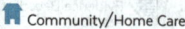 Community/Home Care Cultural

risk for [adult, child] FALL

[Diagnostic Division: Safety]

Definition: Susceptible to an unexpected, bodily descent that may cause physical or emotional injury.

Recognizing Cues

Related/Risk Factors
Decreased muscle strength; decreased coordination; impaired mobility, motor skill development/decline

Altered lower extremity sensation, numbness/tingling, paresthesia; neurological impairment

Musculoskeletal pain

Syncope; orthostatic vital signs; glucose imbalance

Urinary urgency/frequency; diarrhea; stool incontinence

Vision impairment; dim lighting

Dementia; changes in mentation

Pharmaceuticals (e.g., anxiolytics, analgesics, anesthetics, antihypertensives, etc.)

Substance misuse; intoxication

Inappropriately sized clothing; inappropriate footwear

Uneven walking surface; cluttered pathway; slippery surface

Elevated bed/care surface; caregiver fatigue; lack of supervision; lack of safety barriers

Device misuse or failure (i.e., wheelchair, walker, cane, baby stroller, bassinet, etc.)

Clinical Connections
Anemia, amputation, arthritis, osteoporosis, fractures, joint replacement procedure; seizure disorder, cerebrovascular disease, cataracts, dementia, paralysis, hypotension, cardiac dysrhythmias, inner ear dysfunction, alcohol abuse/intoxication, trauma, surgery

Generate Solutions

Plan Desired Outcomes

Client Will (Include Specific Time Frame)
- Verbalize understanding of individual risk factors that contribute to the possibility of falls.
- Demonstrate behaviors and lifestyle changes to reduce risk factors and protect self from injury.

Information that appears in brackets has been added by the authors to clarify and enhance the use of nursing diagnoses.

- Modify environment as indicated to enhance safety.
- Be free of injury.

Interventions/Take Action

Nursing Priority No. 1.

To evaluate source/degree of risk:

- Review client's general health status, **noting multiple factors that might affect safety, such as chronic or debilitating conditions, use of multiple medications, recent trauma (especially a fall within the past year), prolonged bedrest/immobility, unstable balance on standing, or a sedentary lifestyle.**
- Evaluate client's current disorders/conditions that could enhance the risk potential for falls. **Acute, even short-term, situations, such as sudden dizziness, positional blood pressure changes, new medication, change in glasses prescription, improperly fitted clothing that can cause tripping, developmentally inappropriate bed, recent use of alcohol/other drugs, can affect client safety.**
- Note factors associated with age, gender, and developmental level. **Infants, young children, young adults (e.g., sports activities, risk-taking behaviors), and elderly (e.g., significant vision, cognitive, or mobility impairments; osteoporosis; loss of muscle, fat, and subcutaneous tissue) are at greater risk because of developmental issues and impaired or lack of ability to self-protect.**
- Evaluate the client's cognitive status (e.g., presence of brain injury, congenital or neurological disorders; depression, visual/hearing/other sensory impairments). **Affects the client's ability to perceive own limitations or recognize danger.**
- Evaluate the client's general and hip muscle strength, postural stability, gait and standing balance, and gross and fine motor coordination. Review client's history of past or current physical injuries (e.g., musculoskeletal injuries; orthopedic surgery) **altering coordination, gait, and balance.**
- Review the client's ongoing medication regimen, noting the number and type of drugs that could impact fall potential. **Studies have confirmed that use of five to nine medications (polypharmacy) increases the risk of falls and that use of more than nine medications (heightened polypharmacy) greatly increases fall risk.**
- Evaluate use, misuse, or failure to use assistive aids, when indicated. **The client may have an assistive device but is at high risk for falls while adjusting to altered body state**

Information that appears in brackets has been added by the authors to clarify and enhance the use of nursing diagnoses.

and use of unfamiliar device; or the client might refuse to use devices for various reasons (e.g., "waiting for help" or perception of weakness).
- Assess mood, coping abilities, and personality styles. **The client's temperament, typical behavior, stressors, and level of self-esteem can affect attitude toward safety issues, resulting in carelessness or increased risk taking without consideration of consequences.**
- Determine client's/significant other's (SO's) level of knowledge about and attendance to safety needs. **May reveal a lack of understanding, insufficient resources, simple disregard for personal safety (e.g., "I can't watch him every minute," "We can't hire a home assistant," "It's not manly"), a lack of appreciation for effects of current condition (e.g., positional dizziness, onset of macular degeneration, newly replaced hip joint), or a lack of resources to attend to safety issues in all settings.**
- Ascertain the caregiver's expectations of client (whether cognitively impaired, child, and/or elderly family member) and compare with actual abilities. **The reality of client's abilities and needs may be different from the perception or desires of caregivers.**
- Assess family/caregiver for fatigue and ability to provide safe care. **The incidence of parental/caregiver fatigue may play a significant role in increased risk for client falls.**
- Identify hazards in the care setting and/or home/other environment. **Determining needs or deficits provides opportunities for intervention and/or instruction (e.g., concerning clearing of hazards, intensifying client supervision, obtaining safety equipment, or referring for vision evaluation).**
- Assess and document client's fall risk using an age and developmentally appropriate fall-risk scale upon admission, change in status, transfer, and discharge. **Adult fall-risk scales (e.g., Morse Fall Scale [MFS], Functional Ambulation Profile, Tinetti Balance and Gait Assessment, Timed Up-and-Go [TUG]) are widely used in acute care and long-term settings and include numbered rating scales that place the client in risk categories (from low to high). Various pediatric assessment tools have been developed including the General Risk Assessment for Pediatric In-patient Falls (GRAFPIF); the Cummings Scale (measures change in mental status, history of falls, age less than 36 months, mobility impairment,**

Information that appears in brackets has been added by the authors to clarify and enhance the use of nursing diagnoses.

 Diagnostic Studies 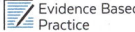 Evidence Based Practice Medications 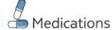 Pediatric/Geriatric/Lifespan and parental involvement and safety [CHAMPS]); The Humpty Dumpty Falls Scale (HDFS); and the I'M SAFE tool (measures impairment, medications, sedation/anesthesia, admitting diagnosis, fall history, and environment of care).

- Note socioeconomic status and availability and use of resources in other circumstances. **Can affect current coping abilities.**
- Note the proximity of client belongings, toileting, and/or supplies. **Reaching for supplies has been associated with falls.**
- Ascertain the responsibilities of the client's caregiver (i.e., work or school schedule, number of children being cared for in addition to the client, additional home responsibilities, etc.). **Heavy workload and the stress of caring for multiple children may increase the risk of client falls as caregivers attempt to fulfill multiple family roles.**

Nursing Priority No. 2.

To assist client/caregiver to reduce or correct individual risk factors:

- Collaborate in treatment of disease or condition(s) (e.g., acute illness, dementia, incontinence, neurological or musculoskeletal conditions) **to improve client's overall health and thereby reduce the potential for falls.**
- Review consequences of previously determined risk factors (e.g., falls caused by failure to make provisions for previously identified impairments or safety needs) **for follow-up instruction or interventions.**
- Discuss medication regimen and how it affects client. Instruct in the monitoring of effects and side effects. **The use of certain medications (e.g., multiple-medication daily regimen; benzodiazepines, antidepressants, antipsychotics, antihypertensives, diuretics) can contribute to weakness, confusion, balance and gait disturbances.** Review medications with client and primary care provider **to determine if changes (e.g., different medication or dosage) could reduce the client's fall risk.**
- Model safe practices during client interactions **to demonstrate behaviors for client/caregiver(s) to emulate.**
- Participate in communicating fall risk status when client is in care facility to (1) client/SO/caregiver (e.g., verbal reminders of fall-prevention interventions in place to reduce client's risk; visible signage); (2) staff (e.g., consistent use of fall-assessment tool; shift-to-shift report;

Information that appears in brackets has been added by the authors to clarify and enhance the use of nursing diagnoses.

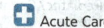 Acute Care 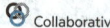 Collaborative 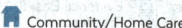 Community/Home Care   Cultural

documentation in client record); and (3) within unit/across units (e.g., hand-off communication to report client's fall risk to the receiving unit/facility). **These interventions are found to be part of best-practice interventions to reduce fall risk in clients while in acute care (e.g., hospital, short-stay or rehabilitation unit; extended care and long-term care units).**

- Recommend or implement needed interventions and safety devices **to manage conditions that could contribute to falling and to promote a safe environment for individual and others:**

  Evaluate vision and encourage use of prescription eyewear, as needed. **Note: The client with bifocals, trifocals, or implanted lenses may have difficulty perceiving steps or uneven surfaces, increasing risk for falls even when wearing glasses.**

  Situate the client's bed to enable the client to exit toward their stronger side whenever possible.

  Place the bed in the lowest possible position, use a raised-edge mattress, pad floor at side of bed, or place mattress on floor as appropriate.

  Use half side rails instead of full side rails or upright pole **to assist individual in arising from bed.**

  Ensure that side rails, when permitted, are raised and properly engaged according to the age, developmental level, and cognitive safety of the client. Note: Avoid beds or cribs with gaps in rails that could allow client to become trapped.

  Avoid use of restraints **to prevent excessive agitation and struggling.**

  Arrange for sitter/SO to remain with client who is agitated.

  Provide chairs with firm, high, nontipping seats and lifting mechanisms when indicated.

  Provide appropriate day or night lighting, encourage use of prescription eyewear.

  Assist client with transfers and ambulation; show client/SO ways to move safely.

  Provide and instruct in use of mobility devices and safety devices, such as grab bars and call light or personal assistance systems.

  Clear the environment of hazards (e.g., obstructing furniture, small items on the floor, electrical cords, and throw rugs).

  Lock wheels on movable equipment (e.g., wheelchairs and beds).

Information that appears in brackets has been added by the authors to clarify and enhance the use of nursing diagnoses.

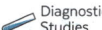 Diagnostic Studies 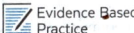 Evidence Based Practice Medications ∞ Pediatric/Geriatric/Lifespan

- Encourage the use of treaded slippers, socks, and shoes, and maintain nonskid floors and floor mats.
  Provide foot and nail hygiene and skin care **to promote foot health and pedal skin sensitivity.**
- Assign client a room close to nurses' station and keep door open as possible. Perform frequent rounding, arrange for a sitter/SO to remain with agitated client, or utilize remote monitoring, if available. **Provides for more frequent supervision to reduce possibility of client getting up without assistance and falling.**
- Provide or encourage the use of analgesics before activity if pain is interfering with desired activities. **Balance and movement can be impaired by pain associated with multiple conditions such as trauma or arthritis.**
- Follow up with client's provider to review usual medication regimen (e.g., narcotics/opiates, psychotropics, antihypertensives, diuretics), **which can contribute to weakness, confusion, and balance and gait disturbances. May benefit from evaluating drug concentrations of certain medications (e.g., anticonvulsants, tricyclic antidepressants, anti-arryhthmics) or may need an adjustment to dose or time of administration, or a change in choice of medication prescribed.**
- Determine the caregiver's expectations of cognitively impaired and/or elderly family members and compare with actual abilities. **The reality of the client's abilities and needs may be different from perception or desires of caregivers.**
- Discuss need for and sources of supervision (e.g., home care provider, elder day care, and personal companions).
- Perform client home visit when appropriate. Observe environment for safety issues (e.g., windows that are low/can be opened; child access to steps or stairs; play areas without soft surfaces; bathtubs without slip-resistant mats or stickers, unlocked beds or wheelchairs, etc.). **Useful in determining that home safety issues are addressed, including supervision, access to emergency assistance, and client's ability to manage self-care in the home.**
- Determine that caregivers are able to perform safe lift and carry practices. **Transfer devices may be available for adult clients or caregivers/SO may be educated on transfer techniques; babies and younger children can be lifted and held in certain positions to prevent accidental falls.**
- Refer to rehabilitation team, physical therapist, or occupational therapist, as appropriate, **to improve the client's balance, strength, or mobility; to improve or relearn**

Information that appears in brackets has been added by the authors to clarify and enhance the use of nursing diagnoses.

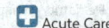 Acute Care 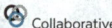 Collaborative 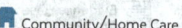 Community/Home Care Cultural

ambulation; and to identify and obtain appropriate assistive devices for mobility, environmental safety, or home modification.

Nursing Priority No. 3.

To promote safety (Teaching/Discharge Considerations) and enhance well-being (long-term goals):

- Refer to other resources as indicated. **Client/caregivers may need financial assistance, home modifications, referrals for counseling, home care, sources for safety equipment, or placement in extended-care facility.**
- Discuss importance of monitoring client and intervening in conditions (e.g., client fatigue; acute illness; depression; objects that block traffic patterns in home; insufficient lighting; unfamiliar surroundings; client attempting tasks that are too difficult for present level of functioning; inability to contact someone when help is needed) **that have been shown to contribute to occurrence of falls.**
- Address client's specific environmental factors associated with falling and create or instruct in a safe physical environment, such as bed height, room lighting, removal of loose carpet or throw rugs, repair of uneven flooring, and installing grab bars in bathrooms.
- Provide educational resources (e.g., home safety checklist, equipment directions for proper use, appropriate websites) **for later review and reinforcement of learning.**
- Connect the client/family with community resources, neighbors, and friends **to assist elderly or clients with disabilities in providing such things as structural maintenance and clearing of snow, gravel, or ice from walks and steps.**
- Promote community awareness about the problems of design of buildings, equipment, transportation, and workplace accidents that contribute to falls.

Documentation Focus

Assessment/Reassessment
- Individual risk factors noting current physical findings (e.g., signs of injury—bruises, cuts; anemia, fatigue; use of alcohol, drugs, and prescription medications)
- Client's/caregiver's understanding of individual risks and safety concerns

Planning
- Plan of care and who is involved in planning
- Teaching plan

Information that appears in brackets has been added by the authors to clarify and enhance the use of nursing diagnoses.

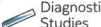 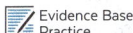 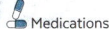 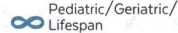

Implementation/Evaluation
- Individual responses to interventions, teaching, and actions performed
- Specific actions and changes that are made
- Attainment of or progress toward desired outcomes
- Modifications to plan of care

Discharge Planning
- Long-term plans for discharge needs, lifestyle, and home setting and community changes, and who is responsible for actions to be taken
- Specific referrals made

Sample Nursing Outcomes & Interventions Classifications NOC/NIC

NOC—Fall Prevention Behavior
NIC—Fall Prevention

---

disrupted FAMILY IDENTITY SYNDROME NANDA-I

[Diagnostic Division: Roles and Relationships]

Definition: Inability to create and maintain an integrated and complete perception of family.

Recognizing Cues

Related/Risk Factors
Ambivalent family relationships; ineffective family communication
Different coping styles among family members; ineffective use of coping strategies
Excessive stress; unrealistic expectations
Disrupted family roles, or rituals
Values incongruent with cultural norms; perceived danger to value system
Inadequate social support; perceived social discrimination
Inconsistent management of therapeutic regimen among family members
Unaddressed domestic violence
Sexual dysfunction

Information that appears in brackets has been added by the authors to clarify and enhance the use of nursing diagnoses.

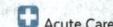 Acute Care   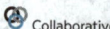 Collaborative   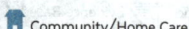 Community/Home Care   Cultural

Defining Characteristics

Author Note: As this is a syndrome diagnosis, the Defining Characteristics are other nursing diagnoses that comprise this syndrome.

impaired Family Processes; disrupted family Interaction Patterns

maladaptive family Coping; impaired Decision-Making

impaired Resilience

impaired Sexual Function; ineffective Childbearing Process

disrupted Personal Identity

Clinical Connections

Acute or chronic mental and physical health (i.e., cardiovascular, kidney, or respiratory diseases; schizophrenia, bipolar, or depression); substance misuse, infertility

Generate Solutions

Plan Desired Outcomes

Client Will (Include Specific Time Frame)
- Communicate, openly sharing thoughts, feelings, concerns.
- Involve members in problem-solving to manage family issues.
- Participate in family traditions/rituals, leisure-time activities.
- Use available support systems, community resources.

Interventions/Take Action

Nursing Priority No. 1.

To assess family roles, beliefs, and relationships:

- Identify family life-cycle changes, actual/potential role and responsibility changes, change in family composition, social interactions, and relationships, including changes with roles and responsibilities. **Helps determine who in the family group is the decision-maker, disciplinarian, caretaker, hero, or scapegoat. Knowing family expectations and responsibilities of each member helps to ascertain who supports or hinders growth and development of individuals or the family.**
- Identify how family members view self and the family related to cultural values, beliefs, and accomplished or unmet goals. **What individuals and families think, believe, and value (based on culture, religion, and ethnicity) is deeply rooted or contributes to a sense of**

Information that appears in brackets has been added by the authors to clarify and enhance the use of nursing diagnoses.

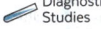 Diagnostic Studies   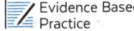 Evidence Based Practice   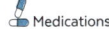 Medications   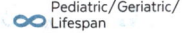 Pediatric/Geriatric/Lifespan

individual and family identity. Assimilation and globalization can bring either interconnectedness or a lack of identity, creating an opportunity for cultures to be lost or undermined.

- Note how family presents their identity to the community or if they are socially isolated. **Ethnic or religious families (outside the community or national norm) may elect to hide or protect their identity because they are not in the "in group" but considered outsiders.**
- Evaluate family members' psychosocial protective factors. **Family protective factors are present with support, socialization, goals, hope, and problem-solving. A lack of protection for the family unit includes individual family members who develop defense mechanisms to protect themselves according to the level of perceived threat and not considering the family unit.**
- Observe family members' body language and verbal content (noting congruence or incongruence) while interacting with others. **Recognizing communication patterns with and between family members helps to identify supportive or dysfunctional communication and relationships.**
- Evaluate the current physical and mental health regime family members have adopted for sick or unhealthy individuals. **Contending with acute or chronic physical or mental health issues can put the family into crisis. Identifying the level of family stress (i.e., emotional, physical, environmental, or economical) helps to determine interventions and needed resources for the plan of care. Beware various cultures use home health remedies to promote curing (e.g., Chinese: moxibustion and cupping therapy; Mexican remedies include herbs in teas and massage ointments).**
- Identify individual's and the family's underlying attitudes, motivation, and readiness to change thinking and behaviors related to family relationships and coping with stressors. **Using approach such as motivational interviewing can help identify what, how, and when clients are ready to change. Attempting interventions before the individual or family is ready to change will result in ambivalence or resistance, as hidden agendas and attitudes contribute to conflict.** NOTE: Refer to NDs: impaired family Coping, impaired Family Process, impaired Parenting, or disrupted family Interaction Patterns as appropriate.

Information that appears in brackets has been added by the authors to clarify and enhance the use of nursing diagnoses.

Nursing Priority No. 2.

To focus on individual stressors:

- Establish a therapeutic relationship with family. **A client-/family-centered approach that builds a therapeutic relationship can help the family to resolve ambivalence or reduce resistance to changing behaviors or improving their lifestyle.**
- Identify family members' primary stressor and family members' awareness and perceptions of the stressor. **Demands placed on adult members of the family can result in financial strain with dual-earner couples or require alternative household arrangements (e.g., living with aging parents, two or more families living together) and overcrowding in home environments. Generations (i.e., baby boomers, generations X and Z, or millennials) view life and work differently, and conflict may arise including domestic or traumatic violence, or self-harming.**
- Determine transitional phase in family life cycle. **Changes in family composition (e.g., death; member moving far away or rejecting family) may cause stress for individuals and impact family identity.**
- Recognize content of family conversations, noting presence/degree of misperceptions, negative or distorted thinking, focusing on limitations or catastrophizing self or others (thinking the worst outcome) rather than focusing on the positive. Determine whether a member's negative thoughts are taken out on family. **Family is a relationship and emotional system where members influence and are influenced by each other, including intergenerational levels. Marital conflict can result in triangulation with one parent aligning with the child against partner, resulting in family dissonance and negative outcomes.**
- Assess how the family presents their identity to the community or if they are socially isolated. **Ethnic or religious families (outside the community or national norm) may elect to hide or protect their identity because they are not in the "in group" but considered outsiders.**
- Identify individuals' contributions or inability to defuse the current family stressor. **Healthy families allow individuals to differentiate self or permit individuals to make independent choices while maintaining their emotional connection. Conflict arises when a member uses emotional cutoff, projects the problem onto another family member, or uses triangulation to temporarily calm the family situation.**

Information that appears in brackets has been added by the authors to clarify and enhance the use of nursing diagnoses.

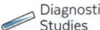 Diagnostic Studies 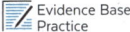 Evidence Based Practice 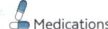 Medications 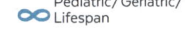 Pediatric/Geriatric/Lifespan

Nursing Priority No. 3.
To assist family members to identify thoughts, feelings, and strengthen relationships:

- Teach family the benefits of working together with an interprofessional team to develop a plan of care for the family using a shared decision-making approach. **Healing of the individuals and the family is a complex dynamic requiring an interprofessional team to meet the family needs and promote development of therapy goals.**
- Encourage family members to express thoughts, feelings (e.g., fears, anxieties, hopefulness) related to current event and family relationships without judgment. **Allows family members to tell their stories while listening for congruence or incongruence with their verbal and body language.**
- Express confidence and provide positive reinforcement to individuals and the family as progress is achieved toward goals. **Confirms that family connectedness is significant for developing and shaping an individual's comfort and security throughout the life span.**

Nursing Priority No. 4.
To promote cohesion and emotional bonding (Teaching/Discharge Considerations) and enhance well-being (long-term goals):

- Assist family members to collaborate with each other and the interprofessional team to identify short- and long-term goals. **Families who begin by expressing their readiness to change and willingness to use the shared decision-making approach benefit from team assistance with the process.**
- Encourage making mealtime a family event with everyone contributing to a pleasant daily experience. **Family time promotes support and guidance for daily living and bonds family members with their unique values, beliefs, and behaviors representing expectations for culture or spiritual beliefs. Time spent together allows individuals to share unconditional love.**
- Recommend family meetings to discuss roles and responsibilities, address issues, and promote positive individual family growth and development. **Regular family meetings can help in coping with a specific problem or concern, communicating schedules or activities of individual members, planning for potential changes such as moving**

Information that appears in brackets has been added by the authors to clarify and enhance the use of nursing diagnoses.

or joyful family event, and determining how members are coping with changes or stressful events.
- Encourage involvement in cultural, spiritual, recreational, and social activities that support the family's identity and family unity. **Individuals and families learn to identify within their community or nation by "intergroup contexts" such as community groups/ethnic clubs, sports, arts, music, or theater that may be significant to their identity.**
- Promote and provide resources for family counseling or therapy, support groups (e.g., Al-Anon, Narcotics Anonymous [NA], Alcoholics Anonymous [AA], National Alliance on Mental Illness [NAMI]). **Family support is variable depending on stress or conflict requiring a variety of resources available for access. Provide individual and family needs in the community or reliable online resources.**

Documentation Focus

Assessment/Reassessment
- Individual relationships and interactions within the family, note precipitating crisis, and individual prescriptions of crisis
- Cultural values, spiritual or religious beliefs, individual family roles
- Current support for family, and resources used
- Family members' readiness to change and the stage of change

Planning
- Plan of care and interprofessional collaboration team members involved in planning
- Family participation in shared decision making
- Teaching/coaching plan

Implementation/Evaluation
- Response to teaching and interventions by individuals and family
- Attainment of or progress toward desired outcome(s)
- Modifications to plan

Discharge Planning
- Long-term needs and who is responsible for actions
- Specific referrals made

Information that appears in brackets has been added by the authors to clarify and enhance the use of nursing diagnoses.

Sample Nursing Outcomes & Interventions Classifications NOC/NIC

NOC—Family Resilience
NIC—Family Integrity Promotion

impaired FAMILY PROCESS ICNP

[Diagnostic Division: Roles/Relationships]

Definition: A lack of family roles, boundaries, or open and honest communication supporting and guiding family members to become self-sufficient. [Authors view this as an ongoing problem affecting family function and well-being]

Recognizing Cues

Related/Risk Factors
Substance misuse/abuse
Extensive use of defense mechanisms; poor problem-solving skills; lack of effective coping strategies
Antisocial, narcissistic, or borderline personality disorder
Schizophrenic disorders, bipolar disorder, or major depression

Defining Characteristics

Subjective
Inability or fear to share thoughts and feeling with family
Loss of personal identify; low self-esteem; loss of confidence
Feels unloved, worthless, helpless, hopeless, and unsupported
Frustration, resentment, tension, denies conflict
Feels alienated, isolated, abandoned, guilty
Interpersonal intimacy problems
Inability to resolve family conflict; poorly defined family roles
Dominant family member is controlling, triangulation, manipulation, scapegoat family members

Objective
Poor academic/work performance; immaturity
Restlessness, agitation; conflict, anger, aggression; conflict avoidance

---

Information that appears in brackets has been added by the authors to clarify and enhance the use of nursing diagnoses.

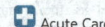 Acute Care 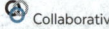 Collaborative 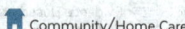 Community/Home Care   Cultural

Argumentative; controlling; inconsistent reactions/
behaviors; dishonest/lying; criticizing; poor communication
skills

Social isolation; disinterest in physical contact; critical
self-judgment/blame

Substance misuse/abuse; enables substance misuse of others

Unable to keep promises; extensive use of defense mechanisms; manipulation; lack responsibilities

Abusive behaviors toward family members

Inconsistent family roles, rules, and boundaries

Clinical Connections
Substance abuse or withdrawal, fetal alcohol syndrome, depression, developmental delay, chronic health condition

Generate Solutions

Plan Desired Outcomes

Client/Family Will (Include Specific Time Frame)
- Verbalize understanding of family roles, relationships, communication, support for all members.
- Attend treatment programs for family and individual members.
- Identify newly learned coping strategies and benefits to individuals and the family.
- Plan and schedule for weekly family meetings to discuss and resolve family issues.
- Develop mental cues to catch self-destructive behaviors prior to taking action.
- Verbalize newly learned parenting skills.

Interventions/Take Action

Nursing Priority No. 1.
To assess contributing factors/underlying problem(s):
- Determine family health history, illness, trauma, or developmental crisis present. **Families with frequent hospitalizations for chronic health conditions or mental illness (e.g., cardiovascular disorders, mood disorders, or personality disorders) can experience disruption in family daily living activities as well as events of individual abuse causing trauma, or a child with developmental delays may experience family chaos.**

Information that appears in brackets has been added by the authors to clarify and enhance the use of nursing diagnoses.

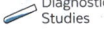 Diagnostic Studies 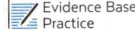 Evidence Based Practice 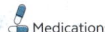 Medications 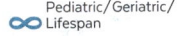 Pediatric/Geriatric/Lifespan

- Identify family members, ages, birth rank, developmental stage (e.g., marriage, birth of a child, children leaving home, retirement), current roles and responsibilities, and relationships of family members. **Information is necessary to understand who is the head of the household and if this person is dominating others. When the subordinate family member upsets the dominant member, blame may be placed on the scapegoat. However, the subordinate and scapegoat may develop an alliance to correct actions of the dominant member. This is known as triangulation. Triangulation or alliances can happen between any of the family members, causing a temporary change in roles and responsibilities, creating a family crisis.**
- Identify family's understanding of current situation; note results of previous involvement in treatment. **Family with a member who is addicted (e.g., substance misuse/abuse, gambling, sexual, or physical abuse), who has often had treatment or been incarcerated, and knowing what has brought about the current situation will determine a starting place for this treatment plan.**
- Determine communication patterns (e.g., who is demanding, controlling thoughts, feelings, or behaviors), history of poor communication skills (e.g., criticizing, anger, blaming, yelling/screaming), and accidents or violent behaviors within family influencing current safety issues. **Poor communication skills in a family put all members at risk of emotional harm; however, special concern for the scapegoat being held accountable for family disruption. The disregard for an individual member can lead to physical and emotional problems (e.g., anxiety, depression, or chronic health conditions). Family members may take out their anger or violence on the vulnerable individual (scapegoat), thus allowing a course of action for further violence.**
- Discuss current and past methods of coping. **Family members have developed skills to cope with behaviors of client or use defense mechanisms that are not helpful with problem-solving or improving the situation. Skills identified as useful can help to change the present situation. Those identified as not helpful (enabling behaviors or defense mechanisms) can be targeted for intervention to bring about desired changes and improve family functioning.**
- Determine extent and understanding of enabling behaviors or defense mechanisms used by family members. **Family**

Information that appears in brackets has been added by the authors to clarify and enhance the use of nursing diagnoses.

324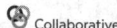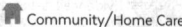

members may have developed behaviors that support the client continuing the pattern of addiction or prevent healing with chronic physical/mental health conditions (e.g., diabetes, cardiovascular disorders, schizophrenia or bipolar disorder). **Awareness, identification, and knowledge of these behaviors provide opportunity for individuals to begin the process of change.**

- Identify sabotage behaviors of family members. **Issues of secondary gain (conscious or unconscious) may impede recovery/growth. Even though family member(s) may verbalize a desire for the individual to be healthy (e.g., free of addiction, function more independently), the reality of interactive dynamics is that they may unconsciously not want the individual to change because this would affect the role(s) of the family member(s) in the relationship.**
- Note presence and extent of behaviors of family, client, and staff that might be enabling or "too helpful," such as client's frequent requests for assistance, excuses for not following through on agreed-on behaviors, and feelings of anger or irritation with others. **Identification of specific behaviors (enabling) can help family members see what they do that complicates acceptance of situation by affected family member and that need to be changed to facilitate resolution of problem.**
- Identify parenting style and expectations. **Ineffective parenting and unrealistic expectations may contribute to abuse. Understanding normal responses and progression of developmental milestones may help parent cope with changes necessitated by current crisis.**

Nursing Priority No. 2.

To assist family to change destructive behaviors:

- Seek mutual agreement on behaviors and responsibilities for nurses/staff and client. **Maximizes understanding of what is expected of each individual.**
- Identify and discuss denial and sabotage behaviors used by family members. **Brings attention to specific behaviors that individuals can be aware of and begin to change so they can move beyond blocks to recovery.**
- Discuss use of anger, defense mechanisms (e.g., rationalization, projection, undoing) and ways in which these interfere with problem resolution. **Client may be unaware of using defense mechanisms to protect self from emotional harm. Developing self-awareness of own feelings can**

Information that appears in brackets has been added by the authors to clarify and enhance the use of nursing diagnoses.

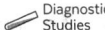 Diagnostic Studies 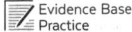 Evidence Based Practice Medications Pediatric/Geriatric/Lifespan

lead to a decision to change; client then has to face the consequences of their own actions and may choose to get well. **Refraining from using defense mechanisms takes time and practice.**

- Encourage family to identify triggers for anger/violence and find solutions to cope with extreme emotions. **Understanding what leads to anger and violence can lead to new behaviors and changes in the family for healthier relationships.**
- Determine family strengths, areas for growth, and individual/family successes. **Family members may not realize they have strengths; as they identify these areas, they can choose to learn and develop new strategies for a more effective family structure.**
- Remain nonjudgmental in approach to family members and to impaired member. **Individual already sees self as unworthy, and judgment by caregivers to family will interfere with ability to be a change agent.**
- Provide information regarding the effects of addiction or chronic health conditions (e.g., cardiovascular disorder, schizophrenia, mood and personality disorders) of the involved family member. **Family members have been struggling with client's situation for a time, and information can help them to understand and cope with negative behaviors without being judgmental or reacting angrily.**
- Discuss differences between destructive aspects of enabling behavior and genuine motivation to aid the client. **Family members often want to help but need to distinguish between helpful and harmful behaviors to solve concerns/problems.**
- Identify use of manipulative behaviors of client/family and discuss ways to avoid or prevent these situations. **The client/family often manipulates the people around them to maintain the status quo. When a client and family begin to interact in a straightforward, honest manner, manipulation is limited or not possible, and healing can begin.**
- Encourage regular/routine family meetings to set new family goals and problem-solve. **Democratic-style family meetings facilitate family unity, support, relationships, and emotional and functional growth for the entire family.**
- Arrange for and encourage family participation in multidisciplinary team conference or group therapy as appropriate. **Participation in family and group therapy for an extended period increases likelihood of success as interactional issues (e.g., marital conflict, "scapegoating"**

Information that appears in brackets has been added by the authors to clarify and enhance the use of nursing diagnoses.

of family members) can be addressed and dealt with. Involvement with group therapy can help family members to experience new ways of interacting and gain insight into their behavior, providing opportunity for change.

Nursing Priority No. 3.

To promote and strengthen family health (Teaching/Discharge Considerations) and enhance well-being (long-term goals):

- Provide factual information to client/family about the effects of addictive or chronic health disorders (e.g., developmental delays, intellectual functioning, respiratory disorders, or mood disorders) and the influence of these behaviors on the family and what to expect after discharge from a program. **Because families may have unrealistic expectations about behavioral changes brought about by therapy (e.g., problem is solved and no further work or change is required), having the information may help them understand that changes made during initial therapy are just the beginning of lifelong changes required for healthy family relationships.**
- Provide information about the enabling behavior of the codependent family member toward the family member with an addictive disease or chronic health condition. **Education is a prime ingredient in treatment of enabling behaviors, addictions, chronic health or mental health conditions that can assist family members to cope realistically with these issues. Changing lifelong patterns of behavior is hard work and may require continued support with a therapist.**
- Discuss the importance of restructuring life activities, work/leisure relationships. **Previous lifestyle/relationships supported substance use, requiring change to prevent relapse.**
- Encourage the family to refocus celebrations excluding alcohol/other drug use, where indicated. **Because celebrations often include the use of alcohol, this is one area where change can be made that can reduce the risk of relapse for substance user.**
- Provide support for family members; encourage participation in group work. **Support is essential to changing client and family behaviors. Participating in group provides an opportunity to practice new skills of communication and behavior. Learning new communication and coping skills takes patience, time, and practice.**

Information that appears in brackets has been added by the authors to clarify and enhance the use of nursing diagnoses.

- Encourage involvement with, and refer to, self-help groups (e.g., Al-Anon, Alateen, Narcotics Anonymous, or family parenting courses, family therapy groups). **Regular attendance at a group can provide support; help client see how others are coping with similar problems; and learn new skills, such as problem-solving, and better methods for handling family disagreements.**
- Provide bibliotherapy as appropriate. **Reading provides helpful information for making desired changes, especially when client/family members are dedicated to making change and willing to learn new ways of interacting within the family.** Refer to websites linked to specific disorders, for example, National Alliance on Mental Illness (NAMI) (www.nami.org) or American Heart Association (www.heart.org).
- Refer to ND impaired family Coping; as appropriate.

Documentation Focus

Assessment/Reassessment
- Assessment findings, including history of substance(s) that have been used and family risk factors and safety concerns
- Family composition and involvement
- Results of prior treatment involvement

Planning
- Plan of care and who is involved in planning
- Teaching plan

Implementation/Evaluation
- Responses of family members to treatment, teaching, and actions performed
- Attainment of or progress toward desired outcome(s)
- Modifications to plan of care

Discharge Planning
- Long-term needs, who is responsible for actions to be taken
- Specific referrals made

Sample Nursing Outcomes & Interventions Classifications NOC/NIC

NOC—Family Functioning
NIC—Counseling

Information that appears in brackets has been added by the authors to clarify and enhance the use of nursing diagnoses.

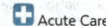 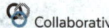 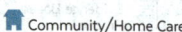

FATIGUE `ICNP`

[Diagnostic Division: Activity/Rest]

Definition: A pervasive, ongoing sense of physical and/or mental lack of energy significantly limiting an individual's ability to perform activities of daily living, maintain social relationships, and/or fulfill desired roles.

Recognizing Cues

Related/Risk Factors
Psychological distress; multiple stressors; depressive symptoms
Inadequate sleep
Physical deconditioning; chronic disease; physical pain
Malnutrition; nutritional deficiency; anemia

Defining Characteristics

Subjective
Frustration; dissatisfaction with self/others
Inability to "catch up on sleep," "so tired," "mental exhaustion"
Loss of pleasure in previously enjoyable activities
Difficulty maintaining usual physical activity or usual routines; feels shame, guilt
Difficulty concentrating

Objective
Socially withdrawn; apathetic; disinterested
Slowed gait; decreased activity tolerance
Drowsy; lethargic
Poor/compromised role performance; lack of attention to appearance/hygiene, environment

Clinical Connections
Anemia, hypothyroidism, cancer, multiple sclerosis (MS), Lyme disease, post-polio syndrome, AIDS, chronic renal failure, chronic fatigue syndrome (CFS), depression, chemotherapy, myasthenia gravis, fibromyalgia

Generate Solutions

Plan Desired Outcomes

Client Will (Include Specific Time Frame)
- Report improved sense of energy.
- Identify basis of fatigue and individual areas of control.

Information that appears in brackets has been added by the authors to clarify and enhance the use of nursing diagnoses.

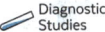 Diagnostic Studies   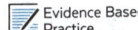 Evidence Based Practice   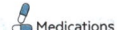 Medications   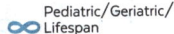 Pediatric/Geriatric/Lifespan

- Perform activities of daily living and participate in desired activities at level of ability.
- Participate in recommended treatment program.

Interventions/Take Action

Nursing Priority No. 1.

To assess causative/contributing factors:

- Identify the presence of physical and/or psychological conditions (e.g., pregnancy; infectious processes; blood loss, anemia; connective tissue disorders [e.g., MS, lupus]; trauma, chronic pain syndromes [e.g., arthritis]; cardiopulmonary disorders; cancer and cancer treatments; hepatitis; AIDS; major depressive disorder; anxiety states; substance use or abuse). **Fatigue is broadly classified as acute/transient fatigue (e.g., after exercise), chronic fatigue (lasting unabated for more than 6 mo) or chronic fatigue syndrome (CFS). Important information can be obtained from knowing (1) if fatigue is a result of an underlying condition or disease process (acute or chronic), (2) the current status of an exacerbating or remitting condition, or (3) whether fatigue has been present over a long time without any identifiable cause.**
- Evaluate possibility of CFS, also sometimes called chronic fatigue immune dysfunction syndrome (CFIDS). **There is no direct test for CFS, it is one of exclusion. CFS has been defined as a distinct disorder (affecting both children and adults) characterized by chronic (often relapsing but always debilitating) fatigue, lasting for at least 6 mo (often for much longer), causing impairments in overall physical and mental functioning and without an apparent etiology.**
- Note age, gender, and developmental stage. **Some studies show a prevalence of fatigue more often in females than males; it most commonly occurs in teens and in young to middle-aged adults, but the condition may be present in any person at any age.**
- Review client's medication regimen/schedule and other drug use. **Many medications have the potential side effect of causing/exacerbating fatigue (e.g., beta blockers, chemotherapy agents, narcotics, sedatives, muscle relaxants, antiemetics, antidepressants, antiepileptics, diuretics, cholesterol-lowering drugs, HIV treatment agents, combinations of drugs and/or substances).**
- Ascertain the client's belief about what is causing the fatigue.

Information that appears in brackets has been added by the authors to clarify and enhance the use of nursing diagnoses.

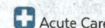 Acute Care 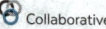 Collaborative 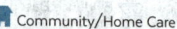 Community/Home Care 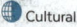 Cultural

- Assess vital signs **to evaluate fluid status and cardiopulmonary response to activity.**
- Determine the presence/degree of sleep disturbances. **Fatigue can be a consequence of, and/or exacerbated by, sleep deprivation.**
- Note recent lifestyle changes, including conflicts (e.g., expanded responsibilities, demands of others, job-related conflicts); maturational issues (e.g., adolescent with an eating disorder); and developmental issues (e.g., new parenthood, loss of spouse/significant other [SO]) **that can be causing or exacerbating level of fatigue.**
- Assess psychological and personality factors that may affect reports of fatigue level. **Client can potentially have issues that affect desire to be active (or work), resulting in over- or underactivity, or concerns of secondary gain from exaggerated fatigue reports.**
- Evaluate client aspects of "learned helplessness" that may be manifested by giving up. **Can perpetuate a cycle of fatigue, impaired functioning, and increased anxiety and fatigue.**

Nursing Priority No. 2.
To determine degree of fatigue/impact on life:
- Obtain client/SO descriptions of fatigue (i.e., lacking energy or strength, tiredness, weakness lasting over length of time). Note the presence of additional concerns (e.g., irritability, lack of concentration, difficulty making decisions, problems with leisure, and relationship difficulties) **to assist in evaluating the impact on the client's life.**
- Have client self-evaluate fatigue (using the Fatigue Assessment Scale or similar scale) and describe its effects on ability to participate in desired activities. **Fatigue may vary in intensity and is often accompanied by irritability, lack of concentration, difficulty making decisions, problems with leisure, and relationship difficulties that can add to stress level and aggravate sleep problems.**
- Assess the severity of client's fatigue using a recognized scale (e.g., Chalder Fatigue Scale, Functional Assessment of Cancer Therapy: Fatigue, Multidimensional Assessment of Fatigue, Piper Fatigue Scale, Global Fatigue Index), as appropriate. **In initial evaluation, these scales can help determine manifestation, intensity, duration, and emotional meaning of fatigue, and reevaluations help estimate response to treatment strategies.**

Information that appears in brackets has been added by the authors to clarify and enhance the use of nursing diagnoses.

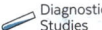 Diagnostic Studies 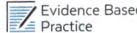 Evidence Based Practice 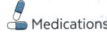 Medications 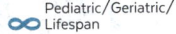 Pediatric/Geriatric/Lifespan

- Discuss with client lifestyle changes or limitations imposed by fatigue state.
- Interview parent/caregiver regarding specific changes observed in child or elder client. **These individuals may not be able to verbalize feelings or relate meaningful information.**
- Note daily energy patterns (i.e., peaks and valleys). **Helpful in determining intensity/timing of activity.**
- Measure the physiological response to activity (e.g., changes in blood pressure or heart and respiratory rate).
- Evaluate the client's need for assistance or assistive devices. **Certain conditions causing fatigue (e.g., post-polio syndrome) worsen with overuse of involved muscles. Client may benefit from support and protection provided by braces, canes, power chairs, and so on.**
- Review the availability and current use of support systems and resources.
- Perform, or review results of, testing, such as the Multidimensional Assessment of Fatigue, Piper Fatigue Scale, and Global Fatigue Index, as appropriate. **Can help determine manifestation, intensity, duration, and emotional meaning of fatigue.**

Nursing Priority No. 3.

To assist client to cope with fatigue and manage within individual limits of ability:

- Treat underlying conditions where possible (e.g., manage pain, depression, or anemia; treat infections; reduce numbers of interacting medications) **to reduce fatigue caused by treatable conditions.**
- Accept the reality of client reports of fatigue and do not underestimate effect on client's quality of life. **Fatigue is subjective and often debilitating. For example, clients with MS or cancer are prone to severe fatigue following minimal energy expenditure and require a longer recovery period.**
- Active-listen client/SO/caregiver concerns and encourage expression of feelings. **Provides support to help client deal with very frustrating and taxing situation.**
- Involve client/SO(s)/caregiver(s) in planning care. Establish realistic activity goals with the client and encourage forward movement. **Incorporating their input, choices, and assistance enhances the commitment to promoting optimal outcomes.**

Information that appears in brackets has been added by the authors to clarify and enhance the use of nursing diagnoses.

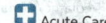 Acute Care 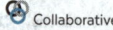 Collaborative 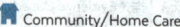 Community/Home Care 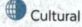 Cultural

- Plan interventions to allow individually adequate rest periods. Schedule activities for periods when the client has the most energy **to maximize participation.**
- Involve the client/SO(s) in schedule planning.
- Encourage the client to do whatever possible (e.g., self-care, sit up in chair, go for walk, interact with family, or play a game). Increase activity level as tolerated.
- Instruct client/caregivers in alternative ways of doing familiar activities and methods to conserve energy, such as the following:
  Sit instead of stand during daily care and other activities.
  Carry several small loads instead of one large load.
  Combine and simplify activities.
  Take frequent, short breaks during activities.
  Delegate tasks.
  Ask for and accept assistance.
  Say "no" or "later."
  Plan steps of activity before beginning so that all needed materials are at hand.
- Encourage the use of assistive devices (e.g., wheeled walker, handicap parking spot, elevator, backpack for carrying objects), as needed, **to extend active time/conserve energy for other tasks.**
- Assist with self-care needs; keep the bed in a low position and keep travelways clear of furniture; assist with ambulation, as indicated.
- Avoid or limit exposure to temperature and humidity extremes, **which can negatively impact energy level.**
- Encourage engagement in diversional activities, avoiding both over- and understimulation (cognitive and sensory). **Participating in pleasurable activities can refocus energy and diminish feelings of unhappiness, sluggishness, and worthlessness that can accompany fatigue.**
- Discuss measures to promote restful sleep if client is experiencing sleep disturbances. (Refer to ND ineffective Sleep Pattern.)
- Encourage nutritionally dense, easy-to-prepare, and easy-to-consume foods and avoidance of caffeine and high-sugar foods and beverages **to promote energy.** Refer to a dietitian as indicated.
- Provide client with supplemental oxygen as needed. **If fatigue is related to anemia or oxygenation/perfusion problems, oxygen may improve energy level and ability**

Information that appears in brackets has been added by the authors to clarify and enhance the use of nursing diagnoses.

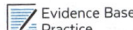

to be active. (Refer to Activity Intolerance for additional interventions.)
- Instruct in/implement stress-management skills of visualization, relaxation, and biofeedback, when appropriate.
- Discuss with client/SO/caregiver alternative therapies (e.g., massage, acupuncture, osteopathic or chiropractic manipulations), if appropriate. **Complementary therapies may be helpful in reducing muscle tension and pain to promote relaxation and rest.**
- Refer client to a comprehensive rehabilitation program, physical and occupational therapy for programmed daily exercises and activities **to improve stamina, strength, and muscle tone and to enhance sense of well-being.**

Nursing Priority No. 4.

To promote vigor (Teaching/Discharge Considerations) and enhance well-being (long-term goals):

- Discuss therapy regimen relating to individual causative factors (e.g., physical and/or psychological illnesses) and explain to client/SO(s) the relationship of fatigue to illness.
- Assist client/SO(s) to develop plan for activity and exercise within individual ability. Emphasize benefits of allowing sufficient time to participate in needed/desired activities.
- Instruct the client in ways to monitor responses to activity and significant signs/symptoms **that indicate the need to alter activity level.**
- Encourage client/SOs to implement measures to preserve energy over longer periods of time. **Client's energy level could benefit from such things as (1) planning and organizing work tasks (e.g., delegating, combining activities, simplifying details; spending energy on important/desired tasks); (2) balancing periods of rest and work and resting before fatigue sets in; (3) pacing self and reducing sudden or prolonged strains; (4) limiting work that increases muscle tension and using good body mechanics; and (5) modifying effects of the environment such as temperature extremes and eliminating smoke and harmful fumes.**
- Promote overall health measures (e.g., nutrition, adequate fluid intake, and appropriate vitamin and iron supplementation).

Information that appears in brackets has been added by the authors to clarify and enhance the use of nursing diagnoses.

- Encourage client to develop assertiveness skills, prioritize goals and activities, learn to delegate duties or tasks, or say "no." Discuss burnout syndrome, when appropriate, and actions client can take to change individual situation.
- Assist client to identify appropriate coping behaviors. **Promotes a sense of control and improves self-esteem.**
- Identify condition-specific support groups and community resources **to provide information, share experiences, and enhance problem-solving.**
- Refer to counseling or psychotherapy, as indicated.
- Identify community resources that can be available to assist with everyday life needs (e.g., Meals on Wheels, homemaker or housekeeper services, yard care).

Documentation Focus

Assessment/Reassessment
- Manifestations of fatigue and other assessment findings
- Degree of impairment and effect on lifestyle
- Expectations of client/SO(s) relative to individual abilities and specific condition

Planning
- Plan of care, specific interventions, and who is involved in the planning
- Teaching plan

Implementation/Evaluation
- Client's response to interventions, teaching, and actions performed
- Attainment of or progress toward desired outcome(s)
- Modifications to plan of care

Discharge Planning
- Discharge needs/plan, actions to be taken, and who is responsible
- Specific referrals made

Sample Nursing Outcomes & Interventions Classifications NOC/NIC

NOC—Fatigue: Disruptive Effects
NIC—Energy Management

Information that appears in brackets has been added by the authors to clarify and enhance the use of nursing diagnoses.

 Diagnostic Studies 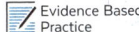 Evidence Based Practice 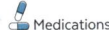 Medications 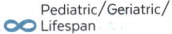 Pediatric/Geriatric/Lifespan

FEAR
ICNP

[Diagnostic Division: Stress Management]

Definition: A protective primitive emotional response to a perceived threat or danger causing a biochemical reaction with an extreme emotional reaction that can negatively impact psychological well-being.

Recognizing Cues

Related/Risk Factors
Specific object or events (e.g., insects, heights, social events, public speaking)
The future and the unknown
Imagined threats
New and different situations/environments

Defining Characteristics

Subjective
Physiological Factors:
Reports chest pain; dry mouth; sweating, upset stomach, nausea, diarrhea, shortness of breath.
Behavioral/Emotional:
Thinking is focused on worry and distress; uneasy feeling, hesitant, expresses intense stress, dread, and apprehension.

Objective
Physiological Factors:
Increased blood pressure, heart rate, respirations; dilated pupils. Diarrhea, nausea and vomiting, and muscle tension.
Behavioral/Emotional:
Impulsivity, irritability, inability to concentrate, focused on fear, decreased self-confidence; impulsive behaviors
Agitation; restlessness/psychomotor agitation

Clinical Connections
Anxiety, panic, post-traumatic stress disorder, phobias, hospitalization/diagnostic procedures, diagnosis of chronic or life-threatening condition

---

Information that appears in brackets has been added by the authors to clarify and enhance the use of nursing diagnoses.

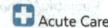 Acute Care 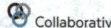 Collaborative 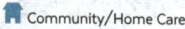 Community/Home Care Cultural

Generate Solutions

Plan Desired Outcomes

Client Will (Include Specific Time Frame)
- Verbalize worries and fears while identifying healthy versus unhealthy thinking.
- Acknowledge accurate sense of safety in current situation.
- Demonstrate ability to use effective coping skills (e.g., deep breathing exercise, problem-solving skills) to find relief of signs/symptoms specific to client.
- Minimize anxiety responses to unrealistic worry and fear.

Interventions/Take Action

Nursing Priority No. 1.
To assess degree of fear and reality of threat perceived by the client:

- Use a calm approach to ask client's/significant other's (SO's) perception of what is occurring and how this affects life. **Fear is a natural reaction to frightening events, and how client views the event will determine how client will react. Fear differs from anxiety in that it is usually unanticipated. Health-related fears may present more like dread and anxiety.**
- Determine the client's age and developmental level. **Helps in understanding usual or typical fears experienced by individuals (e.g., toddler often has different fears than adolescent or older person suffering with dementia being removed from home/usual living situation).**
- Assess family dynamics observing verbal and nonverbal communication actions and responses of family members. **Communication may exacerbate or soothe fears of the client; conversely, if the client is immersed in illness, whether from crisis or fear, it can take a toll on the family/involved others.** (Refer to other NDs, such as difficulty Coping; impaired Family Process; impaired family Coping; Anxiety, for related interventions.
- Observe ability to concentrate, level of attention, degree of incapacitation (e.g., "frozen with fear," inability to engage in necessary activities). **Indicative of extent of anxiety or**

Information that appears in brackets has been added by the authors to clarify and enhance the use of nursing diagnoses.

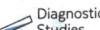 Diagnostic Studies 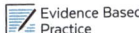 Evidence Based Practice 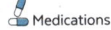 Medications 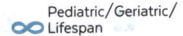 Pediatric/Geriatric/Lifespan

fear related to what is happening and need for specific interventions to reduce physiological reactions. **The presence of a severe reaction (panic or phobias) requires more intensive intervention.**

- Compare verbal and nonverbal responses **to note congruencies or misperceptions of the situation. Client may be able to verbalize what they are afraid of, if asked, providing opportunity to address actual fears.**
- Be alert to signs of denial or depression. **Depression may be associated with fear that interferes with productive life and daily activities.**
- Identify sensory deficits that may be present, such as vision or hearing impairment. **These deficits affect sensory reception and interpretation of the environment. The inability to correctly sense and perceive stimuli leads to misunderstanding, increasing fear.**
- Measure vital signs and note physiological responses to situation. **Provides baseline information of extent of response for comparison as needed. Stabilization can indicate effectiveness of interventions by diminished response to identified fear. Note: Fear and acute anxiety can both involve sympathetic arousal (e.g., increased heart rate, respirations, and blood pressure, hyperalertness, antidiuresis, dilation of skeletal blood vessels, constriction of gut blood vessels, and a surge of catecholamine release). These responses can be blunted (e.g., heart rate may not be increased if client is taking certain beta-blocking medications) and should subside as the fear state is reduced.**
- Investigate the client's reports of subjective experiences, which could be indicative of delusions/hallucinations, **to help clarify the client's interpretation of surroundings and/or stimuli and identify the need for reality orientation and further evaluation.**
- Be alert to and evaluate potential for violence. **Client who is fearful may feel need to protect self and may strike out at closest person. Proactive planning can avert or manage violent behaviors.**

Nursing Priority No. 2.
To assist client/SO(s) in dealing with fear/situation:

- Calmly approach client, use simple sentences, concrete terms, and written materials if appropriate to explain

---

Information that appears in brackets has been added by the authors to clarify and enhance the use of nursing diagnoses.

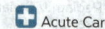 Acute Care   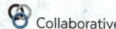 Collaborative   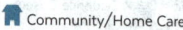 Community/Home Care   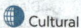 Cultural

assessment process and expectations. **Intense state of fear interferes with reception and interpretation of verbal information; supplementing it with written information facilitates understanding and retention of information. Client's knowledge of the process enhances their ability to respond appropriately.**

- Stay with the very fearful client or make arrangements to have someone else be there. **Presence of a calm, caring person can provide reassurance that individual will be safe. Sense of abandonment can exacerbate fear.**
- Active-listen client's concerns. **Conveys message of belief in competence and ability of client. Promotes understanding of issues when client feels listened to so that problem-solving can begin.**
- Discuss client's perceptions and fearful feelings. **Promotes an atmosphere of caring and permits explanation or correction of misperceptions.**
- Acknowledge normalcy of fear, pain, and despair, and give "permission" to express feelings appropriately and freely. **Promotes an attitude of caring and opens the door for discussion about feelings and/or addressing reality of situation.**
- Provide an opportunity for questions and answer honestly. **Enhances sense of trust and nurse–client relationship.**
- Present objective information when available and allow client to use it freely. Avoid arguing about client's perceptions of the situation. **Limits conflicts when fear response may impair rational thinking.**
- Provide presence and physical contact to provide support as appropriate. **Presence demonstrates support. Use physical contact as needed or accepted by the client to soothe fears and provide assurance. Clients who have experienced physical, sexual, or emotional abuse may be triggered to respond adversely.**
- Modify procedures, if possible (e.g., substitute oral for intramuscular medications, combine blood draws, or use finger-stick method) **to limit the degree of stress and avoid overwhelming a fearful individual.**
- Manage environmental factors, such as loud noises, harsh lighting, changing person's location without knowledge of family/SO(s), strangers in care area, unfamiliar people, and high traffic flow, **which can**

Information that appears in brackets has been added by the authors to clarify and enhance the use of nursing diagnoses.

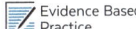 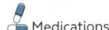 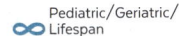

cause or exacerbate stress, especially to very young or older individuals.
- Promote client control, where possible, and help the client identify and accept those things over which control is not possible. **Strengthens the internal locus of control.**
- Encourage attending therapy or therapeutic groups. **Provides opportunity to discuss fearful situations and develop sense of optimism. Individual or group therapy helps the client to work through present issues and how to manage future issues.**

Nursing Priority No. 3.

To assist client in learning to use own responses for problem-solving:

- Acknowledge usefulness of fear for taking care of self. **Provides new idea that can be a motivator to focus on dealing appropriately with situation.**
- Explain the relationship between disease and symptoms, if appropriate, for age and developmental level. **Providing accurate information promotes understanding of why the symptoms occur, allaying anxiety about them.**
- Explain client's responsibility for the solutions while reinforcing that the nurse will be available for help if desired or needed. **Enhances client's sense of control, self-worth, and confidence in own ability, diminishing fear.**
- Determine internal and external resources for assistance (e.g., awareness and use of effective coping skills in the past; SOs who are available for support). **Provides opportunity to recognize and build on resources client/SO may have used successfully in the past.**
- Explain actions and procedures within the level of the client's education and developmental level, being aware of how much information the client wants. **Important to prevent confusion or information overload. Complex and/or anxiety-producing information can be given in manageable amounts over an extended period as opportunities arise and facts are given to assist individual toward acceptance.**

Nursing Priority No. 4.

To support management of self-control and stress response (Teaching/Discharge Considerations):

- Support planning for dealing with reality. **Assists in identifying areas in which control can be exercised and those**

Information that appears in brackets has been added by the authors to clarify and enhance the use of nursing diagnoses.

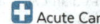 Acute Care 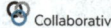 Collaborative 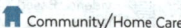 Community/Home Care Cultural

in which control is not possible, thus enabling the client to handle fearful situations/feelings.
- Assist client to learn relaxation, visualization, and guided imagery skills. **Promotes the release of endorphins and aids in developing an internal locus of control, reducing fear and anxiety. May enhance coping skills, allowing the body to go about its work of healing.**
- Encourage regular physical activity within limits of ability. Refer to a physical therapist to develop an exercise program to meet individual needs. **Provides a healthy outlet for energy generated by fearful feelings and promotes relaxation.**
- Provide for and deal with sensory deficits in an appropriate manner (e.g., speak clearly and distinctly, use touch carefully, as indicated by situation). **Recognizing and providing for appropriate contact can enhance communication, promoting understanding.**
- Refer to pastoral care, mental health care providers, support groups, community agencies and organizations, as indicated. **Provides information, ongoing assistance to meet individual needs, and an opportunity for discussing concerns and obtaining further care when indicated.**
- Discuss use of antianxiety medications and reinforce use as prescribed. **Coping with fear, worry, and anxiety requires hard work to overcome. Antianxiety agents may be useful for brief periods in reducing fearful feelings to manageable levels, providing opportunity for initiation of client's own coping skills.**

Documentation Focus

Assessment/Reassessment
- Assessment findings, noting individual factors contributing to current situation, source of fear
- Manifestations of fear

Planning
- Plan of care and who is involved in the planning
- Teaching plan

Implementation/Evaluation
- Client's responses to treatment plan, interventions, and actions performed
- Attainment of or progress toward desired outcome(s)
- Modifications to plan of care

Information that appears in brackets has been added by the authors to clarify and enhance the use of nursing diagnoses.

Discharge Planning
- Long-term needs and who is responsible for actions to be taken
- Specific referrals made

Sample Nursing Outcomes & Interventions Classifications NOC/NIC

NOC—Fear Self-Control
NIC—Anxiety Reduction

---

impaired infant FEEDING BEHAVIOR ICNP

[Diagnostic Division: Food/Fluid]

Definition: Inappropriate caregiver nutritional choices or techniques leading to under or over feeding of child <1 year of age.

Recognizing Cues

Related/Risk Factors
Infant
Difficulty with state regulation (fails to reach state of calm alertness)

Parent/Caregiver
Insufficient/inaccurate information regarding infant nutritional needs, feeding techniques; lack of role model
Failure to accept infant can recognize own hunger/satiety; controlling feeding style
Propping bottle to feed; early introduction of juices, adding cereal to bottle
Food insecurity; neglect/abuse; substance use
Inadequate positive reciprocal interactions between caregiver/infant; multiple caregivers

Defining Characteristics

Subjective
Parent/Caregiver
Anxious; frustrated; concerned; overwhelmed

Objective
Infant
Too sleepy or agitated to feed
Minimal or no interest in eating; refuses to eat adequate amount of food

---

Information that appears in brackets has been added by the authors to clarify and enhance the use of nursing diagnoses.

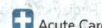 Acute Care 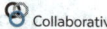 Collaborative 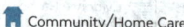 Community/Home Care Cultural

Food refusal—global; food refusal—specific ("picky eater")
Early or delayed progression to spoon or self-feeding
Emotional/stress eating, overeating
Weight deviation from norm less than expected for age, gender, body build
Weight deviation from norm greater than expected for age, gender, body build
Dietary deficiencies (vitamins, iron, zinc, protein)

Parent/Caregiver
Fails to respond appropriately to infant feeding cues
Bribes, forces infant to eat
Impaired infant-caregiver interactions; disconnected

Clinical Connections
Cleft lip/palate, autism spectrum disorder, developmental delays, congenital heart disease, premature infant, enteral nutrition, abuse/neglect

Generate Solutions

Plan Desired Outcomes

Client Will (Include Specific Time Frame)
- Ingest appropriate amount of calories/nutrients to meet metabolic needs.
- Achieve/maintain optimum body weight.

Parents/Caregivers Will (Include Specific Time Frame)
- Verbalize understanding of infant feeding problems.
- Participate in treatment program as able.
- Attend classes to obtain knowledge about infant needs and developmental issues.
- Verbalize knowledge of appropriate methods of feeding infant at each stage of development.

Interventions/Take Action

Nursing Priority No. 1.
To assess causative/contributing factors:

- Identify parent/caregivers' perception of situation and specific needs of infant. **Provides starting point to define needs and develop plan of care.**
- Assess parents' knowledge of infant feeding needs. **The way infant is fed is decisive for the formation of their eating habits. Parents may require basic information or more in-depth support to manage current situation.**

Information that appears in brackets has been added by the authors to clarify and enhance the use of nursing diagnoses.

 Diagnostic Studies
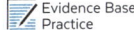 Evidence Based Practice
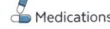 Medications
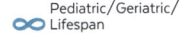 Pediatric/Geriatric/Lifespan

- Determine parents' understanding and recognition of infant cues to feeding needs. **Infants signal appetite through a series of communication cues including facial expressions, gestures/bodily movements, and vocalizations. Responsiveness to infant communication supports effective feeding and can promote self-regulation.**
- Note interaction between parent and infant, and infant's ability to achieve state of calm alertness during feeding. **Parent may need assistance with strategies to stimulate feeding and discourage any maladaptive behavior. Infants who have difficulty with state regulation (e.g., too sleepy or too distressed and agitated) are unable to suckle effectively.**
- Obtain baseline weight and weigh on predetermined schedule. **Weight loss can indicate problems with feeding, inability to suck sufficiently and correctly, insufficient quantity of breast milk.**
- Determine sucking dynamics of the breastfed infant, especially preterm infants. **Breastfeeding is the ultimate nutritional goal, and effective sucking is vital to accomplishing adequate intake.**
- Identify feeding challenges, such as colic, vomiting, slow feeding, or refusal to eat. **Mild to moderately severe issues may be managed by care provider, and more complicated cases may require referral to specialists.**
- Determine timing of food refusal if present. **Consistent refusal to eat foods with specific tastes, textures, smells, and/or appearances can occur during the introduction of a new type or taste of food; however, infant usually eats well when offered preferred foods. This can lead to dietary deficiencies of vitamins, iron, zinc, and protein.**
- Identify family cultural/spiritual beliefs and finances. **Personal beliefs and financial resources affect how family views feeding choice (i.e., breast or bottle) and food choices when solids are introduced.**

Nursing Priority No. 2.
To promote effective infant eating pattern:
- Develop positive nurse/family relationship. **Enables family to feel comfortable discussing issues with nurse, being open and honest about concerns and anxieties.**
- Consult with dietitian. **Provides information and guidance in determining individual nutritional needs incorporating infant's particular issues.**

Information that appears in brackets has been added by the authors to clarify and enhance the use of nursing diagnoses.

- Provide information about normal growth, development, and nutritional needs when no problems are present. **During first 2 years of life, development is rapid and includes dramatic changes in eating behavior. Information helps parents understand what to look for as infant progresses.**
- Discuss needs of infant with structural abnormalities (e.g., naso-oropharynx, larynx, and trachea; cleft lip or palate; esophagus, esophageal atresia, or stenosis; stricture). **Investigation of individual situation can identify specific needs, difficulty with feeding.**
- Provide information about neurodevelopmental disability that has been identified in newborn. **Each situation will need individual assessment: how the problem is manifested, the problems with feeding, weight and development, the emotional climate in the family during feeding or other caregiving.**
- Recommend parent modulate amount of stimulation at mealtime (e.g., calm and low-lighted room for agitated infant or massaging sleeping infant). **Assists infant to achieve a state of calm alertness necessary for effective feeding.**
- Discuss the basic food rules. **Parents control what, when, and where infant is fed. Infant controls how much is eaten in order to learn internal regulation of eating in accordance with physiological signals of hunger and fullness.**
- Discuss principles of responsive feeding as infant progresses from milk-based diet to solid foods. **Responsive feeding is included in the World Health Organization's Global Strategy for Infant and Young Child Feeding to address concerns of childhood underweight, overweight, obesity:**
  Make feeding time pleasurable.
  Minimize distractions during feeding/meal times.
  Be sensitive to infant's signs of hunger and satiety.
  Feed infant directly, slowly.
  Talk to infant during feeding, maintain eye contact.
  Be patient as infant learns to feed self.
  Encourage intake without forcing infant.
  Experiment with different food combinations, tastes, and textures, especially in presence of food refusal.
- Give assistance to parents requiring help with management skills. **Setting time limits for meals, ignoring non-eating behavior, and using positive reinforcement to motivate infant can promote positive feeding behaviors.**

Information that appears in brackets has been added by the authors to clarify and enhance the use of nursing diagnoses.

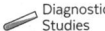 Diagnostic Studies 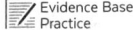 Evidence Based Practice Medications 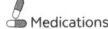 Pediatric/Geriatric/Lifespan

- Discourage behaviors of coaxing, distraction techniques, feeding while playing, or withholding favorite foods to promote desired intake. **May temporize the situation in the short term but may make infant more anxious and lead to oppositional food refusal in general.**
- Refer to ND ineffective infant Suck-Swallow Response; difficulty performing Breastfeeding, inadequate Human Milk Production, as appropriate, for additional interventions.

Nursing Priority No. 3.

To promote nutritional success (Teaching/Discharge Considerations) and enhance well-being (long-term goals):

- Encourage family members to set realistic goals for achieving necessary lifestyle changes. **Depending on the family situation, families will be dealing with problems as infant grows, and having written goals provides reminder of what needs to be accomplished.**
- Discuss methods family can use to make needed changes in family functioning, parenting styles. **Evidence exists to show that associations exist between family characteristics and feeding behavior problems in early childhood.**
- Refer to community resources (e.g., public health visitor program, home care, day care/respite care, nutrition program/food bank, budget counseling). **Additional support and assistance enhance parents' coping abilities and assistance with financial issues such as food insecurity to enhance opportunity for meeting established goals.**
- Refer to support groups, assertiveness or parenting classes, individual and family therapy and/or psychiatric counseling, as indicated. **Involvement with others addressing similar issues or participation in therapy will assist family to problem-solve issues and cope in more positive ways. Treating parental issues such as anxiety or depression can help parent cope more effectively with challenging infant behaviors.**

Documentation Focus

Assessment/Reassessment

- Individual findings, noting specific family problems and infant issues
- Underlying dynamics of current situation
- Infant weight and change over time
- Family support, availability, and use of resources

Information that appears in brackets has been added by the authors to clarify and enhance the use of nursing diagnoses.

Planning
- Plan of care and who is involved in planning
- Teaching plan

Implementation/Evaluation
- Response to interventions, teaching, actions performed, and changes that may be indicated
- Attainment of or progress toward desired outcome(s)
- Modifications to plan of care

Discharge Planning
- Long-term needs and goals and who is responsible for actions
- Specific referrals made

Sample Nursing Outcomes & Interventions Classifications NOC/NIC

NOC—Infant Nutritional Status
NIC—Parenting Promotion

---

risk for FEMALE GENITAL MUTILATION NANDA-I

[Diagnostic Division: Sexuality/Reproduction]

Definition: Susceptible to partial or total removal of or other injury to female external reproductive organs, for nonmedical reasons.

Recognizing Cues

Risk Factors
Inadequate family knowledge about influence of practice on physical, reproductive, or psychosocial health

Generate Solutions

Plan Desired Outcomes

Family/Client Will (Include Specific Time Frame)
- Verbalize understanding of influence of the practice on the health of the child/woman.
- Demonstrate willingness to learn more about the impact of the practice by engaging in conversation with healthcare provider.

Information that appears in brackets has been added by the authors to clarify and enhance the use of nursing diagnoses.

 Diagnostic Studies 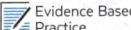 Evidence Based Practice 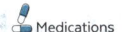 Medications 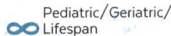 Pediatric/Geriatric/Lifespan

- Review information sources about the effect on physical and psychosocial health of the woman.
- Make the decision not to engage in this practice.
- Develop resources to eliminate the practice of female genital mutilation (FGM).

Interventions/Take Action

Nursing Priority No. 1.

To assess knowledge and beliefs of family/client and cultural/ethnic group:

- Note country of origin of family/client. **Although the practice of FGM has declined in some countries and is banned in a number of others, some type of procedure routinely continues in various regions of Africa and the Middle East. Note: FGM (also known as infibulation) is the full or partial removal of the inner and outer labia, and suturing together of the vulva.**
- Identify cultural/ethnic beliefs of family/client. **FGM has been practiced for over three centuries and may be associated with strong social pressure to continue the practice to conform to tradition, for group identity, marriageability, and right of inheritance.**
- Determine how client views the practice and specific procedure being considered. **Often, women who grow up in a culture that practices FGM view the procedure as "normal," believing it characterizes womanhood and needs to be done, thereby negatively impacting motivation for change and making it harder to give up custom.**
- Determine family/client past experiences with practice, including health consequences. **Often, procedure is performed between first week of life and 8 years of age. Some practices are performed before puberty or at widowhood, and reinfibulation (resuturing after delivery or gynecological procedures of the incised scar tissue resulting from infibulation) may be performed after childbirth. Based on personal experiences, family may have limited understanding of associated risks.**
- Identify prevalence of custom in community and use of nonmedical providers to perform procedure. **Provides insight into needs of the community. Community may or may not support the custom, and nonmedically prepared providers may be utilized, increasing the risk of serious complications/death.**

Information that appears in brackets has been added by the authors to clarify and enhance the use of nursing diagnoses.

Nursing Priority No. 2.
To assist family/client to make informed decision/modify cultural practices:

- Establish a therapeutic relationship with family/client using their terminology in nonjudgmental manner. **Some women do not view the procedure as mutilation, referring to it as "cutting" or "circumcision." Condemning the practice may drive individual(s) away, leading to negative outcome.**
- Provide information about the types of procedures performed in different areas/countries as appropriate. **There are various forms, such as symbolic pricking/piercing or scraping, cutting or removing part or all of the clitoris, or removing the labia minora and majora and suturing the edges closed with only a small hole remaining for urine and menstrual blood to pass (infibulation).**
- Discuss complications that can occur, especially with nonmedical practitioners. **Poor surgical skills of practitioners, absence of anesthesia, and contaminated conditions can result in poor quality of life and even death for the woman. The most common initial complications are bleeding, urine retention, genital tissue swelling, severe pain. Other complications include pelvic inflammatory disease (PID), vaginal and urinary tract infections, dyspareunia (painful sexual intercourse), infertility, anxiety disorder, and post-traumatic stress response. Adverse obstetric outcomes such as postpartum hemorrhage, stillbirth, and cesarean section are not uncommon.**
- Provide detailed information in multiple modes (e.g., pamphlets, models, videos, computer programs) in individual's primary language. Obtain interpreter as indicated. **Information necessary to make informed decision may be better understood in family's/client's primary language.**
- Include client's father/husband in educational sessions as culturally appropriate. **Studies suggest that men who have been educated regarding consequences are less likely to support the practice, whereas those who have not been educated tend to deny reality of physical and obstetrical risks.**
- Refer to community services, if available, for assistance with decision making. **Support groups and/or counseling can provide individual with accurate information, reliable medical care, psychological support.**
- Support client once she has made informed decision. If choice is to proceed, encourage a less invasive or a symbolic

---

Information that appears in brackets has been added by the authors to clarify and enhance the use of nursing diagnoses.

procedure. **In the United States, an individual 18 years of age or older has a legal right to freedom of choice for self, but opting for a less radical procedure can reduce risks and enhance well-being.**

- Refer to competent medical providers who perform genital surgery, as indicated. **If client desires some form of procedure, clinicians who are familiar with the medical sequelae and ramifications of female circumcision will be better able to treat these women knowledgeably and with dignity, while hopefully helping them to make a decision not to have the procedure done. Note: Some argue that FGM is a violation of human rights and against the physician's oath "to do no harm." However, by default, this may drive client to nonmedical providers or to visit country of origin for procedure.**

Nursing Priority No. 3.
To reduce the incidence of FGM:

- Promote the eradication of this practice. **The World Health Organization has declared FGM illegal, and the United Nations calls for its elimination by 2030.**
- Determine additional factors that influence this social change. **Beyond family attitudes, economic benefits to providers, who are often not medically trained but charge substantial fees, cause them to be reluctant to terminate the practice.**
- Encourage religious/community leaders to advocate against practice. **These individuals are generally well respected and influential within their communities.**
- Develop community-based educational programs addressing concepts of sexuality, marriage practices, legal rights, and federal laws. **Necessary to shift community attitudes supporting practice. Note: In some countries, such as the United States and Canada, the procedure cannot be performed on minors below the age of 18. In a number of other countries, it is totally illegal with repercussions for the individual performing the procedure, the client, and on occasion anyone aware of and failing to report the procedure was performed.**
- Educate lawmakers of health and well-being consequences of procedure. **Encourages creation of laws banning practice and allocation of financial resources supporting programs at community level.**
- Assist in developing emergency care resources and referrals to midwives, gynecologist/obstetrician for pregnant women

---

Information that appears in brackets has been added by the authors to clarify and enhance the use of nursing diagnoses.

who have had FGM. **Increases opportunity for a successful delivery of a healthy baby and minimizing injury to the woman. Provides opportunity to discuss reconstructive procedure or at least refrain from reinfibulation.**

Documentation Focus

Assessment/Reassessment
- Assessment findings, including attitudes/expectations of family/client
- Religious and cultural/ethnic factors
- Family/client past experience with practice
- Community prevalence of custom and providers
- Available community resources

Planning
- Plan of care and who is involved in planning
- Teaching plan
- Formulation of community action plan

Implementation/Evaluation
- Client's/family's responses to interventions, teaching, and actions performed
- Attainment of or progress to desire outcome(s)
- Client's/family's decision
- Community's commitment to change

Discharge Planning
- Long-term plans, and who is responsible for actions to be taken
- Specific referrals made

Sample Nursing Outcomes & Interventions Classifications NOC/NIC

NOC—Community Risk Control: Unhealthy Cultural Traditions
NIC—Culture Care Negotiation

---

risk for impaired FLUID VOLUME BALANCE NANDA-I

[Diagnostic Division: Food/Fluid]

Definition: Susceptible to rapid shift from one to the other of intracellular and/or extracellular fluids, not including blood.

Information that appears in brackets has been added by the authors to clarify and enhance the use of nursing diagnoses.

Recognizing Cues

Risk Factors
Excessive, or inadequate fluid intake; excessive sodium intake
Difficulty obtaining fluids
Inadequate knowledge about fluid needs
Ineffective medication self-management
Inadequate muscle mass; malnutrition

Clinical Connections
Major surgical procedures, renal dialysis, conditions requiring IV therapy or parenteral or enteral nutrition, heart failure with use of diuretic therapy, conditions with excessive fluid loss through abnormal or normal routes

Generate Solutions

Plan Desired Outcomes

Client Will (Include Specific Time Frame)
- Demonstrate adequate fluid balance as evidenced by stable vital signs, palpable pulses of good quality, normal skin turgor, moist mucous membranes, individual appropriate urinary output, lack of excessive weight fluctuation (loss or gain), and no edema present.

Client/Caregiver Will (Include Specific Time Frame)
- Identify individual risk factors and plan to prevent/modify occurrence as appropriate.

Interventions/Take Action

Nursing Priority No. 1.
To determine risk/contributing factors:

- Note the presence of conditions associated with fluid imbalance (e.g., severe burns; diabetes insipidus; hyperosmolar nonketotic syndrome; diabetic ketoacidosis [DKA]; vomiting/diarrhea; heart, pancreatitis, sepsis).
- Review current treatment modalities, including (1) major invasive procedures (e.g., surgery or dialysis, plasmapheresis [i.e., apheresis] therapy), (2) use or overuse of certain medications (e.g., diuretics, nephrotoxic agents, sodium-glucose cotransporter-2 inhibitors [SGLT2]), (3) use of IV fluids without a delivery device, (4) too rapid fluid administration, and (5) administration of hyper/hypotonic IV solutions. **These modalities can**

Information that appears in brackets has been added by the authors to clarify and enhance the use of nursing diagnoses.

 Acute Care   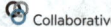 Collaborative   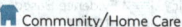 Community/Home Care   Cultural

cause/exacerbate fluid imbalances and must be monitored for complications.
- Note the client's age and current level of hydration. **Assessment of client's current hydration status and concomitant pathophysiological processes (i.e., renal dysfunction, gastrointestinal dysfunction, sepsis, DKA, etc.) provides information regarding the ability to tolerate fluctuations in fluid level. Young and old clients have less robust compensatory fluid balance mechanisms than adults.**
- Note client's mentation. **Provides information regarding risks for potential fluid balance problems (e.g., confused client may have inadequate intake, may disconnect tubing, or may readjust IV flow rate).**

Nursing Priority No. 2.
To prevent fluctuations/imbalances in fluid levels:
- Monitor client's fluid status per protocol. **A physical examination provides cues of the clinical manifestations and compensatory mechanisms of fluid imbalance.**
- Measure and record intake, including all sources such as oral (e.g., food/fluid, liquid medications), IV (e.g., antibiotics, medicated infusions, maintenance fluids), irrigation fluids, etc.
- Measure and record output, including urine output (i.e., per urinal, catheter bag, Purewick, etc.), defecation, vomit, tube drainage (i.e., chest tube, JP drain, Hemovac, nasogastric [NGT], etc.). **Hourly urine output is age dependent, ranging from 0.5 mL/kg/hr to 1.5 mL/kg/hr. Urine output less than expected may indicate deficient fluid volume, cardiac or kidney failure and should be reported to healthcare providers.**
- Observe the color of all excretions. **The color of urine (i.e., clear/pale yellow to amber) may indicate hydration or renal status. Evaluation of fluids for signs of purulence may indicate infection and the opportunity to prevent sepsis.**
- Estimate volume or measure emesis when vomiting.
- Measure or estimate the amount of liquid stool; weigh diapers or continence pads, when indicated.
- Inspect dressing(s), weigh dressings, count dressings or pads saturated per hour. **Note: Small losses can be life-threatening to pediatric clients.**
- Estimate or calculate insensible fluid losses **to include in replacement calculations. Insensible fluid loss (e.g., diaphoresis, respiratory evaporation, wounds, etc.) includes losses of fluid through diffusion through the skin and respiratory tract and are estimated at 400 ml to 800 ml in adults at ambient temperature.**

Information that appears in brackets has been added by the authors to clarify and enhance the use of nursing diagnoses.

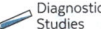 Diagnostic Studies 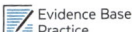 Evidence Based Practice 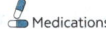 Medications 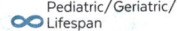 Pediatric/Geriatric/Lifespan

- Calculate 24-hr fluid balance, noting trends (intake more than output or output more than intake).
- Weigh daily, or as indicated, using the same scale, clothing, and equipment in place. **Changes in client weight provide information for early detection and prompt intervention, such as weight gain (may indicate fluid excess) or weight loss (can signify fluid deficit).**
- Monitor vital signs:

  Evaluate vital signs at rest and with activities.

  Measure heart rate. **A heart rate above 90 bpm may indicate an early compensatory response to a hypovolemic state; however, tachycardia may also be caused by a variety of causes (e.g., pain, fever, anxiety).**

  Measure blood pressure. **Falling systolic blood pressure (SBP) is worrisome for inadequate intravascular volume. Tachycardia and declining SBP may indicate impending cardiovascular collapse. Elevated SBP may be an indicator of intravascular volume overload but may also be associated with other etiologies (e.g., hypertension, pain, fever, anxiety). Note: Orthostatic vital signs should be obtained to evaluate the degree of dehydration or investigate the etiology of dizziness or syncope.**

  Measure respiratory rate. **A respiratory rate above 20 bpm in the adult client may indicate inadequate systemic tissue perfusion (with a possible etiology of hypovolemia) and a compensatory response of increased respiratory rate. Adventitious breath sounds (i.e., crackles, rhonchi) may indicate third spacing of fluid from the intravascular space into pulmonary tissue.**
- ∞ Measure and grade peripheral pulses. **In hypovolemic states, pulses may be fast and thready, while in hypervolemic states, pulses will be bounding. Note: Evaluation of the brachial and femoral pulses in infants is a crucial assessment.**
- Measure capillary refill. **Capillary refill time should take less than 3 sec in the fingertips and toes. A refill time greater than 3 sec may indicate compromised perfusion that could be associated with hypovolemia (inadequate intravascular volume).**
- Assess for edema. **Assess client for peripheral edema, grading the edema as indicated. Peripheral edema may be caused by volume overload or the third spacing of intravascular fluid. Note: Intravascular volume depletion**

Information that appears in brackets has been added by the authors to clarify and enhance the use of nursing diagnoses.

can be present at the same time as extravascular fluid excess (seen as edema) is present.

- Measure skin turgor. **In elderly adult, measure skin turgor on the forehead or sternum due to loss of subcutaneous tissue. In severe dehydration, skin tenting will be noted. In infants, a depressed fontanelle may be indicative of dehydration.**
- Assess skin temperature. **Using the dorsa of the hands, palpate skin temperature proximal to distal. While hands and feet often feel cooler bilaterally, cool and clammy skin may indicate the shunting of blood away from superficial blood vessels. This may occur from a variety of causes, including inadequate intravascular volume.**
- Assess oral mucous membranes. **The buccal mucous membranes and the tongue may appear dry in the client with dehydration. In infants and children, assess for the presence of tear production. Ask parents about tear production, or the lack of tears, which can indicate significant dehydration.**
- Evaluate jugular vein appearance. **Jugular vein distention may occur due to cardiac dysfunction (i.e., heart failure). However, while the client may not be considered truly in volume overload, the cardiac dysfunction creates a physiological state that mimics an overload state that warrants follow-up by healthcare provider.**
- Evaluate hemodynamic pressures (e.g., central venous pressure, pulmonary artery, cardiac output, cardiac index, saturation of venous oxygen [SvO_2], stroke volume variability, and pulmonary artery wedge pressure), when available for client in intensive care/perioperative area. **Values may be used in critically ill clients to determine fluid balance and fluid volume responsiveness, and to guide administration of vasoactive medications. Note: Numerous studies in recent years have promoted the benefits of noninvasive monitoring to evaluate fluid status in real time (and thus cardiac output response to fluid challenges such as passive leg raise and the Trendelenburg maneuver).**
- Administer IV fluids on volumetric infusion pumps and rapid infusion devices, as appropriate **to deliver fluids accurately and at desired rates to prevent either underinfusion or overinfusion.**
- Administer enteral fluid solutions as needed. **Clients may be unable or unwilling to take in adequate fluids orally.**

Information that appears in brackets has been added by the authors to clarify and enhance the use of nursing diagnoses.

 Diagnostic Studies 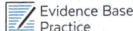 Evidence Based Practice 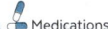 Medications 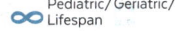 Pediatric/Geriatric/Lifespan

Utilization of the gastrointestinal tract is a preferable method compared to IV route for long-term hydration.
- Note increased lethargy or reports of dizziness, weakness, and muscle cramping. **Electrolyte imbalances (e.g., sodium, potassium, magnesium, calcium) may be present and cause shifts between fluid compartments.**
- Review laboratory data (e.g., blood urea nitrogen/creatinine ratio, transaminases [aspartate aminotransferase/alanine aminotransferase], hemoglobin/hematocrit, serum osmolality, serum sodium, urine osmolality, and urine specific gravity) **to determine changes indicative of electrolyte and/or fluid imbalance and fluid needs.**
- Review x-rays (i.e., chest radiograph, abdominal x-rays) **to determine changes indicative of fluid accumulation.**
- If fluid volume deficit is possible:

Anticipate fluid replacement needs (e.g., major burn injury; person with heat stroke; vomiting, diarrhea, or inability to take fluids). **IV fluid replacement routinely includes crystalloid (i.e., normal saline, half-normal saline, and lactated Ringer solution) or colloid solutions (albumin solutions, hyperoncotic starch, dextran). IV crystalloids are an integral part of client care to maintain and replace body fluids. Note: The pediatric population requires special considerations for fluid maintenance and rehydration. One option for hourly rate of fluid maintenance is the 4-2-1 rule (i.e., first 10 kg: 4 mL/kg/hr, next 10 to 20 kg: 2 mL/kg/hr, and 1mL/kg/hr after that with maximum 100 mL/hr maintenance). Establish and promote oral intake, incorporating beverage preferences when possible. Administer IV fluids (e.g., crystalloids, colloids) to support fluid management.**

Maintain sodium restrictions as needed. Offer fluid consistently over a 24-hr period. **Oral fluids are the preferred route for hydration when possible. As adults age, the thirst mechanism may fail to inspire adequate fluid intake.**

Administer medications (e.g., antidiarrheals, antiemetics, desmopressin) as indicated **to reduce fluid loss.**

Refer to ND inadequate Fluid Volume for additional interventions.

- If fluid volume excess is possible:

Maintain fluid/sodium restrictions as ordered. Offer small amounts of fluid over 24 hr.

Administer medications (e.g., diuretics) **to assist in the management of fluid excess or edema.**

Information that appears in brackets has been added by the authors to clarify and enhance the use of nursing diagnoses.

- Assist with or prepare for procedures (e.g., dialysis, apheresis, ultrafiltration, pacemaker, cardiac assist device) **to correct fluid shifts and prevent overload.** Monitor for complications associated with fluid imbalances.

  Refer to ND excessive Fluid Volume for additional interventions.

Nursing Priority No. 3.

To promote optimum fluid balance (Teaching/Discharge Considerations) and enhance well-being (long-term goals):

- Engage the client, family, and all caregivers in a fluid management plan. **Enhances cooperation with the regimen and achievement of goals.**
- Discuss individual risk factors, potential problems, and specific interventions **to prevent or limit fluid imbalance and complications.**
- Instruct the client/significant other (SO) in how to measure and record I/O as appropriate.
- Discuss use of and provide to the client lidded beverage bottles/containers that show measurements and are easy to hold and keep close. **May be helpful to the child or adult with concerns regarding regulated fluid consumption (e.g., adult may be drinking too much or too little or may have difficulties remembering to drink, or remembering to limit fluids).**
- Instruct client/SO in how to measure and record daily weight, as appropriate.
- Instruct client/SO in dietary changes (e.g., salt limitation, heart healthy choices, weight management), as appropriate. Refer for dietary counseling as indicated.
- Review and instruct on medications or nutritional regimen (e.g., enteral or parenteral) **to alert to potential complications and ways to manage.**
- Identify signs and symptoms indicating the need for prompt evaluation or follow-up by the primary healthcare provider **for timely intervention and correction.**

Documentation Focus

Assessment/Reassessment

- Individual findings, including individual factors influencing fluid needs/requirements
- Baseline weight, vital signs
- Results of laboratory test and diagnostic studies
- Specific client preferences for fluids

Information that appears in brackets has been added by the authors to clarify and enhance the use of nursing diagnoses.

Planning
- Plan of care and who is involved in planning
- Teaching plan

Implementation/Evaluation
- Responses to interventions, teaching, and actions performed
- Attainment of or progress toward desired outcome(s)
- Modifications to plan of care

Discharge Planning
- Individual long-term needs, noting who is responsible for actions to be taken
- Specific referrals made

Sample Nursing Outcomes & Interventions Classifications NOC/NIC

NOC—Fluid Balance
NIC—Fluid Monitoring

---

excessive FLUID VOLUME   NANDA-I

[Diagnostic Division: Food/Fluid]

Definition: Surplus retention of intracellular and/or extracellular fluids, not including blood.

Recognizing Cues

Related/Risk Factors
Excessive fluid intake
Excessive sodium intake
Inadequate knowledge about fluid needs
Ineffective medication self-management

Defining Characteristics

Subjective
Anxiety
[Dyspnea, orthopnea; paroxysmal nocturnal dyspnea]

Objective
Adventitious respiratory sounds; altered respiratory pattern
Altered blood pressure; altered pulmonary artery pressure; increased central venous pressure
Altered mental status; psychomotor agitation
Altered urine specific gravity; intake exceeds output; oliguria

---

Information that appears in brackets has been added by the authors to clarify and enhance the use of nursing diagnoses.

 Acute Care 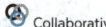 Collaborative 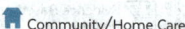 Community/Home Care   Cultural

Azotemia; decreased serum hematocrit or hemoglobin levels
Jugular vein distension; positive hepatojugular reflex; hepatomegaly; pleural effusion; pulmonary congestion
Presence of S_3 heart sound
Edema; weight gain over short period of time

Clinical Connections

Congestive heart failure, renal failure, dialysis, cirrhosis of liver, cancer, toxemia of pregnancy, conditions associated with syndrome of inappropriate antidiuretic hormone (SIADH) secretion (e.g., meningitis, encephalitis, Guillain-Barré syndrome), schizophrenia (where polydipsia is a prominent feature)

Generate Solutions

Plan Desired Outcomes

Client Will (Include Specific Time Frame)

- Stabilize fluid volume as evidenced by balanced input and output (I&O), vital signs within client's normal limits, stable weight, and free of signs of edema.
- Verbalize understanding of individual dietary and fluid restrictions.
- Demonstrate behaviors to monitor fluid status and reduce recurrence of fluid excess.
- List signs that require further evaluation.

Interventions/Take Action

Nursing Priority No. 1.

To assess causative/precipitating factors:

- Note the presence of conditions associated with excess fluid or the risk of excess fluid balance (e.g., inadequate sodium and water excretion as seen in heart failure, chronic kidney disease, Cushing syndrome, SIADH, decreased or loss of serum albumin, severe burns, etc.) **that can contribute to fluid retention.**
- Note current treatment modalities, including (1) major invasive procedures (e.g., surgery, dialysis/continuous renal replacement therapy [CRRT]), (2) use or overuse of certain medications (e.g., diuretics, nephrotoxic agents), (3) fluid resuscitation/fluid bolus/too rapid fluid administration, (4) rapid or liberal administration of hyper/hypotonic IV solutions. **Inattentive administration of hypotonic IV solution may result in intracellular fluid shifts;**

Information that appears in brackets has been added by the authors to clarify and enhance the use of nursing diagnoses.

 Diagnostic Studies   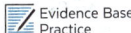 Evidence Based Practice   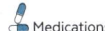 Medications   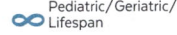 Pediatric/Geriatric/Lifespan

conversely, hypertonic IV fluid administration may result in intravascular fluid shifts. **Note: Knowledge of client pathology, therapeutic strategy, and treatment goals is imperative for successful client outcomes. Consideration should be made in which space(s) the excess is occurring or may occur (i.e., intracellular, interstitial, intravascular).**

- Evaluate amount of fluid intake from all sources, such as oral (e.g., PO, enteral fluid), IV (e.g., antibiotics, medicated infusions, maintenance fluids, parenteral feedings), irrigation, etc., the rate of infusion, and specific conditions that may affect the client's ability to tolerate fluid administration. **The potential exists for fluid overload due to fluid shifts and changes in electrolyte balance. Consequences of fluid overload include cerebral edema, myocardial edema, pulmonary edema, hepatic congestion, cholestasis, gut malabsorption, and tissue edema.**
- Review nutritional issues (e.g., intake of sodium, potassium, and protein). **Imbalances in these areas are associated with fluid imbalances. The severely malnourished client can experience significant fluid shifts and electrolyte imbalances after nutritional support is initiated. This potentially lethal disorder, known as refeeding syndrome, is often associated with parenteral nutrition, but it may also occur with enteral nutrition, oral intake, or dextrose-containing IV fluids.**

Nursing Priority No. 2.
To evaluate degree of excess:

- Weigh daily or as indicated. Compare current weight with admission and/or previously stated weight. **Weigh the client using the same scale, clothing, and equipment in place, which provides a comparative baseline and evaluates the effectiveness of diuretic therapy, when used (i.e., a roughly 1-kg [2.2 lb] change in body weight equates to a 1-L gain or loss in body fluid volume). Note: Volume overload can occur over weeks to months in clients with unrecognized kidney disease/failure where lean muscle mass is lost, and fluid overload occurs with relatively little weight change.**
- Monitor vital signs at rest and with activities. **Blood pressure, heart, and respiratory rate often increase initially when either volume deficit or fluid excess is present.**
- Measure heart rate. **Although no vital sign is a definitive indicator of hypervolemia, tachycardia, hypertension/**

Information that appears in brackets has been added by the authors to clarify and enhance the use of nursing diagnoses.

hypotension, tachypnea, and/or decreased peripheral oxygen saturation (SpO_2) may be suggestive of fluid overload dependent on client history.
- Note presence of tachycardia and irregular rhythms. Auscultate heart tones for S_3 and S_4. **The S_3 heart sound indicates elevated intracardiac filling pressures and reduced ejection fraction suggestive of heart failure, which results in decreased cardiac output and tissue hypoxia. An S_4 heart sound is also suggestive of hypervolemia but less so the S_3.**
- Measure blood pressure. **Tachycardia and declining systolic blood pressure (SBP) may indicate impending cardiovascular collapse. Elevated SBP may be an indicator of intravascular volume overload but may also be associated with other etiologies (e.g., hypertension, pain, fever, anxiety, etc.).**
- Measure respiratory rate. **A respiratory rate above 20 bpm in the adult client may indicate hypoxia associated with pulmonary tissue edema, although the etiology of the tachypnea should be identified.**
- Record occurrence of exertional breathlessness, dyspnea at rest, orthopnea, or paroxysmal nocturnal dyspnea. **The presence of orthopnea or bendopnea (i.e., shortness of breath experienced when the client bends over or leans forward) is highly suspicious for hypervolemia associated with heart failure.**
- Auscultate breath sounds for presence of adventitious breath sounds (i.e., crackles, rhonchi). **Adventitious breath sounds, such as crackles and rhonchi, may indicate third spacing of fluid from the intravascular space into pulmonary tissue and interfere with oxygen–carbon dioxide exchange at the capillary level.**
- Measure and trend invasive hemodynamic parameters (e.g., central venous pressure, pulmonary artery pressure/pulmonary capillary wedge pressure), as needed for critically ill clients. **Pressure trends may reflect elevations associated with excess fluid volume or reductions due to impending cardiac failure.**
- ∞ Measure and grade peripheral pulses. **In hypervolemic states, pulses will be bounding. Note: Evaluation of the brachial and femoral pulses in infants is a crucial assessment.**
- Note the presence, location, and grade of edema (e.g., puffy eyelids, swelling ankles and feet if ambulatory or up in chair, sacrum and posterior thighs when recumbent, scrotum/labia). Determine whether lower extremity edema is new

---

Information that appears in brackets has been added by the authors to clarify and enhance the use of nursing diagnoses.

or increasing. **Dependent edema is often associated with an increase in venous hydrostatic pressure (e.g., heart failure and renal failure). Generalized edema (e.g., upper extremities and eyelids, anasarca) is often associated with a reduction in venous osmotic (oncotic) pull, an increase in venous hydrostatic pressure, and/or a capillary leak. Note: Intravascular volume depletion can be present at the same time extravascular fluid excess (seen as edema) is present.**

- Assess for the presence of neck vein distention, hepatojugular reflux when head of bed is elevated 45 degrees. **Signs of increased intravascular volume.**
- Measure abdominal girth **to evaluate changes that may indicate increasing fluid retention and edema, especially in client with heart failure or cirrhosis.**
- Evaluate mentation for confusion, personality changes. **Signs of decreased cerebral oxygenation (e.g., cerebral edema) or electrolyte imbalance.**
- Assess appetite; note the presence of nausea or vomiting **to determine the presence of problems associated with an imbalance of electrolytes (e.g., glucose, sodium, potassium, or calcium).**
- Observe skin and mucous membranes. **Edematous tissues are prone to ischemia, infection, and breakdown/ulceration.**
- Review laboratory data (e.g., blood urea nitrogen [BUN], creatinine [Cr], hemoglobin/hematocrit, serum albumin, brain natriuretic peptide [BNP] proteins, and electrolytes; urine specific gravity and osmolality, sodium excretion) and chest x-ray **to determine changes indicative of electrolyte and/or fluid imbalance. These tests may be repeated not only to ascertain baseline imbalances but also to monitor response to therapy.**

Nursing Priority No. 3.
To promote mobilization/elimination of excess fluid:

- Restrict fluid intake as indicated (especially when sodium retention is less than water retention or when fluid retention is related to renal failure).
- Provide for sodium restrictions if needed. **Sodium is the primary extracellular electrolyte. Serum sodium levels contribute to the regulation of serum osmolality,**

Information that appears in brackets has been added by the authors to clarify and enhance the use of nursing diagnoses.

intravascular volume, and acid-base balance. Sodium is regulated through dietary intake, renal excretion, and in response to aldosterone and antidiuretic hormone.

- Set an appropriate rate of fluid intake or infusion throughout 24-hr period. Maintain steady rate of all IV infusions **to prevent exacerbation of excess fluid volume and to prevent peaks and valleys in fluid level.**
- Administer medications (e.g., diuretics, cardiac inotropes) in order to improve cardiac output and mobilize excess fluid, thereby **reducing (potential for) congestion and edema. Note: Albumin can be used in conjunction with an IV diuretic to pull fluid into the intravascular space and then facilitate rapid renal excretion of excess fluid.**
- Elevate edematous extremities **to enhance venous return and prevent further edema formation. Note: Caution should be taken in clients with existing dyspnea or impaired cardiac function. Rapid release of fluid from dependent edema back into the general circulation can worsen heart failure or pulmonary edema.**
- Place in semi-Fowler position when at bedrest, as appropriate. **May promote recumbency-induced diuresis and facilitate respiratory effort when movement of the diaphragm is limited/breathing is impaired because of lung congestion.**
- Prepare for and assist with procedures as indicated (e.g., peritoneal or hemodialysis, ultrafiltration; mechanical ventilation, cardiac resynchronization therapy). **May be done to correct volume overload, electrolyte imbalance, acid-base imbalance, and/or to improve cardiac function and support client during shock state.** (Refer to ND risk for Shock.)
- Record I&O accurately; calculate 24-hr fluid balance, noting plus or minus **so that adjustments can be made in the following 24-hr intake if needed.**

Nursing Priority No. 4.
To maintain integrity of skin and oral mucous membranes:

- Refer to NDs impaired Skin Integrity or Tissue Integrity; impaired oral Mucous Membrane; risk for adult/child Pressure Injury for related interventions.

Information that appears in brackets has been added by the authors to clarify and enhance the use of nursing diagnoses.

Nursing Priority No. 5.

To promote euvolemia (Teaching/Discharge Considerations) and enhance well-being (long-term goals):

- Review individual risk factors, potential problems, and specific interventions **to prevent or limit fluid overload and complications.**
- Instruct client/SO in dietary changes (e.g., salt limitation, heart-healthy diet, weight management, renal diet) as appropriate. Review safe substitutes for salt (e.g., lemon juice or spices such as oregano).
- Suggest sugar-free chewing gum, sucking ice chips/hard candy, or lemon slices, and use of lip balm **to help allay thirst and reduce the discomforts of fluid restrictions.**
- Refer for dietary counseling, as indicated **to develop dietary plan and identify foods to be limited or omitted. Note: Suggest avoiding salty or spicy foods, as they increase thirst or fluid retention.**
- Engage the client, family, and caregivers in the fluid management plan, discussing fluid restrictions and "hidden sources" of fluids (e.g., foods high in water content such as fruits, ice cream, sauces, custard). Encourage use of a small drinking cup or glass. **Enhances cooperation with the regimen and achievement of goals.**
- Instruct client/family in ways to keep track of intake. For example, use a marked water bottle or container. Suggest the use of and provide to the client lidded beverage bottles/containers that show measurements. **May be helpful to clients with concerns regarding regulated fluid consumption (e.g., drinking too much or remembering to limit fluids).**
- Measure output, encourage use of voiding record when appropriate, or weigh daily and report gain of more than 2 lb/day (or as indicated by individual situation). **If weight is rising daily, fluid is likely being retained.**
- Instruct client/SO in how to measure and record daily weight, as appropriate.
- Review drug regimen (and side effects) used to increase urine output or manage client conditions (e.g., hypertension, kidney disease, heart failure, etc.) **to alert to potential complications and ways to manage them. Many drugs have an impact on kidney function and fluid balance, especially in the elderly or those with cardiac and kidney impairments.**
- Emphasize the need for mobility, frequent position changes, and early/ongoing ambulation **to promote venous return, prevent stasis, and reduce risk of tissue injury.**

Information that appears in brackets has been added by the authors to clarify and enhance the use of nursing diagnoses.

- Identify client "danger" signs requiring notification of healthcare provider **to ensure timely evaluation/intervention.**

Documentation Focus

Assessment/Reassessment
- Assessment findings, noting existing conditions contributing to and degree of fluid retention (vital signs; amount, presence, and location of edema; and weight changes)
- I&O, fluid balance
- Results of laboratory tests and diagnostic studies

Planning
- Plan of care and who is involved in the planning
- Teaching plan

Implementation/Evaluation
- Response to interventions, teaching, and actions performed
- Attainment of or progress toward desired outcome(s)
- Modifications to plan of care

Discharge Planning
- Long-range needs, noting who is responsible for actions to be taken

Sample Nursing Outcomes & Interventions Classifications NOC/NIC

NOC—Fluid Overload Severity
NIC—Hypervolemia Management

---

inadequate FLUID VOLUME   NANDA-I

[Diagnostic Division: Food/Fluid]

Definition: Decreased intracellular and/or extracellular fluids, not including blood.

Recognizing Cues

Related/Risk Factors
Difficulty obtaining fluids; inadequate fluid intake
Inadequate knowledge about fluid needs
Ineffective medication self-management
Impaired physical mobility, inadequate muscle mass
Malnutrition

Information that appears in brackets has been added by the authors to clarify and enhance the use of nursing diagnoses.

 Diagnostic Studies 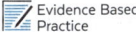 Evidence Based Practice 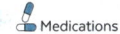 Medications 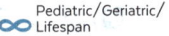 Pediatric/Geriatric/Lifespan

Defining Characteristics

Subjective
Thirst
Weakness

Objective
Altered mental status
Altered skin turgor; decreased tongue turgor; dry mucous membranes or skin
Decreased blood pressure; decreased pulse pressure or pulse volume; decreased venous filling
Decreased urine output
Increased body temperature; increased heart rate
Increased serum hematocrit levels; increased urine concentration
Sudden weight loss; sunken eyes

Clinical Connections

Traumatic injury, surgical procedures; infections; gastroenteritis (with vomiting and diarrhea), gastric intubation, irritable bowel syndrome, malnutrition, anorexia, bulimia, uncontrolled diabetes mellitus, severe burns, draining wounds, fistulas, ascites; depression

Generate Solutions

Plan Desired Outcomes

Client Will (Include Specific Time Frame)

- Maintain fluid volume at a functional level as evidenced by individually adequate urinary output with normal specific gravity, stable vital signs, moist mucous membranes, good skin turgor, prompt capillary refill, and resolution of edema.

Client/Caregiver Will (Include Specific Time Frame)

- Verbalize understanding of causative factors and purpose of individual therapeutic interventions and medications.
- Demonstrate behaviors to monitor and correct deficit, as indicated.

Interventions/Take Action

Nursing Priority No. 1.

To assess causative/precipitating factors:

- Note the presence of conditions associated with inadequate fluid volume or the risk of fluid volume depletion,

---

Information that appears in brackets has been added by the authors to clarify and enhance the use of nursing diagnoses.

 Acute Care 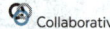 Collaborative 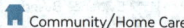 Community/Home Care   Cultural

significant fluid loss (other than blood) such as might occur with severe gastroenteritis, with vomiting and diarrhea, extensive burns, diabetes insipidus, heat stroke, or fluid shifts (e.g., sepsis, anaphylactic shock, cirrhosis with ascites, etc.). **Inadequate fluid volume may result in negative client outcomes such as renal dysfunction, altered mental status, liver injury, hypotension, falls, and impaired tissue perfusion. Note: Be aware of the difference between signs of hypovolemia (e.g., poor skin turgor, dizziness on standing, lethargy, delayed capillary refill, sunken eyeballs, fever, weight loss, little or no urine output) and signs of dehydration (e.g., lethargy, weakness, irritability, nausea, vomiting, hyperreflexia, potentially progressing to coma), which are symptoms of the effect of elevated sodium (hypernatremia) on the central nervous system.**

- Determine fluid space most likely affected **to assist in discerning the etiology of the fluid loss and appropriate treatment strategies:**

  Isotonic (isonatremic) **dehydration occurs when water and sodium are lost in equal amounts. Causes may include vomiting, diarrhea, sweating, burns, intrinsic kidney disease, hyperglycemia, and hypoaldosteronism.**

  Hypertonic (hypernatremic) **dehydration occurs when more water than sodium is lost, leaving the residual serum hypertonic. Causes may include increased respiration and diabetes insipidus.**

  Hypotonic (hyponatremic) **dehydration occurs when more sodium than water is lost, leaving the residual serum hypotonic. Causes may include diuretic use, altered mentation, immobility, impaired thirst mechanism, drug overdose leading to coma, salt-wasting tubular disease, Addison disease, hypoaldosteronism, and hyperglycemia.**

- Note current treatment modalities, including (1) dialysis (e.g., hemodialysis/continuous renal replacement therapy [CRRT], peritoneal dialysis), (2) use or overuse of certain medications (e.g., diuretics, hypertonic/colloidal solutions, vasodilators, beta blockers, aldosterone inhibitors, angiotensin-converting enzyme [ACE] inhibitors, and medications that can cause syndrome of inappropriate antidiuretic hormone secretion [e.g., phenothiazides, vasopressin, some antineoplastic drugs]), (3) wound drainage (fistulas, nasogastric tube [NGT], ileostomy/colostomy, suction devices, etc.),

---

Information that appears in brackets has been added by the authors to clarify and enhance the use of nursing diagnoses.

(4) failure to replace fluid (e.g., fluid restriction, NPO status, inadequate maintenance fluids) **that may contribute to a lack of fluid intake or loss of fluid by various routes.**
- Prepare for and assist with diagnostic evaluations (e.g., imaging studies, x-rays) **to locate cause for hypovolemia.**
- Determine the effects of age and gender **to identify potential factors affecting the client's fluid volume status. In general, men have less risk of dehydration compared to women due to women's higher percentage of body fat and less muscle mass than men. Elderly clients are often at risk for dehydration because of decreased thirst reflex, reduced renal water conservation, chronic comorbidities, polypharmacy, and difficulties with medication self-management. Infants, young children, and other nonverbal clients may not be able to communicate thirst or care for themselves, affecting fluid needs. Worldwide, dehydration (secondary to diarrheal illness) is the leading cause of infant and child mortality.**

Nursing Priority No. 2.

To evaluate degree of fluid deficit:

- Weigh daily or as indicated. Compare current weight with admission or previously stated weight. Weigh the client using the same scale, clothing, and equipment to provide a comparative baseline (i.e., roughly 1 kg [2.2 lb]). **Recent weight changes remain a standard for evaluating fluid accumulation or loss.**
- Measure and record intake. Include all sources such as oral (e.g., food/fluid, liquid medications), IV (e.g., antibiotics, medicated infusions, maintenance fluids), irrigation fluids, etc.
- Measure and record output. Include all sources such as urine output (i.e., per urinal, catheter bag, Purewick, etc.); defecation; vomiting; tube drainage (i.e., chest tube, JP drain, Hemovac, NGT, etc.). Note color (may be dark yellow to greenish-brown because of concentration) and elevated specific gravity (normal range 1.010 to 1.025). **Consideration of client fluid loss should include insensible fluid loss such as diaphoresis, respiratory evaporation, wounds, etc. Note: Hourly urine output is age-dependent, ranging from 0.5 mL/kg/hr to 1.5 mL/kg/hr. Urine output less than expected may indicate deficient fluid volume or cardiac or kidney failure and should be reported to healthcare providers.**
- Monitor vital signs at rest and with activities **to determine degree of intravascular deficit and replacement needs.**

Information that appears in brackets has been added by the authors to clarify and enhance the use of nursing diagnoses.

- Measure heart rate. **A heart rate above 90 bpm may indicate an early compensatory response to a hypovolemic state; however, tachycardia may have a variety of causes (e.g., pain, fever, anxiety).**
- Measure blood pressure (lying/sitting/standing) as appropriate to evaluate orthostatic blood pressure. **Falling systolic blood pressure (SBP) is worrisome for inadequate intravascular volume. Tachycardia and declining SBP may indicate impending cardiovascular collapse. Note: Orthostatic vital signs should be obtained to evaluate the degree of dehydration or investigate the etiology of dizziness or syncope.**
- Note the presence of tachycardic and/or irregular rhythms. **Fluid imbalance and loss can result in electrolyte disturbance, particularly changes in serum potassium, that may cause dysrhythmia.**
- Measure respiratory rate. **A respiratory rate above 20 bpm in the adult client may indicate inadequate systemic tissue perfusion (with a possible etiology of hypovolemia) and a compensatory response of increased respiratory rate.**
- Auscultate breath sounds for presence of adventitious breath sounds (i.e., crackles, rhonchi). **Adventitious breath sounds, such as crackles and rhonchi, may indicate third spacing of fluid from the intravascular space into pulmonary tissue.**
- Measure and trend invasive hemodynamic parameters (e.g., central venous pressure, pulmonary artery pressure/pulmonary capillary wedge pressure) as needed for critically ill clients. **Pressure trends may reflect reductions, possibly indicating decreased intravascular fluid volume or loss of vascular tone.**
- Measure and grade peripheral pulses. **In hypovolemic states, pulses may be fast and thready. Note: Evaluation of the brachial and femoral pulses in infants is a crucial assessment.**
- Measure capillary refill. **Capillary refill time should take less than 3 sec in the fingertips and toes. A refill time greater than 3 sec may indicate compromised perfusion that could be associated with hypovolemia (inadequate intravascular volume).**
- Note the presence, location, and grade of edema (e.g., puffy eyelids, swelling ankles and feet if ambulatory or up in chair, sacrum/posterior thighs when recumbent, scrotum/labia). **Dependent edema is often associated with an**

Information that appears in brackets has been added by the authors to clarify and enhance the use of nursing diagnoses.

increase in venous hydrostatic pressure (e.g., heart failure and renal failure). Generalized edema (e.g., upper extremities and eyelids, anasarca) is often associated with a reduction in venous osmotic (oncotic) pull, an increase in venous hydrostatic pressure, and/or a capillary leak. Note: Intravascular volume depletion can be present at the same time extravascular fluid excess (seen as edema) is present.

- Assess skin temperature. Using the dorsa of the hands, palpate skin temperature proximal to distal. **While hands and feet often feel cooler bilaterally, cool and clammy skin may indicate the shunting of blood away from superficial blood vessels. This may occur from a variety of causes, including inadequate intravascular volume.**
- Assess oral mucous membranes. **The buccal mucous membranes and the tongue may appear dry in the client with dehydration. Note: In infants and children, assess for the presence of tear production. Ask parents about tear production, or the lack of tears. Lack of tear production can indicate significant dehydration.**
- Note change from usual mentation, behavior, or functional abilities (e.g., new confusion, falling, loss of ability to perform usual activities, lethargy, and dizziness). **These signs indicate sufficient dehydration to cause poor cerebral perfusion or can reflect the effects of electrolyte imbalance. In a hypovolemic shock state, mentation changes rapidly, and client may present in coma.**
- Review laboratory data (e.g., hemoglobin/hematocrit, elevated transaminases [aspartate aminotransferase/alanine aminotransferase]; serum electrolytes [sodium, potassium, chloride, bicarbonate] and glucose; blood urea nitrogen [BUN], creatinine [Cr], urine specific gravity, urine osmolality, urine sodium) **to evaluate the body's response to fluid loss and to determine replacement needs. Note: The dehydrated client is not always hypovolemic. An abnormal sodium level is a key marker for salt and water imbalance. For example, in hypertonic dehydration, blood tests may reveal osmolality greater than 300 mOsm/kg and sodium greater than 150 mEq/L. The hypernatremia is the result of dehydration. Hypotonic dehydration may reveal osmolality less than 250 mOsm/kg and sodium less than 130 mEq/L. Hyponatremia is the result of replacing water without sodium.**

Information that appears in brackets has been added by the authors to clarify and enhance the use of nursing diagnoses.

Nursing Priority No. 3.

To correct/replace losses to reverse pathophysiological mechanisms:

- Stop fluid loss (e.g., administer medication to stop vomiting/diarrhea, fever; change antibiotics causing diarrhea; treat fever/infection, malnutrition, or severe depression; discontinue medications contributing to dehydration).
- Administer fluids on volumetric infusion pumps and rapid infusion devices, as appropriate, to deliver fluids accurately at desired rates **to prevent either under-infusion or over-infusion. IV fluid replacement routinely includes crystalloid (i.e., normal saline, half-normal saline, and lactated Ringer solution) or colloid solutions (albumin solutions, hyperoncotic starch, dextran). IV crystalloids are an integral part of client care to maintain and replace body fluids. Note: The pediatric population requires special considerations for fluid maintenance and rehydration. One option for hourly rate of fluid maintenance is the 4-2-1 rule (i.e., first 10 kg: 4 mL/kg/hr, next 10 to 20 kg: 2 mL/kg/hr, and 1mL/kg/hr after that with maximum 100 mL/hr maintenance). Establish and promote oral intake, incorporating beverage preferences when possible.**
- Encourage increased intake of water and other fluids based on individual needs (up to 2.5 L/day or amount determined by physician for client's age, weight, and condition) and/or administer enteral fluid solutions as needed. **Providing a variety of fluids in small frequent offerings and incorporating the client's preferred beverage may enhance cooperation with fluid regimen. Clients may be unable or unwilling to take in adequate fluids orally. Utilization of the gastrointestinal (GI) tract is a preferable method compared to IV route for long-term hydration. Note: Care should be taken to provide a nutritionally balanced diet. Hyperosmolar or excessively high-protein enteral formulas may cause GI upset and require adequate amounts of free water with feedings.**
- Establish and continually evaluate 24-hr fluid replacement needs and routes to be used. **Prevents peaks and valleys in fluid volume.**
- Control humidity and ambient air temperature, as appropriate, especially when major burns are present or in the presence of fever as ordered, **to reduce insensible losses and elevated metabolic rate.** (Refer to ND Hyperthermia.)

Information that appears in brackets has been added by the authors to clarify and enhance the use of nursing diagnoses.

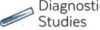 Diagnostic Studies 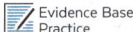 Evidence Based Practice 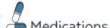 Medications 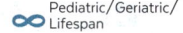 Pediatric/Geriatric/Lifespan

- Reduce bedding or clothes and provide a tepid sponge bath. **Assist with hypothermia to reduce high fever and elevated metabolic rate.** (Refer to ND Hyperthermia or ineffective Thermoregulation as appropriate for additional interventions.)
- Maintain accurate input and output (I&O) documentation **to evaluate the effectiveness of resuscitation measures.**

Nursing Priority No. 4.

To promote comfort and safety:

- Change position frequently **to reduce pressure on fragile skin and tissues and promote mobilization of interstitial fluid.**
- Bathe client using mild cleanser or soap, and provide optimal skin care with emollients **to maintain skin integrity and prevent excessive dryness caused by dehydration.**
- Provide frequent oral as well as eye care **to prevent injury from dryness.**
- Change dressings frequently and use adjunct appliances, as indicated, for draining wounds **to protect skin and monitor losses for replacement needs.**
- Administer medications (e.g., antiemetics, antidiarrheals **to limit gastric or intestinal losses;** antipyretics **to reduce fever**). (Refer to NDs impaired fecal Continence, ineffective Thermoregulation, and Hyperthermia for additional interventions.)
- Observe for sudden or marked elevation of blood pressure, restlessness, moist cough, dyspnea, basilar crackles, and frothy sputum. **Too rapid a correction of fluid deficit may compromise the cardiopulmonary system, causing fluid overload and edema, especially if colloids are used in initial fluid resuscitation.**

Nursing Priority No. 5.

To promote euvolemia (Teaching/Discharge Considerations) and enhance well-being (long-term goals):

- Discuss factors related to occurrence of fluid deficit as individually appropriate (e.g., potential for dehydration in children with fever or diarrhea, inadequate fluid replacement when performing strenuous work or exercise, living in hot climate, improper use of diuretics) **to reduce risk of recurrence.**
- Engage client, family, and caregivers in the fluid management plan, discussing actions (if any) the client/significant

---

Information that appears in brackets has been added by the authors to clarify and enhance the use of nursing diagnoses.

 Acute Care 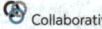 Collaborative 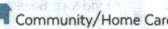 Community/Home Care Cultural

other can take to prevent or correct deficiencies. **Enhances cooperation with the regimen and achievement of goals. Carrying a water bottle when away from home aids in maintaining fluid volume. A client who never takes more than a few sips at a time, even of preferred beverage, may benefit most from being offered frequent small amounts of fluid throughout the day. In cases of mild to moderate dehydration, use of oral solutions (e.g., Gatorade, Rehydralyte), soft drinks, breast milk/ formula, or Pedialyte can provide adequate rehydration.**

- Instruct client/family in ways to keep track of intake. For example, use a marked water bottle or container. Suggest the use of and provide to the client lidded beverage bottles/ containers that show measurements.
- Instruct client/family in ways to keep track of output. Encourage use of voiding record when it is appropriate, and weigh daily, report a gain of more than 2 lb/day (or as indicated by individual situation). **If weight is rising daily, fluid is likely being retained.**
- Instruct the client/significant other(s) in how to monitor the color of urine **(dark urine equates with concentration and dehydration)** or how to measure and record I&O (may include weighing or counting diapers in infant/toddler, or briefs in incontinent client).
- Review medications, interactions, and side effects with client giving attention to medications that can cause or exacerbate fluid loss (e.g., diuretics, laxatives) and those indicated to prevent fluid loss (e.g., antidiarrheals, etc.).
- Discuss signs/symptoms indicating need for emergent or further evaluation and follow-up. **Promotes timely intervention.**

Documentation Focus

Assessment/Reassessment
- Assessment findings, including degree of deficit and current sources of fluid intake
- I&O, urine characteristics, fluid balance, changes in weight, presence of edema, and vital signs
- Results of diagnostic studies

Planning
- Plan of care and who is involved in planning
- Teaching plan

Information that appears in brackets has been added by the authors to clarify and enhance the use of nursing diagnoses.

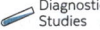 Diagnostic Studies 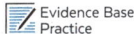 Evidence Based Practice 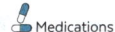 Medications 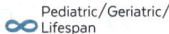 Pediatric/Geriatric/Lifespan

Implementation/Evaluation
- Client's/caregiver's responses to interventions, teaching, and actions performed
- Attainment of or progress toward desired outcome(s)
- Modifications to plan of care

Discharge Planning
- Long-term needs, plan for correction, and who is responsible for actions to be taken
- Specific referrals made

Sample Nursing Outcomes & Interventions Classifications NOC/NIC

NOC—Hydration
NIC—Hypovolemia Management

---

impaired GAS EXCHANGE   NANDA-I

[Diagnostic Division: Respiration]

Definition: Excess or inadequate oxygenation and/or carbon dioxide elimination.

Recognizing Cues

Related/Risk Factors
Ineffective airway clearance; ineffective breathing pattern
Pain

Defining Characteristics

Subjective
[Breathlessness]
Visual disturbance
Headache upon awakening

Objective
Drowsiness; confusion; irritable mood; psychomotor agitation
Abnormal arterial pH; decreased carbon dioxide level; hypercapnea; hypoxemia, hypoxia
Abnormal skin color; diaphoresis; tachycardia
Abnormal respiratory depth, or rhythm; bradypnea; tachypnea
Nasal flaring

Information that appears in brackets has been added by the authors to clarify and enhance the use of nursing diagnoses.

 Acute Care   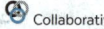 Collaborative   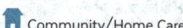 Community/Home Care   Cultural

Clinical Connections

Chronic obstructive pulmonary disease (COPD), asthma, pneumonias, tuberculosis, heart failure, sickle cell anemia, acute respiratory distress syndrome (ARDS), general anesthesia, premature infant, high-altitude pulmonary edema, pulmonary embolus (PE), carbon monoxide poisoning

Generate Solutions

Plan Desired Outcomes

Client Will (Include Specific Time Frame)

- Demonstrate improved ventilation and adequate oxygenation of tissues by arterial blood gases (ABGs) within client's usual parameters and absence of symptoms of respiratory distress (as noted in Defining Characteristics).
- Verbalize understanding of causative factors and appropriate interventions.
- Participate in treatment regimen (e.g., breathing exercises, effective coughing, use of oxygen) within level of ability or situation.

Interventions/Take Action

Nursing Priority No. 1.

To assess causative/contributing factors:

∞ • Identify/ investigate the presence of factors and conditions (e.g., asthma, COPD, pneumonia, heart disease, anemia, prematurity, high altitude, thick secretions, neuromuscular impairment of breathing pattern, pain, etc.) that can cause or be associated in some way with gas exchange problems. **Multiple body systems work simultaneously to facilitate blood oxygenation and carbon dioxide removal through the lungs. The exchange of oxygen and carbon dioxide occurs at the alveolar level. Disease processes or conditions that impair lung tissue, and ventilatory function, or compromise blood quality or quantity may contribute to the body's ability to exchange oxygen for carbon dioxide. Note: Evidence shows compromised lung function in infancy and childhood predicts pulmonary dysfunction, including asthma in adulthood.**

∞ • Consider client's age, gender, and ethnicity **to assess client risk factors. After the age of 35, there is a gradual loss of alveolar surface area, dilation of air spaces, reduced**

Information that appears in brackets has been added by the authors to clarify and enhance the use of nursing diagnoses.

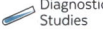 Diagnostic Studies 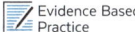 Evidence Based Practice 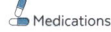 Medications ∞ Pediatric/Geriatric/Lifespan

mucociliary clearance, and changes in lung compliance. Infants born near 28 weeks' gestation (i.e., near the margin of viability) may develop bronchopulmonary dysplasia (BPD), experience chronic lung dysfunction, and have an increased risk of obstructive lung disease in adulthood. While the risk for drug-induced interstitial lung disease (DIILD) increases for the very young or older client, some evidence suggests increased risk for female clients and specific ethnicities associated with specific medications.

- Review client's current medication regimen **to identify medications (e.g., opioids, anesthetic agents, chemotherapy agents, Macrobid, amiodarone, benzodiazepines, barbiturates) that may contribute to DIILD. While the mechanism of injury is not fully understood, alveolar and bronchial chronic inflammation lead to fibrotic changes and scarring.**
- Assist with and review appropriate diagnostic testing (e.g., pulmonary function tests, arterial blood gas [ABG], chest x-ray, chest computed tomography [CT] scan, chest magnetic resonance imaging [MRI], bronchoscopy, hematocrit, hemoglobin) **to evaluate organ systems that impact gas exchange. Note results of pulmonary function studies to evaluate lung mechanics, capacities, and function. Blood studies are useful in revealing systemic reasons for problems with oxygenation and/or the results of hypoxemia and acid-base imbalances to determine response to therapies.**
- Refer to NDs impaired Airway Clearance and ineffective Breathing Pattern for additional assessment interventions as appropriate.

Nursing Priority No. 2.
To evaluate degree of compromise:
- Perform a focused physical examination of the client **to evaluate oxygenation and factors contributing to hypoxia. The examination may include:**
- Evaluate respirations **to provide insight into the work of breathing, adequacy of alveolar ventilation, and potential for pulmonary or cardiac compromise. Observe rate, rhythm, and depth, an increase in both rate and depth of respiration increases alveolar ventilation and occurs in response to exercise and stressors. When both respiratory rate and work of breathing are increased, an in-depth assessment should follow (e.g., dyspnea with activity or at rest, etc.).**

Information that appears in brackets has been added by the authors to clarify and enhance the use of nursing diagnoses.

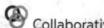 Acute Care 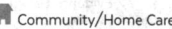 Collaborative 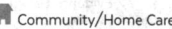 Community/Home Care 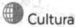 Cultural

- Discuss with client reports/perceptions of breathing ease (i.e., dyspnea) **to ascertain subjective symptoms of "air hunger."** Dyspnea is a subjective client symptom of not getting enough air and, depending on severity, may raise the client's levels of anxiety. The client may report a range of symptoms (e.g., air hunger; shortness of breath with speaking, activity, or at rest).
- Observe client for self-positioning to a position of comfort **to ease breathing and maximize chest expansion and respiratory effort.** The three-point position, or tripod position (i.e., bending forward while supporting self by placing one hand on each knee) raises the shoulders and increases the respiratory volume.
- Observe client for use of accessory muscles (e.g., scalene muscles, pectoralis minor, sternocleidomastoids, external intercostal muscles) **to assist the diaphragm in increasing the volume of the thoracic cavity, which aids in inspiration.**
- ∞ Observe client (e.g., infants/young children, frail, elderly) for nasal flaring and sternal retractions **to indicate increased work of breathing or respiratory distress.**
- Observe client for the use of abdominal muscles during expiration (i.e., normally a passive process) **to reduce thoracic dimensions and overcome airway resistance to expiration.**
- Auscultate and percuss client's chest **to assess the lungs for adventitious breath sounds, describe the presence or absence of breath sounds, or identify areas of decreased airflow or consolidation.** Ventilatory effort may be insufficient to deliver enough oxygen or to get rid of sufficient amounts of carbon dioxide. Abnormal breath sounds are indicative of numerous problems (e.g., hypoventilation such as might occur with atelectasis or presence of secretions, improper endotracheal [ET] tube placement, collapsed lung) and must be evaluated further.
- Note the presence and quality of client's cough, the volume and characteristics of sputum **to determine the impact on client ventilation and the ability to clear airways of secretions.**
- Assess color of client's skin, nailbeds, and mucous membranes **to identify pallor or cyanosis.** The location of cyanosis (i.e., peripheral [nailbeds] versus central [around lips or earlobes] or general duskiness) is significant to the deterioration of the client's condition. Duskiness and central cyanosis are late signs of hypoxemia.

Information that appears in brackets has been added by the authors to clarify and enhance the use of nursing diagnoses.

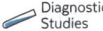 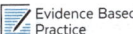 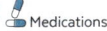 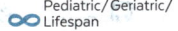

- Assess client's nails for clubbing (i.e., enlargement of the fingertips) **to indicate client conditions of chronic hypoxia (i.e., COPD or congenital deficits in pediatric patients).**
- Assess client's mentation and behavior **to assess for changes in level of consciousness and cerebral hypoxia. A decreased level of consciousness can be an indirect measurement of impaired oxygenation, but it also impairs one's ability to protect the airway, potentially further adversely affecting oxygenation. Note: Carbon dioxide narcosis (e.g., a change in level of consciousness associated with increased CO_2 blood gas levels, flushing, decreased respiratory rate, and headaches) may occur in clients receiving long-term oxygen therapy.**
- Monitor cardiovascular status via vital signs/hemodynamic monitoring and fluid volume status:

    Measure temperature. **A high fever greatly increases metabolic demands and oxygen consumption.**

    Monitor heart rate and rhythm. **Tachycardia and dysrhythmia may be noted as the heart reacts to hypoxemia, especially during activity.**

    Monitor blood pressure (BP). **BP can be variable, depending on underlying condition and cardiopulmonary response.**

    Evaluate hemoglobin oxygen saturation and carbon dioxide at bedside using pulse oximetry and end-tidal CO_2 monitoring (capnography). **Point-of-care testing evaluates ventilation by providing breath-to-breath information. Capnography monitoring improves client outcomes through early recognition of hypoventilation, apnea, and airway obstruction, thus preventing hypoxic episodes. Clients with respiratory failure typically show hypoxemia and metabolic acidosis and are at high risk for developing respiratory acidosis.**

    Note increased pulmonary artery or right ventricular wedge pressures in the critically ill client with central lines. **Indicative of increased pulmonary vascular resistance.**

    Maintain adequate fluid intake **to maintain blood pressure, kidney function, and mobilization of secretions** but avoid fluid overload **that may increase pulmonary congestion.**

Nursing Priority No. 3.
To correct/improve existing deficiencies:
- Assist in the treatment of underlying conditions or factors that may contribute to impaired lung tissue, ventilatory

---

Information that appears in brackets has been added by the authors to clarify and enhance the use of nursing diagnoses.

function, compromised blood quality/quantity, or otherwise compromise the client's ability **to facilitate blood oxygenation and carbon dioxide removal through the lungs.**

- Elevate head of the bed and/or position the client appropriately. **Elevation or an upright position facilitates respiratory function by allowing expansion of the diaphragm; however, clients in severe distress will seek a position of comfort. In ventilated client, prone position may be implemented to improve pulmonary perfusion and increase oxygen diffusion.**
- Provide airway adjuncts and suction, as needed, **to clear secretions or maintain a patent airway.**
- Encourage or assist client with frequent position changes, deep-breathing, directed coughing, use of incentive spirometer, and chest physiotherapy, as indicated **to promote optimal chest expansion, mobilization of secretions, and oxygen diffusion.**
- Educate client/significant other (SO) on pursed-lip breathing **to decrease dyspnea by prolonging the expiratory phase of respiration. By pursing the lips, the client can create a small amount of positive end-expiratory pressure (PEEP) allowing more air to be exhaled. Pursed-lip breathing may also relieve the client's feelings of shortness of breath and help the client regain a sense of control over their breathing while increasing their relaxation.**
- Provide client with supplemental oxygen (i.e., nasal cannula, mask, blow-by, etc.) using the lowest concentration necessary **to improve client oxygenation as indicated by pulse oximetry, ABGs, and client symptoms/underlying condition. Clients at risk for hypercapnia, such as clients with COPD, should have supplemental oxygen administered judiciously within set parameters ("supplemental oxygen to maintain SpO_2 greater than 88%"). Unscrupulous administration of oxygen in these clients may result in carbon dioxide narcosis. Note: Consider the fit of a face mask when applying to a client who is elderly or emaciated. A tight fit may not be achieved, decreasing effectiveness.**
- Ensure the availability of appropriate emergency equipment (e.g., endotracheal/tracheostomy set, suction catheters appropriate for age and size of infant, child, or adult, etc.) at the bedside **to anticipate respiratory emergencies.**
- Prepare for and assist with intubation and mechanical ventilation of client **to facilitate oxygenation and gas exchange**

Information that appears in brackets has been added by the authors to clarify and enhance the use of nursing diagnoses.

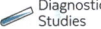 Diagnostic Studies 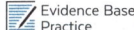 Evidence Based Practice 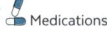 Medications 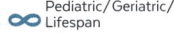 Pediatric/Geriatric/Lifespan

through positive pressure ventilation. A clinical diagnosis of respiratory failure, classified as hypoxemic or hypercapnic, may initiate intubation with mechanical ventilation. Hypoxemic respiratory failure is the most common, associated with acute lung disorders such as pneumothorax, atelectasis, pulmonary edema, pneumonia, ARDS, and smoke inhalation. Hypercapnic respiratory failure can be seen in acute exacerbations of chronic COPD, head trauma, and spinal cord injury. (Refer to ND impaired spontaneous Ventilation for additional interventions.)

- Monitor and trend ventilator readings (e.g., tidal volume, peak inspiratory pressure, spontaneous rate, inspiratory and expiratory ratio, etc.) as indicated when mechanical support is being used. **The mode of ventilation (volume or pressure) and ventilator settings are determined by the specific needs of the client, which are determined by clinical evaluation and blood gas parameters.**

- Address client's/SO's fears and anxiety that may be present **to provide psychological support, active-listen client/SO concerns while maintaining a calm attitude. Anxiety is contagious, and associated agitation can increase oxygen consumption and dyspnea.**

- Cluster client's care, encourage adequate rest, and limit activities to within client tolerance. Promote a calm, restful environment **to facilitate relaxation and help limit oxygen needs and consumption.**

- Administer medications as indicated (e.g., inhaled and systemic glucocorticosteroids, antibiotics, bronchodilators, methylxanthines, antitussives/mucolytics, and vasodilators). **Pharmacological agents are varied, specific to the client, but are used to treat conditions, prevent and control symptoms, reduce the frequency and severity of exacerbations, and improve exercise tolerance.**

- Monitor and instruct client in therapeutic and adverse effects or interactions of drug therapy **to determine efficacy and need for change.**

- Use pain and sedation medication judiciously **to avoid depressant effects on respiratory functioning.**

- Minimize blood loss from procedures (e.g., tests or hemodialysis) **to limit adverse affects of anemia and related gas diffusion impairment.**

- Assist with procedures as indicated (e.g., blood transfusion, bronchoscopy, thoracentesis, etc.) **to improve respiratory function/oxygen-carrying capacity.**

Information that appears in brackets has been added by the authors to clarify and enhance the use of nursing diagnoses.

- Keep client's environment allergen and pollutant free **to reduce the irritant effect of dust and chemicals on airways.**

Nursing Priority No. 4.

To promote maximum gas exchange (Teaching/Discharge Considerations) and enhance well-being (long-term goals):

- Review client risk factors, particularly chronic medical conditions predisposing client to fluid overload resulting in impaired gas exchange (e.g., chronic kidney disease, hepatic insufficiency and cirrhosis, and congestive heart failure [CHF]); or genetic, environmental, or environmental/employment related, **to promote prevention or management of risk.**
- Stress importance of appropriate vaccinations **to prevent client from developing pneumonia. The respiratory syncytial virus (RSV) vaccine is effective to prevent RSV pneumonia in very young and older clients. "The Centers for Disease Control and Prevention's Advisory Committee on Immunization Practices recommends influenza vaccination for persons with COPD, and pneumococcal vaccination for persons 19 to 64 years of age who smoke or have COPD." The influenza vaccine should be received annually.**
- Discuss with client/SO the impact of smoking related to lung function, health, and client's illness or condition. Encourage client and SO to stop smoking and attend cessation programs **to reduce health risks and/or prevent further decline in lung function. Note: Studies confirm an 80% to 90% correlation between smoking and obstructive lung diseases.**
- Discuss with client/SO a pulmonary rehabilitation program **to reduce dyspnea, increase exercise ability, and improve health-related quality of life.**
- Suggest oxygen-conserving techniques (e.g., sitting instead of standing to perform tasks; eating small meals; performing slower, purposeful movements) **to reduce oxygen demands.**
- Discuss with client/SO the importance of adequate rest, while encouraging activity and exercise (e.g., upper and lower extremity endurance, strength training, and flexibility) **to decrease dyspnea and improve quality of life.**
- Discuss the importance of good nutrition **for improving stamina and to maintain a robust immune response.**
- Refer client to dietitian **for nutritional assessment and individual dietary plan as indicated.**

Information that appears in brackets has been added by the authors to clarify and enhance the use of nursing diagnoses.

 Diagnostic Studies 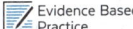 Evidence Based Practice 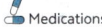 Medications 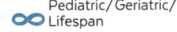 Pediatric/Geriatric/Lifespan

- Instruct client/SO in relaxation and stress-reduction techniques as appropriate.
- Review client's job description and work activities **to identify the need for job modifications or vocational rehabilitation.**
- Discuss safe use of home oxygen therapy when home oxygen is implemented **to ensure client's safety, especially when used in the very young, fragile elderly, or when cognitive or neuromuscular impairment is present.**
- Identify suppliers for supplemental oxygen, necessary respiratory devices, other individually appropriate resources (e.g., home care agencies, Meals on Wheels, etc.) **to facilitate independence.**

Documentation Focus

Assessment/Reassessment
- Assessment findings, including respiratory rate, character of breath sounds; frequency, amount, and appearance of secretions; presence of cyanosis; laboratory findings; and mentation level
- Conditions that may interfere with oxygen supply

Planning
- Plan of care, specific interventions, and who is involved in the planning
- Ventilator settings, liters of supplemental oxygen
- Teaching plan

Implementation/Evaluation
- Client's responses to treatment, teaching, and actions performed
- Attainment of or progress toward desired outcome(s)
- Modifications to plan of care

Discharge Planning
- Long-term needs, identifying who is responsible for actions to be taken
- Community resources for equipment and supplies postdischarge
- Specific referrals made

Sample Nursing Outcomes & Interventions Classifications NOC/NIC

NOC—Respiratory Function: Gas Exchange
NIC—Respiratory Monitoring

Information that appears in brackets has been added by the authors to clarify and enhance the use of nursing diagnoses.

impaired GASTROINTESTINAL MOTILITY   NANDA-I

[Diagnostic Division: Elimination]

Definition: Increased, decreased, ineffective, or lack of peristaltic activity within the gastrointestinal tract.

Recognizing Cues

Related/Risk Factors
Altered water source; eating pattern change; malnutrition
Unsanitary food preparation; exposure to contaminated materials
Anxiety; excessive stress
Impaired physical mobility; sedentary behaviors

Defining Characteristics

Subjective
Abdominal cramping, or pain
Absence of flatulence
Diarrhea; difficulty with defecation; hard, formed stool
Nausea; regurgitation

Objective
Acceleration of gastric emptying
Altered bowel sounds
Bile-colored gastric residual; increased gastric residual
Distended abdomen
Vomiting

Clinical Connections
Abdominal or intestinal surgery, eating disorders, malnutrition, enteral feedings, premature infants, diabetes, celiac disease, anemia, anxiety disorders, biliary cancer, cholecystectomy, Crohn disease, irritable bowel syndrome, gastroesophageal reflux disease (GERD), gastritis, pancreatitis, quadriplegia, peritoneal dialysis, botulism, sepsis, multiple organ dysfunction syndrome, radiation therapy

Generate Solutions

Plan Desired Outcomes

Client Will (Include Specific Time Frame)
- Reestablish and maintain normal pattern of bowel functioning.

Information that appears in brackets has been added by the authors to clarify and enhance the use of nursing diagnoses.

 Diagnostic Studies   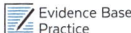 Evidence Based Practice   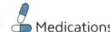 Medications   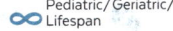 Pediatric/Geriatric/Lifespan

- Verbalize understanding of causative factors and rationale for treatment regimen.
- Demonstrate appropriate behaviors to assist with resolution of causative factors.

Interventions/Take Action

Nursing Priority No. 1.

To assess causative/contributing factors:

- Note the presence of conditions affecting systemic circulation and perfusion (e.g., congestive heart failure, major trauma, chronic conditions, or sepsis) affecting systemic circulation/perfusion **that can result in gastrointestinal (GI) hypoperfusion and short- and/or long-term GI dysfunction.**
- Determine the presence of disorders causing localized or diffuse reduction in GI blood flow (e.g., esophageal varices, GI hemorrhage, intestinal cancer, or obstruction; intestinal surgery, pancreatitis, and intraperitoneal hemorrhage, or strangulated hernia; prior abdominal surgery with adhesions) **to identify a client at higher risk for ineffective tissue perfusion.**
- Note chronic/long-term disorders, such as GI reflux disease (GERD), hiatal hernia, inflammatory bowel disease (e.g., ulcerative colitis, Crohn disease), malabsorption (e.g., dumping syndrome, celiac disease), short-bowel syndrome, as may occur after surgical removal of portions of the small intestine. **These conditions are associated with increased, decreased, or ineffective peristaltic activity.**
- Note client's age and developmental concerns. **Neonates who are premature or have low birth weight are at risk for developing necrotizing enterocolitis (NEC). Children are prone to infections causing gastroenteritis manifested by vomiting and diarrhea. The elderly have problems associated with decreased motility (e.g., constipation, lack of sufficient fiber and fluid intake, polypharmacy, and chronic use of laxatives).**
- Identify lifestyle issues prone to affect GI function. **People who regularly engage in competitive sports such as long-distance running and cycling, have poor sanitary living conditions or who travel to areas with contaminated food or water, overeat or ingest foods associated with gastric distress or intestinal distention, or have anorexia/bulimia may incur temporary or long-term GI difficulties.**
- Ascertain whether client is experiencing anxiety; acute, extreme, or chronic stress; or other psychogenic factors

---

Information that appears in brackets has been added by the authors to clarify and enhance the use of nursing diagnoses.

present in a person with emotional or psychiatric disorders (including anorexia/bulimia, etc.) **that can affect GI function.**
- Review client's medication regimen. **Medications (e.g., laxatives, antibiotics, opiates, sedatives, and iron preparations) may cause or exacerbate intestinal issues. In addition, the likelihood of bleeding increases from the use of medications such as NSAIDs, warfarin, and antiplatelet medications.**
- Review laboratory and other diagnostic studies. **A complete blood count may be done to evaluate for GI problems, such as bleeding, inflammation, toxicity, and infection. Metabolic panel may reveal hepatic dysfunction, electrolyte imbalances, or low albumin levels. Computed tomography (CT) or other scans and abdominal ultrasound can help identify conditions like kidney stones or gallstones. X-rays may show bowel dilation or obstruction and stool and gas patterns. Changes in white blood cell count with x-ray evidence of pneumoperitoneum (air in the abdominal cavity) suggest NEC in the preterm neonate.**

Nursing Priority No. 2.

To note degree of dysfunction or potential for organ involvement:

- Assess vital signs, noting presence of low blood pressure, elevated heart rate, and fever. **May suggest hypoperfusion or developing sepsis. Fever in the presence of bright red blood in stool may indicate ischemic colitis.**
- Ascertain presence of and characteristics of abdominal pain. **Pain is a common symptom of GI disorders and can vary in location, duration, and intensity. Note: Diffuse pain may reflect hypoperfusion of the GI tract, which is particularly vulnerable to even small decreases in circulating volume. Mid-epigastric pain immediately following meals and lasting several hours suggests abdominal angina due to atherosclerotic occlusive disease. Tension pain caused by organ distention may develop in the presence of bowel obstruction, constipation, or accumulation of pus or fluid. Inflammatory pain is deep and initially poorly localized, caused by irritation of either the visceral or the parietal peritoneum, as in acute appendicitis. Ischemic pain (the most serious type of visceral pain) has sudden onset, is intense, is progressive in severity, and is not relieved by analgesics.**

Information that appears in brackets has been added by the authors to clarify and enhance the use of nursing diagnoses.

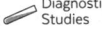 Diagnostic Studies   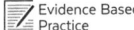 Evidence Based Practice   Medications   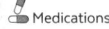 Pediatric/Geriatric/Lifespan

- Assess client's current situation with regard to prior GI history. **Client may have had a prior incident putting them at current risk (e.g., blunt force trauma to abdomen) or be at higher risk for recurrent GI dysfunction associated with prior GI problems.**
- Investigate reports of pain out of proportion to degree of traumatic injury. **May reflect developing abdominal compartment syndrome.**
- Inspect abdomen, noting contour. **Generalized distention may indicate presence of gas or fluid; a localized bulge could indicate a hernia. Distention of bowel may indicate accumulation of fluids (salivary, gastric, pancreatic, biliary, and intestinal) and gases formed from bacteria, swallowed air, or any food or fluid the client has consumed.**
- Auscultate abdomen. **Hypoactive bowel sounds may indicate ileus. Hyperactive bowel sounds may indicate early intestinal obstruction, irritable bowel, or GI bleeding. The presence of a bruit may indicate blood traveling through narrowed arteries.**
- Palpate abdomen **to note masses, enlarged organs (e.g., spleen, liver, or portions of colon), or elicitation of pain with touch that could point to changes in organ size or function.**
- Measure abdominal girth and compare with client's customary waist size or belt length **to monitor development or progression of distention possibly reflecting intra-abdominal bleeding, infection, or edema associated with toxins.**
- Note frequency and characteristics of bowel movements. **Bowel movements by themselves are not necessarily diagnostic but need to be considered in total assessment, as they may reveal an underlying problem or effect of pathology. For example, diarrhea is the cardinal symptom of gastroenteritis, with severity depending on the causative organism. Both diarrhea and constipation can result from medications. Bloody diarrhea may indicate presence of ulcerative colitis, obstruction, or upper or lower GI bleeding.**
- Note presence of nausea, with or without vomiting, and relationship to food intake or other events, if indicated. **History can provide important information about cause (e.g., pregnancy, gastroenteritis, cancers, myocardial infarction, hepatitis, systemic infections, contaminated food, drug toxicity, or eating disorders). The timing of

---

Information that appears in brackets has been added by the authors to clarify and enhance the use of nursing diagnoses.

386   Acute Care   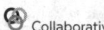 Collaborative   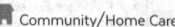 Community/Home Care   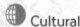 Cultural

vomiting may be important too. For example, vomiting immediately after meals could be indicative of bulimia, or vomiting large amounts several hours after eating can indicate delayed gastric emptying.
- Evaluate client's current nutritional status, noting client's ability to ingest and digest food. Inquire about food intolerances. Observe client's reactions to food, such as reluctance or refusal to eat, anorexia, or anxiety—wants to eat but cannot retain food. **Health depends on the intake, digestion, and absorption of nutrients, which both affect and are affected by GI function.**
- Measure intra-abdominal pressure as indicated. **Tissue edema or free fluid collecting in the abdominal cavity leads to intra-abdominal hypertension, which, if untreated, can cause abdominal compartment syndrome with end-stage organ failure.**

Nursing Priority No. 3.
To reduce risk or improve existing dysfunction:
- Practice and promote hand hygiene and other infection precautions **to prevent transmission of infections that may cause/spread GI illnesses.**
- Collaborate in treatment of underlying conditions **to correct or treat disorders associated with client's current GI dysfunction.**
- Maintain GI rest when indicated—nothing by mouth (NPO), fluids only, or gastric or intestinal decompression **to reduce intestinal bloating and risk of vomiting.**
- Measure GI output periodically and note characteristics of drainage **to manage fluid losses and replacement needs and electrolyte balance.**
- Administer prescribed prophylactic medications (e.g., antiemetics, proton-pump inhibitors, antihistamines, anticholinergics, antibiotics) **to reduce the potential for GI complications such as bleeding, ulceration of stomach mucosa, and viral diarrheas.**
- Administer fluids and electrolytes as indicated **to replace losses and to maintain GI circulation and function.**
- Collaborate with dietitian or nutritionist **to provide diet sufficient in nutrients by best possible route—oral, enteral, or parenteral.**
- Provide small servings of easily digested food and fluids when oral intake is tolerated.
- Encourage rest after meals **to maximize blood flow to the digestive system.**

Information that appears in brackets has been added by the authors to clarify and enhance the use of nursing diagnoses.

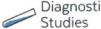 Diagnostic Studies 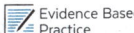 Evidence Based Practice 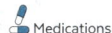 Medications 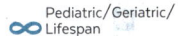 Pediatric/Geriatric/Lifespan

- Emphasize the importance of and assist with early ambulation and ongoing exercise, especially following surgery. Refer to physical therapy as indicated for mobility issues. **Promotes general circulation and stimulates peristalsis and intestinal function to help reduce GI complications associated with immobility and a sedentary lifestyle.**
- Encourage relaxation and distraction techniques **if anxiety is suspected to play a role in GI dysfunction.**
- Encourage client to report changes in nature or intensity of pain. **May indicate worsening of condition, requiring more intensive interventions.**
- Manage pain with medications, as ordered, and nonpharmacological interventions such as positioning, back rub, or heating pad (unless contraindicated) **to enhance muscle relaxation and reduce discomfort.**
- Collaborate with provider for medication management. **Oral medications can be absorbed erratically in the presence of delayed gastric emptying, which can change the therapeutic effect or lead to increased side effects of a particular drug. Dose modification, discontinuation of certain drugs (e.g., laxatives, opioids, antidepressants, iron supplements), or alternative route of administration may be required over a long period of time to improve client's GI function.**
- Prepare client for procedures and surgery, as indicated. **May require a variety of interventions, including endoscopic procedures, appendectomy, bowel resection with/without ostomy, percutaneous transluminal angioplasty, abdominal-aortic bypass graft, mesenteric revascularization, endarterectomy, etc., to treat the problem causing or contributing to severe GI dysfunction.**
- Refer to NDs impaired intestinal Elimination, impaired fecal Continence for additional interventions.

Nursing Priority No. 4.

To promote GI motility (Teaching/Discharge Considerations) and enhance well-being (long-term goals):

- Provide information regarding the cause of GI dysfunction and treatment plans, utilizing best learning methods for client and including written information and bibliography of other resources for postdischarge learning. **May help client/significant other (SO) to manage symptoms in a manner more acceptable to them if this is a long-term issue.**

Information that appears in brackets has been added by the authors to clarify and enhance the use of nursing diagnoses.

- Identify necessary changes in lifestyle and assist client to incorporate disease management into activities of daily living. **Promotes independence and enhances self-concept regarding the ability to deal with change and manage own needs.**
- Discuss normal variations in bowel patterns **to help alleviate unnecessary concern, initiate planned interventions, or seek timely medical care. May prevent the overuse of laxatives or help the client understand when food, fluid, or drug modifications are needed.**
- Review measures to maintain bowel health:
  Use dietary fiber and/or stool softeners to manage constipation and incontinence.
  Ensure fluid intake is appropriate to individual.
  Establish or maintain regular bowel evacuation habits, incorporating privacy needs, assistance to bathroom on regular schedule, and so forth, as indicated.
  Emphasize the benefits of regular exercise in promoting normal GI function.
- Discuss dietary recommendations with client/SO. **The client may need to make adaptations in food choices and eating habits (e.g., may need to avoid overeating in general, schedule mealtime in relation to activities and bedtime, avoid certain foods [or food element, such as wheat or gluten] and/or alcohol).**
- Instruct in healthier variations in preparation of foods, as indicated, e.g., broiled instead of fried, spices/herbs added to foods instead of salt, addition of higher fiber foods, and use of lactose-free dairy products **when these factors are affecting GI health.**
- Recommend maintenance of normal weight, or weight loss if client is overweight, **to decrease risk associated with GI disorders such as GERD or gallbladder disease.**
- Discuss fluid intake appropriate to client's individual situation. **Water is necessary for general health and GI function. Client may need encouragement to increase intake or to make appropriate fluid choices if intake is restricted for certain medical conditions.**
- Discuss medication regimen with client/SO, including reasons for/consequences of failure to take prescribed long-term maintenance therapy (e.g., client with ulcerative colitis may require continuous treatment with 5-aminosalicylates to maintain remission). **Although many reasons are given for failing to take medications as prescribed, including denial of illness, forgetfulness, and costs of prescriptions,**

Information that appears in brackets has been added by the authors to clarify and enhance the use of nursing diagnoses.

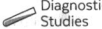 Diagnostic Studies 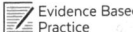 Evidence Based Practice 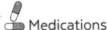 Medications 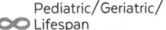 Pediatric/Geriatric/Lifespan

nonadherence negatively affects treatment efficacy and client's quality of life.
- Emphasize to client importance of discussing with the provider current and newly prescribed medications and/or planned use of certain medications (e.g., NSAIDs, antiplatelet medications, corticosteroids, some over-the-counter [OTC] drugs, and herbal supplements). **These medications can be harmful to GI mucosa.**
- Encourage discussion of feelings regarding prognosis and long-term effects of condition. **Major or unplanned life changes can strain coping abilities, impair functioning, jeopardize relationships, and may even result in depression.**
- Discuss the value of relaxation and distraction techniques or counseling **if anxiety or other emotional/psychiatric issues are suspected to play a role in GI dysfunction.**
- Recommend smoking cessation. **Studies have shown various deleterious short- and long-term effects of smoking on the GI circulation and organs. Smoking is a risk factor for acquiring or exacerbating certain GI disorders, such as Crohn disease.**
- Review foodborne and waterborne illnesses, contamination, and hygiene issues, as indicated, and make needed follow-up referrals. **Many different types of viruses, bacteria, and parasites can cause GI illnesses. This can affect a household, a day-care center, a college dorm, international travelers, or a whole segment of population. Information may be given to individuals, groups, and/or the public in general.**
- Refer to appropriate resources (e.g., social services, public health services) **for follow-up if client is at risk for ingestion of contaminated water or food sources or would benefit from education concerning food preparation and storage.**
- Recommend and/or refer to provider for vaccines as indicated. **The Centers for Disease Control and Prevention (CDC) make recommendations for travelers and/or persons in high-risk areas or situations in which client might be exposed to contaminated food or water.**
- Refer to NDs impaired fecal Continence; impaired intestinal Elimination for additional interventions.

Documentation Focus

Assessment/Reassessment
- Individual findings, noting specific risk factors; or nature, extent, and duration of problem, effect on independence and lifestyle

---

Information that appears in brackets has been added by the authors to clarify and enhance the use of nursing diagnoses.

- Dietary pattern, recent intake, food intolerances
- Frequency and characteristics of stools
- Characteristics of abdominal tenderness or pain, precipitators, and what relieves pain

Planning
- Plan of care and who is involved in planning
- Teaching plan

Implementation/Evaluation
- Response to interventions, teaching, and actions performed
- Attainment of or progress toward desired outcome(s)
- Modifications to plan of care

Discharge Planning
- Long-term needs and who is responsible for actions to be taken
- Available resources, specific referrals made

Sample Nursing Outcomes & Interventions Classifications NOC/NIC

NOC—Gastrointestinal Function
NIC—Bowel Management

GRIEF   ICNP

[Diagnostic Division: Stress Management]

Definition: A complex response to an actual, anticipated, or perceived loss through which the individual integrates the change into a new functional reality.

Recognizing Cues

Related/Risk Factors
Anticipated or death of a loved one
Emotional/physical disability
Loss due to natural or environmental catastrophe
Loss of employment, financial status; eviction from home; homelessness

Defining Characteristics

Subjective
Sadness over loss; experiencing relief; feeling at peace that the event is over

---

Information that appears in brackets has been added by the authors to clarify and enhance the use of nursing diagnoses.

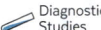 Diagnostic Studies 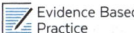 Evidence Based Practice 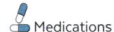 Medications 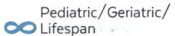 Pediatric/Geriatric/Lifespan

Feeling overwhelmed; difficulty keep track of responsibilites
Competing feelings of anger, despair, guilt, or remorse for no longer caring for a sick loved one
Searching for meaning of loss; seeking purpose, joy, peace in life
Integrating positive feelings/memories of loss or event
Seeking new partner after divorce/loss; changes in lifestyle/responsibilities

Objective
Detachment; disorganization; maintaining attachment to deceased/loss
Fatigue; restlessness
Headache; nausea; tightness in chest or throat; heart palpitations; joint pain
Increase/decrease in appetite
Insomnia, or somnolence

Clinical Connections
Death of significant other (SO), traumatic loss, major health change, depression, suicide

Generate Solutions

Plan Desired Outcomes

Client Will (Include Specific Time Frame)
- Participate in work and self-care and activities, as able.
- Verbalize a sense of progress toward resolution of the grief and hope for the future.

Interventions/Take Action

Nursing Priority No. 1.
To assess causative/contributing factors:
- Determine significance of the loss to client (e.g., death of a loved one, presence of chronic condition leading to divorce, long functional decline followed by death, natural or environmental catastrophe, disruption of family unit and change in lifestyle or financial security). **The more complicated or devastating the loss is to the individual, the more likely the individual will have difficulty reaching resolution.**
- Determine usual ability to manage own affairs. **Provides baseline for understanding client's decision-making process and identify areas of need.**
- Identify availability, dependability, and use of support persons. **Having support for decision making and having**

Information that appears in brackets has been added by the authors to clarify and enhance the use of nursing diagnoses.

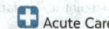 Acute Care 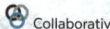 Collaborative 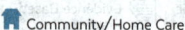 Community/Home Care   Cultural

good information regarding pros and cons of choices helps client to feel comfortable with the decisions made.
- Active-listen and identify client's expectations for change and reason(s) client would like to improve management of grieving. **As client articulates feelings of loss, hope, and goals for the future, the approaches to improve their life become more clear, and direction can be provided. Motivation to improve and high expectations can encourage client to make changes that will improve client's life. However, a negative presence or an external locus of control or unrealistic expectations may hamper efforts.**
- Note presence of physical signs of anxiety. **Client may be excited about the quest for improvement, and excitement may be interpreted as anxiety. It is important to clarify meaning of physical signs.**
- Identify cultural factors and ways individual has dealt with previous loss(es). **Way of expressing self may reflect cultural background and spiritual beliefs. Understanding cultural expectations helps put current behavior and responses in context and guide choice of interventions.**
- Discuss meaning of life, reasons for living, belief in God or higher power, and how these relate to current desire for improvement or growth. **Helps client to clarify beliefs and how they relate to decision-making process.**
- Determine client's readiness to move to a higher level of resolving the grief process. **Moving to a higher level of resolving grief will be met with resistance if the client is not emotionally ready for change.**

Nursing Priority No. 2.

To promote client's progress in dealing appropriately with loss:

- Promote a safe and hopeful environment that helps client identify own inner control. **Will help client understand the control they have with decision making regarding loss (e.g., loss of employment, financial, or environmental catastrophe) and decision making to problem-solve the situation. Professional and organized bereavement groups provide emotional and practical support to clients who have suffered loss of a loved one.**
- Encourage client verbalization of their realities. **It is helpful to listen without correcting misperceptions in the beginning, allowing free flow of expression. Provides opportunity for reflection, aiding resolution, acceptance, and problem-solving.**

Information that appears in brackets has been added by the authors to clarify and enhance the use of nursing diagnoses.

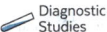 Diagnostic Studies 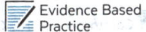 Evidence Based Practice Medications 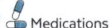 Pediatric/Geriatric/Lifespan

- Give "permission" to be at this point when the client is depressed. **Assures client that feelings are normal and can be a starting point to deal in a positive manner with loss/death that has occurred.**
- Identify positive aspects of this experience, and assist client to view it as an emotional growth opportunity. **As client reframes the negative experience to a learning opportunity for helping to cope with future losses, the client will develop confidence in managing other losses/situations. Working through grief helps coping with the painful feelings of a loss or perceived responsibilities associated with loss.**
- Discuss and clarify spiritual beliefs, accepting client's values in a nonjudgmental manner. **Client may be able to decide what is really acceptable or unacceptable in the choice or situation related to beliefs or values that have been expressed.**
- Reinforce use of previously effective coping skills. Instruct in and encourage use of visualization and relaxation techniques. **Identifying and discussing how client has dealt with loss in the past can provide opportunities in the current situation. Use of these techniques helps client to consider new options for dealing with loss.**
- Encourage family members to participate in support groups or family-focused therapy, as indicated. **Technique of family-focused grief therapy focuses on emotional expression of grief and family functioning to strengthen the family's adaptive capacity and promote cohesiveness. Reminiscence therapy or recalling favorite past experiences, feelings, or thoughts helps finding adaptation to the present being filled with pleasure, and a quality of life recognizing a newly found strength with healing.**
- Refer to mental health provider for counseling if client desires. **Standard individual psychotherapy identifies and addresses symptoms, relationship problems, and their connections to grief. Research suggests the complicated grief therapy technique may be more effective by supporting the idea of dual processing (i.e., alternating attention between the loss and a focus on restoration and the future).**

Nursing Priority No. 3.

To promote emotional healing (Teaching/Discharge Considerations) and enhance well-being (long-term goals):

- Discuss with client/SO alternative healthy ways to coping with difficult situations moving forward. **Identifying ways individual(s) has dealt with losses in the past will help**

Information that appears in brackets has been added by the authors to clarify and enhance the use of nursing diagnoses.

identify strengths and successes and what might be useful in the current situation and into the future. Attempting alternative healthy approaches (e.g., mediation, yoga, or mindfulness) may not have been used in the past but can be helpful for coping with present and future stressors.
- Have individual identify familial, spiritual, and cultural factors that have meaning. **One's family of origin has a major impact on what the individuals learn about these issues and how to deal with losses. Identifying and discussing how they affect the current situation may help bring loss into perspective and facilitate grief resolution.**
- Encourage involvement in usual activities, exercise, and socialization within limits of physical ability and psychological state. **Returning to a regular routine can provide individual(s) with some sense of control.**
- Suggest client keep a journal of experiences and feelings. **As client writes about what is happening, new insights may occur. Reading over what has been written can help individual see progress that has been made and begin to have hope for the future.**
- Advocate planning for the future as appropriate to individual situation (e.g., staying in own home after death of spouse, returning to sporting activities following traumatic amputation, choosing whether to have another child or to adopt, investigating new employment or relocation opportunities, rebuilding home following a disaster).
- Identify volunteer opportunities (e.g., working with children at risk, raising funds for favorite charity, coaching young athletes, mentoring others in educational/career setting, giving time to disaster cleanup/mitigation efforts). **Exercising control in a productive manner empowers individuals and promotes rebuilding of life and community.**
- Refer to other resources (e.g., pastoral care, family counseling, psychotherapy, organized support groups—widows group), as indicated. **Provides additional support to resolve situation and continue grief work.**

Documentation Focus

Assessment/Reassessment
- Assessment findings, including meaning of loss to the client, current stage of the grieving process, and responses of family/SOs
- Cultural or spiritual beliefs and expectations
- Availability and use of resources

Information that appears in brackets has been added by the authors to clarify and enhance the use of nursing diagnoses.

Planning
- Plan of care and who is involved in the planning
- Teaching plan

Implementation/Evaluation
- Client's response to interventions, teaching, and actions performed
- Attainment of or progress toward desired outcome(s)
- Modifications to plan of care

Discharge Planning
- Long-term needs and who is responsible for actions to be taken
- Specific referrals made

Sample Nursing Outcomes & Interventions Classifications NOC/NIC

NOC—Grief Resolution
NIC—Grief Work Facilitation

---

dysfunctional GRIEF ICNP

[Diagnostic Division: Stress Management]

Definition: Persistent, excessive, and overwhelming feelings of loss, sadness, and mourning due to the death of a loved one or significant loss(es) that prevents individual working through the grief process to acceptance/recovery.

Recognizing Cues

Related/Risk Factors
Struggles to cope with simultaneous losses
Overwhelmed with emotional stressors
Denial/delayed response to loss
Lack of social support

Defining Characteristics

Subjective
Expresses sadness, loss, anger, helplessness
Persistent thoughts/rumination of the deceased loved one, significant personal loss

---

Information that appears in brackets has been added by the authors to clarify and enhance the use of nursing diagnoses.

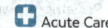 Acute Care 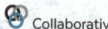 Collaborative 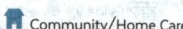 Community/Home Care Cultural

Loneliness; detachment from others
Struggles with daily longing for deceased person/significant loss, living or seeing a future with absence of loss
Somatic complaints (e.g., headache, nausea, changes in bowel habits, shortness of breath, muscle aches, joint pains, impaired memory)

Objective
Fatigue; lack of adequate sleep; decreased concentration
Poor hygiene; inadequate dietary intake
Crying; restlessness or lack of motor activity
Disturbed self-concept, personal identity
Isolation from family/friends
Alcohol/substance misuse

Clinical Connections
Death of significant other (SO), traumatic loss, depression, anxiety disorder, post-trauma stress disorder, suicide

Generate Solutions

Client Will (Include Specific Time Frame)
- Acknowledge persistent and extensive sadness.
- Demonstrate progress working through the stages of grief at their own pace.
- Participate in activities of daily living and family/social activities as able.
- Discuss progress of resolving prolonged and persistent grief while sharing hope for the future.

Interventions/Take Action

Nursing Priority No. 1.
To determine risk/causative/contributing factors.

- Determine what loss has occurred. Note circumstances of death such as sudden or traumatic (e.g., fatal accident, homicide; large-scale natural disaster, global pandemic), related to socially sensitive issue (e.g., AIDS, gun violence in schools, suicide; sexual assault with murder), or associated with unfinished business (e.g., spouse died during time of crisis in marriage, son has not spoken to parent for years) or client's loss of body part/function, personal belongings, financial well-being, community status. **These situations can sometimes cause the individual to become stuck in grief and unable to move forward with life.**
- Determine significance of the loss to the client (life partner, child, home/personal belongings, body part/function,

---

Information that appears in brackets has been added by the authors to clarify and enhance the use of nursing diagnoses.

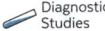 Diagnostic Studies   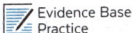 Evidence Based Practice   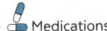 Medications   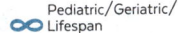 Pediatric/Geriatric/Lifespan

presence of chronic condition leading to divorce or disruption of family unit and change in lifestyle or financial security). **The more complicated or devastating the loss is to the individual (e.g., devastation following a natural disaster/terrorist act), the more likely the individual will have difficulty reaching resolution/acceptance.**

- Identify cultural or spiritual beliefs and expectations that may impact or dictate the client's response to loss. **Different cultures or spiritual beliefs view death and dying in unique ways that may impact or dictate client's response to loss. Understanding and supporting client is a starting point for helping with grief.**
- Discuss the response of the family/SO(s) to the client's situation (e.g., sympathetic or urging client to "just get over it"). **Response of family members will affect how client is dealing with situation—functional families are supportive or conflict resolving in nature, while dysfunctional families tend to be sullen, hostile, or reactionary. Dysfunctional patterns of communication such as avoidance, preaching, and giving advice can block effective communication and isolate family members. A recent study noted that approximately 15% of bereaved persons suffer from complicated grief after the death of their relative.**
- Assess client/family/SO's needs or concerns. **Recognizing the needs of the client/family may not have been addressed prior to or at time of loss and can delay the grieving process.**
- Listen and identify reason(s) client would like to improve management of grieving, and expectations for change. **As client articulates reasons for improvement, they become more clear, and assistance can be provided. Motivation to improve and high expectations can encourage client to make changes that will improve their life. However, presence of external locus of control or unrealistic expectation may hinder efforts.**

Nursing Priority No. 2.
To determine degree of impairment/dysfunction:

- Observe for cues of sadness (e.g., sighing; faraway look; unkempt appearance; inattention to conversation; somatic complaints, such as exhaustion or headaches). **Indicators of the extent of grief and how individual is dealing with situation.**

Information that appears in brackets has been added by the authors to clarify and enhance the use of nursing diagnoses.

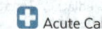 Acute Care   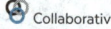 Collaborative   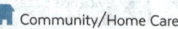 Community/Home Care   Cultural

- Identify stage of grief being expressed: denial, isolation, anger, bargaining, depression, and acceptance. **Helps to establish how client is coping with grieving and degree of difficulty client is having adjusting to the death or loss.**
- Listen to words used in communication as they are indicative of renewed or intense grief (e.g., constantly bringing up death or loss even in casual conversation long after event; outbursts of anger at relatively minor events; expressing desire to die). **Client may be indicating it is impossible or they are unable to adjust/move on from feelings of intense grief and have thoughts of killing themself. Note: Complicated grief therapy utilizes the concept of revisiting the loss through storytelling of the death, especially for individuals prone to avoid thinking about the trauma of the loss.**
- Determine level of functioning, ability to care for self, and use of support systems and community resources. **Individual may be incapacitated by depth of loss and be unable to manage day-to-day activities adequately, necessitating intervention and assistance.**
- Be aware of avoidance behaviors (e.g., anger; withdrawal; long periods of sleeping or refusing to interact with family; sudden or radical changes in lifestyle; inability to handle everyday responsibilities at home, work, or school; conflict). **Additional indicators of depth of grieving being experienced indicate need for more intensive support and monitoring to help client deal effectively with death or loss.**
- Determine if the client is engaging in reckless or self-destructive behaviors (e.g., substance abuse, heavy drinking, promiscuity, or aggression). **Important to identify safety issues.**
- Identify cultural factors and ways individual has dealt with previous loss(es). **Way of expressing self may reflect cultural background and spiritual beliefs. Understanding cultural expectations will help put current behavior and responses in context and determine the nature and degree of dysfunction.**
- Perform or refer for psychological testing, as indicated (e.g., Beck Depression Scale). **Determines degree of depression and possible need for medication.**
- Identify client's stage of readiness to change. **Client's readiness to change (e.g., start the healing process, advance to grief counseling and support groups, etc.) will determine the depth of interventions provided.**

Information that appears in brackets has been added by the authors to clarify and enhance the use of nursing diagnoses.

Clients who are not ready to change will be resistant and ambivalent to moving forward.

Nursing Priority No. 3.

To assist client to cope with loss:

- Encourage verbalization without confrontation about realities. **It is helpful to listen without correcting misperceptions in the beginning, allowing free flow of expression. Provides opportunity for reflection aiding resolution and acceptance.**
- Encourage client to choose topics of conversation and refrain from forcing client to "face the facts." **Talking freely about concerns can help client identify what is important to deal with and how to cope with situation.**
- Active-listen client feelings and be available for support as indicated. Speak in a soft, caring voice. **Communicates acceptance and caring, enabling client to seek own answers to current situation.**
- Encourage expression of anger, fear, and anxiety. (Refer to appropriate NDs.) **These feelings are part of the grieving process, and to accomplish the work of grieving, they need to be expressed and accepted.**
- Permit verbalization of anger with acknowledgment of feelings and setting of limits regarding destructive behavior. **Enhances client safety, promotes resolution of grief process by encouraging expression of feelings that are not usually accepted, and supports self-esteem.**
- Acknowledge reality of feelings of guilt or blame, including hostility toward spiritual power. Do not minimize loss; avoid clichés and easy answers. (Refer to ND impaired Spiritual Well-Being.) **Reinforces that feelings are acceptable and allows client to become aware of own thoughts and begin to deal with feelings.**
- Respect client's desire for quiet, privacy, talking, or silence. **Individual may not be ready to talk about or share grief and needs to be allowed to make own timeline.**
- Give "permission" to be at this point when the client is depressed. **Assures client that feelings are normal and can be a starting point to deal in a positive manner with loss/death that has occurred.**
- Provide comfort and availability as well as caring for physical needs. **Client needs to know they will be supported and helped when not able to care for self.**
- Reinforce use of previously effective coping skills. Instruct in and encourage use of visualization and relaxation

---

Information that appears in brackets has been added by the authors to clarify and enhance the use of nursing diagnoses.

techniques. **Identifying and discussing how client has dealt with loss in the past can provide opportunities in the current situation. Use of these techniques helps client to learn to relax and consider options for dealing with loss.**

- Assist SOs to cope with client's response. Include age-specific interventions. **Family/SO(s) may not understand/be intolerant of client's distress and inadvertently hamper client's progress. Family members, including children, may express their feelings in anger, resulting in punishment for behavior that is deemed unacceptable rather than recognized as the basis of grief.**
- Include family/SO(s) in setting realistic goals for meeting needs of client and family members. **Involving all members enhances the probability that each member will express their needs and hear what the needs of others are, ensuring a more effective outcome.**
- Encourage family members to participate in support group or family-focused therapy as indicated. **Techniques of family-focused grief therapy focus on emotional expression of grief and family functioning to strengthen the family's adaptive capacity and promote cohesiveness.**
- Use sedatives or tranquilizers with caution. **While the use of these medications may be of limited benefit in the short term, too much dependence on them may retard passage through the grief process. Encourage sleep hygiene, progressive relaxation, or imagery to promote sleep.**
- Refer to mental health provider for counseling. **Standard individual psychotherapy identifies and addresses symptoms, relationship problems, and their connections to grief. Research suggests the complicated grief therapy technique may be more effective by supporting the idea of dual processing (i.e., alternating attention between the loss and a focus on restoration and the future).**
- Acknowledge client's sense of relief when death follows a long and debilitating course. **Even when death brings a release, sadness and loss are still there; or client may feel guilty about having a sense of relief.**

Nursing Priority No. 4.

To promote continued growth (Teaching/Discharge Considerations) and enhance well-being (long-term goals):

- Have individual(s) identify familial, spiritual, and cultural factors that have meaning. **One's family of origin has a**

Information that appears in brackets has been added by the authors to clarify and enhance the use of nursing diagnoses.

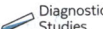 Diagnostic Studies   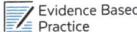 Evidence Based Practice   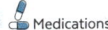 Medications   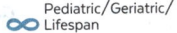 Pediatric/Geriatric/Lifespan

major impact on what the individuals learn about these issues and how to deal with losses. **Identifying and discussing how they affect the current situation may help bring loss into perspective and facilitate grief resolution.**
- Encourage involvement in usual activities, exercise, and socialization within physical and psychological abilities. **Keeping life to a somewhat normal routine can provide individual with some sense of control over events that are not controllable.**
- Suggest client keep a journal of experiences and feelings. **As client writes about what is happening, new insights may occur. Reading over what has been written can help individual see progress that has been made and begin to have hope for the future.**
- Advocate planning for the future, as appropriate, to individual situation (e.g., staying in own home after death of spouse, returning to sporting activities following traumatic amputation, choosing whether to have another child or to adopt, rebuilding home following a disaster). **Provides a sense of control and purpose and ensures that individual's wishes will be heard and respected.**
- Identify volunteer opportunities (e.g., working with children at risk, raising funds for favorite charity, investigating new employment or relocation opportunities, participating in community reorganization or cleanup). **Exercising control in a productive manner empowers individuals and promotes rebuilding of life and community.**
- Refer to other resources (e.g., pastoral care, family counseling, psychotherapy, organized support groups—widow's group). **Provides additional help, when needed, to resolve situation/continue grief work.**

Documentation Focus

Assessment/Reassessment
- Assessment findings, including meaning of loss to the client, current stage of the grieving process, and responses of family/SO(s)
- Cultural or spiritual beliefs and expectations
- Availability and use of resources

Planning
- Plan of care and who is involved in the planning
- Teaching plan

Information that appears in brackets has been added by the authors to clarify and enhance the use of nursing diagnoses.

Implementation/Evaluation
- Client's response to interventions, teaching, and actions performed
- Attainment of or progress toward desired outcome(s)
- Modifications to plan of care

Discharge Planning
- Long-term needs and who is responsible for actions to be taken
- Specific referrals made

Sample Nursing Outcomes & Interventions Classifications NOC/NIC

NOC—Grief Resolution
NIC—Grief Work Facilitation

---

delayed child GROWTH   NANDA-I

[Diagnostic Division: Health Management]

Definition: Inadequate height, length, body mass index, head circumference, and/or height velocity (cm/year) for sex, age, and ethnicity of an individual ≤18 years of age.

Recognizing Cues

Related/Risk Factors
Abnormal eating pattern; inadequate diet for age; inadequate parental feeding techniques
Inadequate parental knowledge regarding nutrition
Inadequate access to safe drinking water; unsanitary housing
Parents inattentive to secondhand smoke
Affectional deprivation

Defining Characteristics

Objective
Body mass index less than –2 standard deviations, or lower than the 30th percentile, compared to the indicators of the reference population
Growth less than –2 standard deviations, or lower than the 30th percentile, compared to the indicators of the reference population

---

Information that appears in brackets has been added by the authors to clarify and enhance the use of nursing diagnoses.

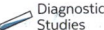 Diagnostic Studies
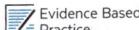 Evidence Based Practice
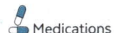 Medications
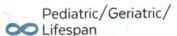 Pediatric/Geriatric/Lifespan

Head circumference less than −2 standard deviations, or lower than the 30th percentile, compared to the indicators of the reference population

Height less than −2 standard deviations, or lower than the 30th percentile, compared to the indicators of the reference population

Height velocity less than −2 standard deviations, or lower than the 30th percentile, compared to the indicators of the reference population

Weight less than −2 standard deviations, or lower than the 30th percentile, compared to the indicators of the reference population

Clinical Connections

Congenital or genetic disorders, premature or low birth weight infant, infection, nutritional problems (malnutrition, anorexia, failure to thrive, excessive intake or obesity), toxic exposures (e.g., lead), abuse or neglect, endocrine disorders, pituitary tumor

Generate Solutions

Plan Desired Outcomes

Client Will (Include Specific Time Frame)
- Receive appropriate nutrition as indicated by individual needs.
- Demonstrate weight and growth velocity stabilizing or progress toward age-appropriate size.
- Participate in plan of care as appropriate for age and ability.

Caregiver Will (Include Specific Time Frame)
- Verbalize understanding of potential for growth delay or deviation and plans for prevention.

Interventions/Take Action

Nursing Priority No. 1.
To assess causative/contributing factors:
- Determine factors or condition(s) existing that could contribute to growth deviation, as listed in Risk Factors, including familial history of pituitary tumors, Marfan syndrome, genetic anomalies, use of certain drugs or substances during pregnancy, maternal diabetes or other chronic illness, poverty or inability to attend to nutritional issues, eating disorders, and so forth.
- Identify nature and effectiveness of parenting and caregiving activities. **Inadequate, inconsistent caregiving; unrealistic**

Information that appears in brackets has been added by the authors to clarify and enhance the use of nursing diagnoses.

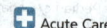 Acute Care 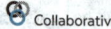 Collaborative 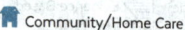 Community/Home Care   Cultural

or insufficient expectations; lack of stimulation; inadequate limit setting; lack of responsiveness **indicate problems in parent-child relationship.**
- Note severity and pervasiveness of situation (e.g., individual showing effects of long-term physical or emotional abuse or neglect versus individual experiencing recent-onset situational disruption or inadequate resources during period of crisis or transition).
- Evaluate nutritional status. **Malnutrition is the most common cause of growth failure worldwide. Even in industrialized nations, children continue to have nutritional deficiencies that can impair growth or development. Overfeeding or malnutrition (protein and other basic nutrients) on a constant basis prevents child from reaching healthy growth potential, even if no disorder/disease exists.**
- Determine cultural, familial, and societal issues **that may impact the situation (e.g., childhood obesity a risk for American children; parental concern for amount of food intake; expectations for "normal growth").**
- Assess significant stressful events, losses, separation, and environmental changes (e.g., abandonment, divorce, death of parent/sibling, aging, move).
- Assess cognition, awareness, orientation, and behavior of the client and caregiver. **Actions such as withdrawal or aggression and reactions to environment and stimuli provide information for identifying needs and planning care.**
- Active-listen concerns about body size and ability to perform competitively (e.g., sports, body building) **to ascertain the potential for use of anabolic steroids or other drugs.**
- Review results of studies such as skull and hand x-rays; bone scans, such as computed tomography or magnetic resonance imaging; and chest or abdominal imaging **to determine bone age and extent of bone and soft tissue overgrowth and the presence of pituitary or other growth hormone–secreting tumor.** Note laboratory studies (e.g., growth hormone levels, glucose tolerance, thyroid and other endocrine studies, serum transferrin, and prealbumin) **that may identify pathology.**

Nursing Priority No. 2.
To prevent/limit deviation from growth norms:
- Determine chronological age and where child should be on growth charts **to determine growth expectations.** Note

---

Information that appears in brackets has been added by the authors to clarify and enhance the use of nursing diagnoses.

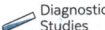 Diagnostic Studies   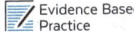 Evidence Based Practice   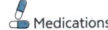 Medications   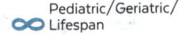 Pediatric/Geriatric/Lifespan

reported losses or alterations in functional level. **Provides a comparative baseline.**
- Note familial factors (e.g., parent's body build and stature) **to help determine individual developmental expectations (e.g., when child should attain a certain weight and height) and how the expectations may be altered by the child's condition.**
- Review expectations for current height and weight percentiles and degree of deviation. Plan for periodic evaluations. **Growth rates are measured in terms of how much a child grows within a specified time (velocity). These rates vary dramatically as a child grows (normal growth is a discontinuous process) and must be evaluated periodically over time to ascertain that child has definite growth disturbance.**
- Investigate deviations from normal (e.g., height and weight, head circumference, hand and feet size, facial features). **Deviations can be multifactorial and require varying interventions (e.g., weight deviation only [increased or decreased] may be remedied by changes in nutrition and exercise; other deviations may require in-depth evaluation and long-term treatment).**
- Determine if child's growth is above 97th percentile (very tall and large) for age. **Suggests a need for evaluation for endocrine or other disorders or pituitary tumor (could result in gigantism). Other disorders may be characterized by excessive weight for height (e.g., hypothyroidism, Cushing syndrome), abnormal sexual maturation, or abnormal body/limb proportions.**
- Determine if child's growth is below fifth percentile (very short and small) for age. **May require evaluation for failure to thrive related to intrauterine growth retardation, prematurity or very low birth weight, small parents, poor nutrition, stress or trauma, or medical condition (e.g., intestinal disorders with malabsorption; diseases of heart, kidneys; diabetes mellitus). Treatment of the underlying condition may alter or improve the child's growth pattern.**
- ∞ Note reports of changes in facial features, joint pain, lethargy, sexual dysfunction, and/or progressive increase in hat, glove, ring, or shoe size in adults, especially after age 40.
- 🅐 Assist with therapies to treat or correct underlying conditions (e.g., Crohn disease, cardiac problems, renal disease);

Information that appears in brackets has been added by the authors to clarify and enhance the use of nursing diagnoses.

endocrine problems (e.g., hyperpituitarism, hypothyroidism, type 1 diabetes mellitus, growth hormone abnormalities); genetic or intrauterine growth retardation; infant feeding problems; and nutritional deficits.

- Include nutritionist and other specialists (e.g., physical and occupational therapist) in developing plan of care. **Helpful in determining specific dietary needs for growth and weight issues as well as child's issues with foods (e.g., child who is sensory overresponsive may be bothered by food textures; child with posture problems may need to stand to eat); the child may require assistive devices and appropriate exercise and rehabilitation programs.**
- Review medications being considered (e.g., appetite stimulant, growth hormone, thyroid replacement, antidepressant), noting potential side effects/adverse reactions **to promote adherence to regimen and reduce risk of untoward responses.**

Nursing Priority No. 3.

To promote appropriate growth (Teaching/Discharge Considerations) and enhance well-being (long-term goals):

- Provide information regarding normal growth, as appropriate, including pertinent reference materials and credible websites.
- Address caregiver issues (e.g., parental abuse, learning deficiencies, environment of poverty) **that could impact the client's ability to thrive.**
- Recommend involvement in regular exercise or sports medicine program **to enhance muscle tone and strength and appropriate body building.**
- Promote a lifestyle that prevents or limits complications (e.g., management of obesity, hypertension, sensory or perceptual impairments); regular medical follow-up; nutritionally balanced meals; and socialization for age and development **to maintain functional independence and enhance quality of life.**
- Discuss with pregnant women and adolescents consequences of substance use or abuse. **Prevention of growth disturbances depends on many factors but includes the cessation of smoking, alcohol, and many drugs that have the potential for causing central nervous system (CNS) or orthopedic disorders in the fetus.**

Information that appears in brackets has been added by the authors to clarify and enhance the use of nursing diagnoses.

- Refer for genetic screening, as appropriate. **There are many reasons for referral, including but not limited to positive family history of a genetic disorder (e.g., fragile X syndrome, muscular dystrophy), woman with exposure to toxins or potential teratogenic agents, women older than 35 years at delivery, previous child born with congenital anomalies, history of intrauterine growth retardation, and so forth.**
- Emphasize the importance of periodic reassessment of growth and development (e.g., periodic laboratory studies to monitor hormone levels, bone maturation, and nutritional status). **Aids in evaluating the effectiveness of interventions over time, promotes early identification of need for additional actions, and helps to avoid preventable complications.**
- Identify available community resources, as appropriate (e.g., public health programs, such as Women, Infants, and Children [WIC]; medical equipment supplies; nutritionists; substance-abuse programs; specialists in endocrine problems/genetics).

Documentation Focus

Assessment/Reassessment
- Assessment findings, individual needs, including current growth status, and trends
- Caregiver's understanding of situation and individual role

Planning
- Plan of care and who is involved in the planning
- Teaching plan

Implementation/Evaluation
- Client's responses to interventions, teaching, and actions performed
- Caregiver response to teaching
- Attainment of or progress toward desired outcome(s)
- Modifications to plan of care

Discharge Planning
- Identified long-term needs and who is responsible for actions to be taken
- Specific referrals made, sources for assistive devices, educational tools

Sample Nursing Outcomes & Interventions Classifications NOC/NIC

NOC—Growth
NIC—Nutritional Monitoring

Information that appears in brackets has been added by the authors to clarify and enhance the use of nursing diagnoses.

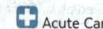 Acute Care 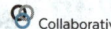 Collaborative 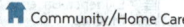 Community/Home Care Cultural

inadequate HEALTH KNOWLEDGE NANDA-I

[Diagnostic Division: Health Management]

Definition: Insufficient acquiring, processing, understanding and/or recalling of information related to specific topic that affects one's well-being.

Recognizing Cues

Related/Risk Factors
Anxiety, depressive symptoms
Inadequate information; misinformation
Inadequate access to, awareness of, or knowledge of resources
Inadequate commitment to learning or interest in learning
Inadequate participation in care planning; inadequate self-efficacy
Inadequate trust in health personnel; difficulty navigating complex healthcare systems

Defining Characteristics

Subjective
Inaccurate statements about a topic
Inability to articulate treatment protocols; inability to engage in knowledge exchange with healthcare team

Objective
Inadequate knowledge about disease process, symptom control, or treatment regimen
Inadequate knowledge about risk factors, modifiable factors, or healthy habits
Inadequate knowledge of healthy habits, or safety precautions; inadequate use of knowledge in everyday decisions to achieve health behavior
Inadequate knowledge of self-care management strategies; inadequate self-knowledge to make healthcare choices for oneself
Inaccurate follow-through of instruction or performance on a test or procedure; inability to repeat an activity to improve performance
Inadequate score on standardized, validated disease knowledge instrument
Absence of knowledge-seeking about one's disease
[Development of preventable complication]

Information that appears in brackets has been added by the authors to clarify and enhance the use of nursing diagnoses.

 Diagnostic Studies
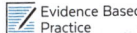 Evidence Based Practice
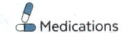 Medications
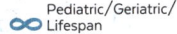 Pediatric/Geriatric/Lifespan

Clinical Connections

Any newly diagnosed disease or traumatic injury, progression of or deterioration in a chronic condition, developmental or neurocognitive disorders, depression

Generate Solutions

Plan Desired Outcomes

Client Will (Include Specific Time Frame)

- Participate in learning process.
- Identify interferences to learning and specific action(s) to cope with them.
- Exhibit increased interest and assume responsibility for own learning by beginning to look for information and ask questions.
- Verbalize understanding of condition, disease process, and treatment.
- Identify relationship of signs/symptoms to the disease process and correlate symptoms with causative factors.
- Perform necessary procedures correctly and explain reasons for the actions.
- Initiate necessary lifestyle changes and participate in treatment regimen.

Interventions/Take Action

Nursing Priority No. 1.

To assess readiness to learn and individual learning needs:

- Ascertain client's capacity to obtain, process, and understand basic health information (health literacy), level of knowledge about current condition, including anticipatory needs. **Learning needs can include many things (e.g., disease cause and process, factors contributing to symptoms, procedures for symptom control, needed alterations in lifestyle, ways to prevent complications). Client may or may not ask for information or may express inaccurate perceptions of health status and needed behaviors to manage self-care.**
- Determine the client's ability, readiness, and barriers to learning. **The individual may not be physically, emotionally, or mentally capable at this time.**
- Be alert to signs of avoidance. **The client may need to suffer the consequences of lack of knowledge before they are ready to accept information.**

Information that appears in brackets has been added by the authors to clarify and enhance the use of nursing diagnoses.

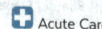 Acute Care 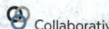 Collaborative 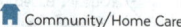 Community/Home Care Cultural

- Identify support individuals/significant other(s) (SO[s]) requiring information (e.g., parent, caregiver, spouse). **Providing appropriate information to others can provide reinforcement for learning, as everyone will understand what is to be expected.**

Nursing Priority No. 2.
To determine other factors pertinent to the learning process:

- Note personal factors (e.g., age and developmental level, gender, social and cultural influences, religion, life experiences, level of education, and emotional stability). **Understanding client's ability and desire to learn and assimilate new information, take control of situation, and accept responsibility for change.**
- Determine blocks to learning: language barriers (e.g., client cannot read; speaks or understands a different language than healthcare provider), physical factors (e.g., cognitive impairment, aphasia, dyslexia), physical stability (e.g., acute illness, activity intolerance), or difficulty of material to be learned. **Many factors affect the client's ability and desire to learn, and expectations of the learning process must be addressed if learning is to be successful.**
- Assess the level of the client's capabilities and the possibilities of the situation. **In presence of client limitation, may need to assist SO(s) or caregivers to learn by introducing one new idea, by building on previous information, by finding pictures to demonstrate an idea, and so forth, to adapt teaching to client's specific needs.**
- Identify motivating factors for the individual (e.g., client needs to stop smoking because of advanced lung cancer, client wants to lose weight because family member died of complications of obesity). **Motivation may be negative (e.g., smoking causes lung cancer) or positive (e.g., client wants to promote health/prevent disease). Level of motivation provides information that can guide content specific to the client's situation and readiness to change.**

Nursing Priority No. 3.
To establish priorities in conjunction with client:

- Determine the client's most urgent need from both client's and nurse's viewpoints **(which may differ and require adjustments in teaching plan).**
- Discuss the client's perception of need. Relate the information to the client's personal desires, needs, values, and beliefs **so that the client feels competent and respected.**

Information that appears in brackets has been added by the authors to clarify and enhance the use of nursing diagnoses.

 Diagnostic Studies   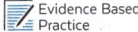 Evidence Based Practice   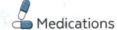 Medications   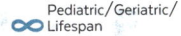 Pediatric/Geriatric/Lifespan

- Differentiate "critical" content from "desirable" content. **Defines information that is essential to understand now as well as content that could be addressed at a later time.**

Nursing Priority No. 4.

To establish the content to be included:

- Identify information that needs to be remembered (cognitive) at client's level of development and education. **Enhances possibility that information will be heard and understood.**
- Identify information having to do with emotions, attitudes, and values (affective). **The affective learning domain addresses a learner's emotions toward learning experiences, and attitudes, interest, attention, awareness, and values are demonstrated by affective behaviors.**
- Identify psychomotor skills that are necessary for learning. **Psychomotor learning involves both cognitive learning and muscular movement. The phases for learning these skills are cognitive (what), associative (how), and autonomous (practice to automaticity).**

Nursing Priority No. 5.

To develop learner's objectives:

- State objectives clearly in learner's terms **to meet learner's (not instructor's) needs.**
- Identify outcomes (results) to be achieved. **Understanding what outcomes will be can help client realize importance of learning the material, providing motivation necessary to learning.**
- Recognize level of achievement, time factors, and short- and long-term goals. **Learning progresses in stages. Stage 1: unconsciously unskilled where we do not know that we do not know. Stage 2: consciously unskilled, we know that we do not know and start to learn. Stage 3: consciously skilled, we know how to do it but need to think and work hard to do it. Stage 4: we become unconsciously skilled, where the new skills are easier and even seem natural.**
- Include the affective goals (e.g., reduction of stress). **The learner's emotional behaviors affect the learning experience and need to be actively addressed for maximum effectiveness.**

Nursing Priority No. 6.

To identify teaching methods to be used:

- Determine the client's method of accessing information (visual, auditory, kinesthetic, gustatory/olfactory) and include in teaching plan **to facilitate learning or recall.**

Information that appears in brackets has been added by the authors to clarify and enhance the use of nursing diagnoses.

 Acute Care 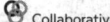 Collaborative 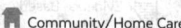 Community/Home Care Cultural

- Involve the client/SO(s) by using age-appropriate materials tailored to the client's literacy skills, questions, and dialogue. **Accesses familiar mental images at client's developmental level to help individual learn more effectively.**
- Involve client/SO(s) with others who have the same problems, needs, or concerns (e.g., group presentations, support groups). **Provides a role model and sharing of information.**
- Use team and group teaching as appropriate.

Nursing Priority No. 7.

To facilitate learning:

- Provide an environment that is conducive to learning. Be aware of factors related to the teacher in the situation (e.g., vocabulary, dress, style, knowledge of the subject, and ability to impart information effectively).
- Provide mutual goal setting and learning objectives. **Clarifies the expectations of teacher and learner.**
- Review information the client already knows and move to what client does not know, progressing from simple to complex. **Can arouse interest/limit sense of being overwhelmed.**
- Use short, simple sentences and concepts. Repeat and summarize at the end of explaining or teaching new concepts, as needed.
- Use gestures and facial expressions that help convey meaning of information.
- Provide information relevant only to the situation, discussing one topic at a time. **Reducing the amount of information at any one given time helps to keep client focused and prevents client from feeling overwhelmed.**
- Provide written information or guidelines and self-learning modules for client to refer to as necessary. **Reinforces the learning process and allows the client to proceed at own pace.**
- Pace and time learning sessions and learning activities to individual's needs. Evaluate the effectiveness of learning activities with client. **Helps to keep the client focused and prevents client from feeling overwhelmed. Client statements, questions, comments provide feedback about ability to grasp information being presented.**
- Deal with the client's anxiety or other strong emotions. Present information out of sequence, if necessary, dealing first with material that is most anxiety producing **when anxiety is interfering with the client's ability to learn.**

Information that appears in brackets has been added by the authors to clarify and enhance the use of nursing diagnoses.

 Diagnostic Studies 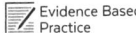 Evidence Based Practice Medications 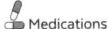 Pediatric/Geriatric/Lifespan

- Provide an active role for the client in the learning process. **Promotes a sense of control over the situation and is a means for determining that the client is assimilating and using new information.**
- Provide for feedback (positive reinforcement) and evaluation of learning and acquisition of skills. **Validates current level of understanding and identifies areas requiring follow-up.**
- Have client paraphrase content in own words, perform return demonstration, and explain how learning can be applied in own situation. **Enhances client's internalization of material and allows teacher to evaluate learning.**
- Be aware of informal teaching and role modeling that takes place on an ongoing basis (e.g., answering specific questions and reinforcing previous teaching during routine care).
- Assist client to use information in all applicable areas (e.g., situational, environmental, personal).

Nursing Priority No. 8.

To support information learned (Teaching/Discharge Considerations) and enhance well-being (long-term goals):

- Provide access information for community resources to client and/or family. **Reinforcement of resources helps client/family validate information postdischarge and engage in follow-up care.**
- Identify available counselors and support groups **to assist with problem-solving, provide role models, and support personal growth/change.**
- Provide information about additional learning resources (e.g., bibliography, reliable websites, audio/visual/digital media). **May assist with further learning and promote learning at own pace.**

Documentation Focus

Assessment/Reassessment
- Individual findings including learning style, identified needs, motivation, presence of learning blocks (e.g., hostility, inappropriate behavior)
- Desire/need to involve SO in learning process.

Planning
- Plan for learning, methods to be used, and who is involved in the planning
- Teaching plan

Information that appears in brackets has been added by the authors to clarify and enhance the use of nursing diagnoses.

Implementation/Evaluation
- Responses of the client/SO(s) to the learning plan and actions performed; how the learning is demonstrated
- Attainment of or progress toward desired outcome(s)
- Modifications to plan of care

Discharge Planning
- Additional learning and referral needs

Sample Nursing Outcomes & Interventions Classifications NOC/NIC

NOC—Knowledge: [specify—76 choices]
NIC—Teaching: Individual

---

inadequate HEALTH LITERACY NANDA-I

[Diagnostic Division: Health Management]

Definition: Unsatisfactory pattern of obtaining, appraising and applying basic health information and services needed to make health decisions.

Recognizing Cues

Related/Risk Factors
Inadequate information regarding healthcare options
Inadequate trust in health personnel; perceived complexity of healthcare information, or of healthcare system
Inadequate self-efficacy; hesitancy to ask questions; dependent on other's opinions
Inadequate communication skills; defensive behavior; depressive symptoms; hopelessness
Inadequate social activities, or social support
Inadequate information available to support person; inadequate understanding of information by support person
Unaddressed inadequate vision

Defining Characteristics

Subjective
Difficulty implementing, or delayed implementation of health-related course of action
Difficulty navigating complex healthcare systems
Inadequate willingness to participate in social interaction

Information that appears in brackets has been added by the authors to clarify and enhance the use of nursing diagnoses.

 Diagnostic Studies 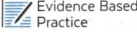 Evidence Based Practice 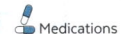 Medications 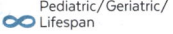 Pediatric/Geriatric/Lifespan

Objective

Inadequate understanding of health information, or healthcare options

Inadequate knowledge of healthy habits, or healthcare practices

Difficulty with personal healthcare decision making

Inappropriate seeking of healthcare services; absence of health-seeking behavior

Clinical Connections

Any acute illness or chronic health condition

Generate Solutions

Plan Desired Outcomes

Client Will (Include Specific Time Frame)

- Identify personal health needs/goals.
- Identify quality informational resources to enhance knowledge and support decision making.
- Verbalize understanding of health information received/accessed.
- Make informed healthcare decisions relevant to needs.
- Engage in preventive health practices.

Interventions/Take Action

Nursing Priority No. 1.

To determine level of health literacy and motivation for change:

- Determine client's health status, client's perception of health, and willingness to change at this time. **Client may perceive self as healthy when actually the client has some serious symptoms client is not aware of, or is minimizing/denying health issues or not willing to make healthcare changes. Keep in mind the family/significant other (SO) may have brought them in for treatment. Finesse the assessment showing patience, support, and understanding of the client concerns while learning more regarding the client's health status, needs, and what they think is needed to improve their health.**
- Identify current ability and knowledge of healthcare system, including how client/SO contacts and interacts with healthcare providers and where to go for emergent/urgent needs. **Ability to verbalize health needs, report symptoms, know where to get healthcare, and follow guidance from the caregiver is vital in accomplishing health goals.**

Information that appears in brackets has been added by the authors to clarify and enhance the use of nursing diagnoses.

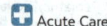 Acute Care 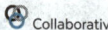 Collaborative 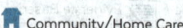 Community/Home Care Cultural

- Listen for client's desire and belief in the ability to accomplish health literacy, which is predictive of their performance. **Client's perception of their abilities to improve is a positive attitude toward learning.**
- Identify cultural beliefs that may influence client's view of the healthcare system and own care. **These beliefs can have strong influence on client's desire to change.**
- Active-listen client's concerns and issues that may be affecting client's desire to make changes. **Factors such as attitudes about health, health insurance, access to care, family problems, and economic situation may motivate client as well as interfere with plan for change.**
- Determine sources client currently uses to access information and how client actually uses the information. **Sources used vary widely depending on multiple factors such as client's age, language proficiency, accessibility of technology. Individual may be very adept at getting information but may not know how to use it in the context of own health, understand insurance papers, or pay bills.**
- Assess client's ability to understand the medical information and instructions provided and client is accessing. **Many adults are challenged by a low health literacy. A significant number of clients read at a fifth-grade level, are economically disadvantaged, are elderly, have a low English proficiency, or are nonnative speakers of English requiring help with medical terms and instructions. Collaboration with social workers/occupational therapy can help with clients requesting their needs/options.**
- Note the Social Determinants of Health (e.g., inadequate access to healthcare, educational disparities, socioeconomic status, or a lack of transportation) that can influence client's behavior regarding healthcare. **Access, transportation, participation in health resources and education programs are not spread evenly across underserved populations and affect their choice or ability to take action on interventions. Nurse's knowledge of these disparities can collaborate with other providers such as social workers/occupational therapy to facilitate access to care, transportation, and/or other needs as identified.**

Nursing Priority No. 2.
To assist client to develop plan for change:
- Provide guidance that fits with client's cultural, dietary, and/or spiritual values. During interactions with client,

---

Information that appears in brackets has been added by the authors to clarify and enhance the use of nursing diagnoses.

 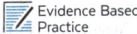 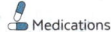 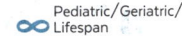

be sensitive to body language, mode of dress, and gender "rules" (e.g., female shaking hands with male, direct eye contact), and when asking sensitive questions to clarify understanding or dispel preconceived ideas. **These strategies help put client at ease, enhance trust, and can improve nurse–client relationship.**

- Assist client to develop a plan addressing individual strengths, weaknesses, threats, and opportunities (personal SWOT Analysis) to improve health literacy and health status. **Identifying specific areas for improvement aids in choice of interventions based on client's desires.**
- Discuss with client/family what areas of their life client has control over, such as choosing foods, cooking, safe place to exercise. **Making these decisions promotes sense of self-esteem, helping to improve health practices. Keep in mind the Social Determinants of Health may influence transportation to shop for groceries, a safe place to exercise, or recreation.**
- Focus energies on promoting informed lifestyle choices, preventive health programs, risk-factor modification, as appropriate. **Patient self-management relies on these factors to improve health, especially in management of chronic diseases.**
- Educate client/family in the use of web portals and public access resource sites as needed. **Persons with limited health literacy are less likely to use these resources, which may be due to ethnic/cultural or racial differences or level of comfort in sharing private health information.**
- Acknowledge efforts the client is making to maintain consistent positive outcomes of interventions. **These actions improve self-care efforts, client satisfaction, coping skills, and perceptions of social support.**

Nursing Priority No. 3.
To promote optimum health literacy (Teaching/Discharge Considerations) and enhance well-being (long-term goals):

- Reduce the use of health industry jargon, provide health materials in several languages, and provide interpreters when needed. **These changes will help client to understand the information the client is given.**
- Deliver health information in a clear, engaging, and personally relevant manner. Have client repeat back what they understand. **Can help client to understand, feel empowered and respected. Provides an opportunity to clarify learning and correct misunderstandings.**

Information that appears in brackets has been added by the authors to clarify and enhance the use of nursing diagnoses.

- Improve print communication by using plain and clear language, organizing ideas clearly, and using logical layout and design. **Facilitates reading and comprehension of potentially complicated consumer health information.**
- Promote client/family involvement in consumer education and health literacy. **Low literacy and numeracy (basic math skills) means that health communication is poorly understood. Individuals who are actively involved in seeking, understanding, and acting on health information learn how to navigate the system for maximum well-being.**
- Provide information about other community resources that can enhance learning and improve health literacy. **Programs such as smoking cessation, nutrition/weight loss, healthy exercise provide opportunities for skill training, problem-solving.**
- Encourage client to do breast self-examination/mammogram, testicular and prostate examinations, regular dental examination, keep immunizations current. **These actions contribute to maintaining wellness and encourage health literacy.**
- Assist client to prepare for healthcare encounters—write list of questions, list of all medications taken (prescription, over-the-counter, vitamins/herbals), and obtain results of diagnostic testing. **Role-playing and collecting necessary information can improve client confidence and facilitate meaningful interaction with provider.**
- Suggest SO/trusted family member accompany client to healthcare appointments, as appropriate. **Helpful for writing down/remembering information presented.**
- Review with client/SO the recently gained knowledge regarding health status, access to healthcare, and communicating their needs with the healthcare providers. **Reminding client/SO of knowledge gained builds self-esteem and self-confidence in communicating their needs and concerns with healthcare providers.**

Documentation Focus

Assessment/Reassessment
- Personal health status
- Goals and motivation for change
- Pertinent social factors, cultural beliefs, and spiritual values impacting health and use of healthcare system
- Primary language, literacy/reading level
- Availability and use of resources/health services

Information that appears in brackets has been added by the authors to clarify and enhance the use of nursing diagnoses.

 Diagnostic Studies 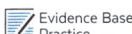 Evidence Based Practice 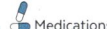 Medications 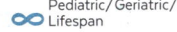 Pediatric/Geriatric/Lifespan

Planning
- Plan of care and who is involved in planning
- Individual learning needs

Implementation/Evaluation
- Response to interventions, teaching, and actions performed
- Attainment of or progress toward desired outcome(s)
- Modifications to plan

Discharge Planning
- Short- and long-term needs and who is responsible for actions
- Available resources, specific referrals made

Sample Nursing Outcomes & Interventions Classifications NOC/NIC

NOC—Health Literacy Behavior
NIC—Health Literacy Enhancement

---

ineffective HEALTH MAINTENANCE BEHAVIORS NANDA-I

[Diagnostic Division: Health Management]

Definition: Management of health knowledge, attitudes, and practices underlying health actions that is unsatisfactory for maintaining or improving well-being, or preventing illness and injury.

Recognizing Cues

AUTHOR NOTE: This diagnosis contains components of other NDs. We suggest subsuming health maintenance interventions under the "basic" nursing diagnosis when a single causative factor is identified (e.g., inadequate Health Knowledge; ineffective Health Self-Management; chronic Confusion; impaired verbal Communication; difficulty Coping; impaired family Coping; impaired child Development).

Related/Risk Factors

Competing demands, or lifestyle preferences; cultural beliefs
Conflict between cultural, or spiritual beliefs and health practices; conflict between health behaviors and social norms

---

Information that appears in brackets has been added by the authors to clarify and enhance the use of nursing diagnoses.

 Acute Care   Collaborative 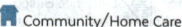 Community/Home Care 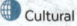 Cultural

Inadequate knowledge about basic health practices
Excessive stress; inability to maintain control; fear of institutionalization
Depressive symptoms; maladaptive grieving
Difficulty with decision making; impaired executive functioning skills
Difficulty accessing community resources
Difficulty navigating complex healthcare systems; inadequate health literacy
Inadequate health resources; inadequate trust in health personnel
Inadequate social support; spiritual distress
Ineffective communication skills; inadequate self-efficacy
Ineffective use of coping strategies
Social anxiety; perceived prejudice or victimization
Perceived constipation; substance misuse
Confusion; disturbed thought processes

Defining Characteristics

Objective

Failure to take action that prevents health problems, or that reduces risk factors; risk-prone health behavior
Inadequate commitment to plan of action; inadequate interest in improving health; inadequate choices in daily living for meeting health goals
Pattern of inadequate health-seeking behavior
Inadequate personal, or environmental hygiene
Inappropriate use of bowel stimulation methods

Clinical Connections

Chronic conditions (e.g., multiple sclerosis [MS], rheumatoid arthritis, chronic pain), brain injury or stroke, spinal cord injury or paralysis, laryngectomy, dementia, Alzheimer disease, developmental delay

Generate Solutions

Plan Desired Outcomes

Client Will (Include Specific Time Frame)

- Identify necessary health maintenance activities.
- Verbalize understanding of factors contributing to current situation.
- Assume responsibility for own healthcare needs within level of ability.
- Adopt lifestyle changes supporting individual healthcare goals.

Information that appears in brackets has been added by the authors to clarify and enhance the use of nursing diagnoses.

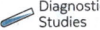 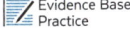 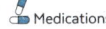

Significant Other/Caregiver Will (Include Specific Time Frame)
- Verbalize the ability to cope adequately with existing situation, provide support/monitoring as indicated.

Interventions/Take Action

Nursing Priority No. 1.
To assess causative/contributing factors:

- Recognize differing perceptions regarding health issues between healthcare providers and clients. Explore ways to partner. **Awareness that healthcare provider's goals may not be the same as client's goals can provide opportunities to explore and communicate. If left undone, the door is open for frustration on both sides, affecting client care experience and/or perceived outcome of care.**
- Identify health practices and beliefs in client's personal and family history, including health values, spiritual or cultural beliefs, and expectations regarding healthcare. **Clients and healthcare providers do not always view a health risk in the same way. The client may not view current situation as a problem or may be unaware of routine health maintenance practices and needs.**
- Note the client's age (e.g., very young or elderly); cognitive, emotional, physical, and developmental status; and level of dependence and independence. **The client's abilities and status may range from complete dependence to partial or relative independence and determine type of interventions/support needed.**
- Determine whether impairment is an acute or sudden onset situation, progressive illness, long-term health problem, or exacerbation or complication of chronic illness. **Determines type and intensity and length of time support may be required.**
- Evaluate medication regimen and also for substance use or abuse (e.g., alcohol or other drugs). **Can affect the client's understanding of information or desire and ability to help self.**
- Ascertain recent changes in lifestyle (e.g., widowed man who has no skills for taking care of his own/family's health needs; loss of independence; changing support systems).
- Note the setting where the client lives (e.g., long-term/other residential care facility, rural versus urban setting; homebound, homeless). **Socioeconomic status and geographic location contribute to an individual's ability to achieve or maintain good health.**

Information that appears in brackets has been added by the authors to clarify and enhance the use of nursing diagnoses.

- Note desire and level of ability to meet health maintenance needs, as well as self-care activities of daily living. **Care may begin with helping client make a decision to improve situation as well as identifying factors that are currently interfering with meeting needs.**
- Determine level of adaptive behavior, knowledge, and skills about health maintenance, environment, and safety. **Determines the beginning point for planning and interventions to assist the client in addressing needs.**
- Assess the client's ability and desire to learn. Determine barriers to learning (e.g., cannot read, speaks or understands different language than is used in the present setting, is overcome with grief or stress, has no interest in subject). **The client may not be physically, emotionally, or mentally capable at present because of current situation or may need information in small, manageable increments.**
- Assess communication skills and ability or need for interpreter. Identify support person requesting or willing to accept information. **The ability to understand is essential to identification of needs and planning care. The information may need to be provided to another individual if the client is unable to comprehend.**
- Note the client's use of professional services and resources (e.g., appropriate or inappropriate/nonexistent).

Nursing Priority No. 2.

To assist client/caregiver(s) to maintain and manage desired health practices:

- Discuss with client/significant other(s) (SO[s]) beliefs about health and reasons for not following prescribed plan of care. **Determines the client's view of current situation and potential for change.**
- Evaluate environment **to note individual adaptation needs.**
- Identify realistic health goals and develop plan with client/SO(s) for self-care. **Allows for incorporating existing disabilities with client's/SO's desires and ability to adapt and organize care activities.**
- Involve comprehensive specialty health teams when indicated (e.g., pulmonary, psychiatric, enterostomal, IV therapy, nutritional support, substance abuse counselors).
- Provide time to active-listen concerns of client/SO(s). **Provides opportunity to clarify expectations and misconceptions.**
- Provide anticipatory guidance **to maintain and manage effective health practices during periods of wellness,**

Information that appears in brackets has been added by the authors to clarify and enhance the use of nursing diagnoses.

 Diagnostic Studies 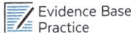 Evidence Based Practice 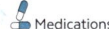 Medications 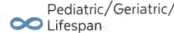 Pediatric/Geriatric/Lifespan

and identify ways the client can adapt when progressive illness/long-term health problems occur.
- Encourage socialization and personal involvement **to enhance support system, provide pleasant stimuli, and prevent permanent regression.**
- Provide for communication and coordination between the healthcare facility team and community healthcare providers **to provide continuation of care and maximize outcomes.**
- Monitor adherence to prescribed medical regimen **to problem-solve difficulties in adherence and alter the plan of care, as needed.**

Nursing Priority No. 3.

To achieve health goals (Teaching/Discharge Considerations) and enhance well-being (long-term goals):

- Provide information about individual healthcare needs, using the client's/SO's preferred learning style (e.g., pictures, words, video, Internet) **to assist the client in understanding own situation and enhance interest/involvement in meeting own health needs.**
- Limit the amount of information presented at one time, especially when dealing with the elderly or cognitively or developmentally impaired client. Present new material through self-paced instruction when possible. **Allows the client time to process and store new information.**
- Help client/SO(s) develop realistic healthcare goals. Provide a written copy to those involved in the planning process **for future reference and revision, as appropriate. Promotes planning to enable the client to maintain a healthy and productive lifestyle.**
- Assist client/SO(s) to develop stress management skills. **Knowing ways to manage stress can help individual to develop and maintain a healthy lifestyle.**
- Identify ways to adapt things in current circumstances **to meet the client's changing needs and abilities and environmental concerns.**
- Identify signs and symptoms requiring further medical screening, evaluation, and follow-up care. **Essential to identify developing problems that could interfere with maintaining well-being.**
- Make referrals, as needed, for community support services (e.g., homemaker/home attendant, Meals on Wheels, skilled nursing care, well-baby clinic, senior citizen healthcare activities). **The client may need additional assistance to maintain self-sufficiency.**

Information that appears in brackets has been added by the authors to clarify and enhance the use of nursing diagnoses.

- Refer to social services, as indicated, **for assistance with financial, housing, or legal concerns (e.g., conservatorship).**
- Refer to support groups, as appropriate (e.g., senior citizens, Salvation Army shelter, homeless clinic, Alcoholics or Narcotics Anonymous).
- Assist with referral for hospice service for client with terminal illness, where indicated, **to help client and family deal with end-of-life issues in a positive manner.**

Documentation Focus

Assessment/Reassessment
- Assessment findings, including individual abilities; family involvement; support factors, and availability of resources
- Cultural or spiritual beliefs and healthcare values

Planning
- Plan of care and who is involved in planning
- Teaching plan

Implementation/Evaluation
- Responses of client/SO(s) to plan, specific interventions, teaching, and actions performed
- Attainment of or progress toward desired outcome(s)
- Modifications to plan of care

Discharge Planning
- Long-range needs and who is responsible for actions to be taken
- Specific referrals made

Sample Nursing Outcomes & Interventions Classifications NOC/NIC

NOC—Health Promoting Behavior
NIC—Health System Guidance

---

ineffective community HEALTH MANAGEMENT NANDA-I

[Diagnostic Division: Health Management]

Definition: Unsatisfactory handling of health problems or factors that deter wellness or increase the risk of health problems experienced by a population.

Information that appears in brackets has been added by the authors to clarify and enhance the use of nursing diagnoses.

 Diagnostic Studies 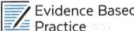 Evidence Based Practice 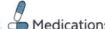 Medications ∞ Pediatric/Geriatric/Lifespan

Recognizing Cues

Related/Risk Factors
Inadequate access to health personnel

Inadequate consumer satisfaction with programs; inadequate expertise within the community; inadequate program budget, or program evaluation plan; inadequate program outcome data

Inadequate health resources; inadequate community support for programs

Programs incompletely address health problems

Defining Characteristics

Subjective
[Community members/agencies verbalize overburdening of resources or inability to meet therapeutic needs of all members]

Objective
Health problems experienced by a population

Programs unavailable to prevent, reduce, or eliminate health problems of a population

Program unavailable to enhance wellness of a group or population

Risk of hospitalization to a population

Risk of physiological or psychological manifestations to a population

Clinical Connections
HIV/AIDS, substance abuse, sexually transmitted infections, teen pregnancy, prematurity, acute lead poisoning, influenza, severe acute respiratory syndromes (SARS-CoV-2)

Generate Solutions

Plan Desired Outcomes

Community Will (Include Specific Time Frame)
- Identify both strengths and limitations affecting community treatment programs for meeting health-related goals.
- Participate in problem-solving of factors interfering with regulating and integrating community programs.
- Develop plans to address identified community health needs.

Information that appears in brackets has been added by the authors to clarify and enhance the use of nursing diagnoses.

Interventions/Take Action

Nursing Priority No. 1.
To identify causative/precipitating factors:

- Evaluate healthcare providers' understanding, terminology, and practice policies relating to community (populations and aggregate). **Population-based practice considers the broad determinants of health, such as income/social status, housing, nutrition, employment/working conditions, social support networks, education, neighborhood safety/violence issues, physical environment, personal health practices and coping skills, cultural customs and values, and community capacity to support family and economic growth.**
- Investigate health problems, unexpected outbreaks or acceleration of illness, and health hazards in the community. **Identifying specific problems allows for population-based interventions emphasizing primary prevention, promoting health, and preventing problems before they occur. Current available resources provide a starting point to determine needs of the community and plan for future needs.**
- Evaluate strengths and limitations of community healthcare resources for wellness, illness, or sequelae of illness. **Knowledge of currently available resources and ease of access provide a starting point to determine needs of the community and plan for future needs.**
- Note reports from members of the community regarding ineffective or inadequate community functioning. **Provides feedback from people who live in the community and avail themselves of resources, thus presenting a realistic picture of problem areas.**
- Determine areas of conflict among members of community. **Cultural or spiritual beliefs, values, social mores, and lack of a shared vision may limit dialogue or creative problem-solving if not addressed.**
- Ascertain effect of related factors on community. **Issues of safety, poor air quality, lack of education or information, and lack of sufficient healthcare facilities affect citizens and how they view their community—whether it is a healthy, positive environment in which to live or lacks adequate healthcare or safety resources.**
- Determine knowledge and understanding of treatment regimen. **Citizens need to know and understand what is being proposed to correct the identified deficiencies**

Information that appears in brackets has been added by the authors to clarify and enhance the use of nursing diagnoses.

before they are willing to be involved and actively support goals of the treatment regimen.
- Note use of resources available to community for developing and funding programs.

Nursing Priority No. 2.

To assist community to develop strategies to improve community functioning/management:

- Foster cooperative spirit of community without negating individuality of members/groups. **As individuals feel valued and respected, they are more willing to work together with others to develop plan for identifying and improving healthcare for the community.**
- Involve the community in determining and prioritizing healthcare goals **to facilitate the planning process.**
- Link people to needed services (e.g., food-distribution sites, rent assistance, transition in and out of shelters; help navigating health systems; facilitate prescription refills; navigate resources for undocumented immigrants), and assure the provision of healthcare to extent possible. **Interventions may be directed at an entire population within a community, the systems that affect the health of those populations, and/or the individuals and families within at-risk populations. Working together promotes a sense of involvement and control, helping people implement more effective problem-solving.**
- Plan together with community health and social agencies **to problem-solve solutions to identified and anticipated problems and needs.**
- Identify specific populations at risk or underserved (e.g., chronically ill or disabled persons; elder adults; mentally ill persons; substance abusers; veterans; economically disadvantaged families; rural, migrant, immigrant, and homeless persons; racial and ethnic minorities) **to actively involve them in the planning and evaluation process. These groups are often marginalized and frequently lack knowledge of available services, may be suspicious or lack interest in available programs, or lack resources to access services. Being part of the solution enhances sense of being heard, empowering these groups and promoting continued participation in the process.**
- Create teaching plan; form speakers' bureau **to disseminate information to community members regarding value of treatment and preventive programs.**

Information that appears in brackets has been added by the authors to clarify and enhance the use of nursing diagnoses.

- Network with others involved in educating healthcare providers and healthcare consumers regarding community needs. Present information in a culturally appropriate manner. **Disseminating information to community members regarding value of treatment or preventive programs helps people to know and understand the importance of these actions and be willing to support the programs.**

Nursing Priority No. 3.
To promote healthy community (Teaching/Discharge Considerations) and enhance well-being (long-term goals):

- Assist the community to develop a plan for continuing assessment of community needs (e.g., access to adequate healthcare; education regarding disease prevention, public health threats, and immunization; local warning system and evacuation plan in event of disaster; planning for community members with special needs [elderly, handicapped, low-income]; violence prevention; water, sanitation, toxic substance management; mobilization of resources) and the functioning and effectiveness of the plan. **Promotes a proactive approach in planning for the future and continuation of efforts to improve healthy behaviors and necessary services.**
- Encourage community to form partnerships within the community and between the community and the larger society **to aid in long-term planning for anticipated or projected needs and concerns.**

Documentation Focus

Assessment/Reassessment
- Assessment findings, including members' perceptions of community problems, healthcare resources
- Community use of available resources

Planning
- Plan of care and who is involved in planning
- Teaching plan

Implementation/Evaluation
- Community's response to plan, teaching, and interventions performed
- Attainment of or progress toward desired outcome(s)
- Modifications to plan of care

Information that appears in brackets has been added by the authors to clarify and enhance the use of nursing diagnoses.

Discharge Planning
- Long-term goals and who is responsible for actions to be taken
- Specific referrals made

Sample Nursing Outcomes & Interventions Classifications NOC/NIC

NOC—Community Competence
NIC—Community Health Development

---

ineffective family HEALTH MANAGEMENT NANDA-I

[Diagnostic Division: Health Management]

Definition: Unsatisfactory handling of symptoms, treatment regimen, and lifestyle changes that is unsatisfactory for meeting specific health goals of the family unit.

Recognizing Cues

Related/Risk Factors
Competing demands on family unit; competing lifestyle preferences within family unit

Conflict between health behaviors and social norms; conflict between spiritual beliefs and treatment regimen; family conflict; unsupportive family relationships

Difficulty accessing community resources; difficulty navigating complex healthcare systems

Difficulty with decision making; difficulty dealing with role changes associated with condition

Difficulty managing complex treatment regimen; inadequate knowledge of treatment regimen; inadequate commitment to plan of action

Negative feelings toward treatment regimen; perceived barrier to treatment regimen

Inadequate number of cues to action; difficulty performing aspects of treatment regimen

Inadequate health literacy of caregiver; ineffective communication skills; inadequate self-efficacy

Inadequate social support; ineffective coping skills; perceived social stigma associated with condition

Substance misuse

Information that appears in brackets has been added by the authors to clarify and enhance the use of nursing diagnoses.

 Acute Care 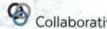 Collaborative 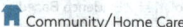 Community/Home Care   Cultural

Unrealistic perception of seriousness of condition; nonacceptance of condition

Unrealistic perception of treatment benefit, or of susceptibility to sequelae

Defining Characteristics

Subjective
One or more family members report dissatisfaction with quality of life

Objective
Caregiving burden; depressive symptoms of caregiver

Decrease in attention to illness in one or more family members

Exacerbation of disease signs or symptoms of one or more family members

Failure to take action to reduce risk factors in one or more family members

Ineffective choices in daily living for meeting health goal of family unit

Clinical Connections
Chronic conditions (e.g., chronic obstructive pulmonary disease, multiple sclerosis, arthritis, chronic pain, depression, substance abuse, end-stage liver or renal failure) or new diagnoses/events necessitating lifestyle changes

Generate Solutions

Plan Desired Outcomes

Client/Family Will (Include Specific Time Frame)
- Identify individual factors affecting regulation/integration of treatment program.
- Participate in problem-solving of identified concerns.
- Engage in mutual goal setting for care/treatment plan.
- Verbalize acceptance of need or desire to change actions to achieve agreed-on outcomes or health goals.
- Demonstrate behaviors and changes in lifestyle necessary to maintain therapeutic regimen.

Interventions/Take Action

Nursing Priority No. 1.
To identify causative/precipitating factors:

- Determine family's perception of efforts to date. **Perceptions are more important than facts, and by getting**

Information that appears in brackets has been added by the authors to clarify and enhance the use of nursing diagnoses.

 Diagnostic Studies 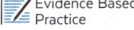 Evidence Based Practice 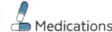 Medications 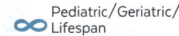 Pediatric/Geriatric/Lifespan

family's point of view, realistic goals can be set and family can look to the future.
- Evaluate family functioning and activities—looking at frequency and effectiveness of family communication, promotion of autonomy, adaptation to meet changing needs, health of home environment and lifestyle, problem-solving abilities, and ties to community. **Understanding the family and the context in which it lives allows for more personalized support of the family and choosing coping strategies in partnership with the family to meet individualized goals.**
- Note family health goals and agreement of individual members. **The presence of conflict interferes with problem-solving and needs to be addressed before family can move forward to meet goals.**
- Determine understanding of and value of the treatment regimen to the family. **Individual members may misunderstand either the cause of the illness or the prescribed regimen and may disagree with what is happening, thereby promoting dissension within the family group and causing distress for the client.**
- Identify cultural values or spiritual beliefs affecting view of situation and willingness to make necessary changes. **These concepts affect a person's health beliefs and practices.**
- Identify availability and use of resources. **Knowing who is available to help and support the family will help in planning care to maximize positive outcomes.**

Nursing Priority No. 2.
To assist family to develop strategies to improve management of therapeutic regimen:
- Provide family-centered education addressing management of condition/chronic illness and incorporation of strategies into family's lifestyle. **Helps the family to make informed decisions and see the connection between illness and treatment; it also facilitates treatment adherence and improved client outcomes. Assisting family to manage needs on a daily basis can instill confidence, decrease anxiety, and provide a degree of predictability to daily life.**
- Assist family members to recognize inappropriate family activities. Help the members identify both togetherness and individual needs and behavior **so that effective interactions can be enhanced and perpetuated.**

Information that appears in brackets has been added by the authors to clarify and enhance the use of nursing diagnoses.

- Make a plan jointly with family members to deal with the complexity of the healthcare regimen or system and other related factors. **Enhances commitment to the plan, optimizing outcomes.**
- Identify community resources, as needed, using the three strategies of education, problem-solving, and resource linking **to address specific deficits.**

Nursing Priority No. 3.

To support family health progress (Teaching/Discharge Considerations) and enhance future well-being (long-term goals):

- Help family identify criteria to promote ongoing self-evaluation of situation and effectiveness and family progress. **Involvement promotes sense of control and provides an opportunity to be proactive in meeting needs.**
- Assist family to plan for potential problems or complications. **Helping families anticipate likely challenges allows them to plan more effective coping strategies.**
- Make referrals to and/or jointly plan with other health, social, and community resources. **Problems are often multifaceted, requiring involvement of numerous providers and agencies.**
- Encourage involvement in disease/condition support groups. **Family resiliency is gained through contact with other families dealing with similar challenges.**
- Provide a contact person or case manager for one-to-one assistance, as needed, **to coordinate care, provide support, assist with problem-solving, and so forth.**
- Refer to NDs excessive Caregiving Burden; ineffective Health Self-Management, as indicated.

Documentation Focus

Assessment/Reassessment
- Individual findings, including nature of problem and degree of impairment; family values, health goals, and level of participation and commitment of family members
- Cultural values, spiritual beliefs
- Availability and use of resources

Planning
- Plan of care and who is involved in planning
- Teaching plan

Information that appears in brackets has been added by the authors to clarify and enhance the use of nursing diagnoses.

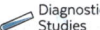 Diagnostic Studies 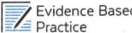 Evidence Based Practice 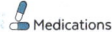 Medications 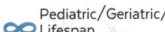 Pediatric/Geriatric/Lifespan

Implementation/Evaluation
- Response to interventions, teaching, and actions performed
- Attainment of or progress toward desired outcome(s)
- Modifications of plan of care

Discharge Planning
- Long-term needs, plan for meeting, and who is responsible for actions
- Specific referrals made

Sample Nursing Outcomes & Interventions Classifications NOC/NIC

NOC—Family Health Status
NIC—Family Involvement Promotion

ineffective HEALTH SELF-MANAGEMENT NANDA-I

[Diagnostic Division: Health Management]

Definition: Unsatisfactory handling of symptoms, treatment regimen, and lifestyle changes associated with living with a chronic condition.

Recognizing Cues

Related/Risk Factors
Competing demands, or lifestyle preferences
Conflict between cultural beliefs and health practices; conflict between health behaviors and social norms; conflict between spiritual beliefs and treatment regimen
Decreased quality of life; excessive stress
Depressive symptoms; inadequate self-efficacy
Difficulty with decision making
Difficulty accessing community resources; difficulty navigating complex healthcare systems
Difficulty managing complex treatment regimen; inadequate commitment to a plan of action; negative feelings toward treatment regimen; perceived barrier to treatment regimen; nonacceptance of condition
Inadequate knowledge of treatment regimen; inadequate number of cues to action; difficulty performing aspects of treatment regimen
Inadequate health literacy

Information that appears in brackets has been added by the authors to clarify and enhance the use of nursing diagnoses.

 Acute Care   Collaborative 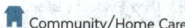 Community/Home Care   Cultural

Inadequate role models, or social support; perceived social stigma associated with condition
Confusion
Substance misuse
Unawareness of seriousness of condition, or of susceptibility to sequelae; unrealistic expectation of treatment benefit

Defining Characteristics

Subjective
Dissatisfaction with quality of life

Objective
Exacerbation of disease signs, or symptoms; exhibits disease sequelae
Failure to attend appointments with health personnel, or to include treatment regimen in daily living, or to take action that reduces risk factors
Inattentive to disease signs, or symptoms; ineffective choices in daily living for meeting health goals

Clinical Connections
Chronic conditions (e.g., cancer; chronic obstructive pulmonary disease; multiple sclerosis; arthritis; chronic pain; end-stage heart, liver, or renal failure), developmental delays, or new diagnoses necessitating lifestyle changes

Generate Solutions

Plan Desired Outcomes

Client Will (Include Specific Time Frame)
- Verbalize acceptance of need and desire to change actions to achieve agreed-on health goals.
- Verbalize understanding of factors or blocks involved in individual situation.
- Participate in problem-solving of factors interfering with integration of therapeutic regimen.
- Demonstrate behaviors and changes in lifestyle necessary to maintain therapeutic regimen.
- Identify and use available resources.

Interventions/Take Action

Nursing Priority No. 1.
To identify causative/contributing factors:
- Determine whether client has acute or chronic illness; if chronic, note comorbidities and assess the complexity of

---

Information that appears in brackets has been added by the authors to clarify and enhance the use of nursing diagnoses.

 Diagnostic Studies 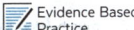 Evidence Based Practice Medications 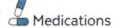 Pediatric/Geriatric/Lifespan care needs. **These factors affect how the client views and manages self-care. The client may be overwhelmed, in denial, depressed, or have complications exacerbating care needs. Furthermore, people tend to become passive and dependent in long-term, debilitating illnesses and may find it difficult to expend energy to follow through with therapeutic regimen.**

- Identify client's knowledge and understanding of condition and treatment needs. **Provides a baseline so planning care can begin where the client is in relation to condition or illness and current regimen.**
- Determine client's/family's health goals and patterns of healthcare. **Provides information about current behaviors and misperceptions that may be potential areas of conflict, values, or financial considerations.**
- Identify health practices and beliefs in the client's personal and family history, including health values, spiritual or cultural beliefs, and expectations regarding healthcare. **The client may not view current situation as a problem or may be unaware of health management needs. Expectations of others may dictate client's adaptation to the situation and willingness to modify life. Note: In one study, researchers found that information designed to meet unique characteristics of the individual through culturally relevant tailoring significantly increased adherence rate with interventions.**
- Identify client locus of control. **Those with an internal locus of control (e.g., expressions of responsibility for self and ability to control outcomes, such as "I did quit smoking") are more likely to take charge of the situation. Individuals with an external locus of control (e.g., expressions of lack of control over self and environment, such as "What bad luck to get lung cancer") may perceive difficulties as beyond their control and will likely look to others to solve their problems.**
- Determine individual perceptions and expectations of treatment regimen. Active-listen client's concerns and comments. **May reveal client's thinking about regimen, misinformation, unrealistic expectations, resistance to change, being overwhelmed with diagnosis, using the problem/condition as a device for avoiding activities, or other factors that may be interfering with the client's willingness to follow a therapeutic regimen.**
- Assess issues of secondary gain for the client/significant others (SOs). **Marital/family concern or attention, school**

Information that appears in brackets has been added by the authors to clarify and enhance the use of nursing diagnoses.

or work issues, or financial considerations may cause client to subconsciously desire to remain ill or disabled, which can interfere with complying with prescribed treatment plans, prolong recovery time, and create frustrating medical-legal issues.
- Review complexity of treatment regimen (e.g., number of expected tasks, such as taking medication several times/day; visiting multiple healthcare providers with treatment or follow-up appointments; abundant, often conflicting, information sources). Evaluate how difficult tasks might be for client (e.g., must stop smoking or must follow strict dialysis diet even when feeling well and manage limitations while remaining active in life roles). **These factors are often involved in lack of participation in treatment plan.**
- Determine who (e.g., client, SO, other) manages the medication regimen, whether individual knows what the medications are and why they are prescribed, and any factors that interfere with taking medications or lead to lack of adherence (e.g., depression, active alcohol or other drug use, low literacy, lack of support, lack of belief in treatment efficacy). **Forgetfulness is the most common reason given for not complying with the treatment plan. In addition, poor patient-provider communication has been identified as a main source of medication nonadherence.**
- Note availability and use of support systems, resources for assistance, caregiving, and respite care. **The client may not have, be aware of, or know how to access available resources.**

Nursing Priority No. 2.
To assist client/SO(s) to develop strategies to improve management of therapeutic regimen:
- Use therapeutic communication skills **to assist client to problem-solve solution(s). Active-listening promotes accurate identification of the problem, ensuring that problem-solving is directed to the correct solution.**
- Explore client involvement in or lack of mutual goal setting. **Understanding client's willingness to be involved (or not) provides insight into the reasons for actions and suggests appropriate interventions.**
- Have client identify consequences of current behaviors/ineffective management of condition. **May help client visualize the "cost" of lack of commitment to therapeutic regimen.**

Information that appears in brackets has been added by the authors to clarify and enhance the use of nursing diagnoses.

 Diagnostic Studies 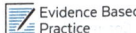 Evidence Based Practice 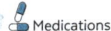 Medications 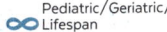 Pediatric/Geriatric/Lifespan

- Use the client's locus of control to develop an individual plan to adapt to regimen. **Encourage the client with internal control to take control of own care; for those with external control, begin with small tasks and add as tolerated.**
- Establish graduated goals or modified regimen as necessary. **Specifying steps to take requires discussion and the use of critical-thinking skills to determine how to best reach the agreed-on goals.**
- Encourage client to participate in care, as appropriate. **By making a contract, client commits self to therapeutic regimen and is more likely to follow through because of commitment.**
- Accept client's evaluation of own strengths and limitations while working together to improve abilities. State belief in client's ability to cope and/or adapt to situation. **Individuals may minimize own strengths or exaggerate limitations when faced with the difficulties of a chronic illness. Stating your belief in positive terms lets the client hear someone else's evaluation and begin to accept that client can manage the situation.**
- Provide positive reinforcement for efforts **to encourage continuation of desired behaviors.**
- Provide information and encourage client to know where and how to find it on own. Reinforce previous instructions and rationale, using a variety of learning modalities, including role-playing, demonstration, and written materials. **Incorporating multiple modalities promotes retention of information. Developing client's skill at finding own information encourages self-sufficiency and sense of self-worth.**

Nursing Priority No. 3.

To promote optimum health (Teaching/Discharge Considerations) and enhance well-being (long-term goals):

- Emphasize the importance of client knowledge and understanding of the need for treatment or medication as well as consequences of actions and choices. **Reinforces client's role in success of therapeutic regimen, encouraging continuation of competent behaviors.**
- Promote client/caregiver/SO(s) participation in planning and evaluating process. **Enhances commitment to the plan and promotes competent self-management, optimizing outcomes.**

Information that appears in brackets has been added by the authors to clarify and enhance the use of nursing diagnoses.

 Acute Care 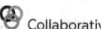 Collaborative 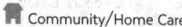 Community/Home Care 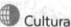 Cultural

- Assist client to develop strategies for monitoring symptoms and response to therapeutic regimen. **Promotes early recognition of changes, allowing a proactive response.**
- Mobilize support systems, including family/SO(s), social services, and financial assistance. **Success of a therapeutic regimen is enhanced by using support systems effectively, avoiding or reducing stress and worry of dealing with unresolved problems.**
- Provide for continuity of care in and out of the hospital or care setting, including long-range plans. **Supports trust and facilitates progress toward goals as client illness is dealt with over time.**
- Refer to counseling or therapy (group and individual), as indicated. **Client may need additional help to deal with stress and anxiety of chronic condition or illness.**
- Identify home- and community-based nursing services **for assessment, follow-up care, and education in the client's home.**

Documentation Focus

Assessment/Reassessment
- Findings, including underlying dynamics of individual situation, client's perception of problem or needs, locus of control
- Cultural values, spiritual beliefs
- Family involvement and needs
- Individual strengths and limitations
- Availability and use of resources

Planning
- Plan of care and who is involved in planning
- Teaching plan

Implementation/Evaluation
- Response to interventions, teaching, and actions performed
- Attainment or progress toward desired outcome(s)
- Modifications to plan of care

Discharge Planning
- Long-term needs and who is responsible for actions to be taken
- Available resources, specific referrals made

Information that appears in brackets has been added by the authors to clarify and enhance the use of nursing diagnoses.

Sample Nursing Outcomes & Interventions Classifications NOC/NIC

NOC—Health Promoting Behavior
NIC—Health Coaching

---

readiness for enhanced HEALTHY AGING — NANDA-I

[Diagnostic Division: Health Management]

Definition: Pattern of developing or maintaining physical, mental, social, spiritual well-being and function with advancing age, which can be strengthened.

Recognizing Cues

Defining Characteristics

Subjective

Desires to enhance:
   Quality of life; healthy lifestyle
   Knowledge to make appropriate choices to promote health; condition management
   Psychological well-being, or resilience
   Functional capacity; independence for self-care
   Autonomy; family dynamics
   Social engagement
   Spirituality

Clinical Connections

Elder individuals with chronic conditions, extended-care residents

Generate Solutions

Plan Desired Outcomes

Client Will (Include Specific Time Frame)

- Schedule routine appointment to see medical or mental healthcare professionals.
- Verbalize readiness to participate in regular exercise.
- Make commitment to eating healthy foods.
- Engage in healthy sleep habits.
- Make a plan to quit smoking and misusing drugs and alcohol.

Information that appears in brackets has been added by the authors to clarify and enhance the use of nursing diagnoses.

 Acute Care 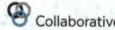 Collaborative 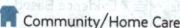 Community/Home Care Cultural

Interventions/Take Action

Nursing Priority No. 1.
To determine desire, motivation to enhance healthy lifestyle:

- Assess health history and present health status. **Age, height, weight, vital signs, and physical and mental health history influence the present health status of a client. Recognizing past health behaviors influence the present and is a starting point to improve the present.**
- Determine client's health concerns and needs. **Client's desires set the stage to plan for their specific needs. Client-centered care acknowledges that client understands their body and what helps them to improve. Healthcare providers collaborating with the client's desires can help to improve their health.**
- Identify communication patterns, coping strategies to problem-solve, or the use of defense mechanism to protect self-esteem. **Promoting self-awareness of what client thinks and feels about themselves is demonstrated in verbal/nonverbal communication and is reflected by using coping skills or defense mechanism.**
- Apply motivational interviewing to identify stage of readiness to change. **motivational interviewing allows client to feel the respect of the interviewer and helps the client express their desire, ability, reason, and need to change behaviors as well as define their stage of readiness to change.**
- Identify current medications, herbals, and illicit substances used. **A comprehensive list of prescribed, over-the-counter medications, herbals, or street drugs taken define their medical needs or the possibility of interactions/overusing medications.**
- Identify level of exercise and physical activity. **Physical activity is paramount to healthy living. The benefits of exercise include maintaining a healthy weight, not under- or overweight, and maintaining muscle mass.**
- Review eating habits and food choices. **Eating patterns determine weight status, protect your immune system, protect brain function, reduce the risk of type 2 diabetes and heart disease. Eating fresh fruit, vegetables, whole grains, healthy fats, and more fish, Mediterranean-style eating, has a positive influence on health.**
- Determine client's level or readiness to change health behaviors. **Knowing the stage of readiness to change (e.g., pre-contemplation, contemplation, preparation, action,**

Information that appears in brackets has been added by the authors to clarify and enhance the use of nursing diagnoses.

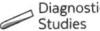 Diagnostic Studies 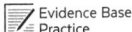 Evidence Based Practice 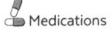 Medications 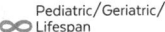 Pediatric/Geriatric/Lifespan

and maintenance) determines the level of interventions required to meet the client's needs. Interventions applied prior to the correct stage of readiness will be met with resistance.

Nursing Priority No. 2.

To assist client to make required changes:

- Establish a nurse–client therapeutic relationship. **Nurses using a care and therapeutic communication develop a trusting relationship to help the client approach their desired health status.**
- Allow time for client to process self-reflection and recognize how they respond/behave to their lifestyle. **Self-reflection contributes to self-awareness and can influence how client may react opposed to thinking about a response.**
- Use role-playing to practice newly learned communication and coping skills. **Practicing new learned communication skills with healthcare providers develops self-esteem and confidence moving forward.**

Nursing Priority No. 3.

To maintain healthy aging (Teaching/Discharge Considerations) and enhance well-being (long-term goals):

- Review new communication patterns and coping skills learned. **Clients are more likely to continue use of open and honest communication and coping skills with a summary of new knowledge.**
- Discuss progress obtained during treatment. **When client recognizes the goals obtained during treatment, their self-esteem and self-confidence promote lasting changes.**
- Provide community health and online health resources for continued support with diet and exercise. **Lifestyle changes are challenging to maintain and require continued support to move to higher stages of readiness to change.**
- Emphasize importance of maintaining healthcare provider visits. **Follow-up visits with healthcare providers monitor improvement obtained and may require making changes to the plan of care due to metabolic improvement (e.g., blood pressure or blood glucose).**

Documentation Focus

Assessment/Reassessment

- Assessment findings, including readiness to change, client's perceptions, and desires for enhancing life

---

Information that appears in brackets has been added by the authors to clarify and enhance the use of nursing diagnoses.

- Cultural and spiritual belief
- Motivation and expectations for improvement

Planning
- Plan of care and who is involved in planning
- Teaching plan

Implementation/Evaluation
- Response to interventions, teaching, and action performed
- Attainment or progress toward desired outcome(s)
- Modifications to plan of care

Discharge Planning
- Identified long-term needs, individual goals for change, and who is responsible for actions to be taken
- Specific referral made

Sample Nursing Outcomes & Interventions Classifications NOC/NIC

NOC—Successful Aging
NIC—Health Coaching

---

ineffective HOME MAINTENANCE BEHAVIORS NANDA-I

[Diagnostic Division: Self-Care]

Definition: ineffective Home Maintenance Behaviors: Unsatisfactory pattern of knowledge and activities for the safe upkeep of one's residence.

Recognizing Cues

Related/Risk Factors
Competing demands; difficulty with decision making; inadequate organizational skills

Depressive symptoms; powerlessness; psychological distress; confusion

Unaddressed environmental constraints

Impaired physical mobility, or postural balance; inadequate physical endurance

Inadequate knowledge of home maintenance, or social resources

Inadequate role models, or social support

Information that appears in brackets has been added by the authors to clarify and enhance the use of nursing diagnoses.

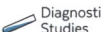 Diagnostic Studies 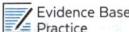 Evidence Based Practice 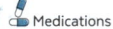 Medications ∞ Pediatric/Geriatric/Lifespan

Defining Characteristics

Subjective
Difficulty maintaining a comfortable [safe] environment
Home task-related anxiety, or stress; negative affect toward home maintenance

Objective
Cluttered, or unsanitary environment; neglected laundry; trash accumulation
Failure to request assistance with home maintenance
Impaired ability to regulate finances
Pattern of hygiene-related diseases
Unsafe cooking equipment

Clinical Connections
Chronic conditions (e.g., cardiovascular disorders, AIDS, multiple sclerosis [MS], rheumatoid arthritis, Parkinson disease), depression, dementia, developmental delay

Generate Solutions

Plan Desired Outcomes

Client Will (Include Specific Time Frame)
- Identify individual factors related to potential difficulty in maintaining a safe environment.
- Verbalize plan to eliminate health and safety hazards.
- Adopt behaviors reflecting lifestyle changes to create and sustain a healthy and growth-promoting environment.
- Demonstrate appropriate, effective use of resources.

Interventions/Take Action

Nursing Priority No. 1.
To assess contributing factors:

- Identify presence of or potential for conditions such as diabetes, fractures, spinal cord injury, amputation, MS, arthritis, stroke, Parkinson disease, dementia, mental illness, and poverty, **which can compromise client's/ significant other's (SO's) functional abilities in taking care of home.**
- Note personal or environmental factors (e.g., family member with multiple care tasks, addition of family member[s] [e.g., new baby, ill parent moving in]; substance abuse; poverty/ inadequate financial resources; absence of family/support systems; lifestyle of self-neglect; client comfortable with

---

Information that appears in brackets has been added by the authors to clarify and enhance the use of nursing diagnoses.

 Acute Care   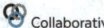 Collaborative   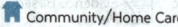 Community/Home Care   Cultural

home environment or has no desire for change) **that can contribute to neglect of home cleanliness or repair. Daily living and the home environment require routine cleaning and scheduled maintenance for health and safe living conditions.**

- Determine problems in the household and degree of discomfort or unsafe conditions noted by client/SO. **Some safety problems may be immediately obvious (lack of heat, water; need for laundry, garbage disposal, etc.), whereas other problems may be more subtle and difficult to manage (e.g., lack of sufficient finances for home repairs, lack of knowledge about food storage, indoor air and fire safety, rodent control).**
- Assess client's/SO's level of developmental, cognitive, emotional, and physical functioning **to ascertain client's needs and caregiver's capabilities when developing plan of care for preventive, supportive, and therapeutic care.**
- Identify lack of interest or knowledge or misinformation **to determine need for health education/home safety program or other intervention.**
- Identify support systems available to client/SO(s) **to determine needs and initiate referrals (e.g., companionship, daily care, respite care, homemaking, running errands, meal preparation or meal-service program, financial assistance).**
- Determine financial resources to meet needs of individual situation. **May need referral to social services for funds, necessary equipment, home repairs, transportation, and so forth.**

Nursing Priority No. 2.

To help client/SO(s) to create a safe, growth-promoting environment:

- Coordinate planning with multidisciplinary team and client/SO as appropriate. **Coordination and cooperation of team improve motivation and maximize outcomes.**
- Assist client/SO(s) to develop plan for restoring/maintaining a clean, healthful environment. **Activities such as sharing of household tasks or repairs among family members, contract services, exterminators, and trash removal can promote ongoing maintenance.**
- Educate and assist client/family to address lifestyle adjustments that may be required, such as personal/home hygiene practices, elimination of substance abuse or unsafe smoking habits, proper food storage, stress management, and so forth. **Individuals may not be aware of impact of these**

Information that appears in brackets has been added by the authors to clarify and enhance the use of nursing diagnoses.

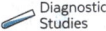 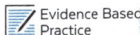 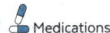 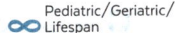

factors on their health or welfare; they may be overwhelmed and in need of specific assistance for varying periods of time.

- Discuss home environment or perform home visit, as indicated, **to determine client's ability to care for self, to identify potential health and safety hazards, and to determine adaptations that may be needed (e.g., wheelchair-accessible doors and hallways, safety bars in bathroom, safe place for child to play, clean water available, working cook stove or microwave; ability to control pests; safe food storage).**
- Assist client/SO(s) to identify and acquire necessary equipment and services (e.g., food delivery; bath assistance; aids for hearing, seeing, mobility; trash removal; cleaning supplies).
- Identify resources available for appropriate assistance (e.g., visiting nurse, social services, budget counseling, homemaker, Meals on Wheels, physical or occupational therapy, social services).
- Discuss options for financial assistance with housing needs. **Client may be able to stay in home with minimal assistance or may need significant assistance over a wide range of possibilities, including removal from the home.**

Nursing Priority No. 3.

To maintain safe environment (Teaching/Discharge Considerations) and enhance well-being (long-term goals):

- Evaluate client at each community contact or before facility discharge **to determine if home maintenance needs are ongoing in order to initiate appropriate referrals.**
- Discuss environmental hazards **that may negatively affect health or ability to perform desired activities.**
- Develop long-term plan **for taking care of environmental needs (e.g., assistive personnel, specialized controls for electrical equipment, trash removal, and pest control services).**
- Provide information necessary for the individual situation. **Helps client/family decide what can be done to improve situation.**
- Identify ways to access/use community resources and support systems (e.g., extended family, neighbors, church group, seniors' program).
- Refer to NDs excessive Caregiving Burden, impaired family Coping, difficulty Coping, risk for physical Injury, inadequate Health Knowledge, and Self-Care deficit [specify] for related interventions as appropriate.

Information that appears in brackets has been added by the authors to clarify and enhance the use of nursing diagnoses.

 Acute Care 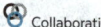 Collaborative 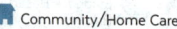 Community/Home Care 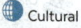 Cultural

Documentation Focus

Assessment/Reassessment
- Assessment findings, include individual (developmental, cognitive, emotional, and physical functioning) and environmental factors, specific safety concerns
- Availability and use of support systems

Planning
- Plan of care and who is involved in planning; support systems and community resources identified
- Teaching plan

Implementation/Evaluation
- Client's/SO's responses to interventions, teaching, and actions performed.
- Attainment or progress toward desired outcome(s).
- Modifications to plan of care.

Discharge Planning
- Long-term needs and who is responsible for actions to be taken.
- Specific referrals made, equipment needs/resources.

Sample Nursing Outcomes & Interventions Classifications NOC/NIC

NOC—Safe Home Environment
NIC—Home Maintenance Assistance

---

readiness for enhanced HOPE NANDA-I

[Diagnostic Division: Self-Perception/Self-Concept]

Definition: Pattern of expectations and desires for mobilizing energy to achieve positive outcomes, which can be strengthened.

Recognizing Cues

Defining Characteristics

Subjective
Desires to enhance initiative
Desires to enhance ability to set achievable goals, congruency of expectation with goal, problem-solving to meet goal

---

Information that appears in brackets has been added by the authors to clarify and enhance the use of nursing diagnoses.

Desires to enhance belief in possibilities, deep inner strength, spirituality, sense of meaning in life, positive outlook on life

Desires to enhance giving and receiving love

Desires to enhance response to unwanted health events, involvement with self-care, giving and receiving care

Clinical Connections

Any acute or chronic condition, or healthy individual looking to improve well-being

Generate Solutions

Plan Desired Outcomes

Client Will (Include Specific Time Frame)

- Identify and verbalize desire, ability, reason, and need to change lifestyle behaviors to improve mental and physical health expectations.
- Verbalize belief in possibilities for the future.
- Discuss current situation and desire to enhance hope.
- Set short-term goals that will lead to behavioral changes to meet desire and need for enhanced hope.

Interventions/Take Action

Nursing Priority No. 1.

To determine needs and desire for improvement:

- Review client's familial and social history to identify past situations (e.g., illness, emotional conflicts, alcoholism) that have led to decision to improve life. **When trials of life have been resolved, individuals may be optimistic about making life better.**
- Determine current physical/mental health condition of client/significant other(s) (SO[s]). **The treatment regimen and indicators of healing can influence and promote positive feelings of hope.**
- Identify client's perception of current state and expectations/goals for the future (e.g., general well-being, prosperity, independence).
- Identify spiritual beliefs and cultural values that influence sense of hope and connectedness and give meaning to life.
- Determine meaning of life or reasons for living, and belief in God or higher power. **Helps client to clarify beliefs and how they relate to desire for improvement in life.**
- Assess motivation and expectations for change. Note congruency of expectations with desires for change. **Motivation**

Information that appears in brackets has been added by the authors to clarify and enhance the use of nursing diagnoses.

to improve and high expectations can encourage client to make changes that will improve their life. However, presence of unrealistic expectations may hamper efforts.
- Determine degree of involvement in activities and relationships with others. **Superficial interactions with others can limit sense of connectedness and reduce enjoyment of relationships.**
- Using motivational interviewing, identify the stage of readiness to change behaviors (e.g., pre-contemplation, contemplation, preparation, action, and maintenance) for a healthy lifestyle. **Knowing client's current stage of readiness guides specific choice of interventions.**

Nursing Priority No. 2.

To assist client to achieve goals and strengthen sense of hope:

- Establish a therapeutic relationship (e.g., speaking respectfully, honoring and regarding the client as worthy of being a human being) showing hopefulness for the client. **Enhances feelings of worth and comfort, inspiring client to continue pursuit of goals.**
- Help client recognize areas that are in own control versus those that are not. **To be most effective, the client needs to expend energy in those areas where they have control/can make changes and let the others go.**
- Assist client to develop manageable short-term goals.
- Identify activities to achieve goals and facilitate contingency planning. **Promotes dealing with situation in manageable steps, enhancing chances for success and sense of control.**
- Explore interrelatedness of unresolved emotions, anxieties, fears, and guilt. **Provides an opportunity to address issues that may be limiting the individual's ability to improve own life situation.**
- Assist client to acknowledge current coping behaviors and defense mechanisms that are not helping the client move toward goals. **Allows client to focus on coping skills that are more successful in problem-solving.**
- Encourage the client to concentrate on progress not perfection. **If client can accept that perfection is difficult or not always the desirable outcome, they may be able to view accomplishments with pride.**
- Involve the client in care and explain all procedures, answering questions truthfully. **Enhances trust and relationship, promoting hope for a positive outcome.**

Information that appears in brackets has been added by the authors to clarify and enhance the use of nursing diagnoses.

- Express hope to client and encourage SO(s) and other health team members to do so. **Enhances client's sense of hope and belief in the possibility of a positive outcome.**
- Identify ways to strengthen a sense of interconnectedness or harmony with others **to support sense of belonging and connection that promotes feelings of wholeness and hopefulness.**

Nursing Priority No. 3.

To promote continued growth (Teaching/Discharge Considerations) and enhance well-being (long-term goals):

- Demonstrate and encourage the use of relaxation techniques, guided imagery, and meditation activities. **Learning to relax can decrease tension, resulting in refreshment of body and mind, enabling individual to perform and think more successfully.**
- Provide positive feedback for actions taken to improve problem-solving skills and for setting achievable goals. **This acknowledges the client's efforts and reinforces gains.**
- Explore how beliefs give meaning and value to daily living. **As the client's understanding of these issues improves, hope for the future is strengthened.**
- Encourage life-review by client. **Client acknowledging own successes while identifying opportunities for change and clarify meaning in life leads to positive outcomes.**
- Identify ways for client to express and strengthen spirituality. **There are many options for enhancing spirituality through connectedness with self/others (e.g., volunteering, mentoring, involvement in religious activities).**
- Encourage the client to join groups with similar or new interests. **Expanding knowledge and making friendships with new people will broaden horizons for the individual.**
- Refer to community resources and support groups, spiritual advisor, as indicated.

Documentation Focus

Assessment/Reassessment
- Assessment findings, including client's perceptions of current situation, relationships, sense of desire for enhancing life
- Motivation and expectations for improvement

Planning
- Plan of care and who is involved in planning
- Teaching plan

Information that appears in brackets has been added by the authors to clarify and enhance the use of nursing diagnoses.

 Acute Care  Collaborative 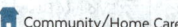 Community/Home Care Cultural

Implementation/Evaluation
- Responses to interventions, teaching, and actions performed
- Attainment of or progress toward desired outcome(s)
- Modifications to plan of care

Discharge Planning
- Long-term needs and goals for change, and who is responsible for actions to be taken
- Specific referrals made

Sample Nursing Outcomes & Interventions Classifications NOC/NIC

NOC—Hope
NIC—Hope Inspiration

---

inadequate HUMAN MILK PRODUCTION NANDA-I

[Diagnostic Division: Food/Fluid]

Definition: Insufficient lactation to exclusively meet the nutritional needs of an infant in the first 6 months of life.

Recognizing Cues

Related/Risk Factors
Parent Factors:
Inadequate fluid intake; inadequate knowledge about essential nutrients; inadequate vitamin intake

Inadequate behaviors to support human milk production; early introduction of formula

Provides inadequate opportunity for suckling; inadequate chestfeeding technique counseling

Inadequate knowledge of importance of initiating early chestfeeding; delayed initiation of chestfeeding

Inadequate chestfeeding opportunities in the workplace

Excessive stress; inadequate chestfeeding self-efficacy; inadequate family, or social support

Tobacco use; alcohol consumption; malnutrition

Ineffective overweight self-management

Difficulty managing complex treatment regimen [e.g., medication side effects—contraceptives, diuretics]

Information that appears in brackets has been added by the authors to clarify and enhance the use of nursing diagnoses.

 Diagnostic Studies 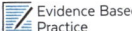 Evidence Based Practice 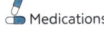 Medications ∞ Pediatric/Geriatric/Lifespan

Infant Factors:
Ineffective latching on; resisting latching on to nipple
Ineffective suckling reflex; inadequate suckling time at breast
Ineffective infant suck-swallow response
Refusal to chestfeed

Defining Characteristics

Objective
Parent:
Absence of milk duct engorgement despite sufficient stimulation; absence of milk production despite sufficient nipple stimulation
Expressed human milk is less than prescribed volume
Delayed milk production

Infant:
Feeding more than 12 times within a 24-hr period; prolonged chestfeeding time
Suckling is too rapid, or shallow; suckling without pause; unsustained suckling at breast
Crying at breast when positioned to chestfeed; frequent crying episodes shortly after chestfeeding
Urine output less than 2 mL/kg/hr in full-term infant; urine output less than 1 mL/kg/hr in preterm infant; urine specific gravity greater than 1.030
Constipation; feces that have not turned yellow by fifth day of life
Inadequate weight gain for age and gender

Clinical Connections
Postpartum hemorrhage; malnutrition; premature infant; infant cleft lip/pallet, adolescent mother; substances misuse

Generate Solutions

Plan Desired Outcomes

Client Will (Include Specific Time Frame)
- Develop plan to correct/change contributing factors.
- Demonstrate techniques to enhance milk production.
- Achieve mutually satisfactory breastfeeding pattern with infant content after feedings and gaining weight appropriately.

Information that appears in brackets has been added by the authors to clarify and enhance the use of nursing diagnoses.

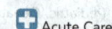 Acute Care 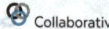 Collaborative 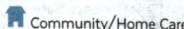 Community/Home Care Cultural

Interventions/Take Action

Nursing Priority No. 1.
To identify maternal causative or contributing factors:

- Engage in therapeutic nurse/client relationship. **Research reveals that a respectful professional relationship with client is an essential bridge to improving communication, encouraging sharing of feelings and concerns, detecting human milk insufficiency early, and implementing appropriate interventions.**
- Assess the mother's knowledge about breastfeeding and the extent of instruction that has been provided. **Lack of knowledge, unresolved problems, or stories told by others may cause client to doubt abilities and chances for success. Concern about insufficient milk supply is identified as a prevalent concern in 60% to 90% of mothers in low- and middle-income countries and is a primary reason for early breastfeeding cessation.**
- Identify cultural expectations and conflicts about breastfeeding and beliefs or practices regarding lactation, letdown techniques, and maternal food preferences. **Understanding the impact of culture and idiosyncrasies of specific feeding practices is important to determine the effect on infant breastfeeding success.**
- Note myths/misunderstandings, especially in teenage mothers, **who are more likely to have limited knowledge and more concerns about body image issues.**
- Identify maternal support systems and presence/response of significant others (SOs)/extended family. **Lack of support of partner/family or negative attitudes and comments interfere with efforts and may cause client to prematurely abandon attempt to breastfeed.**
- Perform a physical examination, noting the appearance of breasts and nipples, marked asymmetry of breasts, obvious inverted or flat nipples, and minimal or no breast enlargement during pregnancy. **Inadequate mammary gland tissue, breast surgery that has damaged the nipple, and areola enervation result in irremediable primary lactation failure.**
- Assess for other causes of primary lactation failure. **Maternal prolactin deficiency/serum prolactin levels, pituitary or thyroid disorders, and anemia may be corrected with medication.**
- Review lifestyle for common causes of secondary lactation failure. **Smoking, caffeine/alcohol use, lack of adequate**

Information that appears in brackets has been added by the authors to clarify and enhance the use of nursing diagnoses.

 Diagnostic Studies   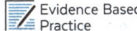 Evidence Based Practice   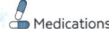 Medications   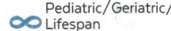 Pediatric/Geriatric/Lifespan

healthy food, becoming pregnant again, stress, and fatigue are known to inhibit milk production.
- Note medication/drug use. **Use of birth control pills containing estrogen or of medications such as antihistamines, decongestants, diuretics also inhibit milk production.**
- Determine the desire/motivation to breastfeed. **Increasing the milk supply can be intense, requiring commitment to therapeutic regimen and possible lifestyle changes.**

Nursing Priority No. 2.
To identify infant causative or contributing factors:

- Observe the infant at breast to evaluate latching-on skill and the presence of suck/swallow difficulties. **Poor latching on and lack of audible swallowing/gulp are associated with inadequate intake. The infant gets substantial amounts of milk when drinking with an open-pause-close type of suck. Note: Open-pause-close is one suck; the pause is not a pause between sucks.**
- Evaluate the signs of inadequate infant intake. **Infant arching and crying at the breast with resistance to latching on, decreased urinary output/frequency of stools, and inadequate weight gain indicate the need for further evaluation and intervention.**
- Review the feeding schedule—frequency, length of feeding, and taking one or both breasts at each feeding.

Nursing Priority No. 3.
To increase mother's milk supply:

- Instruct on how to differentiate between perceived and actual insufficient milk supply. **Normal breastfeeding frequencies, suckling times, and amounts not only vary among mothers but also are based on infant's needs/moods. Milk production is likely to be a reflection of the infant's appetite rather than the mother's ability to produce milk.**
- Provide emotional support to the mother. Use one-to-one instruction with each feeding during the hospital stay and clinic or home visits. Refer adoptive mothers choosing to breastfeed to a lactation consultant **to assist with induced lactation techniques.**
- Encourage unrestricted frequency and duration of breastfeeding. **Provides stimulation of breast tissue and may increase milk supply naturally.**
- Inform the mother how to assess and correct a latch if needed. Demonstrate an asymmetric latch aiming the

---

Information that appears in brackets has been added by the authors to clarify and enhance the use of nursing diagnoses.

infant's lower lip as far from the base of the nipple as possible, then bringing the infant's chin and lower jaw in contact with the breast while the mouth is wide open and before the upper lip touches the breast. **Correct latching on is the most effective way to stimulate milk supply.**

- Demonstrate the breast massage technique to increase milk supply naturally. **Gently massaging the breast while the infant feeds from it can improve the release of higher-calorie hindmilk from the milk glands.**
- Recommend using the breast pump 8 to 12 times a day. **Expressing with a hospital-grade, double (automatic) pump is ideal for stimulating/reestablishing milk supply.**
- Suggest using a breast pump or hand expression after the infant finishes breastfeeding. **Continued breast stimulation cues the mother's body that more milk is needed, increasing supply.**
- Monitor increased filling of breasts in response to nursing and/or pumping **to help evaluate the effectiveness of interventions.**
- Recommend reducing or stopping supplemental feedings if used. **Gradual tapering off of supplementation can increase frequency/duration of infant's breastfeeding, stimulating maternal milk production.**
- Discuss appropriate/safe use of herbal supplements. **Herbs such as sage, parsley, oregano, peppermint, jasmine, and yarrow may have a negative effect on milk supply if taken in large quantities. A number of herbs have been used for centuries to stimulate milk production, such as fenugreek (*Trigonella foenum-graecum*), the most commonly recommended herbal galactagogue to facilitate lactation.**
- Discuss the possible use of prescribed medications (galactagogue) to increase milk production. **Metoclopramide (Reglan) has been shown to increase milk supply by 72% to 110%, depending on how many weeks the mother is postpartum.**

Nursing Priority No. 4.

To promote optimal success and satisfaction of breastfeeding process for mother and infant:

- Encourage frequent rest periods, sharing household and childcare tasks. **Having assistance can limit fatigue (known to impact milk production) and facilitate relaxation at feeding time.**

Information that appears in brackets has been added by the authors to clarify and enhance the use of nursing diagnoses.

- Discuss with the spouse/SO the mother's requirement for rest, relaxation, and time together with family members. **Enhances understanding of mother's needs, and family members feel included and are therefore more willing to support breastfeeding activity/treatment plan.**
- Arrange a dietary consult to review nutritional needs and vitamin/mineral supplements, such as vitamin C, as indicated. **During lactation, there is an increased need for energy, requiring supplementation of protein, vitamins, and minerals to provide nourishment for the infant.**
- Emphasize the importance of adequate fluid intake. **Alternating types of fluids (e.g., water, juice, decaffeinated tea/coffee, and milk) enhances intake, promoting milk production. Note: Beer and wine are not recommended for increasing lactation.**
- Promote peer counseling for teen mothers. **Provides a positive role model that the teen can relate to and feel comfortable with discussing concerns and feelings.**
- Recommend monitoring the number of infant's wet and soiled diapers. **Stools should be yellow in color, and the infant should have at least six wet diapers a day to determine that the infant is receiving sufficient intake.**
- Weigh the infant every 3 days, or as directed by the primary provider/lactation consultant, and record. **Monitors weight gain, verifying the adequacy of intake or the need for additional interventions.**
- Identify products/programs for cessation of smoking. **Smoking can interfere with the release of oxytocin, which stimulates the letdown reflex.**
- Refer to support groups (e.g., La Leche League, parenting support groups, stress reduction, or other community resources), as indicated.

Documentation Focus

Assessment/Reassessment
- Identified maternal assessment factors—hydration level, medication use, lifestyle choices
- Infant assessment factors—latching-on technique, hydration level/number of wet diapers, weight gain/loss
- Use of supplemental feedings

Planning
- Plan of care, specific interventions, and who is involved in planning
- Individual teaching plan

Information that appears in brackets has been added by the authors to clarify and enhance the use of nursing diagnoses.

Implementation/Evaluation
- Mother's/infant's responses to interventions, teaching, and actions performed
- Change in infant's weight
- Attainment of or progress toward desired outcomes
- Modification to plan of care

Discharge Planning
- Specific referrals made

Sample Nursing Outcomes & Interventions Classifications NOC/NIC

NOC—Breastfeeding Maintenance
NIC—Lactation Counseling

---

neonatal HYPERBILIRUBINEMIA — NANDA-I

[Diagnostic Division: Safety]

Definition: Accumulation of unconjugated bilirubin in the circulation above the 95th percentile for age during first week of life.

Recognizing Cues

Related/Risk Factors
Inadequate fluid intake, or fluid volume
Inadequate meconium passage
Inadequate parental feeding behavior; malnourished infants

Defining Characteristics

Objective
Abnormal liver function test results
Bruised skin
Yellow mucous membranes or sclera; yellow-orange skin color

Clinical Connections
Newborns, premature infant

Information that appears in brackets has been added by the authors to clarify and enhance the use of nursing diagnoses.

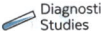 Diagnostic Studies 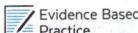 Evidence Based Practice 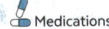 Medications Pediatric/Geriatric/Lifespan

Generate Solutions

Plan Desired Outcomes

Client Will (Include Specific Time Frame)
- Display decreasing bilirubin levels with resolution of jaundice.
- Be free of central nervous system (CNS) involvement or complications associated with therapeutic regimen.

Parent/Caregiver Will (Include Specific Time Frame)
- Verbalize an understanding of cause, treatment, and possible outcomes of hyperbilirubinemia.
- Demonstrate appropriate care of infant.

Interventions/Take Action

Nursing Priority No. 1.
To assess causative/contributing **or risk** factors:

- Evaluate presence of, potential for jaundice. Determine infant and maternal blood group and blood type, as indicated. **Jaundice is not uncommon in newborns. ABO incompatibility is more often seen in newborns who have type A blood (higher frequency of type A compared to type B in most populations). Incidence figures are difficult to compare because authors of different studies do not use the same definitions for significant neonatal hyperbilirubinemia or jaundice.**
- Note gender, race, and place of birth. **The risk of developing jaundice is higher in males and infants born at high altitudes and areas around the Mediterranean Sea, especially Greece. An increased prevalence of physiological jaundice is observed in infants of Southeast and East Asian ancestry (e.g., Chinese, Japanese, Korean), and Native American descent as well.**
- Review intrapartal record for specific factors, such as low birth weight (LBW) or intrauterine growth retardation (IUGR), prematurity, abnormal metabolic processes, vascular injuries, abnormal circulation, sepsis, or polycythemia. **The risk of significant neonatal jaundice is increased in LBW or premature infants, presence of congenital infection, or maternal diabetes.**
- Note the use of instruments or vacuum extractor for delivery. Assess the infant for the presence of birth trauma, cephalhematoma, and excessive ecchymosis or petechiae.

Information that appears in brackets has been added by the authors to clarify and enhance the use of nursing diagnoses.

Resorption of blood trapped in fetal scalp tissue and excessive hemolysis may increase the amount of bilirubin being released.

- Review infant's condition at birth, noting the need for resuscitation or evidence of excessive ecchymosis or petechiae, cold stress, asphyxia, or acidosis. **Asphyxia and acidosis reduce affinity of bilirubin to albumin, increasing the amount of unbound circulating (indirect) bilirubin, which may cross the blood-brain barrier, causing CNS toxicity.**
- Evaluate feeding patterns in newborn, noting if breastfed or formula-fed, and length of time breastfeeding, when indicated. **Jaundice occurs more frequently in breastfed infants than in formula-fed infants, possibly associated with poor caloric intake and dehydration. Therefore, increasing the frequency of breastfeeding may decrease the likelihood of significant hyperbilirubinemia.**
- Evaluate maternal and prenatal nutritional levels; note possible neonatal hypoproteinemia, especially in a preterm infant. **One gram of albumin carries 16 mg of unconjugated bilirubin; therefore, lack of sufficient albumin (hypoproteinemia) in the newborn increases the risk of jaundice.**
- Assess the infant for signs of hypoglycemia, such as jitteriness, irritability, and lethargy. Obtain heel-stick glucose levels as indicated. **Hypoglycemia necessitates the use of fat stores for energy-releasing fatty acids, which compete with bilirubin for binding sites on albumin.**
- Evaluate the infant for pallor, edema, or hepatosplenomegaly. **These signs may be associated with hydrops fetalis, Rh incompatibility, and in utero hemolysis of fetal red blood cells (RBCs).**
- Evaluate infant for jaundice in natural light, noting sclera and oral mucosa, yellowing of skin immediately after blanching, and specific body parts involved. Assess oral mucosa, posterior portion of hard palate, and conjunctival sacs in dark-skinned newborns.
- Note the infant's age at onset of jaundice, which aids in differentiating the type of jaundice (i.e., physiological, breast milk induced, or pathological). **Physiological jaundice usually appears between the second and third days of life, breast milk jaundice between the fourth and seventh days of life, and pathological jaundice occurs within the first 24 hr of life, or when the total serum bilirubin level rises by more than 5 mg/dL per day.**

Information that appears in brackets has been added by the authors to clarify and enhance the use of nursing diagnoses.

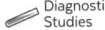 Diagnostic Studies 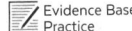 Evidence Based Practice Medications 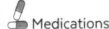 Pediatric/Geriatric/Lifespan

Nursing Priority No. 2.

To evaluate degree of compromise/prevent complications:

- Review laboratory studies, including total serum bilirubin and albumin levels, hemoglobin and hematocrit, and reticulocyte count.
- Calculate plasma bilirubin-albumin binding capacity. **Aids in determining the risk of kernicterus (a condition marked by the deposit of bile pigments in the nuclei of the brain and spinal cord and by degeneration of nerve cells) and treatment needs.**
- Assess the infant for progression of signs and behavioral changes associated with bilirubin toxicity. **Early-stage toxicity involves neuro-depression-lethargy, poor feeding, high-pitched cry, diminished or absent reflexes; late-stage toxicity signs may include hypotonia, neuro-hyperreflexia-twitching, convulsions, opisthotonos, and fever.**
- Evaluate the appearance of skin and urine, noting brownish-black color. **An uncommon side effect of phototherapy involves exaggerated pigment changes (bronze baby syndrome) that may last for 2 to 4 months but are not associated with harmful sequelae.**

Nursing Priority No. 3.

To **prevent onset of** or correct hyperbilirubinemia:

- Keep the infant warm and dry; monitor skin and core temperature frequently. **Prevents cold stress and the release of fatty acids that compete for binding sites on albumin, thus increasing the level of freely circulating bilirubin.**
- Initiate early oral feedings within 4 to 6 hr following birth, especially if infant is to be breastfed. **Establishes proper intestinal flora necessary for reduction of bilirubin to urobilinogen and decreases reabsorption of bilirubin from bowel.**
- Encourage frequent breastfeeding—8 to 12 times per day. Assist the mother with pumping of breasts, as needed, **to maintain/increase milk production.**
- Apply transcutaneous jaundice meter, as indicated. **Provides noninvasive screening of jaundice, quantifying skin color in relation to total serum bilirubin. Note: Although transcutaneous bilirubin (TcB) monitoring has gained widespread use in clinical settings, research is ongoing about whether TcB measurements are accurate during and after phototherapy.**

Information that appears in brackets has been added by the authors to clarify and enhance the use of nursing diagnoses.

 Acute Care 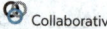 Collaborative 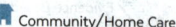 Community/Home Care Cultural

- Initiate phototherapy per protocol, using fluorescent blue lights placed above the infant or fiberoptic pad or blanket underneath (except for newborns with Rh disease). **Phototherapy is the primary therapy for neonates with unconjugated hyperbilirubinemia.**
- Apply eye patches, ensuring correct fit during periods of phototherapy, to prevent retinal injury. Remove eye covering during feedings or other care activities, as appropriate, **to provide visual stimulation and interaction with caregivers/parents.**
- Avoid application of lotion or oils to skin of infant receiving phototherapy **to prevent dermal irritation or injury.**
- Reposition the infant every 2 hr **to ensure that all areas of skin are exposed to bili light when fiberoptic pad or blanket is not used.**
- Cover male groin with small pad **to protect from heat-related injury to testes.**
- Monitor the infant's weight loss, urine output and specific gravity, and fecal water loss from loose stools associated with phototherapy **to determine adequacy of fluid intake.** *Note:* **The infant may sleep for longer periods in conjunction with phototherapy, increasing the risk of dehydration.**
- Administer IV immunoglobulin (IVIG) to neonates with Rh or ABO isoimmunization. **IVIG inhibits antibodies that cause red cell destruction, helping to limit the rise in bilirubin levels.**
- Administer enzyme induction agent (phenobarbital) as appropriate. **May be used on occasion to stimulate hepatic enzymes to enhance the clearance of bilirubin.**
- Assist with preparation and administration of exchange transfusion. **Exchange transfusions are occasionally required in cases of severe hemolytic anemia unresponsive to other treatment. Note: Although exchange transfusion in the preterm infant was common before 1980, recent data suggest that it is now rare (occurs currently in less than 0.5% of preterm infants).**
- Document events during transfusion, carefully recording amount of blood withdrawn and injected (usually 7 to 20 mL at a time). **Helps prevent errors in fluid replacement.**

Nursing Priority No. 4.
To promote wellness (Teaching/Discharge Considerations):

- Provide information about types of jaundice and pathophysiological factors and future implications of

---

Information that appears in brackets has been added by the authors to clarify and enhance the use of nursing diagnoses.

hyperbilirubinemia. **Promotes understanding, corrects misconceptions, and can reduce fear and feelings of guilt.**

- Review means of assessing infant status (feedings, intake and output, stools, temperature, and serial weights if scale available) and monitoring increasing bilirubin levels (e.g., observing blanching of skin over bony prominence or behavior changes), especially if the infant is to be discharged early. **Enables parents to monitor infant's progress and to recognize signs of increasing bilirubin levels.** *Note:* **Persistence of jaundice in formula-fed infant beyond 2 wk, or 3 wk in breastfed infant, requires further evaluation.**
- Review proper formula preparation/storage and demonstrate feeding techniques, as indicated, **to meet nutritional and fluid needs.**
- Refer to lactation specialist **to enhance or reestablish breastfeeding process.**
- Provide parents with 24-hr emergency telephone number and name of contact person, emphasizing importance of reporting increased jaundice or changes in behavior. **Promotes independence and provides for timely evaluation and intervention.**
- Arrange appropriate referral for home phototherapy program, if necessary.
- Provide a written explanation of home phototherapy, safety precautions, and potential problems. **Home phototherapy is recommended only for full-term infants after the first 48 hr of life, if serum bilirubin levels are between 14 and 18 mg/dL, with no increase in direct-reacting bilirubin concentration.**
- Make appropriate arrangements for follow-up testing of serum bilirubin at the same laboratory facility. **Treatment is discontinued once serum bilirubin concentrations reach 13 to 14 mg/dL. Untreated or chronic hyperbilirubinemia can lead to permanent CNS damage, demonstrated by conditions such as high-pitch hearing loss, cerebral palsy, or developmental difficulties.**
- Discuss possible long-term effects of hyperbilirubinemia and the need for continued assessment and early intervention, if indicated. **Neurological damage associated with kernicterus includes cerebral palsy, developmental delays, sensory difficulties, delayed speech, poor muscle coordination, learning difficulties, and death.**

Information that appears in brackets has been added by the authors to clarify and enhance the use of nursing diagnoses.

Documentation Focus

Assessment/Reassessment
- Assessment findings, risk or related factors
- Adequacy of intake—hydration level, character and number of stools
- Laboratory results and bilirubin trends

Planning
- Plan of care, specific interventions, and who is involved in the planning
- Teaching plan and resources provided

Implementation/Evaluation
- Client's responses to treatment and actions performed
- Parents' understanding of teaching
- Attainment of or progress toward desired outcome(s)
- Modifications to plan of care

Discharge Planning
- Long-range needs, identifying who is responsible for actions to be taken
- Community resources for equipment and supplies post discharge
- Specific referrals made

Sample Nursing Outcomes & Interventions Classifications NOC/NIC

NOC—Newborn Adaptation
NIC—Infant Care: Newborn
NIC—Photography: Neonate

HYPERTHERMIA NANDA-I

[Diagnostic Division: Safety]

Definition: Abnormal elevation of body temperature, usually as a result of inability to regulate core body temperature due to non-pathologic factors.

Information that appears in brackets has been added by the authors to clarify and enhance the use of nursing diagnoses.

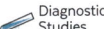 Diagnostic Studies 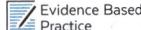 Evidence Based Practice 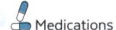 Medications 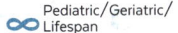 Pediatric/Geriatric/Lifespan

Recognizing Cues

Related/Risk Factors
Indoor temperatures greater than 26°C (78.8°F); continuous environmental heat stress
Inadequate fluid volume
Inappropriate clothing for environmental temperature; over-wrapping of infant for environmental temperature; inadequate moisture-wicking clothing
Vigorous activity; inadequate heat acclimation prior to increased physical activity

Defining Characteristics
Core Body Temperature
37.4°C (99.3°F) or higher in neonates
37.5°C (99.5°F) or higher in children
38.3°C (100.9°F) or higher in adults
Mild to Moderate Manifestations

Subjective
Feels feverish; intermittently hot and cold
Lightheadedness; headache
Nausea; muscle cramps
Fatigue; altered sleep-wake cycle

Objective
Flushed skin; skin warm to touch; pruritic erythematus
Excessive sweating; chilling
Dehydration; tachycardia
Irritability; decrease in cognition; impaired coordination
Mild peripheral edema
Infant does not maintain suck
Severe Manifestations

Subjective
Altered mental status; impaired judgment; increased anxiety symptoms; short-term memory loss
Inappropriate behavior; combativeness
Cold clammy skin; severe chills with violent shivering
Hypotension; vasodilation; altered cardiac output
Apnea; tachypnea
Coma; stupor; delirium; seizure
Electrolyte abnormalities; dysglycemia; lactic acidosis

Clinical Connections
Head trauma, hyperthyroidism, heat exhaustion or heatstroke, surgical procedure, anesthesia

---

Information that appears in brackets has been added by the authors to clarify and enhance the use of nursing diagnoses.

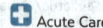 Acute Care 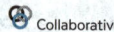 Collaborative 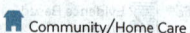 Community/Home Care Cultural

Generate Solutions

Plan Desired Outcomes

Client Will (Include Specific Time Frame)
- Maintain core temperature within normal range.
- Be free of complications, such as irreversible brain or neurological damage and acute renal failure.
- Identify underlying cause or contributing factors and importance of treatment, as well as signs/symptoms requiring further evaluation or intervention.
- Demonstrate behaviors to monitor and promote normothermia.
- Be free of seizure activity.

Interventions/Take Action

Nursing Priority No. 1.
To assess causative/contributing factors:

- Identify underlying cause. **Hyperthermia is defined as a body temperature greater than 40°C/104°F. The spectrum of heat-related illnesses includes heatstroke, heat exhaustion, heat syncope, heat edema, heat cramps, and heat rash; heatstroke is the most serious. Manifestation of heat-related illness can be associated with** *excessive heat production* **such as occurs with strenuous exercise, fever, shivering, tremors, convulsions, hyperthyroid state, malignant hyperpyrexia, and sympathomimetic drugs;** *impaired heat dissipation* **such as occurs with dermatologic diseases, burns, and inability to perspire such as occurs with spinal cord injury and certain medications (e.g., diuretics, sedatives, certain heart and blood pressure medications, and prescription amphetamines for attention deficit-hyperactivity disorder (ADHD); and** *loss of thermoregulation* **such as may occur in infections, brain lesions, and drug overdose.**
- Note chronological and developmental age of client. **People older than 65 years of age, young children, infants, pregnant women, clients with certain preexisting medical conditions (i.e., obesity, cardiovascular disease, cognitive impairment) or disabilities, outdoor workers, and athletes are at increased risk, as are persons living in lower-income households. Infants, young children, and elderly persons are most susceptible to damaging hyperthermia.**

Information that appears in brackets has been added by the authors to clarify and enhance the use of nursing diagnoses.

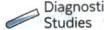 Diagnostic Studies 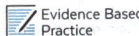 Evidence Based Practice 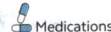 Medications 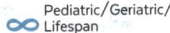 Pediatric/Geriatric/Lifespan

Environmental factors can produce a much higher temperature in infants and young children than in older children and adults. Infants, children, or impaired individuals are not able to protect themselves and cannot recognize and/or act on symptoms of hyperthermia. Elderly persons have age-related risk factors (e.g., poor circulation, inefficient sweat glands, skin changes caused by normal aging, chronic diseases, multiple medications [may include diuretics and blood pressure medications]). In the United States, youth football is significantly associated with emergency department evaluation for heat-related illness in clients ≤19 years of age. Nearly two-thirds of these incidents occur in the month of August. Medications, such as prescribed amphetamines and dietary creatine, may contribute to dehydration and heatstroke in client population.

- Determine recent client exposure to anesthetic drugs. **Malignant hyperthermia is an autosomal dominant genetic disorder often triggered by client exposure to volatile anesthetics or depolarizing muscle relaxants (e.g., sevoflurane, isoflurane; and succinylcholine, respectively).**
- ∞ Note diagnosis of traumatic brain injury (TBI). **Fever is a common symptom in TBI, often occurring in 20% to 50% of clients. However, advanced age has been identified as an independent predictor of poor outcomes of TBI-associated fever, possibly related to increased and accelerated rates of cerebral edema.**

Nursing Priority No. 2.
To evaluate effects/degree of hyperthermia:

- ∞ ✚ Monitor core temperature by appropriate route (e.g., rectal, esophageal, bladder probe). Note the presence of temperature elevation (>98.6°F [37°C]). **The hallmark indicators of heatstroke are the combination of central nervous system dysfunction and core body temperature greater than 104°F/40°C. The initial client assessment should include history, including recent heat exposure and exertion (i.e., client's occupation, degree of recent physical exertion, home environment) as well as individual risk factors (i.e., coexisting conditions, use of medications or other drugs). Heat-related illness may mimic other illnesses (e.g., sepsis, ischemic stroke, toxicological emergencies), and other etiologies should be considered; however, treatment for heatstroke should not be delayed.**

Information that appears in brackets has been added by the authors to clarify and enhance the use of nursing diagnoses.

- Assess whether body temperature reflects heatstroke. **Heatstroke is characterized by elevated body temperature higher than 104°F (40°C), hot, red, dry or damp skin; rapid, strong pulse; and neurological changes including confusion, agitation, slurred speech, seizures, and coma. "Heat stroke often presents in three phases: an hyperthermic–neurological acute phase, a hematologic–enzymatic phase (characterized by inflammation and coagulopathy and peaking at 24 to 48 hours after onset), and a late hepatic–renal phase (characterized by organ failure and occurring 96 hours or longer after onset)" (Sorensen & Hess, 2022).**
- Assess neurological responses, noting level of consciousness and orientation, reaction to stimuli, reaction of pupils, and presence of posturing or seizures. **High fever accompanied by changes in mentation (from confusion to delirium) may indicate heatstroke. A change in level of consciousness (e.g., confusion or delirium) "best differentiates heat stroke from heat exhaustion and other milder forms of heat-related illness" (Sorensen & Hess, 2022). Early signs include behavior changes, confusion, delirium, syncope, weakness, agitation, combativeness, slurred speech, nausea, and vomiting. Seizures and incontinence may occur.**
- Monitor blood pressure and invasive hemodynamic parameters if available (e.g., cardiac output, arterial pressures). **In heatstroke, tachycardia, tachypnea, and hypotension are common. Central hypertension or postural hypotension can occur, especially in person with preexisting cardiovascular disease if heat-related illness (e.g., heatstroke or malignant hyperthermia reaction to anesthesia) has rendered the client critically ill.**
- Monitor heart rate and rhythm. **Dysrhythmias and electrocardiogram (ECG) changes are common due to electrolyte and acid-base imbalances, dehydration, specific action of catecholamines, and direct effects of hyperthermia on blood and cardiac tissue.**
- Monitor respirations. **Hyperventilation may initially be present, but ventilatory effort may eventually be impaired by seizures or hypermetabolic state (shock and acidosis).**
- Auscultate breath sounds **to note presence and progression of adventitious sounds (rales), especially when heart failure is present.**

Information that appears in brackets has been added by the authors to clarify and enhance the use of nursing diagnoses.

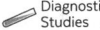 Diagnostic Studies   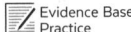 Evidence Based Practice   Medications   Pediatric/Geriatric/Lifespan

- Monitor and record all sources of fluid loss such as urine **(oliguria and/or renal failure may occur due to hypotension, dehydration, shock, and tissue necrosis),** vomiting and diarrhea, wounds, fistulas, and insensible losses, **which can potentiate fluid and electrolyte losses.**
- Note the presence or absence of sweating as the body attempts to increase heat loss by evaporation, conduction, and diffusion. **Evaporation is decreased by environmental factors of high humidity and high ambient temperature, as well as body factors producing loss of ability to sweat or sweat gland dysfunction (e.g., spinal cord transection, cystic fibrosis, dehydration, vasoconstriction).**
- Monitor laboratory studies, such as arterial blood gas (ABG) levels, electrolytes, and cardiac and liver enzymes **(may reveal tissue degeneration);** glucose; urinalysis **(myoglobinuria, proteinuria, and hemoglobinuria can occur as products of tissue necrosis);** and coagulation profile **(for presence of disseminated intravascular coagulation [DIC]).**

Nursing Priority No. 3.

To assist with measures to reduce body temperature/restore normal body/organ function:

- Administer antipyretics, orally or rectally (e.g., ibuprofen, acetaminophen), as ordered for non-heat-related conditions. Refrain from use of aspirin products in children **which may cause Reye syndrome or liver failure. For heat-related illness, "Antipyretic agents such as aspirin, ibuprofen, and acetaminophen are not recommended in heat stroke because fever and heat stroke raise core temperature through different physiological mechanisms. In addition, nonsteroidal anti-inflammatory agents theoretically risk exacerbating coagulopathy and renal injury. Acetaminophen (paracetamol) similarly risks exacerbating hepatic injury."**
- Manage mild heat-related illness with passive cooling (e.g., limited and lightweight, loose-fitting clothes [conduction] and cooling the environment with air-conditioning or fans [convection]) and rehydration. Provide active management with convective cooling (e.g., use of fans) and infusion of cold fluids for moderate heat-related cases. Other interventions include cooling blankets, ice-water slurry client saturation, urinary catheter irrigation, ice water sheets/towels (i.e., whole-body conductive cooling). **Critical rescue for heatstroke starts with removal of the client from the**

Information that appears in brackets has been added by the authors to clarify and enhance the use of nursing diagnoses.

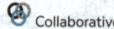 Acute Care 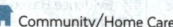 Collaborative 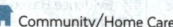 Community/Home Care 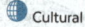 Cultural

heat source and supportive care of airway, breathing, and circulation (ABCs). Once the client's ABCs have been stabilized, rapid cooling should begin quickly with a target temperature reduction to 39°C to 39.2°C (102°F to 102.5°F) within 30 min of symptom onset (preferably 0.20°C to 0.35°C per minute). Cold water immersion is the preferred strategy for rapid temperature reduction but is not always feasible.

- Provide evaporative cooling (e.g., spraying child with cold water/fan utilization). **Preferred treatment for hospitalized child because of limited interference with monitoring and ongoing resuscitation while achieving rapid temperature reduction to prevent end-organ damage and mortality related to the duration of hyperthermia. Note: Preadmission care of child with heatstroke includes cold water immersion after stabilization of ABCs.**
- Monitor for shivering and continue monitoring vital signs and hemodynamic values. Perform skin assessment during the cooling process and cover ice packs with a towel or sheet and regularly adjust application site. **Shivering may cause significant client discomfort and may increase heat retention. Critically ill clients may further decompensate during initial cooling interventions. Additionally, if a client's body temperature drops below normal (36°C), they will be at risk for the sequelae of hypothermia, including dysrhythmias and coagulopathy. Skin is susceptible to damage from prolonged exposure to ice and covering ice packs and adjusting application site will decrease this risk.**
- Turn off hypothermia blanket when core temperature is within 1 to 3 degrees of desired temperature. **Allow for downward drift. Current guidelines suggest a target temperature of 38.3°C to 38.8°C (100.9°F to 101.8°F) when actively cooling heatstroke victims.**
- Administer medications (e.g., chlorpromazine or diazepam) as ordered **to control shivering and seizures.**
- Assist with internal cooling methods to treat malignant hyperthermia such as cool IV fluids, urinary bladder irrigation **to promote rapid core cooling.**
- Promote client safety (e.g., maintain patent airway; padded side rails; quiet environment; mouth care for dry mucous membranes; skin protection from cold; observation of equipment safety measures).
- Provide supplemental oxygen **to offset increased oxygen demands and consumption.**

Information that appears in brackets has been added by the authors to clarify and enhance the use of nursing diagnoses.

- Administer medications, as indicated to treat underlying cause, such as dantrolene **(for malignant hyperthermia)** or beta-adrenergic blockers **(for thyroid storm).**
- Administer replacement fluids and electrolytes **to support circulating volume and tissue perfusion.**
- Maintain bedrest **to reduce metabolic demands and oxygen consumption.**
- Provide high-calorie diet, enteral nutrition, or parenteral nutrition **to meet increased metabolic demands.**

Nursing Priority No. 4.

To maintain normothermia (Teaching/Discharge Considerations) and enhance well-being (long-term goals):

- Instruct the parents in how to measure the child's temperature, at what body temperature to give antipyretic medications, and what symptoms to report to the physician. **Fever may be treated at home to relieve the general discomfort and lethargy associated with fever. Fever is reportable, however, especially in infants or very young children with or without other symptoms and in older children or adults if it is unresponsive to antipyretics and fluids, because it often accompanies a treatable infection (viral or bacterial).**
- Review specific risk factor or cause, such as (1) underlying conditions (hyperthyroidism, dehydration, neurological diseases, nausea, vomiting, sepsis); (2) use of certain medications (diuretics, blood pressure medications, alcohol or other drugs [cocaine, amphetamines]); (3) environmental factors (exercise or labor in hot environment, lack of air-conditioning, lack of acclimatization); (4) reaction to anesthesia (malignant hyperthermia); or (5) other risk factors (salt or water depletion, elderly living alone).
- Identify those factors that the client can control (if any), such as (1) treating underlying disease process (e.g., thyroid control medication), (2) protecting oneself from excessive exposure to environmental heat (e.g., proper clothing, restriction of activity, scheduling outings during cooler part of day, use of fans/air-conditioning where possible), and (3) understanding family traits (e.g., malignant hyperthermia reaction to anesthesia is often familial).
- Instruct families/caregivers (of young children, persons who are outdoors in very hot climate, elderly living alone) in the dangers of heat exhaustion and heatstroke and ways to manage hot environments. Caution parents to avoid leaving young children in an unattended car, emphasizing the

---

Information that appears in brackets has been added by the authors to clarify and enhance the use of nursing diagnoses.

extreme hazard to the child in a very short period of time **to prevent heat injury and death.**
- Discuss importance of adequate fluid intake at all times and ways to improve hydration status when ill or when under stress (e.g., exercise, hot environment) **to prevent dehydration.**
- Review signs/symptoms of hyperthermia (e.g., flushed skin, increased body temperature, increased respiratory and heart rate, fainting, loss of consciousness, seizures). **Indicates a need for prompt intervention.**
- Recommend avoidance of hot tubs and saunas, as appropriate (**e.g., clients with multiple sclerosis and cardiac conditions; during pregnancy, as the high temperature may affect fetal development or increase cardiac workload**).
- Identify community resources, especially for elderly clients, to address specific needs (**e.g., provision of fans for individual use, location of cooling rooms—usually in a community center—during heat waves, daily telephone contact to assess wellness**).

Documentation Focus

Assessment/Reassessment
- Temperature and other assessment findings, including vital signs and state of mentation

Planning
- Plan of care, specific interventions, and who is involved in the planning
- Teaching plan

Implementation/Evaluation
- Responses to interventions, teaching, and actions performed
- Attainment of or progress toward desired outcome(s)
- Modifications to plan of care

Discharge Planning
- Referrals that are made, those responsible for actions to be taken

Sample Nursing Outcomes & Interventions Classifications NOC/NIC

NOC—Thermoregulation
NIC—Hyperthermia Management:

Information that appears in brackets has been added by the authors to clarify and enhance the use of nursing diagnoses.

 Diagnostic Studies 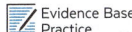 Evidence Based Practice 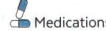 Medications 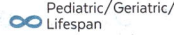 Pediatric/Geriatric/Lifespan

risk for disrupted **IMMIGRATION TRANSITION**

NANDA-I

[Diagnostic Division: Stress Management]

Definition: Susceptible to negative feelings and consequences during the process of relocation and adjustment from country of origin.

Recognizing Cues

Related/Risk Factors
Available work below educational preparation
Communication or cultural barriers; parent-child conflicts related to enculturation
Inadequate knowledge about accessing resources; inadequate social support; overt social discrimination
Overcrowded housing; inadequate environmental hygiene

Generate Solutions

Plan Desired Outcomes

Client Will (Include Specific Time Frame)
- Verbalize understanding of current situation.
- Develop plan to address identified issues.
- Engage in activities to overcome issues impacting transition to new life.
- Express optimism about outcome of transition.

Interventions/Take Action

Nursing Priority No. 1.
To determine underlying dynamics of individual situation:
- Determine circumstances of migration, nature of the voluntary/involuntary move, acculturation since arrival, and ability to maintain self-identity. **These individuals/families face multiple consequences and barriers that are specific to their situation and require unique solutions.**
- Note age and gender of immigrant. **A growing number of older people are immigrating and face economic disadvantages. Midlife women who immigrate show more depressive symptoms than nonimmigrants. Young children are more likely to have health rated as "poor" or "fair," and their health tends to decline more rapidly as they age versus citizens by birth in economically stable countries.**

Information that appears in brackets has been added by the authors to clarify and enhance the use of nursing diagnoses.

 Acute Care    Collaborative   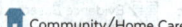 Community/Home Care   Cultural

- Determine primary language and ability to speak, read, and understand the language of the host country. **Acculturation is slowed when dominant language is not understood by client/family members.**
- Identify level of stress being experienced (e.g., anxiety, inadequate housing, difficulty sleeping, changes in eating habits, language barriers, social rejection, poverty, and substance misuse). **Difficulties encountered with relocation can impair coping and general well-being. Substance misuse, frustration, anger, hostility, and violence may occur in the family unit. Note: A recent study addressed the emotional stress and possibility of mental illness brought on by immigration stress, especially in those forced to migrate and experiencing the trauma of leaving their home country, unemployment issues and other difficulties in the new country resulting in higher rates of mental illness in certain refugee communities.**
- Identify current coping strategies and past skills used. **Bringing to mind previous situations in which the individual functioned successfully can help client to use these skills in the current situation and provides opportunity to learn new skills.**
- Determine financial situation and access to and use of available resources. **Provides insight for client/family needs and possible options to lessen stressors and facilitate integration into community/society.**

Nursing Priority No. 2.

To promote integration of immigrants into new environment:

- Obtain services of an interpreter and bilingual written materials/videos, as indicated. **Note: An interpreter working in healthcare must be trained to understand differences in colloquialisms used in the native language and be aware of providing respectful interactions and maintain Health Insurance Portability and Accountability Act regulations.**
- Allow sufficient time for discussions, information exchanges, and teaching. **Lack of/weak language skills may impede communications. If client feels rushed, they may falsely indicate understanding.**
- Identify resources for English as second language classes.
- Designate a primary nurse or "family nurse" who can coordinate the team, aiding the family as appropriate. **Additional services lead to empowering family to develop a well-functioning daily life and adaptation to their new environment.**

Information that appears in brackets has been added by the authors to clarify and enhance the use of nursing diagnoses.

- Make home visits, as appropriate, noting family identity, communication pattern/interactions, relationships, parenting style, family member roles, socialization of family members, conflicts/conflict resolution, and safety concerns. **Provides opportunity to observe client/family in more relaxed surroundings, identify issues to be addressed, answer questions, and impart needed information.**
- Discuss changes from previous life to new circumstances and expectations for the future. **Acculturation is a complex social and psychological process implying cultural learning, and behavioral adaptation to a nonnative country takes time, tolerance, persistence, and patience.**
- Identify cultural differences, value conflicts, and similarities. **Transition is complicated when long-held beliefs/values and traditional family roles are in conflict with those of host country. Recognizing and addressing conflicts while accepting that differences will exist allow client to build on similarities, facilitating adaptation while maintaining their identity.**
- Provide useful resources as desired for immigrants to learn new lifestyle (e.g., food, dress, language, manner of interacting). **Can assist in efforts to "blend in" and relate to others.**
- Encourage participation in community activities, sporting events, neighborhood gatherings, and governmental affairs as interested. **Provides opportunity to socialize and learn various aspects of new society.**
- Assist immigrants, especially seniors and children, to navigate language barriers and improve health literacy. **While these problems affect most immigrants, seniors 65 years or older are a growing proportion of immigrants (an estimated 34.3 million) with all the resultant problems of managing how to survive on limited resources. In addition, globally there is an increase of 230% in young migrants 15 to 24 years of age who have been forced into exile from their country of origin (Migration Data Portal). These two groups especially tend to have greater healthcare needs.**
- Identify cultural/spiritual resources, ethnic organizations, and support groups. **Provides mentors in new culture to introduce immigrants to local business, engage in spiritual practices, and visit other facilities where immigrants can find support and guidance as they progress toward acculturation.**

Information that appears in brackets has been added by the authors to clarify and enhance the use of nursing diagnoses.

🅲 Acute Care   ⓒ Collaborative   🏠 Community/Home Care   🌐 Cultural

Nursing Priority No. 3.

To assist immigrants to improve quality of life (Teaching/Discharge Considerations) and enhance well-being (long-term goals):

- Encourage client/family to identify positives in life to build on. **Assists client/family to find hope for the future.**
- Identify community resources/programs such as emergency housing, utilities, transportation, Supplemental Nutrition Assistance Program (SNAP)/pantries, and clothing/home goods assistance.
- Refer to vocational counselor/resources as indicated. **Helpful for evaluating marketable skills, developing resume, preparing for interview, and obtaining additional education as appropriate to gain employment and provide for family.**
- Provide assistance with health/behavioral issues that may occur, identifying healthcare and counseling resources available to client/family. **The changes incurred with the transition from the old to the new country markedly increase stressors, impacting role performance of family members and family cohesiveness, negatively affecting both physical and psychological well-being of client/family. Families leaving a war-torn country may have experienced trauma that will require specialized counseling depending on their experiences.**

Documentation Focus

Assessment/Reassessment
- Individual findings regarding immigrant's circumstances
- Immigrant's perception of what has happened, specific stressors
- Language(s) spoken, fluency with language of host country
- Perceived cultural barriers
- Safety concerns

Planning
- Plan of care and who is involved in planning
- Teaching plan

Implementation/Evaluation
- Response to interventions, teaching, actions performed
- Attainment of or progress toward desired outcome(s)
- Modifications to plan of care

Information that appears in brackets has been added by the authors to clarify and enhance the use of nursing diagnoses.

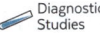 Diagnostic Studies   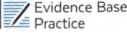 Evidence Based Practice   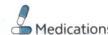 Medications   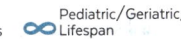 Pediatric/Geriatric/Lifespan

Discharge Planning
- Long-term needs and goals, and who is responsible for actions to be taken
- Specific referrals made

Sample Nursing Outcomes & Interventions Classifications NOC/NIC

NOC—Relocation Adaptation
NIC—Relocation Stress Reduction

IMMUNOLOGIC IMPAIRMENT ICNP

[Diagnostic Division: Safety]

Definition: Increased risk of infection and failure to regain a state of health due to quantitative or qualitative immune system dysfunction.

Recognizing Cues

Related/Risk Factors
Autoimmune disorders (primary or secondary)
Chemotherapy, immunosuppressive therapy
Radiation therapy/treatment
Malnutrition
Significant burn injury

Defining Characteristics

Subjective
Fatigue; malaise
Depressive symptoms; hopelessness; low self-efficacy
Gastrointestinal upset, anorexia
Autoimmune disorders

Objective
Frequent/protracted infection
Unexplained fever, weight loss, or night sweats
Rashes, pruritus, or redness; hair loss
Swollen lymph nodes
Constipation, gas, diarrhea
Hematologic abnormalities; low platelet count, anemia
Delayed growth and development

Information that appears in brackets has been added by the authors to clarify and enhance the use of nursing diagnoses.

 Acute Care 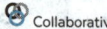 Collaborative 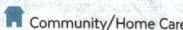 Community/Home Care   Cultural

Clinical Connections
HIV positive, AIDS, cancer, chemotherapy, malnutrition, long-term use of steroids (e.g., asthma, rheumatoid arthritis, systemic lupus erythematosus [SLE]), diabetes mellitus, substance abuse, burns, tuberculosis

Generate Solutions

Plan Desired Outcomes

Client Will (Include Specific Time Frame)
- Be free of infection.
- Maintain effective response in presence of pathogen exposure or injury.

Caregiver Will (Include Specific Time Frame)
- Verbalize understanding of client risk and provide supportive measures to keep client free of infection

Interventions/Take Action

Nursing Priority No. 1.
To determine risk/contributing factors:
- Assess client for host-specific factors that affect immunity: Presence of underlying disease or dysfunction: Altered immunocompetence can be subdivided into primary or secondary. *Primary immunodeficiency* is typically characterized by congenital deficiencies of cellular, humoral, or both components of adaptive immunity (e.g., severe combined immunodeficiency [SCID], ataxia-telangiectasia, DiGeorge syndrome, X-linked agammaglobulinemia, etc.). *Secondary immunodeficiency* is acquired and characterized by loss or deficiency in cellular or humoral immune components that occur as a result of disease or its therapy (e.g., AIDS, severe malnutrition, major burns, diabetes, nephrotic syndrome, asplenia, measles, certain cancers [i.e., leukemia, lymphoma, multiple myeloma]).

∞ Extremes of age: Newborns and the elderly are more susceptible to disease and infection than the general population. **The immune system of infants and young children (i.e., less than 24 months old) are developmentally immature and lack sufficient exposure for a robust adaptive immune response. Production and function of T cells begin to wane at age 40 years. Physiological changes in the aging client's immune function associated with client comorbidities create a specific risk profile for each client.**

Information that appears in brackets has been added by the authors to clarify and enhance the use of nursing diagnoses.

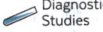 Diagnostic Studies   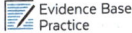 Evidence Based Practice   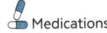 Medications   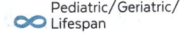 Pediatric/Geriatric/Lifespan

- Certain medications: Steroids, immunosuppressive agents (e.g., tacrolimus, cyclosporine), antimetabolites (e.g., methotrexate, 5-fluorouracil [5-FU]), phenytoin, and chemotherapeutic agents **affect the immune system and may compromise the client's ability to ward off and fight infection. Long-term or improper antibiotic treatment can be detrimental by disrupting the client's normal flora, causing an overgrowth of endogenous organisms and/or increased susceptibility to antibiotic-resistant organisms.**
- Certain treatment settings/modalities: Clients in an acute/critical-care setting may have additional infection risk based on the use of invasive monitoring and supportive devices (e.g., extracorporeal membrane oxygenation [ECMO], continuous renal replacement therapy [CRRT], mechanical ventilation, urinary catheter, central venous access, ventriculostomy tubes, chest tubes, etc.) and conditions compromising breathing, circulation, gastrointestinal motility, mobility, etc. **Client condition and the required treatment or monitoring strategies require vigilant and judicious nursing care to prevent client harm.**
- Trauma: Loss of skin or tissue via invasive surgical or diagnostic procedures, pressure injury, premature rupture of amniotic membranes, urinary catheterizations, etc.
- Nutritional status: Malnutrition weakens the immune system; poor oral intake, insufficient essential nutrients, inadequate food preparation, improper handling of tube feedings/infant formula; elevated serum glucose levels (e.g., administration of total parenteral nutrition or poorly controlled diabetes mellitus) **increase the risk for pathogen proliferation.**
- Lifestyle: Personal habits or living situations, such as persons sharing close quarters and/or equipment (e.g., college dorm, group home, long-term care facility, day care, large public assembly facilities, correctional facility); persons/groups with inadequate vaccination protection; and IV drug use, shared needles, and unprotected sex **can increase susceptibility to infections.**
- Presence or absence of immunity: Natural immunity may be acquired by development of antibodies to a specific agent following infection or vaccination, preventing the recurrence of the specific disease or infecting agent (e.g., chickenpox, measles, etc.). **Clients with immunologic impairment may be unable to produce an adequate or quality response to antigen exposure, thus, in the immunologically impaired client, exposure may not equate to immunity.**

Information that appears in brackets has been added by the authors to clarify and enhance the use of nursing diagnoses.

Nursing Priority No. 2.

To reduce/correct existing risk factors:

- Wear gloves to minimize hand contamination and perform hand hygiene after glove removal.
- Instruct client/significant other (SO)/visitors to wash hands, as indicated.
- Follow universal precautions and provide for isolation needs as indicated (e.g., contact, droplet, airborne precautions, etc.). Educate staff in infection-control procedures. **Reduces risk of cross-contamination.**
- Emphasize proper use of personal protective equipment (PPE) by staff/visitors as dictated by agency policy for particular exposure risk (e.g., airborne, droplet, contact).
- Institute neutropenic precautions, as appropriate.
- Ensure adequate supply and easy access to appropriate PPE (i.e., gloves, face masks, goggles, and isolation gowns) **to facilitate and promote PPE utilization.**
- Provide a single-client clean, well-ventilated environment.
- Ensure client's environment is cleaned and disinfected regularly, per agency policy, including bed rails, over-bed tables, doorknobs, bathroom, toys in pediatric areas, etc.
- Monitor client's visitors/caregivers for illness. Restrict interpersonal contact when necessary **to limit exposures and reduce cross-contamination.**
- Provide hand sanitizer, tissues, and no-touch receptacles (e.g., foot-pedal-operated lid, open, plastic-lined wastebasket) **for disposal of potentially infectious material.**
- Post signs in public areas (e.g., entrances, cafeterias, elevators) with instructions for visitors **to limit visitation if symptoms of respiratory infection, cough, or sneezing.**
- Discuss with client limiting exposure to pediatric visitors while in the acute care setting.
- Encourage early ambulation, deep breathing, coughing, position changes, and early removal of endotracheal and/or nasal or oral feeding tubes **to mobilize respiratory secretions and prevent aspiration and respiratory infections.**
- Monitor and assist client with use of prophylactic devices (e.g., incentive spirometry, flutter valve, etc.) to prevent infection.
- Perform or assist client/SO with daily mouth care and personal hygiene. **Utilization of routine antimicrobial hygiene (e.g., daily bathing with chlorhexidine gluconate [CHG], antiseptic mouthwash) for individuals in acute or long-term care settings at high risk for healthcare-associated infections, has a significant impact.**

Information that appears in brackets has been added by the authors to clarify and enhance the use of nursing diagnoses.

- Provide client with preoperative measures (i.e., bowel prep, pre-op hygiene, etc.) and teaching (e.g., respiratory measures to prevent pneumonia, wound or dressing care, avoidance of others with infection) **to reduce the potential for postoperative infection.**
- Administer and monitor medication regimen, as ordered (e.g., antimicrobials, immunizing agents, etc.) **for treatment and/or infection prophylaxis.**
- Administer enteral or parenteral nutrition **to ensure adequate nutritional support and client healing.**
- Maintain adequate hydration and electrolyte balance **to prevent imbalances that would predispose to infection.**
- Maintain aseptic technique for administration of parenteral medications, handling of IV lines, and invasive interventions (e.g., bedside insertion of central lines or parenteral access, wound care, urinary catheterization, etc.) and discontinue devices as soon as indicated.
- Monitor and trend laboratory values (e.g., complete blood cell count [i.e., granulocyte count and differential results], blood glucose, cultures [i.e., blood, urine, sputum, or wound]), immunoglobulin levels, etc., **to identify the presence of pathogens and treatment options. Clients with altered immunocompetence often require peripheral blood smears to evaluate the components of cell-mediated and humoral immunity.**
- Monitor client for systemic and localized signs/symptoms of infection, and promptly report findings to healthcare provider. (Refer to ND risk for Infection for related assessments and interventions.)
- Offer client/SO/caregiver(s) vaccinations as indicated and appropriate **to prevent infection and reduce infection exposure. Note: Clients with compromised immune function may need vaccinations delayed to prevent illness or promote an opportunity for a more robust immune response and subsequent client protection.**
- Emphasize the necessity of taking medications such as antivirals or antibiotics as directed (e.g., dosage and length of therapy). **Premature discontinuation of treatment when client begins to feel well may result in the return of infection and potentiate drug-resistant strains.**
- Provide education to client/SO regarding signs and symptoms of infection and when to report them to healthcare provider.

Information that appears in brackets has been added by the authors to clarify and enhance the use of nursing diagnoses.

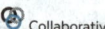 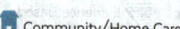

- Encourage client/SO/caregiver(s) to participate in immunization/vaccination programs, as indicated and appropriate **to prevent infection and reduce infection exposure. Note: Clients with compromised immune function may need to receive attenuated vaccines.**
- Encourage client/SO/caregiver(s) to contact their healthcare provider for prophylactic therapy as indicated following exposure to individuals with infectious disease (e.g., tuberculosis, hepatitis, influenza).
- Provide education to client/SO/caregiver(s) how to avoid infections:

    Cleanse incisions/breaks in client's skin with appropriate antimicrobial **to prevent the growth of microorganisms.**

    Encourage client to wear a face mask in a crowded environment.

    Recommend client avoid self-serve buffets/salad bars.

    Provide education to client/SO/caregiver to avoid uncooked or undercooked foods (e.g., eggs, rare burgers and steaks), soft cheeses, and uncooked deli meats.

    Discourage client from sharing towels, eating utensils, or drinking cups with anyone, even family members—especially children.

    Discourage the use of humidifiers or vaporizers.

    Provide education and instruct client to avoid animal exposure (e.g., litter box, bird cage, etc.).

    Provide education to client/SO/caregiver to protect from insect bites/stings (e.g., wear loose-fitting clothing, use insect repellant, remove standing water from near client's home, etc.).

Nursing Priority No. 3.

To promote effective immunologic function (Teaching/Discharge Considerations) and enhance well-being (long-term goals):

- Review and educate client/SO/caregiver regarding client's specific nutritional needs, appropriate exercise program, and need for rest **to enhance immune system function and healing.**
- Instruct client/SO(s) in techniques to protect the integrity of skin, care for lesions, measure temperature, and prevent spread of infection in the home setting **to provide basic knowledge for self-help and self-protection.**
- Discuss the role of smoking and secondhand smoke in respiratory infections and postoperative healing. Refer to smoking cessation programs as indicated.

Information that appears in brackets has been added by the authors to clarify and enhance the use of nursing diagnoses.

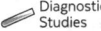 Diagnostic Studies 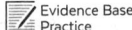 Evidence Based Practice 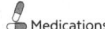 Medications 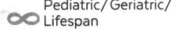 Pediatric/Geriatric/Lifespan

- Promote safer sex practices to prevent the spread of HIV or other sexually transmitted infections.
- Promote childhood immunization program. Encourage adults to update immunizations as appropriate.
- Review client's need for prophylactic antibiotics (e.g., before dental work for clients with a history of rheumatic fever, heart valve replacements).
- Identify resources available to client (e.g., substance abuse or rehabilitation, needle-exchange program as appropriate; available or free condoms).
- Provide client/SO with information regarding appropriate community and national education programs **to increase awareness and prevention of communicable diseases.**
- Refer to NDs ineffective Health Maintenance Behaviors and ineffective Home Maintenance Behaviors for additional interventions as appropriate.

Documentation Focus

Assessment/Reassessment
- Individual risk factors present, including recent and current medication and/or treatment therapies
- Significant failure of immune response associated with congenital or acquired conditions
- Signs/symptoms of infectious process

Planning
- Plan of care, specific interventions, and who is involved in planning
- Teaching plan

Implementation/Evaluation
- Responses to interventions, teaching, and actions performed
- Attainment or progress toward desired outcome(s)
- Modifications to plan of care

Discharge Planning
- Discharge needs and who is responsible for actions to be taken
- Specific referrals made

Sample Nursing Outcomes & Interventions Classifications NOC/NIC

NOC—Immune Status
NIC—Risk Identification: Infectious Disease

Information that appears in brackets has been added by the authors to clarify and enhance the use of nursing diagnoses.

ineffective IMPULSE CONTROL NANDA-I

[Diagnostic Division: Self-Perception/Self-Concept]

Definition: Pattern of unsatisfactory, rapid, unplanned, and uncontrolled reactions to internal or external stimuli without regard for the negative consequences.

Recognizing Cues

Related/Risk Factors
Confusion; impaired memory
Impaired verbal communication
Hopelessness; mood disorders
Tobacco use; substance misuse

Defining Characteristics

Subjective
Asking personal questions despite discomfort of others
Impaired ability to regulate finances

Objective
Inappropriate sharing of personal details; overly familiar with strangers
Irritable mood, temper tantrums, verbally and physically aggressive
Gambling addiction; sensation seeking; sexual promiscuity
Irritable mood; bedtime procrastination

Clinical Connections
Eating disorders, addictions—substance/sexual, anxiety, depression, bipolar disorders, schizophrenic disorders, dementia, attention deficit-hyperactivity disorder (ADHD), antisocial, borderline and narcissistic personality disorders, oppositional defiant and conduct disorders, traumatic brain injury, Down syndrome, autism spectrum disorder (ASD), Parkinson disease, obsessive-compulsive disorder; developmental delays

Generate Solutions

Plan Desired Outcomes

Client Will (Include Specific Time Frame)
- Acknowledge problem with impulse control.
- Identify thoughts and feelings that precede desire to engage in impulsive actions.

Information that appears in brackets has been added by the authors to clarify and enhance the use of nursing diagnoses.

 Diagnostic Studies 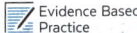 Evidence Based Practice 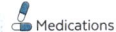 Medications 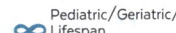 Pediatric/Geriatric/Lifespan

- Verbalize desire to learn new ways of controlling impulsive behavior.
- Participate in anger management therapy.

Interventions/Take Action

Nursing Priority No. 1.

To assess causative/contributing factors:

- Investigate causes/individual factors that may be involved in the client's situation. Note co-occurring emotional, psychiatric, and medical conditions. **Current theory suggests unbalanced neurotransmitters, as well as the hormone imbalances implicated in violent and aggressive behavior, may cause ineffective impulse control. The presence of comorbidities has treatment implications and, if left untreated, will complicate and/or limit successful outcomes for impulse control therapy.**
- Evaluate for underlying neurological conditions. **Presence of traumatic brain injury, strokes, brain tumors, and so forth, may result in poor impulse control, affecting therapeutic choices.**
- Explore the individual's inability to control actions. **Healthy people are aware of an impulse and are able to make a decision about following the urge or not. The key differentiation between healthy impulsiveness and an impulse disorder is the negative consequences that follow.**
- Document negative consequences incurred by client's impulsive actions, such as repeat detentions or suspensions from school, loss of employment, financial ruin, arrests/convictions, or civil litigation. **Those with lack of control engage in the behavior even if the individual knows that there will be a negative consequence such as incarceration, poverty, homelessness.**
- Determine the degree of anxiety the client experiences when having an impulse to act on the desire. **Not acting on the impulse creates intense anxiety or arousal in the individual, whereas engaging in the behavior produces a release of the anxiety and possibly pleasure or gratification. This may be followed by remorse, regret, or, conversely, satisfaction.**
- Identify current prescribed and over-the-counter medications used. **Critical to understand medications taken for specific psychiatric or medical conditions preventing overprescribing. Some antipsychotic medications may be a contributing factor to movement disorders causing**

Information that appears in brackets has been added by the authors to clarify and enhance the use of nursing diagnoses.

 Acute Care 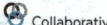 Collaborative 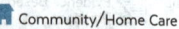 Community/Home Care   Cultural

physical distressing symptoms for the client. Anticholinergic medications can help to reduce involuntary movements, or a medication change may be necessary. **Some over-the-counter herbals are contraindicated with antipsychotic medications.**

Nursing Priority No. 2.

To assist client to develop strategies to manage impulsive behaviors:

- Collaborate with treatment team and client regarding plan of care, as indicated. **Complex health issues require an interprofessional treatment team to coordinate care with and for the client.**
- Empower client to participate in shared decision making and to set personally achievable goals according to ability and developmental level. Include family members, teachers, other providers, as appropriate, to assist client. **Client involvement in decision making helps with selecting interventions based on client's stage of readiness to change encouraging client to engage and commit to therapy.**
- Encourage client to identify negative consequences of behavior by expressing own feelings and anxieties regarding the adverse impact on client's life. **Helps the individual begin to understand problems of impulsive behavior.**
- Engage in therapies/approaches such as cognitive-behavioral therapy, including exposure and response prevention, mindfulness, yoga, and meditation. **Choices in therapeutic interventions provide opportunity to address client's specific needs/preferences.**
- Debrief after physical or emotional outbursts, encouraging client to express their thoughts, feelings, and anxieties regarding the adverse impact on own life. **Helps individual to recognize negative consequences of impulsive behavior and begin to manage problems.**
- Manage milieu (e.g., structure, safety, norms, balance, limit setting), as needed. **Therapeutic milieu helps guide client to calmness and intellectual engagement, and promotes learning to live at home/in community setting, functioning as a capable individual.**
- Organize a routine schedule for all clients (e.g., especially for clients with ADHD and ASD). **Milieu management is required in healthcare environments. Deficits in cognitive functioning and disorganized thinking make it difficult for clients to organize their activities of daily**

Information that appears in brackets has been added by the authors to clarify and enhance the use of nursing diagnoses.

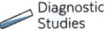 Diagnostic Studies   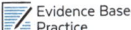 Evidence Based Practice   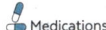 Medications   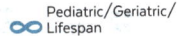 Pediatric/Geriatric/Lifespan

living. Therefore, it is a challenge for them to understand how an action interacts with another action or the consequence of an action, process information, and understand the concept of time.

- Assist client to identify and plan for early physical or emotional signs that trigger a loss of control and to take responsibility to act to resolve situation. **Parents/caregivers with a plan for meltdowns, tantrums, or rage in children with ASD and other impulse disorders must remain calm, remove child in a nonpunitive approach to a quieter environment by moving in closer to the child/client speaking softly, redirecting their behavior while removing them from the present environment.**
- Develop a treatment plan for a child with ADHD/ASD in conjunction with parents, teachers, counselor, and physician/psychiatrist. **Medications and behavioral therapy can be helpful along with monitoring the child and setting realistic and achievable goals.**
- Discuss the issue of substance misuse, hypersexuality, gambling, self-injury, or aggression. **Clients tend to lack the understanding of harm to self or others. The impulse to seek gratification, arousal, or pleasure may develop into a compulsive behavior to limit discomfort or anxiety.**

Nursing Priority No. 3.

Operationalize self-control (Teaching/Discharge Considerations) and enhance well-being (long-term goals):

- Review newly learned coping skill and practice response to situations when thoughts/feelings could lead to loss of self-control. **Role-playing in a safe environment facilitates how to respond to communications that might escalate to unwanted behaviors/actions.**
- Review medications and side effects (i.e., extrapyramidal symptoms to tardive dyskinesia) and what to do when side effects are noticed or felt with client/family. **Education about movement disorder, medication benefits, and side effects empowers clients to actively participate with treatment plan and seek timely intervention as indicated.**
- Identify counseling/therapy resources, support group, or community activities. **Clients experiencing ineffective impulse control require ongoing support to help control impulses, learn new social skills, and feel better about self.**
- Apply positive reinforcement for family member and self-reward for successful outcomes (e.g., praise, rewards). **Words of encouragement and praise have a lasting impression to continue/repeat behaviors.**

Information that appears in brackets has been added by the authors to clarify and enhance the use of nursing diagnoses.

Documentation Focus

Assessment/Reassessment
- Individual findings, including type of situation involved in client's loss of control
- Negative consequences incurred due to behavior
- Client awareness of consequences of actions

Planning
- Plan of care, specific interventions, and who is involved in planning
- Individual teaching plan

Implementation/Evaluation
- Responses to interventions, teaching, and actions performed
- Attainment of or progress toward desired outcome(s)
- Any modifications to plan of care

Discharge Planning
- Long-term needs and who is responsible for actions to be taken
- Specific referrals made

Sample Nursing Outcomes & Interventions Classifications NOC/NIC

NOC—Impulse Self-Control
NIC—Impulse Control Training

---

disability-associated urinary INCONTINENCE NANDA-I

[Diagnostic Division: Elimination]

Definition: Inability to reach the toilet after sensation of urge to avoid unintentional loss of urine due to physical or cognitive condition.

Recognizing Cues

Related/Risk Factors
Avoidance of nonhygienic toilet use; embarrassment regarding toilet use in social situations
Caregiver inappropriately implements bladder training techniques
Difficulty finding a toilet or obtaining timely assistance to toilet

---

Information that appears in brackets has been added by the authors to clarify and enhance the use of nursing diagnoses.

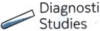 Diagnostic Studies 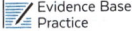 Evidence Based Practice 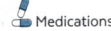 Medications 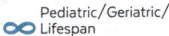 Pediatric/Geriatric/Lifespan

Unaddressed environmental constraints
Habitually suppresses urge to urinate; inadequate motivation to maintain continence; confusion
Impaired physical mobility or postural balance; weakened pelvic floor
Increased fluid intake

Defining Characteristics

Subjective

Difficulty reaching toilet after sensation of urge; voiding prior to reaching toilet
Use of techniques to prevent urination
Adaptive behaviors to avoid others' recognition of urinary incontinence
Mapping routes to public bathrooms prior to leaving home

Clinical Connections

Diabetes mellitus, congestive heart failure (CHF) (diuretic use), arthritis, multiple sclerosis (MS); Parkinson disease; bladder prolapse or cystocele, stroke, dementia, depression; developmental delays

Generate Solutions

Plan Desired Outcomes

Client Will (Include Specific Time Frame)

- Verbalize understanding of condition and identify interventions to prevent incontinence.
- Alter environment to accommodate individual needs.
- Report voiding in individually appropriate amounts.
- Urinate at acceptable times and places.

Interventions/Take Action

Nursing Priority No. 1.

To assess causative/contributing factors:

- Identify/investigate the client's clinical signs and symptoms to differentiate between types of urinary incontinence (i.e., urge incontinence, disability incontinence, stress incontinence, or mixed incontinence). The client with disability-associated (also known as functional) incontinence has normal bladder and urethral function but either cannot get to the toilet or fails to recognize the need to urinate in time to get to the toilet. **Many causes are transient and reversible but may also occur chronically in the elderly client.**

Information that appears in brackets has been added by the authors to clarify and enhance the use of nursing diagnoses.

Note: A mnemonic to help remember the functional contributors to disability-associated incontinence is as follows: DIAPPERS: D—delirium; I—infection (urinary); A—atrophic urethritis or vaginitis; P—pharmacological agents; P—psychiatric illness; E—excess urine output (due to excess fluid intake, alcoholic or caffeinated beverages, diuretics, peripheral edema, CHF, metabolic disorders such as hyperglycemia or hypercalcemia); R—reduced mobility; S—stool impaction.

- Consider the client's gender and age **to assess the client's risk factors.** The incidence of disability-associated incontinence continues to increase with age and is more prevalent in women. Current evidence supports the correlation between more frequent and increased volume of urine leakage with the degree of client disability, particularly in the domains of mobility and communication.
- Review the client's current medication regimen **to identify medications that may contribute to incontinence symptoms** (e.g., alpha-adrenergic agonists/antagonists, angiotensin-converting enzyme inhibitors, anticholinergic drugs, calcium channel blockers, cholinesterase inhibitors, diuretics, lithium, psychotropic medications, sedatives, hypnotics, selective serotonin reuptake inhibitors, and opioid analgesics).
- Discuss the client's dietary patterns and identify the presence of bladder irritants (e.g., alcohol, caffeine, acidic, or spicy food) **to ascertain the potential impact of the client's diet on urinary incontinence.**
- Identify/investigate client conditions that may interfere with the client's ability **to recognize or meet toileting needs** such as impaired cognition (e.g., dementia, acute confusion, etc.), functional impairments (e.g., physical trauma, arthritis, poor eyesight, mobility difficulties, dexterity problems, self-care deficits, etc.), and environmental conditions (e.g., access to bathroom, unfamiliar surroundings, poor lighting, improperly fitted chair/walker, low toilet seat, absence of safety bars, travel distance to the toilet, etc.).
- Review the client's medical history for comorbid conditions known **to increase urine output or alter bladder tone.** For example, diabetes mellitus, prolapsed bladder, and MS can affect the frequency of urination and the ability to hold urine until the client can reach the bathroom.

Information that appears in brackets has been added by the authors to clarify and enhance the use of nursing diagnoses.

 Diagnostic Studies 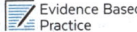 Evidence Based Practice 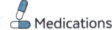 Medications 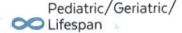 Pediatric/Geriatric/Lifespan

- Evaluate cognition. **Delirium or acute confusion or psychiatric illness can affect mental status, orientation to place, recognition of urge to void, and/or its significance.**
- Determine if the client is voluntarily postponing urination. **Often the demands of the work setting (e.g., restrictions on bathroom breaks, heavy workload, and inability to find time for bathroom breaks) make it difficult for individuals to go to the bathroom when the need arises, resulting in incontinence.**
- Measure the amount of urine voided, especially noting amounts less than 100 mL or greater than 550 mL, **to determine bladder capacity and effectiveness of bladder contractions to facilitate emptying.**
- Collaborate with the healthcare provider to perform a focused physical examination **to identify causes or factors contributing to urinary incontinence. The examination may include:**

  Pelvic/genitourinary examination **to assess vaginal atrophy, incontinence-associated dermatitis, and extraurethral urine loss/fistula. A digital examination may be performed to evaluate the tone and strength of the client's pelvic floor. Having a client perform a Valsalva maneuver for more than 6 sec may provide evidence of pelvic organ prolapse. A postvoid residual should be measured via sonography to assess bladder emptying.**

  Abdominal examination **to reveal costovertebral angle tenderness, pelvic masses, and a palpable bladder.**

  Neurological examination **to assess the client's mental status, perineal reflexes and sensation, patellar reflexes, gait, and mobility.**

  Body mass index assessment.
- Assess for cloudy, odorous urine associated with acute, painful urgency symptoms. **Incontinence often reflects presence of infection.**
- Assist with appropriate diagnostic testing (e.g., urinalysis, noninvasive bladder scanning, urine culture, urine and serum glucose, voiding cystometrogram). **Accurate assessment and diagnosis can determine voiding patterns and identify pathology that may lead to the development of incontinence. Additional bedside examinations, such as the cough stress test and the cotton swab test, may be used to discern incontinence causes. Note: Routine imaging should not be performed in the initial assessment of uncomplicated urge incontinence other than sonography to assess postvoid residual. Urinalysis should be used**

Information that appears in brackets has been added by the authors to clarify and enhance the use of nursing diagnoses.

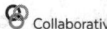 Acute Care 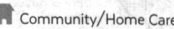 Collaborative Community/Home Care 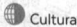 Cultural

to evaluate for the presence of urinary tract infection and to exclude hematuria, proteinuria, and glycosuria. Renal function should be assessed if there is concern for obstruction. The presence of glucose in the urine may cause polyuria, resulting in overdistention of the client's bladder and difficulty in holding urine.
- Refer to NDs mixed, stress, or disability-associated urinary Incontinence for related assessments and interventions.

Nursing Priority No. 2.

To assess degree of interference/disability:

- Record client fluid intake, urinary frequency, and volume of incontinence during a typical day and night **to gather data on fluid intake, client symptoms, situations associated with incontinence symptoms, and voiding patterns (e.g., client is voiding every 3 hr). A voiding diary can facilitate timed voiding (e.g., every 2 hr).**
- Provide client/caregiver with a validated questionnaire (e.g., Pelvic Floor Distress Inventory, Pelvic Floor Impact Questionnaire, Urogenital Distress Inventory (UDI), King Health Questionnaire, or Urge UDI) **to quantify the impact of bladder symptoms on the client's quality of life. There is a considerable impact on the quality of life of individuals with an incontinence problem, affecting socialization and view of themselves as sexual beings and sense of self-esteem. Clients with incontinence problems are often embarrassed, withdraw from social activities and relationships, and hesitate to discuss the problem—even with their healthcare provider.**

Nursing Priority No. 3.

To assist in treating/preventing incontinence:

- Assist in treatment of the underlying conditions that may contribute to disability-associated urinary incontinence. **Symptoms may resolve with treatment of the problem (e.g., physical injury, acute confusion, return to familiar surroundings, etc.).**

- Implement continence management interventions:
  Establish a voiding schedule based on the client's usual voiding pattern. Encourage the client to resist ignoring the urge to urinate or have a bowel movement. **Emptying the bladder on a regular schedule or when feeling an urge reduces the risk for incontinence. Since the urge to void may be difficult to differentiate from the urge to defecate, advise the client to respond to the urge.**

Information that appears in brackets has been added by the authors to clarify and enhance the use of nursing diagnoses.

- Encourage regular pelvic floor strengthening exercises (Kegel exercises) **to improve pelvic musculature, tone, and strength, thus preventing or halting incontinence. Combining pelvic floor strengthening with biofeedback may enhance the effectiveness of training and success at controlling incontinence.**
- Instruct client to tighten pelvic floor muscles before arising from bed or chair **to help prevent loss of urine as abdominal pressure changes.**
- Help client manage fluid and ensure adequate intake (e.g., 50 to 70 oz daily) in smaller increments, such as 10 to 12 servings daily, **to prevent dehydration and promote good urine flow. Clients on fluid restriction may require additional guidance from their healthcare provider. Monitor intake and output and reduce fluid if indicated. Too much water can also increase bladder irritation, so the amount of intake needs to be determined by the client's response.**
- Limit liquid intake 2 to 3 hr prior to bedtime **to promote a predictable voiding pattern and limit nocturia.**
- Suggest diet modifications (e.g., reduce acidic/citrus juices, chocolate and caffeine-containing drinks, carbonated beverages, spicy foods, artificial sweeteners) **to reduce bladder irritants. Note: Using a food/drink diary may help identify which foods/food groups/beverages cause bladder pain, and/or urgency.**
- Assist client in managing bowel elimination **to prevent urinary incontinence associated with constipation or fecal impaction.** (Refer to NDs chronic functional Constipation and impaired intestinal Elimination.)
- Administer prescribed diuretics in the morning **to lessen nighttime voidings. The effect of these medications diminishes over time, possibly reducing nighttime incontinence. Note: Client taking diuretics multiple times during the day has the potential for repeated episodes of incontinence, which may carry over into the night.**
- Reduce or eliminate the use of hypnotics, if possible, **as the client may be too sedated to recognize or respond to the need to void.**
- Provide assistance or devices (e.g., raised toilet seat, bedside commode, urinal, or bedpan), as indicated, for clients who are mobility impaired. **Providing summoning assistance and an accessible urinary device within the client's reach can promote a sense of control in self-managing voiding. Additionally, prompt response to client summons can promote continence.**

Information that appears in brackets has been added by the authors to clarify and enhance the use of nursing diagnoses.

- Use night-lights to indicate bathroom location. **Elderly clients may become confused and be unable to locate the bathroom in the dark. Lighting facilitates access, reducing the possibility of accidents.**
- Adapt client clothing to facilitate quick and easy removal. **Velcro fasteners, full skirts, crotchless panties or no panties, and suspenders or elastic waists may be easier to remove quickly without assistance once urge to void is noted.**
- Collaborate with physical/occupational therapist in determining ways **to alter the client's environment and identify appropriate assistive devices to meet the client's individual needs.**
- Refer client to a urologist or continence specialist, as indicated, for interventions such as pelvic floor strengthening exercises, biofeedback techniques, and/or vaginal weight training, as needed **to meet the individual needs of client.**

Nursing Priority No. 4.

To promote urinary continence (Teaching/Discharge Considerations) and enhance well-being (long-term goals):

- Discuss with client/significant other(s) the need for prompted and scheduled voiding **to manage continence when the client is unable to respond immediately to the urge to void.**
- Encourage comfort measures (e.g., use of incontinence pads or adult briefs, wearing loose-fitting, or adapted clothing) **to manage disability-associated incontinence symptoms over the long term as well as to enhance the client's sense of security and confidence in the ability to be socially active.**
- Maintain positive regard **to reduce embarrassment associated with incontinence, need for assistance, or use of bedpan.**
- Recommend limiting intake of coffee, tea, and alcohol. **These substances have an irritating effect on the bladder and may contribute to incontinence.**
- Discuss with client/caregiver the importance of perineal care after each voiding **to prevent skin irritation and reduce the potential for bladder infection and incontinence-related dermatitis.**
- Promote client/caregiver participation in developing a long-term plan of care **to encourage the possibility of success and confidence in the client's own ability to manage the program.**

Information that appears in brackets has been added by the authors to clarify and enhance the use of nursing diagnoses.

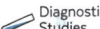 Diagnostic Studies 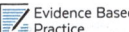 Evidence Based Practice 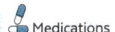 Medications 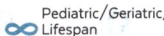 Pediatric/Geriatric/Lifespan

- Refer to NDs mixed, stress, urge urinary Incontinence for additional interventions, as appropriate.

Documentation Focus

Assessment/Reassessment
- Current elimination pattern and assessment findings
- Effect on lifestyle and self-esteem

Planning
- Plan of care and who is involved in planning
- Teaching plan

Implementation/Evaluation
- Response to interventions, teaching, and actions performed
- Attainment of or progress toward desired outcome(s)
- Modifications to plan of care

Discharge Planning
- Long-term needs and who is responsible for actions to be taken
- Specific referrals made

Sample Nursing Outcomes & Interventions Classifications NOC/NIC

NOC—Urinary Continence
NIC—Urinary Habit Training

---

mixed urinary INCONTINENCE   NANDA-I

[Diagnostic Division: Elimination]

Definition: Involuntary loss of urine in combination with or following a strong sensation or urgency to void, and also with activities that increase intra-abdominal pressure.

Recognizing Cues

Related/Risk Factors
Incompetence of the bladder neck or urethral sphincter
Ineffective overweight self-management
Weakened pelvic floor
Skeletal muscle atrophy
Tobacco use

Information that appears in brackets has been added by the authors to clarify and enhance the use of nursing diagnoses.

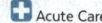 Acute Care 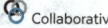 Collaborative 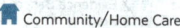 Community/Home Care   Cultural

Defining Characteristics

Subjective
Incomplete bladder emptying; urinary urgency
Involuntary loss of urine upon coughing, effort, physical exertion, or sneezing
Nocturia

Clinical Connections
Multiple sclerosis (MS), Parkinson disease, diabetes, stroke, spinal cord or pelvic injury, pregnancy, menopause, benign prostatic hyperplasia

Generate Solutions

Plan Desired Outcomes

Client Will (Include Specific Time Frame)
- Verbalize understanding of condition and identify interventions to prevent or manage incontinence.
- Alter environment to accommodate individual needs.
- Report voiding in individually appropriate amounts.

Interventions/Take Action

Nursing Priority No. 1.
To assess causative/contributing factors:
- Identify/investigate the client's clinical signs and symptoms **to differentiate between types of urinary incontinence (i.e., urge incontinence, disability incontinence, stress incontinence, or mixed incontinence).** Urge urinary incontinence **is characterized by a sudden urge to void that often results in involuntary leakage of urine, nocturia, and increased urinary frequency.** Stress urinary incontinence **is characterized by involuntary loss of urine due to an increase in intra-abdominal pressure yet not associated with an urge to void.** Mixed urinary incontinence **is a complex clinical problem represented by characteristics of both stress and urge urinary incontinence simultaneously.**
- Consider client's gender and age **to assess client risk factors. The incidence of urge and stress incontinence is higher in women and increases with age. Older women often have a mix of stress and urge incontinence, whereas individuals with dementia or disabling neurological disorders tend to have urge and disability-associated incontinence.**

Information that appears in brackets has been added by the authors to clarify and enhance the use of nursing diagnoses.

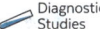 Diagnostic Studies   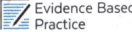 Evidence Based Practice   Medications   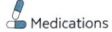 Pediatric/Geriatric/Lifespan

- Discuss client's current medication regimen **to identify medications that may contribute to incontinence symptoms (e.g., alpha-adrenergic agonists/antagonists, angiotensin-converting enzyme inhibitors, anticholinergic drugs, calcium channel blockers, cholinesterase inhibitors, diuretics, lithium, psychotropic medications, sedatives, hypnotics, selective serotonin reuptake inhibitors, and opioid analgesics).**
- Review client's dietary patterns and identify the presence of bladder irritants (e.g., alcohol, caffeine, acidic, or spicy food) **to ascertain the potential impact of the client's diet on urinary incontinence.**
- Review medical and incontinence history with client/significant other (SO)/caregiver. **Mixed incontinence can involve any two (or more) types of incontinence but typically shares the symptoms and the causes of both stress incontinence and urge incontinence. Stress incontinence often results from conditions (1) that cause weakening of the muscles supporting and controlling the bladder (e.g., childbirth, surgery or radiation to the vagina [women], rectum, or prostate [men]); or (2) that increase pressure on the bladder (e.g., coughing, sneezing), causing urine to leak.**
- Note presence of conditions often associated with urgent voiding (e.g., bladder dysfunction associated with nerves damaged by various diseases [diabetes, stroke, MS, Parkinson disease], spinal cord injury). Other comorbidities associated with overactive bladder include recent/ongoing urinary tract infection (UTI), fecal incontinence, chronic constipation; obesity; postmenopausal hormonal changes. **These conditions affect bladder innervation, musculature tone, and storage. Additionally, triggering factors (e.g., feeling of running water, lifting, bending, sexual activity, movement, changes in position) should be evaluated to obtain a comprehensive assessment of relevance to the client's urinary incontinence. Refer to ND urge Incontinence for related assessments.**
- Identify physiological causes of increased intra-abdominal pressure (e.g., obesity, gravid uterus; repeated heavy lifting [occupational risk]), contributing history (e.g., multiple births, bladder or pelvic trauma/fractures), surgery (e.g., hysterectomy, prostatectomy, other bladder or pelvic surgeries that may damage sphincter muscles), radiotherapy, neurological conditions, and participation in high-impact athletic or military field activities (particularly women).

Information that appears in brackets has been added by the authors to clarify and enhance the use of nursing diagnoses.

 Acute Care 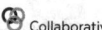 Collaborative 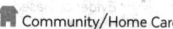 Community/Home Care 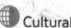 Cultural

Identification of specifics of the client's situation provides for developing an accurate plan of care. Refer to ND stress Incontinence for related assessments.

- Measure the amount of urine voided, especially noting amounts less than 100 mL or greater than 550 mL, **to determine bladder capacity and effectiveness of bladder contractions to facilitate emptying. Bladder capacity may be impaired, or bladder contractions facilitating emptying may be ineffective.** Refer to ND risk for urinary Retention.
- Collaborate with the healthcare provider to perform a focused physical examination **to identify causes or factors contributing to urinary incontinence. The examination may include:**

  Pelvic/genitourinary examination **to assess vaginal atrophy, incontinence-associated dermatitis, and extraurethral urine loss/fistula. A digital examination may be performed to evaluate the tone and strength of the client's pelvic floor. Having a client perform a Valsalva maneuver for more than 6 sec may provide evidence of pelvic organ prolapse. A postvoid residual should be measured via sonography to assess bladder emptying.**

  Abdominal examination **to reveal costovertebral angle tenderness, pelvic masses, and a palpable bladder.**

  Neurological examination evaluation **to assess the client's mental status, perineal reflexes and sensation, patellar reflexes, gait, and mobility.**

  Body mass index assessment, weight-adjusted waist index, etc.

- Assess for cloudy, odorous urine associated with acute, painful urgency symptoms. **Incontinence often reflects presence of infection.**
- Assist with appropriate diagnostic testing (e.g., urinalysis, noninvasive bladder scanning, urine culture, urine and serum glucose, voiding cystometrogram). **Accurate assessment and diagnosis can determine voiding patterns and identify pathology that may lead to the development of incontinence. Additional bedside examinations, such as the cough stress test and the cotton swab test, may be used to discern incontinence causes. Note: Routine imaging should not be performed in the initial assessment of uncomplicated urge incontinence other than sonography to assess postvoid residual. Urinalysis should be used to evaluate for the presence of UTI and to exclude hematuria, proteinuria, and glycosuria. Renal function should be assessed if there is concern for obstruction.**

Information that appears in brackets has been added by the authors to clarify and enhance the use of nursing diagnoses.

The presence of glucose in the urine may cause polyuria, resulting in overdistention of the client's bladder and difficulty in holding urine.
- Refer to NDs stress urinary Incontinence; urge urinary Incontinence for related assessments.

Nursing Priority No. 2.
To assess degree of interference/disability:

- Record client fluid intake, urinary frequency, and degree of urgency during a typical day and night **to identify the degree of difficulty being experienced by the client. A voiding diary gathers data on fluid intake, client symptoms, and situations associated with incontinence symptoms, and may identify the degree of difficulty being experienced by the client.**
- Provide client/caregiver with a validated questionnaire (e.g., Pelvic Floor Distress Inventory, Pelvic Floor Impact Questionnaire, Urogenital Distress Inventory (UDI), King Health Questionnaire, or Urge UDI) **to quantify the impact of bladder symptoms on the client's quality of life. There is a considerable impact on the quality of life of individuals with an incontinence problem, affecting socialization and view of themselves as sexual beings and sense of self-esteem.**
- Discuss skin concerns with client/caregiver **to identify what measures the client is using to manage incontinence. Constant moisture can cause skin to be irritated and to break down. Absorbent pads with wicking materials help keep moisture away from the body and avoid irritation, while moisture barrier creams can help protect skin from coming into contact with urine. The client may already be limiting liquid intake, voiding before any activity, or using undergarment protection.**

Nursing Priority No. 3.
To assist in treating/preventing incontinence:

- Assist in treatment of the underlying conditions that may contribute to stress incontinence (e.g., UTI; recovery from pelvic surgery, childbirth, or pelvic trauma; use of estrogen-based oral or topical products for atrophic vaginitis) or urge incontinence (e.g., nerve damage [stroke, spinal cord injury, diabetes]; weakened pelvic floor muscles; bladder irritation [infection/inflammation]; and overactive bladder).

Information that appears in brackets has been added by the authors to clarify and enhance the use of nursing diagnoses.

 Acute Care 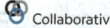 Collaborative 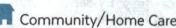 Community/Home Care   Cultural

- Implement continence management interventions:
  - Establish voiding schedule (habit and bladder training) based on client's usual voiding pattern. **A bladder retraining program may be successful in alleviating urge incontinence. Note: A review of multiple studies revealed a strongly positive effect on continence using a combination of behavioral interventions (including bladder control strategies, fluid management, and pelvic floor muscle exercises) and medications in older women. However, clients may have difficulty sustaining the effort of behavioral modification, and thus the positive effect is lost.**
  - Practice timed voiding (e.g., 3-hr intervals during the day) **to keep the bladder relatively empty.**
  - Extend the time between voiding to 3- to 4-hr intervals **to improve bladder capacity and retention time.**
  - Void before physical exertion such as exercise or sports activities **to reduce the potential for incontinence.**
  - Recommend consciously delaying voiding by using distraction (e.g., slow, deep breathing), self-statements (e.g., "I can wait"), and contracting pelvic muscles when exposed to triggers. **Behavioral techniques that are sometimes helpful for urge suppression, especially in younger clients.**
  - Encourage regular pelvic floor strengthening exercises (Kegel exercises) **to improve pelvic musculature, tone, and strength, thus preventing or halting incontinence. Combining pelvic floor strengthening with biofeedback may enhance the effectiveness of training and success at controlling incontinence. Note: These exercises should be done numerous times throughout the day.**
  - Recommend client start and stop the urinary stream two or three times during voiding **to isolate and strengthen muscles involved in the voiding process.**
  - Instruct client to tighten pelvic floor muscles before arising from bed or chair **to help prevent loss of urine as abdominal pressure changes.**
  - Incorporate "bent-knee sit-ups" into the exercise program **to increase abdominal muscle tone and help prevent/alleviate stress incontinence.**
  - Avoid or limit heavy lifting and high-impact aerobics or sports **to decrease incontinence associated with elevated intra-abdominal pressure.**

mixed urinary INCONTINENCE

Information that appears in brackets has been added by the authors to clarify and enhance the use of nursing diagnoses.

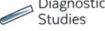 Diagnostic Studies   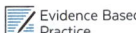 Evidence Based Practice   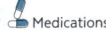 Medications   Pediatric/Geriatric/Lifespan

Help client manage fluid and ensure adequate intake (e.g., 50 to 70 oz daily) in smaller increments, such as 10 to 12 servings daily **to prevent dehydration and promote good urine flow. Clients on fluid restriction may require additional guidance from their healthcare provider. Monitor intake and output and reduce fluid, if indicated. Too much water can also increase bladder irritation, so the amount of intake needs to be determined by the client's response.**

Limit liquid intake 2 to 3 hr prior to bedtime **to promote a predictable voiding pattern and limit nocturia.**

Suggest diet modifications (e.g., reduce acidic/citrus juices, chocolate and caffeine-containing drinks, carbonated beverages, spicy foods, artificial sweeteners), **to reduce bladder irritants and limit nocturia. Note: Using a food/drink diary may help identify which foods/food groups/beverages cause bladder pain, and/or urgency.**

Encourage weight loss as indicated **to reduce pressure on intra-abdominal and pelvic organs.**

Assist client in managing bowel elimination **to prevent urinary incontinence associated with constipation or fecal impaction. (Refer to ND chronic functional Constipation and impaired intestinal Elimination.)**

Provide assistance or devices, as indicated, for clients who are mobility impaired. **Providing a means of summoning assistance and placing a bedside commode, urinal, or bedpan within the client's reach can promote a sense of control in self-managing voiding.**

Set an alarm to awaken during the night, if indicated. **May be useful in maintaining continence during training schedule.**

Offer assistance to the cognitively impaired client (e.g., prompt client or take to the bathroom on regularly timed schedule) **to reduce the frequency of incontinence episodes and promote comfort.**

Refer client to a specialist or treatment program, as indicated, for additional or specialized interventions (e.g., use of vaginal cones, electronic stimulation therapy, etc.). **Significant reduction in incontinence episodes is reported with the use of combined therapies (e.g., electronic stimulation therapy plus pelvic muscle exercises).**

Discuss with client/caregiver the use of medications such as antimuscarinic agents (e.g., darifenacin [Enablex], fesoterodine [Toviaz], oxybutynin [Ditropan],

---

Information that appears in brackets has been added by the authors to clarify and enhance the use of nursing diagnoses.

solifenacin [VESIcare], tolterodine [Detrol], trospium [Sanctura], or beta-3 adrenoceptor agonists (e.g., mirabegron [Myrbetriq]), **which may improve bladder tone, capacity, and increase the effectiveness of bladder sphincter and proximal urethra contractions, particularly in mixed urinary incontinence. However, in the United States, no medications are Food and Drug Administration (FDA) approved to specifically treat stress urinary incontinence. Unlabeled uses of alpha-adrenergic agonists (e.g., pseudoephedrine and phenylephrine) are based on the urethral smooth-muscle response to alpha stimulation, resulting in improved control of the internal sphincter and reduced urine loss. Lack of proven efficacy with these agents and concerns with adverse effects, including insomnia, anxiety, hypertension, arrhythmias, and stroke, limit their utility.**

- Discuss possible surgical interventions with client/caregiver. **Surgical treatments may be required or desired when conservative treatments fail. Some of these include Burch colposuspension, pubovaginal slings, and urethral bulking. Additional surgical interventions (e.g., intradetrusor onabotulinum toxin A, acupuncture, electroacupuncture (EA), or sacral neuromodulation) are specific to urge urinary incontinence.**
- Refer to NDs stress urinary Incontinence; urge urinary Incontinence for related nursing interventions and treatments.

Nursing Priority No. 4.

To promote urinary continence (Teaching/Discharge Considerations) and enhance well-being (long-term goals):

- Provide information to client/caregiver about the potential for stress or urge incontinence and lifestyle measures **to prevent or limit incontinence.**
- Suggest the use of incontinence pads or undergarments **considering the client's activity level, amount of urine loss, physical size, manual dexterity, and cognitive ability to determine products best suited to the client's situation and needs when leakage continues to occur despite other measures.**
- Discuss with client/caregiver the importance of perineal care following voiding and frequent changing of incontinence pads. Recommend application of oil-based emollient **to prevent infection and protect skin from irritation.**

Information that appears in brackets has been added by the authors to clarify and enhance the use of nursing diagnoses.

 Diagnostic Studies 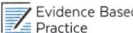 Evidence Based Practice 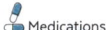 Medications 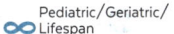 Pediatric/Geriatric/Lifespan

- Review with client/caregiver signs/symptoms indicating urinary complications and the need for medical follow-up care **to help the client seek intervention promptly to prevent more serious problems from developing.**
- Recommend to client/caregiver limiting the client's intake of coffee, tea, and alcohol. **These substances have an irritating effect on the bladder and may contribute to incontinence.**
- Discuss with client/caregiver participation in incontinence management for activities such as heavy lifting and strenuous sports activities that increase intra-abdominal pressure. **Substituting swimming or other low-impact exercises may help reduce the frequency of incontinence while still maintaining an active lifestyle.**
- Recommend or refer client for behavioral training, as indicated. **An important part of pelvic floor biofeedback therapy is the consistent practice of pelvic floor muscle exercises at home. With biofeedback, an individual can learn to stop using the incorrect muscles and start using the correct ones.**
- Recommend or refer for specialist interventions as indicated.

Documentation Focus

Assessment/Reassessment
- Findings including pattern of incontinence and physical factors present
- Effect on lifestyle and self-esteem
- Client understanding of condition

Planning
- Plan of care and who is involved in the planning
- Teaching plan

Implementation/Evaluation
- Responses to interventions, teaching, actions performed, and changes that are identified
- Attainment of or progress toward desired outcome(s)
- Modifications to plan of care

Discharge Planning
- Long-term needs, referrals, and who is responsible for specific actions
- Specific referrals made

Information that appears in brackets has been added by the authors to clarify and enhance the use of nursing diagnoses.

Sample Nursing Outcomes & Interventions Classifications NOC/NIC

NOC—Urinary Elimination
NIC—Urinary Habit Training

stress urinary INCONTINENCE NANDA-I

[Diagnostic Division: Elimination]

Definition: Involuntary loss of urine with activities that increase intra-abdominal pressure, which is not associated with urgency to void.

Recognizing Cues

Related/Risk Factors
Ineffective overweight self-management
Weakened pelvic floor

Defining Characteristics

Subjective or Objective
Urine leakage:
   In the absence of detrusor contraction, or overextended bladder
   Upon coughing, laughing, physical exertion, or sneezing

Clinical Connections
Multiple sclerosis, Parkinson disease, diabetes, stroke, spinal cord or pelvic injury, pregnancy, menopause, benign prostatic hyperplasia, prostatectomy

Generate Solutions

Plan Desired Outcomes

Client Will (Include Specific Time Frame)
- Verbalize understanding of condition and interventions for bladder conditioning.
- Demonstrate behaviors or techniques to strengthen pelvic floor musculature.
- Remain continent even with increased intra-abdominal pressure.

Information that appears in brackets has been added by the authors to clarify and enhance the use of nursing diagnoses.

Interventions/Take Action

Nursing Priority No. 1.
To assess causative/contributing factors:

- Identify/investigate client's clinical signs and symptoms **to differentiate between types of urinary incontinence (i.e., urge incontinence, disability incontinence, stress incontinence, or mixed incontinence).** Stress urinary incontinence is characterized by involuntary loss of urine due to an increase in intra-abdominal pressure yet not associated with an urge to void. **Often due to weakened support of pelvic floor musculature, connective tissue, and urethral hypermobility (e.g., connective tissue disorders, obesity, pelvic floor trauma, pregnancy/[traumatic] vaginal delivery, pelvic or vaginal surgery, chronic constipation, heavy lifting). Other causes include urinary sphincter dysfunction (e.g., cauda equina, sacral/severe pelvic fractures, nerve injury, prostatectomy); and decreased estrogen stimulation of the urogenital tissue (e.g., vaginal atrophy, hypoestrogenic state [postpartum period, lactation, hypothalamic amenorrhea, or use of antiestrogenic drugs]. Note: Some cases of stress urinary incontinence are idiopathic and have no discernible cause.**
- Consider the client's gender and age **to assess client risk factors. The incidence of stress incontinence continues to increase with age and primarily affects women, although men who undergo surgical prostatectomy are at increased risk for developing stress incontinence. The cumulative effect of age, obesity, and the number of vaginal births increases the risk and prevalence of stress incontinence.**
- Discuss client's current medication regimen **to identify medications that may contribute to incontinence symptoms (e.g., alpha-adrenergic agonists/antagonists, angiotensin-converting enzyme inhibitors, anticholinergic drugs, calcium channel blockers, cholinesterase inhibitors, diuretics, lithium, psychotropic medications, sedatives, hypnotics, selective serotonin reuptake inhibitors, and opioid analgesics).**
- Review client's dietary patterns and identify the presence of bladder irritants (e.g., alcohol, caffeine, acidic, or spicy food) **to ascertain the potential impact of the client's diet on urinary incontinence.**

Information that appears in brackets has been added by the authors to clarify and enhance the use of nursing diagnoses.

 Acute Care 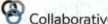 Collaborative 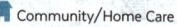 Community/Home Care 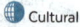 Cultural

- Identify causes of increased intra-abdominal pressure **physiological** (e.g., obesity, gravid uterus; repeated heavy lifting [occupational risk]), contributing history (e.g., multiple births, bladder or pelvic trauma/fractures), surgery (e.g., in women, hysterectomy, prolapse, or other incontinence surgery) or other urological surgery (e.g., prostate surgery/other bladder or pelvic surgeries **that may damage sphincter muscles**), radiotherapy, neurological problems, and participation in high-impact athletic or military field activities (particularly women). Note: Women who have an overactive bladder may also have mixed incontinence, when both urgency and stress incontinence occur. **Identification of specifics of individual situation provides for developing an accurate plan of care.**
- Measure the amount of urine voided, especially noting amounts less than 100 mL or greater than 550 mL, **to determine bladder capacity and effectiveness of bladder contractions to facilitate emptying. Bladder capacity may be impaired, or bladder contractions facilitating emptying may be ineffective.** (Refer to ND risk for urinary Retention.)
- Collaborate with the healthcare provider to perform a focused physical examination **to identify causes or factors contributing to urinary incontinence. The examination may include:**
  - Pelvic/genitourinary examination **to assess vaginal atrophy, incontinence-associated dermatitis, and extraurethral urine loss/fistula. A digital examination may be performed to evaluate the tone and strength of the client's pelvic floor. Having a client perform a Valsalva maneuver for more than 6 sec may provide evidence of pelvic organ prolapse. A postvoid residual should be measured via sonography to assess bladder emptying.**
  - Abdominal examination **to reveal costovertebral angle tenderness, pelvic masses, and a palpable bladder.**
  - Neurological examination evaluation **to assess the client's mental status, perineal reflexes and sensation, patellar reflexes, gait, and mobility.**
  - Body mass index assessment, weight-adjusted waist index, etc.
- Assess for cloudy, odorous urine associated with acute, painful urgency symptoms. **Incontinence often reflects presence of infection.**
- Assist with appropriate diagnostic testing (e.g., urinalysis, noninvasive bladder scanning, urine culture, urine and

---

Information that appears in brackets has been added by the authors to clarify and enhance the use of nursing diagnoses.

serum glucose, voiding cystometrogram). **Accurate assessment and diagnosis can determine voiding patterns and identify pathology that may lead to the development of incontinence. Additional bedside examinations, such as the cough stress test and the cotton swab test, may be used to discern incontinence causes. Note: Routine imaging should not be performed in the initial assessment of uncomplicated urge incontinence other than sonography to assess postvoid residual. Urinalysis should be used to evaluate for the presence of urinary tract infection (UTI) and to exclude hematuria, proteinuria, and glycosuria. Renal function should be assessed if there is concern for obstruction. The presence of glucose in the urine may cause polyuria, resulting in overdistention of the client's bladder and difficulty in holding urine.**
- Refer to NDs mixed urinary Incontinence; urge urinary Incontinence for related assessments and interventions.

Nursing Priority No. 2.

To assess the degree of interference/disability:

- Record client fluid intake, urinary frequency, and degree of urgency during a typical day and night. **A voiding diary gathers data on fluid intake, client symptoms, and the stimulus provoking the incontinence episode.**
- Provide client/caregiver with a validated questionnaire (e.g., Pelvic Floor Distress Inventory, Pelvic Floor Impact Questionnaire, Urogenital Distress Inventory (UDI), King Health Questionnaire, or Urge UDI) **to quantify the impact of bladder symptoms on the client's quality of life. There is a considerable impact on the quality of life of individuals with an incontinence problem, affecting socialization and view of themselves as sexual beings and sense of self-esteem.**
- Ascertain current methods of self-management. **The client may already be limiting liquid intake, voiding before any activity, or using undergarment protection.**

Nursing Priority No. 3.

To assist in treating/preventing incontinence:

- Assist in treatment of the underlying conditions that may contribute to stress incontinence. Symptoms may resolve with treatment/resolution of the medical problem (e.g., recovery from pelvic surgery, childbirth, or pelvic trauma; use of estrogen-based oral or topical products for atrophic vaginitis).

Information that appears in brackets has been added by the authors to clarify and enhance the use of nursing diagnoses.

 Acute Care 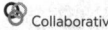 Collaborative 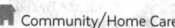 Community/Home Care 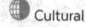 Cultural

- Implement nonsurgical treatment techniques:
  - Establish voiding schedule based on client's usual voiding pattern. **The use of a frequency/volume chart is helpful in bladder training. A review of urine output in relation to fluid intake records can reveal the need to modify fluid intake in clients who are resistant to fluid management efforts.**
  - Practice timed voiding (e.g., every 3-hr intervals during the day) **to keep the bladder relatively empty.**
  - Extend time between voiding to 3- to 4-hr intervals **to improve bladder capacity and retention time.**
  - Void before physical exertion, such as exercise or sports activities **to reduce potential for incontinence.**
  - Encourage regular pelvic floor strengthening exercises (Kegel exercises) **to improve pelvic musculature, tone, and strength, thus preventing or halting incontinence. Combining pelvic floor strengthening with biofeedback may enhance the effectiveness of training and success at controlling incontinence. Note: These exercises should be done numerous times throughout the day.**
  - Recommend client start and stop the urinary stream two or three times during voiding **to isolate and strengthen muscles involved in the voiding process.**
  - Instruct client to tighten pelvic floor muscles before arising from bed or chair **to help prevent loss of urine as abdominal pressure changes.**
  - Incorporate "bent-knee sit-ups" into the exercise program **to increase abdominal muscle tone and help prevent/alleviate stress incontinence.**
  - Avoid or limit heavy lifting and high-impact aerobics or sports **to decrease incontinence associated with elevated intra-abdominal pressure.**
  - Help client manage fluid and ensure adequate intake (e.g., 50 to 70 oz daily) in smaller increments, such as 10 to 12 servings daily **to prevent dehydration and promote good urine flow. Clients on fluid restriction may require additional guidance from their healthcare provider. Monitor intake and output and reduce fluid, if indicated. Too much water can also increase bladder irritation, so the amount of intake needs to be determined by the client's response.**
  - Limit liquid intake 2 to 3 hr prior to bedtime **to promote a predictable voiding pattern and limit nocturia.**

Information that appears in brackets has been added by the authors to clarify and enhance the use of nursing diagnoses.

- Suggest diet modifications (e.g., reduce acidic/citrus juices, chocolate and caffeine-containing drinks, carbonated beverages, spicy foods, artificial sweeteners) **to reduce bladder irritants and limit nocturia. Note: Using a food/drink diary may help identify which foods/food groups/beverages cause bladder pain and/or urgency.**
- Encourage weight loss, as indicated, **to reduce pressure on pelvic organs.**
- Assist client in managing bowel elimination **to prevent urinary incontinence associated with constipation or fecal impaction.** (Refer to ND chronic functional Constipation and impaired intestinal Elimination.)
- Assist with medical treatment of underlying urological condition, as indicated. **Stress incontinence may be treated with surgical intervention (e.g., bladder neck suspension, pubovaginal sling to reposition bladder and strengthen pelvic musculature, prostate surgery) or nonsurgical therapies (e.g., behavioral modification, pelvic muscle exercises, medications, use of pessary, vaginal cones, electrical stimulation, biofeedback).**
- Discuss with client/caregiver the use of medications such as antimuscarinic agents (e.g., darifenacin [Enablex], fesoterodine [Toviaz], oxybutynin [Ditropan], solifenacin [VESIcare], tolterodine [Detrol], trospium [Sanctura], or beta-3 adrenoceptor agonists (e.g., mirabegron [Myrbetriq]), **which may improve bladder tone, capacity, and increase effectiveness of bladder sphincter and proximal urethral contractions. However, in the United States, no medications are Food and Drug Administration (FDA) approved to specifically treat stress incontinence. Unlabeled uses of alpha-adrenergic agonists (e.g., pseudoephedrine and phenylephrine) are based on the urethral smooth-muscle response to alpha stimulation, resulting in improved control of the internal sphincter and reduced urine loss. Lack of proven efficacy with these agents and concerns with adverse effects including insomnia, anxiety, hypertension, arrhythmias, and stroke limit their utility.**

Nursing Priority No. 4.

To promote urinary continence (Teaching/Discharge Considerations) and enhance well-being (long-term goals):

- Provide information to client/caregiver about the potential for stress or urge incontinence and lifestyle measures **to prevent or limit incontinence.**

Information that appears in brackets has been added by the authors to clarify and enhance the use of nursing diagnoses.

- Suggest to client/caregiver use of incontinence pads or undergarments **considering client's activity level, amount of urine loss, physical size, manual dexterity, and cognitive ability to determine products best suited to client's situation and needs when leakage continues to occur despite other measures.**
- Discuss with client/caregiver the importance of perineal care following voiding and frequent changing of incontinence pads. Recommend application of oil-based emollient **to prevent infection and protect skin from irritation.**
- Recommend to client/caregiver limiting client's intake of coffee, tea, and alcohol. **These substances have an irritating effect on the bladder and may contribute to incontinence.**
- Discuss with client/caregiver participation in incontinence management for activities such as heavy lifting and strenuous sports that increase intra-abdominal pressure. **Substituting swimming or other low-impact exercises may help reduce the frequency of incontinence while still maintaining an active life.**
- Recommend or refer client for behavioral training, as indicated. **An important part of pelvic floor biofeedback therapy is the consistent practice of the pelvic floor muscle exercises at home. With biofeedback, an individual can learn to stop using the incorrect muscles and start using the correct ones.**

Documentation Focus

Assessment/Reassessment
- Individual findings including pattern of incontinence and physical factors present
- Effect on lifestyle and self-esteem
- Client understanding of condition

Planning
- Plan of care and who is involved in the planning
- Teaching plan

Implementation/Evaluation
- Responses to interventions, teaching, actions performed, and changes that are identified
- Attainment of or progress toward desired outcome(s)
- Modifications to plan of care

Information that appears in brackets has been added by the authors to clarify and enhance the use of nursing diagnoses.

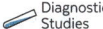 Diagnostic Studies 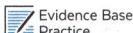 Evidence Based Practice 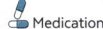 Medications 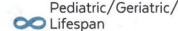 Pediatric/Geriatric/Lifespan

Discharge Planning
- Long-term needs and who is responsible for specific actions
- Specific referrals made

Sample Nursing Outcomes & Interventions Classifications NOC/NIC

NOC—Urinary Continence
NIC—Pelvic Muscle Exercise

---

urge urinary INCONTINENCE — NANDA-I

[Diagnostic Division: Elimination]

Definition: urge urinary Incontinence: Involuntary loss of urine associated with an abrupt and strong desire to void.

Recognizing Cues

Related/Risk Factors
Alcohol, caffeine, or carbonated beverage consumption
Anxiety
Ineffective overweight self-management
Fecal impaction; involuntary sphincter relaxation
Ineffective toileting habits
Weakened pelvic floor

Defining Characteristics

Subjective or Objective
Decreased bladder capacity
Feeling of urgency with triggered stimulus; urine leakage before reaching toilet, with bladder contractions, or bladder spasms
Increased urinary frequency; loss of varying volumes of urine between voids, with urgency
Nocturia

Clinical Connections
Abdominal trauma/surgery, pelvic inflammatory disease; pregnancy; childbirth; pelvic surgery; overweight; enlarged prostate, prostate surgery; recurrent urinary tract infections (UTIs), diabetes, stroke, multiple sclerosis (MS), Parkinson disease, spinal cord injury, depression

---

Information that appears in brackets has been added by the authors to clarify and enhance the use of nursing diagnoses.

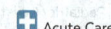 Acute Care 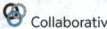 Collaborative 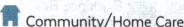 Community/Home Care Cultural

Generate Solutions

Plan Desired Outcomes

Client Will (Include Specific Time Frame)
- Identify individual risk factors and appropriate interventions.
- Verbalize understanding of condition.
- Demonstrate behaviors or techniques to control or correct situation.
- Report increase in interval between urge and involuntary loss of urine.
- Void every 3 to 4 hr in individually appropriate amounts.

Interventions/Take Action

Nursing Priority No. 1.
To assess causative/contributing factors:
- Identify/investigate the client's clinical signs and symptoms **to differentiate between types of urinary incontinence (i.e., urge incontinence, disability incontinence, stress incontinence, or mixed incontinence).** Urge urinary incontinence **is characterized by a sudden urge to void that often results in involuntary leakage of urine, nocturia, and increased urinary frequency. Causes of urge incontinence include detrusor muscle dysfunction (i.e., involuntary contraction, neurogenic dysfunction, poor compliance), bladder hypersensitivity (i.e., inflammation, infection), or idiopathic causes.**
- Consider client's gender and age **to assess client risk factors. The incidence of urge incontinence continues to increase with age. Older women often have a mix of stress and urge incontinence, whereas individuals with dementia or disabling neurological disorders tend to have urge and disability-associated incontinence.**
- Discuss client's current medication regimen **to identify medications that may contribute to incontinence symptoms (e.g., alpha-adrenergic agonists/antagonists, angiotensin-converting enzyme inhibitors, anticholinergic drugs, calcium channel blockers, cholinesterase inhibitors, diuretics, lithium, psychotropic medications, sedatives, hypnotics, selective serotonin reuptake inhibitors, and opioid analgesics).**
- Review client's dietary patterns and identify the presence of bladder irritants (e.g., alcohol, caffeine, acidic, or spicy

---

Information that appears in brackets has been added by the authors to clarify and enhance the use of nursing diagnoses.

food) **to ascertain the potential impact of the client's diet on urinary incontinence.**
- Note presence of conditions often associated with urgent voiding (e.g., bladder dysfunction associated with nerves damaged by various diseases [diabetes, stroke, MS, Parkinson disease], spinal cord injury). Other comorbidities associated with overactive bladder include recent/ongoing UTI, fecal incontinence, chronic constipation; obesity; postmenopausal hormonal changes. **These conditions affect bladder innervation, musculature tone, and storage. Additionally, triggering factors (e.g., feeling of running water, lifting, bending, sexual activity, movement, changes in position) should be evaluated to obtain a comprehensive assessment of relevance to the client's urinary incontinence.**
- Discuss the degree of urgency and length of warning time between the initial urge and loss of urine. **Bladder overactivity or irritability shortens the length of time between urge and urine loss and helps clarify the type of incontinence.**
- Measure the amount of urine voided, especially noting amounts less than 100 mL or greater than 550 mL, **to determine bladder capacity and effectiveness of bladder contractions to facilitate emptying.** Refer to ND risk for urinary Retention.
- Collaborate with the healthcare provider to perform a focused physical examination **to identify causes or factors contributing to urinary incontinence. The examination may include:**
  Pelvic/genitourinary examination **to assess vaginal atrophy, incontinence-associated dermatitis, and extraurethral urine loss/fistula. A digital examination may be performed to evaluate the tone and strength of the client's pelvic floor. Having a client perform a Valsalva maneuver for more than 6 sec may provide evidence of pelvic organ prolapse. A postvoid residual should be measured via sonography to assess bladder emptying.**
  Abdominal examination **to reveal costovertebral angle tenderness, pelvic masses, and a palpable bladder.**
  Neurological examination evaluation **to assess the client's mental status, perineal reflexes and sensation, patellar reflexes, gait, and mobility.**
  Body mass index assessment.
- Assess for cloudy, odorous urine **associated with acute, painful urgency symptoms. Incontinence often reflects presence of infection.**

Information that appears in brackets has been added by the authors to clarify and enhance the use of nursing diagnoses.

- Assist with appropriate diagnostic testing (e.g., urinalysis, noninvasive bladder scanning, urine culture, urine and serum glucose, voiding cystometrogram). **Accurate assessment and diagnosis can determine voiding patterns and identify pathology that may lead to the development of incontinence. Additional bedside examinations, such as the cough stress test and the cotton swab test, may be used to discern incontinence causes. Note: Routine imaging should not be performed in the initial assessment of uncomplicated urge incontinence other than sonography to assess postvoid residual. Urinalysis should be used to evaluate for the presence of UTI and to exclude hematuria, proteinuria, and glycosuria. Renal function should be assessed if there is concern for obstruction. The presence of glucose in the urine may cause polyuria, resulting in overdistention of the client's bladder and difficulty in holding urine.**
- Refer to NDs mixed, stress, or disability-associated urinary Incontinence for related assessments and interventions.

Nursing Priority No. 2.
To assess degree of interference/disability:

- Record client fluid intake, urinary frequency, and degree of urgency during a typical day and night **to identify the degree of difficulty being experienced by the client. A voiding diary gathers data on fluid intake, client symptoms, and situations associated with incontinence symptoms, and may identify the degree of difficulty being experienced by the client.**
- Provide client/caregiver with a validated questionnaire (e.g., Pelvic Floor Distress Inventory, Pelvic Floor Impact Questionnaire, Urogenital Distress Inventory (UDI), King Health Questionnaire, or Urge UDI) **to quantify the impact of bladder symptoms on the client's quality of life. There is a considerable impact on the quality of life of individuals with an incontinence problem, affecting socialization and view of themselves as sexual beings and sense of self-esteem.**
- Interview client/caregiver regarding their perceptions and concerns about urinary incontinence **to discern the degree of concern client is experiencing and the need for preventive measures to be instituted.**

Information that appears in brackets has been added by the authors to clarify and enhance the use of nursing diagnoses.

Nursing Priority No. 3.
To assist in **treating** incontinence:

- Assist in treatment of the underlying conditions that may contribute to urge incontinence. **Urgency symptoms may resolve with treatment of the medical problem (e.g., UTI; recovery from pelvic surgery, childbirth, or pelvic trauma; use of estrogen-based oral or topical products for atrophic vaginitis).**
- Implement continence management interventions:

Establish voiding schedule (habit and bladder training) based on client's usual voiding pattern. **A bladder retraining program may be successful in alleviating urge incontinence. Note: A review of multiple studies revealed a strongly positive effect on continence using a combination of behavioral interventions (including bladder control strategies, fluid management, and pelvic floor muscle exercises) and medications in older women. However, clients may have difficulty sustaining the effort of behavioral modification, and thus, the positive effect is lost.**

Recommend consciously delaying voiding by using distraction (e.g., slow, deep breathing), self-statements (e.g., "I can wait"), and contracting pelvic muscles when exposed to triggers. **Behavioral techniques are sometimes helpful for urge suppression, especially in younger clients.**

Encourage regular pelvic floor strengthening exercises (Kegel exercises) **to improve pelvic musculature, tone, and strength, thus preventing or halting incontinence. Combining pelvic floor strengthening with biofeedback may enhance the effectiveness of training and success at controlling incontinence.**

Instruct client to tighten pelvic floor muscles before arising from bed or chair **to help prevent loss of urine as abdominal pressure changes.**

Help client manage fluid and ensure adequate intake (e.g., 50 to 70 oz of fluid daily in smaller increments, such as 10 to 12 servings daily) **to prevent dehydration and promote good urine flow. Clients on fluid restriction may require additional guidance from their healthcare provider.** Monitor I/O and reduce fluid if indicated. **Too much water can also increase bladder irritation, so amount of intake needs to be determined by the client's response.**

Limit liquid intake 2 to 3 hr prior to bedtime **to promote a predictable voiding pattern and limit nocturia.**

Information that appears in brackets has been added by the authors to clarify and enhance the use of nursing diagnoses.

Suggest diet modifications (e.g., reduce acidic/citrus juices, chocolate and caffeine-containing drinks, carbonated beverages, spicy foods, artificial sweeteners) **to reduce bladder irritants. Note: Using a food/drink diary may help identify which foods/food groups/beverages cause bladder pain and/or urgency.**

Assist client in managing bowel elimination **to prevent urinary incontinence associated with constipation or fecal impaction.** (Refer to ND risk for [chronic/functional] Constipation and impaired intestinal Elimination.)

- Provide assistance or devices, as indicated, for clients who are mobility impaired. **Providing means of summoning assistance and placing bedside commode, urinal, or bedpan within client's reach can promote a sense of control in self-managing voiding.**

- Offer assistance to cognitively impaired client (e.g., prompt client or take to bathroom on regularly timed schedule) **to reduce frequency of incontinence episodes and promote comfort.**

- Refer client to specialists or treatment program, as indicated, for additional and specialized interventions (e.g., use of vaginal cones, electronic stimulation therapy). **Significant reduction in incontinence episodes is reported with use of combined therapies (e.g., electronic stimulation therapy plus pelvic muscle exercises).**

- Administer medications such as antimuscarinic agents (e.g., darifenacin [Enablex], fesoterodine [Toviaz], oxybutynin [Ditropan], solifenacin [VESIcare], tolterodine [Detrol], trospium [Sanctura], or beta-3 adrenoceptor agonists (e.g., mirabegron [Myrbetriq]) **to treat urge incontinence. Although these medications are effective in reducing voiding frequency and urgency, common adverse events associated with these drugs include dry mouth, blurred vision, tachycardia, constipation, impaired cognition, and urinary retention. The high incidence of adverse effects has caused many clients to be noncompliant with these medication regimens.**

- Discuss possible surgical interventions with client/caregiver. **Surgical treatments may be required or desired when conservative treatments fail. Some of these include percutaneous tibial nerve stimulation; intravesical onabotulinum toxin A (Botox) injection delivered via cystoscopy; surgically implanted sacral, pudendal, and paraurethral nerve stimulators.**

Information that appears in brackets has been added by the authors to clarify and enhance the use of nursing diagnoses.

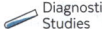 Diagnostic Studies 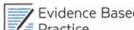 Evidence Based Practice 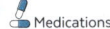 Medications 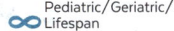 Pediatric/Geriatric/Lifespan

Nursing Priority No. 4.

To promote urinary continence (Teaching/Discharge Considerations) and enhance well-being (long-term goals):

- Provide information to client/significant other (SO)(s) about potential for urge incontinence and lifestyle measures **to prevent or limit incontinence.**
- Encourage comfort measures (e.g., use of incontinence pads or undergarments, wearing loose-fitting or especially adapted clothing) **to prepare for and manage urge incontinence symptoms over the long term and enhance sense of security and confidence in abilities to be socially active.**
- Discuss with client/caregiver the importance of regular perineal care after each voiding **to prevent skin irritation and reduce the potential for bladder infection and incontinence-related dermatitis.**
- Review with client/caregiver signs/symptoms indicating urinary complications and the need for medical follow-up care **to help the client seek intervention promptly to prevent more serious problems from developing.**
- Recommend limiting intake of coffee, tea, and alcohol. **These substances have an irritating effect on the bladder and may contribute to incontinence.**

Documentation Focus

Assessment/Reassessment
- Individual findings, including specific risk factors and pattern of voiding or incontinence effect on lifestyle, and self-esteem

Planning
- Plan of care, specific interventions, and who is involved in planning
- Teaching plan

Implementation/Evaluation
- Response to interventions, teaching, and actions performed
- Attainment of or progress toward desired outcome(s)
- Modifications to plan of care

Discharge Planning
- Discharge needs and who is responsible for actions to be taken
- Specific referrals made

Information that appears in brackets has been added by the authors to clarify and enhance the use of nursing diagnoses.

Sample Nursing Outcomes & Interventions Classifications NOC/NIC

NOC—Urinary Continence
NIC—Urinary Bladder Training

risk for INFECTION NANDA-I

[Diagnostic Division: Safety]

Definition: Vulnerable to invasion and multiplication of pathogenic organisms.

Recognizing Cues

Risk Factors

Difficulty managing long-term invasive devices, or wound care
Dysfunctional gastrointestinal motility; status of body fluid
Malnutrition; ineffective overweight self-management
Impaired skin integrity
Inadequate access to personal protective equipment; inadequate adherence to public health recommendations; inadequate environmental hygiene; inadequate personal hygiene, or oral hygiene practices
Inadequate health literacy; inadequate knowledge to avoid pathogen exposure; inadequate vaccination
Tobacco use

Clinical Connections

Immune-suppressed conditions (e.g., HIV positive, AIDS, cancer), chronic obstructive pulmonary disease, long-term use of steroids (e.g., asthma, rheumatoid arthritis, systemic lupus erythematosus), diabetes mellitus, malnutrition, anemia, surgical or invasive procedures, substance abuse, burns, wounds, pregnancy—preterm labor, premature/prolonged rupture of amniotic membranes

Generate Solutions

Plan Desired Outcomes

Client Will (Include Specific Time Frame)
- Verbalize understanding of individual risk factor(s).
- Identify interventions to prevent or reduce risk of infection.

Information that appears in brackets has been added by the authors to clarify and enhance the use of nursing diagnoses.

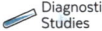 Diagnostic Studies 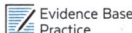 Evidence Based Practice 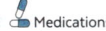 Medications 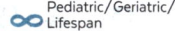 Pediatric/Geriatric/Lifespan

- Demonstrate techniques and lifestyle changes to promote safe environment.
- Achieve timely wound healing; be free of purulent drainage or erythema; be afebrile.

Interventions/Take Action

Nursing Priority No. 1.
To assess risk factors:

- Assess for presence of host-specific factors that affect immunity:

    Extremes of age. **Newborns and the elderly are more susceptible to disease and infection than the general population.**

    Presence of underlying disease. **The client may have a disease that directly impacts the immune system (e.g., cancer, AIDS, autoimmune disorder) or may be weakened by prolonged disease conditions (e.g., diabetes, kidney disease, heart failure) or their treatments.**

    Certain treatment settings/modalities. **The client in an acute care/critical care setting and/or on mechanical ventilation may have a prolonged exposure to risk factors for infection, including problems with breathing, circulation, gastrointestinal motility disorders, and use of analgesics and sedatives, causing a higher rate of acquired infections. Acute/critical-care settings often include use of invasive monitoring and supportive devices (e.g., mechanical ventilation, urinary catheter, central venous access, ventriculostomy tubes, chest tubes). The addition of these treatment or monitoring strategies to the acutely/critically ill client requires vigilant and judicious nursing care to prevent client harm.**

    Lifestyle. **Personal habits or living situations such as persons sharing close quarters and/or equipment (e.g., college dorm, group home, long-term care facility, day care, large public assembly facilities, correctional facility), persons/groups with inadequate vaccination protection, IV drug use and shared needles, and unprotected sex can increase susceptibility to infections.**

    Nutritional. **Malnutrition weakens the immune system (particularly in infants, young children, elderly sick, and individuals with chronic conditions). Poor oral intake, insufficient essential nutrients, inadequate**

Information that appears in brackets has been added by the authors to clarify and enhance the use of nursing diagnoses.

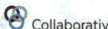 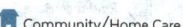

food preparation, improper handling of tube feedings/infant formula, or elevated serum glucose level (e.g., administration of total parenteral nutrition, glucocorticoid use, or poorly controlled diabetes mellitus) **increases the risk for pathogen proliferation.**

Trauma. **Loss of skin and tissue integrity, invasive diagnostic procedures or surgery, premature rupture of amniotic membrane, urinary catheterizations, parenteral injection, sharps, and needlesticks are common paths of pathogen entry.**

Certain medications. **Steroids, immunosuppressives, and chemotherapeutic agents directly affect the immune system. Long-term or improper antibiotic treatment can disrupt the body's normal flora and result in increased susceptibility to antibiotic-resistant organisms.**

Presence or absence of immunity. **Natural immunity may be acquired as a result of the development of antibodies to a specific agent following infection, preventing recurrence of a specific disease (e.g., chickenpox). Active immunity (via vaccination, e.g., measles, polio) and passive immunity (e.g., antitoxin or immunoglobulin administration) can prevent certain communicable diseases. Note: Passive immunity does not provide permanent protection from an antigen.**

Environmental exposure, **which may be accidental or intentional. Exposure can occur in different ways, such as the use of specific microorganisms (in laboratories, biotechnological industries, or acts of bioterrorism). Accidental exposures can result from exposure to contaminants arising from commonplace processes (e.g., wastewater recycling), through animal contact (e.g., agriculture, animal food processing), or through contact with humans (e.g., healthcare, education, mass transit, close contact living).**

- Observe at-risk client for:

  Changes in skin color and warmth at insertion sites of invasive lines, sutures, surgical incisions, and wounds **that could be signs of developing localized infection.**

  Changes in mental status, skin warmth and color, heart and respiratory rate, oxygen saturation, temperature **that could be signs of developing systemic infection.**

  Changes in color and/or odor of secretions (e.g., sputum), drainage (e.g., wound drains or invasive tubes), and excretions (e.g., urine) **that could indicate onset of infection.**

Information that appears in brackets has been added by the authors to clarify and enhance the use of nursing diagnoses.

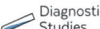 Diagnostic Studies
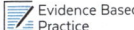 Evidence Based Practice
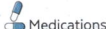 Medications
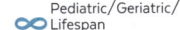 Pediatric/Geriatric/Lifespan

Skin conditions around insertions of orthopedic pins, wires, and tongs. **Direct connection to bone increases the risk of infections in bone sites that can lead to osteomyelitis, bone loss, and long-term delays of healing.**

- Review laboratory values (e.g., complete white blood cell count and with differential, cultures [i.e., blood, urine, sputum, or wound]) **to identify presence of anemia, leukopenia, type of pathogens and treatment options.**
- Refer to NDs risk for Aspiration; Contamination Exposure; risk for urinary tract Injury; impaired oral Mucous Membrane; impaired Skin Integrity; impaired Tissue Integrity for related assessments and interventions.

Nursing Priority No. 2.
To reduce/correct existing risk factors:

Healthcare Environment—General Concerns

- Practice and emphasize consistent and proper hand hygiene by all caregivers between therapies and clients. Wear gloves when appropriate to minimize contamination of hands, and discard gloves after each client. Wash hands after glove removal. Instruct the client/significant other (SO)/visitors to wash hands, as indicated. **This is a first-line defense against healthcare-associated infections (HAIs).**
- Provide clean, well-ventilated environment (may require turning off central air-conditioning and opening window for good ventilation; room with negative air pressure, etc.).
- Monitor the client's visitors and caregivers for respiratory illnesses. Limit interpersonal contact when necessary. Offer masks and tissues to client/visitors who are at risk for acquiring or transmitting infections **to limit exposures, thus reducing cross-contamination.**
- Post visual alerts in healthcare settings instructing clients/SO(s) to inform healthcare providers if they have symptoms of respiratory infections or influenza-like symptoms.
- Provide for isolation, as indicated (e.g., contact, droplet, airborne precautions). Educate staff in infection control procedures. **Reduces the risk of cross-contamination.**
- Emphasize proper use of personal protective equipment by staff and visitors, as dictated by agency policy, **for particular exposure risk (e.g., airborne, droplet, splash risk), including appropriate mask or respiratory filter, gowns, aprons, head covers, face shields, and protective eyewear.**
- Include information in preoperative teaching about ways to reduce potential for postoperative infection (e.g., respiratory

---

Information that appears in brackets has been added by the authors to clarify and enhance the use of nursing diagnoses.

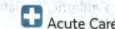 Acute Care 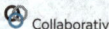 Collaborative 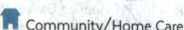 Community/Home Care   Cultural

measures to prevent pneumonia, wound or dressing care, avoidance of others with infection).
- Encourage early ambulation, deep breathing, coughing, position changes, early removal of endotrachial tube and/or nasal or oral feeding tubes **for mobilization of respiratory secretions and prevention of aspiration/respiratory infections.**
- Maintain adequate hydration and electrolyte balance **to prevent imbalances that would predispose to infection.**
- Provide or encourage a balanced diet, emphasizing proteins to support the immune system. **Immune function is affected by protein intake; the balance between omega-6 and omega-3 fatty acid intake; and adequate amounts of vitamins A, C, and E, and the minerals zinc and iron.**
- Handle and properly package used tissues and fluid specimens.
- Assist with medical procedures (e.g., wound or joint aspiration, incision and drainage of abscess, bronchoscopy), as indicated.
- Administer/monitor medication regimen (e.g., antimicrobials, drip infusion into osteomyelitis, subeschar clysis, topical antibiotics) and note the client's response **to determine effectiveness of therapy or presence of side effects.**
- Administer prophylactic antibiotics and immunizations, as ordered.
- Encourage or assist with use of adjuncts (e.g., respiratory aids, such as incentive spirometry, flutter valve) **to prevent pneumonia.**

Medical Devices
- Maintain sterile technique for all invasive procedures (e.g., IV, urinary catheter, pulmonary suctioning).
- Fill bubbling humidifiers and nebulizers with *sterile* water, not distilled or tap water. Avoid use of room-air humidifiers unless unit is sterilized daily and filled with sterile water.
- Use disposable equipment whenever possible. Disinfect or sterilize reusable equipment and surfaces according to manufacturer recommendations.
- Dispose of needles and sharps in approved containers **to reduce risk of needlestick or sharps injury.**
- Assist with monitoring client on the ventilator for signs of bacterial infections and weaning from mechanical ventilator as soon as possible **to reduce risk of ventilator-associated pneumonia (VAP).**

Information that appears in brackets has been added by the authors to clarify and enhance the use of nursing diagnoses.

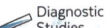 Diagnostic Studies 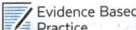 Evidence Based Practice 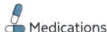 Medications 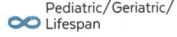 Pediatric/Geriatric/Lifespan

- Choose a proper vascular access device based on anticipated treatment duration, solution/medication to be infused, and best available aseptic insertion techniques; cleanse incisions and insertion sites daily/per facility protocol with the appropriate solution **to reduce the potential for catheter-related bloodstream infections.**

Skin/Tissues
- Change surgical or other wound dressings, as indicated, using proper technique for changing/disposing of contaminated materials.
- Cleanse incisions and insertion sites per facility protocol with appropriate antimicrobial topical or solution **to prevent the potential for catheter-related bloodstream infections and to prevent the growth of bacteria.**
- Separate touching surfaces when skin is excoriated, such as in herpes zoster, burns, weeping dermatitis, and apply appropriate skin barriers. Use gloves when caring for open lesions **to minimize auto-inoculation or transmission of viral diseases.**
- Cover perineal and pelvic region dressings or casts with plastic when using bedpan **to prevent contamination.**
- Perform or instruct client/SO in daily mouth care. Include use of antiseptic mouthwash for individuals in acute or long-term care settings **at high risk for HAIs, especially in client on a ventilator.**
- Provide regular urinary catheter and perineal care. **Reduces the risk of ascending urinary tract infection.**
- Recommend or assist client with routine or preoperative antiseptic body shower or scrubs when indicated (e.g., orthopedic, plastic surgery) **to reduce bacterial colonization.**

Community
- Encourage parents of sick children to keep them away from childcare settings and school until afebrile for 24 hr.
- Recommend individuals/staff isolate themselves at home when ill to prevent the spread of infection to others, including coworkers.
- Alert infection control officer/proper authorities to the presence of specific infectious agents and number of cases, as required by individual state/Centers for Disease Control and Prevention, such as sexually transmitted infections (STIs), tuberculosis (TB), measles, chickenpox, foodborne illnesses,

---

Information that appears in brackets has been added by the authors to clarify and enhance the use of nursing diagnoses.

arboviral disease (e.g., viruses spread by mosquitoes, ticks), viral hepatitis. **Provides for case finding and helps curtail outbreaks.**
- Group/cohort individuals with the same diagnosis or exposure as resources require. **Limited resources (as may occur with an outbreak or epidemic) may dictate a wardlike environment.**
- Encourage client/SO/caregiver(s) to contact healthcare provider for prophylactic therapy as indicated following exposure to individuals with infectious disease (e.g., TB, hepatitis, influenza).

Nursing Priority No. 3.

To promote uncomplicated healing (Teaching/Discharge Considerations) and enhance well-being (long-term goals):

- Review client's nutritional needs, appropriate exercise program, and need for rest.
- Instruct the client/SO(s) in techniques to protect the integrity of the skin, care for lesions, and prevent spread of infection.
- Emphasize the necessity of taking antivirals or antibiotics, as directed (e.g., dosage and length of therapy). **Premature discontinuation of treatment when client begins to feel well may result in return of infection and potentiation of drug-resistant strains.**
- Discuss the importance of not taking antibiotics or of using "leftover" drugs unless specifically instructed by a healthcare provider. **Inappropriate use can lead to development of drug-resistant strains or secondary infections.**
- Discuss the role of smoking in respiratory infections and in postoperative healing. Refer to smoking cessation programs as indicated.
- Promote safer-sex practices and report sexual contacts of infected individuals **to prevent the spread of HIV and other STIs.**
- Encourage high-risk persons, including healthcare workers, to have influenza, and pneumonia, and other appropriate vaccinations **to reduce individual risk as well as help prevent the spread of flu and viral pneumonia to others.**
- Provide client/SO with information and involve the client in appropriate community and national education programs **to increase awareness of and prevention of communicable diseases.**

Information that appears in brackets has been added by the authors to clarify and enhance the use of nursing diagnoses.

- Discuss precautions with the client engaged in domestic or international travel, and refer for restrictions/immunizations **to reduce incidence and transmission of global infections.**
- Promote childhood immunization program. Encourage adults to obtain/update immunizations as appropriate.
- Review the use of prophylactic antibiotics, if appropriate (e.g., prior to dental work for clients with a history of immunosuppressive conditions, rheumatic fever, or valvular heart disease).
- Encourage contacting healthcare provider for prophylactic therapies, as indicated, following exposure to individuals with infectious disease (e.g., TB, hepatitis, influenza).
- Identify resources available to the individual (e.g., substance abuse rehabilitation or needle exchange program, as appropriate; free condoms).
- Refer to NDs ineffective Home Maintenance Behaviors; ineffective Health Maintenance Behaviors.

Documentation Focus

Assessment/Reassessment
- Individual risk factors, including recent or current antibiotic therapy
- Wound and/or insertion sites, character of drainage or body secretions
- Signs and symptoms of infectious process

Planning
- Plan of care, specific interventions, and who is involved in planning
- Teaching plan

Implementation/Evaluation
- Responses to interventions, teaching, and actions performed
- Attainment of or progress toward desired outcome(s)
- Modifications to plan of care

Discharge Planning
- Discharge needs, referrals made, and who is responsible for actions to be taken
- Specific referrals made

Sample Nursing Outcomes & Interventions Classifications NOC/NIC

NOC—Knowledge: Infection Management
NIC—Infection Protection

Information that appears in brackets has been added by the authors to clarify and enhance the use of nursing diagnoses.

risk for burn INJURY

NANDA-I

[Diagnostic Division: Safety]

Definition: Susceptible to skin or tissue damage by heat, steam, chemicals, electricity, or the like.

Recognizing Cues

Risk Factors
Inattentive to environmental safety

Inadequate knowledge of safety precautions; inadequate caregiver knowledge of safety precautions

Inadequate protective clothing (e.g., flame-retardant sleepwear, gloves, ear coverings); inappropriate use of protective clothing

Inappropriate use of heating pad, hot water bottle, or electric blanket

Inadequate supervision; unsafe cooking equipment

Smoking in bed, or near oxygen

Clinical Connections
Head trauma, stroke, spinal cord injury, peripheral neuropathy, surgical procedure, radiation therapy, neonatal jaundice therapy, dementia/Alzheimer disease, substance misuse, attempted suicide

Generate Solutions

Plan Desired Outcomes

Client Will (Include Specific Time Frame)
- Be free of damage to skin or mucous membranes associated with extreme temperatures.
- Demonstrate behaviors, lifestyle changes to reduce risk factors and protect from injury.

Interventions/Take Action

Nursing Priority No. 1.
To identify causative/precipitating factors related to risk:
- Identify client at risk (e.g., chronic illness conditions with weakness or prolonged immobility; acute or chronic confusion, mental illness, dementia, head injury; use of multiple medications; use of alcohol or other drugs; cultural, familial, and socioeconomic factors adversely affecting lifestyle and home; exposure to environmental chemicals).

Information that appears in brackets has been added by the authors to clarify and enhance the use of nursing diagnoses.

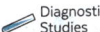 Diagnostic Studies 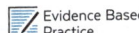 Evidence Based Practice 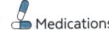 Medications 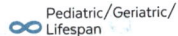 Pediatric/Geriatric/Lifespan

- Note chronological and developmental age of client. **Infants, young children, disabled, debilitated, aged, or impaired individuals are not able to protect themselves and may not recognize and/or react appropriately in dangerous situations. Fire-/burn-related injuries are among the leading 10 causes of unintentional injury in children ages 0 to 5, with children aged 2 years and younger at greatest risk.**
- Evaluate client's/significant other's (SO's) level of cognition, competence, decision-making ability, and independence.
- Ascertain if client is using alcohol/other drugs or medications **that could impair ability to act in best interest of self or others.**
- Evaluate client's lifestyle practices, noting reports of risk-prone behavior (e.g., smoking in bed, failure to use safety equipment when working with chemicals, allowing child to play with matches, unprotected exposure to sun or hot environment) **that can place client or others at high risk for injury.**
- Ascertain knowledge of safety needs and injury prevention as well as motivation to prevent injury. **Information may reveal areas of misinformation, lack of knowledge, need for teaching.**

Nursing Priority No. 2.

To assist client/caregiver to reduce or correct individual risk factors:

- Provide client/SO information regarding client's specific situation and consequences of continuing unsafe behaviors **to enhance decision making, clarify expectations and individual needs.**
- Review client's physical and psychological abilities or limitations **to determine adaptations that may be required by current situation.**
- Provide for client's safety while in facility care (e.g., apply hot treatments judiciously; prevent/monitor smoking; exercise care in use of all electrical equipment in presence of oxygen; supervise shower/bath temperature in confused individuals, young children, or elderly adults) **to reduce risk of dermal injury.**
- Be mindful of skin safety issues during surgical procedures:
    Conduct a fire risk assessment at beginning of each surgical procedure and continuously monitor for changes in

---

Information that appears in brackets has been added by the authors to clarify and enhance the use of nursing diagnoses.

risk during procedure. **The highest risks involve an ignition source (e.g., electrocautery device), delivery of supplemental oxygen, and the operation of the ignition source near the oxygen (e.g., head, neck, or upper chest surgery).**

- Provide supplemental oxygen safely, using the lowest concentration possible, **to reduce amount of oxygen flowing into surgical field.**
- Verify electrical safety of equipment including intact cords, grounds, and medical engineering verification labels.
- Place dispersive electrode (electrocautery pad) over largest available muscle mass closest to surgical site, ensuring its contact **to prevent electrical burns.**
- Ascertain that alcohol-containing skin prep solutions are not pooled under client or in surgical drapes and had sufficient drying time **to prevent sparking when electrocautery equipment activated.**
- Protect surrounding skin and tissues appropriately when laser equipment is used in surgical procedures. **Prevents inadvertent skin integrity disruption, hair ignition, and adjacent anatomy injury in area of laser beam use.**

Apply eye protection before laser activation. **Eye protection for specific laser wavelength must be used to prevent injury.**

- Implement skin care protocol for client receiving radiation therapy:

Assess skin frequently for side effects of therapy; note breakdown and delayed wound healing. Emphasize importance of reporting open areas to caregiver. **A reddening and/or tanning effect (radiation dermatitis) may develop within the field of radiation.**

Avoid rubbing the skin or use of soap, lotions, creams, ointments, powders, or deodorants on area; avoid applying heat or attempting to wash off marks/tattoos placed on skin to pinpoint location for radiation therapy. **These factors can potentiate or otherwise interfere with radiation delivery and may increase dermal reaction.**

- Follow skin-care guidelines in infants receiving **phototherapy** for hyperbilirubinemia **to prevent dermal injury:**

Note type of phototherapy light source, and follow manufacturer's recommendations for safe use. **Each light source has unique specifications regarding the intensity of the light and distance between the light and**

Information that appears in brackets has been added by the authors to clarify and enhance the use of nursing diagnoses.

 Diagnostic Studies   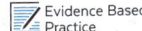 Evidence Based Practice   Medications   Pediatric/Geriatric/Lifespan the infant's skin. Note: **Halogen lamps emit more heat than fluorescent bulbs and therefore increase the risk of a burn.**

Cover male genitals. **Protects testes against chromatic radiant damage.**

Cover eyes completely with protective shields during use of overhead lights **to protect against retinal damage.**

Avoid application of lotion or oils to skin **to prevent dermal injury.**

- Provide or instruct in proper care of skin surfaces during exposure to sun or hot weather. **Although everyone is at risk for sunburn, individuals with impaired sensation or cognition and infants/young children require special attention to deal with exposure (e.g., limit/avoid exposure to sun between 10 a.m. and 2 p.m. when ultraviolet rays are most intense, using sunscreen as appropriate, limiting time in sun, and wearing light clothing and hat shading ears and neck to protect from dermal injury in summer).**

- Review proper use of sunscreen and avoiding use in infants less than 6 months of age. **The U.S. Food and Drug Administration and American Academy of Pediatrics recommend keeping infants in shade out of direct sunlight and avoiding use of sunscreen in this age group due to greater risk of side effects such as rash.**

- Discuss importance of self-monitoring of factors that can contribute to occurrence of injury (e.g., fatigue, anger). **Client/SO may be able to modify risk through monitoring of actions, especially during times when client is likely to be highly stressed/agitated.**

- Perform home assessment, if indicated, **to address safety issues. Concerns vary widely and may include evaluation of fire alarms or extinguisher function; safe use of oxygen; checking hot water temperature for elderly confused person; proper storage of chemicals; obtaining medical alert device or home health service, and so forth.**

- Review specific employment concerns or worksite issues and needs (e.g., properly fitting safety equipment, regular use of safety glasses or goggles, safe storage of hazardous substances).

- Discuss need for and sources of supervision (e.g., before- and after-school programs for children, elder day programs, home care assistance) **when client or care provider is unable or unwilling to attend to safety concerns.**

Information that appears in brackets has been added by the authors to clarify and enhance the use of nursing diagnoses.

Nursing Priority No. 3.

To promote continued vigilance (Teaching/Discharge Considerations) and enhance well-being (long-term goals):

- Identify individual needs and resources for safety education.
- Prevent burn injuries (flame, scalding, chemical, electrical, sunburn):

  Install smoke alarms in kitchen, in every sleeping area, and on every floor of home.

  Keep space heaters away from flammable materials and from at-risk persons.

  Check all fuel-burning appliances including fireplaces for proper function and install safety screens.

  Store combustibles away from all heat-producing appliances.

  Prepare and practice an emergency escape plan.

  Avoid smoking in bed. Dispose of used cigarettes carefully.

  Prevent small children from playing with matches or near open flame or stove.

  Turn handles of pots and pans toward side of stove or use back burners, do not leave stove unattended.

  Set the temperature on water heater to 120°F or use the "low-medium" setting.

  Test water temperature before allowing child/impaired person into tub or shower.

  Use cool-water humidifiers instead of hot-steam vaporizers.

  Store cleaning supplies and other chemicals out of the reach of children.

  Wear gloves, safety glasses, and other protective clothing when handling chemicals.

  Avoid storing chemicals in easily accessible locations or in food or drink containers; store in original containers with intact labels **to reduce risk of chemical burns.**

  Check electrical appliances for proper function and follow manufacturer's safety instructions. Discard frayed or damaged electrical cords. Avoid using electrical appliances while showering or in other wet environmental conditions **to reduce risk of electrical burns. Note: Most electrical injuries that occur in the home are low-voltage burns and almost exclusively involve either the hands or oral cavity.**

  Use child safety plugs in all electrical outlets.

  Avoid lengthy or unnecessary sun exposure/ultraviolet tanning, especially with specific disease conditions or treatments (e.g., systemic lupus, tetracycline or psychotropic drug use, radiation therapy) **to reduce risk of sunburn/ dermal injury.**

Information that appears in brackets has been added by the authors to clarify and enhance the use of nursing diagnoses.

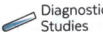 Diagnostic Studies 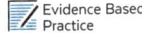 Evidence Based Practice 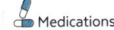 Medications 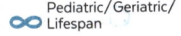 Pediatric/Geriatric/Lifespan

- Start protecting child from the sun when a baby, dressing infants in lightweight long pants, long-sleeved shirts, and brimmed hats that shade the neck/ears to prevent sunburn. **Note: Sunscreen is not recommended in babies under the age of 6 months; however, when used, sun protection factor (SPF) of 30 or higher is needed to protect babies' and children's sensitive skin.**
- Supervise child at play, identify environmental safety hazards and instruct child in safe play. **For example, playground equipment (e.g., slides, metal surfaces/monkey bars) and hardscape surfaces can heat up quickly, resulting in serious burns. Powerlines present risk of electrical injury when kite flying, climbing towers.**
- Refrain from use of fireworks by/near child. **In 2023, there were an estimated 9,700 hospital visits for firework-related injuries. Note: The tip of a sparkler can burn at up to 1,800°F.**
- Provide telephone numbers and other contact information as individually indicated (e.g., fire, police, physician).
- Refer to community resources/classes as indicated (e.g., smoking cessation, substance recovery, anger management, and parenting classes) **to address conditions that could exacerbate risk of injury to self or others.**
- Refer to or assist with community education programs **to increase awareness of safety measures and available resources, including First Aid and CPR.**
- Identify emergency escape plans and routes for home and community to be **prepared in the event of natural or man-made disaster (e.g., fire, toxic chemical release).**

Documentation Focus

Assessment/Reassessment
- Individual risk factors identified, knowledge of safety concerns/needs
- Client's concerns or difficulty making and following through with plan

Planning
- Plan of care and who is involved in planning
- Teaching plan

Implementation/Evaluation
- Response to interventions, teaching, and actions performed
- Attainment of or progress toward outcome(s)

Information that appears in brackets has been added by the authors to clarify and enhance the use of nursing diagnoses.

Discharge Planning
- Referrals to other resources
- Long-term need and who is responsible for actions

Sample Nursing Outcomes & Interventions Classifications NOC/NIC

NOC—Tissue Integrity: Skin & Mucous Membrane
NIC—Skin Surveillance

---

risk for cold INJURY NANDA-I

[Diagnostic Division: Safety]

Definition: Susceptible to skin or tissue damage by low environmental temperatures.

Recognizing Cues

Risk Factors
Inadequate knowledge of safety precautions
Inadequate caregiver knowledge of safety precautions; inadequate supervision
Inadequate use of ice pack
Inattentive to environmental safety; prolonged exposure to low temperature
Wet clothing in low-temperature environment
Inadequate protective clothing; inappropriate use of protective clothing
Inadequate nutritional intake
Tobacco use

Generate Solutions

Plan Desired Outcomes

Client Will (Include Specific Time Frame)
- Display body temperature within normal range.
- Be free of tissue damage or associated complication.

Client/Caregiver Will (Include Specific Time Frame)
- Identify underlying cause or contributing factors that are within client/caregiver control.
- Verbalize understanding of specific interventions to prevent hypothermia/cold injury.
- Maintain safe environment.

Information that appears in brackets has been added by the authors to clarify and enhance the use of nursing diagnoses.

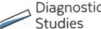 Diagnostic Studies   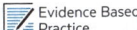 Evidence Based Practice   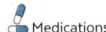 Medications   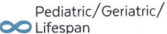 Pediatric/Geriatric/Lifespan

Interventions/Take Action

Nursing Priority No. 1.
To assess specific risks and contributing factors:

- Note the underlying risks (e.g., exposure to cold weather, winter outdoor activities; cold water drenching or immersion; improper clothing, shelter; and overtreatment of hyperthermia).
- Identify contributing factors: age of client (e.g., premature infant, child, elderly person), other factors (e.g., alcohol or other drug use or abuse), nutrition status (e.g., thin, tall person loses heat easier than short stature, overweight person), and living condition and relationship status (e.g., aged or cognitive impaired client living alone, homelessness).

Nursing Priority No. 2.
To assess the degree of injury/cold exposure:

- Assess client's skin/affected areas **for indications of tissue injury or death:**

  Color may be reddened, pale, white-gray, or bluish in color, indicating degree of tissue injury and compromised perfusion. **Skin palpation may demonstrate firm, waxy, consistency.**

  Swelling/edema may be present.

  Pain may accompany skin injury. **However, depending on the degree of injury, client sensation of the affected area may range from stinging/aching to numbness and paresthesia.**

  Ulceration and blisters may be noted in frostbitten tissue, including thickened wound drainage.

  Dysfunction of the affected area/extremity, **as hypothermia may cause joint stiffening and compromised muscle function.**

- Measure core temperature with low register thermometer (measuring below 94°F [34.4°C]).
- Monitor vital signs. **Cold stress reduces pacemaker function, and bradycardia (unresponsive to atropine), atrial fibrillation, atrioventricular blocks, and ventricular tachycardia can occur.**
- Measure urine output. **Cold injury/frostbite can cause muscle damage due to reduced blood flow and tissue ischemia and increases client risk for kidney injury (i.e., rhabdomyolysis).**

Information that appears in brackets has been added by the authors to clarify and enhance the use of nursing diagnoses.

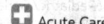 Acute Care 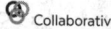 Collaborative 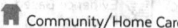 Community/Home Care 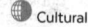 Cultural

- Monitor laboratory studies such as electrolytes (hyperkalemia initially, followed by hypokalemia after hypothermia-induced diuresis), complete blood count (increased hematocrit, decreased white blood cell count), cardiac enzymes (myocardial infarct may occur owing to electrolyte imbalance, cold stress catecholamine release, hypoxia, or acidosis), and glucose (hyperglycemia occurs initially, followed by hypoglycemia), as well as pharmacological profile (for toxicology [alcohol/other drugs]).

Nursing Priority No. 3.
To prevent/minimize injury and promote rewarming:

- Remove client from causative or contributing factors.
- Dry the skin, cover client with blankets or vapor barrier, and provide shelter with warm ambient temperature; use radiant lights.
- Warm the client's trunk first, not hands and feet. **Warming extremities first can cause shock.**
- Avoid exposing skin/the affected area to direct heat (e.g., uninsulated hot water bottles, heating pad, etc.). **Compromised sensation may prevent awareness of injury to tissue from direct heat.**
- Remove tight clothing or jewelry (e.g., rings or watches) **to prevent tissue constriction, prevent comprised perfusion, and prevent further injury.**
- Administer oxygen, as needed, **to support client's tissue oxygenation.**
- Collaborate with a wound specialist to dress injured and affected area(s). **Clients may require specialized treatment to promote revitalization of damaged tissue.**
- Administer medications, as indicated (e.g., antibiotics, analgesia, etc.).
- Offer and encourage warmed oral fluids (e.g., coffee, hot chocolate, hot tea, warm soup, etc.).
- Provide well-balanced, high-calorie diet or feedings **to replenish glycogen stores and nutritional balance.**

Nursing Priority No. 4.
To promote normothermia (Teaching/Discharge Considerations) and enhance well-being (long-term goals):

- Identify and discuss factors that client can control (if any), such as having protection from environment and adequate heat in home, layering clothing and blankets, minimizing heat loss from head with hat or scarf, having appropriate cold weather clothing, avoiding alcohol or other drugs

---

Information that appears in brackets has been added by the authors to clarify and enhance the use of nursing diagnoses.

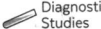 Diagnostic Studies 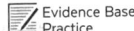 Evidence Based Practice 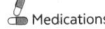 Medications 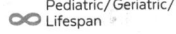 Pediatric/Geriatric/Lifespan

if anticipating exposure to cold, potential risks for future hypersensitivity to cold, etc.
- Discuss signs/symptoms of early cold injury/frostbite (e.g., paresthesia in the affected area, skin discoloration, etc.) **to facilitate recognition of problem and timely intervention. Information may be especially important if client works or plays outdoors (e.g., camping, skiing, hiking).**
- Emphasize the importance of follow-up with healthcare providers, as needed (e.g., wound care, physical therapy, etc.) **to ensure optimal wound healing and reduce the incidence of complications.**
- Educate client/caregiver to avoid alcohol, caffeine, and tobacco **to prevent cold-related injury.**
- Identify assistive community resources, as indicated (e.g., social services, emergency shelters, rewarming center, clothing suppliers, food bank, public service company, and financial resources). **Individual/significant other may need numerous resources if cold exposure was associated with inadequate housing, homelessness, or malnutrition.**
- Discuss client needs for counseling, and make referrals as appropriate.

Documentation Focus

Assessment/Reassessment
- Findings, noting degree/effects of hypothermia
- Graph temperature

Planning
- Plan of care and who is involved in planning
- Teaching plan

Implementation/Evaluation
- Responses to interventions, teaching, and actions performed
- Attainment or progress toward desired outcome(s)
- Modifications to plan of care

Discharge Planning
- Long-term needs, identifying who is responsible for each action
- Specific referrals made

Sample Nursing Outcomes & Interventions Classifications NOC/NIC

NOC—Personal Safety Behavior
NIC—Hypothermia Treatment

Information that appears in brackets has been added by the authors to clarify and enhance the use of nursing diagnoses.

risk for corneal INJURY   NANDA-I

[Diagnostic Division: Safety]

Definition: Susceptible to damage or trauma inflicted to the clear front surface of the eye by external means.

Recognizing Cues

Risk Factors
Exposure of the eyeball; exposure to chemical, biological, or physical agents
Excessive wind; low humidity
Inadequate knowledge of modifiable factors
Inappropriate use of contact lenses
Inadequate access to, or improper use of personal protective equipment
Omega-3 fatty acids deficiency; unaddressed vitamin A deficiency

Clinical Connections
Any condition where client is unable to protect self from injury to eye tissues, including facial or general trauma or surgery; mechanical ventilation; brain injury, cerebrovascular accident; neurological conditions such as Parkinson disease, Bell palsy; diabetic retinopathy; lupus; rheumatoid arthritis

Generate Solutions

Plan Desired Outcomes

Client/Caregiver Will (Include Specific Time Frame)
- Identify/monitor personal risk factors.
- Engage in risk-control strategies.

Client Will (Include Specific Time Frame)
- Be free of discomfort or damage to corneal tissues.

Interventions/Take Action

Nursing Priority No. 1.
To identify causative/precipitating factors related to risk:
- Obtain history of eye conditions when assessing client concerns overall. Listen for reports of eye pain, foreign body sensation, watery eye(s), light sensitivity (photophobia),

---

Information that appears in brackets has been added by the authors to clarify and enhance the use of nursing diagnoses.

and blurring or distorted vision. **These symptoms can be associated with corneal injury and, if present, require further evaluation and possible treatment.**
- Note the presence of conditions (e.g., recent neurological event, facial trauma or burns; use of contact lenses, failure to use safety glasses in high-risk employment situation) or treatment environments (e.g., intubated client on mechanical ventilation; use of therapeutic hypothermia; sedated, anesthetized, or obtunded client with absent blink reflex) **to identify client at high risk for corneal injury. Note: It has been reported that more than half of sedated/paralyzed clients on mechanical ventilation in the intensive care unit have incomplete closure of the eyelids (lagophthalmos), predisposing them to corneal dryness and inflammation.**
- Obtain a history of events from client/others when trauma (e.g., facial blunt force trauma, car crash with airbag deployment, accidental or intentional gunshot wounds; accidents with fireworks or hot metal) has occurred. **Eye injury (including corneal abrasions and lacerations) may not be immediately discovered but should be suspected.**
- Evaluate current drug regimen, noting pharmaceutical agents (e.g., topical drugs and preservatives in eyedrops; beta blockers, antihistamines, phenothiazides; diuretics, steroids, sedatives, neuromuscular blocking agents, antiparkinsonian agents, topical anesthetics), **which can contribute to dry eye, thereby increasing risk of corneal inflammation or injury in high-risk clients.**

Nursing Priority No. 2.
To promote eye health/comfort:

- Refer for diagnostic evaluation and interventions as indicated. **Standard eye examination and visual acuity testing may be performed, and other diagnostic studies (e.g., radiography, computed tomography, or magnetic resonance imaging may be indicated to locate foreign bodies or associated orbital, cranial, or facial trauma).**
- Assist in/refer for treatment of underlying conditions that might be affecting corneal health.
- Perform routine assessment of eyes and preventive interventions in critically ill client:
  Evaluate the client's ability to maintain eyelid closure on a daily basis and as needed.
  Perform actions to maintain eyelid closure in a client who cannot do it for self (e.g., taping).
  Observe for developing complications.

Information that appears in brackets has been added by the authors to clarify and enhance the use of nursing diagnoses.

- Perform eye care (e.g., cleaning with saline-soaked gauze and administration of eye-specific lubricant, when indicated).
- Refer for medical assessment and intervention, as indicated.
- Ascertain that the client undergoing anesthesia has proper eye protection (e.g., lubricant, eyelids taped, goggles), especially when placed in prone position. **The cornea is easily abraded because of reduced lacrimation during anesthesia or if face masks are improperly applied. In some positions, such as prone, a significant amount of pressure can be applied to the eyes.**

Nursing Priority No. 3.

To promote eye safety (Teaching/Discharge Considerations) and enhance well-being (long-term goals):

- Instruct high-risk client/caregivers in self-management interventions **to prevent corneal inflammation symptoms:**
  Avoid rubbing eyes with fingers or harsh cloths.
  Protect eyes from blowing air or oxygen; discuss benefit of redirecting airflow.
  Wear protective eyewear in situations or sports where objects may fly into eyes or face, including shooting sports.
  Wear protective eyewear that gives 180-degree protection while using power tools, a grinding wheel, or hammering on metal; or wear welding helmet when using welding torch.
  Wear protective goggles when handling chemical solutions. Immediately flush the eye with large amount of clean water if chemical splash occurs.
  Wear sunglasses that block ultraviolet radiation when in bright sunlight or under sunlamps, and especially during outdoor activities such as snow-/waterskiing. **The reflection of sunlight off the snow, water, or light sand in combination with direct sunlight causes a doubling of sunlight exposure.**
  Follow prescribed wear time for contact lenses. Remove with care **to prevent scratching eye with fingernail.**
  Use caution when applying eye makeup with mascara brush.
  Add moisture to indoor air, especially in winter. **Reduces corneal irritation associated with dryness.**
  Blink repeatedly for a few seconds at intervals when using the computer for any length of time **to prevent dryness and help spread tears evenly over eye.**

Information that appears in brackets has been added by the authors to clarify and enhance the use of nursing diagnoses.

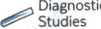 Diagnostic Studies 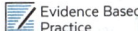 Evidence Based Practice 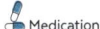 Medications 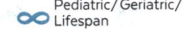 Pediatric/Geriatric/Lifespan

- Instruct in use of eyedrops or ointments, as indicated, **to prevent inflammation/infection, or to protect corneal surface.**
- Refer to appropriate healthcare provider concerning glasses, contact lenses, or other safety eyewear and resources.

Documentation Focus

Assessment/Reassessment
- Individual risk factors identified

Planning
- Plan of care and who is involved in planning
- Teaching plan

Implementation/Evaluation
- Response to interventions, teaching, and actions performed
- Attainment of or progress toward outcome(s)
- Difficulty following through with plan

Discharge Planning
- Referrals to other resources
- Long-term need and who is responsible for actions

Sample Nursing Outcomes & Interventions Classifications NOC/NIC

NOC—Risk Control: Visual Impairment
NIC—Eye Care

---

risk for occupational physical **INJURY** NANDA-I

[Diagnostic Division: Safety]

Definition: Susceptible to work-related bodily harm.

Recognizing Cues

Risk Factors
Individual:
Distraction from interpersonal relations
Excessive stress; ineffective use of coping strategies; overconfident behaviors
Improper use of personal protective equipment; unhealthy habits; unsafe work behaviors

---

Information that appears in brackets has been added by the authors to clarify and enhance the use of nursing diagnoses.

Inadequate knowledge; inadequate time management skills; misinterpretation of information

Psychological distress

Environmental Factors:

Unaddressed environmental constraints; exposure to environmental temperature extremes

Exposure to biological or chemical agents; exposure to radiation or teratogenic agents

Exposure to physical agents; pathogen exposure

Exposure to excessive noise; prolonged or excessive physical workload

Repetitive movements; exposure to vibration

Inadequate access to individual protective equipment; inadequate physical environment

Conflicted labor relationships

Clinical Connections

Any occupation and/or job setting has the potential for causing/aggravating injury

Generate Solutions

Plan Desired Outcomes

Client Will (Include Specific Time Frame)

- Develop/engage in plan to address individual risk factors and safety hazards.
- Demonstrate proper body alignment to prevent injury when performing work-related activities.
- Conform to safety guidelines in the workplace.
- Be free of injury.

Interventions/Take Action

Nursing Priority No. 1.

To evaluate degree/source of risk inherent in work setting:

- Determine factors related to individual situation and extent of risk for injury/illness. **Influences scope and intensity of interventions to manage threats to safety, which are dynamic and constants in every life and situation.**
- Note client's age, gender, developmental stage, decision-making ability, level of cognition, and competence **to determine client's ability to recognize danger and to protect self. Note: Younger workers (14 to 24 years) are twice as likely to incur injuries than older workers, and women are three times more likely than men, which may reflect**

Information that appears in brackets has been added by the authors to clarify and enhance the use of nursing diagnoses.

 Diagnostic Studies   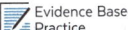 Evidence Based Practice   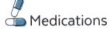 Medications   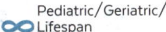 Pediatric/Geriatric/Lifespan

client's ability or desire to protect self, and influences choice of interventions or teaching.

- Identify client's history of injuries, medical conditions, and medications—prescribed, over-the-counter, vitamins, and herbals. **Can impact client's ability to safely perform certain movements/activities and suggests possible choice of interventions. Note: Research suggests cannabis abuse can increase severity of/time away from work following injury.**
- Evaluate visual, auditory, tactile, and kinesthetic perception. **Ability to correctly perceive and respond to one's environment greatly impacts worker's safety and well-being. Note: Blue-collar workers, older workers, and Hispanic workers have highest rates of uncorrected visual and/or hearing impairment, creating safety issues.**
- Identify employment/job specifics (e.g., works with dangerous tools/machinery, electricity, explosives, hazardous chemicals, first responder, healthcare worker, computer data entry, works alone or above ground). **Aids in identifying risks and individual safety needs.**
- Determine client's perception of individual safety and view of hazards in workplace including exposure to violence. **Lack of knowledge of safety needs or appreciation of significance of individual hazards increases risk of injury. Lack of focus on specific problem(s) can result in no change or may even result in increased injuries.**
- Clarify client's awareness of Occupational Safety and Health Administration (OSHA) standards applicable to client. **Lack of awareness can limit client's ability to make best decisions to promote personal safety.**
- Have client demonstrate routine work activities. **Musculoskeletal injuries are estimated to account for 33% of all workplace injuries. Proper body mechanics is vital for safe lifting, bending, reaching, stooping, pushing/pulling, repetitive motions, and so forth. Note: Hospital workers experience injuries at nearly three times the rate of professional and business services. Even physical therapists incur musculoskeletal injuries, especially low back injury, in spite of their knowledge of body mechanics.**
- Determine workplace environmental hazards and stressors (e.g., physical, biological, psychological, chemical, ergonomic) and their interrelationships. **May impair/negatively impact client's judgment and increase potential for injury. Furthermore, at a time of cost cutting and reorganization to sustain business profits/viability,**

Information that appears in brackets has been added by the authors to clarify and enhance the use of nursing diagnoses.

organizational culture may deflect responsibility of occupational injuries onto the worker without adequately considering all factors contributing to the situation.

Nursing Priority No. 2.

To assist client to reduce/correct individual risk factors:

- Review pertinent job-related safety regulations with client. **Provides information necessary for client to make informed decisions.**
- Develop plan with client to address individual needs and goals. **Being part of the solution increases likelihood of client commitment to the plan.**
- Identify facility/company resources available to decrease risk factors. **Solutions may be available at limited or no additional cost.**
- Modify work space as appropriate. **For example, for office worker, consider ergonomic chair, elevated computer desk, headset/Bluetooth device, voice recognition computer program; industrial site might require better lighting, handrails on stairs, reflective paint marking floor step-downs, containment barrier around chemical storage/mixing station; healthcare worker may need ceiling-mounted lifts to facilitate transfers, redesign of workstations with adjustable-height computer monitors.**
- Instruct in safety techniques/procedures specific to client's situation; for example:

  Wear appropriate protective gear—clothing/gowns, safety glasses/goggles, ear protectors, closed toe/steel-toed footwear, gloves, mask/respirator, safety harness, helmet.

  Avoid operating mechanical equipment/vehicle when using substances, including over-the-counter and prescription, that may impair functioning.

  Maintain adequate hydration/cooling in hot environments.

  Use proper body mechanics, frequent change of work position.

  Practice safe handling of sharps, double gloving during needlesticks, precautions with flammable materials, including oxygen.

  Practice proper handling of biologic materials/body fluids, chemical spills.

  Avoid mixing chemicals if possible; use in well-ventilated area.

  Practice situational awareness or being aware of what is happening around oneself and recognizing unsafe situations.

Information that appears in brackets has been added by the authors to clarify and enhance the use of nursing diagnoses.

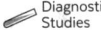 Diagnostic Studies 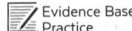 Evidence Based Practice Medications Pediatric/Geriatric/Lifespan

- Encourage client to read chemical labels or Material Safety Data Sheets (MSDS notebook) **to be aware of primary hazards, safe storage and handling.**
- Identify location of eye wash station/shower, first-aid kit, and safe use of automated external defibrillator.

Nursing Priority No. 3.
To promote optimum safety and well-being:
- Emphasize importance of adherence to lunch/break policy and using vacation or personal time regularly. **Too often, workers feel compelled to work through break time or postpone time away because of short staffing or to meet deadlines.**
- Refer to trainer or physical therapist for regular exercise program, including focus on core strength/stability and flexibility. **Research suggests decreased core strength contributes to injuries of back and extremities.**
- Encourage participation in wellness programs/monitoring of chronic conditions. **Stress management, weight loss, smoking cessation, and monitoring of long-term health issues such as hypertension and diabetes can help reduce illness and time away from work.**
- Recommend keeping vaccinations up to date, obtaining yearly flu shots and immunizations recommended for occupational risks. **Reduces risk of acquiring illness in workplace.**
- Support modified or light-duty work options as indicated. **Provides time for recovery while keeping worker engaged and reducing sense of isolation.**
- Emphasize importance of reporting injuries/completing reports in timely manner. **Although it is not unusual for minor injuries to go unreported, violence in the workplace can be accepted as "part of the job" and not reported but can cause significant psychological trauma and stress. Note: Workplace violence incidents requiring days off for worker to recuperate have been reported to be four times more common in healthcare than in private industry.**
- Obtain preventive screening/testing and initiate referrals to healthcare providers as appropriate. **Some chronic illnesses, such as respiratory, some cancers, and birth defects, have long latencies between occupational exposure and clinical findings.**

Information that appears in brackets has been added by the authors to clarify and enhance the use of nursing diagnoses.

Nursing Priority No. 4.

To promote safety in workplace:

- Identify applicable OSHA standards and workplace compliance with standards. **Knowledge keeps clients informed to potential hazards.**
- Provide OSHA or facility safety poster(s), copies of standards, and informational placards **to inform workers of their rights and responsibilities.**
- Inform workers of hazardous substances to which they may be exposed. **Promotes self-responsibility for personal safety.**
- Use problem-solving framework such as Public Health Model **to systematically identify and prioritize problems or risks, identify interventions or develop new strategies to prevent injury/illness, implement activities, and evaluate and monitor results of interventions.**
- Bring unsafe working conditions to employer's attention. **Advises employers of safety hazards and potential harm to employees requiring intervention.**
- Develop corrective plan with all parties involved. **Effectiveness of program requires commitment of management and participation of employees to analyze safety data and identify appropriate solutions.**
- Initiate workplace health promotion programs based on identified health risk assessment (e.g., smoking cessation, weight loss, stress management).
- Provide incentives for meeting individual/group goals. **Rewards/bonuses for health and safety behaviors or number of injury-free days encourages continuation of efforts.**
- Repair, replace, or correct unsafe equipment. Provide adaptive devices (e.g., step stool, handrails on movable stairs, safety guard/shield on mechanical equipment).
- Provide protective devices such as locked external doors, gates at stairwells, emergency alarms/phone stations, metal detectors, trained security personnel.
- Initiate screening programs for environmental hazards, such as noise, pollutants, allergens, dust, asbestos, lead/other heavy metals, vapor intrusion, radon, diesel emissions.
- Collaborate with appropriate agencies, such as public health and Environmental Protection Agency, to improve environmental hazards.
- Develop plan for long-term monitoring of health risks and evaluation of risk reduction strategies. **Provides evidence of effectiveness of interventions, possible need for revision. Information also adds to the body of knowledge in the field.**

Information that appears in brackets has been added by the authors to clarify and enhance the use of nursing diagnoses.

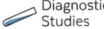 Diagnostic Studies 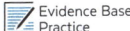 Evidence Based Practice 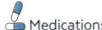 Medications 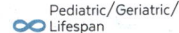 Pediatric/Geriatric/Lifespan

Documentation Focus

Assessment/Reassessment
- Medical history including past injuries, current medications; sensory abilities
- Client's awareness of safety needs, view of individual hazards in workplace
- Specific requirements of client's job
- Evaluation of workplace environmental hazards and stressors

Planning
- Plan of care and who is involved in the planning, including outside/public partners
- Teaching plan

Implementation/Evaluation
- Responses to interventions, teaching, and actions performed
- Attainment of or progress toward desired outcome(s)
- Modifications to plan of care

Discharge Planning
- Long-term needs and who is responsible for actions to be taken
- Available resources, specific referrals made

Sample Nursing Outcomes & Interventions Classifications NOC/NIC

NOC—Risk Control: Environmental Hazards
NIC—Environmental Management: Worker Safety

---

risk for perioperative positioning INJURY NANDA-I

[Diagnostic Division: Safety]

Definition: Susceptible to inadvertent bodily harm as a result of required posture or positioning equipment during an invasive and/or surgical procedure.

Recognizing Cues

Risk Factors
Inadequate fluid volume
Factors identified by standardized validated screening tool

Information that appears in brackets has been added by the authors to clarify and enhance the use of nursing diagnoses.

 Acute Care 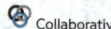 Collaborative 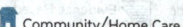 Community/Home Care   Cultural

Inadequate access to appropriate equipment, or support surfaces; rigid support surface

Inadequate availability of equipment for individuals with obesity

Prolonged inappropriate positioning of limbs

Clinical Connections
Surgical procedures, arthritis, diabetes, obesity, malnutrition, peripheral vascular disease

Generate Solutions

Plan Desired Outcomes

Client Will (Include Specific Time Frame)
- Be free of injury related to perioperative disorientation or altered consciousness.
- Be free of untoward skin and tissue or nerve injury or changes lasting beyond 24 to 48 hr postprocedure.
- Be free of nerve injury.

Interventions/Take Action

Nursing Priority No. 1.
To identify individual risk factors/needs:

- ∞ Review client's history, noting age, weight and height, nutritional status, physical limitations, or preexisting conditions (e.g., elderly person with arthritis; extremes of weight; diabetes or other conditions affecting peripheral vascular health; nutrition and hydration impairments). **Affects choice of perioperative positioning and affects skin and tissue integrity during surgery.**
- Evaluate and document client's preoperative reports of neurological, sensory, or motor deficits **for comparative baseline of perioperative and postoperative sensations.**
- Note anticipated length and type of procedure, type of anesthesia to be used, and customary position **to increase awareness of potential postoperative complications (e.g., supine position may cause low back pain and skin pressure at heels, elbows, and sacrum; lateral chest position can cause shoulder and neck pain, or eye and ear injury on the client's downside).**
- Evaluate environmental conditions/safety issues surrounding the sedated client (e.g., client alone in holding area, side rails up on bed and cart, use of tourniquets and arm boards, need for local injections) **that predispose client to potential tissue injury.**

Information that appears in brackets has been added by the authors to clarify and enhance the use of nursing diagnoses.

 Diagnostic Studies   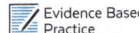 Evidence Based Practice   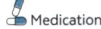 Medications   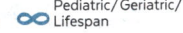 Pediatric/Geriatric/Lifespan

- Assess the individual's responses to preoperative sedation/medication, noting level of sedation and/or adverse effects (e.g., drop in blood pressure) and report to surgeon, as indicated. **Hypotension is a common factor associated with nerve ischemia.**

Nursing Priority No. 2.

To position client to provide protection for anatomical structures and to prevent client injury:

- Stabilize and lock transport cart or bed in place; support client's body and limbs; use adequate number of personnel during transfer **to prevent client fall or shear and friction injuries.**
- Position client on operating surface, using sufficient staff, appropriate positioning equipment or devices, and padding **to provide protection for anatomical structures and to prevent injury:**

  Apply padding and other safety devices depending on the particular position needed for procedure (not a comprehensive list):

  Place padding under all pressure points (e.g., skin and bony prominences over the occiput, scapulae, elbows, sacrum, coccyx, and heels); avoid overstretching shoulders when placing arms at 90 degrees **when client is in *supine* position.**

  Maintain neck alignment and provide protection or padding for forehead, eyes, nose, chin, breasts, genitalia, knees, and feet **when client is in *prone* position. Associated risks include increased abdominal pressure, bleeding, compartment syndrome, nerve injuries, cardiovascular compromise, ocular injuries/vision loss, and venous air embolism.**

  Protect bony prominences and pressure points on dependent side (e.g., axillary roll for dependent axilla; lower leg flexed at hip, upper leg straight; padding between knees, ankles, and feet) **when client is in *lateral* position. Risks include pressure to points on the dependent side as well as brachial plexus injury, venous pooling, diminished lung capacity, and deep venous thrombosis.**

  Place legs in stirrups simultaneously, adjusting stirrup height to client's legs, maintaining symmetrical position, and pad popliteal space as indicated **to reduce risk of peroneal and tibial nerve damage, prevent muscle strain, and reduce risk of hip dislocation when *lithotomy* position is used.**

Information that appears in brackets has been added by the authors to clarify and enhance the use of nursing diagnoses.

Secure client and pad shoulder braces to avoid sliding toward head on the surgical table. Avoid position for extremely obese clients **when *Trendelenburg* position is used. Note: This position may also result in respiratory compromise and eye injury.**
- Place safety straps strategically to secure client for specific procedure **to prevent unintended movement.**
- Apply and periodically reposition padding of pressure points and bony prominences (e.g., arms, elbows, sacrum, ankles, heels) and neurovascular pressure points (e.g., breasts, knees) **to maintain position of safety, especially when repositioning client and/or table attachments.**
- Position extremities to facilitate periodic evaluation of hands, fingers, and toes **to reduce risk of neurovascular injuries from prolonged pressure due to static position, compression, or stretch.**
- Protect body from contact with metal parts of the operating table, **which could produce burns or electric shock injury.**
- Prevent pooling of prep and irrigating solutions and body fluids. **Pooling of liquids in areas of high pressure under client increases risk of pressure injury development and presents electrical hazard.**
- Ascertain that eyelids are closed and secured **to prevent corneal abrasions.**
- Check peripheral pulses and skin color and temperature periodically **to monitor circulation.**
- Reposition slowly at transfer and in bed (especially halothane-anesthetized client) **to prevent severe drop in blood pressure, dizziness, or unsafe transfer.**
- Protect airway and facilitate respiratory effort following extubation.
- Determine specific position reflecting procedure guidelines (e.g., head of bed elevated following spinal anesthesia, **to prevent headache;** turn to unoperated side following pneumonectomy) **to facilitate maximal respiratory effort.**

Nursing Priority No. 3.
To promote well-being (Teaching/Discharge Considerations):

- Maintain equipment in good working order **to identify potential hazards in the surgical suite/recovery and implement corrections as appropriate.**
- Review perioperative teaching relative to client safety issues, including not crossing legs during procedures

---

Information that appears in brackets has been added by the authors to clarify and enhance the use of nursing diagnoses.

performed under local or light anesthesia, postoperative needs and limitations, and signs/symptoms requiring medical evaluation **to reduce incidence of preventable complications.**
- Inform client and postoperative caregivers of expected/transient reactions (e.g., low backache, localized numbness, and reddening or skin indentations, all of which should disappear in 24 hr).
- Assist with therapies and perform routine nursing actions, including skin care measures, application of elastic stockings, early mobilization **to enhance circulation and promote skin and tissue integrity.**
- Encourage range-of-motion exercises, especially when joint stiffness occurs.
- Refer to appropriate resources (e.g., pharmacy, medical supply, therapy, home health care), as needed.

Documentation Focus

Assessment/Reassessment
- Findings, including individual risk factors for problems in the perioperative setting or need to modify routine activities or positions
- Periodic monitoring activities

Planning
- Plan of care and who is involved in planning
- Teaching plan

Implementation/Evaluation
- Response to interventions and actions performed
- Attainment of or progress toward desired outcome(s)
- Modifications to plan of care

Discharge Planning
- Immediate needs and who is responsible for actions to be taken

Sample Nursing Outcomes & Interventions Classifications NOC/NIC

NOC—Risk Control
NIC—Positioning: Intraoperative

Information that appears in brackets has been added by the authors to clarify and enhance the use of nursing diagnoses.

risk for physical INJURY NANDA-I

[Diagnostic Division: Safety]

Definition: Susceptible to bodily harm due to trauma, electrical discharges, changes in pressure, and/or radiation.

Recognizing Cues

Risk Factors
Exposure to toxic chemicals
Inadequate knowledge of safety precautions, or modifiable factors
Inadequate safety protocol; inaccurate follow-through of safety protocols; inadequate safety equipment
Inattentive to environmental safety; inadequate safety rails; inattentive to safety devices during sports activities
Malnutrition
Psychomotor agitation; confusion
Inadequate caregiver knowledge of safety precautions
Cluttered environment; physical barrier
Unsafe mode of transportation

Clinical Connections
Head injury, stroke, seizure disorder, dementia, AIDS, cataracts, glaucoma, Parkinson disease, substance abuse, malnutrition, developmental delay, para-/quadriplegia, neuropathy, radiation therapy

Generate Solutions

Plan Desired Outcomes

Client Will (Include Specific Time Frame)
- Be free of injury.
- Verbalize understanding of individual factors that contribute to possibility of injury.
- Demonstrate behaviors, lifestyle changes to reduce risk factors and protect self from injury.
- Modify environment as indicated to enhance safety.

Information that appears in brackets has been added by the authors to clarify and enhance the use of nursing diagnoses.

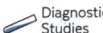 Diagnostic Studies 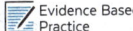 Evidence Based Practice 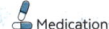 Medications 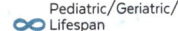 Pediatric/Geriatric/Lifespan

Interventions/Take Action

Nursing Priority No. 1.

To evaluate degree/source of risk inherent in the individual situation:

- ✚ Perform thorough assessments regarding safety issues when planning for client care and/or preparing for discharge from care. **Failure to accurately assess and intervene or refer these issues can place the client at needless risk and creates negligence issues for the healthcare practitioner. Note: Research has identified more than 30 safe practices that evidence shows can work to reduce or prevent adverse events and medical errors regarding client safety, including but not limited to adequate numbers of nursing personnel; evaluating each person on admission, and regularly thereafter, for the risk of developing pressure injuries; employing clinically appropriate strategies to prevent malnutrition; vaccinating healthcare workers against influenza to protect both them and clients; and standardizing methods for labeling, packaging, and storing medications.**
- Ascertain client's knowledge of safety needs, injury prevention, and motivation to prevent injury in home, community, and work settings.
- ∞ Note the client's age, gender, developmental stage, decision-making ability, and level of cognition/competence. **May affect the client's ability to protect self and/or others, and influence choice of interventions and teaching.**
- ∞ Review expectations caregivers have of children, cognitively impaired, and/or elderly family members.
- Assess mood, coping abilities, personality styles (e.g., temperament, aggression, impulsive behavior, level of self-esteem) **that may result in carelessness or increased risk taking without consideration of consequences.**
- ∞ Assess client's muscle strength and gross and fine motor coordination **to identify risk for falls. Note: The frequency of falls increases with age and frailty level. Risk factors for falls lie in four categories: (1) biological, (2) behavioral, (3) environmental, and (4) socioeconomic. In each of these areas, some risk factors can be modified to decrease fall risk.**
- Note socioeconomic status and availability and use of resources. **May limit their ability to access safety equipment, required services.**

Information that appears in brackets has been added by the authors to clarify and enhance the use of nursing diagnoses.

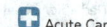 Acute Care 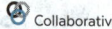 Collaborative 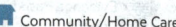 Community/Home Care   Cultural

- Evaluate the individual's emotional and behavioral response to violence in environmental surroundings (e.g., home, neighborhood, peer group, media). **May affect the client's view of and regard for own/others' safety.**
- Determine the potential for abusive behavior by family members/significant other(s) (SO[s])/peers.
- Observe for signs of injury and age (current, recent, and past such as old or new bruises, history of fractures, frequent absences from school or work) **to determine need for evaluation of intentional injury or abuse in client relationship or living environment.**
- Identify knowledge of safety needs and injury prevention and motivation to prevent injury in home, community, and work settings. **Information may reveal areas of misinformation, lack of knowledge, and need for improved communication or teaching.**

Nursing Priority No. 2.

To assist client/caregiver to reduce or correct individual risk factors:

- Provide healthcare within a culture of safety (e.g., adherence to nursing standards of care and facility safe-care policies) **to prevent errors resulting in client injury, promote client safety, and model safety behaviors for client/SO(s):**
  Practice hand hygiene at all times and device safety when client has IV lines and catheters **to prevent healthcare-associated infections and potential for bloodborne pathogens.**
  Administer medications and infusions using "six rights" system (right client, right medication, right route, right dose, right time, right documentation).
  Inform and educate client/SO regarding all treatments and medications.
  Monitor the environment for potentially unsafe conditions or hazards and modify as needed.
  Adhere to measures to prevent blood clots, especially in client with abnormal blood profile; surgical procedures, immobility.
- Prevent falls:
  Orient or reorient client to environment, as needed.
  Place confused elderly client or young child near the nurses' station **to provide for frequent observation.**
  Instruct the client/SO to request assistance, as needed; make sure call light is within reach and client knows how to operate.

Information that appears in brackets has been added by the authors to clarify and enhance the use of nursing diagnoses.

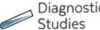 Diagnostic Studies 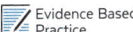 Evidence Based Practice 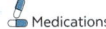 Medications 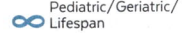 Pediatric/Geriatric/Lifespan

Utilize bed/chair alarms (if allowed) **that alert when client is trying to get up alone.**

Maintain bed or chair in lowest position with wheels locked. Provide netted bed for agitated clients with traumatic brain injury.

Provide seat raisers for chairs; use stand-assist, repositioning, or lifting devices, as indicated, **to prevent injury to both client and care providers.**

Ensure that all floors are clear of tripping hazards and that pathway to bathroom is unobstructed and properly lighted.

Place assistive devices (e.g., walker, cane, glasses, hearing aid) within reach, and ascertain that the client is using them appropriately.

Safety-lock exit and stairwell doors **when the client can wander away.**

Avoid the use of restraints as much as possible when the client is confused. **Restraints can increase the client's agitation and risk of entrapment and death.**

- Develop plan of care with family to meet client's and SO's individual needs.
- Provide information regarding disease or condition(s) that may result in increased risk of injury (e.g., weakness, dementia, head injury, immunosuppression, use of multiple medications, use of alcohol or other drugs, exposure to environmental chemicals or other hazards).
- Identify interventions and safety devices **to promote safe physical environment and individual safety.**
- Refer to physical or occupational therapist, as appropriate, **to identify high-risk tasks; conduct site visits; select, create, and modify equipment or assistive devices; and provide education about body mechanics and musculoskeletal injuries, in addition to providing therapies as indicated.**
- Demonstrate and encourage the use of techniques to reduce or manage stress and vent emotions, such as anger and hostility.
- Review consequences of previously determined risk factors that client is reluctant to modify. **Many consequences could occur (e.g., oral cancer in teenager using smokeless tobacco, fetal alcohol syndrome or neonatal addiction in prenatal woman using drugs, fall related to failure to use assistive equipment, toddler getting into medicine cabinet, binge drinking while skiing, health and legal implications of illicit drug use).**

Information that appears in brackets has been added by the authors to clarify and enhance the use of nursing diagnoses.

- Discuss the importance of self-monitoring of condition or emotions that can contribute to occurrence of injury (e.g., fatigue, anger, irritability). **Client/SO may be able to modify risk through monitoring of actions or postponement of certain actions, especially during times when client is likely to be highly stressed.**
- Encourage participation in self-help programs, such as assertiveness training, anger management, and positive self-image, **to enhance self-esteem and sense of self-worth.**
- Perform home assessment and identify safety issues, such as:
  Locking up medications and poisonous substances
  Using window grates or locks; using safety gates at top and bottom of stairs
  Installing handrails, ramps, bathtub safety tapes
  Using electrical outlet covers or lockouts
  Locking exterior doors
  Removing matches, smoking materials, and knobs from the stove
  Properly placing lights, alarms (e.g., fire, carbon monoxide, and intruder), and fire extinguishers
  Discussing safe use of oxygen
  Obtaining medical alert device or home monitoring service
- Review specific employment concerns or worksite issues and needs (e.g., ergonomic chairs and workstations; properly fitted safety equipment, footwear; regular use of safety glasses or goggles and ear protectors; safe storage of hazardous substances; number of hours worked per shift/week).
- Discuss the need for and sources of supervision (e.g., before- and after-school programs, elder day care).
- Discuss concerns about childcare, discipline practices.

Nursing Priority No. 3.

To maintain safety (Teaching/Discharge Considerations) and enhance well-being (long-term goals):

- Identify individual needs and resources for safety education, such as first aid/CPR classes, babysitter class, water or gun safety, smoking cessation, substance abuse program, weight and exercise management, and industry and community safety courses. **Client's knowledge is vital for preventing, rescuing family/friends from harm, or providing first aid.**
- Provide telephone numbers and other contact numbers, as individually indicated (e.g., doctor, 911, poison control, police, lifeline, hazardous materials handler).

Information that appears in brackets has been added by the authors to clarify and enhance the use of nursing diagnoses.

- 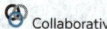 Refer to other professional resources, as indicated (e.g., counseling, psychotherapy, budget counseling, parenting classes).
- Provide bibliotherapy or written resources **for later review and self-paced learning.**
- 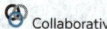 Promote community education programs geared to increasing awareness of safety measures and resources available to the individual. **Many evidence-based programs are being implemented nationally to promote safe environments for children, adolescents, and adults (e.g., correct use of child safety seats, home hazard information, firearm safety, fall prevention, CPR and first aid; education about bullying, internet safety issues; suicide prevention; use of helmets when riding bicycles or skateboarding; drowning prevention; substance abuse, intimate partner violence, and anger management).**
- Promote community awareness about the problems of design of buildings, equipment, transportation, and workplace practices that contribute to accidents.
- Identify community resources/neighbors/friends to assist elderly/handicapped individuals in providing such things as structural maintenance and removal of snow and ice from walks and steps.
- Identify emergency escape plans and routes for home and community **to be prepared in the event of natural or man-made disaster (e.g., fire, hurricane, earthquake, toxic chemical release).**

Documentation Focus

Assessment/Reassessment
- Individual risk factors, noting current physical findings (e.g., bruises, cuts)
- Client's/caregiver's understanding of individual risks and safety concerns
- Availability and use of resources

Planning
- Plan of care and who is involved in planning
- Teaching plan

Implementation/Evaluation
- Individual responses to interventions, teaching, and actions performed
- Specific actions and changes that are made
- Attainment of or progress toward desired outcome(s)
- Modifications to plan of care

Information that appears in brackets has been added by the authors to clarify and enhance the use of nursing diagnoses.

Discharge Planning
- Long-range plans for discharge needs, lifestyle and community changes, and who is responsible for actions to be taken
- Specific referrals made

Sample Nursing Outcomes & Interventions Classifications NOC/NIC

NOC—Personal Safety Behavior
NIC—Environmental Management: Safety

---

risk for urinary tract INJURY   NANDA-I

[Diagnostic Division: Elimination/Safety]

Definition: Susceptible to inadvertent damage of lower genitourinary structures.

Recognizing Cues

Risk Factors
Confusion
Inadequate knowledge, or caregiver knowledge regarding urinary catheter care
Ineffective overweight self-management

Clinical Connections
Pelvic trauma/surgical procedure, pregnancy labor/delivery, benign prostatic hyperplasia, prostatectomy, spinal cord injury, multiple sclerosis (MS)

Generate Solutions

Plan Desired Outcomes

Client Will (Include Specific Time Frame)
- Be free of injury.

Client/Caregivers Will (Include Specific Time Frame)
- Verbalize an understanding of individual factors that contribute to the possibility of injury.
- Demonstrate behaviors, lifestyle changes to reduce risk factors and protect from injury.

Information that appears in brackets has been added by the authors to clarify and enhance the use of nursing diagnoses.

Interventions/Take Action

Nursing Priority No. 1.
To assess causative/contributing factors:

- Identify conditions potentially affecting client need for/response to catheterization (e.g., acute illness, presence of infection, surgery, trauma including skin and tissue problems; chronic illness, including neurological conditions with paralysis or weakness; prolonged immobility; acute or chronic confusion, dementia, sedation, or use of multiple medications affecting mental acuity). **These conditions could require indwelling catheter for varying lengths of time with attendant potential for complications. Risk factors include longer duration of catheterization, bacterial colonization of the drainage bag, errors in catheter care, catheterization late in the hospital course, and immunocompromised or debilitated states.**
- Determine type of catheterization client is likely to require. **The client might require one-time or intermittent long-term single catheterization for any number of reasons (e.g., relief of acute urinary retention, management of voiding issues associated with MS or spinal cord injury). Indwelling urinary catheters are generally used when longer-term urinary management issues are expected.**
- Note client's age, developmental level, decision-making ability, level of cognition, competence, and independence. **These factors determine the client's/significant other's (SO's) ability to attend to safety issues and influences choice of interventions or teaching about catheterization.**
- Check for allergies to latex and select appropriate catheter (e.g., coated). **Latex allergic reactions are implicated in the development of urethritis and urethral stricture or anaphylaxis.**

Nursing Priority No. 2.
To reduce potential for complications:

- Avoid catheterization when possible. Refer to NDs pertaining to impaired urinary Elimination and Incontinence for related interventions. **Studies have shown that urinary catheters often are placed unnecessarily, remain in use without physician awareness, and are not removed promptly when no longer needed.**
- Perform catheterization using best practices:
  Use strict aseptic technique when inserting indwelling catheter (clean technique may be implemented for long-term

---

Information that appears in brackets has been added by the authors to clarify and enhance the use of nursing diagnoses.

 Acute Care 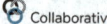 Collaborative 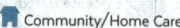 Community/Home Care Cultural

intermittent catheterization). **Note: The Centers for Disease Control and Prevention (CDC; 2009) recommended using aseptic technique and sterile equipment in the acute care setting, but clean (i.e., nonsterile) technique is acceptable and more practical in the community care setting for patients requiring chronic intermittent catheterization.**

∞ Select the smallest-bore catheter possible that will allow for adequate drainage, using size guidelines. **Appropriate catheter size helps reduce the likelihood of bladder spasm. Adult sizes are typically 14 Fr or 16 Fr. Guidelines are available for each pediatric age group from neonate (5 to 6 Fr) to adolescent (10, 12, 14 Fr).**

Refrain from inflating the balloon without first establishing urine flow. **Assures that catheter has been correctly inserted into the bladder. Note: If balloon is opened before catheter is completely inserted into the bladder, bleeding, damage, and even rupture of the urethra can occur.**

Inflate the balloon, using the correct amount of sterile liquid (usually 10 mL but check actual balloon size). **Balloon size is relevant to levels of bladder irritation. Although balloons are thin walled to reduce irritation to the bladder, it is still important to use the smallest size possible, usually with a 5- to 10-mL capacity.**

Secure catheter to thigh or abdomen, as indicated. Inspect the skin underneath the securement device with each reapplication to monitor for irritation or dermatitis. **Indwelling catheters should be secured to avoid traction on the catheter (which can cause irritation and trauma to the urethra, e.g., urethritis, necrosis, erosion, or stricture). Note: Caution should be exercised in high-risk individuals (e.g., those with bleeding disorders, fragile skin, sensitivities to adhesives, impaired circulation, and diabetes) who are at higher risk for skin disruptions.**

Perform an ongoing evaluation of catheter function and monitor color and characteristics of urine **to assess for developing complications. A properly maintained closed-drainage system and unobstructed urine flow are essential for prevention of urinary tract infection (UTI).**

• Ascertain if the client is experiencing discomfort or pain (e.g., bladder spasms). **Bladder spasms are distressing**

Information that appears in brackets has been added by the authors to clarify and enhance the use of nursing diagnoses.

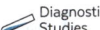 Diagnostic Studies 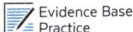 Evidence Based Practice Medications 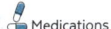 Pediatric/Geriatric/Lifespan

but are usually self-limiting when procedure is followed (e.g., proper size and insertion of catheter as well as appropriate size and inflation of balloon).

Nursing Priority No. 3.

To promote wellness (Teaching/Discharge Considerations):

- Review individual needs regarding catheter self-management with client/SO **to reduce the risk of complications:**

  Wash hands before and after handling the catheter.

  Make sure that urine is flowing out of the catheter into the collection bag.

  Keep the urine collection bag below the level of the bladder.

  Make sure that catheter tubing does not get twisted or kinked.

  Check for inflammation or signs of infection (e.g., pus or irritated, swollen, red, or tender skin) in the area around the catheter.

  Clean the area around the catheter twice a day using soap and water. Dry with a clean towel afterward.

  Avoid applying powder or lotion to the skin around the catheter.

  Refrain from tugging or pulling on the catheter.

  Follow physician instructions regarding catheter cleaning and/or replacement (if long-term indwelling).

  Follow physician instructions regarding frequency of catheterization (if intermittent).

- Instruct client/caregiver in techniques to protect the integrity of the skin. Refer to NDs impaired Skin Integrity; impaired Tissue Integrity; Pressure Injury for related interventions.

- Instruct client/caregiver in reportable problems, such as leaking, sediment in urine, absence of urine, presence of pain, and so on. **In the 2000s, studies regarding healthcare-associated infections (HAIs) reported a high percentage of UTIs related to urethral catheterization. However, recent reports on progress toward the prevention of HAIs have noted a significant decrease in catheter-associated urinary tract infections (CAUTIs). (This decrease may be a result of reduced utilization of indwelling catheters as well as improved catheter care).**

- Identify resources available to the individual (e.g., urinary catheters, samples and supplies, and various types of assistance and support)

Information that appears in brackets has been added by the authors to clarify and enhance the use of nursing diagnoses.

Documentation Focus

Assessment/Reassessment
- Individual risk factors, noting current physical findings
- Client's/caregiver's understanding of individual risks and safety concerns

Planning
- Plan of care and who is involved in planning
- Teaching plan

Implementation/Evaluation
- Individual responses to interventions, teaching, and actions performed
- Specific actions and changes that are made
- Attainment of or progress toward desired outcome(s)
- Modifications to plan of care

Discharge Planning
- Long-term plans for discharge needs, lifestyle changes, and who is responsible for actions to be taken
- Specific referrals made

Sample Nursing Outcomes & Interventions Classifications NOC/NIC

NOC—Physical Injury Severity
NIC—Urinary Catheterization

---

disrupted family INTERACTION PATTERNS NANDA-I

[Diagnostic Division: Roles/Relationships]

Definition: Disturbance in family organization and structure which fails to support the well-being of its members. [Authors view this as a break in pattern of support.]

Recognizing Cues

Related/Risk Factors
Difficulty dealing with altered community interaction; perceived social discrimination
Difficulty dealing with altered family role; excessive stress

---

Information that appears in brackets has been added by the authors to clarify and enhance the use of nursing diagnoses.

 Diagnostic Studies 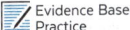 Evidence Based Practice 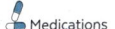 Medications ∞ Pediatric/Geriatric/Lifespan

Difficulty dealing with hierarchical, power, or social role shift among family members
Unaddressed domestic or community violence
Substance misuse

Defining Characteristics

Subjective
Altered family satisfaction
Decreased emotional support availability; decreased mutual support; decreased emotional support availability; decreased mutual support
Assigned tasks change; power alliance change; ritual change
Decreased contact among family members; family reports altered interaction
Altered intimacy; altered sexual partner relations
Conflict with or isolation from community resources

Objective
Altered:
  Affective responsiveness or communication pattern
  Family conflict resolution, or interpersonal relations
  Participation in decision making; problem-solving
  Somatization; stress-reduction behavior
Limited family interaction; limited familial affection; limited cooperative co-parenting
Disordered, stressed, or collusive alliance within family
Ineffective task completion
Unstable family alliance score using standardized, validated instrument

Clinical Connections
Chronic illness, cancer, surgical procedures, traumatic injury, substance abuse, Alzheimer disease, pregnancy, adolescent rebellion, conduct disorder, depression, schizophrenia

Generate Solutions

Plan Desired Outcomes

Client Will (Include Specific Time Frame)
- Express feelings freely and appropriately.
- Demonstrate individual involvement in problem-solving processes directed at appropriate solutions for the situation or crisis.
- Direct energies in a purposeful manner to plan for resolution of the crisis.

Information that appears in brackets has been added by the authors to clarify and enhance the use of nursing diagnoses.

 Acute Care 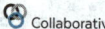 Collaborative 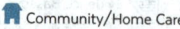 Community/Home Care Cultural

- Verbalize understanding of condition, treatment regimen, and prognosis.
- Encourage and allow affected member to handle situation in their own way, progressing toward independence.

Interventions/Take Action

Nursing Priority No. 1.

To assess individual situation for causative/contributing factors:

- Determine if a chronic health condition exists (e.g., cardiovascular, respiratory, cancer), trauma (e.g., sexual assault, a violent attack, or automobile accident), and/or presence of a developmental issue (e.g., intellectual disability, autism spectrum disorder). **Identifies areas of need for planning care for this family.**
- Identify family developmental stage (e.g., marriage, birth of a child, child entering school, child leaving home for college or marriage, retirement, or death of a spouse). **Developmental stage will affect family functioning; for instance, a newly married couple will be coping with issues of learning how to live with each other, children leaving home may result in problems related to "empty nest syndrome," adjusting to retirement and being home full-time may create stress between family members, or death of a spouse radically changes life for the survivor.**
- Note components and availability of the family: parent(s), children, male/female, and extended family. **Relationships among members may be supportive or strained depending on members' roles, boundaries, communication patterns, and how the family copes with stress.**
- Identify family relationships with immediate or extended family. **Family tensions may cause an emotional cutoff from immediate or extended family due to unresolved conflict. The cutoff may be moving away or not speaking or having any contact with a family member. Also, sibling position may influence relationships. For example, the firstborn child may take the role of leadership of younger siblings. Middle child may take both role of leadership for the youngest sibling and follower with the oldest sibling. Note recent changes in family relationships.**
- Observe patterns of communication in the family unit. **Healthy families have open, honest communication that**

Information that appears in brackets has been added by the authors to clarify and enhance the use of nursing diagnoses.

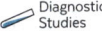 Diagnostic Studies 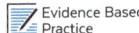 Evidence Based Practice 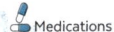 Medications 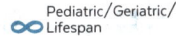 Pediatric/Geriatric/Lifespan

allows for emotions to be expressed freely. **Communication that is demeaning, demanding, and controlling limits family unity. The dominant family member attempts to control thoughts, feelings, and behaviors of all other family members. The controlled family members may not verbalize the oppression but demonstrate with their body language the fear or lack of self-confidence to speak. Note changes in family alliances and support or lack of support for others.**

- Assess boundaries of family members. **Has a shift recently taken place with a shared family identity, and do others have a sense of individuality? What precipitated the shift in boundaries, and is the family emotionally distant from others causing a lack of emotional support? These factors are critical to understanding family dynamics, who is being supported/not supported, and developing strategies to reconnect and change. Boundaries need to be clear so individual family members are free to be responsible for themselves.**

- Identify role expectations of family members. Who is the head of household, nurturer, peacemaker, or who challenges the rules? How do the roles interact and collaborate with others? **Understanding family roles provides guidance of who is responsible for specific tasks. Sometimes responsibilities may overlap with a specific role causing a misunderstanding as to who is responsible, thus causing a problem with expectations.**

- Determine "family rules"; for example, how adult concerns (finances, illness, etc.) are kept from the children. **Rules may be imposed by adults rather than through a democratic process involving all family members, leading to conflict and angry confrontations. Understanding the family's defined set of rules, or lack of rules, sets the stage for all interactions. Setting positive family rules with all family members participating can promote a more functional family.**

- Identify parenting skills and expectations. **Ineffective parenting and unrealistic expectations may contribute to abuse. Understanding normal responses and progression of developmental milestones may help parent cope with changes necessitated by current crisis. Positive reinforcement conditions family members to think, feel, and behave according to family expectations. The outcomes of reinforcement can be positive or negative behaviors according to cultural norms.**

Information that appears in brackets has been added by the authors to clarify and enhance the use of nursing diagnoses.

- Discuss current and past methods of coping. **Family members have developed patterns of giving positive reinforcement to promote desired repetitive behaviors. When positive regard/support is limited to individuals, they may be confused about family expectations, thus returning to past behaviors that were considered undesirable and using defense mechanisms to protect their self-esteem.**
- Listen for expressions of despair or helplessness (e.g., "I don't know what to do"). **Such feelings may contribute to difficulty adjusting to situation (e.g., teenage independence, change in health status of household breadwinner, dependence of aging parent on grown child) and ability to cooperate with plan of care or treatment regimen required. Generally, parents learn parenting from their parents. Not understanding the power of positive/ negative communication or relationship effects on roles, rules, and boundaries can create a lack of guidance and support for family members.**
- Note cultural and/or spiritual factors that may affect perceptions/expectations of family members. **These factors affect client/SO reactions and adjustment to situation and may limit choice of interventions and potential for successful resolution. For example, Arab American family relationships often include nuclear and extended family, with families making collective decisions. Men are expected to be responsible for carrying out decisions. Women are usually delegated care for daily needs of the family, while children may have little independence, and birth control may not be allowed for teenagers.**
- Determine extent and understanding of enabling behaviors used by family members. **Family members may have developed a protective pattern of oversupporting an individual (e.g., only child, youngest child, physically/ mentally/intellectually disabled individual). Thus, giving too much praise or support is enabling undesirable behaviors.**
- Determine if family holds regular family meetings to set goals, address individual/family problems, plus support and problem-solve issues as a family. **Open and honest discussion supports each family member and keeps family goals at the forefront of work to achieve success as well as helps to address problems that may require making changes to the goals or creating a new goal.**

Information that appears in brackets has been added by the authors to clarify and enhance the use of nursing diagnoses.

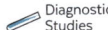 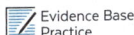 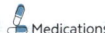 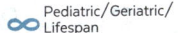

- Assess support systems available internally and externally for the family. **Having these resources can help the family begin to pull together and deal with current problems they are facing.**
- Determine family's readiness to improve family interactions. **Attempting to implement interventions prior to the family's readiness to change will be met with resistance.**

Nursing Priority No. 2.

To assist family to deal with situation/crisis:

- Interact with family members in a warm, caring, honest, and respectful manner. **Provides feelings of empathy and promotes individual's sense of worth and competence in ability to handle current situation.**
- Acknowledge difficulties and realities of the situation. **Communicates message of understanding and reinforces that some degree of conflict is to be expected and can be used to promote growth. Learning successful parenting and family strategies to guide and support members results in family resilience and connections.**
- Introduce styles and strategies for parenting. **Learning successful parenting and family strategies to guide and support members results in family resilience and connections.**
- Encourage expressions of anger. Avoid taking comments personally, as the client is usually angry at the situation over which they have little or no control. **Feelings of anger are to be expected when individuals are coping with a difficult situation. Appropriate expression enables progress toward problem resolution.**
- Emphasize the importance of continuous, open dialogue between family members to facilitate ongoing problem-solving. **Scheduling regular family meetings is an avenue to promote family cohesion, problem-solving conflicts, and guiding and supporting individuals. Promotes understanding and assists family members to maintain clear communication and resolve problems effectively.**
- Provide information, verbal and written, and reinforce as necessary. **Promotes learning, understanding, and opportunity to review as needed.**
- Assist the family to identify and encourage their use of previously successful coping behaviors and recognize the use of defense mechanisms. **Generally, people have developed effective coping skills, but some use defense mechanisms,**

Information that appears in brackets has been added by the authors to clarify and enhance the use of nursing diagnoses.

which are counterproductive to problem-solving. **Encouraging use of past effective coping skills facilitates positive problem-solving.**
- Recommend contact by family members on a regular, frequent basis. **Promotes feelings of warmth, caring, support, and brings family closer to one another, enabling them to manage current difficult situation.**
- Arrange for and encourage family participation in multidisciplinary team conference or group therapy, as appropriate. **Participation in family and group therapy for an extended period increases likelihood of success as interactional issues (e.g., marital conflict, "scapegoating" of members) can be addressed and dealt with. Involvement with others can help family members to experience new ways of interacting and gain insight into their behavior, providing opportunity for change.**
- Involve the family in social support and community activities of their interest and choice. **Involvement with others outside of family constellation provides opportunity to observe how others handle problems and deal with conflict.**

Nursing Priority No. 3.

To promote healthy family interactions and support for all members (Teaching/Discharge Considerations) and enhance well-being (long-term goals):

- Encourage the use of stress-management techniques (e.g., appropriate expression of feelings, relaxation exercises). **The relaxation response helps members think more clearly, deal more effectively with conflict, and promote more effective relationships to enhance family interactions.**
- Provide educational materials and information. **Learning about the problems they are facing can assist family members in resolution of current crisis.**
- Refer to classes (e.g., parent effectiveness, specific disease/disability support groups, self-help groups, clergy, psychological counseling, and family therapy), as indicated. **Can assist family to effect positive change and enhance conflict-resolution skills. Presence of substance abuse problems requires all family members to seek support and assistance in dealing with situation to promote a healthy outcome.** Refer to ND impaired Family Process for additional interventions, as appropriate.

Information that appears in brackets has been added by the authors to clarify and enhance the use of nursing diagnoses.

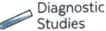 Diagnostic Studies 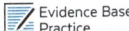 Evidence Based Practice 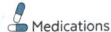 Medications 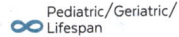 Pediatric/Geriatric/Lifespan

- Assist the family with identifying situations that may lead to fear or anxiety (e.g., diagnosis of chronic debilitating condition, decline in mental functioning of aging spouse/parent, sexually active teenager). **When parents have knowledge, they can plan for prevention.** (Refer to NDs Fear; Anxiety.)
- Involve the family in planning for future and mutual goal setting. **Promotes commitment to goals/continuation of plan.**
- Identify community agencies (e.g., Meals on Wheels, visiting nurse, trauma support group, American Cancer Society, Veterans Administration, Boys and Girls Club). **Provides for both immediate and long-term support.**

Documentation Focus

Assessment/Reassessment
- Assessment findings, including family composition, developmental stage of family, and role expectations
- Family communication patterns

Planning
- Plan of care, specific interventions, and who is involved in planning
- Teaching plan

Implementation/Evaluation
- Each individual's response to interventions, teaching, and actions performed
- Attainment of or progress toward desired outcome(s)
- Modifications to plan of care

Discharge Planning
- Long-term needs, noting who is responsible for actions to be taken
- Specific referrals made

Sample Nursing Outcomes & Interventions Classifications NOC/NIC

NOC—Family Functioning
NIC—Family Process Maintenance

Information that appears in brackets has been added by the authors to clarify and enhance the use of nursing diagnoses.

 Acute Care 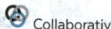 Collaborative 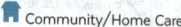 Community/Home Care Cultural

risk for LATEX ALLERGY　　　　　　　　　ICNP

[Diagnostic Division: Safety]

Definition: Susceptible to a mild to life-threatening immunologic response after exposure to natural latex or latex-protein-containing foods.

Recognizing Cues

Risk/Related Factors
Repeated latex exposure via occupational exposure
Repeated latex exposure via medical/surgical procedures (e.g., clients with spina bifida, recurrent urinary catheterizations)
Food allergies (e.g., avocado, banana, chestnut, kiwi, passion fruit, strawberry, plum, tomato

Clinical Connections
Neural tube defects (e.g., spina bifida, myelomeningoceles), multiple surgeries (at an early age), chronic urological conditions (e.g., neurogenic bladder, exstrophy of bladder), spinal cord trauma

Generate Solutions

Plan Desired Outcomes

Client Will (Include Specific Time Frame)
- Be free of signs of hypersensitive response.
- Identify and correct potential risk factors in the environment.
- Verbalize understanding of individual risks and responsibilities in avoiding exposure.
- Identify signs/symptoms requiring prompt intervention.
- Identify resources to assist in promoting a safe environment.

Interventions/Take Action

Nursing Priority No. 1.
To assess contributing risk factors:

- Question client regarding latex allergy on admission to healthcare facility, especially when procedures are anticipated (e.g., laboratory, emergency department, operating room, wound care management, one-day surgery, dentist). **This basic safety information helps healthcare providers prepare a safe environment for client and themselves while providing care.**

Information that appears in brackets has been added by the authors to clarify and enhance the use of nursing diagnoses.

 Diagnostic Studies 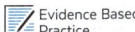 Evidence Based Practice 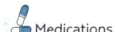 Medications 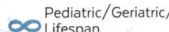 Pediatric/Geriatric/Lifespan

- Identify persons in high-risk categories, such as (1) those with history of certain **food allergies** (e.g., melons, tomatoes, bell peppers, certain nuts, wheats [not a comprehensive list]); (2) prior **allergies, asthma, and skin conditions** (e.g., eczema and other dermatitis); (3) those **occupationally exposed** to latex products (e.g., healthcare workers, police, firefighters, emergency medical technicians [EMTs], food handlers, hairdressers, cleaning staff, factory workers in plants that manufacture latex-containing products); (4) those with **neural tube defects** (e.g., spina bifida); or (5) those with **congenital urological conditions** requiring frequent surgeries and/or catheterizations (e.g., exstrophy of the bladder). **The most severe reactions tend to occur with latex proteins contacting internal tissues during invasive procedures and when they touch mucous membranes of the mouth, lungs, vagina, urethra, or rectum.**

Nursing Priority No. 2.

To assist in correcting factors that could lead to latex allergy:

- Discuss the necessity of avoiding/limiting latex exposure if sensitivity is suspected/family history of reaction. **Avoidance of latex is the only way to prevent the allergic reaction.**
- Recommend that client/family survey environment and remove any medical or household products containing latex.
- Create latex-safe healthcare environments in care settings (e.g., substitute nonlatex products, such as natural rubber gloves; polyvinyl chloride [PVC] IV tubing; latex-free tape, thermometers, electrodes, oxygen cannulas) **to enhance client safety by reducing exposure.**
- Ascertain that facilities and/or employers have established policies and procedures **to address safety and reduce risk to workers and clients.**
- Promote good skin care when latex gloves may be preferred for barrier protection in specific disease conditions such as HIV or during surgery. Use powder-free gloves, wash hands immediately after glove removal, and refrain from use of oil-based hand cream. **Reduces dermal and respiratory exposure to latex proteins that bind to the powder in gloves.**

Nursing Priority No. 3.

To promote safety/manage exposure (Teaching/Learning) and enhance well-being (long-term goals):

- Instruct client/caregivers to survey and routinely monitor the environment for latex-containing products, and replace as needed. **Reaction may be gradual but progressive,**

Information that appears in brackets has been added by the authors to clarify and enhance the use of nursing diagnoses.

affecting multiple body systems, or may be sudden, requiring lifesaving treatment.
- Instruct the client and caregivers about the potential for sensitivity reactions, how to recognize symptoms of latex allergy (e.g., skin rash; hives; flushing; itching; nasal, eye, or sinus symptoms; asthma; and [rarely] shock).
- Identify measures to take if reactions occur.
- Refer to allergist/other provider **for testing, as appropriate, such as challenge test with latex gloves, a skin patch test, or a blood test for IgE.**
- Provide a list of suppliers of products that can replace latex (e.g., rubber grip utensils/toys/hoses, rubber-containing pads, undergarments, carpets, shoe soles, computer mouse pad, erasers, and rubber bands).
- Emphasize the necessity of wearing a medical ID bracelet and informing all new care providers of hypersensitivity **to reduce preventable exposures.**
- Advise client to be aware of the potential for related food allergies (e.g., bananas, kiwis, melons, tomatoes, avocados, nuts [among others]). **These foods can trigger a latex-like allergic reaction because the proteins in them mimic latex proteins as they break down in the body.**
- Provide worksite review/recommendations to prevent exposure. **Latex allergy can be a disabling occupational disorder. Education about the problem promotes the prevention of allergic reaction, facilitates timely intervention, and helps the nurse to protect clients, latex-sensitive colleagues, and themselves.**
- Refer to resources, including but not limited to the American Latex Allergy Association, Latex Allergy News, Spina Bifida Association, National Institute for Occupational Safety and Health (NIOSH), medical supply websites **for further information about common latex products in the home, latex-free products, and assistance.**

Documentation Focus

Assessment/Reassessment
- Assessment findings, pertinent history of contact with latex products, and frequency of exposure
- Type and extent of symptomatology

Planning
- Plan of care and interventions, and who is involved in planning
- Teaching plan

Information that appears in brackets has been added by the authors to clarify and enhance the use of nursing diagnoses.

 Diagnostic Studies 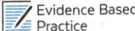 Evidence Based Practice 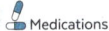 Medications 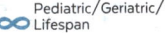 Pediatric/Geriatric/Lifespan

Implementation/Evaluation
- Response to interventions, teaching, and actions performed
- Attainment of or progress toward desired outcome(s)
- Modifications to plan of care

Discharge Planning
- Discharge needs and referrals made, additional resources available

Sample Nursing Outcomes & Interventions Classifications NOC/NIC

NOC—Risk Control
NIC—Latex Precautions

---

risk for impaired LIVER FUNCTION Ref. NANDA-I

[Diagnostic Division: Food/Fluid]

Definition: Susceptible to acute liver dysfunction and progressive deterioration following liver injury or infection.

Recognizing Cues

Risk Factors
Substance misuse
[Exposure to hepatic pathogens (e.g., hepatitis, Epstein-Barr virus [EBV], cytomegalovirus [CMV])]
[Hepatotoxic pharmaceutical agents; chemotherapy]
[Hepatotoxic exposure (e.g., carbon tetrachloride, paraquat, polychlorinated biphenyls)]
[Chronic excess caloric intake]
[Pancreatic/biliary injury, inflammation; hepatic ischemia]

Clinical Connections
Hepatitis, HIV, substance abuse, drug overdose (acetaminophen; NSAIDs), Epstein-Barr infection, poisoning

Generate Solutions

Plan Desired Outcomes

Client Will (Include Specific Time Frame)
- Verbalize understanding of individual risk factors that contribute to possibility of liver damage/failure.

Information that appears in brackets has been added by the authors to clarify and enhance the use of nursing diagnoses.

- Demonstrate behaviors, lifestyle changes to reduce risk factors and protect self from injury.
- Be free of signs of liver failure as evidenced by liver function studies within normal levels, and absence of jaundice, hepatic enlargement, or altered mental status.

Interventions/Take Action

Nursing Priority No. 1.

To identify individual risk factors/needs:

- Determine presence of disease condition(s), noting whether problem is acute (e.g., viral hepatitis, acetaminophen overdose) or chronic (e.g., alcoholic hepatitis or cirrhosis). **These factors influence choice of interventions.**
- Note client history of known/possible exposure to virus, bacteria, or toxins **that can damage the liver:**

    Works in high-risk occupation (e.g., performs tasks that involve contact with blood, blood-contaminated body fluids, other body fluids, or sharps)

    Injects drugs, especially if client shared a needle or received a tattoo or a piercing with an unsterile needle

    Received blood or blood products prior to 1989

    Ingested contaminated food or water or experienced poor sanitation practices by food-service workers

    Has close contact (e.g., lives with or has sex with infected person or carrier; infant born to infected mother)

    Is regularly exposed to toxic chemicals (e.g., carbon tetrachloride cleaning agents, bug spray, paint fumes, and tobacco smoke)

    Has history of gallbladder and biliary disease; pancreatic injury or disease

    Uses prescription drugs (e.g., sulfonamides, phenothiazines, isoniazid)

    Ingests certain herbal remedies or megadoses of vitamins

    Uses alcohol with medications (including over-the-counter medications)

    Consumes alcohol heavily and/or over long period of time

    Ingested acetaminophen (accidentally, as may occur when a client takes too large a dose or has several medications containing acetaminophen over time; or intentionally, as may occur with suicide attempt)

    Travels internationally to or immigrates from areas/countries such as Africa, Southeast Asia, Korea, China, Vietnam, Eastern Europe, Mediterranean countries, or the Caribbean

---

Information that appears in brackets has been added by the authors to clarify and enhance the use of nursing diagnoses.

 Diagnostic Studies 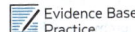 Evidence Based Practice 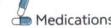 Medications 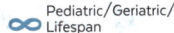 Pediatric/Geriatric/Lifespan

- Review results of laboratory tests (e.g., abnormal liver function studies, international normalized ratio [INR], drug toxicity, hepatitis B virus positive) and other diagnostic studies (e.g., ultrasonography, computed tomography [CT] scanning; magnetic resonance imaging [MRI]) **that indicate presence of a hepatotoxic condition and the need for medical treatment.**

Nursing Priority No. 2.

To assist client to reduce or correct individual risk factors:

- Assist with medical treatment of underlying condition (e.g., hepatitis, alcoholism, drug overdose, gallbladder/biliary disease; pancreatic injury/disease) **to support organ function and minimize liver damage.**
- Educate the client on way(s) to prevent exposure to/incidence of hepatitis infections and limit damage to liver:
  Practice safer sex (e.g., avoid multiple-partner sex, wear condoms, avoid sex with partners known to be infected).
  Wash hands well after using the bathroom or changing soiled diapers/briefs.
  Avoid injecting drugs or sharing needles.
  Avoid sharing razors, toothbrushes, or nail clippers.
  Make sure needles and inks are sterile for tattooing and body piercing.
  Use proper precautions and appropriate protective equipment when working in high-risk occupations, such as healthcare, police and fire departments, emergency services, day-care services, and chemical manufacturing, **where one is most at risk for inhalation of toxins, needlesticks, or body fluid exposure.**
  Avoid tap water and practice good hygiene and sanitation when traveling internationally.
  Use harsh cleansers and aerosol products in well-ventilated room; wear mask and gloves, cover skin, and wash well afterward. **Chemicals can reach the liver through skin and destroy liver cells.**
  Obtain vaccinations when appropriate. **Some hepatitis strains (e.g., A and B) are preventable, thus minimizing the risk of liver damage.**
- Emphasize the importance of responsible drinking or avoiding alcohol, when indicated, **to reduce the incidence of cirrhosis or severity of liver damage or failure.**
- Encourage the client with liver dysfunction to avoid fatty foods. **Fat interferes with normal function of liver cells**

Information that appears in brackets has been added by the authors to clarify and enhance the use of nursing diagnoses.

and can cause additional damage and permanent scarring to liver cells when they can no longer regenerate.
- Encourage smoking cessation. **The additives in cigarettes pose a challenge to the liver by reducing the liver's ability to eliminate toxins.**
- Refer to a nutritionist, as indicated, for dietary needs, including intake of calories, proteins, vitamins, and trace minerals, **to promote healing and limit effects of deficiencies.**
- Discuss safe use and concerns about client's medication regimen (e.g., acetaminophen; nonsteroidal anti-inflammatory drugs; herbal or vitamin supplements; phenobarbitol; cholesterol-lowering drugs, such as "statins"; some antibiotics [e.g., sulfonamides, isoniazid (INH)]; certain cardiovascular drugs [e.g., amiodarone, hydralazine]; antidepressants [e.g., tricyclics]) **known to cause hepatotoxicity, either alone or in combination, or in an overdose situation.**
- Emphasize importance of responsible drinking or avoidance of alcohol when indicated (if client has any kind of liver disease) **to avoid or reduce risk of liver damage. Refer for professional treatment, where indicated.**
- Encourage smoking cessation. **The additives in cigarettes pose a challenge to the liver by reducing its ability to eliminate toxins.**
- Identify signs/symptoms that warrant prompt notification of healthcare provider (e.g., increased abdominal girth; rapid weight loss or gain; increased peripheral edema; dyspnea, fever; blood in stool or urine; excess bleeding of any kind; jaundice). **These are indicators of severe liver dysfunction, possible organ failure.**
- Refer to specialist or liver treatment center, as indicated. **Referral may be beneficial for a person with chronic liver disease when decompensating, or a client with hepatitis and other coexisting disease condition (e.g., HIV) or intolerance to treatment due to side effects.**

Nursing Priority No. 3.

To promote hepatic health and prevent liver injury (Teaching/Discharge Considerations) and enhance well-being (long-term goals):

- Encourage the client routinely taking acetaminophen for pain management to read labels, determine strength of medication, note safe number of doses over 24 hr,

---

Information that appears in brackets has been added by the authors to clarify and enhance the use of nursing diagnoses.

 Diagnostic Studies 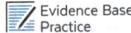 Evidence Based Practice 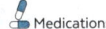 Medications 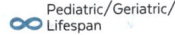 Pediatric/Geriatric/Lifespan

become familiar with "hidden" sources of acetaminophen (e.g., Nyquil, Vicodin), and limit alcohol intake **to avoid/limit risk of liver damage.**
- Emphasize the importance of hand hygiene and avoidance of fresh produce, use of bottled water, and avoidance of raw meat and seafood **if client is traveling to an area where hepatitis A and E are endemic or foodborne or waterborne illness is a risk.**
- Instruct in measures including protection from blood and other body fluids, sharps safety, safer sex practices, avoiding needle sharing and body tattoos or piercings **to prevent occupational and nonoccupational exposures to hepatitis.**
- Discuss need and refer for vaccination, as indicated (e.g., healthcare and public safety worker, children under 18, international traveler, recreational drug user, men who have sexual relationships with other men, client with clotting disorders or liver disease, anyone sharing household with an infected person), **to prevent exposure and transmission of blood or body fluid hepatitis and limit risk of liver injury.**
- Discuss appropriateness of prophylactic immunizations. **Although the best way to protect against hepatitis B and C infections is to prevent exposure to viruses, postexposure prophylaxis should be initiated promptly to prevent or limit the severity of the infection.**
- Provide information regarding the availability of gamma globulin, immune serum globulin, HepB immunoglobulin, and HepB vaccine (Recombivax HB, Engerix-B) through the health department or family physician.
- Emphasize the necessity of follow-up care (in client with chronic liver disease) and adherence to therapeutic regimen **to monitor liver function and effectiveness of interventions** and importance of adherence to therapeutic regimen **to prevent or minimize permanent liver damage.**
- Refer to community resources, drug and alcohol treatment program, as indicated.

Documentation Focus

Assessment/Reassessment
- Assessment findings, including individual risk factors
- Results of laboratory tests and diagnostic studies

Planning
- Plan of care and who is involved in planning
- Teaching plan

Information that appears in brackets has been added by the authors to clarify and enhance the use of nursing diagnoses.

Implementation/Evaluation
- Response to interventions, teaching, and actions performed
- Attainment of or progress toward desired outcome(s)
- Modifications to plan of care

Discharge Planning
- Long-term needs, plan for follow-up, and who is responsible for actions to be taken
- Specific referrals made

Sample Nursing Outcomes & Interventions Classifications NOC/NIC

NOC—Knowledge: Disease Process
NIC—Substance Use Treatment

---

excessive LONELINESS NANDA-I

[Diagnostic Division: Roles/Relationships]

Definition: Overwhelming feeling of sadness, dejection or discomfort associated with lack of companionship or being separated from others.

Recognizing Cues

Related/Risk Factors
Difficulty establishing social interaction; inadequate positive social interaction
Inadequate informational, instrumental, or emotional support
Impaired physical mobility; physical isolation

Defining Characteristics

Subjective
Anxiety; physical, psychological discomfort
Altered, inadequate appetite
Fatigue; altered sleep-wake cycle
Decreased social interaction; disconnected from others; overwhelming feeling of isolation
Longing for meaningful connections

Objective
Inadequate self-esteem; negative thought patterns
Depressive symptoms; rumination

Information that appears in brackets has been added by the authors to clarify and enhance the use of nursing diagnoses.

Self-neglect
Addictive behaviors; excessive use of interactive electronic devices

Clinical Connections
Debilitating conditions (e.g., multiple sclerosis [MS], chronic obstructive pulmonary disease [COPD], renal failure), cancer, AIDS, major depression, long-term care residents

Generate Solutions

Plan Desired Outcomes

Client Will (Include Specific Time Frame)
- Identify individual difficulties causing sadness and isolation and ways to address socialization.
- Engage in social activities.
- Report involvement in interactions and relationships client views as meaningful.

Parent/Caregiver Will (Include Specific Time Frame)
- Provide infant/child with consistent and loving caregiving.
- Participate in programs for adolescents and families.
- Promote caring milieu for elderly and institutionalized individuals.

Interventions/Take Action

Nursing Priority No. 1.
To identify causative/precipitating factors:
- Differentiate between ordinary loneliness and a state or constant sense of loneliness due to a mental health disorder (e.g., schizophrenic disorders or mood disorders). **Loneliness is a subjective feeling about relationships and being emotionally and socially disconnected from family and friends. Individuals with a mental illness may be isolated from family/friends/society creating anxiety, depression, or fear of being mistreated in society; thus, they often select social isolation. Influences the type and intensity of interventions.**
- Note the client's age and duration of the problem, and whether situational or chronic. **Situational loneliness (e.g., leaving home for college, retirement, death of a loved one) appears across the life span. Chronic loneliness (e.g., married couples no longer share emotions or feelings, decline in physical health) increases health**

Information that appears in brackets has been added by the authors to clarify and enhance the use of nursing diagnoses.

 Acute Care 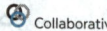 Collaborative 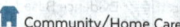 Community/Home Care   Cultural

risks including cardiovascular disease and less effective immune system.
- Determine degree of distress, tension, anxiety, or restlessness present and the frequency of illnesses, accidents, or crises. **Identifies somatic complaints that can result from loneliness. Individuals under stress tend to have more illnesses and accidents related to inattention and anxiety. A recent study about loneliness in older home-dwelling people identified six factors independently associated with loneliness: living alone, not being satisfied with life, having mental problems, a weak sense of coherence, not having contact with friends, and being at risk for undernourishment. However, other studies also reported that at least 60% of older married people also reported feeling lonely.**
- Note the presence and proximity of family/significant other(s) (SO[s]), and whether or not they are helpful. **Family may live near and be available to help with planning care and socialization. Or client may be estranged from family members, and they may not be willing to be involved with client. Loneliness may not be related to being alone. Clients may have family and friends yet feel disconnected emotionally, socially, and feel lonely.**
- Discuss with client whether there is a person or persons in their life who can be trustworthy and who will listen with empathy to the feelings that are expressed.
- Determine how the individual perceives and copes with solitude. **The client may see being alone as positive, allowing time to pursue own interests, or may view solitude as sad and long for lost people, lifestyle patterns, or events.**
- ∞ Review issues of separation from parents as a child, loss of SO(s)/spouse. **Early separation from parents often affects the individual as other losses occur throughout life, leading to feelings of inadequacy and inability to deal with current situation.**
- Assess sleep and appetite disturbances and ability to concentrate. **These are indicators of distress related to feelings of loneliness and low self-esteem. Identifies client's ability to care for self and meet own needs.**
- Note expressions of "yearning" for an emotional partnership. **For example, widows and widowers are particularly prone to feelings of loneliness. Going from being a couple to being alone is often a difficult transition, and these feelings are indicative of a desire to return to the couple state.**

excessive LONELINESS

Information that appears in brackets has been added by the authors to clarify and enhance the use of nursing diagnoses.

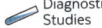 Diagnostic Studies   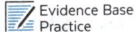 Evidence Based Practice   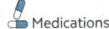 Medications   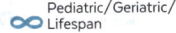 Pediatric/Geriatric/Lifespan

577

- Assess feelings of loneliness in a client who is receiving palliative/hospice care. **These individuals often feel alienated and lonely as they face the end of their life and may need additional socialization to help them feel valued.**

Nursing Priority No. 2.

To assist client to identify feelings and situations in which they experience loneliness:

- Establish a nurse–client relationship. **The client may feel free to talk about feelings in the context of an empathetic relationship.**
- Accept client's expressions of loneliness as a primary condition and not necessarily as a symptom of some underlying condition. **Provides a beginning point, which will allow the client to look at what loneliness means in life without having to search for deeper meaning.**
- Discuss individual concerns about thoughts and feelings of loneliness and relationship between loneliness and lack of SO(s). Note desire and willingness to change situation. **Motivation can facilitate while a lack of motivation can impede achieving desired outcomes. Often, feelings of loneliness arise from underlying depression related to loss, thus affecting individual's coping abilities.**
- Support expression of negative perceptions of others and note whether the client believes they are true. **Provides opportunity for the client to clarify reality of the situation and recognize own denial or distorted thoughts. Individual's view of the world is colored by thoughts and feelings of being disconnected emotionally and socially, causing loneliness, anxiety, and depression.**

Nursing Priority No. 3.

To assist client to become involved:

- Discuss reality versus perceptions of situation. Have client identify people with whom client interacts on a regular basis. **Provides opportunity for reality check and beginning to understand own feelings of loneliness related to what is happening in own life.**
- Discuss importance of emotional bonding (attachment) between infants or young children and parents/caregivers when appropriate. **Understanding the importance of attachment provides parents with information that will help them take measures to ensure that this bonding occurs.**

Information that appears in brackets has been added by the authors to clarify and enhance the use of nursing diagnoses.

 Acute Care 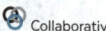 Collaborative 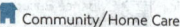 Community/Home Care  Cultural

- Involve client in classes, such as assertiveness, language and communication, and social skills, **to address individual needs and potential for enhanced socialization.**
- Role-play situations that are new or are anxiety provoking for client. **Practicing new situations helps develop self-confidence and provides client with information about what to expect and how to deal with the unexpected in a positive manner.**
- Discuss positive health habits, including personal hygiene and exercise activity of client's choosing. **Improves feelings of self-esteem, thus enabling client to feel more confident in social situations.**
- Identify individual strengths and areas of interest (e.g., volunteering, recreational activities, or classes related to special interest) that client identifies and is willing to pursue. **Provides opportunities for involvement with others.**
- Encourage attendance at support group activities to meet individual needs (e.g., therapy, separation/grief, spiritual). **Helps client begin to deal with feelings of loneliness.**
- Help client establish a plan for progressive involvement, beginning with a simple activity (e.g., call an old friend or speak to a neighbor; schedule weekly Zoom/FaceTime with family, Snapchat, Facebook or similar social media contacts (reminding client to be careful about sharing personal information on social media) and then leading to more complicated interactions and activities. **Taking small steps promotes success, and confidence is gained as each step is taken, thus helping the client to be more involved and to resolve feelings of loneliness.**
- Provide opportunities for interactions in a supportive environment (e.g., have client accompanied, as in a buddy system) during initial attempts to socialize. **Helps to reduce stress, provides positive reinforcement, and facilitates a successful outcome.**

Nursing Priority No. 4.

To promote healthy social connections (Teaching/Discharge Considerations) and enhance well-being (long-term goals):

- Inform client that loneliness can be overcome. **Although it is up to the individual to begin to feel good about self, hearing that loneliness does not have to be permanent can provide hope in early days.**
- Encourage involvement in special-interest groups (e.g., computers, gardening club, reading circles, bird watchers, puzzles/other gaming groups) and charitable

services (e.g., serving in a soup kitchen, youth groups, animal shelter). **When the client is willing to become involved in these kinds of activities, the perception of loneliness fades into the background; even though the individual may still be lonely, the sense of loneliness is not so pervasive.**

- Suggest volunteering for church committee or choir, attending community events with friends and family, becoming involved in political issues or campaigns, or enrolling in classes at local college or continuing education programs, as able. **When client is willing to become involved in these kinds of activities, perception of loneliness fades into the background, and even though individual may still be lonely, the sense of loneliness is not so pervasive.**
- Refer to appropriate counselors for help with relationships or other identified needs.
- Refer to NDs Anxiety; inadequate Social Connectedness; readiness for enhanced Hope for related interventions, as appropriate.

Documentation Focus

Assessment/Reassessment
- Assessment findings, including client's perception of problem, availability of resources and support systems
- Client's desire and commitment to change

Planning
- Plan of care and who is involved in planning
- Teaching plan

Implementation/Evaluation
- Response to interventions, teaching, and actions performed
- Attainment of or progress toward desired outcome(s)
- Modifications to plan of care

Discharge Planning
- Long-term needs, plan for follow-up, and who is responsible for actions to be taken
- Specific referrals made

Sample Nursing Outcomes & Interventions Classifications NOC/NIC

NOC—Loneliness Severity
NIC—Socialization Enhancement

Information that appears in brackets has been added by the authors to clarify and enhance the use of nursing diagnoses.

ineffective LYMPHEDEMA SELF-MANAGEMENT

NANDA-I

[Diagnostic Division: Circulation]

Definition: Unsatisfactory handling of treatment regimen, consequences associated with edema related to obstruction or disorders of lymph vessels or nodes.

Recognizing Cues

Related/Risk Factors

Competing demands or lifestyle preferences; decreased quality of life

Conflict between health behaviors and social norms; nonacceptance of condition; unaware of seriousness of condition, or of susceptibility to sequelae

Difficulty managing complex treatment regimen, or navigating complex healthcare systems; difficulty accessing community resources

Inadequate health literacy or knowledge of treatment regimen; inadequate commitment to a plan of action; inadequate number of cues to action

Difficulty performing aspects of treatment regimen; negative feelings toward treatment regimen; perceived barrier to treatment regimen; unrealistic perception of treatment benefit

Inadequate role models or social support; perceived social stigma associated with condition

Difficulty with decision making; inadequate self-efficacy; confusion

Defining Characteristics

Lymphedema Symptoms

Subjective
Feeling of discomfort, pain, heaviness, or tightness in affected limb

Lymphedema Signs

Objective
Decreased range of motion of affected limb
Fibrosis in affected limb; swelling in affected limb
Recurring infections

Information that appears in brackets has been added by the authors to clarify and enhance the use of nursing diagnoses.

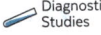 Diagnostic Studies   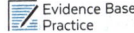 Evidence Based Practice   Medications   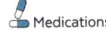 Pediatric/Geriatric/Lifespan

Behaviors
Average daily physical activity is less than recommended for age and gender; inappropriate dietary habits

Inadequate manual lymph drainage; inattentive to lymphedema signs or symptoms; inadequate protection of affected area; inappropriate skin care

Inappropriate application of nighttime bandaging; refuses to apply nighttime bandaging; inappropriate use of compression garments; refuses to use compression garments

Inattentive to carrying heavy objects; inattentive to extreme temperatures or to sunlight exposure

Clinical Connections
Mastectomy, various cancers, cancer therapies (chemotherapy, radiotherapy), cellulitis, rheumatoid or psoriatic arthritis, trauma, deep vein thrombosis, venous insufficiency, obesity

Generate Solutions

Plan Desired Outcomes

Client Will (Include Specific Time Frame)
- Demonstrate behaviors to manage lymphedema.
- Engage in risk-reduction strategies, or strategies to cope with impact of condition.
- List signs/symptoms that require further evaluation.

Interventions/Take Action

Nursing Priority No. 1.
To assess for causative/contributing factors:

 • Determine presence of underlying condition (e.g., any cancer or its treatment that affects lymph drainage, deep vein thrombosis [DVT], cellulitis, rheumatoid arthritis). **Lymphedema can occur slowly over time, typically as a late effect of cancer treatment. However, it can also be suddenly provoked by an infection (e.g., cellulitis), a limb injury, or DVT. Upper-extremity lymphedema most often occurs after breast cancer; lower-extremity edema most often occurs with uterine or vulvar cancers, prostate cancer, bladder or ovarian cancer, lymphoma, or melanoma. Other risk factors include (1) extent of surgery, (2) local radiation, (3) delayed healing, (4) tumor causing lymphatic obstruction. Note: Lymphedema in children can be primary (due to congenital lymphatic abnormalities) or secondary (acquired). Lymphedema in**

Information that appears in brackets has been added by the authors to clarify and enhance the use of nursing diagnoses.

 Acute Care 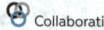 Collaborative 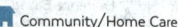 Community/Home Care Cultural

children is relatively rare but carries with it the significant and lifelong burden of having to manage chronic swelling and prevent secondary complications.
- Document client's report of symptoms. **Heaviness or fullness, puffiness, swelling (nonpitting edema), and aching of the limb; tight sensation of the skin; decreased flexibility of nearby joint. Client may report difficulty fitting affected limb into sleeve or pants leg or problems wearing jewelry on affected hand. Other symptoms may include itching of legs or toes, burning sensation in legs.**
- Assist with measurements of affected extremity. **The most widely used method to diagnose extremity lymphedema is circumferential measurement using specific anatomical landmarks.**
- Prepare for/assist with imaging of the lymphatic system (lymphoscintigraphy; MRI), infrared scanning or bioelectrical impedance measures, as required.
- Identify stage of severity. **Stage I is spontaneously reversible and typically is marked by pitting edema, increase in extremity girth, and heaviness. Stage II is characterized by a spongy consistency of the tissue without signs of pitting edema. Tissue fibrosis can then cause the limbs to harden and increase in size. At stage III, the affected limb or area of the body becomes very large and misshapen, and the skin takes on a leathery, wrinkled appearance.**
- Examine skin and compare to unaffected limb. **Various skin manifestations can occur (e.g., tight, shiny, warm, or red skin; hardened skin, thicker skin; orange peel appearance [swollen with small indentations]; or small blisters that leak clear fluid).**
- Note current weight and usual dietary intake. **Excessive weight/obesity can be a significant risk factor for development of secondary lymphedema. Note: Morbid obesity can cause primary lymphedema.**
- Determine ability to navigate healthcare system, commitment to management of condition. **Perceived barrier to care or inadequate commitment to treatment plan increases likelihood for failure in managing condition.**

Nursing Priority No. 2.

To ascertain scope of problem:
- Determine how current situation is affecting client's quality of life (e.g., difficulty with activities of daily living, walking, or performing usual work tasks; relationships).

Information that appears in brackets has been added by the authors to clarify and enhance the use of nursing diagnoses.

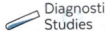 Diagnostic Studies 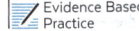 Evidence Based Practice 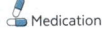 Medications 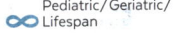 Pediatric/Geriatric/Lifespan

Condition can affect ability to function as well as client's self-image and relationships with others.
- Discuss client's current self-management:
  If wearing compression garment, does it fit appropriately? Is client using appropriate type of compression garment (e.g., sleeve or stocking, bandages, gradient pressure garment)? Is client compliant with wearing garment for prescribed time?
  If engaged in regular exercise, is program nonfatiguing but sufficient to cause muscle contraction in lymph system?

Nursing Priority No. 3.

To promote lymphedema management/reduce potential complications:

- Assist with/instruct client/caregiver in standard lymphedema treatments. **In early lymphedema (stage I), swelling can be partially or fully eliminated by elevating a limb. Standard treatment for later stage (or unresolved) lymphedema is complex (or combined) decongestive therapy (CDT), which includes (1)** *manual lymphatic drainage (massage), compression wrapping, compression garments, pneumatic compression;* **and (2)** *education on skin safety and exercise.*
- Instruct/reinstruct client in skin/tissue care:
  Use cream or lotion to keep the skin moist.
  Treat small cuts or breaks in the skin with an antibacterial ointment.
  Avoid needlesticks of any type, including injections or blood tests, into the limb (arm or leg) with lymphedema.
  Avoid testing bath or cooking water using the limb with lymphedema. There may be less feeling (touch, temperature, pain) in the affected arm or leg, increasing risk of thermal injury.
  Wear gloves when gardening and cooking.
  Wear sunscreen and shoes when outdoors.
  Cut toenails straight across. See a podiatrist (foot doctor) as needed to prevent ingrown nails and infections. Keep feet clean and dry and wear cotton socks.
- Instruct/reinstruct client in techniques to avoid blocking flow of fluid through the body or to keep blood from pooling in affected limb:
  Avoid crossing legs while sitting.
  Change sitting position frequently (e.g., every 30 min).
  Avoid carrying heavy objects on affected arm.

Information that appears in brackets has been added by the authors to clarify and enhance the use of nursing diagnoses.

Avoid swinging limb quickly in circles or letting limb hang down.
- Refer to lymphedema specialist **to provide guidance to client/caregiver for management, including wrapping and pressure garment use, manual lymphatic drainage exercises, as well as education on skin care and on preventing flare-ups and secondary complications.**
- Prepare for more aggressive interventions, as indicated. **When conservative treatment fails or delivers suboptimal outcomes, low-level laser therapy may be used to increase lymph fluid mobility and vessel regeneration, or client may need surgical interventions (reconstructive or ablative) where applicable.**

Nursing Priority No. 4.
To promote lymphatic drainage (Teaching/Discharge Considerations) and enhance well-being (long-term goals):
- Instruct client/family in ways to keep track of edema.
- Emphasize need for mobility, frequent position changes, and early/ongoing ambulation **to prevent stasis and reduce risk of worsening edema and complications associated with immobility.**
- Identify "danger" signs requiring notification of healthcare provider **to ensure timely evaluation and intervention.**
- Review nutritional intake. Discuss weight loss as appropriate. Refer to NDs ineffective Overweight Self-Management; Body Weight Problem.
- Identify community resource such as support groups, reputable chat rooms. **Provides opportunity to interact with others facing similar issues and may assist in problem-solving challenges.**
- Refer for individual/group counseling as indicated. **May require assistance in dealing with body image issues, intimacy concerns.**

Documentation Focus

Assessment/Reassessment
- Assessment findings, noting existing conditions contributing to risk; or stage and location of lymphedema, when present
- Results of laboratory tests and diagnostic studies
- Self-care management

Planning
- Plan of care and who is involved in the planning

Information that appears in brackets has been added by the authors to clarify and enhance the use of nursing diagnoses.

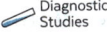 Diagnostic Studies 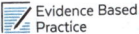 Evidence Based Practice 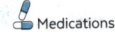 Medications 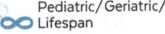 Pediatric/Geriatric/Lifespan

Implementation/Evaluation
- Response to interventions, teaching, and actions performed
- Attainment of or progress toward desired outcome(s)
- Modifications to plan of care

Discharge Planning
- Long-term needs, noting who is responsible for actions to be taken
- Community referrals

Sample Nursing Outcomes & Interventions Classifications NOC/NIC

NOC—Knowledge: Lymphedema Management
NOC—Self-Management: Lymphedema
NIC—Circulatory Precautions

---

risk for impaired MATERNAL-FETAL DYAD NANDA-I

[Diagnostic Division: Sexuality/Reproduction]

Definition: Susceptible to a disruption of the symbiotic mother-fetal relationship affecting physiological exchange and affective-emotional interactions during pregnancy as a result of comorbid or pregnancy-related conditions.

Recognizing Cues

Risk Factors
Inadequate prenatal care
Inadequate partner or social support
Tobacco use during pregnancy; alcohol consumption during pregnancy
Unaddressed abuse (e.g., physical, psychological, sexual)
Substance misuse

Clinical Connections
High-risk pregnancy, adolescent pregnancy, prenatal substance abuse, gestational hypertension, maternal diabetes mellitus, prenatal hemorrhage, prenatal infection, premature dilatation of cervix, abdominal trauma, maternal depression, domestic violence

---

Information that appears in brackets has been added by the authors to clarify and enhance the use of nursing diagnoses.

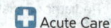 Acute Care 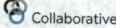 Collaborative 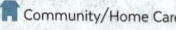 Community/Home Care 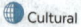 Cultural

Generate Solutions

Plan Desired Outcomes

Client Will (Include Specific Time Frame)

- Verbalize understanding of individual risk factors or condition(s) that may impact pregnancy.
- Engage in necessary alterations in lifestyle and daily activities to manage risks.
- Participate in screening procedures as indicated.
- Identify signs/symptoms requiring medical evaluation or intervention.
- Display fetal growth within normal limits and carry pregnancy to term.

Interventions/Take Action

Nursing Priority No. 1.

To identify individual risk/contributing factors:

- Review history of previous pregnancies for presence of complications, such as premature rupture of membranes (PROM), placenta previa, miscarriage or pregnancy losses due to premature dilation of the cervix, preterm labor or deliveries, previous birth defects, hyperemesis gravidarum, or repeated urinary tract or vaginal infections.
- Obtain history about prenatal screening and amount and timing of care. **Lack of prenatal care can place both mother and fetus at risk.**
- Note conditions potentiating vascular changes/reduced placental circulation (e.g., diabetes, gestational hypertension, cardiac problems, smoking) or those that alter oxygen-carrying capacity (e.g., asthma, anemia, Rh incompatibility, hemorrhage). **Extent of maternal vascular involvement and reduction of oxygen-carrying capacity have a direct influence on uteroplacental circulation and gas exchange.**
- Note maternal age. **Maternal age greater than 35 years is associated with increased risk of spontaneous abortions, preterm delivery or stillbirths, fetal chromosomal abnormalities and malformations, and intrauterine growth retardation (IUGR). In pregnant adolescents (younger than 15), the most common high-risk conditions include gestational hypertension, anemia, labor dysfunction, cephalopelvic disproportion, low birth weight, and preterm delivery.**

Information that appears in brackets has been added by the authors to clarify and enhance the use of nursing diagnoses.

 Diagnostic Studies   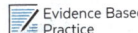 Evidence Based Practice   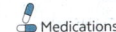 Medications   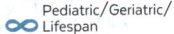 Pediatric/Geriatric/Lifespan

- Ascertain current/past dietary patterns and practices. **Client may be malnourished, obese, or underweight (weight less than 100 lb or greater than 200 lb) or may reveal preconception of eating disorders that can have a negative impact on fetal organ development—especially brain tissue in the early weeks of pregnancy.**
- Assess for severe, unremitting nausea and vomiting, especially when it persists after the first trimester (hyperemesis gravidarum). **Hyperemesis gravidarum places the mother at risk for substantial weight loss and fluid and electrolyte imbalances, and exposes the developing fetus to acidotic state and malnutrition. Development of hyperemesis gravidarum may require hospitalization.**
- Note history of exposure to teratogenic agents, infectious diseases (e.g., tuberculosis, influenza, measles); high-risk occupations; exposure to toxic substances such as lead, organic solvents, carbon monoxide; use of certain over-the-counter or prescription medications; and substance use or abuse (including illicit drugs and alcohol).
- Identify family or cultural influences in pregnancy. **Family history may include multiple births or congenital diseases, generational abuse, or lack of support or finances. Cultural background may identify health risks associated with nationality (e.g., sickle cell in people of African descent or Tay-Sachs disease in people of Eastern European Jewish ancestry) or religious practices (e.g., exclusion of dairy products, no maternal immunizations for rubella) that can impact the health of the mother or fetal development.**
- Review laboratory studies. **Low hemoglobin suggests anemia, which is associated with hypoxia. Blood type and Rh group may reveal incompatibility risks; elevated serum glucose may be seen in gestational diabetes mellitus (GDM); elevated liver function studies suggest hypertensive liver involvement; drop in platelet count may be associated with gestational hypertension and HELLP (hemolysis, elevated liver enzymes, and low platelet) syndrome. Nutritional studies may reveal decreased levels of serum proteins, electrolytes, minerals, or vitamins essential to maternal health and fetal development.**
- Review vaginal, cervical, or rectal cultures and serology results. **May reveal presence of sexually transmitted**

Information that appears in brackets has been added by the authors to clarify and enhance the use of nursing diagnoses.

- infections (STIs) or identify active or carrier state of hepatitis or HIV.
- Assist in screening for and identifying genetic or chromosomal disorders. **Disorders such as phenylketonuria (PKU) or sickle cell disease necessitate special treatment to prevent negative effects on fetal growth.**
- Investigate current home situation. **Client may have history of unstable relationships or inadequate/lack of housing that affects safety as well as general well-being.**

Nursing Priority No. 2.
To monitor maternal/fetal status:

- Weigh client and compare current weight with pregravid weight. Have client record weight between visits. **Underweight clients are at risk for anemia, inadequate protein and calorie intake, vitamin or mineral deficiencies, and gestational hypertension. Overweight women are at increased risk for development of gestational hypertension, gestational diabetes, and hyperinsulinemia of the fetus.**
- Assess fetal heart rate (FHR), noting rate and regularity. Have the client monitor fetal movement daily as indicated. **Tachycardia in a term infant may indicate a compensatory mechanism to reduced oxygen levels and/or presence of sepsis. A reduction in fetal activity occurs before bradycardia.**
- Test urine for presence of ketones. **Indicates inadequate glucose utilization and breakdown of fats for metabolic processes.**
- Provide information and assist with procedures as indicated, for example:
  Amniocentesis: **May be performed for genetic purposes or to assess fetal lung maturity. Spectrophotometric analysis of the fluid may be done to detect bilirubin after 26 weeks' gestation.**
  Ultrasonography: **Assesses gestational age of fetus; detects presence of multiples or fetal abnormalities; locates placenta (and amniotic fluid pockets before amniocentesis, if performed); and monitors clients at risk for reduced or inadequate placental perfusion (such as adolescents, clients older than 35 years, and clients with diabetes, gestational hypertension, cardiac or kidney disease, anemia, or respiratory disorders).**

Information that appears in brackets has been added by the authors to clarify and enhance the use of nursing diagnoses.

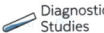 Diagnostic Studies 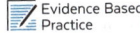 Evidence Based Practice 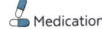 Medications 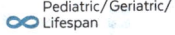 Pediatric/Geriatric/Lifespan

Biophysical profile: **Assesses fetal well-being through ultrasound evaluation to measure amniotic fluid index (AFI), FHR, nonstress test (NST) reactivity, fetal breathing movement, body movement (large limbs), and muscle tone (flexion and extension).**

Contraction stress test (CST): **A positive CST with late decelerations indicates a high-risk client and fetus with possible reduced uteroplacental reserves.**

- Screen for abuse during pregnancy. **Prenatal abuse is correlated with a low maternal weight gain, infections, anemia, delay in seeking prenatal care until the third trimester, and preterm delivery.**
- Screen for preterm uterine contractions, which may or may not be accompanied by cervical dilatation. **May result in delivery of a preterm infant if tocolytic management is not successful in reducing uterine contractility and irritability.**

Nursing Priority No. 3.

To correct/improve maternal/fetal well-being:

- Instruct client in reportable symptoms and monitor for unusual symptoms at each prenatal visit (e.g., vaginal bleeding, headache along with blurred vision and ankle swelling, faintness, persistent vomiting). **Provides opportunity for early intervention in event of developing complications.**
- Assist in treatment of underlying medical condition(s) that have potential for causing maternal or fetal harm.
- Assess perceived impact of complication on client and family members. Encourage verbalization of concerns. **Family stress is amplified in a high-risk pregnancy, where concerns focus on the health of both the client and the fetus. Family is strengthened if all members have a chance to express fears openly and work cooperatively.**
- Facilitate positive adaptation to situation through active-listening, acceptance, and problem-solving. **Helps in successful accomplishment of the psychological tasks of pregnancy.**
- Develop dietary plan with client that provides necessary nutrients (calories, protein, vitamins, and minerals) **to create new tissue and to meet increased maternal metabolic needs.**
- Promote fluid intake of at least 2 quarts of noncaffeinated fluid per day **to prevent dehydration, which may**

Information that appears in brackets has been added by the authors to clarify and enhance the use of nursing diagnoses.

compromise optimal uterine and placental functioning and increase uterine irritability.

- Encourage client to participate in individually appropriate adaptations and self-care techniques, such as scheduling rest periods two to three times a day, avoiding overexertion or heavy lifting, or maintaining contact with family and daily life if bedrest is required. **Preventive problem-solving promotes participation in own care and enhances self-confidence, sense of control, and client/couple satisfaction.**
- Review medication regimen. **Prepregnancy treatment for chronic conditions (e.g., hypertension, diabetes mellitus, HIV, STI) may require alteration for maternal and fetal safety.**
- Review availability and use of resources. **Presence or absence of supportive resources can make the difference for the client and family in being able to manage the situation.**
- Administer Rh immunoglobulin (RhIgG) to client at 28 weeks' gestation in Rh-negative clients with Rh-positive partners or following amniocentesis, if indicated. **RhIgG helps reduce the incidence of maternal isoimmunization in nonsensitized mothers and helps prevent erythroblastosis fetalis and fetal red blood cell (RBC) hemolysis.**
- Encourage modified or complete bedrest, as indicated. **Activity level may need modification, depending on symptoms of uterine activity, cervical changes, or bleeding. Side-lying position increases renal and placental perfusion, which is effective in preventing supine hypotensive syndrome.**
- Provide supplemental oxygen as appropriate. **Increases the oxygen available for fetal uptake, especially in clients with severe anemia or sickle cell crisis.**
- Prepare for and assist with intrauterine fetal exchange transfusion as indicated by titers (Kleihauer-Betke test). **If excess fetal RBC hemolysis occurs, RhO-negative blood may be transfused into fetal peritoneal cavity (replaces hemolyzed RBCs) when fetus is determined at risk of dying before 32 weeks' gestation.**

Nursing Priority No. 4.

To promote successful pregnancy (Teaching/Discharge Considerations) and enhance well-being (long-term goals):

- Emphasize the normalcy of pregnancy; focus on pregnancy milestones and "countdown to birth." **Avoids or**

Information that appears in brackets has been added by the authors to clarify and enhance the use of nursing diagnoses.

 Diagnostic Studies 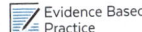 Evidence Based Practice 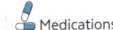 Medications 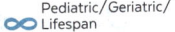 Pediatric/Geriatric/Lifespan limits perception of "sick role"; promotes sense of hope that modifications or restrictions serve a worthwhile purpose.

- Discuss implications of preexisting condition and possible impact on pregnancy. **Pregnancy may have no effect or may reduce or exacerbate severity of symptoms of chronic conditions.**
- Provide information about risks of weight reduction during pregnancy and about nourishment needs of client and fetus. **Prenatal calorie restriction and resultant weight loss may result in nutrient deficiency or ketonemia, with negative effects on fetal central nervous system and possible IUGR.**
- Encourage smoking cessation; refer to community program or support group as indicated. **Severe adverse effects of smoking on the fetus may be reduced if mother quits smoking early in pregnancy, and pregnancy outcomes can still be improved if mother stops smoking as late as 32 weeks' gestation.**
- Help client/couple plan restructuring of roles and activities necessitated by complication of pregnancy. **Education, support, and assistance in maintenance of family integrity help foster growth of its individual members and reduce stress that the client may feel from her dependent role.**
- Encourage client to demonstrate new behaviors and therapeutic techniques. **During pregnancy, control of condition may require specific modified or new behaviors.**
- Recommend client assess uterine tone and contractions for 1 hr, once or twice a day, as indicated, **to monitor uterine irritability or early indication of premature labor.**
- Encourage close monitoring of blood glucose levels, as appropriate. **Clients who have type I (insulin-dependent) diabetes mellitus generally need to check blood glucose levels 4 to 12 times/day because insulin needs may increase two to three times above pregravid baseline.**
- Demonstrate technique and specific equipment used when FHR monitoring is done in the home setting.
- Identify danger signals requiring immediate notification of healthcare provider (e.g., PROM, preterm labor, vaginal drainage or bleeding). **Recognizing risk situations encourages prompt evaluation and intervention, which may prevent or limit untoward outcomes.**

Information that appears in brackets has been added by the authors to clarify and enhance the use of nursing diagnoses.

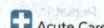 Acute Care 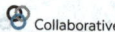 Collaborative 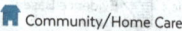 Community/Home Care Cultural

- Review availability and use of resources. **Presence or absence of supportive resources can make the difference for the client and family in being able to manage the situation.**
- Refer to community service agencies (e.g., visiting nurse, social service) or resources, such as Sidelines. **Community supports may be needed for ongoing assessment of medical problem, family status, coping behaviors, and financial stressors.** *Note:* Sidelines is a national support group for high-risk pregnant women. Email or phone support may be available for women on bedrest.
- Refer for counseling if family does not sustain positive coping and growth. **May be necessary to promote growth and to prevent family disintegration.**

Documentation Focus

Assessment/Reassessment
- Assessment findings, including weight, signs of pregnancy, safety concerns
- Specific risk factors, comorbidities, and treatment regimen
- Results of screening laboratory tests and diagnostic studies
- Participation in prenatal care
- Cultural beliefs and practices

Planning
- Plan of care, specific interventions, and who is involved in the planning
- Community resources for equipment and supplies
- Specific referrals made
- Teaching plan

Implementation/Evaluation
- Client/fetal response to treatment and actions performed
- Client's response to teaching provided
- Attainment of or progress toward desired outcome(s)
- Modifications to plan of care

Discharge Planning
- Specific referrals made and follow-up plan

Sample Nursing Outcomes & Interventions Classifications NOC/NIC

NOC—Prenatal Health Behavior
NIC—High-Risk Pregnancy Care

Information that appears in brackets has been added by the authors to clarify and enhance the use of nursing diagnoses.

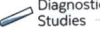 Diagnostic Studies   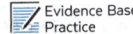 Evidence Based Practice   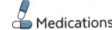 Medications   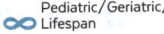 Pediatric/Geriatric/Lifespan

impaired MEMORY

NANDA-I

[Diagnostic Division: Neurosensory]

Definition: Persistent inability to acquire, remember, or recall bits of information or skills while maintaining the capacity to independently perform activities of daily living.

Recognizing Cues

Related/Risk Factors
Depressive symptoms
Inadequate intellectual stimulation; decreased motivation; decreased social interaction; inadequate social support
Water-electrolyte imbalance
[Substance use/abuse; effects of medications (e.g., sedatives, narcotics)]

Defining Characteristics

Subjective
Forgetfulness
Feeling overwhelmed with decision making
Difficulty with thought processes; difficulty with concentrating
Depression

Objective
Consistently forgets to perform a behavior at the scheduled time; difficulty recalling if a behavior was performed
Difficulty performing a previously learned skill
Difficulty acquiring or retaining a new skill; difficulty acquiring or retaining new information
Difficulty recalling events or factual information
Difficulty recalling familiar names, objects, or words

Clinical Connections
Brain injury, stroke, dementia, Alzheimer disease, hypoxia (e.g., chronic obstructive pulmonary disease [COPD], anemia, altitude sickness), alcohol or substance abuse

Generate Solutions

Plan Desired Outcomes

Client Will (Include Specific Time Frame)
- Verbalize awareness of memory problems.
- Establish methods to help in remembering essential things when possible.

Information that appears in brackets has been added by the authors to clarify and enhance the use of nursing diagnoses.

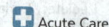 Acute Care   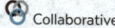 Collaborative   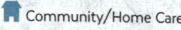 Community/Home Care   Cultural

- Accept limitations of condition and use resources effectively.

Interventions/Take Action

Nursing Priority No. 1.
To assess causative factor(s)/degree of impairment:
- Determine physical, biochemical, and environmental factors (e.g., systemic infections; brain injury/neurological disorders, cardiopulmonary disorders with hypoxia; diabetes, urinary tract infections; use of multiple medications, exposure to toxic substances; smoking, use or abuse of alcohol or other drugs; traumatic event; removal from known environment). **May be associated with confusion and loss of memory.**
- Assess client's age and potential for depression. **Depressive disorders affecting memory and concentration are particularly prevalent in older adults; however, impairments can occur in depressed persons of any age.**
- Note presence of stressful situation(s) and degree of anxiety. **Can increase client's confusion and disorganization, further interfering with attempts at recall. Stress may also accelerate memory decline in person whose cognitive function is already impaired.** (Refer to ND Anxiety for additional interventions, as indicated.)
- Collaborate with medical and psychiatric providers in evaluating orientation, attention span, ability to follow directions, send/receive communication, and appropriateness of response. **Helps to determine presence and/or severity of impairment.**
- Perform or review results of cognitive screening/testing (e.g., General Practitioner Assessment of Cognition [GPCOG], short Informant Questionnaire on Cognitive Decline in the Elderly [IQCODE], Blessed Information-Memory-Concentration [BIMC] test, Mini-Mental State Examination [MMSE]). **Although the etiology for some memory impairments may be obvious or established by client/significant other (SO)/caregiver report, a combination of tests may be needed to demonstrate that the client is below some cut-point on standardized memory tests that represents a significant change from the client's baseline to obtain a complete picture of the client's overall condition and prognosis.**
- Evaluate skill proficiency levels. **Evaluation may include many self-care activities (e.g., daily grooming, steps in preparing a meal, participating in a lifelong hobby,**

Information that appears in brackets has been added by the authors to clarify and enhance the use of nursing diagnoses.

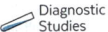 Diagnostic Studies 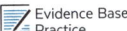 Evidence Based Practice 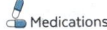 Medications 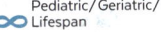 Pediatric/Geriatric/Lifespan

balancing a checkbook, and driving ability) to determine level of independence or needed assistance.
- Ascertain how client/family views the problem (e.g., practical problems of forgetting and/or role and responsibility impairments related to loss of memory and concentration). **Helps determine significance and impact of problem and suggest interventions, especially as they relate to basic safety issues.**

Nursing Priority No. 2.
To maximize level of function:

- Assist with treatment of underlying conditions (e.g., electrolyte imbalances, infection, anemia, drug interactions/reaction to medications; alcohol or other drug intoxication; malnutrition, vitamin deficiencies; pain), **where treatment can improve memory processes.**
- Orient/reorient client as needed. Introduce self with each client contact. **Important for meeting client's safety and comfort needs.** (Refer to NDs acute/chronic Confusion, for additional interventions.)
- Implement appropriate memory-retraining techniques (e.g., keeping calendars and to-do lists, memory cue games, mnemonic devices, computer programs for cognitive retraining). **Provides restorative or compensatory training.**
- Assist with and instruct client and family in associate-learning tasks, such as practice sessions recalling personal information, reminiscing, and locating a geographic location (stimulation therapy). **Practice may improve performance and integrate new behaviors into the client's coping strategies.**
- Encourage ventilation of feelings of frustration and helplessness. Refocus attention to areas of control and progress. **Helps to diminish feelings of powerlessness/hopelessness.**
- Provide for and emphasize importance of pacing learning activities and getting sufficient rest. **Helps to avoid fatigue and frustration that may further impair cognitive abilities.**
- Monitor client's behavior and assist in use of stress-management techniques (e.g., music therapy, reading, television, games, socialization). **Reduces boredom and enhances enjoyment of life.**
- Structure teaching methods and interventions to client's level of functioning. **Teaching at the client's level of functioning potential increases the opportunity for improvement of learning.**

Information that appears in brackets has been added by the authors to clarify and enhance the use of nursing diagnoses.

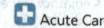 Acute Care 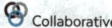 Collaborative 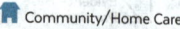 Community/Home Care Cultural

- Determine client's response to and effects of medications prescribed to improve attention, concentration, memory processes, and to lift spirits or modify emotional responses. **Medication for cognitive enhancement can be effective, but benefits need to be weighed against whether quality of life is improved after side effects and cost of drugs are considered.**

Nursing Priority No. 3.
To sustain improvements (Teaching/Discharge Considerations) and enhance well-being (long-term goals):

- Assist client/SO(s) to establish compensation strategies (e.g., menu planning with a shopping list, timely completion of tasks on a daily planner, checklists at the front door to ascertain that lights and stove are off before leaving). **Improves functional lifestyle and safety.** (Refer to NDs acute/chronic Confusion for additional interventions.)
- Instruct client and family/caregivers in memory involvement tasks, such as reminiscence and memory exercises. **Activities are geared toward improving client's functional ability.**
- Refer for follow-up with counselors, rehabilitation programs, job coaches, social or financial support systems. **Provides support for client/SO to cope with persistent or difficult problems.**
- Refer to rehabilitation services as appropriate. **Allows for matching needs, strengths, and capacities of individual and modified as needs change over time.**
- Discuss and encourage safety interventions, as indicated (e.g., assistance with meal preparation, evaluation of driving abilities, cessation of tobacco use or its use only under supervision, removal of guns and other weapons). **Prevents injury to client/others.**
- Assist client to deal with functional limitations (e.g., loss of driving privileges) and identify resources. **Facilitates maximizing independence.**

Documentation Focus

Assessment/Reassessment
- Individual findings, testing results, and perceptions of significance of problem
- Actual impact on lifestyle and independence

Planning
- Plan of care and who is involved in planning process
- Teaching plan

Information that appears in brackets has been added by the authors to clarify and enhance the use of nursing diagnoses.

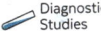 Diagnostic Studies 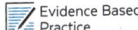 Evidence Based Practice 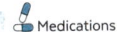 Medications 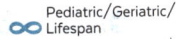 Pediatric/Geriatric/Lifespan

Implementation/Evaluation
- Responses to interventions, teaching, and actions performed
- Attainment of or progress toward desired outcome(s)
- Modifications to plan of care

Discharge Planning
- Long-term needs and who is responsible for actions to be taken
- Specific referrals made

Sample Nursing Outcomes & Interventions Classifications NOC/NIC

NOC—Memory
NIC—Memory Training

---

impaired bed MOBILITY   NANDA-I

[Diagnostic Division: Activity/Rest]

Definition: Limitation in independent movement from one bed position to another.

Recognizing Cues

Related/Risk Factors
Decreased flexibility; impaired postural balance; inadequate muscle strength; prolonged immobility
Unaddressed environmental constraints (e.g., bed size or type, equipment, restraints); inadequate angle of headboard
Inadequate knowledge of mobility strategies
Ineffective overweight self-management
Pain

Defining Characteristics

Objective
Difficulty moving between long sitting and supine positions, or between prone and supine positions, or between sitting and supine positions
Difficulty reaching objects on the bed
Difficulty repositioning self in bed, rolling in the bed, or sitting on edge of bed

---

Information that appears in brackets has been added by the authors to clarify and enhance the use of nursing diagnoses.

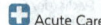 Acute Care 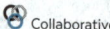 Collaborative 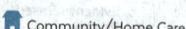 Community/Home Care   Cultural

Clinical Connections

Paralysis (e.g., spinal cord injury, stroke), traumatic brain injury, neuromuscular disorders (e.g., amyotrophic lateral sclerosis), surgery, mechanical ventilation, Parkinson disease, major chest or back surgery, severe depression, dementia, catatonic schizophrenia

Generate Solutions

Plan Desired Outcomes

Client Will (Include Specific Time Frame)

- Verbalize willingness to participate in repositioning program.
- Verbalize understanding of situation and risk factors, individual therapeutic regimen, and safety measures.
- Demonstrate techniques and behaviors that enable safe repositioning.
- Maintain position of function and skin integrity as evidenced by absence of contractures, footdrop, decubitus, and so forth.
- Maintain or increase strength and function of affected and/or compensatory body part.

Interactions/Take Action

Nursing Priority No. 1.

To identify causative/contributing factors:

- Determine diagnoses that contribute to immobility (e.g., multiple sclerosis, arthritis, Parkinson disease, hemi-/para-/tetraplegia, fractures [especially hip joint and long bone fractures], multiple trauma, burns, head injury, depression, dementia) **to identify interventions specific to client's mobility impairment and needs.**
- Note individual risk factors and current situation, such as surgery, casts, amputation, traction, pain, age, general weakness, or debilitation, **which can contribute to problems associated with immobility.**
- Determine degree of perceptual or cognitive impairment and/or ability to follow directions. **Impairments related to age, acute or chronic conditions (including severe depression or dementia), trauma, surgery, or medications require alternative interventions or changes in plan of care.**
- Review results of testing (e.g., Lower Extremity Functional Scale, Harris Hip Score; the self-paced walk, timed up-and-go tests) **to determine limitations in body activity, function, and structure.**

Information that appears in brackets has been added by the authors to clarify and enhance the use of nursing diagnoses.

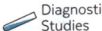 Diagnostic Studies   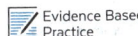 Evidence Based Practice   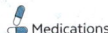 Medications   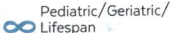 Pediatric/Geriatric/Lifespan

Nursing Priority No. 2.
To assess functional ability:
- Determine functional level classification 0 to 4. (**The client at level 0 is completely independent; level 1 requires use of equipment or device; level 2 requires help from another person for assistance; level 3 requires help from another person and equipment or device; level 4 dependent, does not participate in activity.**)
- Note emotional and behavioral responses to problems of immobility. **Can negatively affect self-concept and self-esteem, autonomy, and independence.**
- Note presence of complications related to immobility. **The effects of immobility are rarely confined to one body system and can include decline in cognition, muscle wasting, contractures, pressure sores, constipation, aspiration pneumonia, and so forth.**

Nursing Priority No. 3.
To promote optimal level of function and prevent complications:
- 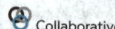 Assist with treatment of underlying condition(s) **to maximize potential for mobility and optimal function.**
- Determine that dependent client is placed in best bed for situation (e.g., correct size, support surface, and mobility functions) **to promote mobility and enhance environmental safety.**
- Instruct client/caregiver in bed capabilities (e.g., mobility functions and set positions), encouraging client to participate as much as possible, even if only to move head or run bed controls. **Promotes independence and purposeful movement.**
- Change client's position, moving individual parts of the body (e.g., legs, arms, head) using appropriate support and proper body alignment. Encourage periodic changes in head of bed (if not contraindicated by conditions such as an acute spinal cord injury), with client in supine, sitting, and prone positions at intervals **to improve circulation, reduce tightening of muscles and joints, normalize body tone, and more closely simulate body positions an individual would normally use.**
- Turn dependent client frequently, utilizing bed and mattress positioning settings to assist movements; reposition in good body alignment, using appropriate supports.
- Instruct client and caregiver in methods of moving client relative to specific situations (e.g., turning side to side,

---

Information that appears in brackets has been added by the authors to clarify and enhance the use of nursing diagnoses.

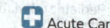 Acute Care 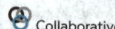 Collaborative 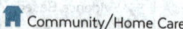 Community/Home Care   Cultural

prone, or sitting) **to provide support for the client's body and to prevent injury to the lifter.**
- Instruct caregiver on proper positions for certain conditions (e.g., paralyzed client) as well as the safe movement and positioning of body parts (e.g., rolling, bridging, scooting, sitting) **to prevent injury to both client and caregiver.**
- Perform and encourage regular skin examination for reddened or excoriated areas. Use a pressure-risk assessment scale (e.g., Braden, Waterlow, Ramstadius), as appropriate. Provide frequent skin care (e.g., cleansing, moisturizing, gentle massage) **to reduce pressure on sensitive areas and prevent development of problems with skin or tissue integrity.** (Refer to NDs impaired Skin Integrity; impaired Tissue Integrity.)
- Use pressure-relieving devices (e.g., egg crate, alternating air pressure, or water mattress) and padding and positioning devices (e.g., foam wedge, pillows, hand rolls) for bony prominences, feet, hands, elbows, head **to prevent dermal injury or stress on tissues and reduce potential for disuse complications.** Refer to ND risk for impaired peripheral Neurovascular Function for additional interventions.
- Provide or assist with daily range-of-motion interventions (active and passive) **to maintain joint mobility, improve circulation, and prevent contractures.**
- Assist with activities of hygiene, feeding, and toileting, as indicated. Assist on and off bedpan and into sitting position (or use cardioposition bed or foot-egress bed) to facilitate elimination.
- Administer medication prior to activity as needed for pain relief **to permit maximal effort and involvement in activity.**
- Observe for change in strength to do more or less self-care **to promote psychological and physical benefits of self-care and to adjust level of assistance, as indicated.**
- Provide diversional activities (e.g., television, books, games, music, visiting), as appropriate, **to decrease boredom and potential for depression.**
- Ensure telephone/cell phone and call bell are within reach **to promote safety and timely response.**
- Provide individually appropriate methods to communicate adequately with client.
- Provide extremity protection (padding, exercises, etc.). (Refer to NDs impaired Skin Integrity; risk for peripheral Neurovascular Dysfunction for additional interventions.)

Information that appears in brackets has been added by the authors to clarify and enhance the use of nursing diagnoses.

 Diagnostic Studies 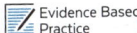 Evidence Based Practice 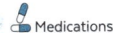 Medications 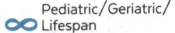 Pediatric/Geriatric/Lifespan

- Collaborate with rehabilitation team, physical therapists, or occupational therapists to create exercise and adaptive program designed specifically for client, identifying assistive devices (e.g., splints, braces, boots) and equipment (e.g., transfer board, sling, trapeze, hydraulic lift, specialty beds).
- Refer to ND Activity Intolerance; impaired physical Mobility; impaired wheelchair Mobility; impaired Transferring Ability; impaired Walking Ability for additional interventions.

Nursing Priority No. 4.

To promote safety and maintain function (Teaching/Discharge Considerations) and enhance well-being (long-term goals):

- Involve client/significant other(s) in determining activity schedule. **Promotes commitment to plan, maximizing outcomes.**
- Instruct all caregivers in safety concerns regarding body mechanics, as well as client's required positions and exercises, **to prevent injury to both and to minimize potential for preventable complications.**
- Encourage continuation of regular exercise regimen **to maintain and enhance gains in strength and muscle control.**
- Obtain, or identify sources for, assistive devices. Demonstrate safe use and proper maintenance.

Documentation Focus

Assessment/Reassessment
- Individual findings, including level of function, ability to participate in specific or desired activities

Planning
- Plan of care and who is involved in the planning

Implementation/Evaluation
- Responses to interventions, teaching, and actions performed
- Attainment of or progress toward desired outcome(s)
- Modification to plan of care

Discharge Planning
- Discharge and long-term needs, noting who is responsible for each action to be taken
- Specific referrals made
- Sources for, and maintenance of, assistive devices

Information that appears in brackets has been added by the authors to clarify and enhance the use of nursing diagnoses.

Sample Nursing Outcomes & Interventions Classifications NOC/NIC

NOC—Body Position: Self-Initiated
NIC—Bed Rest Care

impaired physical MOBILITY NANDA-I

[Diagnostic Division: Activity/Rest]

Definition: Limitation in independent, purposeful movement of the body or of one or more extremities.

Recognizing Cues

Related/Risk Factors
Anxiety; reluctance to initiate movement; sedentary behaviors
Ineffective overweight self-management; malnutrition
Cultural belief regarding acceptable activity; inadequate knowledge of physical activity benefit
Decreased muscle control; inadequate muscle mass, or strength; disuse; inadequate physical endurance; joint stiffness; prolonged immobility
Inadequate environmental support
Pain; unaddressed physical discomfort

Defining Characteristics

Subjective
Discomfort with movement

Objective
Altered gait; decreased range of motion; postural instability
Decreased fine or gross motor skills; engages in substitutions for movement; prolonged reaction time
Difficulty turning from side to side

Clinical Connections
Neuromuscular disorders (e.g., multiple sclerosis [MS], amyotrophic lateral sclerosis, Parkinson disease), traumatic injuries (e.g., fractures, spinal cord or brain injuries), osteoarthritis, rheumatoid arthritis, developmental delays, severe depression

---

Information that appears in brackets has been added by the authors to clarify and enhance the use of nursing diagnoses.

 Diagnostic Studies 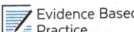 Evidence Based Practice 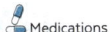 Medications 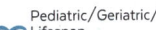 Pediatric/Geriatric/Lifespan

Specify level of independence using a standardized functional scale [such as]

[0—Full self-care
I—Requires use of equipment or device
II—Requires assistance or supervision of another person
III—Requires assistance or supervision of another person and equipment or device
IV—Is dependent and does not participate]

Generate Solutions

Plan Desired Outcomes

Client Will (Include Specific Time Frame)

- Verbalize understanding of situation and individual treatment regimen and safety measures.
- Demonstrate techniques or behaviors that enable resumption of activities.
- Participate in activities of daily living (ADLs) and desired activities.
- Maintain position of function and skin integrity as evidenced by absence of contractures, footdrop, decubitus, and so forth.
- Maintain or increase strength and function of affected and/or compensatory body part.

Interventions/Take Action

Nursing Priority No. 1.

To identify causative/contributing factors:

- Determine diagnosis that contributes to immobility (e.g., MS, arthritis, Parkinson disease, cardiopulmonary disorders, hemi- or paraplegia, depression). **These conditions can cause physiological and psychological problems that can seriously impact physical, social, and economic well-being.**
- Identify factors affecting current situation (e.g., surgery, fractures, amputation, tubings [chest tube, Foley catheter, IV tubes, pumps]) and potential time involved (e.g., few hours in bed after surgery versus serious trauma requiring long-term bedrest or debilitating disease limiting movement). **Identifies potential impairments and determines types of interventions needed to provide for client's safety.**
- Assess client's developmental level, motor skills, ease and capability of movement, posture, and gait **to determine**

Information that appears in brackets has been added by the authors to clarify and enhance the use of nursing diagnoses.

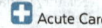 Acute Care 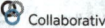 Collaborative 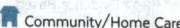 Community/Home Care Cultural

presence of characteristics of client's unique impairment and to guide choice of interventions.

- Note older client's general health status. **Mobility has been identified as the most important component of functional abilities determining client's degree of independence. While aging, per se, does not cause impaired mobility, several predisposing factors in addition to age-related changes can lead to immobility (e.g., diminished body reserves of musculoskeletal system, chronic diseases, sedentary lifestyle, decreased ability to quickly and adequately correct movements affecting center of gravity).**
- Evaluate for presence and degree of pain, listening to client's description about manner in which pain limits mobility **to determine if pain management can improve mobility.**
- Determine client's perception of activity and exercise needs and impact of current situation. Identify cultural beliefs and expectations affecting recovery or response to long-term limitations. **Helps to determine client's expectations and beliefs related to activity and potential long-term effect of current immobility. Also identifies barriers that may be addressed (e.g., lack of safe place to exercise, focus on pre-illness or disability activity, controlling behavior, depression, cultural expectations, distorted body image).**
- Determine history of falls and relatedness to current situation. **Client may be restricting activity because of weakness or debilitation, actual injury during a fall, or from psychological distress (i.e., fear and anxiety) that can persist after a fall.** (Refer to ND risk for Fall for additional interventions.)
- Assess nutritional status and client's report of energy level. **Deficiencies in nutrients and water, electrolytes, and minerals can negatively affect energy and activity tolerance.**

Nursing Priority No. 2.
To assess functional ability:

- Determine degree of immobility in relation to 0 to 4 scale, noting muscle strength and tone, joint mobility, cardiovascular status, balance, and endurance. **Identifies strengths and deficits (e.g., ability to ambulate with or without assistive devices, inability to transfer safely from bed to wheelchair) and may provide information regarding potential for recovery.**

Information that appears in brackets has been added by the authors to clarify and enhance the use of nursing diagnoses.

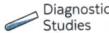 Diagnostic Studies 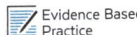 Evidence Based Practice 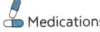 Medications 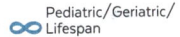 Pediatric/Geriatric/Lifespan

- Determine degree of perceptual or cognitive impairment and ability to follow directions. **Impairments related to age, chronic or acute disease condition, trauma, surgery, or medications require alternative interventions or changes in plan of care.**
- Observe movement when client is unaware of observation **to note any incongruency with reports of abilities.**
- Note emotional/behavioral responses to problems of immobility. **Feelings of frustration or powerlessness may impede attainment of goals.**
- Determine presence of complications related to immobility. **Effects of immobility are rarely confined to one body system and can include muscle wasting, contractures, pressure sores, constipation, aspiration pneumonia, thrombotic phenomena, and weakened immune system functioning. Studies have shown that healthy individuals who were subjected to immobility experienced a 1.3% to 3% loss in muscle strength per day, and overall postural muscle strength decreased by 10% during 1 week of bedrest.**

Nursing Priority No. 3.

To promote optimal level of function and prevent complications:

- Assist with treatment of underlying condition causing pain and/or dysfunction **to maximize the potential for mobility and function.**
- Discuss discrepancies in movement noted when client is unaware of observation and address methods for dealing with identified problems. **May be necessary when the client is using avoidance or controlling behavior or is not aware of own abilities due to anxiety or fear.**
- Assist or have client reposition self on a regular schedule as dictated by individual situation (including frequent shifting of weight when client is wheelchair bound).
- Review and encourage use of proper body mechanics. **Helps client prevent injury to self and caregiver.**
- Instruct in use of side rails, overhead trapeze, roller pads, walker, cane **for position changes, transfers, and to facilitate safe ambulation.**
- Support affected body parts or joints using pillows, rolls, foot supports or shoes, gel pads, foam, and so on, **to maintain position of function and reduce risk of pressure ulcers.**

Information that appears in brackets has been added by the authors to clarify and enhance the use of nursing diagnoses.

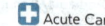 Acute Care 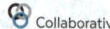 Collaborative 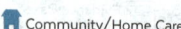 Community/Home Care Cultural

- Perform and encourage regular skin examination and care **to reduce pressure on sensitive areas and to prevent development of problems with skin integrity.** (Refer to NDs impaired Skin Integrity; impaired Tissue Integrity for additional interventions.)
- Provide or recommend pressure-reducing mattress, such as egg crate, or pressure-relieving mattress, such as alternating air pressure or water. **Reduces tissue pressure and aids in maximizing cellular perfusion to prevent dermal injury.**
- Use padding and positioning devices (e.g., foam wedge, pillows, hand rolls) for bony prominences, feet, hands, elbows, head **to prevent stress on tissues and reduce potential for disuse complications.**
- Encourage adequate intake of fluids and nutritious foods. **Promotes well-being and maximizes energy production.**
- Administer medications prior to activity as needed for pain relief **to permit maximal effort and involvement in activity.**
- Schedule activities with adequate rest periods during the day **to reduce fatigue.**
- Provide client with ample time to perform mobility-related tasks.
- Identify energy-conserving techniques for ADLs, **which limit fatigue, maximizing participation.**
- Encourage participation in self-care; occupational, diversional, or recreational activities. **Enhances self-concept and sense of independence.**
- Note change in strength to do more or less self-care (e.g., hygiene, feeding, toileting, therapies) **to promote psychological and physical benefits of self-care and to adjust level of assistance as indicated.**
- Provide for safety measures as indicated by individual situation, including environmental management and fall prevention.
- Collaborate with physical medicine specialist and occupational or physical therapists in providing range-of-motion exercise (active or passive), isotonic muscle contractions (e.g., flexion of ankles, push-and-pull exercises), assistive devices, and activities (e.g., early ambulation, transfers, stairs) **to develop individual exercise and mobility program, to identify appropriate mobility devices, and to limit or reduce effects and complications of immobility.**
- Refer to NDs Activity Intolerance, risk for Fall; impaired bed Mobility; impaired wheelchair Mobility;

Information that appears in brackets has been added by the authors to clarify and enhance the use of nursing diagnoses.

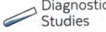 Diagnostic Studies 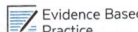 Evidence Based Practice 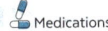 Medications 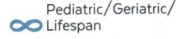 Pediatric/Geriatric/Lifespan

impaired Transferring Ability; impaired Sitting Ability; impaired Standing Ability; impaired Walking Ability; adult/child Pressure Injury for additional interventions.

Nursing Priority No. 4.

To maintain function and safety (Teaching/Discharge Considerations) and enhance well-being (long-term goals):

- Encourage client's/significant other's (SO's) involvement in decision making as much as possible. **Enhances commitment to plan, optimizing outcomes.**
- Review importance and purpose of regular exercise (**e.g., increased cardiovascular and respiratory tolerance; improved flexibility, balance, and muscle strength and tone; enhanced sense of well-being). Client/family may be overwhelmed with information, and reminders can help retain that information.**
- Discuss safe ways that client can exercise. **Multiple options provide client choices and variety (e.g., walking around the block with companion or in a mall during bad air days, participating in a water aerobics class, attending regular rehabilitation sessions).**
- Review safety measures as individually indicated (e.g., use of heating pads, locking wheelchair before transfers, removal or securing of scatter/area rugs).
- Involve client and SO(s) in care, assisting them to learn ways of managing problems of immobility. **May need referral for support and community services to provide care, supervision, companionship, respite services, nutritional and ADLs assistance, adaptive devices or changes to living environment, financial assistance, and so on.**
- Demonstrate use of standing aids and mobility devices (e.g., walkers, strollers, scooters, braces, prosthetics), and have client/care provider demonstrate knowledge about and safe use of device. Identify appropriate resources for obtaining and maintaining appliances and equipment. **Promotes safety and independence and enhances quality of life.**

Documentation Focus

Assessment/Reassessment

- Individual findings, including level of function and ability to participate in specific or desired activities

Planning

- Plan of care and who is involved in the planning
- Teaching plan

Information that appears in brackets has been added by the authors to clarify and enhance the use of nursing diagnoses.

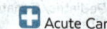 Acute Care 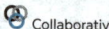 Collaborative 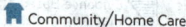 Community/Home Care Cultural

Implementation/Evaluation
- Responses to interventions, teaching, and actions performed
- Attainment of or progress toward desired outcome(s)
- Modifications to plan of care

Discharge Planning
- Discharge and long-term needs, noting who is responsible for each action to be taken
- Specific referrals made
- Sources for and maintenance of assistive devices

Sample Nursing Outcomes & Interventions Classifications NOC/NIC

NOC—Mobility
NIC—Exercise Therapy: [specify]

---

impaired wheelchair MOBILITY — ICNP

[Diagnostic Division: Activity/Rest]

Definition: Difficulty independently operating wheelchair within environment.

Recognizing Cues

Related/Risk Factors
Lack of knowledge of safe wheelchair use, maintenance
Lack of muscle strength/control, physical endurance; pain
Improper wheelchair size or adjustment; obesity
Environmental barriers
Impaired vision; confusion; substance misuse

Defining Characteristics

Subjective
Reports frustration, stress, anger, depression

Objective
Difficulty transferring to/from wheelchair
Difficulty operating motorized wheelchair
Difficulty maneuvering wheelchair indoors, outdoors

Clinical Connections
Neuromuscular disorders (e.g., multiple sclerosis [MS], amyotrophic lateral sclerosis [ALS]), paralysis (e.g., brain injury/stroke, spinal cord injury [SCI]), muscular dystrophy, cerebral palsy, fractures

---

Information that appears in brackets has been added by the authors to clarify and enhance the use of nursing diagnoses.

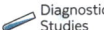 Diagnostic Studies   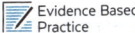 Evidence Based Practice   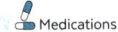 Medications   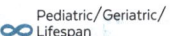 Pediatric/Geriatric/Lifespan

Generate Solutions

Plan Desired Outcomes

Client Will (Include Specific Time Frame)
- Move safely within environment, maximizing independence.
- Identify and use resources appropriately.

Caregiver Will (Include Specific Time Frame)
- Provide safe mobility within environment and community.

Interventions/Take Action

Nursing Priority No. 1.
To identify causative/contributing factors:
- Determine diagnosis that contributes to immobility (e.g., ALS, SCI, spastic cerebral palsy, brain injury) and client's functional level and individual abilities.
- Identify factors in environments frequented by the client that contribute to inaccessibility (e.g., uneven floors or surfaces, lack of ramps, steep incline or decline, narrow doorways or spaces).
- Ascertain access to and appropriateness of public and/or private transportation.

Nursing Priority No. 2.
To promote optimal level of function and prevent complications:
- Determine that client's underlying physical, cognitive, and emotional impairment(s) (e.g., brain injury or SCI, fractures/other trauma, pain, depression, vision deficits) are treated or being managed **to maximize ability, desire, and motivation to participate in wheelchair activities.**
- Ascertain that wheelchair provides the base mobility to maximize function. **Wheelchair must be matched with client's age and size/body type; developmental level and diagnosis, or reason to use wheelchair; desired activities; and unique functional needs (e.g., proper seating and support for people in wheelchairs is critical to their ability to travel, work, participate in sports, learn at school, play, and interact socially). If a spouse or family member will be assisting the person using the wheelchair, their needs may also need to be considered in the wheelchair selection.**
- Perform periodic assessments of client and wheelchair to monitor chair usage and function as well as changes in

---

Information that appears in brackets has been added by the authors to clarify and enhance the use of nursing diagnoses.

client's postural, behavioral, and functional status. **Helps to identify problems (e.g., abnormal wear patterns on the chair requiring mechanical adjustments/repair; loss of client's strength where power add-ons to the chair would improve mobility; or alternative methods of mobility that might be needed).**
- Provide for, and instruct client in, safety while in a wheelchair (e.g., adaptive cushions, supports for all body parts, repositioning and transfer assistive devices, and height adjustment).
- Note evenness of surfaces client would need to negotiate and refer to appropriate sources for modifications. Clear pathways of obstructions.
- Recommend or refer for modifications to home, work, or school and recreational settings frequented by client **to provide safe and suitable environments.**
- Determine need for and capabilities of assistive persons. Provide training and support as indicated.
- Monitor client's use of joystick, sip and puff, sensitive mechanical switches, and so forth, **to provide necessary equipment if condition or capabilities change.**
- Collaborate with physical medicine and physical or occupational therapists in planning activities to improve client's ability to independently operate wheelchair within limits of tolerance and various environments. **May require individual instruction and encouragement, strengthening exercises, assistance with various tasks, and close supervision.**
- Monitor client for adverse effects of immobility (e.g., contractures, muscle atrophy, deep venous thrombosis, pressure ulcers). (Refer to NDs risk for peripheral Neurovascular Dysfunction for additional interventions.)

Nursing Priority No. 3.

To maintain safe mobility (Teaching/Discharge Considerations) and enhance well-being (long-term goals):

- Identify or refer to medical equipment suppliers **to customize client's wheelchair and accessories (e.g., side guards, headrests, heel loops, brake extensions, tool packs) and electronics suited to client's ability (e.g., sip and puff, head movement, sensitive switches).**
- Encourage client's/significant other's (SO's) involvement in decision making as much as possible. **Enhances commitment to plan, optimizing outcomes.**

Information that appears in brackets has been added by the authors to clarify and enhance the use of nursing diagnoses.

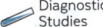 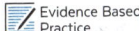 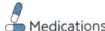 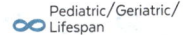

- Involve client/SO(s) in care, assisting them in managing immobility problems. **Promotes independence in self-evaluation and self-care, including managing the type of wheelchair and other assistive devices best for client, how the user's needs and abilities change over time, and modifications that might be made (e.g., number and placement of ramps around the home; modifications to rooms, doors, and vehicles).**
- Demonstrate, discuss, and provide information regarding wheelchair safety as individually appropriate, including safe transfers, dealing with uneven surfaces, ramps, and curbs; programming speed on power chairs, and so forth. Include information and refer for wheelchair preventative maintenance measures (e.g., for wheelchair locks, tires, axles, casters, metal parts, batteries), as indicated. **Wheelchair safety involves people and equipment, including not only acquiring the best chair but also provision for obtaining relief when chair malfunctions.**
- Refer to support groups relative to specific medical condition or disability; independence or political action groups focused on access/disability needs. **Provide role modeling, assistance with problem-solving, and social change.**
- Identify community resources. **Persons with disabilities have the right to achieve the quality of life each believes is personal best. This places as much emphasis on community regarding integration as on physical rehabilitation and functional capabilities.**

Documentation Focus

Assessment/Reassessment
- Individual findings, including level of function, ability to participate in specific or desired activities
- Type of wheelchair and equipment needs

Planning
- Plan of care and who is involved in the planning
- Teaching plan

Implementation/Evaluation
- Responses to interventions, teaching, and actions performed
- Attainment of or progress toward desired outcome(s)
- Modifications to plan of care

Information that appears in brackets has been added by the authors to clarify and enhance the use of nursing diagnoses.

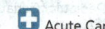 Acute Care 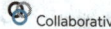 Collaborative 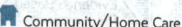 Community/Home Care   Cultural

Discharge Planning
- Discharge and long-term needs, noting who is responsible for each action to be taken
- Specific referrals made
- Sources for, and maintenance of, assistive devices

Sample Nursing Outcomes & Interventions Classifications NOC/NIC

NOC—Ambulation: Wheelchair
NIC—Positioning: Wheelchair

---

impaired MOOD REGULATION   NANDA-I

[Diagnostic Division: Self-Perception/Self-Concept]

Definition: Mental state characterized by shifts in mood or affect and which is composed of a constellation of affective, cognitive, somatic, physiological and/or behavioral manifestations.

Recognizing Cues

Related/Risk Factors
Hypervigilance; external factors influencing self-concept
Difficulty establishing social interaction
Pain; substance misuse

Defining Characteristics

Subjective
Inadequate appetite; inadequate sleep pattern; altered sleep-wake cycle
Excessive guilt, self-blame; religious thought content
Loneliness; hopelessness
Altered libido; sexual thought content; altered sexual behaviors
Recurrent thoughts of death, or suicide

Objective
Affect inadequacy; affective blunting, or distancing; sad affect; apathy
Slowed mental processes; impaired attention; altered quality, or tempo of thoughts; blocking of thoughts

---

Information that appears in brackets has been added by the authors to clarify and enhance the use of nursing diagnoses.

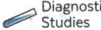 Diagnostic Studies   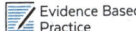 Evidence Based Practice   Medications   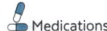 Pediatric/Geriatric/Lifespan

Decreased logical coherence of thoughts; delusions; grandiose thought content; euphoria; dysphoria; derogatory thought content; rumination

Tangential speech; pressured speech; neologisms; loosening of associations; poverty of speech

Psychomotor agitation, or retardation; irritable mood

Childishness; disinhibition; difficulty functioning socially; social alienation; persecutory thought content; inadequate self-concept

Dysthymia; hypomodulation

Clinical Connections

Depression, bipolar disorder, anxiety states, schizophrenia, autism spectrum disorder, dysthymia, postpartum psychosis, chronic disease, substance misuse/abuse

Generate Solutions

Plan Desired Outcomes

Client Will (Include Specific Time Frame)

- Acknowledge reality of mood problems/needs.
- Identify areas of concern.
- Participate in treatment program or therapy regimen.
- Maintain physical health as evidenced by adequate nutrition, weight within normal limits, good sleep habits.

Interventions/Take Action

Nursing Priority No. 1.

To assess causative/contributing factors:

- Determine specific reasons for client's mood swings/difficulties and specific manifestations. (Refer to related factors and defining characteristics.) **Allows for accurate planning of care for individual.**
- Assess ability to understand current situation. **Mood disturbances are prevalent in many disorders and may affect individual's cognitive functioning and understanding of events.**
- Review history, evaluate for underlying neurological disorders. **Presence of traumatic brain injuries, tumors, stroke, and autism may result in variations of mood and emotional processing deficits.**
- Identify degree of depression or mood swings individual is experiencing. **Impaired mood regulation is known to be a factor in vulnerability to depression, bipolar disorders, schizophrenia. When providers avoid using clinical tools**

Information that appears in brackets has been added by the authors to clarify and enhance the use of nursing diagnoses.

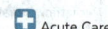 Acute Care 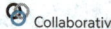 Collaborative 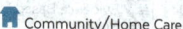 Community/Home Care Cultural

(e.g., PHQ-9 for depression, Mood Disorder Questionnaire), an improper diagnosis may result in serious harm due to treating with antidepressants and eliminating a mood stabilizer that may activate a manic episode.
- Identify behaviors that interfere with person's daily activities (e.g., hallucinations, delusions, situational stress, grief and loss). **Awareness of impairments in behaviors such as sleep, appetite, concentration, and effect on functioning facilitates identification of treatment options for change.**
- Directly ask the client if they have thoughts of harming self or others. **Clients experiencing depression, mood swings, or other mental health disorders may have disturbed thinking causing suicidal ideation or thoughts of harming others, requiring immediate precautions/interventions to keep the client and others safe from harm.**

Nursing Priority No. 2.

To assist client to regulate mood changes more effectively:
- Administer medications prescribed. **Depending on the mental diagnosis, specific medications will be prescribed. For example, depression—antidepressants such as selective serotonin reuptake inhibitors, anxiety—benzodiazepines or BuSpar, bipolar—mood stabilizers or lithium, schizophrenia—antipsychotics such as Haldol or Zyprexa.**
- Discuss how client perceives the current situation and how it is affecting emotions using straightforward and uncomplicated language. **A negative outlook is associated with difficulty in cognitive control and emotional regulation strategies. Communicating with client at their psychosocial developmental/educational level helps foster a nurse–client relationship.**
- Assist client to recognize the extent of negative thinking, rumination, reappraisal, and expressive suppression. **As the individual goes over and over the negative thoughts, it is more difficult to effect cognitive control, and depression can worsen.**
- Encourage client to pay attention to emotional states and feelings, identify when they occur (e.g., sleepless night, complex decision making, relational conflict), and record in a journal or notebook. **Awareness of one's emotions helps the individual to cope appropriately with them.**
- Clarify meanings of feelings by checking meaning with client and provide feedback. **Validates and ensures accuracy of meaning of the communication.**

Information that appears in brackets has been added by the authors to clarify and enhance the use of nursing diagnoses.

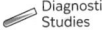 Diagnostic Studies 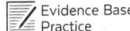 Evidence Based Practice 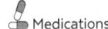 Medications 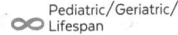 Pediatric/Geriatric/Lifespan

- Help client understand that programs, policies, and procedures are designed to promote emotional growth and development. **The components of milieu (structure, limit setting, balance, norms, client safety) are designed for staff to promote a therapeutic environment for all clients.**
- Provide information regarding use of electroconvulsive therapy (ECT), as indicated. **It is not known exactly how this treatment helps; it is thought to alter brain chemistry and function that relieves depression in 80% to 90% of clients. Clients with severe depression who do not respond to medication may benefit from ECT along with psychotherapy.**

Nursing Priority No. 3.

To minimize mood swings (Teaching/Discharge Considerations) and enhance well-being (long-term goals):

- Involve in cognitive/behavioral, mindful-based, assertiveness training, or individual psychotherapy. **Having the client identify thinking patterns that result in depression allows the individual to recognize and avoid them and improve the ability to recover.**
- Discuss the use of and administer medications, as indicated. **Antidepressants and/or mood stabilizers can be useful in mood disorders along with psychotherapy, and can help the client maintain usual activities.**
- Provide information about individual/group therapy, community resources, and associations supporting impaired mood regulations such as Depression and Bipolar Support Alliance (dbsalliance.org), National Institute of Mental Health (NIMH.nih.gov), or Substance Abuse and Mental Health Services Administration (SAMHSA.gov). **Group discussions promote awareness of others who are experiencing similar difficulties and promote new ideas for coping with own concerns.**
- Encourage client to become involved in community activities (e.g., recreational, educational, or spiritual groups). **Provides opportunity to develop social skills and interests outside of own concerns.**

Documentation Focus

Assessment/Reassessment

- Individual findings, including client's specific situation, impact on functioning/life
- Description of negative thinking patterns

Information that appears in brackets has been added by the authors to clarify and enhance the use of nursing diagnoses.

Planning
- Treatment plan and individual responsibility for activities
- Teaching plan

Implementation/Evaluation
- Client involvement and response to interventions, teaching, and actions performed
- Attainment of or progress toward desired outcome(s)
- Modification to plan of care

Discharge Planning
- Specific referrals made and follow-up plan

Sample Nursing Outcomes & Interventions Classifications NOC/NIC

NOC—Mood Equilibrium
NIC—Mood Management

MORAL DISTRESS ICNP

[Diagnostic Division: Values/Beliefs]

Definition: A challenging situation requiring a decision that creates psychological conflict resulting in moral distress.

Recognizing Cues

Related/Risk Factors
Controversy regarding provision of care for the client by the client/family/significant other (SO), healthcare providers, healthcare organization, insurance providers, or regulatory agencies
Challenge addressing end-of-life care
Conflicting information impedes decision making
Time limitations for decision making
Values and cultural norms are misaligned

Defining Characteristics

Subjective
Emotional conflict with making a decision; feels anxious, stressed
Reports GI distress; difficulty sleeping

Objective
Appears exhausted
Angry outbursts

Information that appears in brackets has been added by the authors to clarify and enhance the use of nursing diagnoses.

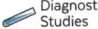 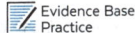 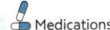

Clinical Connections
Anyone involved in making a healthcare decision

Generate Solutions

Plan Desired Outcomes

Client Will (Include Specific Time Frame)
- Verbalize understanding of causes for conflict in own situation.
- Be aware of own moral values conflicting with desired/required course of action.
- Identify positive ways or actions necessary to deal with situation.
- Express sense of satisfaction with or acceptance of resolution.

Interventions/Take Action

Nursing Priority No. 1.
To identify cause/situation in which moral distress is occurring:

- Note events/situations and individuals at risk for conflicted problem-solving and decisions to be made. **For example, family members not agreeing on proper course of action for comatose loved one, parents faced with expectation of taking ventilator-dependent child home and effect on family as a whole. Or, the inability to save the life of an infant/child or a colleague. Recognizing potential for moral distress allows for timely intervention and support for involved parties.**
- Determine client's perceptions and specific factors resulting in a sense of distress or a lack of control with all parties involved in event/situation. **Conflict may be personal, health, or job related. Moral resilience focuses on healing and provides a sense of control in how the client may have struggled with decisions (e.g., financial constraints; chronic medical condition; or scarcity of resources); however, client feels satisfied with the decision.**
- Identify use of sarcasm, avoidance, apathy, crying, or reports of depression or loss of meaning. **Individuals may not understand or may feel conflicted with their feelings of uneasiness/distress or know that the emotional basis for moral distress is anger.**
- Determine response of family/SO(s) to client's situation or healthcare choices. **May provide clues to emotional or conflictual problems individual is experiencing.**

Information that appears in brackets has been added by the authors to clarify and enhance the use of nursing diagnoses.

 Acute Care 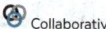 Collaborative 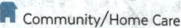 Community/Home Care Cultural

- Identify healthcare goals and expectations. **New treatment options or technology can prolong life or postpone death based on the individual's personal viewpoint, increasing the possibility of conflict with others, including healthcare providers. Moral judgments can include reviewing the risks versus the benefits to the client.**
- Identify cultural beliefs and values and degree of importance to client. **Cultural diversity may lead to disparate views or expectations between clients, SO/family members, and healthcare providers. When tensions between conflicting values cannot be resolved, persons experience moral distress.**
- Detect attitudes and expressions of dissatisfaction of caregivers/staff. **Client may feel pressure or disapproval if own views are not congruent with expectations of those perceived to be more knowledgeable or in "authority." The client may begin to question their values and beliefs regarding the event/situation, creating moral distress and conflict. Nurses may feel conflicted with the client's decision (e.g., female without children elects to be sterilized or places her infant up for adoption) and become judgmental or disrespect the client's rights or decision.**
- Determine if the client/nurse is aware of the problem causing emotional and physical distress (e.g., fatigue, headaches, forgetfulness, anger, guilt, resentment) the individual(s) are experiencing and impact on ability to function. **Moral distress can be very destructive, affecting one's ability to carry out daily tasks or care for self or others, and may lead to a crisis of faith.**
- Assess sleep habits of involved parties. **Evidence suggests that sleep deprivation can harm a person's physical health and emotional well-being, hindering the ability to integrate emotion and cognition to guide moral judgments.**
- Use a moral distress tool, such as the Moral Distress-Appraisal Scale or the Moral Distress Scale, **to help measure degree of involvement and identify possible actions to improve situation.**
- Note availability of family/friends/coworkers for support and encouragement.
- Assess client/provider commitment to address moral distress. **Attempting to make changes prior to a readiness to change will be met with resistance. However, addressing moral distress may start the thought process of solving the problem.**

Information that appears in brackets has been added by the authors to clarify and enhance the use of nursing diagnoses.

Diagnostic Studies | Evidence Based Practice | Medications | Pediatric/Geriatric/Lifespan

Nursing Priority No. 2.

To assist client/involved individuals to develop and/or effectively use problem-solving skills:

- Encourage involved individuals to recognize and name the experience resulting in moral sensitivity. **Allows for an open and honest discussion of values and beliefs related to the event/situation.**
- Affirm the distress, and ask client to commit to thinking about possibilities for solutions. **Validates the thoughts and feelings of the client and provides a sense of control.**
- Use skills, such as active-listening, I-messages, and problem-solving to assist individual(s) **to clarify feelings of anxiety and conflict.**
- Make time available for support and provide information as desired **to help individuals understand the ethical dilemma that led to moral distress.**
- Provide time for nonjudgmental discussion of care issues or questions about impact of conflict leading to moral questioning of current situation. **It is not possible to accurately read another's mind, and open discussion helps those involved in conflict to better understand the situation and begin to look at options.**
- Provide for privacy when discussing sensitive or personal issues **to show regard and concern for individual's self-worth.**
- Determine coping strategies/behaviors client has used successfully in the past that may be helpful in dealing with current situation.
- Involve facility/local ethics committee or ethicist, as appropriate, **to educate client/family, make recommendations, and facilitate mediation/resolution of issues.**

Nursing Priority No. 3.

To promote responsible and moral decision making (Teaching/Discharge Considerations) and enhance well-being (long-term goals):

- Encourage client/family/SO to discuss the issues with making a difficult decision causing moral distress. **Provides opportunity to address family values, spiritual and cultural beliefs, and how to cope with conflicting healthcare needs or requirements for the care of a loved one. Resolving one's moral distress requires making changes or compromises while preserving one's integrity and authenticity.**

Information that appears in brackets has been added by the authors to clarify and enhance the use of nursing diagnoses.

- Refer client/family/SO to a spiritual or cultural leader, counseling, organized support groups, or classes where they can learn approaches for decision making when confronted with resolving moral or ethical issues. **Spiritual and cultural leaders can give support to the family while allowing them to make their decision.**
- Assist individuals to recognize that if they follow their moral decisions, they may clash with the legal system. Suggest referral to appropriate resource for legal opinion/options. **Moral or ethical dilemmas may be difficult to resolve depending on the complexity of the situation. In a hospital setting, an ethics committee may review the situation and provide feedback to the client/family and healthcare providers.**

Documentation Focus

Assessment/Reassessment
- Individual findings, including nature of moral conflict, individuals involved in conflict
- Physical and emotional responses to conflict
- Individual cultural or religious beliefs and values, healthcare goals
- Responses and involvement of family/SOs

Planning
- Plan of care and who is involved in planning
- Teaching plan

Implementation/Evaluation
- Responses to interventions, teaching
- Attainment of or progress toward desired outcome(s)
- Modifications to plan of care

Discharge Planning
- Long-term needs and who is responsible for actions to be taken
- Available resources
- Specific referrals made

Sample Nursing Outcomes & Interventions Classifications NOC/NIC

NOC—Decision-Making
NIC—Decision-Making Support

Information that appears in brackets has been added by the authors to clarify and enhance the use of nursing diagnoses.

 Diagnostic Studies 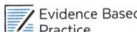 Evidence Based Practice 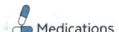 Medications 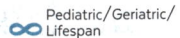 Pediatric/Geriatric/Lifespan

delayed infant MOTOR DEVELOPMENT   NANDA-I

[Diagnostic Division: Activity/Rest]

Definition: Consistent failure to achieve developmental milestones related to the normal strengthening of bones, muscles, and ability to move and touch one's surroundings in an individual 29 days to 1 year of age.

Recognizing Cues

Related/Risk Factors
Infant Factors:
Difficulty with sensory processing
Inadequate curiosity, initiative, or persistence

Caregiver Factors:
Anxiety about infant care; birth parent postpartum depressive symptoms; negative opinion of infant temperament; perceived infant care incompetence
Carries infant in arms for excessive time; limits infant experiences in the prone position
Does not allow infant to choose physical activities, or toys
Does not encourage infant to grasp, or reach; does not teach movement words
Does not encourage sufficient play with other children
Does not engage infant in games about body parts
Does not supply fine or gross motor toys for infant
Inadequate time between periods of infant stimulation; overstimulation of infant

Defining Characteristics
Objective
Difficulty lifting head, or maintaining head position
Difficulty picking up blocks; difficulty transferring objects
Difficulty rolling over, sitting with or without support, or hand-and-knee crawling; difficulty pulling self to stand, or standing with assistance
Does not engage in or initiate activities

Clinical Connections
Premature infant, hospitalization, low birth weight, failure to thrive, infection, abuse/neglect, neonatal abstinence syndrome, cerebral palsy, Down syndrome

---

Information that appears in brackets has been added by the authors to clarify and enhance the use of nursing diagnoses.

 Acute Care 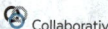 Collaborative 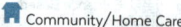 Community/Home Care   Cultural

Generate Solutions

Plan Desired Outcomes

Client Will (Include Specific Time Frame)
- Perform motor skills appropriate for age.

Parent/Caregiver Will (Include Specific Time Frame)
- Verbalize an understanding of age-appropriate development and expectations.
- Identify individual developmental delay or deviation if present.
- Initiate interventions and lifestyle changes promoting appropriate development.

Interventions/Take Action

Nursing Priority No. 1.
To assess for causative/contributing or **risk** factors:

- Identify condition(s) that could contribute to developmental deviations. **Potential for developmental issues might be apparent at birth (neonatal brain injury, especially that occurring before or at time of birth; prematurity; extremes of maternal age; unwanted or complicated pregnancy; known prenatal substance abuse, etc.). However, risks are not confined to the infant's birth events but also encompass parent/family issues and environment (e.g., family history of developmental disorders; mother with mental illness or impairment; infant with acute or chronic severe illness and lengthy hospitalizations; family poverty with inadequate living quarters, nutrition, nurturing, or supervision; family instability or violence; shaken baby syndrome and other maltreatment or child abuse; institutional home or foster system during early life or prior to adoption).**
- Participate in screening infant's development level by means of observation and history related by concerned parents/significant others. **Key elements of motor development can be identified with these screening questions: (1) Is your baby *not* doing something that you think they should be doing? (e.g., delayed acquisition of skill); (2) Is there anything your baby *is* doing that you are concerned about? (e.g., involuntary movements or impaired coordination); (3) Is there anything your baby *used* to do but is no longer doing? (loss/regression of skill); (4) Is there**

Information that appears in brackets has been added by the authors to clarify and enhance the use of nursing diagnoses.

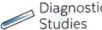 Diagnostic Studies 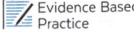 Evidence Based Practice Medications Pediatric/Geriatric/Lifespan

anything *other babies (the same age as yours) can do that is difficult for your baby?* (e.g., evaluating strength, coordination, endurance).

- Obtain information from variety of sources. **Parents are often the first ones to think that there is a problem with their baby's development and should be encouraged to have routine well-baby checkups and screening for developmental delays. However, others (e.g., grandparents, babysitters, clinic nurses) may have valuable input on baby's progress over time.**
- Identify cultural beliefs, norms, and values, as they may impact parent/caregiver view of situation. **Culture shapes parenting practices, understanding of health and illness, perceptions, and beliefs about individuals affected by developmental disorders.**
- Ascertain nature of required parent/caregiver activities and evaluate caregiver's abilities to perform needed activities.
- Note severity and pervasiveness of situation (e.g., potential for long-term stress).
- Evaluate environment in which long-term care will be provided. **The physical, emotional, financial, and social needs of a family are impacted and intertwined with the needs of the infant. Changes may be needed in the family roles, resulting in disruption and stress, placing everyone at risk.**
- Refer for and assist with in-depth evaluation, if indicated, using screening/assessment tools (e.g., Ages and Stages Questionnaire, Parents' Evaluation of Developmental Status, Temperament and Atypical Behavior Scale). **Provides guide for comparative measurement as infant progresses. Note: The most commonly used developmental screening instruments have not been validated on children with motor delays.**

Nursing Priority No. 2.

To assist in managing infant with motor delays (**delayed infant Motor Development**):

- Note chronological age and review with parents the expectations for "normal development" in infancy at clinic visits **to help determine developmental expectations (e.g., when infant should roll over, sit up alone, speak first words, attain a certain weight or height) and how the expectations may be altered by infant's medical condition(s).**
- Describe realistic, age-appropriate patterns of development to parent/caregiver and promote activities and interactions

---

Information that appears in brackets has been added by the authors to clarify and enhance the use of nursing diagnoses.

that consider infant's behavioral style and temperament patterns and support developmental tasks where infant is at this time. **Important for planning interventions in keeping with the individual's current status and potential.**

- Note severity and pervasiveness of situation (e.g., potential for long-term stress leading to abuse or neglect versus situational disruption during period of crisis or transition that may eventually level out). **Situations require different interventions in terms of the intensity and length of time that assistance and support may be critical to the parent/caregiver.**
- Collaborate with related professional resources, as indicated (e.g., pediatrician, physical, rehabilitation, speech therapists; home health agencies; social services, nutritionist; family therapists). **Multidisciplinary team care increases the likelihood of developing a well-rounded plan of care that meets infant's/family's specialized and varied needs, minimizing identified risks.**
- Stress importance of parents/caregivers routinely carrying out plan of care:
  Review developmentally appropriate toys and activities, items available in the home that can be used as toys
  Assist to identify infant readiness cues and responses to stimulation, protect from overstimulation
  Reposition infant every hour while awake
  Encourage visual following of objects, play hide-and-seek, peekaboo
  Encourage infant to reach for/grasp objects, position on back under mobile/floor gym
  Place infant on stomach while awake to encourage head lifting, reaching for toys, moving legs in crawling motion
  Stand infant on lap, swaying side to side
  Assist infant to stand, holding on to hands for stabilization
  Encourage infant to walk holding infant by hands
  Discuss safe spaces in home for infant exploration

Nursing Priority No. 3.

To promote optimal development (Teaching/Discharge Considerations) and enhance well-being (long-term goals):

- Evaluate infant's motor development progress at each well-baby visit. Identify for parents target symptoms requiring intervention **to make referrals in a timely manner and/or to make adjustments in plan of care, as indicated.**
- Emphasize importance of follow-up appointments with healthcare/rehabilitation providers, as recommended, **to**

Information that appears in brackets has been added by the authors to clarify and enhance the use of nursing diagnoses.

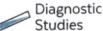 Diagnostic Studies 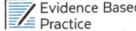 Evidence Based Practice 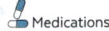 Medications 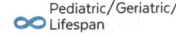 Pediatric/Geriatric/Lifespan

promote ongoing evaluation, support, or management of situation.
- Discuss proactive wellness actions (e.g., periodic laboratory studies to monitor nutritional status, getting immunizations on schedule to prevent serious infections) **to avoid preventable complications.**
- Provide information, as appropriate, including pertinent reference materials and reliable internet sites, being sensitive to parent's/caregiver's health literacy, cultural and socioeconomic concerns. **Provides opportunity to learn at own pace, enhancing likelihood of retention.**
- Encourage attendance at educational programs (e.g., parenting classes, infant stimulation sessions; food buying, cooking, and nutrition; home and family safety, anger management, seminars on life stresses, aging process) **to address specific learning need or desires and interact with others with similar life challenges.**
- Refer to available community and national resources if appropriate (e.g., early intervention programs, disabled children's services, medical equipment and supplier, caregiver support and respite services).

Documentation Focus

Assessment/Reassessment
- Assessment findings, individual needs, including current motor and general developmental level
- Caregiver's understanding of situation and individual role

Planning
- Plan of care and who is involved in the planning
- Teaching plan

Implementation/Evaluation
- Infant's response to interventions and actions performed
- Caregiver response to teaching
- Attainment of or progress toward desired outcome(s) by infant/caregiver
- Modifications to plan of care

Discharge Planning
- Identified long-term needs and who is responsible for actions to be taken
- Specific referrals made, sources for assistive devices, educational tools

---

Information that appears in brackets has been added by the authors to clarify and enhance the use of nursing diagnoses.

Sample Nursing Outcomes & Interventions Classifications NOC/NIC

NOC—Child Development: [specify age]
NOC—Knowledge: Infant Care
NIC—Developmental Enhancement: Infant

impaired oral MUCOUS MEMBRANE ICNP

[Diagnostic Division: Food/Fluid]

Definition: The presence of injury to structures of the mouth and oral mucosa.

Recognizing Cues

Related/Risk Factors
Alcohol consumption; smoking/vaping; tobacco use
Decreased salivation; mouth breathing
Malnutrition, nutrient deficiency; inadequate fluid intake
Depressive symptoms
Inability/difficulty performing oral self-care; inadequate oral hygiene habits, or knowledge of oral care
Avoids/inadequate access to dental care
Oral/facial trauma
Injuring agents (e.g., chemotherapy, radiation); medication regimen

Defining Characteristics

Subjective
Dysgeusia (bad/altered taste in mouth); decreased taste perception
Dysphagia (difficulty eating or swallowing); anorexia
Oral discomfort or pain
Xerostomia (dry mouth)

Objective
Bleeding; erythema/pallor; edema
Leukoplakia (spongy or white patches or plaque in mouth)
Ulceration; fissure; nodule; papule; vesicles
Halitosis; purulent oral-nasal drainage or exudates; white, curd-like oral exudate

---

Information that appears in brackets has been added by the authors to clarify and enhance the use of nursing diagnoses.

 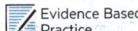

Cheilitis, coated tongue; smooth atrophic or geographic tongue
Dysphonia (difficulty speaking)
Tonsillar inflammation; presence of mass
Gingival hyperplasia, pallor, recession, or pocketing deeper than 4 mm

Clinical Connections

Oral trauma, nil per os (NPO) greater than 24 hr, cancer, chemo/radiation therapy, malnutrition, allergies, infection, oral surgery, cleft lip/palate, conditions requiring endotracheal (ET) intubation (e.g., brain injury, stroke, spinal cord injury, chronic obstructive pulmonary disease, acute respiratory distress syndrome, amyotrophic lateral sclerosis)

Generate Solutions

Plan Desired Outcomes

Client Will (Include Specific Time Frame)
- Verbalize understanding of causative factors.
- Identify specific interventions to promote healthy oral mucosa.
- Demonstrate techniques to restore/maintain integrity of oral mucosa.

Interventions/Take Action

Nursing Priority No. 1.

To identify causative/contributing factors that are affecting **or may affect** oral health:

- Perform oral screening or comprehensive assessment upon admission to facility care using tool (e.g., Beck Oral Assessment Score, Bedside Oral Exam [validated tool], mucosal plaque score, the BRUSHED assessment model, Oral Health Assessment Tool [OHAT] for Long-term Care [or similar tool]), as indicated. **Standardized tool is beneficial in evaluating health of entire mouth, including lips, tongue, gums, and other soft tissues, as well as condition of natural teeth or dentures and status of oral hygiene.**
- Note presence of systemic or local conditions (e.g., oral infections; dehydration, malnutrition, facial fractures, head or neck cancers or treatment including chemotherapy or radiation; pancreatic enzyme replacement therapy; systemic lupus erythematosus, rheumatoid arthritis, Sjögren syndrome, scleroderma, sarcoidosis, amyloidosis,

---

Information that appears in brackets has been added by the authors to clarify and enhance the use of nursing diagnoses.

 Acute Care 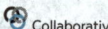 Collaborative 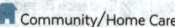 Community/Home Care Cultural

hypothyroidism, diabetes) **that can affect health of buccal tissues. Note: Oral mucositis is a major complication of chemotherapy and/or radiation therapy.**
- Note presence of illness, disease, or trauma (e.g., gingivitis, periodontal disease; presence of oral ulcerations; bacterial, viral, fungal, or oral infections; gum or palate malformations; facial fractures; generalized debilitating conditions) **that affect health of oral tissues.**
- Note client's age and functional status upon admission to facility care. **The very young, the elderly client, or any client with functional deficits (e.g., age-related dependency needs, cognitive or physical impairments, trauma, or complex treatments) may require daily assistance with oral care.**
- Determine if client is resistant to oral care. **Clients with behavioral and/or communication difficulties (e.g., dementia, client will not open mouth or is agitated or lethargic, client does not understand/respond to instructions) may require special equipment, timing of efforts, and/or referral for professional services.**
- Investigate reports of oral pain to determine possible source (e.g., oral lesion, gum disease, tooth abscess, ill-fitting dentures) **to identify needed interventions and reduce risk of complications such as systemic infection.**
- Obtain history of client's medications **to identify those medications that can impact health of buccal tissues or cause immunosuppression, which can impact oral health. Note: Many drugs (e.g., anticholinergics, antidepressants, antiparkinsonian drugs, antihistamines or decongestants, urinary antispastics, antipsychotics, hypnotics, systemic bronchodilators, muscle relaxants, reserpine, narcotics) can impair salivary function and promote xerostomia.**
- Observe for abnormal lesions of mouth, tongue, and cheeks (e.g., white or red patches, ulcers). **White ulcerated spots may be canker sores, especially in children; white curd patches (thrush) are common in infants. Reddened, swollen bleeding gums may indicate infection, poor nutrition, or poor oral hygiene. A red tongue may be related to vitamin deficiencies. Malignant lesions are more common in elderly than in younger clients (especially if there is a history of tobacco, alcohol, or denture use [ill fitting]), or in persons who rarely visit a dentist.**
- Observe for chipped, sharp-edged or malpositioned teeth. Note fit of dentures or other prosthetic devices

---

Information that appears in brackets has been added by the authors to clarify and enhance the use of nursing diagnoses.

when used. **These factors increase the risk of injury to delicate tissues.**
- Note client lifestyle factors including use of tobacco (including smokeless), vaping, and alcohol/other drugs (e.g., methamphetamines), **which may predispose gums and mucosa to effects of nutritional deficiencies, infection, cell damage, and cancer.**
- Determine nutrition and fluid intake and reported changes (e.g., avoiding eating, reports change in taste, difficulty chewing, painstakingly swallows numerous times for even small bites, insufficient fluid intake/dehydration; unexplained weight loss). **Malnutrition and dehydration are associated with problems with oral mucosa.**
- Determine allergies to food, drugs, oral care products, or other substances **that may result in irritation or disruption of oral mucosa.**
- Review oral hygiene practices, noting frequency and type (e.g., brushing, flossing, water appliances). Inquire about client's professional dental care, regularity and date of last dental examination.
- Evaluate client's ability to provide self-care and the availability of necessary equipment or assistance. **Client's age (very young or elderly) impacts client's habits and lifestyle, ability to provide self-care, as well as current health issues (e.g., disease condition or treatment, weakness).**

Nursing Priority No. 2.
To correct identified/developing problems:

- Collaborate in treatment of underlying conditions (e.g., structural defects, infections) **that may correct or limit problem with oral tissues.**
- Inspect client's oral cavity and throat routinely for inflammation, sores, lesions, and/or bleeding. **Can help with early identification and management of mucous membrane concerns.**
- Discuss the safe use of products used to treat xerostomia. **Artificial saliva/moisturizing treatments mimic natural saliva to relieve soft tissue discomfort and are more effective and longer lasting than simple rinses but do not stimulate natural salivary gland production; cholinergic agonist preparations (e.g., pilocarpine, cevimeline) do stimulate saliva production.**
- Encourage adequate fluids **to prevent dry mouth and dehydration.**

Information that appears in brackets has been added by the authors to clarify and enhance the use of nursing diagnoses.

- Encourage frequent sips of cool drinks, sugar-free chewing gum; sucking hard candy or frozen fruits **to stimulate saliva. Use citrus foods and liquids with caution as they may irritate mucosa, increase pain, and injure enamel.**
- Lubricate lips as needed using facility-approved products.
- Provide for increased humidity, if indicated, by vaporizer or room humidifier if client is mouth-breather or ambient humidity is low.
- Provide dietary modifications (e.g., food of comfortable texture, temperature, density—soft or pureed) **to reduce discomfort and improve intake,** and adequate nutrients **to promote healing.**
- Avoid sharp, hard, coarse, spicy, salty, and acidic foods **that can irritate or damage fragile mucosa and existing ulcers.**
- Provide or encourage regular oral care (e.g., after meals and at bedtime) for all clients and more frequently for critically ill clients. **Note: Oral care has been determined to be a nursing intervention that decreases colonization of oropharynx and saliva, thereby reducing the incidence of ventilator-associated pneumonia (VAP) in the critically ill client:**

   Use bland rinses, or sodium bicarbonate solutions; mucosal coating and moisturizing agents **for oral hydration and cleansing of mouth, gums, and mucous membrane surfaces.**

   Avoid mouthwashes containing alcohol (**drying effect**) or hydrogen peroxide (**drying and foul tasting**). **These substances can worsen dryness or cause irritation. Note: Anti-infective solutions like hydrogen peroxide can be utilized to relieve sore throat and/or clean minor mouth ulcers.**

   Use soft-bristle brush (on suction if needed), electric toothbrush, or sponge/cotton-tip applicators to cleanse teeth and tongue. **Brushing the teeth is the most effective way to reduce plaque and manage periodontal disease.**

   Floss gently or use Waterpik **to remove food particles that promote bacterial growth and gum disease.**

   Use foam sticks dipped in standard oral rinse (containing antifungal and antibacterial ingredients) mouthwash where indicated **to swab mouth, tongue, and gums when client is intubated or has no teeth. Note: Sponge/cotton-tip applicators should not be left soaking in solution as soaking may loosen applicator head, creating a choking hazard.**

Information that appears in brackets has been added by the authors to clarify and enhance the use of nursing diagnoses.

 Diagnostic Studies 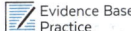 Evidence Based Practice 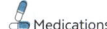 Medications 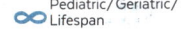 Pediatric/Geriatric/Lifespan

- Avoid/limit use of lemon/glycerin swabs, which are generally discouraged **as the acidity of the swabs may injure client's tooth enamel and worsen xerostomia. Follow facility policy as end-of-life care discussions mention the use of glycerin swabs.**
- Provide or assist with denture care, as needed. **Evidence-based protocol for denture care states that dentures are to be removed and washed at least once daily, removed and rinsed after every meal, and kept in an appropriate solution at night.**
- Refer for evaluation of dentures or other prosthetics and structural defects **when impairments are affecting oral health.**
- Adjust medication regimen where possible **to reduce the use of drugs with the potential for causing or exacerbating painful dry mouth.**
- Provide anesthetic lozenges or analgesics such as viscous lidocaine (Xylocaine), mouthwash containing lidocaine, magic mouthwash, and sucralfate slurry, as indicated, **to provide protection and reduce oral discomfort or pain. Note: Pain of mucositis associated with anticancer therapies has been found to be controlled by mouthwashes containing lidocaine to coat the oral cavity.**
- Administer medications, as indicated (e.g., antibiotics, antifungal agents, antimicrobial mouth rinse or spray), **to treat oral infections or reduce potential for bacterial overgrowth.**
- Assist with ET tube position change or airway per facility protocol **to minimize pressure on fragile tissues and improve access to all areas of oral cavity.**
- Suction oral cavity if client cannot swallow secretions. **Note: Saliva contains digestive enzymes that may be erosive to exposed tissues (such as might occur because of heavy drooling following radical neck surgery).**

Nursing Priority No. 3.

To promote oral health and hygiene (Teaching/Discharge Considerations) and enhance well-being (long-term goals):

- Review current oral hygiene patterns and provide information about oral health, as required or desired, **to correct deficiencies and encourage proper care.**
- Recommend regular dental checkups and care, as well as episodic evaluation of oral health prior to certain medical treatments (e.g., chemotherapy, radiation), **to maintain oral health and reduce risks associated with impaired tissues.**

Information that appears in brackets has been added by the authors to clarify and enhance the use of nursing diagnoses.

- Instruct parents in oral hygiene techniques and proper dental care for infants/children (e.g., safe use of a pacifier, brushing of teeth and gums, avoidance of sweet drinks and candy, recognition and treatment of thrush). **Encourages early initiation of good oral health practices and timely intervention for treatable problems.**
- Discuss mouth care required during and after illness, trauma, or following surgical repair (e.g., cleft lip or palate) **to prevent injury or infection and to facilitate healing.**
- Discuss need for and demonstrate use of special "appliances" (e.g., power toothbrushes, dental water jets, flossing instruments, applicators) **to perform own oral care.**
- Discuss and instruct caregiver(s) in mouth care during end-of-life care/hospice **to promote optimal comfort in client who has stopped eating or drinking and who has dry mouth and feeling of thirst.**
- Active-listen client concerns about appearance and provide accurate information about possible treatments and outcomes. Discuss effect of condition on self-esteem and body image, noting withdrawal from usual social activities or relationships and/or expressions of powerlessness. **May reveal need for more formal intervention (e.g., psychological counseling).**
- Adjust medication regimen **to reduce use of drugs with potential for causing or exacerbating painful dry mouth.**
- Promote good general health and mental health habits including stress management. **Promotes healthy immune function, which can positively affect the oral mucosa.**
- Provide/refer for nutritional information **to correct deficiencies, reduce gum irritation or disease, and prevent dental caries.**
- Recommend avoiding alcohol, smoking/vaping, or chewing tobacco, **which can contribute to mucosal inflammation and gum disease.**
- Identify community resources (e.g., low-cost dental clinics, smoking cessation resources, cancer information services or support groups, Meals on Wheels, Supplemental Nutrition Assistance Program (SNAP), home-care aide) **to meet individual needs.**

Documentation Focus

Assessment/Reassessment
- Condition of oral mucous membranes, routine oral care habits and interferences
- Availability of oral care equipment and products

Information that appears in brackets has been added by the authors to clarify and enhance the use of nursing diagnoses.

- Knowledge of proper oral hygiene and care
- Availability and use of resources

Planning
- Plan of care and who is involved in planning
- Teaching plan

Implementation/Evaluation
- Responses to interventions, teaching, and actions performed
- Attainment of or progress toward desired outcome(s)
- Modifications to plan of care

Discharge Planning
- Long-term needs and who is responsible for actions to be taken
- Specific referrals made, resources for special appliances

Sample Nursing Outcomes & Interventions Classifications NOC/NIC

NOC—Oral Health
NIC—Oral Health Restoration

NAUSEA ICNP

[Diagnostic Division: Food/Fluid]

Definition: A subjective, abdominal experience of malaise with an urge to vomit, which may or may not result in vomiting.

Recognizing Cues

Related/Risk Factors
Autonomic dysfunction (e.g., postural orthostatic tachycardia syndrome [POTS], orthostatic intolerance)
Impaired gastrointestinal (GI) motility, obstruction
Anxiety; fear
Exposure to toxin, chemical, biological; medication
Noxious taste; unpleasant sensory stimuli; motion sickness

Defining Characteristics

Subjective
Food aversion; anorexia
Dysgeusia (bad taste in mouth); water brash (sour taste, gastric reflux)
Dysphagia, gagging sensation

Information that appears in brackets has been added by the authors to clarify and enhance the use of nursing diagnoses.

 Acute Care 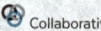 Collaborative 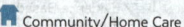 Community/Home Care  Cultural

Objective
Increased salivation; frequent swallowing
Retching

Clinical Connections
Functional dyspepsia, gastroparesis, pregnancy, surgery, cancer, chemo/radiation therapy, AIDS, gastritis, peptic ulcer disease, dumping syndrome, renal failure, brain injury, meningitis, Ménière disease, panic disorders, phobias

Generate Solutions

Plan Desired Outcomes

Client Will (Include Specific Time Frame)
- Be free of nausea.
- Manage chronic nausea, as evidenced by acceptable level of dietary intake.
- Maintain or regain weight as appropriate.

Interventions/Take Action

Nursing Priority No. 1.
To determine causative/contributing factors:

- Assess for presence of conditions of the GI tract (e.g., peptic ulcer disease, bleeding into the stomach, cholecystitis, pancreatitis, appendicitis, gastritis, constipation, intestinal blockage, ingestion of "problem" foods, eating disorders, food poisoning, excessive alcohol/other drugs intake) **that may cause or exacerbate nausea.**
- Note systemic conditions that may result in nausea (e.g., pregnancy, cancer treatment, myocardial infarction, hepatitis, systemic infections, toxins, drug toxicity, presence of neurogenic causes [stimulation of the vestibular system], central nervous system trauma/tumor). **Helps in determining appropriate interventions or need for treatment of underlying condition.**
- Identify situations that client perceives as anxiety inducing, threatening, or distasteful (e.g., "This is nauseating"), such as might occur if client is having multiple diagnostic studies, surgery, or anticipating chemotherapy that has previously induced nausea or other stressful situations. **May be able to limit or control exposure to situations or take medication prophylactically.**
- Note psychological factors, including those that are culturally determined (e.g., eating certain foods considered

---

Information that appears in brackets has been added by the authors to clarify and enhance the use of nursing diagnoses.

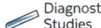 Diagnostic Studies 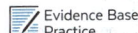 Evidence Based Practice 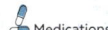 Medications 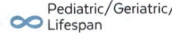 Pediatric/Geriatric/Lifespan

repulsive in one's own culture; seeing or smelling something "gross"; eating disorders such as anorexia and bulimia).
- Determine if nausea is potentially (1) **mild/self-limiting** (e.g., first trimester of pregnancy, 24-hr GI viral infection); (2) **severe and prolonged** (e.g., advanced cancer with multiple medications accompanied by anorexia, constipation, imbalances of calcium/other blood salts; certain cancer treatments; hyperemesis gravidarum); (3) **occurs in patterns. Suggests severity of effect on fluid and electrolyte balance and nutritional status.**
- Ascertain/document pattern of client's nausea (e.g., anticipatory, acute, delayed). **Dictates type and intensity of interventions to manage/treat client's condition.**
- Note client age and developmental level. **Vomiting may occur along with nausea, especially in children (often a part of a short-lived viral infection). Nausea can occur with food intolerances, inner ear problems, pain, or medication reactions in client of any age. Nausea in the elderly (in the absence of acute disease/condition) may be associated with GI motility dysfunction, or medications, pain, or end-of-life issues. Nausea in a female of childbearing age may indicate pregnancy or hormonal influences associated with menstruation, anorexia, or migraine headaches.**
- Record client's food intake and changes in symptoms **to help identify food intolerances or eating disorders when nausea is chronic or related to psychological issues with food.**
- Review medication regimen, especially in client on multiple drugs (polypharmacy). **Drug interactions and side effects may cause or exacerbate nausea.**
- Review results of diagnostic studies. **Various studies may be done depending on the clinical suspicion of cause, such as blood tests (to check electrolytes, blood cell count), urinalysis (to check for dehydration and infection), and x-rays, ultrasound, or computed tomography scan to help identify or localize cause.**

Nursing Priority No. 2.
To promote comfort and enhance intake:
- Collaborate with provider to treat client's underlying medical condition **when cause of nausea is known (e.g., infection, adverse effect of medications, recent anesthesia, chemotherapy or radiotherapy treatments; food allergies, GI reflux).**

Information that appears in brackets has been added by the authors to clarify and enhance the use of nursing diagnoses.

- Administer and monitor client's response to medications used to treat nausea (e.g., vestibular, bowel obstruction, dysmotility of upper gut, infection, inflammation, toxins, cancer treatments) **to determine effectiveness of treatment and to monitor for adverse effects of added medication (e.g., oversedation with risk of aspiration).**
- Select route of medication administration best suited to client's needs (i.e., oral, sublingual, injectable, rectal, transdermal).
- Review pain control regimen when client is experiencing nausea. **Converting to long-acting opioids or combination drugs may decrease stimulation of the chemotactic trigger zone, reducing the occurrence of opioid-related nausea.**
- Administer antiemetic on regular schedule before, during, and after administration of antineoplastic agents **to prevent or control side effects of medication.**
- Time chemotherapy doses **for least interference with food intake.**
- Manage food and fluids:

    Recommend client try dry foods such as toast, crackers, dry cereal before arising when nausea occurs in the morning or throughout the day, as appropriate.

    Encourage client to begin with ice chips or sips/small amounts of fluids—4 to 8 oz for adult; 1 oz or less for child.

    Advise client to drink liquids 30 min before or after meals instead of with meals.

    Suggest sipping fluids slowly and using cool, clear liquids (e.g., water, ginger ale or lemon-lime soda, electrolyte drinks).

    Provide diet and snacks of preferred or bland foods (including skinless chicken, rice, toast, pasta, potatoes) and fluids (including caffeine-free nondiet carbonated beverages, clear soup broth, nonacidic fruit juice, gelatin, sherbet, or ices) **to reduce gastric acidity and improve nutrient intake.**

    Recommend that client avoid milk/dairy products, overly sweet or fried and fatty foods, gas-forming vegetables (e.g., broccoli, cauliflower, cucumbers) **that may increase nausea or be more difficult to digest.**

    Encourage client to eat small meals spaced throughout the day instead of large meals **so stomach does not feel excessively full.**

    Instruct client to eat slowly, chewing food well **to enhance digestion.**

Information that appears in brackets has been added by the authors to clarify and enhance the use of nursing diagnoses.

- Advise client to suck on ice cubes, sugarless, or hard candies. **Keeps mucous membranes moist and can provide some fluid and nutrient intake.**
- Monitor infusion rate of enteral feeding, if present, **to prevent rapid administration that can cause gastric distention and produce nausea.**
- Recommend client remain seated after meal or with head well elevated above feet if in bed.
- Provide clean, peaceful environment and fresh air with fan or open window. Avoid offending odors, such as cooking smells, smoke, perfumes, and mechanical emissions when possible, **as they may stimulate or worsen nausea.**
- Implement nonpharmacological measures:

  Encourage deep, slow breathing **to promote relaxation and refocus attention away from nausea.**

  Use distraction with music, connecting with family/friends, and watching TV **to refocus attention away from unpleasant sensations.**

  Provide frequent oral care (especially after vomiting) **to cleanse mouth and minimize "bad tastes."**

  Avoid sudden changes in position or excessive motion; move to an aisle seat on plane or front seat of car. Focus on distance; face forward when riding. **The actions may help prevent or limit severity of nausea associated with labyrinthitis or motion sickness.**
- Investigate use of electrical nerve stimulation or acupressure point therapy (e.g., may be performed by hands-on technique or application of device against the acupressure point). **Some clients with chronic nausea or history of motion sickness report this to be helpful, without the sedative effect of medication.**

Nursing Priority No. 3.

To promote GI comfort (Teaching/Discharge Considerations) and enhance well-being (long-term goals):

- Review individual factors or triggers causing client's nausea and ways to avoid problem. **Provides necessary information for client to manage own care. Some individuals develop anticipatory nausea (a conditioned reflex) that recurs each time they encounter the situation that triggers the reflex.**
- Instruct client/SO/caregiver in proper use, side effects, and adverse reactions of antiemetic medications. **Enhances client safety and effective management of condition.**

Information that appears in brackets has been added by the authors to clarify and enhance the use of nursing diagnoses.

- Discuss appropriate use of over-the-counter medications and herbal products (e.g., chlorpromazine, metoclopramide, ondansetron, Dramamine, antacids, antiflatulents, ginger) or the use of cannabis or THC compounds (Marinol).
- Encourage use of nonpharmacological interventions. **Activities such as self-hypnosis, progressive muscle relaxation, biofeedback, guided imagery, and systemic desensitization promote relaxation, refocus client's attention, increase client's sense of control, and decrease feelings of helplessness.**
- Advise client/SO to prepare and freeze meals in advance, have someone else cook, or use microwave or oven instead of stove-top cooking **for days when nausea is severe or cooking is impossible.**
- Suggest wearing loose-fitting clothing **to reduce external pressure on client's abdomen.**
- Recommend recording weight weekly, if appropriate, **to help monitor fluid and nutritional status.**
- Discuss potential complications and possible need for medical follow-up or alternative therapies. **Timely recognition and intervention may limit severity of complications (e.g., dehydration).**
- Review signs of dehydration and emphasize importance of replacing fluids and/or electrolytes with products such as Gatorade or other electrolyte drinks for adults or Pedialyte for children. **Increases likelihood of preventing potentially serious electrolyte depletion.**
- Review signs (e.g., hematemesis [emesis appears bloody, black, or like coffee grounds]; feeling faint, syncope, palpitations) that require immediate notification of healthcare provider **for needed interventions to prevent serious complications.**

Documentation Focus

Assessment/Reassessment
- Individual findings, including individual factors causing nausea
- Baseline and periodic weight, vital signs
- Specific client preferences for nutritional intake
- Response to medication

Planning
- Plan of care and who is involved in planning
- Teaching plan

Information that appears in brackets has been added by the authors to clarify and enhance the use of nursing diagnoses.

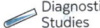 Diagnostic Studies   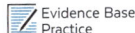 Evidence Based Practice   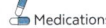 Medications   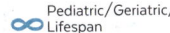 Pediatric/Geriatric/Lifespan

Implementation/Evaluation
- Response to interventions, teaching, and actions performed
- Attainment of or progress toward desired outcome(s)
- Modifications to plan of care

Discharge Planning
- Individual long-term needs, noting who is responsible for actions to be taken
- Specific referrals made

Sample Nursing Outcomes & Interventions Classifications NOC/NIC

NOC—Nausea & Vomiting Control
NIC—Nausea Management

NEONATAL ABSTINENCE SYNDROME Ref. NANDA-I

[Diagnostic Division: Safety]

Definition: A constellation of withdrawal symptoms as a result of in utero exposure to addicting substances, or as a consequence of postnatal pharmacological pain management [in neonate up to 28 days of age].

Recognizing Cues

Related/Risk Factors
[Maternal prenatal substance misuse]
[Postnatal pain management]

Defining Characteristics

Objective
Disorganized infant behavior; neurobehavioral stress; risk for impaired attachment
Ineffective sleep pattern; impaired comfort
Risk for aspiration
Impaired intestinal elimination
Risk for ineffective thermoregulation
Risk for impaired skin integrity
Risk for [physical] injury

Clinical Connections
Prenatal substance misuse, premature, acute condition/surgery pain management

---

Information that appears in brackets has been added by the authors to clarify and enhance the use of nursing diagnoses.

 Acute Care  Collaborative   Community/Home Care   Cultural

Generate Solutions

Plan Desired Outcomes

Client Will (Include Specific Time Frame)
- Be free of adverse effects of substance withdrawal (e.g., irritability, tremors, vomiting, diarrhea, difficulty sleeping).
- Demonstrate feeding tolerance, appropriate weight gain, physiological stability with normal vital signs.
- Display neurobehavioral recovery as evidenced by reaching full alert state, responding to social stimuli, being consoled with appropriate measures.

Parent(s) Will (Include Specific Time Frame)
- Engage in behavior/lifestyle changes to eliminate substance use.
- Use available personal, professional, and community resources.
- Provide safe/growth promoting environment for child.

Interventions/Take Action

Nursing Priority No. 1.
To determine degree of impairment:

- Note maternal risks for fetal well-being, including substance(s) used, dose, duration (especially last week before delivery), route, and presence of infections. **Maternal IV drug use associated with increased risk of infections (e.g., HIV, hepatitis B, hepatitis C) requiring additional testing/surveillance and treatment. Note: Maternal self-report of substance use may significantly understate fetal exposure.**
- Review maternal urine/drug screen. **Maternal use is likely to include more than one substance, complicating treatment. Neonate symptoms and timing of occurrence depend on type of substance(s) used and last dose. Note: Use of opiates within 1 week of delivery causes withdrawal in more than half of infants exposed prenatally.**
- Note fetal status—full-term or premature birth. **Preterm infants have lower risk or less severe symptoms and tend to recover more quickly than full-term infants, if no other complications are present. Longer gestation with increased permeability of placental barrier can increase fetal exposure to drugs prior to delivery.**
- Obtain urine and/or meconium samples for toxicology screen. **Urine sample reflects last several days of exposure; meconium is more sensitive with longer window of detection—from 20 weeks' gestation.**

Information that appears in brackets has been added by the authors to clarify and enhance the use of nursing diagnoses.

 Diagnostic Studies 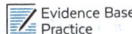 Evidence Based Practice Medications 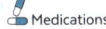 Pediatric/Geriatric/Lifespan

- Monitor for signs/symptoms such as excessive high-pitched cry, problems with sleep, feeding difficulties, tremors, frequent yawning/sneezing, vomiting, and diarrhea. **Symptoms reflecting dysregulation in central and autonomic nervous systems and gastrointestinal system are varied based on substance(s) used (e.g., symptoms can appear as early as 24 hr or be delayed) and require supportive interventions.**
- Screen neonate at birth using a standardized tool such as Finnegan Neonatal Abstinence Scoring Tool (FNAST). Repeat evaluation every 3 to 4 hr when infant is awake. **Baseline is used for comparison of subsequent tests, with usually two or three consecutive scores of 8 or higher indicating need for pharmacological therapy. Scores assist in monitoring, titrating, and determining termination of therapy. Note: Scoring may not be useful in preterm infants, as delayed central nervous system development impacts score.**

Nursing Priority No. 2.

To facilitate safe withdrawal from substance(s):

- Develop nurse/mother relationship; projecting an accepting attitude about drug use that will support mother/infant bonding. **A nonthreatening attitude by nurse encourages maternal participation, provides client a sense of humanness, and helps to decrease paranoia and distrust. (Client will be able to detect biased or condescending attitude of caregivers, negatively impacting relationship.) May help client to accept the negative effects of drugs on her infant and contemplate making a change in her behavior.**
- Coordinate/interact with interdisciplinary team (e.g., neonatologist, pediatrician, nutritionist). **Addresses immediate needs of infant during withdrawal process.**
- Encourage rooming-in as appropriate. **Promotes attachment and greater maternal involvement in infant's care, improves breastfeeding outcomes, may reduce need for pharmacological therapy, and shortens length of hospital stay.**
- Support breastfeeding efforts. Refer to lactation consultant as needed. **Confers immunological benefits to neonate, enhances bonding, and may lower Finnegan scores during first 9 days of life. Note: Not recommended in presence of HIV infection or presence of drug use, except in maternal methadone therapy.**

Information that appears in brackets has been added by the authors to clarify and enhance the use of nursing diagnoses.

- Provide comfort measures based on individual needs. **Eat, Sleep, Console (ESC) is generally first option in treatment, includes parents in maximizing treatment for their infant, and may be sufficient in cases of mild withdrawal:**

    Swaddling in blanket **provides containment boundaries and enhances sleep.**

    Kangaroo (skin-to-skin) care **may enhance neurophysiological organization.**

    Gentle rocking of infant.

    Lower light and noise levels **can minimize excess environmental stimuli.**

    Frequent, demand feedings.

    Pacifier for nonnutritive sucking.

    Water bed, but avoid oscillating bed.

    Complementary therapies (e.g., massage, auricular acupressure, acupuncture, aromatherapy, music therapy).

    Avoidance of unnecessary handling or awakening of sleeping infant.

- Monitor vital signs, intake/output, and weight. **Poor feeding efforts, vomiting, and excessive diarrhea may result in dehydration.**
- Provide high-calorie (150–250 Kcal/kg per 24 hr), small, more frequent feedings if infant is not breastfeeding. **May be necessary to minimize weight loss and promote growth during significant withdrawal.**
- Provide meticulous skin care. **Skin irritation from restlessness/agitation and excessive diarrhea requires careful cleaning and skin barrier creams to prevent breakdown.**
- Administer IV fluids as needed. **May be required to prevent dehydration or electrolyte imbalance.**
- Administer medication(s) for withdrawal when supportive measures fail to improve or correct symptoms, withdrawal scores remain high, seizures develop, or severe dehydration or vomiting and/or diarrhea are present:

    Morphine (i.e., dilute tincture of opium)—administered orally, most commonly preferred medication for treatment of opioid withdrawal

    Methadone—alternative to morphine and may shorten length of opioid withdrawal

    Buprenorphine—may have shorter duration and require shorter hospital stay than treatment with oral morphine; approved for outpatient/postdischarge therapy due to

---

Information that appears in brackets has been added by the authors to clarify and enhance the use of nursing diagnoses.

characteristics of decreased respiratory and cardiovascular side effects

Phenobarbital—preferred for treatment of nonopiate and polydrug exposure

Clonidine—second-line treatment for symptoms refractory to opioid therapy

- Wean from medication as indicated. **Once withdrawal scores decline and symptoms can be managed by comfort measures, a modified protocol can be initiated to decrease pharmacological therapy. Note: Protocol can be extended for 3 weeks or more depending on infant's needs.**

Nursing Priority No. 3.

To promote continued recovery (Teaching/Discharge Considerations) and enhance well-being (long-term goals):

- Interact with expanded interdisciplinary team to include substance abuse counselor, social worker, child development specialist, and other professionals as needed. **Provides support for mother/family in preparation for discharge and future care needs of infant.**

- Determine parents' understanding of current situation. **Provides information about degree of denial, acceptance of personal responsibility, and commitment to change.**

- Provide information to parents in multiple modes, reviewing general infant care and long-term needs specific to substances used. **For example, methadone exposure associated with increased motor rigidity and dysregulated motor patterns can persist into toddlerhood with decreased attention span, impaired social responsibility with poor social engagement. Cocaine use can result in poor fetal growth, developmental delays, learning disabilities, and lower IQ.**

- Stress importance/develop schedule for follow-up monitoring. **Necessary evaluations include neurodevelopmental assessments to monitor motor deficits, cognitive delays, or relative microcephaly; psychobehavioral assessments for hyperactivity, impulsivity, attention deficit in preschool-aged children, and behavioral problems in school-aged children; growth/nutritional assessment for short stature and failure to thrive.**

Information that appears in brackets has been added by the authors to clarify and enhance the use of nursing diagnoses.

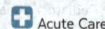 Acute Care 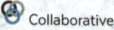 Collaborative 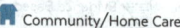 Community/Home Care 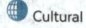 Cultural

- Perform home visit to determine safety of environment. **Optimum home environment required for global development and well-being of infant.**
- Encourage continued involvement of mother in peer group therapy, individual/family counseling, drug recovery education programs. **Provides follow-up support to maintain mother's sobriety.**
- Identify community/social assistance resources (e.g., safe housing, food pantry, licensed day care, transportation, medical care). **Provides for basic human needs of infant and family, enhances maternal coping abilities, and decreases risk of relapse and possible abusive situation.**

Documentation Focus

Assessment/Reassessment
- Individual findings including general health status of infant, comorbidities, signs/stage of withdrawal
- Maternal substance(s) used, route, dose, frequency, last dose
- Results of laboratory tests/diagnostic studies
- Parental attachment, involvement in care

Planning
- Plan of care and who is involved in planning
- Teaching plan
- Plan for maternal sobriety

Implementation/Evaluation
- Response to interventions, teaching, and actions performed
- Attainment of or progress toward desired outcome(s)
- Modifications to plan

Discharge Planning
- Long-term needs and who is responsible for actions to be taken
- Specific referrals made

Sample Nursing Outcomes & Interventions Classifications NOC/NIC

NOC—Substance Withdrawal Severity
NIC—Substance Use Treatment: Drug Withdrawal

Information that appears in brackets has been added by the authors to clarify and enhance the use of nursing diagnoses.

impaired infant NEURODEVELOPMENTAL ORGANIZATION

[Diagnostic Division: Neurosensory]

Definition: Diminished coordination of cognitive, motor, and sensory skills, which may lead to delays in reaching developmental milestones in individuals <1 year of age.

Recognizing Cues

Related/Risk Factors
Inadequate caregiver knowledge, or recognition of behavioral cues; inadequate caregiver responsiveness to infant

Environmental overstimulation; inadequate environmental sensory stimulation; sensory deprivation/overstimulation

Feeding intolerance; malnutrition

Inadequate physical environment; inadequate containment within environment; inadequate environmental supportive positioning

Unaddressed pain; unaddressed poor sleep quality

Defining Characteristics (disorganized infant Behavior)

Objective
Attention-interaction system:
Impaired response to sensory stimuli

Motor system:
Altered primitive reflexes; exaggerated startle response; fidgeting

Finger splaying; fisting; hands-to-face behavior; maintains hands-to-face position; hyperextension of extremities

Impaired motor tone; tremor, twitching; uncoordinated extremity movement

Physiological:
Abnormal skin color (e.g., pale, dusky); oxygen desaturation

Cardiac arrhythmia; bradycardia; tachycardia

Inability to tolerate rate, or volume of feeding

Time-out signals (e.g., gaze, hiccup, sigh, slack jaw, tongue thrust)

Regulatory problems:
Impaired ability to inhibit startle reflex; irritable mood

State-Organization system:
Active-awake or quiet-awake state

Information that appears in brackets has been added by the authors to clarify and enhance the use of nursing diagnoses.

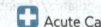 Acute Care 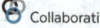 Collaborative 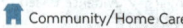 Community/Home Care 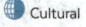 Cultural

Diffuse alpha-electroencephalogram (EEG) activity with eyes closed; state-oscillation

Irritable crying

Clinical Connections

Prematurity, congenital or genetic disorders, meconium aspiration, respiratory distress syndrome, small for gestational age, brain trauma, neonatal abstinence syndrome

Generate Solutions

Plan Desired Outcomes

Client Will (Include Specific Time Frame)

- Exhibit organized behaviors that allow the achievement of optimal potential for growth and development as evidenced by modulation of physiological, motor, state, and attentional-interactive functioning.
- Engage in some self-regulatory measures.

Parent/Caregiver Will (Include Specific Time Frame)

- Recognize cues reflecting infant's stress threshold and current status.
- Identify appropriate responses (including environmental modifications) to infant's cues.
- Engage in responses to promote infant adaptation and development.
- Verbalize readiness to assume caregiving independently.

Interventions/Take Action

Nursing Priority No. 1.

To assess causative/contributing factors:

- Determine the infant's chronological and developmental age; note the length of gestation. **Note: Small-for-gestational-age (SGA) premature infants are at higher risk for developmental and cognitive delays, and those born at extremely low birth weight are at double risk.**
- Observe for cues suggesting the presence of situations that may result in pain/discomfort. **Some behavior that appears to be disorganized may be caused by a pain source that, once identified, may be alleviated.**
- Determine the adequacy of physiological support.
- Evaluate level and appropriateness of environmental stimuli. **Infant behavior is affected by a wide range of stimuli. Careful assessment narrows focus of concerns.**

Information that appears in brackets has been added by the authors to clarify and enhance the use of nursing diagnoses.

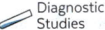 Diagnostic Studies 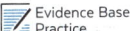 Evidence Based Practice 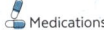 Medications ∞ Pediatric/Geriatric/Lifespan

- Ascertain the parents' understanding of infant's needs and abilities.
- Active-listen parents' concerns about their capabilities to meet infant's needs. **Active-listening can reassure parents, pinpoint areas to be addressed, and provide an opportunity to correct misconceptions.**

Nursing Priority No. 2.

To assist parents in providing coregulation to the infant:

- Provide a calm, nurturing physical and emotionally supportive environment.
- Encourage parents to hold the infant, including skin-to-skin contact, using kangaroo care (KC) as appropriate. **Research suggests KC may have a positive effect on infant development by enhancing neurophysiological organization, as well as an indirect effect by improving parental mood, perceptions, and interactive behavior.**
- Model gentle handling of baby and appropriate responses to infant behavior. **Provides cues to the parent.**
- Support and encourage parents to be with the infant and participate actively in all aspects of care. **The situation may be overwhelming, and support may enhance coping and strengthen attachment.**
- Encourage parents to refrain from social interaction during feedings, as appropriate. **The infant may have difficulty/lack necessary energy to manage feeding and social stimulation simultaneously.**
- Provide positive feedback for progressive parental involvement in the caregiving process. **Transfer of care from staff to parents progresses along a continuum as parents' confidence level increases and they are able to take on more complex care activities.**
- Discuss infant growth and development, pointing out current status and progressive expectations, as appropriate. **Augments parents' knowledge of coregulation.**
- Incorporate the parents' observations and suggestions into the plan of care. **Demonstrates valuing of parents' input and encourages continued involvement.**

Nursing Priority No. 3.

To deliver care within the infant's stress threshold:

- Provide a consistent caregiver. **Facilitates recognition of infant cues or changes in behavior.**
- Identify the infant's individual self-regulatory behaviors (e.g., sucking, mouthing, grasp, hand to mouth, face

---

Information that appears in brackets has been added by the authors to clarify and enhance the use of nursing diagnoses.

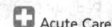 Acute Care 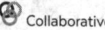 Collaborative 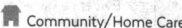 Community/Home Care 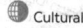 Cultural

- behaviors, foot clasp, brace, limb flexion, trunk tuck, or boundary seeking).
- Support hands to mouth and face; offer pacifier or nonnutritive sucking at the breast with gavage feedings. **Provides opportunities for the infant to suck.**
- Avoid aversive oral stimulation, such as routine oral suctioning; suction endotracheal tube only when clinically indicated.
- Use oxyhood large enough to cover the infant's chest so arms will be inside the hood if oxygen support required. **This allows for hand-to-mouth activities during this therapy.**
- Provide opportunities for the infant to grasp. **Helps with development of motor function skills and can have a calming effect.**
- Provide boundaries and/or containment during all activities. Use swaddling, nesting, bunting, and caregiver's hands as indicated.
- Allow adequate time and opportunities to hold the infant. Handle the infant very gently, move the infant smoothly and slowly, and keep it contained, avoiding sudden or abrupt movements.
- Maintain normal alignment, position the infant with limbs softly flexed and with shoulders and hips adducted slightly. Use appropriate-sized diapers.
- Evaluate the chest for adequate expansion, placing rolls under the trunk if a prone position is indicated.
- Avoid restraints, including at IV sites. If IV board is necessary, secure to limb positioned in normal alignment.
- Provide a sheepskin, egg-crate mattress, water bed, and/or gel pillow or mattress for the infant who does not tolerate frequent position changes. **Minimizes tissue pressure and lessens the risk of tissue injury.**
- Assess color, respirations, activity, and invasive lines visually **to avoid disturbing the infant.** Assess with "hands on" every 4 hr as indicated and prn. **Allows for undisturbed rest and quiet periods.**
- Schedule care activities to allow time for rest and organization of sleep and wake states to maximize tolerance of the infant. Defer routine care to when the infant is in quiet sleep.
- Provide care with the baby in side-lying position. Begin by talking softly to the baby, then place hands in a containing hold on the baby, **which allows baby to prepare.** Proceed with least-invasive manipulations first.

Information that appears in brackets has been added by the authors to clarify and enhance the use of nursing diagnoses.

- Respond promptly to infant's agitation or restlessness. Provide a "time out" when the infant shows early cues of overstimulation. Comfort and support the infant after stressful interventions.
- Remain at the infant's bedside for several minutes after procedures and caregiving **to monitor the infant's response and provide necessary support.**
- Administer analgesics as individually appropriate.

Nursing Priority No. 4.

To modify the environment to provide appropriate stimulation:
- Introduce stimulation as a single mode and assess individual tolerance:

Light/Vision

Reduce lighting perceived by the infant; introduce diurnal lighting (and activity) when infant achieves physiological stability. (Daylight levels of 20 to 30 candles and night-light levels of less than 10 candles are suggested.) Change light levels gradually **to allow the infant time to adjust.**

Protect the infant's eyes from bright illumination during examinations and procedures, as well as from indirect sources, such as neighboring phototherapy treatments, **to prevent retinal damage.**

Deliver phototherapy (when required) with biliblanket devices, if available. **Alleviates need for eye patches.**

Provide caregiver's face (preferably parent's) as visual stimulus when infant shows readiness (awake, attentive).

Evaluate/readjust placement of pictures, stuffed animals, and so on, within the infant's immediate environment. **Promotes state maintenance and smooth transition by allowing the infant to look away easily when visual stimuli become stressful.**

Sound

- Identify sources of noise in the environment and eliminate/reduce them (e.g., speak in a low voice; reduce volume on alarms and telephones to quieter [but audible] levels; pad metal trash can lids; open paper packages, such as IV tubing and suction catheters, slowly and at a distance from the bedside; conduct rounds or report away from bedside; place soft, thick fabric, such as blanket rolls and toys, near infant's head to absorb sound).
- Keep all incubator portholes closed, closing with two hands **to avoid a loud snap and associated startle response.**
- Refrain from playing musical toys or tape players inside the incubator.

Information that appears in brackets has been added by the authors to clarify and enhance the use of nursing diagnoses.

- Avoid placing items on top of the incubator; if necessary to do so, pad the surface well.
- Conduct regular decibel (dB) checks of interior noise level in incubator (recommended not to exceed 60 dB). **Verifies that decibel levels are within acceptable/safe range.**
- Provide auditory stimulation **to console and support infant before and through handling or to reinforce restfulness.**

Olfactory

- Be cautious in exposing the infant to strong odors (e.g., alcohol, Betadine, perfumes), **as olfactory capability of the infant is very sensitive.**
- Place a cloth or gauze pad scented with milk near the infant's face during gavage feeding. **Enhances association of milk with act of feeding and gastric fullness.**
- Invite parents to leave near the infant a handkerchief that they have scented by wearing close to their body. **Strengthens infant recognition of parents.**

Vestibular

- Move and handle the infant slowly and gently. Do not restrict spontaneous movement.
- Provide vestibular stimulation (e.g., water bed [with or without oscillation], a motorized or moving bed or cradle, or rocking in the arms of a caregiver) **to console, stabilize breathing and heart rate, or enhance growth.**

Gustatory

- Dip pacifier in milk and offer to infant during gavage feeding **for sucking and to stimulate tasting.**

Tactile

- Maintain skin integrity and monitor closely. Limit the frequency of invasive procedures.
- Minimize the use of chemicals on the skin (e.g., alcohol, Betadine, solvents) and remove afterward with warm water, **because skin is very sensitive/fragile.**
- Limit the use of tape and adhesives directly on skin. Use DuoDerm under tape **to prevent dermal injury.**
- Touch the infant with a firm containing touch; avoid light stroking. Provide a sheepskin pad or soft linen. **Note: Tactile experience is the primary sensory mode of the infant.**
- Encourage frequent parental holding of the infant (including skin-to-skin). Supplement activity with extended family, staff, and volunteers.

Information that appears in brackets has been added by the authors to clarify and enhance the use of nursing diagnoses.

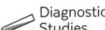 Diagnostic Studies 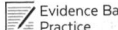 Evidence Based Practice 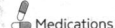 Medications 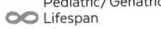 Pediatric/Geriatric/Lifespan

Nursing Priority No. 5.

To continue appropriate stimulation and developmental growth (Teaching/Discharge Considerations) and enhance well-being (long-term goals):

- Evaluate the home environment **to identify appropriate modifications.**
- Provide information about current and projected developmental needs as infant advances. **Visual, auditory, tactile, and kinetic stimulation needs will change over time. Note: Premature and SGA infants often display neurodevelopmental delay at 1 year of age.**
- Discuss structuring care and interactions (including play) around infant's behavioral style and temperament patterns. **Stimulation that is appropriate in complexity and intensity allows infant to maintain a stable balance of their subsystems and enhances development.**
- Assess family stability, and effectiveness of coping strategies for dealing with infant's needs. **Family stressors such as socioeconomic challenges, low educational level, substance use, can lead to attachment difficulties, developmental delays, and increased risk of abuse/neglect.**
- Identify community resources (e.g., early stimulation programs, qualified childcare facilities, respite care, visiting nurse, home-care support, specialty organizations).
- Determine sources for equipment and therapy needs.
- Refer to support or therapy groups, as indicated, **to provide role models, facilitate adjustment to new roles/responsibilities, and enhance coping.**
- Provide contact number, as appropriate (e.g., primary nurse), **to support adjustment to home setting.**
- Stress importance in regular medical follow-up. **Periodic evaluation and screening promote appropriate changes in treatment plan, improving neurodevelopmental outcomes.**
- Refer to additional NDs, such as impaired Caregiver Child Attachment; impaired family Coping; delayed child Growth; delayed child Development; excessive Caregiving Burden.

Documentation Focus

Assessment/Reassessment

- Findings, including infant's cues of stress, self-regulation, and readiness for stimulation, and chronological and developmental age
- Parents' concerns/level of knowledge

Information that appears in brackets has been added by the authors to clarify and enhance the use of nursing diagnoses.

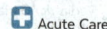 Acute Care 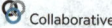 Collaborative 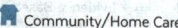 Community/Home Care   Cultural

Planning
- Plan of care and who is involved in the planning
- Teaching plan

Implementation/Evaluation
- Infant's responses to interventions and actions performed
- Parents' participation and response to interactions and teaching
- Attainment of or progress toward desired outcome(s)
- Modifications of plan of care

Discharge Planning
- Long-term needs and who is responsible for actions to be taken
- Specific referrals made

Sample Nursing Outcomes & Interventions Classifications NOC/NIC

NOC—Preterm Infant Organization
NIC—Developmental Enhancement: Infant

---

risk for impaired peripheral NEUROVASCULAR FUNCTION   NANDA-I

[Diagnostic Division: Circulation]

Definition: Susceptible to disruption in the circulation, sensation, and motion of an extremity.

Recognizing Cues

Risk Factors
Prolonged inappropriate positioning of limbs
Prolonged pressure on peripheral nerves, or blood vessels; unaddressed nerve entrapment
Inattentive to peripheral neurovascular symptoms
Difficulty cooperating with instructions
Inadequate knowledge of modifiable factors

Clinical Connections
Traumatic injuries, fractures, burns, joint replacement, laminectomy, deep vein thrombosis (DVT), peripheral vascular obstruction, compartment syndrome

---

Information that appears in brackets has been added by the authors to clarify and enhance the use of nursing diagnoses.

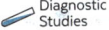 Diagnostic Studies 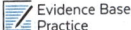 Evidence Based Practice 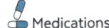 Medications 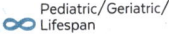 Pediatric/Geriatric/Lifespan

Generate Solutions

Plan Desired Outcomes

Client Will (Include Specific Time Frame)
- Maintain function as evidenced by sensation and movement within normal range for the individual.
- Develop plan to address individual risk factors.
- Demonstrate and participate in behaviors and activities to prevent complications.
- Relate signs/symptoms that require medical reevaluation.

Interventions/Take Action

Nursing Priority No. 1.
To determine significance/degree of potential for compromise:

- Assess for individual risk factors: (1) **trauma to extremity(ies)** that causes internal tissue damage (e.g., high-velocity and penetrating trauma); fractures (especially long-bone fractures) with hemorrhage, or external pressures from burn eschar; (2) **tissue compression** (e.g., tight dressings, splints, or casting); (3) presence of **conditions affecting peripheral circulation,** such as atherosclerosis, diabetes, cardiovascular or cerebrovascular disease, sickle cell disease; (4) **smoking, obesity, and sedentary lifestyle;** and (5) presence of **coagulation disorders,** or use of anticoagulants, **which potentiate risk of circulatory disruption, insufficiency, and occlusion.**
- Monitor for tissue bleeding and spread of hematoma formation, **which can compress blood vessels and raise compartment pressures.**
- Note the position and location of casts, braces, and traction apparatus **to ascertain the potential for pressure on tissues.**
- Review client's recent and current drug regimen, noting the use of anticoagulants and vasoactive agents.

Nursing Priority No. 2.
To prevent deterioration/maximize circulation:

- Conduct a comprehensive upper or lower extremity assessment in at-risk client, including color, sensation, and functional ability. **Early detection of circulatory issues may prevent the onset or severity of functional impairments associated with arterial or venous disorders of the extremities.**

Information that appears in brackets has been added by the authors to clarify and enhance the use of nursing diagnoses.

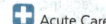 Acute Care 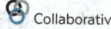 Collaborative 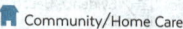 Community/Home Care   Cultural

- Perform neurovascular assessment of affected extremities in clients with suspected neurovascular problems (e.g., surgery, diabetic neuropathy, or fractures), noting differences in the affected limb as compared with the unaffected limb. Use the six Ps of neurovascular assessment (**provides a baseline for future comparisons**):

  Pain: Using 0 to 10 (or a similar pain scale), assess for presence, location, severity, and duration of pain. **Pain may be intermittent (e.g., intermittent claudication) or more constant (e.g., compartment syndrome or arterial occlusion). Pain may range from muscle tension/tenderness and burning to severe pain. Pain may be present with active or passive movement or at rest.**

  Pulses: Monitor presence (or absence) and quality of peripheral pulses (distal to injury or impairment) via palpation and/or Doppler. **An intact pulse usually indicates adequate circulation. However, occasionally a pulse may be palpated even though circulation is blocked by a soft clot; also, perfusion through larger arteries may continue after increased compartment pressure has collapsed the arteriole and venule circulation in the muscle.**

  Pallor: Evaluate skin temperature, capillary refill, and color changes to assess perfusion to the affected area. **Pallor with cool, shiny, taut skin and slow venous refill is indicative of circulatory impairment. Cold, pale, bluish color with purpura indicates arterial insufficiency.**

  Paresthesia: Assess sensation (e.g., test peroneal nerve by pinch or pinprick in the dorsal web between first and second toe, and assess client's ability to dorsiflex toes in the presence of leg fracture). **Changes in sensation cover a wide continuum and may include feelings of tingling, numbness, "pins and needles," burning, or diminished or absent sensation.**

  Paralysis: Evaluate for range of motion of the affected area. **Movement may be limited or absent because of tissue edema and nerve compression or nerve impingement such as would occur with spinal nerve compression.**

  Pressure: Evaluate the affected area by palpating the extremity. **Swelling or tightness may indicate obstruction, such as might occur with compartment syndrome.**

- Assist with diagnostic studies (e.g., blood studies, Doppler, ultrasound, angiography, segmental arterial pressures,

---

Information that appears in brackets has been added by the authors to clarify and enhance the use of nursing diagnoses.

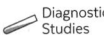 Diagnostic Studies 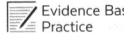 Evidence Based Practice Medications 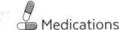 Pediatric/Geriatric/Lifespan

intracompartmental pressures, ankle-brachial index [ABI], transcutaneous oximetry), as indicated. **Numerous diagnostic tests may be needed in view of the multitude of medical and surgical conditions associated with peripheral vascular dysfunction.**

Nursing Priority No. 3.

To minimize elevated tissue pressure and maximize circulation:

- Minimize edema formation:

  Maintain elevation of injured extremity(ies) unless contraindicated by confirmed presence of compartment syndrome **where elevation can impede arterial flow, decreasing perfusion.**

  Apply cold packs to affected area as indicated **to limit tissue swelling and hematoma formation.**

  Remove jewelry and constrictive clothing from affected limb.

  Avoid or limit the use of restraints. Pad affected area and evaluate status frequently if restraints are required.

  Observe position and location of the supporting ring of orthopedic splints or sling. Readjust, as indicated.

- Maximize circulation:

  Use protective techniques such as repositioning and padding **to prevent or relieve pressure.**

  Encourage client to routinely exercise digits or joints distal to injury.

  Encourage ambulation as soon as possible.

  Administer IV fluids and blood products, as needed, **to maintain circulating volume and tissue perfusion.**

  Administer anticoagulants or antithrombic agents, as indicated, **to prevent or treat thrombotic vascular obstructions.**

  Split or bivalve cast, or reposition traction or restraints, as appropriate, **to quickly release pressure.**

  Prepare for surgical intervention or other therapies (e.g., fibulectomy or fasciotomy, revascularization surgery), as indicated, **to relieve pressure and restore circulation.**

- Monitor for the development of complications:

  Inspect tissues around cast edges for rough places and pressure points. Investigate reports of "burning sensation" under cast.

  Monitor hemoglobin/hematocrit, coagulation studies (e.g., prothrombin time).

Information that appears in brackets has been added by the authors to clarify and enhance the use of nursing diagnoses.

Investigate sudden signs of limb ischemia (e.g., decreased skin temperature, pallor, or increased pain), reports of pain that are extreme for the type of injury, increased pain on passive movement of extremity, development of paresthesia, muscle tension or tenderness with erythema, or change in pulse quality distal to the affected area. Place the limb in a neutral position, avoiding elevation. Report symptoms to physician immediately **to provide for timely intervention/limit the severity of problem.**

Nursing Priority No. 4.

To promote peripheral circulation (Teaching/Discharge Considerations) and enhance well-being (long-term goals):

- Educate client on proper body alignment and elevation of limbs, as appropriate.
- Keep linens off the affected extremity with bed cradle or cut-out box, as indicated.
- Discuss the necessity of avoiding constrictive clothing, sharp angulation of legs, and crossing legs.
- Review safe use of heat or cold therapy, as indicated.
- Instruct client/significant other(s) to check shoes and socks for proper fit and/or wrinkles.
- Discuss the need for/promote benefits of smoking cessation and regular exercise **to maintain function and improve circulation of limbs.**
- Review the proper use and monitoring of medication regimen and safety concerns associated with anticoagulant use **to ensure maximum benefit and avoid complications and bleeding problems.**
- Recommend regular follow-up with a healthcare provider **to monitor status of client condition(s), to monitor treatment efficacy, and to provide timely intervention when needed.**

Documentation Focus

Assessment/Reassessment

- Specific risk factors, nature of injury to limb
- Assessment findings, including comparison of affected and unaffected limb, characteristics of pain in involved area
- Use of anticoagulants and vasoactive agents

Planning

- Plan of care and who is involved in the planning
- Teaching plan

Information that appears in brackets has been added by the authors to clarify and enhance the use of nursing diagnoses.

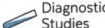 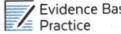 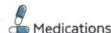 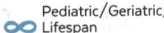

Implementation/Evaluation
- Response to interventions, teaching, and actions performed
- Attainment of or progress toward desired outcome(s)
- Modification of plan of care

Discharge Planning
- Long-term needs, referrals made, and who is responsible for actions to be taken
- Specific referrals made

Sample Nursing Outcomes & Interventions Classifications NOC/NIC

NOC—Neurological Function: Peripheral
NIC—Peripheral Sensation Management

---

impaired NIPPLE-AREOLAR COMPLEX INTEGRITY NANDA-I

[Diagnostic Division: Food/Fluid]

Definition: Localized damage to the pigmented area of the breast as a result of excessive moisture and/or repetitive micro-traumas during chestfeeding.

Recognizing Cues

Related/Risk Factors
Parent Factors:
Anxiety about chestfeeding
Use of products that remove the natural protection of the nipple; prolonged exposure to moisture
Chestfeeding individual withdraws infant from nipple without breaking suction
Breast engorgement; mastitis; hardened areola; postprocedural pain
Supplemental feeding
Improper fit of milk pump
Infant or Child Factors:
Inadequate latching on; ineffective sucking reflex
Nipple confusion due to use of artificial nipple; ineffective nonnutritive sucking

---

Information that appears in brackets has been added by the authors to clarify and enhance the use of nursing diagnoses.

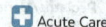 Acute Care 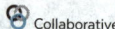 Collaborative 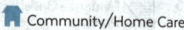 Community/Home Care   Cultural

Defining Characteristics

Subjective
Localized nipple pain

Objective
Altered skin thickness of nipple-areolar complex; hyperkeratosis

Altered skin color; discolored skin patches; erythema; ecchymosis; hematoma; swelling

Abraded skin; disrupted skin surface; macerated skin; excessive exudate

Blistered skin; milk blister; skin vesicles; scabbed skin; skin ulceration, or fissure

Eroded skin; tissue exposure below the epidermis

Classification of nipple and areolar complex lesions using standardized, validated instrument

Clinical Connections
Postpartum women, premature infants, neonates/infants with special needs, maxillofacial abnormalities

Generate Solutions

Plan Desired Outcomes

Client Will (Include Specific Time Frame)
- Verbalize understanding of causative/contributing or risk factors.
- Engage in techniques/behavior changes to promote healthy/healing of breast tissue.
- Maintain/reestablish mutually satisfactory breastfeeding regimen.

Interventions/Take Action

Nursing Priority No. 1.
To identify maternal causative/contributing or risk factors:

 • Assess client knowledge about breastfeeding, expectations, prior experience. **Provides baseline information for identifying needs and developing plan of care. New/recurring difficulties may affect client's commitment to change behaviors. Best practices include breastfeeding education both in prenatal care and postpartum, which increases favorable breastfeeding patterns contributing to the prevention of nipple injury.**

Information that appears in brackets has been added by the authors to clarify and enhance the use of nursing diagnoses.

 Diagnostic Studies   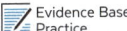 Evidence Based Practice   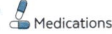 Medications   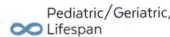 Pediatric/Geriatric/Lifespan

- Perform physical assessment, noting appearance of breasts and nipples, including swelling, erythema, rashes, lumps/lesions, cracked nipples, marked asymmetry of breasts, obvious inverted or flat nipples, and minimal or no breast enlargement during pregnancy. **Identifies existing problems that may interfere with successful breastfeeding experience and provides opportunity to correct them when possible. Note: The presence of nipple damage is more frequent in the first postpartum week and affects approximately 29% to 76% of women who breastfeed and is a common cause for the early cessation of exclusive breastfeeding.**
- Ascertain mother's age, number of children at home, and additional responsibilities. **These factors may have a detrimental effect on desire to breastfeed or manage difficulties. Immaturity may influence mother to give up breastfeeding or may cause her to be insensitive to the infant's needs. The stress of the responsibility of other children or the need to return to work can affect the ability to manage effective breastfeeding.**
- Observe breastfeeding process. Inspect infant oral anatomy. **Determines maternal or infant issues to be corrected/improved. For example, infant may have poor latch, high arched palate, ankyloglossia (tongue-tie).**

Nursing Priority No. 2.
To promote breast tissue/nipple integrity:

- Provide appropriate teaching addressing contributing factors (e.g., infant latch and positioning, maternal and infant anatomy, breast care practices, and improper use of breast pumps):

  Wear supportive bra, 100% cotton fabric; dry nipples after feeding, change breast pads frequently. **Prolonged exposure to moisture can lead to maceration, infection.**

  Avoid use of soap/alcohol/drying agents on nipples, and rough towels. **Use of these products removes the natural protection of the nipple tissue.**

  Recommend relaxation techniques before nursing (e.g., maintain quiet atmosphere, have beverage available, assume position of comfort with back/neck/arms/feet well supported).

  Inform client how to assess and correct a latch if needed. Demonstrate asymmetric latch by aiming infant's lower lip as far from base of the nipple as possible and then bringing infant's chin and lower jaw in contact with

---

Information that appears in brackets has been added by the authors to clarify and enhance the use of nursing diagnoses.

breast while mouth is wide open and before upper lip touches breast. **This position allows infant to use both tongue and jaw more effectively to obtain milk from the breast.**

- Administer a mild pain reliever as appropriate.
- Refer to breastfeeding support provider such as certified lactation consultant, La Leche League. **Vital in identifying and problem-solving issues to facilitate successful breastfeeding.**

Nursing Priority No. 3.

To promote management of breast issues:

- Engage in actions/interventions relevant to specific problem:

  Nipple Pain: Wear 100% cotton fabrics, avoid use of drying agents on nipples, and avoid use of nipple shields or nursing pads that contain plastic; cleanse and pat dry with a clean cloth; apply thin layer of highly purified anhydrous (HPA) lanolin on nipple. (This cream is edible and does not need to be removed before breastfeeding.) Infant should latch on least sore side, or begin with hand expression to establish letdown reflex. Break suction carefully after breastfeeding is complete. **Nipple pain can occur without signs of damage (average rated 2.7/10) and is responsible for approximately 30% of women in the United States introducing formula or ceasing breastfeeding in the first month. Over half of affected clients go on to develop visible damage with pain rated 6.2/10.**

  Engorgement: Wear supportive bra; apply heat or cool applications to the breasts and massage from chest wall down to nipple; soothe "fussy baby" before latching on the breast, and properly position baby on breast/nipple; alternate the side on which baby starts nursing; nurse around the clock or pump with piston-type electric breast pump with bilateral collection chambers at least 8 to 12 times/day; and avoid using bottle, pacifier, or supplements.

  Clogged ducts: Use larger bra or extender to avoid pressure on site; use moist or dry heat and gently massage from above plug down to nipple; nurse infant, hand express, or pump after massage; and nurse more often on affected side.

  Inhibited letdown: Use relaxation techniques before nursing (e.g., maintain quiet atmosphere, massage, apply heat to breasts, have beverage available, assume position of

---

Information that appears in brackets has been added by the authors to clarify and enhance the use of nursing diagnoses.

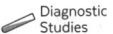 Diagnostic Studies 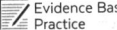 Evidence Based Practice 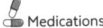 Medications 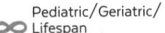 Pediatric/Geriatric/Lifespan

comfort, place infant on mother's chest, skin-to-skin). Encourage mother to relax and enjoy her baby.

Mastitis: Promote bedrest (with infant) for several days; administer antibiotics; provide warm, moist heat before and during nursing; and empty breasts completely, continuing to nurse baby at least 8 to 12 times/day or pumping breasts for 24 hr, and then resuming breastfeeding as appropriate.

Nipple dermatoses: Reduce identifiable triggers; apply an emollient, short-course low- to medium-strength steroid ointment (immediately after a breastfeed to maximize contact time before the next breastfeed).

Use nonsedating antihistamines for pruritus.

Flat/inverted nipples: Instruct in proper use of breast pump when indicated. **Breast pump may be used to pull out flat or inverted nipple and help break up any underlying adhesions.**

- Refer to breastfeeding support provider such as certified lactation consultant, La Leche League. **Vital in identifying and problem-solving issues to facilitate successful breastfeeding.**

Nursing Priority No. 4.

To promote successful breastfeeding (Teaching/Discharge Considerations) and enhanced well-being (long-term goals):

- Discuss and demonstrate breastfeeding aids (e.g., infant sling, nursing footstool, or pillows) and suggest using a variety of nursing positions. **Inappropriate positioning of the infant or mother during breastfeeding may result in breast tissue injury. Positions particularly helpful for plus-sized women or those with large breasts include the "football" hold, with infant's head to mother's breast and body curved around behind her, or lying down to nurse.**

- Recommend avoidance or overuse of supplemental bottle feedings and pacifiers (unless specifically indicated). **The shape of the mouth and lips and the sucking mechanism are different for breast and bottle, and the infant may be confused by the difference, causing interference in the breastfeeding process and increasing risk of not emptying breast, leading to engorgement.**

- Restrict use of nipple shields (i.e., only temporarily to help draw the nipple out, deal with sore nipples), and then place baby directly on nipple. **Temporary use of properly sized shield may be beneficial in the presence of severe nipple**

Information that appears in brackets has been added by the authors to clarify and enhance the use of nursing diagnoses.

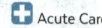 Acute Care 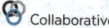 Collaborative 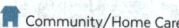 Community/Home Care Cultural

cracking. Hand pumps can also help draw a flat nipple out before latching.
- Demonstrate proper use of breast pump, ensure the pump flange is the correct fit, and if using an electric pump, verify the suction is comfortable and not turned too high. **Prevents breast tissue trauma.**
- Refer to community breastfeeding support group as desired/available. **Provides role modeling, ongoing support, and problem-solving suggestions.**

Documentation Focus

Assessment/Reassessment
- Maternal physical assessment findings (e.g., breast engorgement, flat/inverted nipples)
- Infant assessment findings (e.g., latching on, oral anatomy)
- Maternal knowledge and expectations

Planning
- Plan of care, specific interventions, and who is involved in planning
- Teaching plan

Implementation/Evaluation
- Mother's/infant's responses to interventions, teaching, and actions performed
- Attainment of or progress toward desired outcome(s)
- Modifications to plan of care

Discharge Planning
- Referrals that have been made and mother's choice of participation
- Sources for equipment/supplies

Sample Nursing Outcomes & Interventions Classifications NOC/NIC

NOC—Knowledge: Breastfeeding
NIC—Lactation Counseling

---

inadequate NUTRITIONAL INTAKE NANDA-I

[Diagnostic Division: Food/Fluid]

Definition: Insufficient nutrient consumption to meet metabolic needs.

Information that appears in brackets has been added by the authors to clarify and enhance the use of nursing diagnoses.

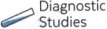 Diagnostic Studies 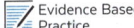 Evidence Based Practice 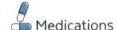 Medications 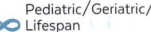 Pediatric/Geriatric/Lifespan

Recognizing Cues

Related/Risk Factors

Altered taste perception; inadequate appetite; food aversion; satiety immediately upon ingesting food

Inadequate physical activity for nutrient absorption

Depressive symptoms; inadequate social support; difficulty establishing social interaction

Impaired swallowing; weakened muscles required for mastication, or swallowing; dry mouth; impaired oral mucous membrane integrity; unaddressed inadequate dentition

Inaccurate information; unrealistic expectation of ability to ingest food

Inadequate food supply; food insecurity; inadequate interest in food, or knowledge of nutrient requirements

Difficulty independently performing activities of daily living, or instrumental activities of daily living; inadequate cooking skills; inappropriate utensils

Unattractive food presentation; unpleasant ambient environment

Inappropriate management of food allergies

Inadequate caregiver knowledge of metabolic, feeding strategies, or strategies to manage appetite

Interrupted chestfeeding

Defining Characteristics

Subjective
Abdominal cramping, or pain
Constipation; diarrhea

Objective

Underweight for age and gender; unintended weight loss with adequate food intake

Inadequate head circumference growth for age and gender; neonatal weight gain less than 30 g/day; low Z-score for individual anthropometric measurement in children (less than 30 g/day)

Altered metabolism with elevation of resting energy expenditure

Capillary fragility; pale mucous membranes; inflammation; delayed wound healing

Food intake less than recommended daily allowance, or estimated requirements; unaddressed hypoglycemia

Hyperactive bowel sounds

Lethargy; muscle hypotonia; increased muscle catabolism

Information that appears in brackets has been added by the authors to clarify and enhance the use of nursing diagnoses.

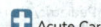 Acute Care 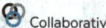 Collaborative 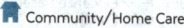 Community/Home Care   Cultural

Excessive hair loss (or increased growth of hair on body [lanugo])
[Cessation of menses]
[Abnormal laboratory studies (e.g., decreased albumin, total proteins; iron deficiency; electrolyte imbalances)]

Clinical Connections
Cancer, AIDS, anorexia or bulimia nervosa, burns, facial trauma, brain injury, coma, stroke, Parkinson disease, cleft lip/palate, anemia, dementia, Alzheimer disease, major depression, schizophrenia

Generate Solutions

Plan Desired Outcomes

Client Will (Include Specific Time Frame)
- Demonstrate progressive weight gain toward goal.
- Display normalization of laboratory values and be free of signs of malnutrition as reflected in Defining Characteristics.
- Verbalize understanding of causative factors when known and necessary interventions.
- Demonstrate behaviors and lifestyle changes to regain and/or maintain appropriate weight.

Interventions/Take Action

Nursing Priority No. 1.
To assess causative/contributing factors:

- ∞ Identify client at risk for malnutrition (e.g., institutionalized or hospitalized elderly; client with chronic illness; child or adult living in poverty/low-income area; client with jaw or facial injuries; intestinal surgery, postmalabsorptive or restrictive surgical interventions for weight loss; hypermetabolic states [e.g., burns, hyperthyroidism]; malabsorption syndromes, lactose intolerance; cystic fibrosis; pancreatic disease; prolonged time of restricted intake; prior nutritional deficiencies).
- Obtain dietary history noting:
  Current diagnosis/condition with increased caloric requirements and with difficulty ingesting sufficient calories (e.g., cancer, burns).
- ∞ Maturational or developmental issues (e.g., premature baby with sucking difficulties, child with lack of emotional stimulation, frail elderly living alone, hospitalized, or in long-term care).

Information that appears in brackets has been added by the authors to clarify and enhance the use of nursing diagnoses.

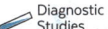 Diagnostic Studies 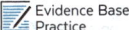 Evidence Based Practice Medications 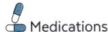 Pediatric/Geriatric/Lifespan

- Swallowing difficulties (e.g., stroke, Parkinson disease, cerebral palsy, dementia [especially Alzheimer disease]; other neuromuscular/neurodevelopmental disorders).
- Poor dentition (damaged or missing teeth, ill-fitting dentures, gum disease).
- Decreased absorption (e.g., lactose intolerance, Crohn disease).
- Diminished desire or refusal to eat (e.g., anorexia nervosa, cirrhosis, pancreatitis, alcoholism, bipolar disorder, depression, chronic fatigue).
- Treatment-related issues (e.g., chemotherapy, radiation, stomatitis, facial surgery, wired jaw).
- Personal or situational factors (e.g., inability to procure or prepare food, social isolation, grief, loss).

- Assess nutritional needs related to age and growth phase, presence of congenital anomalies (e.g., tracheoesophageal fistula, cleft lip/palate), or metabolic or malabsorption problems (e.g., diabetes, phenylketonuria, cerebral palsy; chronic infections).
- Evaluate client's ability to feed self, and document presence of interfering factors. **Difficulties such as paralysis, tremor, or injury to hands or arms with inability to grasp or lift utensils to mouth; cognitive impairments affecting coordination or remembering to eat; age; and/or developmental issues may require input of multiple providers and therapists to develop individualized plan of care.**
- Determine older or impaired client's ability to chew, swallow, and taste food. Evaluate teeth and gums for poor oral health, and note denture fit, as indicated. **All are factors that affect ingestion and/or digestion of nutrients.**
- Ascertain client's understanding of individual nutritional needs and ways client is meeting those needs **to determine informational needs of client/significant other (SO).**
- Note availability and use of financial resources and support systems. **These factors affect or determine ability to acquire, prepare, and store food. Lack of support or socialization may impact client's desire to eat.**
- Determine lifestyle factors that may affect weight. **Socioeconomic resources, amount of money available for purchasing food, proximity of grocery store, and available storage space for food are all factors that may impact food choices and intake.**

Information that appears in brackets has been added by the authors to clarify and enhance the use of nursing diagnoses.

- Explore lifestyle factors such as specific eating habits, the meaning of food to client (e.g., never eats breakfast, snacks throughout entire day, fasts for weight control, no time to eat properly), and individual food preferences and intolerances/aversions. **Identifies eating practices that may need to be corrected and provides insight into dietary interventions that may appeal to client.**
- Assess drug interactions, disease effects, allergies, and use of laxatives or diuretics **that may be affecting appetite, food intake, or absorption.**
- Evaluate impact of cultural, ethnic, or spiritual desires and influences. **Foods are used for prevention or treatment of disease (e.g., client may believe in use of "hot" or "cold" foods to treat certain conditions or use low-fat, low-sodium foods to prevent heart disease). Certain foods may be thought to cause a disease condition (e.g., upset stomach caused by eating too many cold foods). Special diets or food preparation may be based in cultural or spiritual beliefs (e.g., kosher preparation for Jewish client; followers of Buddhism, Hinduism, and Jainism are vegetarians, in part, because of spiritual beliefs).**
- Determine psychological factors, perform psychological assessment, as indicated, **to assess body image and congruency with reality.**
- Assess for occurrence of amenorrhea, tooth decay, swollen salivary glands, and report of constant sore throat, **suggesting eating disorders (e.g., bulimia) and affecting ability to eat.**
- Review usual activities and exercise program, noting repetitive activities (e.g., constant pacing) or inappropriate exercise (e.g., prolonged jogging). **May reveal obsessive nature of weight-control measures.**

Nursing Priority No. 2.
To evaluate degree of deficit:

- Assess current weight compared to usual weight and norms for age, gender, and body size. Measure muscle mass or calculate body fat by means of anthropometric measurements and growth scales **to identify deviations from the norm and to establish baseline parameters.**
- Obtain weights using same scale, same time of day, and same clothing as much as possible. **Provides for accurate comparison to evaluate effectiveness of therapeutic regimen.**

Information that appears in brackets has been added by the authors to clarify and enhance the use of nursing diagnoses.

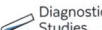 Diagnostic Studies 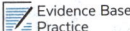 Evidence Based Practice 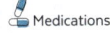 Medications 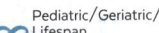 Pediatric/Geriatric/Lifespan

- Calculate growth percentiles in infants/children using growth chart **to identify deviations from the norm.**
- Observe for absence of subcutaneous fat and muscle wasting, loss of hair, fissuring of nails, delayed healing, gum bleeding, swollen abdomen, and so on, **which indicate protein-energy malnutrition.**
- Auscultate presence and character of bowel sounds **to determine ability and readiness of intestinal tract to handle digestive processes (e.g., hypermotility accompanies vomiting or diarrhea, whereas absence of bowel sounds may indicate bowel obstruction).**
- Assist in nutritional status assessment, using screening tools (e.g., Mini Nutritional Assessment [MNA], the Malnutrition Universal Screening Tool [MUST], or similar tool). **Among hospitalized elderly, low MNA scores have been associated with longer hospitalizations and higher rates of discharge to nursing homes and death.**
- Review indicated laboratory data (e.g., serum albumin/prealbumin, transferrin, amino acid profile, iron, BUN, nitrogen balance studies, glucose, liver function, electrolytes, total lymphocyte count, indirect calorimetry).

Nursing Priority No. 3.

To establish a nutritional plan that meets individual needs:

- Collaborate with interdisciplinary team **to set nutritional goals when client has specific dietary needs, malnutrition is profound, or long-term feeding problems exist.**
- Calculate client's energy and protein requirements using basal energy expenditure and the Harris-Benedict (or similar) formula. **Various factors may be considered in choosing a useful formula, including age, sex, disease state, stress associated with current illness, body size (e.g., obesity), and activity (e.g., bedbound versus out of bed).**
- Provide dietary, environmental, and behavioral modifications, as indicated:
  Optimization of client's intake of protein, carbohydrates, fats, calories within eating style and needs
  Several small meals and snacks daily
  Mechanical soft or blenderized tube feedings
  Appetite stimulants (e.g., wine), if indicated
  High-calorie, nutrient-rich dietary products such as meal-replacement shake or supplements
  Formula tube feedings; parenteral nutrition infusion

Information that appears in brackets has been added by the authors to clarify and enhance the use of nursing diagnoses.

Determine whether client prefers or tolerates more calories in a particular meal.

Use flavoring agents (e.g., lemon and herbs) if salt is restricted **to enhance food satisfaction and stimulate appetite.**

Encourage use of sugar or honey in beverages if carbohydrates are tolerated well.

Encourage client to choose foods or have family member bring foods that seem appealing **to stimulate appetite.**

Avoid foods that cause intolerances or increase gastric motility (e.g., foods that are gas forming, hot/cold, or spicy; caffeinated beverages; milk products), according to individual needs.

Limit fiber or bulk, if indicated, **because it may lead to early satiety.**

Promote pleasant, relaxing environment, including socialization when possible **to enhance intake.**

Prevent or minimize unpleasant odors or sights. **May have a negative effect on appetite and eating.**

Assist with or provide oral care before and after meals and at bedtime.

Encourage use of lozenges and so forth **to stimulate salivation when dryness is a factor.**

Promote adequate and timely fluid intake. Limit fluids 1 hr prior to meal **to reduce possibility of early satiety.**

Weigh regularly and graph results **to monitor effectiveness of efforts.**

- Administer pharmaceutical agents, as indicated:
  Digestive drugs or enzymes
  Vitamin and mineral (iron) supplements, including chewable multivitamin
  Medications (e.g., antacids, anticholinergics, antiemetics, antidiarrheals)

- Develop individual strategies when problem is mechanical (e.g., wired jaws or paralysis following stroke). Consult occupational therapist **to identify appropriate assistive devices** or speech therapist **to enhance swallowing ability.** (Refer to ND impaired Swallowing.)

- Refer to structured (behavioral) program of nutrition therapy (e.g., documented time and length of eating period, blenderized food or tube feeding, administered parenteral nutritional therapy) per protocol, **particularly when problem is anorexia nervosa or bulimia.**

- Refer for/support hospitalization **for controlled environment in severe malnutrition or life-threatening situations.**

inadequate NUTRITIONAL INTAKE

Information that appears in brackets has been added by the authors to clarify and enhance the use of nursing diagnoses.

 Diagnostic Studies   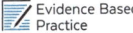 Evidence Based Practice   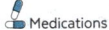 Medications   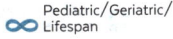 Pediatric/Geriatric/Lifespan

- Refer to social services or other community resources **for possible assistance with client's limitations in buying and preparing foods.**

Nursing Priority No. 4.

To maintain appropriate nutrient intake (Teaching/Discharge Considerations) and enhance well-being (long-term goals):

- Emphasize importance of well-balanced, nutritious intake. Provide information regarding individual nutritional needs and ways to meet these needs within financial constraints.
- Discuss myths client/SO(s) may have about weight and weight gain **to address misconceptions and perhaps improve motivation for needed behavior changes.**
- Provide positive regard, love, and acknowledgment of "voice within" guiding client with eating disorder. **These efforts encourage the client to recognize maladaptive eating patterns as defense mechanisms to ease the emotional pain and begin to resolve underlying issues and develop more adaptive coping strategies for dealing with stressful situations.**
- Develop consistent, realistic weight goal with client.
- Weigh at regular intervals and document results **to monitor effectiveness of dietary plan.**
- Involve client in developing behavior modification program appropriate to specific needs based on consistent, realistic weight gain goal. **Enhances commitment to change and likelihood of accomplishing desired outcomes.**
- Involve SO(s) in treatment plan as much as possible. **Provides ongoing support for client and increases likelihood of accomplishing dietary goals.**
- Consult with dietitian or nutritional support team, as necessary, **for long-term and special needs.**
- Discuss with client/caregiver ways to develop regular exercise and stress reduction program. **Enhances general well-being, improves organ function/muscle tone, and increases appetite.**
- Review drug regimen, side effects, and potential interactions with other medications and over-the-counter drugs. **Medication education empowers client to manage side effects.**
- Review medical regimen and provide information and assistance, as necessary.
- Assist client to identify and access resources, such as way to obtain nutrient-dense, low-budget foods, Supplemental Nutrition Assistance Program, Meals on Wheels, community food banks, and/or other appropriate assistance programs.

Information that appears in brackets has been added by the authors to clarify and enhance the use of nursing diagnoses.

- Refer for dental hygiene or other professional care, including counseling or psychiatric care, family therapy, as indicated.
- Provide and reinforce client teaching regarding preoperative and postoperative dietary needs when surgery is planned.
- Assist client/SO(s) to learn how to blenderize food and/or perform tube feeding.
- Refer to home health resources **for initiation and supervision of parenteral nutrition therapy when used.**

Documentation Focus

Assessment/Reassessment
- Baseline and subsequent assessment findings to include signs/symptoms, as noted in Defining Characteristics, and laboratory diagnostic findings
- Caloric intake
- Individual cultural or spiritual restrictions, personal preferences
- Availability and use of resources
- Personal understanding or perception of problem

Planning
- Plan of care and who is involved in planning
- Teaching plan

Implementation/Evaluation
- Client's responses to interventions, teaching, and actions performed
- Results of periodic weigh-in
- Attainment of or progress toward desired outcome(s)
- Modifications to plan of care

Discharge Planning
- Long-term needs, and who is responsible for actions to be taken
- Specific referrals made

Sample Nursing Outcomes & Interventions Classifications NOC/NIC

NOC—Nutritional Status
NIC—Nutrition Management

Information that appears in brackets has been added by the authors to clarify and enhance the use of nursing diagnoses.

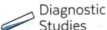 Diagnostic Studies
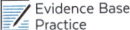 Evidence Based Practice
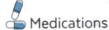 Medications
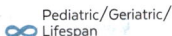 Pediatric/Geriatric/Lifespan

risk for OCCUPATIONAL ILLNESS — NANDA-I

[Diagnostic Division: Safety]

Definition: Susceptible to work-related condition or disorder resulting from a non-instantaneous event or exposure.

Recognizing Cues

Risk Factors

Individual Factors:

Inaccurate follow-through of employee health, or safety protocol; inadequate vaccination

Inadequate knowledge of modifiable factors; inadequate action to address modifiable factors

Improper use of personal protective equipment (PPE); inadequate understanding of importance of PPE

Inattentive to ergonomic principles; ineffective weight management

Excessive stress; inadequate communication skills; inadequate social support

Difficulty with decision making

Environmental Factors:

Inadequate employee health, or safety protocol

Exposure to chemical, or biological agents; pathogen exposure

Inadequate biological, or dosimetry monitoring; exposure to intermittent impacts

Inadequate placement of collective protective equipment; inadequate access to PPE

Ineffective workload management; excessive workload

Inadequate adoption of ergonomic principles; exposure to repetitive motion activities

Exposure to psychosocial agents

Conflicted labor relationships

Clinical Connections

Muscle strain/injury, carpal/cubital tunnel syndrome, herniated disk, poisoning (e.g., lead, mercury, asbestos, carbon monoxide), radiation injury, depression, pregnancy

Generate Solutions

Plan Desired Outcomes

Client Will (Include Specific Time Frame)

- Be free of signs/symptoms of occupational-related illness.

Information that appears in brackets has been added by the authors to clarify and enhance the use of nursing diagnoses.

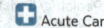 Acute Care 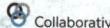 Collaborative 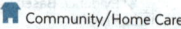 Community/Home Care Cultural

- Develop/engage in plan to address individual risk factors and health hazards.
- Conform to safety guidelines in the workplace.

Interventions/Take Action

Nursing Priority No. 1.

To evaluate degree/source of client exposure:

- Ascertain type of risk to which client may be exposed **to identify potential injuring agents and develop a mitigation strategy:**
  Occupational infections
  Injury (e.g., carpal tunnel, asbestos exposure, hepatic injury, etc.)
  Occupational hazardous chemicals and exposure route
  Occupational radiation
  Psychological trauma/violence and harassment
  Occupational environmental hazards (e.g., inadequate sanitation, unsafe water supply)
- Administer a client occupational history screening (e.g., the Healthy Work Survey [HWS]) **to anticipate, identify, quantify, and control occupational hazards.**
- Investigate factors that increase client's risk for occupational illness or injury (e.g., substance use/abuse, inadequate client training, comorbid conditions, etc.).
- Assess client coping abilities and personality style (e.g., temperament, impulsive behavior, level of self-esteem) **that may result in carelessness and increased risk-taking without consideration of consequences.** (Refer to ND risk for Suicide.)
- Ascertain client's knowledge of work-related hazards.
- Refer to ND Contamination Exposure and risk for Poisoning for additional actions and interventions.

Nursing Priority No. 2.

To assist in correcting factors that can lead to occupational exposures:

- Educate client regarding adequate ventilation and utilization of respiratory adjuncts (i.e., masks, respirators, etc.) **to prevent inhalation exposure to occupational risks.**
- Encourage client to follow organizational policies/safety standards for water supply, sanitation, and waste facilities.
- Encourage client to follow organizational policies/safety standards for utilization and discarding outdated or expired chemicals and equipment.

Information that appears in brackets has been added by the authors to clarify and enhance the use of nursing diagnoses.

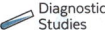 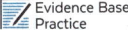 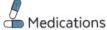

- Provide education regarding the use of occupational equipment and safe body mechanics **to prevent musculoskeletal injury.**
- Provide opportunities for client to discuss occupational stressors (e.g., time pressure, workload, moral distress, workplace incivility/violence, etc.) **to promote client coping and mental health.** Refer for counseling as indicated. Refer to ND difficulty Coping for additional assessments and interventions.
- Refer to NDs Contamination Exposure and risk for Poisoning for additional assessments and interventions.

Nursing Priority No. 3.

To promote client knowledge and safety (Teaching/Discharge Considerations) and enhance well-being (long-term goals):

- Encourage client to place safety stickers on dangerous products (drugs and chemicals) **to warn of harmful contents.**
- Provide client with a list of emergency numbers (i.e., local or national poison control numbers) **to be placed in prominent location if poisoning occurs.**
- Instruct client in the event of poisoning to have product container on hand when contacting the emergency provider.
- Encourage client to maintain immunizations, as indicated, **to promote client resistance to infectious exposures.**
- Refer clients with substance abuse issues to detoxification programs, inpatient/outpatient rehabilitation, counseling, support groups, and psychotherapy as appropriate.
- Encourage client participation in safety awareness and first aid programs (e.g., cardiopulmonary resuscitation, workplace safety, hazardous materials, and old medications disposal) **to assist client in timely and effective responses to workplace hazards.**
- Refer client to an occupational medicine specialist, as needed, **for additional resources or assistance.**
- Refer to Contamination Exposure and risk for Poisoning for additional interventions.

Documentation Focus

Assessment/Reassessment
- Identified client risk factors
- Drug allergies or sensitivities
- Identified occupational hazards

Planning
- Plan of care and who is involved in the planning
- Teaching plan including how to be safe with occupational and environmental hazards

---

Information that appears in brackets has been added by the authors to clarify and enhance the use of nursing diagnoses.

Implementation/Evaluation
- Response to interventions, teaching, and actions performed
- Attainment or progress toward desired outcome(s)
- Modification to plan of care

Discharge Planning
- Long-term needs and who is responsible for actions to be taken
- Specific referrals made

Sample Nursing Outcomes & Interventions Classifications NOC/NIC

NOC—Knowledge: Health Behavior
NIC—Environmental Management: Worker Safety

---

ineffective OVERWEIGHT SELF-MANAGEMENT NANDA-I

[Diagnostic Division: Food/Fluid]

Definition: Unsatisfactory handling of treatment regimen, consequences, and lifestyle changes associated with accumulation of excessive fat for age and gender.

Recognizing Cues

Related/Risk Factors
Competing demands; conflicting information sources; self-defeating thoughts; inadequate intrinsic motivation

Excessive stress; depressive symptoms; inadequate autonomy; inadequate self-confidence, or self-efficacy

Inappropriate dietary intake; inadequate eating plan, or meal planning; unhealthy family meals

Decreased awareness of available nutrition services

Unaddressed absence of affordable, or local availability of healthy food options

Inappropriate weight-loss targets; inconsistent recording in a food diary

Inadequate knowledge of appropriate nutritional requirements, or weight management strategies

Inadequate recommendations regarding management obstacles to weight loss; inadequate social support network

Inadequate access to accurate weight management information, or programs; inadequate structured lifestyle support

---

Information that appears in brackets has been added by the authors to clarify and enhance the use of nursing diagnoses.

 Diagnostic Studies 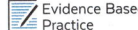 Evidence Based Practice Medications 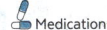 Pediatric/Geriatric/Lifespan

Inadequate activity program; inadequate commitment to recommended physical activity level; inadequate access to safe exercise facilities, or adaptive equipment to enable physical activity

Ineffective fatigue self-management; unaddressed sleep deprivation

Inadequate caregiver knowledge of appropriate nutritional requirements, or of weight management strategies

Defining Characteristics

Subjective
Overweight Complications:
Musculoskeletal pain
Difficulty maintaining usual physical activity
Shortness of breath; obstructive sleep apnea
Overweight Behaviors:
Stress eating; disinhibited eating; binge eating
Prioritizing other's meal preferences
Average daily physical activity is less than recommended for age and gender

Objective
Overweight Signs:
Body mass index (BMI) greater than 25 kg/m^2 in individuals older than 18 years of age
BMI greater than 85th percentile or greater than 25 kg/m^2 or 30 kg/m^2 for age and gender in individuals 2 to 18 years of age
Weight-for-length greater than 95th percentile in individuals 2 years of age
Overweight Complications:
Increased blood pressure
Excessive sweating; frequent skin diseases
Increased fasting plasma glucose; insulin resistance
Increased serum low-density, or decreased serum high-density lipoprotein levels; increased serum triglyceride levels
Overweight Behaviors:
Inadequate participation in weight management program; difficulty with realistic goal-setting
Ineffective medication self-management

Clinical Connections
Bulimia nervosa, diseases requiring long-term steroid use (e.g., chronic obstructive pulmonary disease [COPD]), conditions associated with immobility (e.g., stroke/paralysis, multiple sclerosis [MS], amputation), depression, developmental delay, abuse

---

Information that appears in brackets has been added by the authors to clarify and enhance the use of nursing diagnoses.

 Acute Care 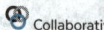 Collaborative 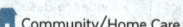 Community/Home Care  Cultural

Generate Solutions

Plan Desired Outcomes

Client Will (Include Specific Time Frame)

- Verbalize a realistic self-concept or body image (congruent mental and physical picture of self).
- Participate in development of, and commit to, a personal weight loss program.
- Demonstrate appropriate changes in lifestyle and behaviors, including eating patterns, food quantity/quality, and exercise program.
- Attain desirable body weight with optimal maintenance of health.

Interventions/Take Action

Nursing Priority No. 1.

To identify contributing factors:

- Obtain client nutrition history using a validated screening tool (e.g., Mini Nutritional Assessment [MNA], short form [MNA-SF]). **The MNA provides valuable adult client information regarding potential malnutrition and causative factors. Poor nutrition may be present despite the amount of calories consumed daily.**
- Obtain weight history, noting if client has weight gain out of character for self or family, is or was an obese child, or used to be much more physically active than is now **to identify trends. Note: According to Centers for Disease Control and Prevention (CDC) 2018 statistics: (1) About 40% of young adults between ages 20 and 39 years are obese; (2) 42.8% of those aged 60 and older are obese; (3) 18.4% of children between ages 6 and 11 are obese, and 20.6% of those between 12 and 19 are obese.**
- Assess risk and presence of factors or conditions associated with obesity (e.g., familial pattern of obesity; decreased basal metabolic rate or hypothyroidism; type 2 diabetes; reproductive dysfunction; menopause; chronic disorders, such as heart disease, kidney disease, chronic pain; food or other substance addictions; stressful or sedentary lifestyle; depression; use of certain medications such as steroids, birth control pills; physical disabilities or limitations; lack of socioeconomic resources for obtaining or preparing healthy foods) **to determine treatments and interventions that may be indicated in addition to weight management. Note: Studies have shown that the strongest correlate of**

Information that appears in brackets has been added by the authors to clarify and enhance the use of nursing diagnoses.

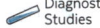 Diagnostic Studies   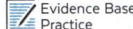 Evidence Based Practice   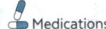 Medications   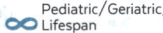 Pediatric/Geriatric/Lifespan

weight gain over 20 years was susceptibility to overeating in response to everyday cues within the environment (habitual disinhibition); susceptibility to overeating in response to emotional states such as depression (emotional disinhibition).

- Assess client's knowledge of own body weight, nutritional needs, and determine cultural expectations regarding size. **Although nutritional needs are not always understood, being overweight or having large body size may not be viewed negatively by a client, because it aligns with family eating patterns and peer and cultural influences.**
- Identify familial and cultural influences regarding food. **People of many cultures place a high importance on food and food-related events, while some cultures routinely observe fasting days (e.g., Muslim, Greek, Irish, Jewish) that may be done for health or spiritual purposes.**
- Ascertain how the client perceives food and the act of eating. **The client may be eating to satisfy an emotional need rather than physiological hunger, not only because food plays a significant role in socialization but also because food can offer comfort, a sense of security, and acceptance.**
- Evaluate the client's routine medications. **Some medications can contribute to weight gain (e.g., cortisol and other glucocorticoids; sulfonylureas, tricyclic antidepressants, monoamine oxidase inhibitors; oral contraceptives; insulin [in excessive doses]; risperidone).**
- Assess dietary practices through collection of a client food diary recalling 3 to 7 days. **Recall of foods and fluids ingested; times, patterns, and places of eating; whether alone or with other(s); and feelings before, during, and after eating can increase the client's understanding of eating behaviors and serve as the basis for dietary modifications.**
- Ascertain previous dieting history. **The client may report normal or excessive food intake, but calories and intake of certain food groups (e.g., sweets and fats) are often underestimated. The client may report experimentation with numerous types of diets, repeated dieting efforts ("yo-yo" dieting) with varying results, or may never have attempted a weight-management program.**
- Collaborate in assessment of client with disordered eating habits or eating perceptions:
  Obtain comparative body drawing having client draw self on wall with chalk, then standing against it and having actual

---

Information that appears in brackets has been added by the authors to clarify and enhance the use of nursing diagnoses.

Acute Care   Collaborative   Community/Home Care   Cultural

body outline drawn to note the difference between the two. **Determines whether the client's view of self-body image is congruent with reality.**

Ascertain occurrence of negative feedback from significant other(s) (SO[s]). **May reveal control issues and may impact motivation for change.**

- Review client's daily activity and assess for a regular exercise program **for a comparative baseline and to identify areas for modification. Note: According to 2020 state maps of adult physical inactivity, all states and territories had more than 15% of adults who were physically inactive. Inactivity levels vary among adults by race/ethnicity and location.**
- Review laboratory test results (e.g., complete blood count with differential, full lipid panel, fasting glucose, A_{1C}, and insulin levels; thyroid and leptins; proteins, vitamin levels) **that may reveal medical conditions associated with obesity and identify problems that may be treated with alterations in diet or medications.**

Nursing Priority No. 2.

To determine weight loss goals:

- Obtain client anthropometric measurements **to determine the presence and severity of weight concerns:**

  Calculate BMI **to estimate the percentage of client body fat. The CDC has standardized BMI calculations, removing age and sex differences for adults, with 25 to 29.9 kg/m² defining "overweight." The CDC has recommended that children (over age 2) and adolescents be considered overweight if the BMI exceeds the 85th percentile (and is less than the 95th percentile) on growth curves or exceeds 25 kg/m² at any age.**

  Determine waist circumference, if indicated. **Some studies support that waist circumference (WC) is more closely linked to cardiovascular risk factors than BMI alone, because a high WC can occur in persons with normal or near-normal BMIs.**

- Evaluate body fat, body water, and muscle mass via scale skin caliper measurements and scale weight (**direct** measurement), bioelectric impedance analysis, dual-energy x-ray absorptiometry, and hydrostatic weighing (**indirect** measurement) per facility protocol. **Note: These methods to measure body weight are not recommended over estimates of BMI as they are not readily available and require highly trained personnel.**

Information that appears in brackets has been added by the authors to clarify and enhance the use of nursing diagnoses.

 Diagnostic Studies 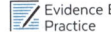 Evidence Based Practice 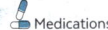 Medications 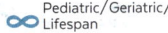 Pediatric/Geriatric/Lifespan

- Determine client's motivation for weight loss (e.g., for own satisfaction or self-esteem, to improve health status, or to gain approval from another person). **The client is more likely to succeed and maintain the desired weight when change is for self (e.g., acceptance of self "as is," general well-being) rather than to please others.**
- Discuss myths client/SO may have about weight and weight loss **to address misconceptions and possibly enhance motivation for needed behavior changes.**

Nursing Priority No. 3.
To establish a weight-reduction program:

- Obtain commitment for weight loss. **Verbal agreement to goals or a written contract formalizes the plan and may enhance efforts and maximize outcomes.**
- Involve SO(s) in the treatment plan as much as possible **to provide ongoing support and increase the likelihood of success.**
- Set realistic goals (short and long term) for weight loss. **Reasonable weight loss (1 to 2 lb/wk) has been shown to have more lasting effects than rapid weight loss. A loss of 5% to 10% of total body weight can reduce many of the health risks associated with obesity in adults.**
- Collaborate with physician and dietitian **to develop and implement comprehensive weight-loss program that includes food, activity, behavior alteration, and support.**
- Calculate calorie requirements based on physical factors and activity. **Although many weight-reduction programs focus on portion size and food components (e.g., low-fat, high-protein, low-glycemic foods), reducing calorie intake is essential for weight loss.**
- Provide information regarding nutritional plan and incorporating client's desires and specific needs. **Client may be deficient in needed nutrients (e.g., proteins, vitamins, or minerals) or may eat too much of one food group (e.g., fats or carbohydrates) and not enough of another food group (e.g., vegetables).**
- Discuss modifications to achieve **(or maintain)** a healthy body weight:
  Eat from each food group (fruits, vegetables, whole grains, lean meats, low-fat dairy, and oils).
  Start with small changes, such as adding one more vegetable/day, and introducing healthier versions of favorite foods.

Information that appears in brackets has been added by the authors to clarify and enhance the use of nursing diagnoses.

- Choose nutrient-dense foods that provide substantial amounts of fiber, vitamins, electrolytes, and minerals.
- Avoid saturated fats, trans fats, cholesterol, excess salt (sodium), and added sugars.
- Focus on portion sizes. **Calorie-dense foods (high in fat and/or sugar) should be eaten in smaller quantities, whereas high-fiber foods can be eaten in larger quantities.**
- Discuss smart snacks (e.g., low-fat yogurt with fruit, nuts, apple slices with peanut butter, low-fat string cheese).
- Emphasize the need for adequate fluid intake and taking fluids between meals rather than with meals to provide fluid while leaving more room for food intake at meals **to assist in the digestive process and to quench thirst, which is often mistakenly identified as hunger.**
- Educate client on availability of digital applications (e.g., MyFitnessPal, Fitbit, MyFitnessBuddy, etc.) **to assist with food and activity tracking, and progression toward established goals.**
- Encourage involvement in planned activity program of client's choice and within physical abilities. Refer to formal exercise program, if desired. **Moderately increased physical activity can support both loss of pounds and maintenance of lower weight. Children should participate in vigorous physical activity throughout adolescence and limit time spent watching television and playing computer games, to facilitate weight control.**
- Recommend weighing only once/week, at the same time, wearing the same clothes, and graph on a chart. Measure and monitor body fat when possible **to track progress while focusing on health conscious and responsible rather than what the scale may reveal.**
- Provide positive reinforcement and encouragement for efforts as well as actual weight loss. **Enhances commitment to the program and enhances the client's sense of self-worth.**
- Administer medication(s), as indicated. *The U.S. Food and Drug Administration has approved medications (e.g., glucagon-like peptide-1 [GLP-1] agonist) for the treatment of weight management concerns.*
- Refer to bariatric physician/surgeon when indicated. **Evaluation for special measures may be needed (e.g., supervised fasting or bariatric surgery) for obese or severely obese persons.**

Information that appears in brackets has been added by the authors to clarify and enhance the use of nursing diagnoses.

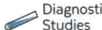 Diagnostic Studies
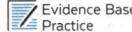 Evidence Based Practice
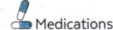 Medications
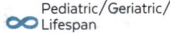 Pediatric/Geriatric/Lifespan

Nursing Priority No. 4.

To promote a healthy weight (Teaching/Discharge Considerations) and enhance well-being (long-term goals) **(Overweight or risk for Overweight):**

- Assist in and encourage periodic evaluation of nutritional status and modification of dietary plan. **May be desired or needed for addressing special needs (e.g., diabetes mellitus, age considerations, very low calorie or fasting) and monitoring health status.**
- Emphasize the importance of avoiding fad diets **that may be harmful to health and often do not produce long-term positive results.**
- Identify and encourage finding ways to reduce tension when eating. **Promotes relaxation to permit focusing on the act of eating and awareness of satiety.**
- Identify unhelpful eating behaviors (e.g., eating over the sink, "gobbling, nibbling, or grazing") and address kinds of activities associated with eating (e.g., watching television or reading, being unmindful of eating or food) **that result in taking in too many calories as well as eliminating the joy of food because of failure to notice flavors or sensation of fullness or satiety.**
- Review and discuss strategies to deal appropriately with stressful events **to avoid overeating as a means of coping.**
- Discuss importance of an occasional treat by planning for inclusion in diet **to avoid feelings of deprivation arising from self-denial.**
- Advise planning for special occasions (birthday or holidays) by reducing intake before event and/or eating "smart" **to redistribute or reduce calories and allow for participation in food events.**
- Discuss normalcy of ups and downs of weight loss: plateau, set point (at which weight is not being lost), hormonal influences, and so forth. **Prevents discouragement when progress stalls.**
- Encourage buying personal items and clothing **as a reward for weight loss or other accomplishments.**
- Suggest disposing of "fat clothes" **to encourage positive attitude of permanent change and remove "safety valve" of having wardrobe available "just in case" weight is regained.**
- Review prescribed drug regimen (e.g., appetite suppressants, hormone therapy, vitamin and mineral supplements) **for benefits or adverse side effects and drug interactions.**
- Recommend reading labels of nonprescription diet aids if used. **Herbals containing diuretics or ma huang (product**

Information that appears in brackets has been added by the authors to clarify and enhance the use of nursing diagnoses.

similar to ephedrine) **may cause adverse side effects in vulnerable persons.**

- Encourage parents and school dietitians to model and offer good nutritional choices (e.g., offer vegetables, fruits, and lower-fat foods in daily meals and snacks) **to assist child in accepting healthy eating styles. Note: Studies have shown a high correlation between parents and children regarding patterns of food intake and food choices.**
- Refer to community support groups or psychotherapy, as indicated, **to provide role models, address issues of body image or self-worth.**
- Provide contact number for dietitian and/or audiovisual materials, reliable internet sites for resources **to address ongoing nutritional needs and dietary changes.**
- Refer to NDs disturbed Body Image; difficulty Coping, Body Weight Problem for additional interventions, as appropriate.

Documentation Focus

Assessment/Reassessment
- Individual findings, including current weight, dietary pattern; perceptions of self, food, and eating; motivation for loss; support or feedback from SO(s)
- Results of laboratory and diagnostic testing
- Results of interval weigh-ins

Planning
- Plan of care, specific interventions, and who is involved in planning
- Teaching plan

Implementation/Evaluation
- Responses to interventions, weekly weight, and actions performed
- Attainment of or progress toward desired outcome(s)
- Modifications to plan of care

Discharge Planning
- Long-term needs and who is responsible for actions to be taken
- Plan for monitoring weight
- Specific referrals made

Sample Nursing Outcomes & Interventions Classifications NOC/NIC

NOC—Weight Loss [or] Maintenance Behavior
NIC—Weight Reduction Assistance

Information that appears in brackets has been added by the authors to clarify and enhance the use of nursing diagnoses.

 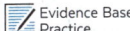 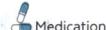 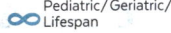

acute PAIN
NANDA-I

[Diagnostic Division: Comfort]

Definition: Unpleasant sensory and emotional experience associated with, or resembling that associated with, actual or potential tissue damage, with a duration of less than 3 months.

Recognizing Cues

Related/Risk Factors
Biological injury agent (e.g., infection, ischemia, neoplasm)
Inappropriate use of chemical agent
Physical injury agent (e.g., trauma, operative procedure, burn, heavy lifting, overtraining)

Defining Characteristics

Subjective
Inadequate appetite; hopelessness
Verbal report of pain
Pain characteristics/intensity assessed using standardized, validated assessment instrument
Proxy report of pain activity/behavior changes

Objective
Altered physiological parameter (e.g., blood pressure, heart rate, respiratory rate, oxygen saturation); pupil dilation; diaphoresis
Distraction behavior; expressive behavior
Evidence of pain using standardized pain behavior checklist for those unable to communicate verbally (e.g., Neonatal Infant Pain Scale, Pain Assessment Checklist for Seniors With Limited Ability to Communicate)
Positioning to ease pain; protective behavior
Facial expression of pain
Hypervigilance to pain

Clinical Connections
Traumatic injuries, surgical procedures, infections, cancer, burns, skin lesions, gangrene, thrombophlebitis, pulmonary embolus, angina, renal stones, neuralgia

---

Information that appears in brackets has been added by the authors to clarify and enhance the use of nursing diagnoses.

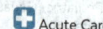 Acute Care   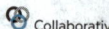 Collaborative   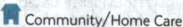 Community/Home Care   Cultural

Generate Solutions

Plan Desired Outcomes

Client Will (Include Specific Time Frame)
- Report pain is relieved or controlled.
- Follow prescribed pharmacological regimen.
- Verbalize nonpharmacological methods that provide relief.
- Demonstrate use of relaxation skills and diversional activities, as indicated, for individual situation.
- Verbalize sense of control of response to acute situation and positive outlook for the future.

Interventions/Take Action

Nursing Priority No. 1.
To assess etiology/precipitating contributory factors:
- Note possible pathophysiological and psychological causes of pain (e.g., inflammation; tissue trauma, burns, fractures; surgery; infections; heart attack or angina; abdominal conditions [e.g., appendicitis, cholecystitis]; grief; fear, anxiety; depression). **Acute pain is that which follows an injury, trauma, or procedure such as surgery, or occurs suddenly with the onset of a painful condition (e.g., herniated disk, migraine headache, pancreatitis).**
- Assess for potential types of pain that may be affecting client (i.e., nociceptive pain or neuropathic pain). **Can aid in understanding reason for severity of pain associated with client's condition and point toward needed interventions for pain management.** Note: *Nociceptive* **pain results from actual tissue damage or potentially tissue-damaging stimuli. Subsets of nociceptive pain include (1) somatic (localized, and usually stemming from muscle, joint, bone, or connective tissue) and (2) visceral (caused by problem in internal organs, such as abdomen, pelvis) with localized pain occurring from obstruction, distension, or ischemia.** *Neuropathic* **pain is complex and caused by a variety of problems with nerves or the processing of nerve impulses. Neuropathic pain can become chronic (e.g., diabetic neuropathy) or have an acute onset related to direct nerve injury (e.g., severe trauma, surgery, certain types of cancer).**
- Note client's age and developmental level and current condition (e.g., infant/child, critically ill, ventilated, sedated, or cognitively impaired client) **affecting ability to report pain**

Information that appears in brackets has been added by the authors to clarify and enhance the use of nursing diagnoses.

 Diagnostic Studies 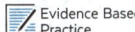 Evidence Based Practice 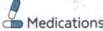 Medications 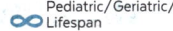 Pediatric/Geriatric/Lifespan

parameters or response to pain and pain management interventions. Note: Appropriate pain management in childhood is imperative because children's early pain experiences can shape their response to pain as adults.
- Determine history or presence of chronic conditions (e.g., multiple sclerosis, stroke, diabetes, sickle cell disease, depression) **that may also be associated with acute and chronic pain simultaneously, be associated with an exacerbation of pain symptoms, or interfere with accurate assessment of acute pain.**
- Note anatomical location of surgical incisions, **as this can influence the amount of postoperative pain experienced; for example, vertical or diagonal incisions are more painful than transverse or S-shaped.**
- Assess client's perceptions of pain, along with behaviors and cultural expectations regarding pain. **Client's perception of and expression of pain are influenced by age, developmental stage, underlying problem causing pain, cognitive, and behavioral and sociocultural factors.**
- Note client's attitude toward pain and use of pain medications, including any history of substance use/abuse. **Client may have beliefs restricting use of medications, may have a high tolerance for drugs because of recent or current use, or may not be able to take pain medications at all if participating in a substance abuse recovery program.**
- Note client's perception of their pain and sense of control over situation. **Individuals with feelings of powerlessness (external locus of control) may take little or no responsibility for pain management.**
- Determine medications (e.g., muscle relaxants, antibiotics, antidepressants, anticoagulants, opioids), alcohol or other drugs currently being used, and any medication allergies **that may affect choice of analgesics.**
- Collaborate with medical providers in pain assessment, including neurological and psychological factors (pain inventory, psychological interview) as appropriate when pain persists.
- Assist with and review results of laboratory tests and diagnostic studies depending on results of history and physical examination.

Nursing Priority No. 2.
To evaluate client's response to pain:
- Obtain client's/significant other's (SO's) assessment of pain to include location, characteristics, onset, duration,

---

Information that appears in brackets has been added by the authors to clarify and enhance the use of nursing diagnoses.

frequency, quality, and intensity. Identify precipitating or aggravating and relieving factors **in order to fully understand client's pain symptoms. Note: Experts agree that attempts should always be made to obtain self-reports of pain. When that is not possible, credible information can be received from another person who knows the client well (e.g., parent, spouse, caregiver). Note: Some special populations may have difficulty communicating pain, such as neonates, toddlers and young children, persons with intellectual disabilities, critically ill/unconscious patients, older adults with advanced dementia, and clients at the end of life.**

- Perform pain assessment each time pain occurs. Document and investigate changes from previous reports and evaluate results of pain interventions **to demonstrate improvement in status or to identify worsening of underlying condition/developing complications.**

- Select and utilize a pain scale appropriate for client (e.g., 0 to 10 scale, facial expression or Wong-Baker FACES pain rating scale [pediatric, nonverbal], Adolescent Pediatric Pain Tool, Checklist of Nonverbal Pain Indicators). **Utilization of a pain scale and tracking client pain measurement facilitates nurse-client communication and optimizes goal-directed pain control interventions.**

- Accept client's description of pain. Be aware of the terminology client uses for pain experience (e.g., young child may say "owie" or "hurt"; elderly may say "it aches so bad"). **Pain is a subjective experience and cannot be felt by others. Note: Some elderly clients experience a reduction in perception of pain or have difficulty localizing or describing pain, and pain may be manifested as a change in behavior (e.g., restlessness, loss of appetite, increased confusion or wandering, acting out, change in functional abilities).**

- Note cultural and developmental influences affecting pain response. **Verbal and/or behavioral cues may have no direct relationship to the degree of pain perceived (e.g., client may deny pain even when feeling uncomfortable, or reactions can be stoic or exaggerated, reflecting cultural or familial norms).**

- Observe nonverbal cues and pain behaviors (e.g., diaphoresis; how client walks or sits, body position; facial expression; distraction behaviors, narrowed focus; crying, poor feeding, lethargy in infants) and other objective Defining Characteristics, as noted, especially in persons who cannot

---

Information that appears in brackets has been added by the authors to clarify and enhance the use of nursing diagnoses.

communicate verbally. **Observations may not be congruent with verbal reports or may be only indicator present when client is unable to verbalize.**
- Assess for referred pain, as appropriate, **to help determine possibility of underlying condition or organ dysfunction requiring treatment.**
- Monitor skin color and temperature and vital signs (e.g., heart rate, blood pressure, respirations), **which are usually altered in acute pain.**
- Ascertain client's knowledge of and expectations about pain management. **Provides baseline for interventions and teaching, provides opportunity to allay common fears and misconceptions, or to address expected side effects of analgesics.**
- Review client's previous experiences with pain and methods found either helpful or unhelpful for pain control in the past.
- Be aware of client's "Right to Treatment" with regard to pain management, **which includes prevention of and adequate relief from pain. Failure to meet the standard of assessing for pain can be legally interpreted as nursing negligence.**

Nursing Priority No. 3.

To assist client to explore methods for alleviation/control of pain:

- Use an appropriate pain scale to determine client's acceptable level of pain and pain control goals. **Client may not be 100% pain free but may feel that a "3" is a manageable level of discomfort, while another may require medication for pain at the same level because the experience is subjective.**
- Determine factors in client's lifestyle (e.g., alcohol or other drug use or abuse) **that can affect responses to analgesics and/or choice of interventions for pain management.**
- Note when pain occurs (e.g., only with ambulation, every night, painful procedure) **to medicate prophylactically, as appropriate.**
- Collaborate in treatment of underlying condition or disease processes causing pain and proactive management of pain (e.g., epidural analgesia, nerve blockade for postoperative pain).
- Work with client to prevent rather than "chase" pain. Use flow sheet to document pain, therapeutic interventions, response, and length of time before pain recurs. Instruct client to report pain prior to reaching personal level of

---

Information that appears in brackets has been added by the authors to clarify and enhance the use of nursing diagnoses.

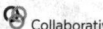 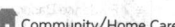

NURSES POCKET MINDER
Convert Client Problem Into Nursing Diagnosis
Quickly · Easily · Accurately

Following is an index of the more commonly used nursing diagnoses from NANDA-I (2024–2026) and ICNP (2019) categorized according to Diagnostic Divisions.

Author Note: We believe that most of the problems listed here can also be stated as a risk for, or an opportunity for, enhancement.

ACTIVITY/REST—*Ability to engage in necessary/desired activities of life (work and leisure) and to obtain adequate sleep/rest*
Activity Intolerance, 5–11
Diversional Activity Engagement, decreased, 237–242
Fatigue, 329–335
Mobility, impaired bed, 598–603
Mobility, impaired physical, 603–609
Mobility, impaired wheelchair, 609–613
Motor Development, delayed infant, 622–626
Sedentary Behaviors, excessive, 813–818
Sitting Ability, impaired, 877–882
Sleep Pattern, ineffective, 893–897
Standing Ability, impaired, 920–923
Transferring Ability, impaired, 1006–1010
Walking Ability, impaired, 1051–1055

CIRCULATION—*Ability to transport oxygen and nutrients necessary to meet cellular needs*
Autonomic Dysreflexia, risk for, 41–45
Bleeding, risk for excessive, 45–50
Blood Pressure, risk for imbalanced, 58–63
Cardiac Output, impaired, 111–121
Cardiovascular Function, risk for impaired, 122–126
Lymphedema Self-Management, ineffective, 581–586
Neurovascular Function, risk for impaired peripheral, 653–658
Shock, risk for, 872–877
Thrombosis, risk for, 977–980
Tissue Perfusion, ineffective peripheral, 992–1000
Tissue Perfusion, risk for ineffective cerebral, 1000–1006

COMFORT—*Ability to control internal/external environment to maintain comfort*
Chronic Pain Syndrome, 692–702
Discomfort, [specify physical, psychological], 229–237
Dry Eye, risk for, 242–245
Dry Mouth Self-Management, ineffective, 246–250
End-of-Life Comfort Syndrome, impaired, 297–300
Pain, acute, 684–692
Pain, chronic, 692–702
Pain, labor, 702–708
Pain Self-Management, ineffective, 709–717

ELIMINATION—*Ability to excrete waste products (bowel, bladder)*
Constipation, chronic functional, 171–176
Continence, impaired fecal, 185–192
Elimination, impaired intestinal, 267–275
Elimination, impaired urinary, 276–283
Gastrointestinal Motility, impaired, 383–391
Incontinence, disability-associated urinary, 487–494
Incontinence, mixed urinary, 494–503
Incontinence, stress urinary, 503–510
Incontinence, urge urinary, 510–517
Injury, risk for urinary tract, 555–559
Retention, urinary, risk for, 802–808

FOOD/FLUID—*Ability to maintain intake of and utilize nutrients and liquids to meet physiological needs*
Blood Glucose Within Normal Limits, 51–58
Body Weight Problem, 83–89
Breastfeeding, difficulty performing, 90–98
Breastfeeding, interrupted, 98–105
Eating Dynamics, ineffective adolescent, 251–255
Eating Dynamics, ineffective child, 256–260
Feeding Behavior, impaired infant, 342–347
Fluid Volume, excessive, 358–365
Fluid Volume, inadequate, 365–374
Fluid Volume Balance, risk for impaired, 351–358
Human Milk Production, inadequate, 451–457
Liver Function, risk for impaired, 570–575
Mucous Membrane, impaired oral, 627–634
Nausea, 634–640
Nipple-Areolar Complex Integrity, impaired, 658–663
Nutritional Intake, inadequate, 663–671
Overweight Self-Management, ineffective, 675–683
Suck-Swallow Response, ineffective infant, 924–928
Swallowing, impaired, 956–963
Underweight Self-Management, ineffective, 1010–1019
Water-Electrolyte Balance, risk for impaired, 1056–1064
Weight Self-Management, readiness for enhanced, 1064–1068

HEALTH MANAGEMENT—*Ability to incorporate and act on information to achieve healthy lifestyle/optimal wellness*
Development, impaired child, 220–225
Elder Frailty Syndrome, 261–267
Emancipated Decision-Making, impaired, 289–293
Exercise Engagement, readiness for enhanced, 305–308
Growth, delayed child, 403–408
Health Knowledge, inadequate, 409–415
Health Literacy, inadequate, 415–420
Health Maintenance Behaviors, ineffective, 420–425
Health Management, ineffective community, 425–430
Health Management, ineffective family, 430–434
Health Self-Management, ineffective, 434–440
Healthy Aging, readiness for enhanced, 440–443
Surgical Recovery, impaired, 945–951

NEUROSENSORY—*Ability to perceive, integrate, and respond to internal and external cues*
Confusion, acute, 160–166
Confusion, chronic, 166–170
Memory, impaired, 594–598
Neurodevelopmental Organization, impaired infant, 646–653

Sensory Deficit [specify: visual, auditory, kinesthetic, gustatory, tactile, olfactory], 858–864
Thought Process, disrupted, 968–977

RESPIRATION—*Ability to provide and use oxygen to meet physiological needs*

Airway Clearance, impaired, 18–24
Aspiration, risk for, 35–40
Breathing Pattern, ineffective, 105–111
Gas Exchange, impaired, 374–382
Ventilation, impaired spontaneous, 1019–1026
Ventilatory Weaning Response, impaired adult, 1027–1034
Ventilatory Weaning Response, impaired child, 1034–1041

ROLES/RELATIONSHIPS—*Ability to accomplish role development and establish and maintain relationships*

Caregiver Child Attachment, impaired, 126–132
Caregiving Burden, excessive, 133–140
Communication, impaired verbal, 151–160
Coping, impaired community, 200–203
Coping, impaired family, 203–208
Disrupted Family Identity Syndrome, 316–322
Family Process, impaired, 322–328
Interaction Patterns, disrupted family, 559–566
Loneliness, excessive, 578–580
Parenting, impaired, 718–725
Relationship, ineffective intimate partner, 773–777
Relationship problem, 778–782
Role Performance, impaired, 808–812
Social Connectedness, inadequate, 897–907
Social Support Network, inadequate, 908–913

SAFETY—*Ability to provide safe, growth-promoting environment*

Acute Substance Withdrawal Syndrome, 11–18
Allergy Reaction, risk for, 24–28
Body Temperature, decreased, 70–76
Body Temperature, decreased neonatal, 76–80
Body Temperature, risk for decreased perioperative, 80–83
Contamination Exposure, 176–185
Elopement, risk for, 283–288
Fall, risk for [adult, child], 309–316
Hyperbilirubinemia, neonatal, 457–463
Hyperthermia, 463–471
Immunologic Impairment, 476–482
Infection, risk for, 517–524
Injury, risk for burn, 525–531
Injury, risk for cold, 531–534
Injury, risk for corneal, 535–538
Injury, risk for occupational physical, 538–544
Injury, risk for perioperative positioning, 544–548
Injury, risk for physical, 549–555
Latex Allergy, risk for, 567–570
Neonatal Abstinence Syndrome, 640–645
Occupational Injury, risk for, 672–675
Poisoning, risk for, 732–737
Pressure Injury, adult, 751–758
Pressure Injury, child, 758–766
Pressure Injury, neonatal, 767–772
Skin Integrity, impaired, 882–892
Sudden Infant Death, risk for, 928–933
Suffocation, risk for accidental, 933–938
Surgical Wound Infection, risk for, 952–956
Thermoregulation, ineffective, 964–968
Tissue Integrity, impaired, 981–992

SELF-CARE—*Ability to perform activities of daily living*

Home Maintenance Behaviors, ineffective, 443–447
Self-Care Deficit: bathing, dressing, grooming, feeding, toileting, 818–830

SELF-PERCEPTION/CONCEPT—*Ability to develop and use skills and behaviors to understand own attitudes and beliefs to integrate and manage life experiences*

Body Image, disturbed, 63–70
Dignity, risk for compromised, 225–229
Hope, readiness for enhanced, 447–451
Impulse Control, ineffective, 483–487
Mood Regulation, impaired, 613–617
Personal Identity, disturbed, 726–731
Resilience, lack of, 795–802
Self-Compassion, inadequate, 830–834
Self-Concept, readiness for enhanced, 834–838
Self-Esteem, chronic inadequate, 838–845
Self-Esteem, situational inadequate, 845–851
Social Identity, readiness for enhanced transgender, 904–908

SEXUALITY/REPRODUCTION—*Ability to meet requirements/characteristics of male/female role [component of Self-Perception/Concept and Roles/Relationships]*

Childbearing Process, ineffective, 141–151
Female Genital Mutilation, risk for, 347–351
Maternal-Fetal Dyad, risk for impaired, 586–593
Sexual Functioning, impaired, 865–872

STRESS MANAGEMENT—*Preventing or adapting to life changes, managing individual response to stressors*

Anxiety [mild, moderate, severe, panic], 28–35
Coping, difficulty, 192–199
Death Anxiety, 209–214
Emotional Regulation, ineffective, 293–297
Energy Field, disrupted, 301–305
Fear, 336–342
Grief, 391–396
Grief, dysfunctional, 396–403
Immigration Transition, risk for disrupted, 472–476
Post-Trauma Syndrome, 738–751
Relocation Stress, risk for, 789–795
Self-Injurious Behavior, non-suicidal, 851–858
Suicide, risk for, 935–945
Violence, risk for other-directed, 1041–1051

VALUES/BELIEFS—*Ability to use personal values, beliefs (including spiritual), and goals to guide life choices/decisions*

Decision-Making, impaired, 215–220
Moral Distress, 617–621
Religiosity, impaired, 783–789
Spiritual Well-Being, impaired, 913–920

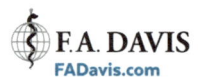

F.A. DAVIS
FADavis.com
1915 Arch Street · Philadelphia, Pennsylvania 19103 · Call Toll Free 800.323.3555
(In Canada, call 800.665.1148)

tolerance, **as timely intervention is more likely to be successful in alleviating pain.**
- Encourage verbalization of feelings about the pain, such as concern about tolerating pain, anxiety, and pessimistic thoughts **to evaluate coping abilities and to identify areas of additional concern.**
- Review procedures and expectations and inform client when treatments will hurt. Discuss pain management methods that will be used **to reduce concerns of the unknown and muscle tension associated with anxiety or fear.**
- Use puppets or dolls for explanations and teaching, when indicated, **to demonstrate procedures for child and enhance understanding to reduce level of anxiety or fear.**
- Provide or promote nonpharmacological pain management:
  Quiet environment, calm activities
  Comfort measures (e.g., back rub, change of position, use of heat or cold compresses)
  Use of relaxation exercises (e.g., focused breathing, visualization, guided imagery)
  Diversional or distraction activities, such as television and radio, video games, socialization with others, commercial or individualized tapes (e.g., "white" noise, music)
- Encourage presence of parent during painful procedures **to comfort child.**
  Identify ways to avoid or minimize pain. **Splinting incision during cough, keeping body in good alignment and using proper body mechanics, and resting between activities can reduce occurrence of muscle tension or spasms, or undue stress on incision.**
- Establish collaborative approach for pain management based on client's understanding about and acceptance of available treatment options. **Pharmacological management is based on client's symptomatology and mechanism of pain as well as tolerance for pain and for the various analgesics. Multimodal pain medications may include pills/liquids or suckers/lozenges, skin patch, suppository; injections, IV dosing; patient-controlled analgesia (PCA) or regional analgesia (e.g., epidural and spinal blocking).**
- Administer analgesics, as ordered up to maximum dosage **to maintain "acceptable" level of comfort, starting with the lowest dose possible to achieve safe pain control. The type of medication(s) ordered depends on the type and severity of pain (e.g., acetaminophen and NSAIDs are commonly used to treat mild to moderate pain, while opiates [e.g., morphine, oxycodone, hydromorphone,**

Information that appears in brackets has been added by the authors to clarify and enhance the use of nursing diagnoses.

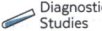 Diagnostic Studies   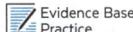 Evidence Based Practice   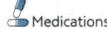 Medications   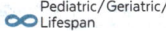 Pediatric/Geriatric/Lifespan

fentanyl] are used to treat moderate to severe pain). Combinations of medications may be used on prescribed intervals. Note: The American Academy of Pediatrics (AAP) guidelines suggest restricting the use of codeine or tramadol among children under age 12; teens aged 12 to 18 with obesity, obstructive sleep apnea, or severe lung disease; and clients under age 18 with postsurgical pain after tonsillectomy or adenoidectomy. Also, codeine or tramadol should be avoided in clients who are breastfeeding.

- Notify physician/healthcare provider if regimen is inadequate to meet pain control goal. Assist client to prevent (rather than treat pain) and alter drug regimen based on individual needs. **Once established, pain is more difficult to suppress. Increasing dosage, changing medication, or using a stepped program (e.g., switching from injection to oral route, or lengthening time interval between doses) helps in self-management of pain.**
- Evaluate and document client's response to analgesia and assist in transitioning or altering drug regimen, based on individual needs and planned interventions. **Limits adverse effects, reduces risk of drug dependence, and deals with barriers to adequate use of analgesics.**
- Evaluate for adverse medication effects (e.g., bradypnea, decreased oxygen saturation, decrease in mental acuity, change in thought processes, confusion or delirium, urinary retention, severe nausea, vomiting, pruritus). **Intolerable symptoms may require a change of medication(s).**
- Demonstrate, educate, and monitor use of self-administration/PCA that involves client in plan **to administer own IV pain medication.**
- Provide information and monitor use of site-specific medications (e.g., spinal, epidural, regional anesthesia) **that might be used for certain procedures such as back surgery, amputation, or labor and delivery.**
- Instruct client in use of transcutaneous electrical stimulation unit, when ordered.

Nursing Priority No. 4.

To promote optimal pain control (Teaching/Discharge Considerations) and enhance well-being (long-term goals):

- Acknowledge the pain experience and convey acceptance of client's response to pain. **Reduces defensive responses, promotes trust, and enhances cooperation with regimen.**
- Encourage adequate rest periods **to prevent fatigue that can impair client's ability to manage or cope with pain.**

Information that appears in brackets has been added by the authors to clarify and enhance the use of nursing diagnoses.

- Review additional nonpharmacological measures for lessening pain. **Relaxation skills and techniques such as Therapeutic Touch (TT), biofeedback, and self-hypnosis have no detrimental side effects.**
- Provide information and discuss pain management before planned procedures. **The primary concern of most clients/families is pain and discomfort following surgery or invasive procedure.**
- Discuss impact of pain on lifestyle/independence and ways to maximize level of functioning.
- Encourage performance of individualized physical therapy or exercise program that can be continued by the client after discharge. **Promotes active role in preventing muscle spasms or contractures and enhances sense of control.**
- Discuss with SO(s) ways in which they can assist client with pain management. **Family members/SOs may provide assistance by transporting client to prevent walking long distances, or by taking on client's strenuous chores, supporting timely pain control, encouraging eating nutritious meals to enhance wellness, and providing gentle massage to reduce muscle tension.**
- Identify specific signs/symptoms and changes in pain characteristics requiring medical follow-up. **Provides opportunity to modify pain management regimen and allows for timely intervention for developing complications.**
- Educate caregivers to identify a potential overdose and the proper administration of naloxone followed by notification of emergency responders. **Quick reversal of overdose may be lifesaving and requires medical follow-up.**

Documentation Focus

Assessment/Reassessment
- Individual assessment findings, including client's description of response to pain, specifics of pain inventory, expectations of pain management, and acceptable level of pain
- Prior medication use; substance abuse

Planning
- Plan of care and who is involved in planning
- Teaching plan

Implementation/Evaluation
- Response to interventions, teaching, and actions performed
- Attainment of or progress toward desired outcome(s)
- Modifications to plan of care

Information that appears in brackets has been added by the authors to clarify and enhance the use of nursing diagnoses.

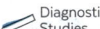 Diagnostic Studies 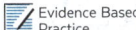 Evidence Based Practice 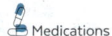 Medications 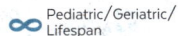 Pediatric/Geriatric/Lifespan

Discharge Planning
- Long-term needs, noting who is responsible for actions to be taken
- Specific referrals made

Sample Nursing Outcomes & Interventions Classifications NOC/NIC

NOC—Pain Level
NIC—Pain Management: Acute

chronic PAIN and CHRONIC PAIN SYNDROME NANDA-I

[Diagnostic Division: Comfort]

Definition: chronic Pain: Unpleasant sensory and emotional experience associated with, or resembling that associated with, actual or potential tissue damage with a duration of greater than 3 months.

Definition: Chronic Pain Syndrome: Recurrent or persistent pain that has lasted at least 3 months, and that significantly affects daily functioning or well-being.

Recognizing Cues

AUTHOR NOTE: Pain is a signal that something is wrong. Chronic pain may be recurrent and periodically disabling (e.g., migraine headaches, kidney stones, prostatitis) or may be unremitting. It is a complex entity, combining elements from many other NDs, such as excessive Sedentary Behaviors; decreased Diversional Activity Engagement; disturbed Body Image; impaired family Coping; impaired Family Process; lack of Resilience; Self-Care Deficit [specify]; impaired Sexual Functioning; inadequate Social Connectedness. The nurse is encouraged to refer to other NDs as indicated.

Related/Risk Factors (chronic Pain)
Ineffective fatigue self-management; malnutrition
Ineffective overweight self-management
Ineffective sexuality pattern
Injury agent; repeated handling of heavy loads; whole-body vibration
Psychological distress; difficulty establishing social interaction
Prolonged computer use

Information that appears in brackets has been added by the authors to clarify and enhance the use of nursing diagnoses.

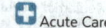 Acute Care 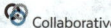 Collaborative 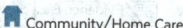 Community/Home Care   Cultural

Defining Characteristics

Subjective
Altered ability to continue activities; altered sleep-wake cycle; fatigue; inadequate appetite
Verbal report of pain; pain characteristic and intensity assessed using standardized, validated assessment instrument
Proxy report of activity changes or pain behavior

Objective
Evidence of pain using standardized pain behavior checklist for those unable to communicate verbally (e.g., Neonatal Infant Pain Scale, Pain Assessment Checklist for Seniors with Limited Ability to Communicate)
Facial expression of pain
Hypervigilance to pain

Related/Risk Factors (Chronic Pain Syndrome)
Ineffective chronic pain self-management
Fear of pain; fear-avoidance beliefs
Inadequate knowledge of pain management behaviors
Ineffective overweight self-management
Negative affect
Unaddressed sleep disturbances

Defining Characteristics

Subjective
Excessive anxiety, excessive fear; excessive stress
Impaired intestinal elimination
Ineffective sleep pattern

Objective
Impaired mood regulation; inadequate social connectedness
Impaired physical mobility

Clinical Connections
Traumatic injuries, migraines, repetitive motion injury (carpal or cubital tunnel syndrome), osteoarthritis, rheumatoid arthritis; peripheral neuropathies in diabetes or AIDS, cancer, burns, endometriosis, neuralgia, gangrene, kidney disorders/diseases

Generate Solutions

Plan Desired Outcomes

Client Will (Include Specific Time Frame)
- Verbalize and demonstrate (nonverbal cues) relief and/or control of pain or discomfort.

Information that appears in brackets has been added by the authors to clarify and enhance the use of nursing diagnoses.

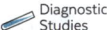 Diagnostic Studies 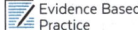 Evidence Based Practice 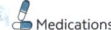 Medications 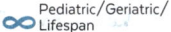 Pediatric/Geriatric/Lifespan

- Verbalize recognition of interpersonal and family dynamics and reactions that affect the pain situation.
- Demonstrate and initiate behavioral modifications of lifestyle and appropriate use of therapeutic interventions.
- Verbalize increased sense of control and enhanced enjoyment of life.

Family/Significant Other(s) Will (Include Specific Time Frame)
- Cooperate in pain management and rehabilitation program.

Interventions/Take Action

Nursing Priority No. 1.
To assess etiology/precipitating factors:

- Identify contributing physical factors, where known. **These factors associated with chronic pain (defined by the International Association for the Study of Pain [IASP] as pain that persists or continues to recur longer than 3 months, i.e., longer than the expected healing time) and Chronic Pain Syndrome (CPS) appear to include (1) musculoskeletal disorders such as osteoarthritis, rheumatoid arthritis, and fibromyalgia; (2) back pain from various causes such as disk herniation, vertebral fractures, muscular strains/sprains, overuse syndromes such as tendonitis, and bursitis, as well as pelvic disorders; (3) neurological disorders, such as spinal/other conditions causing nerve impingement, and radiculopathies and neuropathies with direct or referred pain; (4) urological disorders such as bladder neoplasms, chronic urinary tract infections or stones, testicular torsion, prostatitis; (5) gastrointestinal disorders such as colitis, gastroesophageal reflux, inflammatory bowel disease, and pancreatitis; (6) reproductive/gynecological disorders including endometriosis, disorders of ovaries, prolapse, etc.; and (7) miscellaneous/other causes including trauma (including childhood physical and sexual abuse), cardiovascular disease, peripheral vascular disease, and complications of medical treatments such as chemotherapy, radiation, or surgery.**

- Assess for type of pain client is experiencing. **Chronic pain types include (1) *neuropathic path* (e.g., burning, tingling, shooting, electric shocks) caused by damage to or dysfunction of the nervous system, such as might occur with sciatica, diabetic peripheral neuropathy, trigeminal neuralgia, and postherpetic neuralgia; (2) *nociceptive pain* (e.g., sharp, dull, aching) that is caused by tissue damage**

Information that appears in brackets has been added by the authors to clarify and enhance the use of nursing diagnoses.

and/or inflammation. Inflammatory pain can include sources like arthritis, infection, tissue injury, and postoperative pain; (3) *nociplastic pain*, which is pain without evidence of tissue damage. This type of pain may reflect changes in how the nervous system processes pain. Nociplastic pain has no clear correlation with injury, tissue damage, inflammation, or disease, and this kind of pain sensation varies widely. Examples of nociplastic pain include fibromyalgia, irritable bowel syndrome, and chronic low back pain.

- Note/document treatments that have been provided currently and in the past **to determine effectiveness.**
- Assist in and/or review diagnostic testing, including physical (e.g., selected tests for identifying and/or monitoring suspected known disease states; urine or blood toxicology for drug detoxification or therapy; and imaging studies); neurological, psychological evaluation (e.g., Minnesota Multiphasic Personality Inventory [MMPI], pain inventory, psychological interview). **Note: While additional diagnostic studies may be indicated when advanced treatment of the client with CPS is initiated, care should be exercised to avoid duplication of tests. This prevents unnecessary costs as well as inadvertent reinforcement of client's psychological need for "something to be physically wrong."**
- Determine presence of suspected psychological disorders. **Psychological factors may include (but are not limited to) depression, anxiety, somatization, post-traumatic stress disorders, substance abuse, compulsive sexual behaviors, eating disorders, and bipolar personality disorders. Testing may be indicated if organic cause of pain cannot be found, when psychological factors are known to exist, or when pain problems are prolonged and/or life-limiting.**
- Evaluate emotional/psychological components of individual situation. **Individuals with certain psychological syndromes (e.g., major depression, somatic symptom disorder, hypochondriasis) are prone to develop CPS. Note: People with chronic pain tend to report much higher rates of having experienced trauma in their past, when compared to people without chronic pain. The high rate of past trauma (e.g., domestic violence, sexual assault, childhood neglect, physical/sexual abuse, terrorism/combat) in people with chronic pain suggests an association with the development of chronic pain. Abuse in childhood is a strong predictor of depression and**

Information that appears in brackets has been added by the authors to clarify and enhance the use of nursing diagnoses.

 Diagnostic Studies   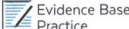 Evidence Based Practice   Medications   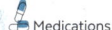 Pediatric/Geriatric/Lifespan physical complaints, both expanded and unexplained, in adulthood.

- Evaluate client's pattern of coping and locus of control (internal or external). **Fear and avoidance or lack of active engagement in self-management activities can contribute to perpetuation of chronic pain. Individuals with external locus of control may take little or no responsibility for pain management.**
- Determine relevant cultural and spiritual factors affecting pain response. **Pain is accepted and expressed in different ways (e.g., moaning aloud or enduring in stoic silence). Some may magnify symptoms to convince others of the reality of pain or may believe that suffering in silence helps atone for past wrongdoing. Note: A person with chronic pain who identifies self as a spiritual being may report the link to divine help as empowering client to use strategies for healing.**
- Note gender and age of client. **There may be differences between how women and men perceive and/or respond to pain. Pain in children or in cognitively impaired clients is often underestimated and undertreated; effective pain management may be compromised due to communication difficulties and the lack of effective scales to measure pain in clients with special needs. The prevalence of chronically painful conditions (e.g., arthritis) and illnesses (e.g., cancers) is common in the elderly, and they may be reluctant to report pain. These clients may demonstrate more nonverbal clues (e.g., guarding, changes in behavior, eating and sleeping poorly, crying, moaning).**
- Evaluate current and past analgesic, opioid, other drug use (including alcohol, marijuana/CBD products). **Provides clues to options to try or to avoid; identifies need for changes in medication regimen as well as possible need for detoxification program.**

Nursing Priority No. 2.
To determine client response to chronic pain situation:

- Evaluate pain behavior, noting past and current pain experience. *Pain* **that (1) is more generalized (although clients may complain of specific areas of pain), (2) that continues or is intermittently recurring for 3 months or more, (3) is unresponsive to conventional treatment, and (4) is experienced by clients who have an existing condition that may result in ongoing pain.** *Non-pain* **related factors**

Information that appears in brackets has been added by the authors to clarify and enhance the use of nursing diagnoses.

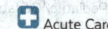 Acute Care 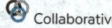 Collaborative 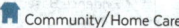 Community/Home Care Cultural

such as (1) sleep disturbance, chronic fatigue despite sleep; (2) poor concentration, memory impairment; (3) hypersensitivity to audio, visual, and tactile stimulation; and (4) anxiety, depression, feelings. *Medical history such as comorbid conditions and/or multiple allergies.*

- Utilize pain rating scale or diary, including functional effects and psychological factors. **Pain behaviors can include the same ones present in acute pain (e.g., crying, grimacing, withdrawal, narrowed focus) but may also include other behaviors (e.g., dramatization of complaints, depression, drug misuse). Pain complaints may be exaggerated because of client's perception that pain reports are not believed or because client believes caregivers are discounting reports of pain.**

- Acknowledge and assess pain matter-of-factly, avoiding undue expressions of concern as well as expressions of disbelief about client's suffering. **Conveying an attitude of empathic understanding of client's disabling distress can have a beneficial impact on client's perception of health and healthcare providers.**

- Ascertain who has been consulted and what therapies (including alternative/complementary) have been used. **If medical treatments are ongoing for painful conditions (e.g., spinal stenosis, pancreatitis, endometriosis, arthritis), consultations with specialists may be helpful in finding curative or palliative treatments. If pain is present without a clear etiology or continues unabated, complex rehabilitation techniques may be required, incorporating physical, occupational, psychological, and recreational therapies.**

- Note effects of pain on lifestyle. **Major effects of chronic pain on the client's life can include weight loss or gain, reduced activity and libido, excessive use of drugs and alcohol, dependent behavior, and disability seemingly out of proportion to impairment.**

- Assess degree of personal maladjustment of the client, such as isolationism, anger, irritability, loss of work time or employment, and school absenteeism. **Chronic pain reduces client's coping abilities and psychological well-being, often resulting in problems with relationships and life functioning.**

- Determine issues of secondary gain for the client/significant other(s) (SO[s]) (e.g., financial or insurance compensation pending, legal or marital or family concern, school or work issues), **which may be present if there is marked**

Information that appears in brackets has been added by the authors to clarify and enhance the use of nursing diagnoses.

 Diagnostic Studies 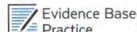 Evidence Based Practice 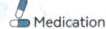 Medications 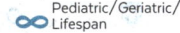 Pediatric/Geriatric/Lifespan

discrepancy between claimed distress and objective findings or there is a lack of cooperation during evaluation and in complying with prescribed treatment.
- Note codependent components, enabling behaviors of caregivers/family members **that support continuation of the status quo and may interfere with progress in pain management or resolution of situation.**
- Assess availability and use of personal and community resources. **Client/SO may need many things (e.g., equipment, financial resources, vocational training, respite services, or placement in rehabilitation facility) in order to manage painful conditions and/or concerns or difficulties associated with condition.**
- Make home visit when indicated, observing such factors as client's safety, equipment, adequate lighting, or family interactions **to note impact of home environment on the client and to determine changes that might be useful in improving client's life (e.g., grab bars in bathrooms and hallways, wider doors, ramps, assistance with activities of daily living [ADLs], housekeeping, yard work).**

Nursing Priority No. 3.

To assist client to cope with pain:

- Encourage participation in multidisciplinary pain management plan. **Comprehensive team may include physical medicine specialist; physical, occupational, recreational, and vocational therapists; and emotional or behavioral therapists to address complex issues of unresolved pain issues, to set goals for pain relief, and to develop an individualized treatment and evaluation plan. Treatments could involve extended-relief oral pain medications or dermal patches, nerve-blocking injections or an implanted pump, and massage and other hands-on therapies, as well as counseling and home exercise programs.**
- Discuss pain management goals and review client expectations versus reality **because it may be that while pain cannot be completely resolved, it can be significantly reduced or managed to the degree that client can participate in desired or needed life activities, thus improving quality of life.**
- Discuss the physiological dynamics of tension and anxiety and how this affects pain.
- Administer or encourage client use of analgesics, as indicated. **Medications may be available in pills, liquids, or**

Information that appears in brackets has been added by the authors to clarify and enhance the use of nursing diagnoses.

suckers to take by mouth, and in injection, skin patch, and suppository forms. Different medications or combinations of drugs may be used such as opioids/narcotics, nonopioids, and adjuvant medications (e.g., muscle relaxants, anticonvulsants, antidepressants, serotonin and norepinephrine reuptake inhibitors) to manage persistent pain so that client may find relief and increase level of function. **Note: Studies support that people with intense pain can take very high doses of opioids without experiencing side effects/euphoria.**

- Provide consistent and sufficient medication for pain relief, tailored to the individual, especially in one who tends to be undermedicated (e.g., elderly, cognitively impaired, person with lifelong pain, those with terminal cancer). **For clients aged 65 and older, the American Geriatrics Society (AGS) Beers Criteria should be considered when making an analgesic selection. For some clients, medications may need to be scheduled around the clock, doses titrated up or down, and doses maximized to optimize pain relief while managing side effects.**

- Recommend or employ nonpharmacological interventions, methods of pain control (e.g., heat or cold applications, progressive muscle relaxation, biofeedback, deep breathing, meditation, visualization or guided imagery, posture correction and muscle strengthening exercises, water therapy, electrical stimulation, massage, acupuncture, therapeutic touch [TT]) **to obtain comfort, improve healing, and decrease dependency on analgesics.**

- Assist with/educate client/SO on medical devices or procedures to alleviate pain, such as transcutaneous electrical nerve stimulation (TENS), peripheral nerve stimulation, spinal cord stimulation, nerve blocks, radiofrequency ablation, and surgery.

- Address medication misuse with client/SO and refer for appropriate counseling or interventions **when addiction is known or suspected to be interfering with client's well-being. Clients may misrepresent their pain levels and their activities in order to obtain pain medications or progressively higher doses of medications, and they require specialized evaluation and interventions.**

- Assist family in developing a program of coping strategies (e.g., staying active even when modified activities are required, living a healthy lifestyle). **Positive reinforcement, encouraging client to use own control can aid in focusing energies on more productive activities.**

Information that appears in brackets has been added by the authors to clarify and enhance the use of nursing diagnoses.

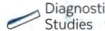 Diagnostic Studies 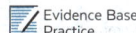 Evidence Based Practice 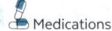 Medications 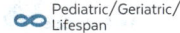 Pediatric/Geriatric/Lifespan

- Encourage limiting attention to pain behaviors, when appropriate (e.g., discussing pain for only a specified time; or acknowledging "I'm sorry your pain returned today, but you need to go to school"; or actively practicing relaxation or coping skills). **Reduces focus on pain, especially if client is highly dependent on pain for secondary gain issues or is addicted to medications.**
- Encourage client to use positive affirmations: "I am healing." "I am relaxed." "I love this life." Have client be aware of internal-external dialogue. Say "cancel" when negative thoughts develop. **Negative thinking can exacerbate feelings of hopelessness, and replacing those thoughts with positive ones can be helpful to pain management.**
- Encourage right-brain stimulation with activities such as love, laughter, and music. **These actions can release endorphins, enhancing sense of well-being.**
- Encourage use of subliminal tapes **to bypass logical part of the brain by reinforcing:** "I am becoming a more relaxed person." "It is all right for me to relax." Stress hormones (e.g., cortisol) can cause sensations of pain to feel more intense, thus finding helpful ways to cope with stress can help lower pain intensity.
- Use anxiolytics, narcotics, and analgesics sparingly. **These drugs are physically and psychologically addicting and promote sleep disturbances, especially interference with deep rapid eye movement (REM) sleep. Client may need to be detoxified if many medications are currently used.**
- Be alert to changes in pain characteristics **that may indicate a new physical problem or developing complication.**

Nursing Priority No. 4.

To promote optimal pain control (Teaching/Discharge Considerations) and enhance well-being (long-term goals):

- Provide anticipatory guidance to client with condition in which pain is common and educate about when, where, and how to seek intervention or treatments.
- Discuss potential for developmental delays in child with chronic pain. Identify current level of function and review appropriate expectations for individual child.
- Instruct client/SO in medication administration, including safe use of patient-controlled analgesia (PCA) pumps, as indicated. Review safe use of analgesics, including side effects requiring home management (e.g., constipation) or adverse effects requiring medical intervention (e.g., possible drug reactions). **Appropriate instruction in home**

Information that appears in brackets has been added by the authors to clarify and enhance the use of nursing diagnoses.

management increases the accuracy and safety of medication administration.
- Instruct client/SO on tapering/discontinuing opioids as directed. **Clients who have been prescribed/taken opioids long-term have an increased risk of adverse effects, particularly if opioids are discontinued rapidly.**
- Encourage and assist family member(s)/SO(s) to learn home-care interventions. **Massage and other nonpharmacological pain management techniques benefit the client through reduction of pain level and sense that client is not alone/has support of SO.**
- Incorporate desired safe cultural/folk healthcare practices and beliefs into regimen whenever possible. **Has been shown to increase compliance with pain management treatment plan.**
- Identify and discuss potential hazards of unproved or nonmedical therapies or remedies.
- Assist client and SO(s) to learn how to heal **by developing sense of internal control, by being responsible for own treatment, and by obtaining the information and tools to accomplish this.**
- Recommend client and SO(s) take time for themselves. **Provides opportunity to reenergize and refocus on living/tasks at hand.**
- Address client's preferences and wishes for incurable pain or end-of-life pain management via advance directives **in order to assist family/SO in attending to client's needs.** (Refer to impaired End-of-Life Comfort Syndrome for appropriate interventions.)
- Identify community support groups and resources to meet individual needs (e.g., yard care, home maintenance, transportation). **Proper use of resources may reduce negative pattern of "overdoing" heavy activities and then spending several days in bed recuperating.**
- Refer for counseling (e.g., individual, family, marital therapy, parent effectiveness classes) as needed. **Presence of chronic pain affects all relationships and family dynamics.**
- Refer to NDs impaired family Coping, difficulty Coping.

Documentation Focus

Assessment/Reassessment
- Individual findings, including duration of problem, specific contributing factors, previously and currently used interventions

---

Information that appears in brackets has been added by the authors to clarify and enhance the use of nursing diagnoses.

 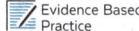 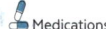 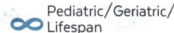

- Perception of pain, effects on lifestyle, and expectations of therapeutic regimen
- Locus of control and cultural beliefs affecting response to pain
- Family's/SO's response to client, and support for change
- Availability and use of resources

Planning
- Plan of care and who is involved in planning
- Teaching plan

Implementation/Evaluation
- Responses to interventions, teaching, and actions performed
- Attainment of or progress toward desired outcome(s)
- Modifications to plan of care

Discharge Planning
- Long-term needs and who is responsible for actions to be taken
- Specific referrals made

Sample Nursing Outcomes & Interventions Classifications NOC/NIC

NOC—Pain Control
NIC—Pain Management: Chronic

labor PAIN NANDA-I

[Diagnostic Division: Comfort]

Definition: Sensory and emotional experience that varies from pleasant to unpleasant, associated with labor and childbirth.

Recognizing Cues

Related/Risk Factors
Behavioral Factors:
Insufficient fluid intake
Supine position
Cognitive Factors:
Perceives pain as meaningful
Inadequate self-efficacy

Information that appears in brackets has been added by the authors to clarify and enhance the use of nursing diagnoses.

Inadequate knowledge about childbirth; inadequate preparation to deal with labor pain

Fear of childbirth; perceives labor pain as: nonproductive, unnatural, negative, threatening

Social Factors:
Unsupportive companionship
Interference in decision making

Unmodified Environmental Factors:
Noisy, overcrowded delivery room; turbulent environment

Defining Characteristics

Subjective

Verbal report of pain; uterine contraction; perineal pressure
Inadequate appetite; nausea; vomiting
Anxiety
Altered urinary functioning; altered sleep-wake cycle

Objective

Altered blood pressure/heart rate/respiratory rate
Distraction/expressive behavior; protective behavior; positioning to ease pain
Altered muscle tension; diaphoresis
Altered neuroendocrine functioning
Hypervigilance to pain; self-focused attention; pupil dilation
Facial expression of pain

Clinical Connections

Stages of labor and delivery, preterm labor, dysfunctional labor, induced labor, spontaneous or elective termination

Generate Solutions

Plan Desired Outcomes

Client Will (Include Specific Time Frame)
- Participate in decision making for pain management plan to include personal preferences and cultural beliefs.
- Engage in nonpharmacological measures to reduce discomfort/pain.
- Report pain at manageable level.

Partner/Labor Coach Will (Include Specific Time Frame)
- Participate in labor process providing client's desired level of support.

Information that appears in brackets has been added by the authors to clarify and enhance the use of nursing diagnoses.

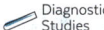 Diagnostic Studies 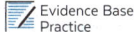 Evidence Based Practice Medications 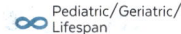 Pediatric/Geriatric/Lifespan

Interventions/Take Action

Nursing Priority No. 1.
To determine client's individual needs:

- Identify stage and phase of labor; perform vaginal examination noting nature and amount of vaginal show, cervical dilation, effacement, fetal station, and fetal descent. **Choice and timing of medications are affected by degree of dilation and contractile pattern.**
- Note timing of initiation of prenatal care and participation in childbirth education classes. **Economic, emotional, and cultural concerns can limit the mother's access or involvement in preparation for labor, increasing her need for information and support.**
- Evaluate degree of discomfort through verbal and nonverbal cues; note cultural influences on pain response. **Attitudes and reactions to pain are individual and based on past experiences, understanding of physiological changes, and familial/cultural expectations.**
- Ascertain presence of a birth plan, individual expectations, and cultural or spiritual beliefs affecting the labor and delivery process. **Cultural influences may include how the laboring mother views pain management, as well as who attends the mother during the birth process.**
- Determine availability and preparation of support person(s). **Presence of a supportive partner, family/friend, or doula can provide emotional support and enhance level of comfort. Labor coaching and support provided by a doula have been shown to decrease use of pharmacological analgesia and decrease rates of assisted vaginal delivery.**

Nursing Priority No. 2.
To engage client in nonpharmacological pain management techniques:

- Provide/encourage use of comfort measures (e.g., back/leg rubs, sacral pressure, back rest, mouth care, repositioning; shower/hot tub use; cool, moist cloths to face and neck; hot compresses to perineum, abdomen; perineal care, linen changes). **Promotes relaxation and hygiene, which enhance feeling of well-being and may reduce the need for analgesia or anesthesia. Position changes can also enhance circulation, reduce muscle tension. Note: Clients positioned with their head above their hips, rather than recumbent, during the first stage of labor are less likely**

Information that appears in brackets has been added by the authors to clarify and enhance the use of nursing diagnoses.

 Acute Care 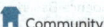 Collaborative Community/Home Care Cultural

to require epidural analgesia and shorten the first stage of labor by more than 1 hr.
- Assess client's desire for physical touch during contractions. **Touch may serve as a distraction, provide supportive reassurance and encouragement, and may aid in maintaining sense of control and reducing pain. Note: Remain respectful of client's preferences regarding touch.**
- Coach use of appropriate breathing/relaxation techniques and abdominal effleurage based on stage of labor. **May block pain impulses within the cerebral cortex through conditioned responses and cutaneous stimulation and gives client a means of coping with and controlling the level of discomfort.**
- Encourage client to void every 1 to 2 hr. **Reduces bladder distention, which can increase discomfort and prolong labor.**
- Review birth plan periodically. Provide information about stage of labor and projected delivery, available analgesics, usual responses/side effects (client and fetal), and duration of analgesic effect in light of current situation. **Empowers client to be actively involved and make informed decisions about means of pain control, enhancing client's sense of control.**
- Assist with complementary therapies as indicated (e.g., acupressure/acupuncture, moxibustion, hypnosis, reflexology). **Some clients and healthcare providers may prefer a trial of therapies theorized to stimulate/regulate contractions, reduce muscle tension, and mediate perception of pain before pursuing pharmacological interventions. Note: Differences in cultural and regional acceptance of these options as well as provider technique can impact the effectiveness of these interventions.**
- Provide for a quiet environment that is adequately ventilated, dimly lit, and free of unnecessary personnel. Offer soothing music, aromatherapy as appropriate. **Nondistracting environment provides optimal opportunity for rest and relaxation between contractions. Aromatherapy using essential oils for massage, warm bath, or air diffusion stimulates the limbic system, releasing serotonin and endorphins and reducing anxiety and tension.**
- Discuss appropriateness/timing of hydrotherapy (shower, hot tub) as client desires. **Warm water during the first stage of labor, or second stage as appropriate, stimulates**

labor PAIN

Information that appears in brackets has been added by the authors to clarify and enhance the use of nursing diagnoses.

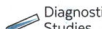 Diagnostic Studies   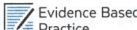 Evidence Based Practice   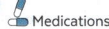 Medications   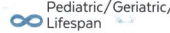 Pediatric/Geriatric/Lifespan

705

the release of endorphins and relaxes muscles, enhancing circulation and tissue oxygenation with reduction in use of analgesia.
- Provide opportunity to engage in cultural practices such as using a Mexican rebozo; praying, reciting the Quran or Islamic meditation (dhikr). **Wrapping a rebozo snugly around the midsection of the body provides abdominal support, facilitating laboring in a squatting position, relaxing pelvic muscles and ligaments, and promoting fetal descent. Religious practices offer mental comfort and distraction as client focuses attention away from discomfort.**
- Offer encouragement, provide information about labor progress, and provide positive reinforcement for client's/couple's efforts. **Provides emotional support, which can reduce fear, lower anxiety levels, and help minimize pain.**

Nursing Priority No. 3.
To provide more intensive pain management measures:
- Time and record the frequency, intensity, and duration of uterine contractile pattern per protocol. **Information necessary for choosing appropriate interventions and preventing or limiting undesired side effects of medication.**
- Review birth plan, provide positive feedback for efforts to date, and be supportive of client's decisions regarding pain management. **Each labor and delivery experience is different and can challenge prenatal expectations. Acceptance and support from the nurse can enhance coping and promote a more positive birth experience.**
- Provide safety measures (e.g., encourage client to move slowly, bed in low position, raise side rails) as indicated postmedication administration. **Regional block anesthesia produces vasomotor paralysis, so sudden movement may precipitate hypotension and risk for fall.**
- Discuss option of inhaled medication (nitrous oxide, fluranes), if desired. **Self-administered medication provides noninvasive pharmacological pain relief, improving pain scores, and has rapid clearance once mask is removed. Note: Possible environmental concern as this is a potent greenhouse gas.**
- Administer analgesic, such as butorphanol tartrate (Stadol), remifentanil (Ultiva), or morphine, by IV during contractions or deep intramuscular (IM) if indicated during active phase of stage I labor. **IV route provides more rapid and equal absorption of analgesic, and IM route may require**

Information that appears in brackets has been added by the authors to clarify and enhance the use of nursing diagnoses.

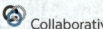
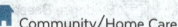

up to 45 min to reach adequate plasma levels. Administering IV drug during uterine contraction decreases amount of medication that immediately reaches fetus. **Note: Clients with opioid use disorder require attention to individualized pain management plans for judicious use of analgesia.**

- Monitor maternal vital signs noting drug's effectiveness and the physiological response. **Maternal side effects include nausea, vomiting, dizziness, respiratory depression–oxygen desaturation, and sedation.**
- Prepare for/assist with neuraxial anesthesia (i.e., epidural or caudal block anesthesia) using an indwelling catheter. **Provides relief once active labor is established unless delivery is imminent. Note: Use of ultra–low dose epidural is being promoted to achieve pain control without negative effect on client's ability to sense contractions and push effectively.**
- Monitor fetal heart rate (FHR) electronically, and note decreased variability or bradycardia. **Decreased FHR variability is a common side effect of many anesthetics/analgesics. These side effects can begin 2 to 10 min after administration of anesthetic and may last for 5 to 10 min on occasion. Narcotics can have a depressant effect on fetus, particularly when administered 2 to 3 hr before delivery.**
- Monitor level of block per protocol. **Migration of decreased sensation from belly button (dermatome T10) to tip of breastbone (approximately T6) increases risk of respiratory depression and profound hypotension.**
- Turn client side to side periodically during continuous infusions. **Promotes even distribution of drug to prevent "one-sided" or unilateral block.**
- Inform client of onset of contractions as appropriate. **Client may "sleep" and/or encounter partial amnesia between contractions, impairing her ability to recognize contractions as they begin and her ability to initiate pain management techniques.**
- Provide information about type of regional analgesia/anesthesia available at stage II specific to the delivery setting (e.g., local, pudendal block, lumbar epidural reinforcement, spinal block). **Local perineal infiltration may be performed immediately before delivery for episiotomy/laceration repair if needed. While pudendal blocks are used less often now, may be used to facilitate use of forceps or vacuum extraction assisted delivery.**

Information that appears in brackets has been added by the authors to clarify and enhance the use of nursing diagnoses.

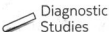 Diagnostic Studies   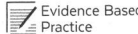 Evidence Based Practice   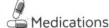 Medications   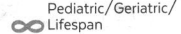 Pediatric/Geriatric/Lifespan

Nursing Priority No. 4.

To support delivery process:

- Note perineal bulging or vaginal show. **Discomfort levels increase as cervix dilates, fetus descends, and small blood vessels rupture.**
- Assist client in assuming optimal position for bearing down (e.g., squatting or lateral recumbent). **Proper positioning with relaxation of perineal tissue optimizes bearing-down efforts, facilitates labor progress, and reduces discomfort.**
- Assist with reinforcement of medication via indwelling lumbar epidural catheter when caput is visible. **Reduces discomfort associated with episiotomy, forceps application if needed, and fetal expulsion.**
- Assist as needed with administration of local anesthetic just before episiotomy, if performed. **Anesthetizes perineum tissue for incision/repair purposes.**

Documentation Focus

Assessment/Reassessment
- Stages of labor, results of vaginal examination, status of fetus/fetal monitoring
- Client's degree of preparation and expectations for labor process
- Choice/effectiveness of support person(s)

Planning
- Specifics of birth plan
- Plan of care and who is involved in planning

Implementation/Evaluation
- Response to actions and interventions performed
- Attainment of or progress toward desired outcome(s)

Discharge Planning
- Postpartal pain management choices

Sample Nursing Outcomes & Interventions Classifications NOC/NIC

NOC—Pain Control
NIC—Labor Pain Management

Information that appears in brackets has been added by the authors to clarify and enhance the use of nursing diagnoses.

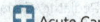 Acute Care  Collaborative 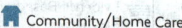 Community/Home Care 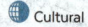 Cultural

ineffective PAIN SELF-MANAGEMENT   NANDA-I

[Diagnostic Division: Comfort]

Definition: Unsatisfactory handling of treatment regimen, consequences, and lifestyle changes related to an unpleasant sensory and emotional experience resembling that associated with actual or potential tissue damage.

Related/Risk Factors

Competing demands, or lifestyle preferences; conflict between health behaviors and social norms

Nonacceptance of condition; unaware of seriousness of condition; unaware of susceptibility to sequelae

Difficulty managing complex treatment regimen; difficulty navigating complex healthcare systems; inadequate health literacy

Negative feelings toward treatment regimen; perceived barrier to treatment regimen; unrealistic expectation of treatment regimen

Inadequate action to address modifiable factors; inadequate commitment to a plan of action

Inadequate knowledge of underlying cause of pain, of pain complications, or of modifiable factors

Inadequate knowledge of treatment regimen, or distraction techniques

Excessive stress; unaddressed environmental constraints

Inadequate self-efficacy; inadequate self-confidence in decision making; learned helplessness

Inadequate caregiver knowledge of modifiable factors

Recognizing Cues

Defining Characteristics

Subjective
Pain Symptoms:
Verbal report of pain; fear of movement
Fatigue; inadequate appetite
Anxiety; hopelessness
Pain Complications:
Altered sleep-wake cycle
Behaviors:
Pain catastrophizing

Information that appears in brackets has been added by the authors to clarify and enhance the use of nursing diagnoses.

 Diagnostic Studies 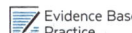 Evidence Based Practice 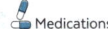 Medications 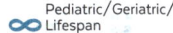 Pediatric/Geriatric/Lifespan

Objective
Pain Signs:
Holding breath; facial expression of pain
Guarding a particular body part; rubbing painful area; pain gestures
Restlessness; moaning with movement; reluctance to move
Altered blood pressure; increased heart rate, respiratory rate; diaphoresis; pupil dilation
Evidence of pain using standardized pain behavior checklist for those unable to communicate verbally

Pain Symptoms:
Irritable mood; hypervigilance to pain
Decreased physical endurance; decreased social interaction
Pain characteristics, intensity assessed using standardized, validated assessment tool

Behaviors:
Inattentive to underlying causes of pain, pain complications, or modifiable factors
Inadequate use of distraction techniques
Nonadherence to recommended treatment; inadequate follow-through on agreed lifestyle modifications
Proxy report of pain behavior

Clinical Connections
Trauma (skeletal, soft tissue/muscle), arthritis, degenerative joint disease; amputation, depression, schizophrenia; developmental delay

Generate Solutions

Plan Desired Outcomes

Client Will (Include Specific Time Frame)
- Report pain is relieved or controlled at acceptable level.
- Follow prescribed pharmacological/treatment regimen.
- Demonstrate or initiate behavioral modifications of lifestyle and appropriate use of therapeutic interventions.
- Engage in use of relaxation skills and diversional activities as indicated for individual situation.
- Verbalize sense of control of response to pain situation and positive outlook for the future.

Interventions/Take Action

Nursing Priority No. 1.
To assess etiology/precipitating contributory factors:
- Note possible pathophysiological and psychological causes of pain (e.g., inflammation, tissue trauma, burns, fractures,

---

Information that appears in brackets has been added by the authors to clarify and enhance the use of nursing diagnoses.

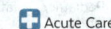 Acute Care 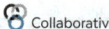 Collaborative 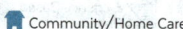 Community/Home Care Cultural

surgery; infections, heart attack, angina; abdominal conditions [e.g., appendicitis, cholecystitis], grief, fear, anxiety, depression, personality disorders).
- Evaluate client/significant other's (SO's) understanding of therapeutic regimen. **Consistent adherence to a medical regimen increases the likelihood of client pain relief and enhanced quality of life.**
- Evaluate for presence of/suspected psychological stress. **Psychological stressors may include (but are not limited to) depression, anxiety, somatization, post-traumatic stress disorders, substance abuse, compulsive sexual behaviors, eating disorders, and bipolar personality disorders. Individuals with certain psychological syndromes (e.g., major depression, somatic symptom disorder, hypochondriasis) are prone to develop Chronic Pain Syndrome (CPS). Note: People with chronic pain tend to report much higher rates of trauma in their past when compared to people without chronic pain. The high rate of past trauma (e.g., domestic violence, sexual assault, childhood neglect, physical/sexual abuse, terrorism/combat) in clients with chronic pain suggests an association with the development of chronic pain. Testing may be indicated if the organic cause of pain cannot be found, when psychological factors are known to exist, or when pain problems are prolonged and/or life-limiting.**
- Note gender and age of client. **There may be differences between women and men as to how they perceive and/or respond to pain. Pain in children, or cognitively impaired clients is often underestimated and undertreated; effective pain management may be compromised due to communication difficulties and the lack of effective scales to measure pain in clients with special needs. The prevalence of chronically painful conditions (e.g., arthritis) and illnesses (e.g., cancers) is common in the elderly; they may be reluctant to report pain. These clients may demonstrate more nonverbal clues (e.g., guarding, changes in behavior, eating and sleeping poorly, crying, moaning).**
- Assess client's perceptions of pain, along with behaviors and cultural expectations regarding pain. **Client's perception of and expression of pain are influenced by age, developmental stage, underlying problem causing pain, and cognitive, behavioral, and sociocultural factors. Pain is accepted and expressed in different ways (e.g., moaning aloud or enduring in stoic silence); some may**

Information that appears in brackets has been added by the authors to clarify and enhance the use of nursing diagnoses.

 Diagnostic Studies   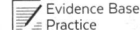 Evidence Based Practice   Medications   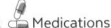 Pediatric/Geriatric/Lifespan

magnify symptoms to convince others of the reality of pain or believe that suffering in silence helps atone for past wrongdoing. A client with chronic pain who identifies as a spiritual being may report the link to divine help as empowering them to use strategies for healing. Studies show that spiritual interventions may include faith healing, laying on of hands, anointing with oil, prayer and meditation, attending church and religious events, Bible and other spiritual readings, listening to gospel music, and ministerial and community service.
- Note client's attitude toward pain and use of specific pain medications, including any history of substance abuse. **Client may have beliefs restricting use of medications, may have a high tolerance for drugs because of recent or current use, or may not be able to take pain medications at all if participating in a substance abuse recovery program.**
- Note client's locus of control (internal or external). **Individuals with external locus of control may take little or no responsibility for pain management.**
- Collaborate with medical providers in pain assessment, including neurological and psychological factors (pain inventory, psychological interview) as appropriate.

Nursing Priority No. 2.
To evaluate client's response to pain:

- Obtain client's/SO's description of pain to include location, characteristics, onset, duration, frequency, quality, and intensity. Identify precipitating or aggravating and relieving factors **to fully understand client's pain symptoms. Note: Experts agree that attempts should always be made to obtain self-reports of pain. When not possible, credible information can be received from another person who knows the client well (e.g., parent, spouse, caregiver). Note: There are six populations in which difficulty communicating pain often exists: neonates, toddlers, and young children; clients with intellectual disabilities; critically ill/unconscious clients; older adults with advanced dementia; and clients at the end of life. Numerous studies have revealed that physicians and nurses need to be aware of their tendency to underestimate client's pain in early postoperative days.**
- Accept client's description of pain. Be aware of the terminology client uses for pain experience (e.g., young child may say "owie" or "hurt"; elderly may say "it aches so bad").

Information that appears in brackets has been added by the authors to clarify and enhance the use of nursing diagnoses.

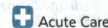 Acute Care 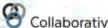 Collaborative 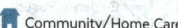 Community/Home Care Cultural

Pain is a subjective experience and cannot be felt by others. Note: Some elderly clients experience a reduction in perception of pain or have difficulty localizing or describing pain, and pain may be manifested as a change in behavior (e.g., restlessness, loss of appetite, increased confusion or wandering, acting out, change in functional abilities).

- Note cultural influences affecting pain response. **Verbal or behavioral cues may not have a direct relationship to the degree of pain perceived (e.g., client may deny pain even when feeling uncomfortable, reactions can be stoic or exaggerated, reflecting cultural and familial norms). These factors affect client's and caregiver's attitudes and beliefs regarding the pain experience, expressions of pain, and expectations regarding pain management.**

- Observe nonverbal cues (e.g., how client walks, holds body, guarding behaviors; sleeplessness; grimacing facial expressions; distraction behaviors, narrowed focus; crying, poor feeding, lethargy in infants). Ask others who know client well (e.g., spouse, parent) to identify behaviors that may indicate pain in persons who cannot communicate verbally. **Helpful in recognizing presence of pain; however, cues not congruent with verbal reports indicate need for further evaluation.**

- Ascertain client's knowledge of and satisfaction with pain management. **Provides baseline for interventions and teaching, provides opportunity to allay common fears and misconceptions (e.g., fears about addiction to opiates, belief that complete pain relief is possible in every situation) or to address expected side effects of analgesics (e.g., constipation).**

- Investigate client's previous experiences with pain and methods found either helpful or unhelpful for pain control in the past. Identify what therapies (including alternative/complementary) have been used. **If medical treatments are ongoing for painful conditions (e.g., spinal stenosis, pancreatitis, endometriosis, arthritis), consultations with specialists may be helpful in finding curative or palliative treatments. If pain is present without a clear etiology or continues unabated, complex rehabilitation techniques may be required, incorporating physical, occupational, psychological, and recreational therapies.**

- Note lifestyle effects of pain. **Major effects of chronic pain on the client's life can include weight loss or gain, reduced activity and libido, excessive use of drugs and**

Information that appears in brackets has been added by the authors to clarify and enhance the use of nursing diagnoses.

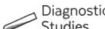 Diagnostic Studies 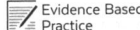 Evidence Based Practice 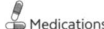 Medications 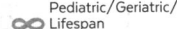 Pediatric/Geriatric/Lifespan

alcohol, dependent behavior, and disability seemingly out of proportion to impairment.
- Assess the degree of personal maladjustment of the client such as isolationism, anger, irritability, loss of work time or employment, and school absenteeism. **Chronic pain reduces client's coping abilities and psychological well-being, often resulting in problems with relationships and life functioning.**
- Note availability and use of personal and community resources. **Client/SO may need many things (e.g., equipment, financial resources, vocational training, respite services, placement in rehabilitation facility) in order to manage painful conditions and/or concerns or difficulties associated with condition.**

Nursing Priority No. 3.

To assist client to explore methods for alleviation/control of pain:

- Determine client's acceptable level of pain and pain control goal. **Client may not be 100% pain free but may feel that a "3" is a manageable level of discomfort, while another may require medication for pain at the same level because the experience is subjective.**
- Determine factors in client's lifestyle (e.g., alcohol or other drug use or abuse) that can affect responses to analgesics and/or choice of interventions for pain management.
- Help client to identify pain patterns (e.g., when pain occurs [only with ambulation, every night]), factors that aggravate or alleviate pain, associated symptoms (e.g., nausea, vomiting, lethargy), etc., **to identify pain trends and optimize pain relief.**
- Encourage participation in multidisciplinary pain management plan. **Comprehensive team may include physical medicine specialist; physical, occupational, recreational, and vocational therapists; and emotional or behavioral therapists to address complex issues of unresolved pain issues, to set goals for pain relief, and to develop an individualized treatment and evaluation plan. Treatments could involve extended-relief oral pain medications or dermal patches, nerve-blocking injections or an implanted pump, and massage and other hands-on therapies, as well as counseling and home exercise programs.**
- Educate client/caregiver to prevent rather than "chase" pain. **Early implementation of pain relief strategies**

Information that appears in brackets has been added by the authors to clarify and enhance the use of nursing diagnoses.

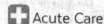 Acute Care 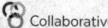 Collaborative 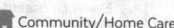 Community/Home Care Cultural

(i.e., before reaching a personal level of tolerance) promotes timely intervention and is more likely to be successful in alleviating pain. Discuss altering drug regimen based on individual needs. **Once established, pain is more difficult to suppress. Increasing dosage, changing medication, or using a stepped program (e.g., switching from injection to oral route, or lengthening time interval between doses) helps in self-management of pain.**

- Educate client and encourage the use of analgesics, as indicated. **Medications may be available in pills, liquids, or suckers to take by mouth, and in injection, skin patch, and suppository forms. Different medications or combinations of drugs may be used, such as opioids/narcotics, nonopioids, and adjuvant medications (e.g., muscle relaxants, anticonvulsants, antidepressants, serotonin and norepinephrine reuptake inhibitors) to manage persistent pain so that client may find relief and increase level of function.** Note: Studies support that people with prolonged intense pain develop tolerance to very high doses of opioids without experiencing adverse side effects. "While that same high dose could be fatal for others, it can control pain and still allow the person to be wide awake enough to do his or her activities of daily living."

- Encourage verbalization of feelings about the pain, such as concern about tolerating pain, anxiety, and pessimistic thoughts, **to evaluate coping abilities and identify areas of additional concern.**

- Provide education and promote nonpharmacological pain management **to obtain comfort, improve healing, and decrease dependency on analgesics, such as:**
  Application of heat or cold
  A quiet environment and calm activities
  Use of relaxation exercises (e.g., progressive muscle relaxation, biofeedback, deep breathing, meditation, yoga, visualization or guided imagery)
  Correct posture/muscle strengthening exercises
  Alternative therapies (e.g., water therapy, electrical stimulation, massage, acupuncture, Therapeutic Touch)
  Supervised physical therapy, multidisciplinary biopsychosocial rehabilitation
  Comfort measures (e.g., back rub, change of position)
  Diversional or distraction activities, such as television and radio, socialization with others, and commercial or individualized tapes (e.g., "white" noise, music, instructional)

Information that appears in brackets has been added by the authors to clarify and enhance the use of nursing diagnoses.

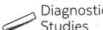 Diagnostic Studies 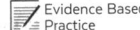 Evidence Based Practice Medications 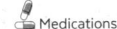 Pediatric/Geriatric/Lifespan

Emotional and social support (e.g., presence of parent during painful procedures to comfort child, family, church visit)

Identification of ways to avoid or minimize pain (e.g., splinting incision during cough, keeping body in good alignment and using proper body mechanics, and resting between activities) **can reduce occurrence of muscle tension or spasms or undue stress on incision.**

- Address medication misuse with client/SO and refer for appropriate counseling or interventions when addiction is known or suspected to be interfering with client's well-being. **Most people (if they do not already have a substance [drug or alcohol] abuse problem) do not become addicted to pain medications even when used on a long-term basis. These individuals will take the pain medications in order to go about the business of their lives. Others may misrepresent their pain levels and their activities in order to obtain pain medications or progressively higher doses of medications, and they require specialized evaluation and interventions.**
- Provide client education to assess for adverse medication effects (e.g., decrease in mental acuity, change in thought processes, confusion or delirium, urinary retention, severe nausea, vomiting, pruritus). **Intolerable symptoms usually require change of medication(s).**
- Educate client/caregiver to notify physician/healthcare provider if pain relief regimen is inadequate **to meet client's pain control goal.**

Nursing Priority No. 4.

To promote improved self-management and pain relief (Teaching/Discharge Considerations) and enhance well-being (long-term goals):

- Acknowledge the pain experience and convey acceptance of client's response to pain. **Reduces defensive responses, promotes trust, and enhances cooperation with regimen.**
- Encourage adequate rest periods **to prevent fatigue that can impair ability to manage or cope with pain.**
- Review nonpharmacological measures for lessening pain. **Relaxation skills and techniques such as self-hypnosis, biofeedback, and Therapeutic Touch have no detrimental side effects.**
- Encourage performance of individualized physical therapy/exercise program. **Promotes active role in preventing muscle spasms or contractures and enhances sense of control.**

Information that appears in brackets has been added by the authors to clarify and enhance the use of nursing diagnoses.

- Discuss ways SO(s) can assist client with pain management. **Family members/SOs may provide assistance by transporting client to prevent walking long distances or by taking on client's strenuous chores, supporting timely pain control, encouraging eating nutritious meals to enhance wellness, and providing gentle massage to reduce muscle tension.**
- Educate client/caregiver regarding specific signs/symptoms and changes in pain requiring evaluation by healthcare provider.
- Encourage client to use positive affirmations (e.g., "I am healing," "I am relaxed," "I love this life"). Have client be aware of internal-external dialogue. Say "cancel" when negative thoughts develop. **Negative thinking can exacerbate feelings of hopelessness, and replacing those thoughts with positive ones can be helpful to pain management.**
- Incorporate desired safe alternative healthcare practices and beliefs into regimen whenever possible **to increase client compliance with pain management treatment plan.**
- Assist client and SO(s) to learn how to heal by developing sense of internal control, by being responsible for own treatment, and by obtaining the information and tools to accomplish this.
- Recommend that client and SO(s) take time for themselves. **Provides opportunity to reenergize and refocus on living/tasks at hand.**
- Identify community support groups and resources to meet individual needs (e.g., emotional support, yard care, home maintenance, Meals on Wheels, transportation). **Proper use of resources may reduce negative pattern of "overdoing" heavy activities and then spending several days in bed recuperating.**
- Refer for counseling (e.g., individual, family, marital therapy, parent effectiveness classes) as needed. **Presence of chronic pain affects all relationships and family dynamics.**
- Refer to NDs impaired family Coping and difficulty Coping.

Documentation Focus

Assessment/Reassessment
- Individual assessment findings, including client's description of response to pain, specifics of pain inventory, expectations of pain management, and acceptable level of pain
- Locus of control and cultural beliefs affecting response to pain
- Prior medication use; substance abuse

Information that appears in brackets has been added by the authors to clarify and enhance the use of nursing diagnoses.

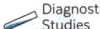 Diagnostic Studies
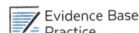 Evidence Based Practice
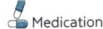 Medications
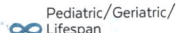 Pediatric/Geriatric/Lifespan

Planning
- Plan of care and who is involved in planning
- Teaching plan

Implementation/Evaluation
- Response to interventions, teaching, and actions performed
- Attainment or progress toward desired outcome(s)
- Modifications to plan of care

Discharge Planning
- Long-term needs, noting who is responsible for actions to be taken
- Specific referrals made

Sample Nursing Outcomes & Interventions Classifications NOC/NIC

NOC—Pain Control
NIC—Pain Management: Acute [or] Chronic

---

impaired PARENTING   ICNP

[Diagnostic Division: Roles/Relationships]

Definition: Primary caregiver fails to foster a loving, encouraging, protective, and supportive environment for optimal growth and development of child.

Recognizing Cues

Related/Risk Factors

Adult

Parental role unclear; deficient parental role modeling; lacks knowledge of child developmental/health needs; adolescent parent

Lacks emotional awareness of self/others; lacks self-confidence

Challenge of managing illness/condition, economic concerns; inadequate sleep-wake cycle

Relocation stress; lack of support; social isolation

Focused on self rather than family/child

Marital conflict/violence; divorce; child maltreatment; separation from child

Depressive symptoms; substance misuse/abuse

Information that appears in brackets has been added by the authors to clarify and enhance the use of nursing diagnoses.

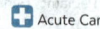 Acute Care   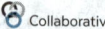 Collaborative   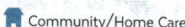 Community/Home Care   Cultural

Child
Major health, developmental, psychological issues
Volatile emotions; uncontrolled anxiety

Defining Characteristics

Subjective
Adult
Frustration; anger
Negative disposition toward child
Social hostility, isolation
Child/Adolescent
Anxiety; feels shame, self-doubt, inferiority
Role confusion; questions self-identity
Somatic complaints; suicidal ideation

Objective
Adult
Limited parent/child interactions; unsatisfactory response to infant's cues; neglects/rejects infant/child
Hostile, or violent parenting methods; impulsive and/or insensitive behaviors; rapid or extreme mood swings
Belittling and disparaging communication
Substance misuse/abuse
Infant
Crying; restlessness; irritability
Nonresponsive to attention/bonding efforts; emotional dysregulation
Child/Adolescent
Lacks trust of others; emotional dysregulation
Behavioral problems; mood swings
Delayed cognitive development; low academic performance; inadequate role development
Poor socialization skills; unable to establish healthy interpersonal relationships
Difficulty controlling weight; depressive symptoms
Somatic complaints
Substance misuse/abuse

Clinical Connections
Prematurity, multiple births, genetic or congenital defects, chronic illness (parent/child), substance misuse/abuse, physical/emotional neglect/abuse, major depression, developmental delay, schizophrenia, bipolar disorder, antisocial, narcissistic and borderline personality disorders

---

Information that appears in brackets has been added by the authors to clarify and enhance the use of nursing diagnoses.

Generate Solutions

Plan Desired Outcomes

Parent/Client Will (Include Specific Time Frame)

- Verbalize knowledge and understanding of how to develop an environment that provides optimal growth and development for child.
- Define a clear role for protecting and supporting child.
- Verbalize value of emotional awareness, and controlling anxiety/mood swings.
- Discuss value of, and participation in classes to improve parenting techniques.
- Identify family members' strengths, need for growth, and where to find community support.

Interventions/Take Action

Nursing Priority No. 1.

To assess causative/contributing factors:

- Note family constellation: nuclear (two-parent), single-parent, extended family (parents living with children, aunts, uncles, or cousins living in same household), stepfamily, or grandparent family. **Helps identify problem areas and strengths to formulate plans to change situation that is currently creating difficulties for the parents.**
- Review type, severity, duration of problem, and contribution of, as well as impact on, individual family members. **Affects choice of interventions; for example, when abuse is the problem, it is an act of commission, whereas neglect is considered an act of omission. These behaviors indicate the presence of problems with relationships and/or parenting skills and individual problems such as inability to deal with stressors, substance abuse, mental illness, cognitive limitations, or criminality.**
- Listen for negative statements about self, child, or other family members, as signs of trauma/failure to thrive, and history of recurring abuse, neglect, unexplained accidents, or chronic health issues. **May reflect physical or psychological abuse or neglect necessitating appropriate actions as legally and professionally indicated if child's safety is a concern. Note: Safety of child is paramount and needs to be dealt with immediately.**
- Determine developmental stage of the family (e.g., new baby, adolescent, child leaving or returning home, parents

---

Information that appears in brackets has been added by the authors to clarify and enhance the use of nursing diagnoses.

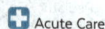 Acute Care 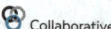 Collaborative 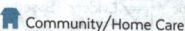 Community/Home Care Cultural

retiring, or death of a child/parent). **These maturational transitions bring changes in the family that can be stressful. Understanding family expectations provides direction for improving parenting skills and family interactions. Note: Important to be sensitive to families experiencing these changes as some may view role transition as a crisis.**

- Assess family relationships between individual members and with others. **These factors are critical to understanding individual family dynamics (e.g., overly connected or disconnected relationships, triangulation: involving child in parental conflict, or scapegoating: unfairly blaming one family member) and developing strategies for change.**
- Assess parenting skill level (e.g., authoritarian, authoritative, permissive, or uninvolved), taking into account the individual's intellectual, emotional, and physical strengths and weaknesses. **Parents with significant impairments may need more education or support. Ineffective parenting and unrealistic expectations contribute to problems of abuse and neglect. Understanding normal responses and progression of developmental milestones can help parents understand and cope with changes.**
- Observe attachment behaviors between parental figure and child, recognizing cultural background. **Failure to bond effectively is thought to affect subsequent parent-child interaction and relationships. Behaviors such as eye-to-eye contact, use of en face position, and talking to the infant in a high-pitched voice are indicative of attachment behaviors in American culture but may not be appropriate in another culture.**
- Identify presence of factors in the child such as unwanted gender, birth defects (e.g., unidentifiable gender, cleft palate), or hyperactivity that may be related to difficulties of parenting. **Unanticipated needs of the child may affect attachment and caretaking needs. Parents have an ideal of what is expected in a child, and when circumstances dictate otherwise, they may experience feelings of sadness and anger.**
- Refer to ND dysfunctional Grief.
- Evaluate physical or mental challenges, educational, or intellectual limitations of parent. **Presence of complicating factors (e.g., visual or hearing impairment, quadriplegia, severe depression, mental illness) may affect ability to**

Information that appears in brackets has been added by the authors to clarify and enhance the use of nursing diagnoses.

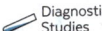 Diagnostic Studies 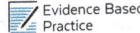 Evidence Based Practice 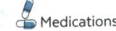 Medications 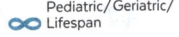 Pediatric/Geriatric/Lifespan

care for a child and indicate need for additional planning to assist the parent.

- Determine presence and effectiveness of support systems, role models, extended family, and community resources available to the parent(s). **Lack of or ineffective use of support systems increases risk of continued inability to parent effectively.**

Nursing Priority No. 2.

To determine level of motivation for improvement:

- Active-listen parents' issues regarding family relationships. **This technique conveys respect and acceptance that enables parent(s) to openly discuss desires, abilities, reasons, and needs to change or deny the current situation as a problem.**
- Determine parent's(s') level of readiness to change parenting behaviors. **Implementing interventions prior to the readiness level of change (e.g., precontemplation: not intending to take action, contemplation: not sure of taking action, preparation: starting to take action) will result in resistance from parent(s).**
- Collaborate with parents to develop realistic goals for family members dependent on the current level of readiness to change. **Individual family member's growth and development is unique requiring different approaches and goals for success.**
- Identify cultural and spiritual influences on parenting, expectations of self/child, and sense of success or failure. **Not considering cultural and spiritual expectations when developing plan of care may be met with resistance because of differences in beliefs. For example, Arab Americans hold children to be sacred, but child-rearing is often based on negative rather than positive reinforcements, and parents are stricter with girls than boys. These beliefs may interfere with the ability to improve parenting skills when there is a conflict between the cultural/spiritual beliefs.**

Nursing Priority No. 3.

To foster development of parenting skills:

- Provide an environment fostering learning to develop parenting skills and relationships. **Learning is more effective when individuals feel safe and free to express feelings and concerns without fear of judgment.**

Information that appears in brackets has been added by the authors to clarify and enhance the use of nursing diagnoses.

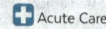 Acute Care 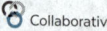 Collaborative 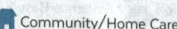 Community/Home Care Cultural

- Active-listen parents' concerns with new or different parenting skill(s). **An open dialogue permits clarity of concepts, enhances learning, and encourages a practical application of skills.**
- Emphasize positive aspects of the family's current situation. **Maintaining a hopeful attitude toward the parent's capabilities and potential for improving the situation will help the parent to manage what is happening more effectively.**
- Encourage expression of feelings, such as helplessness, anger, frustration. **When feelings are expressed openly, they can be acknowledged and dealt with, enabling parent(s) to move forward in dealing with the illness or situation. Individuals may express anger by acting-out behaviors, which need to be restrained before damage is done to self, self-esteem, others, or environment.**
- Acknowledge difficulty of situation and normalcy of feelings. **Individuals feel validated when difficulty is recognized, enhancing feelings of acceptance.**
- Recognize stages of grieving process when the child is disabled or other than anticipated. **Expectation of a "normal" or desired child (e.g., having a girl instead of boy, child with a prominent birthmark or birth defect such as cleft palate) results in grieving for the loss of that expectation.**
- ∞ Provide time for parents to express feelings and deal with the "loss." **Each person grieves at own pace, and allowing this time facilitates the process.**
- Emphasize parenting functions rather than mothering/fathering skills. **By virtue of gender, each person brings something to the parenting role; however, nurturing tasks can be done by both parents.**
- Help parent(s) identify unique temperament(s) of child. **Individual temperament is generally a consistent response to daily living. Appreciating the differences in temperament (e.g., sanguine, choleric, melancholic, phlegmantic) enhances our respect for the diversity and uniqueness of humankind.**
- Assist parent(s) to appropriately respond to emotional or behavioral signals of child/family members. **Nonverbal communication is vital for recognizing congruence and noncongruence of spoken words while body language sends messages.**
- Encourage parents to develop realistic goals for each family member. **Individual family member's growth and development is unique, requiring different approaches**

Information that appears in brackets has been added by the authors to clarify and enhance the use of nursing diagnoses.

 Diagnostic Studies 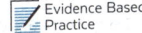 Evidence Based Practice 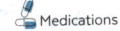 Medications 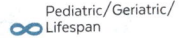 Pediatric/Geriatric/Lifespan

and goals for success. **Using positive discipline is a focus on supporting, encouraging, developing a relationship, problem-solving/decision making, and teaching life skills for success.**
- Provide positive feedback to parent(s) for supporting child's personal growth and development. **Using positive discipline is a focus on supporting, encouraging, developing a relationship, problem-solving/decision making, and teaching life skills for success.**
- Encourage attendance at skill classes, such as parent effectiveness. **Helps parents to develop communication and problem-solving techniques that promote positive relationships between parent and child.**

Nursing Priority No. 4.
To support optimum parenting skills (Teaching/Discharge Considerations) and enhance well-being (long-term goals):
- Involve all available members of the family in learning. **Promotes understanding and effective communication when each individual has the same information and is able to ask questions and clarify what has been heard.**
- Provide information appropriate to the situation, including time management, limit setting, and stress-reduction techniques. **Facilitates satisfactory implementation of plan and new behaviors.**
- Review parental beliefs about child-rearing, punishment, and rewards. **Identifying these beliefs allows opportunity to provide new information regarding not using spanking and/or yelling and what actions can be substituted for more effective parenting.**
- Encourage parents to develop support systems appropriate to the situation. **Engaging extended family, friends, social worker, home-care services may be needed to help parents cope positively with what is happening.**
- Assist parents to plan time and conserve energy in positive ways. **Planning and scheduling for family activities (e.g., family meetings, special time for parent/child activities, doctor, school, therapy appointments, time for self) enables individual to cope more effectively with difficulties as they arise.**
- Encourage parents to identify positive outlets for meeting their own needs. **Going out for dinner or dating and making time for their own interests and each other promotes general well-being and helps reduce burnout.**

Information that appears in brackets has been added by the authors to clarify and enhance the use of nursing diagnoses.

- Refer to appropriate social, support, or therapy groups as indicated. **Underlying issues may interfere with adaptation to situation, and additional support may help individuals to deal more effectively with them.**
- Identify community resources (e.g., child-care services, after-school activities, Boys and Girls Clubs). **Will assist with individual needs to provide respite and support.**
- Report and take necessary actions, as legally and professionally indicated, if child's safety is a concern. **Parents/caregivers who engage in corporal punishment as a technique to ensure desired behavior in a child are at risk for abusive behavior and increase the possibility of childhood depression.**
- Refer to NDs difficulty Coping; impaired family Coping; risk for Other-Directed Violence; Self-Esteem [specific]; and interrupted Family Process for additional interventions as appropriate.

Documentation Focus

Assessment/Reassessment
- Individual findings, including parenting skill level, deviations from normal parenting expectations, family makeup, and developmental stages
- Availability and use of support systems and community resources

Planning
- Plan of care and who is involved in planning
- Teaching plan

Implementation/Evaluation
- Responses by parent(s)/child to interventions, teaching, and actions performed
- Attainment of or progress toward desired outcome(s)
- Modification to plan of care

Discharge Planning
- Long-term needs and who is responsible for actions to be taken
- Specific referrals made

Sample Nursing Outcomes & Interventions Classifications NOC/NIC

NOC—Parenting Performance
NIC—Parenting Promotion

Information that appears in brackets has been added by the authors to clarify and enhance the use of nursing diagnoses.

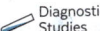 Diagnostic Studies 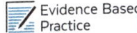 Evidence Based Practice 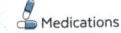 Medications 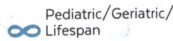 Pediatric/Geriatric/Lifespan

disturbed PERSONAL IDENTITY

ICNP

[Diagnostic Division: Self Perception/Concept]

Definition: disturbed Personal Identity: Personal internal confusion and distress due to a lack of recognizing physical, psychological, interpersonal characteristics, race, ethnicity, or social roles as a part of self.

Recognizing Cues

Related/Risk Factors
Altering social role; goals, beliefs, values, behaviors in constant state of fluctuation
Aging process; serious/chronic medical condition
Stress; trauma; major life changes
Cult indoctrination; impulsive behaviors; emotionally unstable
Abusive, chaotic family history; depression; anxiety; low self-esteem
Gender conflict
Substance misuse/abuse

Defining Characteristics

Subjective
Altered body image
Confusion about cultural and ideological values and goals
Expresses feeling of emptiness, or strangeness; fluctuating feelings about self
Inadequate interpersonal relations; reports social discrimination

Objective
Delusional description of self
Impaired ability to distinguish between internal and external stimuli

Clinical Connections
Traumatic injury (e.g., amputation, spinal cord injury, traumatic brain injury), substance abuse, dementia, schizophrenia, borderline personality disorder, developmental delay, autism, abuse/neglect, gender identity conflict

---

Information that appears in brackets has been added by the authors to clarify and enhance the use of nursing diagnoses.

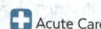 Acute Care 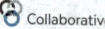 Collaborative 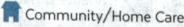 Community/Home Care   Cultural

Generate Solutions

Plan Desired Outcomes

Client Will (Include Specific Time Frame)
- Acknowledge impulsive behaviors and potential threat to identity.
- Identify a set of goals, values, and beliefs guiding the future.
- Describe positive attributes of self.
- Identify strategies to cope with stressful situations.

Interventions/Take Action

Nursing Priority No. 1.
To assess risk/contributing factors:

- Assess mental health and threat to self. **Many factors can impinge on client's life and cause concern about possibility of changes that will make life different. A comprehensive psychiatric assessment will be needed to understand contributing factors to an identity disorder (e.g., childhood trauma, abuse/neglect, adverse life events, attachment problems, or interpersonal conflicts).**
- Identify history of family conflict or abuse. **Chaotic family relationships can contribute to Borderline Personality Disorder that shows signs of identity disturbance.**
- Identify client extensive use of defense mechanisms. **Client extensively uses defense mechanisms to protect their ego and image. Using coping strategies would indicate the client is attempting to accept self as they are.**
- Ask client to define their body image. **The basis of personal identity is body image, and perception of changes may affect client's view in a negative or positive manner.**
- Determine whether issues of gender identity are a concern. **Client may have conflicting feelings about how to deal with realization of an incongruence between sex assigned at birth and their gender identity.**
- Note age of individual. **Changes affect persons differently depending on their stage of life. The maturational changes of adolescence may generally be viewed as positive, while the older person may view aging changes in a negative way.**
- Identify cultural affiliations/discontinuity. **Individuals belonging to subcultures or cults tend to come into conflict with the greater societal views affecting one's perception of self and perception of reality, often resulting**

Information that appears in brackets has been added by the authors to clarify and enhance the use of nursing diagnoses.

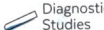 Diagnostic Studies 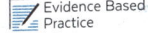 Evidence Based Practice 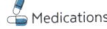 Medications 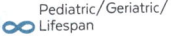 Pediatric/Geriatric/Lifespan

in isolation from outside support groups and reluctance to engage in therapeutic interventions.
- Determine type and speed of changes that are imminent. **The diagnosis of a chronic illness, such as diabetes, versus a terminal illness or a traumatic injury or disfiguring surgery that will change how life is lived, may be threatening, as the thought of how different life will be affects the individual.**
- Ask client to identify goals, values, and beliefs that guide their life and if they have changed periodically. **Compare and contrast the changes in the value system. Clients lacking a sense of self may be struggling with their goals, values, and beliefs and consistently and drastically changing them.**
- Note availability and use of support systems, including attitude of family/significant others. **Having a positive support system can help individual get through difficult situations/illness; however, lack of family support can add to level of distress. Client/family conflict with client's constant changing of thoughts, beliefs, behaviors, or presentation of self can result in isolating from each other.**
- Identify the use of defense mechanism client uses to protect their self-image. **The use of defense mechanisms is common with clients attempting to self-identify and with clients with Borderline Personality Disorder.**
- Assess behaviors such as withdrawal, general behavioral disorganization, and delayed development. **Poor coping skills will affect how client copes with possibility of disturbance in personal identity by changes occurring in life.**
- Note withdrawn or automatic behavior, regression to earlier developmental stage, general behavioral disorganization, or display of self-mutilation behaviors in adolescent or adult, and delayed development, preference for solitary play, and unusual display of self-stimulation in child. **Indicators of poor coping skills and need for specific interventions to help client develop sense of self and identity. Inability to identify self interferes with interactions with others.**
- Discuss use of alcohol and/or other substances. **Individuals often use these substances to avoid painful stressors.**
- Be aware of physical signs of panic state (e.g., heart palpitations, trembling, shortness of breath, chest pressure or pain). **Use of inadequate strategies to cope with changes affecting lifestyle may result in exacerbation of symptoms in anxious client. Presence of severe anxiety state may**

Information that appears in brackets has been added by the authors to clarify and enhance the use of nursing diagnoses.

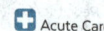 Acute Care 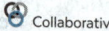 Collaborative 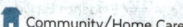 Community/Home Care Cultural

progress to panic when concerns seem overwhelming to client. (Refer to ND Anxiety.)

- Determine presence of hallucinations, delusions, or distortions of reality/symptoms of mental illness. **Indicators of psychosis and need for immediate interventions (e.g., antipsychotic medications) to manage disorganized thoughts.**

Nursing Priority No. 2.
To assist client to manage/cope with stressors:

- Develop a nurse/client relationship. **A therapeutic nurse–client relationship is built on honesty, respect, and valuing the client as a worthy individual.**
- Listen/active-listen, making time to encourage client to express feelings, including anger and hostility. **Conveys a sense of confidence in client's ability to identify extent of threat, how it is affecting sense of identity, and how to cope with feelings in acceptable ways. Possibility of changes in life may affect sense of self and identity. A chaotic/abusive/stressful life may be a contributing factor.**
- Speak softly and calmly, stand in a nonthreatening (e.g., open hands at side, or in front of body) stance when client is irritated to help de-escalate the situation. **May be necessary to help client restore equilibrium when situation escalates because they feel at risk or threatened.**
- Maintain reality orientation without confronting client's irrational beliefs. **Irrational beliefs may interfere with ability to manage situation and maintain reality-based perception of self. Client may become defensive, blocking opportunity to look at other possibilities. Arguing does not change the perceptions and can interfere with or damage nurse–client relationship.**
- Encourage client and family to maintain a calm environment and positive attitude. **Anxiety is contagious and can interfere with client's efforts to maintain control and cope with the situation. Discuss parenting styles, family roles, responsibilities, and communication patterns to help develop positive attitudes and a calm home environment.**
- Discuss client's commitment to an identity. **Those who have made a strong commitment to an identity tend to be more comfortable with self and happier than those who have not.**
- Assist client to develop strategies to cope with threat to identity. **Reduces anxiety, promotes self-awareness, and**

Information that appears in brackets has been added by the authors to clarify and enhance the use of nursing diagnoses.

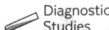 Diagnostic Studies 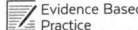 Evidence Based Practice 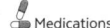 Medications 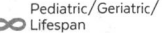 Pediatric/Geriatric/Lifespan

enhances self-esteem, enabling client to deal with threat more realistically.
- Provide for simple decisions, concrete tasks, and calming activities. **Promotes sense of control and positive expectations to enable client to regain sense of self.**
- Allow client to cope with situation in small steps. **May have difficulty coping with larger picture when in stress overload. Taking small steps promotes feelings of success and ability to manage illness or situation.**
- Help client to identify strategies to cope with current situation/possibility of threat. **Having a plan to enhance coping strategies can reduce anxiety and promote self-esteem.**
- Provide groups and activities applicable for client's situation. **For example, the viewing of body part/using a mirror for visual feedback or tactile stimulation to reconnect with parts of the body (i.e., amputation) or participation in monitored social interactions helps client to confront fear and see self as an individual who is still worthwhile. Therapy groups for Borderline Personality Disorders are found to be effective with behavioral changes.**
- Collaborate with client in making decisions and plans for the future. **Provides opportunity for client to feel in control and promotes positive expectations while at the same time the nurse can give suggestions for improvement.**
- Develop an individualized exercise program. **Releases endorphins, reducing stress and promoting a sense of well-being.**
- Provide concrete assistance as needed. **Until basic-level needs, such as activities of daily living and food, are met, individual is unable to cope with higher-level needs. Once these needs are met, client can begin to cope with threat to identity.**
- Take advantage of opportunities to provide information to promote growth. **Alterations in mental status can interfere with ability to process information, and new information can increase confusion and disorientation.**
- Refer to NDs disturbed Body Image, Self-Esteem (specify), and impaired Spiritual Well-being for additional interventions as appropriate.

Nursing Priority No. 3.

To promote self-identity (Teaching/Discharge Considerations) and enhance well-being (long-term goals):

- Provide accurate information/resources for issues client is concerned about. **Worrying about what might happen is counterproductive to coping with reality, and**

Information that appears in brackets has been added by the authors to clarify and enhance the use of nursing diagnoses.

information can help to lessen anxiety, allowing individual to cope with current situation.
- Discuss potential changes in lifestyle that may occur with major diagnosis/accident, gender-affirming procedure. **Planning for these possibilities can enhance self-confidence and allow client to move forward with life. A diagnosis, accident, etc., can require major life changes, such as wearing identification bracelet when prone to mental confusion, a new lifestyle to accommodate change of gender for transgender client, or a diet and medication routine with the diagnosis of diabetes mellitus.**
- Refer to appropriate support groups. **Sharing concerns with others in group settings may help client to be realistic regarding concerns about effects of anticipated changes/life challenges.**
- Explore community resources, as appropriate. **Additional assistance such as day programs, individual/family counseling, and drug/alcohol-cessation programs can strengthen client's coping abilities and sense of control.**

Documentation Focus

Assessment/Reassessment
- Findings, noting degree of impairment or possible changes in lifestyle, and future expectations
- Nature of and client's perception of threat or potential threat
- Degree of commitment to own identity

Planning
- Plan of care and who is involved in the planning
- Teaching plan

Implementation/Evaluation
- Client's response to interventions/teaching and actions performed
- Attainment of or progress toward desired outcome(s)
- Modifications to plan of care

Discharge Planning
- Long-term needs and who is responsible for actions to be taken
- Specific referrals made

Sample Nursing Outcomes & Interventions Classifications NOC/NIC

NOC—Personal Identity
NIC—Self-Esteem Enhancement

Information that appears in brackets has been added by the authors to clarify and enhance the use of nursing diagnoses.

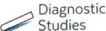 Diagnostic Studies 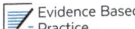 Evidence Based Practice 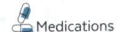 Medications 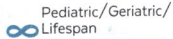 Pediatric/Geriatric/Lifespan

risk for POISONING   ICNP

[Diagnostic Division: Safety]

Definition: Susceptible to injury or death after inadvertent or intentional consumption/exposure to toxic substances.

Recognizing Cues

Risk Factors

External Factors:
Access/exposure to unsafe substances; unsafe storage of toxic substances
Access to illicit drugs, drugs contaminated by poisonous additives
Access to pharmaceutical preparations; polypharmacy
Intentional use of multiple supplements (i.e., megadosing)
Occupational exposure; occupational environment with inadequate safeguards
Inadequate discharge education

Internal Factors:
Neurobehavioral manifestations (e.g., cognitive dysfunction; behavioral disorders; impulse control impairment)
Psychological/emotional discontent
Inadequate knowledge of pharmaceutical preparations, or poisoning prevention
Poor vision

Clinical Connections
Substance abuse, dementia, cataracts, glaucoma, hepatitis, cirrhosis, renal failure, depression, suicidal ideation, developmental delay

Generate Solutions

Plan Desired Outcomes

Client Will (Include Specific Time Frame)
- Verbalize understanding of dangers of poisoning.
- Identify hazards that could lead to accidental poisoning.
- Correct external hazards as identified.
- Demonstrate necessary actions/lifestyle changes to promote safe environment.

Refer to ND Contamination Exposure for additional interventions related to poisoning associated with environmental contaminants.

Information that appears in brackets has been added by the authors to clarify and enhance the use of nursing diagnoses.

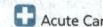 Acute Care   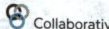 Collaborative   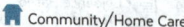 Community/Home Care   Cultural

Interventions/Take Action

Nursing Priority No. 1.
To assess causative/contributing factors:

- Identify internal and external risk factors in client's environment, including presence of infants, young children, or frail elderly (**who are at risk for accidental poisoning**) and teenagers or young adults (**who are at risk for substance experimentation**); confused or chronically ill client on multiple medications; client with potential for suicidal action; client who partakes in illicit drug use/dealing (e.g., opioids, cocaine, heroin); person who manufactures drugs in home (e.g., meth).
- Note client's age, gender, socioeconomic status, developmental stage, decision-making ability, level of cognition, and competence **to identify individuals who could be at higher risk for accidental poisoning. These factors affect client's ability to protect self/others and influence choice of interventions/teaching.**
- Determine client's allergies to medications and foods **in order to avoid exposure to substances causing potentially lethal reaction.**
- Assess mood, coping abilities, personality styles (e.g., temperament, impulsive behavior, level of self-esteem) **that may result in carelessness/increased risk taking without consideration of consequences or suicidal actions.** (Refer to ND risk for Suicide.)
- Assess client's knowledge of safe use of drugs/herbal supplements, safety hazards in the environment, and ability to respond to potential threat. **People may believe "if a little is good, a lot is better," placing them at risk for overdose, adverse drug effects (ADEs), or interactions. Knowledge and use also affect the client's storage (e.g., may not use labeled bottles) and/or taking of medications that look alike (potentiating risk of overdose or adverse drug interactions). The elderly may unintentionally take the wrong medication at the wrong time or "double up," forgetting that they already took their daily dose of a prescription medicine.**
- Determine client's *specific* drug hazards:
- Use of prescription, over-the-counter (OTC) medications and culturally based home remedies. **These have potential for intentional and accidental overdose, as well as dangerous interactions. Note: In 2021, similarities in drug name (and color) of daily medications were**

Information that appears in brackets has been added by the authors to clarify and enhance the use of nursing diagnoses.

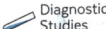 Diagnostic Studies 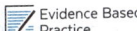 Evidence Based Practice 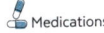 Medications 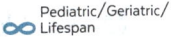 Pediatric/Geriatric/Lifespan

implicated in a large number of unintentional poisonings or ADEs among the elderly.

Availability or regular use of vitamins, minerals, and herbal supplements. **Vitamins (especially A and D) are toxic in large doses, and iron is especially harmful, often fatal to children. Herbal drugs can be a source of poisoning (usually when taken long term) due to toxicity of individual ingredients or from contaminants (e.g., mercury, lead, arsenic).**

Abuse of alcohol or other drugs (e.g., cocaine, methamphetamine, lysergic acid diethylamide, methadone). **Those who abuse street drugs are at high risk for overdose because the purity of these drugs is largely unknown. These substances have potential for adverse reactions, cumulative effects with other substances, and risk for intentional and accidental overdose.**

- Identify environmental hazards:

Storage of household chemicals (e.g., oven, toilet bowl, or drain cleaners; dishwasher products; bleach; hydrogen peroxide; fluoride preparations; essential oils; furniture polish; lighter fluid; lamp oil; kerosene; paints; turpentine; rust remover; lubricant oils; bug sprays or powders; fertilizers). **These products are readily available toxins in various forms that are often improperly stored.**

Review client's home, employment, or work environment **for exposure to chemicals, including vapors and fumes.**

Refer to ND Contamination Exposure and risk for Contamination for environmental issues.

- Review results of laboratory tests and toxicology screening, as indicated. **Guides treatment when overdose or accidental poisoning is known or suspected.**

Nursing Priority No. 2.

To assist in correcting factors that can lead to accidental poisoning:

- Discuss medication safety with client/significant other(s) (SO[s]) **to prevent accidental poisoning:**

Emphasize importance of supervising infant, child, frail elderly, or client with developmental/cognitive limitations.

Keep medicines and supplements out of sight and reach of children or cognitively impaired clients.

Review with client/caregivers medications with similar color or shape, and brainstorm ways to safely identify them in home medication boxes.

Information that appears in brackets has been added by the authors to clarify and enhance the use of nursing diagnoses.

Emphasize environmental safety regarding medications for all situations in which young child may be exposed (e.g., all rooms of the home, grandparents' home, day care, preschool).

Use child-resistant or tamper-resistant caps and lock medication cabinets.

Recap medication containers immediately after obtaining current dosage. Do not leave open container out.

Code medicines for the visually impaired.

Instruct client to turn on light if the room is dark and to put on glasses (if visually impaired) before taking or giving medications.

Refer to/administer children's medications as drugs/medicine, not candy.

Emphasize environmental safety regarding medications for all situations in which a young child may be exposed (e.g., all rooms of the home, grandparents' home, day care, preschool).

Discuss vitamin/supplement use (especially those containing iron) **that can be poisonous to children if taken in large doses or in small doses over time.**

- **Prevent duplication or possible overdose:**

Review analgesic safety (e.g., opioids; acetaminophen [ingredient in many OTC medications, and unintentional overdose can occur]).

Keep an updated list of all medications (prescription, OTC, herbals, supplements) and review with healthcare providers when medications are changed, new ones added, or new healthcare providers are consulted.

Keep prescription medication in the original bottle with label intact. Do not mix with other medication or place in unmarked containers.

Have responsible SO/home health nurse supervise medication regimen/prepare medications for the cognitively or visually impaired client, or obtain prefilled medication box from pharmacy.

Take prescription medications and OTC drugs as prescribed on label.

Do not adjust medication dosage except with direction of the provider.

Retain and read safety information that accompanies prescriptions about expected effects, minor side effects, reportable or adverse effects that require medical intervention, and how to manage forgotten doses.

Information that appears in brackets has been added by the authors to clarify and enhance the use of nursing diagnoses.

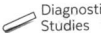 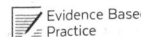

- **Avoid taking medications that interact with one another or OTCs, herbals, or other supplements in an undesired or dangerous manner:**

  Keep a list of medication allergies, including type of reaction, and submit to healthcare providers/pharmacist.

  Wear medical alert bracelet or necklace, as appropriate.

  Do not take outdated or expired medications. Do not save partial prescriptions to use another time.

  Encourage discarding outdated or unused drug safely (disposing in hazardous waste collection areas, not down drain or toilet).

  Do not take medications prescribed for another person.

  Avoid mixing alcohol with medications (**may potentiate effects of many drugs or cause client injury**).

  Coordinate care when multiple healthcare providers are involved **to limit number of prescriptions and dosage levels.**

Nursing Priority No. 3.

To promote client knowledge and safety (Teaching/Discharge Considerations) and enhance well-being (long-term goals):

- Discuss general poison prevention measures:

  Encourage parent/caregiver to place safety stickers on dangerous products (drugs and chemicals) **to warn children of harmful contents.**

  Teach children about the hazards of poisonous substances and to "ask first" before eating or drinking anything.

  Review drug side effects, potential interactions, and possibilities of misuse or overdosing (as with vitamin megadosing, etc.). **Note: Vitamins (especially those containing iron) can be poisonous or lethal to children.**

  Discuss issues regarding drug use in home (e.g., alcohol, marijuana, opioids, heroin) **to provide opportunity to address potential for client's/SO's accidental overdose or accidental ingestion by children when drugs or drug paraphernalia are in the home.**

  Provide list of emergency numbers (i.e., local or national poison control numbers, physician's office) to be placed by telephone **for use if poisoning occurs.**

  Encourage client to obtain regular screening tests at prescribed intervals (e.g., international normalized ratio [INR] for Coumadin; drug levels for Dilantin, digoxin; liver function studies when lipid-lowering agents [statins] are prescribed; or renal and thyroid function and serum glucose levels for antimanics [lithium] use) **to ascertain**

Information that appears in brackets has been added by the authors to clarify and enhance the use of nursing diagnoses.

that circulating blood levels are within therapeutic range and absence of adverse effects.
- Discuss with healthcare provider/pharmacist any considered medications if pregnant, nursing, or planning to become pregnant, **as some drugs are dangerous to fetus or nursing infant.**
- Refer substance abuser to detoxification programs, inpatient/outpatient rehabilitation, counseling, support groups, psychotherapy, as appropriate.
- Encourage participation in community awareness and education programs (e.g., cardiopulmonary resuscitation and first aid class, home and workplace safety, hazardous materials and old medications disposal, access emergency medical personnel) **to assist individuals to identify and correct risk factors in client's environment and be prepared for emergency situation.**

Documentation Focus

Assessment/Reassessment
- Identified risk factors noting internal and external concerns
- Drug allergies or sensitivities
- Current medications prescribed or available to individual, use of OTC medications, herbals or supplements, illicit drug use

Planning
- Plan of care and who is involved in the planning
- Teaching plan, including how to be safe with habitual medications, added/new/deleted medications; substances and environmental hazards

Implementation/Evaluation
- Response to interventions, teaching, and actions performed
- Attainment of or progress toward desired outcome(s)
- Modification to plan of care

Discharge Planning
- Long-term needs and who is responsible for actions to be taken
- Specific referrals made

Sample Nursing Outcomes & Interventions Classifications NOC/NIC

NOC—Knowledge: Medication
NIC—Medication Management

Information that appears in brackets has been added by the authors to clarify and enhance the use of nursing diagnoses.

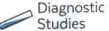 Diagnostic Studies
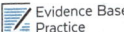 Evidence Based Practice
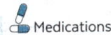 Medications
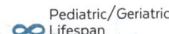 Pediatric/Geriatric/Lifespan

POST-TRAUMA SYNDROME   NANDA-I

[Diagnostic Division: Stress Management]

Definition: Post-Trauma Syndrome: Sustained maladaptive response to a traumatic, overwhelming event.

Definition: A chronic intense and emotional response to a past traumatic/overwhelming event that may reoccur with a reminder/memory of the original trauma/event.

Recognizing Cues

Risk/Related Factors
Diminished ego strength
Environment not conducive to needs; inadequate social support network
Exaggerated sense of responsibility

Defining Characteristics (Post-Trauma Syndrome)

Subjective
Excessive anxiety; excessive fear
Ineffective sleep pattern

Objective
Maladaptive coping; impaired decision making
Inadequate self-compassion; impaired resilience
Impaired mood regulation; disrupted thought processes
Impaired sexual function
NOTE:
[Stages:
Acute: Begins within 6 mo and does not last longer than 6 mo
Chronic: Lasts more than 6 mo
Delayed Onset: Period of latency of 6 mo or more before onset of symptoms]

Clinical Connections
Traumatic injuries, physical/psychological abuse, dissociative disorder, depression

---

Information that appears in brackets has been added by the authors to clarify and enhance the use of nursing diagnoses.

Generate Solutions

Plan Desired Outcomes

Client Will (Include Specific Time Frame)

- Express own feelings or reactions, avoiding projection, denial, or undoing.
- Verbalize a positive self-image.
- Report absence of severe anxiety, or reduced level of anxiety or fear when memories occur.
- Demonstrate ability to cope with emotional reactions appropriately.
- Demonstrate appropriate changes in behavior and lifestyle (e.g., share experiences with those who need to know, seek or get support from significant others [SO(s)] as needed, or change job or residence).
- Report relief or absence of physical manifestations (pain, nightmares or flashbacks, fatigue) associated with event.

Nursing Priority No. 1.
To assess causative factor(s) and individual reaction:

Acute

- Identify client who experienced or witnessed a traumatic event (e.g., sexual assault, robbery at gunpoint, motor vehicle or airplane crash, mass shooting or rioting, fire destroying home, war or violent act). **If event involved loss or injury of loved ones, as well as self, individual is at risk for post-traumatic syndrome.**
- Review informational resources such as police/ambulance/ eyewitnesses/previous medical records if available. **Helpful in determining specifics/duration of precipitating event(s) impacting client to aid in preparing for initial interview with client.**
- Note occupation (e.g., police, fire, emergency responders/ rescue workers, healthcare providers, soldiers, support personnel in combat areas, and family members). **Studies reveal a moderate to high percentage of post-traumatic stress (PTS) cases develop in these populations when they have been exposed to one or more traumatic incidents and their exposure lasts over longer periods of time (e.g., working a plane crash, healthcare worker in pandemic, survivor of abuse/torture). In addition, family members are also at risk because they are subjected to the same trauma as they see the events repeated on TV**

Information that appears in brackets has been added by the authors to clarify and enhance the use of nursing diagnoses.

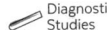 Diagnostic Studies   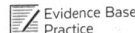 Evidence Based Practice   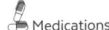 Medications   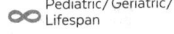 Pediatric/Geriatric/Lifespan

news channels/hear stories repeated by their loved one(s) who were directly involved.
- Encourage client to share their story as able. **Sharing their story verbally (or through role-play, depending on client's age) provides a more personal picture of how client views the event and what may be most important to them.**
- Observe and elicit information regarding physical/somatic complaints (e.g., numbness, headache, tightness in chest, nausea, pounding heart). Investigate reports of symptoms, reactivation or changes in symptoms. Refer for further evaluation as appropriate. **Anxiety is viewed as a normal reaction to a realistic danger or threat, and noting these factors can suggest the severity of the anxiety the client is currently experiencing. In PTS response, this reaction is changed or damaged. The client may feel stressed or frightened even when they are no longer in danger. Physical symptoms (e.g., gastric irritation, anorexia, insomnia, muscle tension, headache), neurobehavioral manifestations (e.g., depression, trouble concentrating, impaired motor skills, diminished memory) may accompany disorganization and need further evaluation and interventions.**
- Assess client's risk for developing PTS using screening tool (e.g., Breslau Short Screening Scale, neurobehavioral symptom inventory [NSI], Trauma Screening Questionnaire [TSQ]). **Short self-report questionnaire or other screening tool helps with early identification of client at risk for post-trauma response. Quantifying client's risk is a first step toward providing timely and appropriate treatment and possibly preventing the development of maladaptive responses.**
- Identify such psychological responses as anger, aggression, shock, acute anxiety, confusion, and denial. Note laughter, crying, calm or agitated, excited (hysterical) behavior, as well as expressions of disbelief, guilt and/or self-blame, and labile emotions. **Indicators of severe response to trauma that client has experienced and need for specific interventions (e.g., quiet room, medications such as Ativan, Benadryl, and Haldol as chemical restraint, and if necessary, a physical restraint to prevent harm to self or others).**
- Assess client's knowledge of and anxiety related to the situation (e.g., shooting in line of duty or viewing body of murdered child); if client is able to respond logically and

---

Information that appears in brackets has been added by the authors to clarify and enhance the use of nursing diagnoses.

coherently, determine the number, duration, and intensity of recurring situations (e.g., emergency medical technician exposed to numerous on-the-job traumatic incidents; rescuers searching for victims of disasters). Note ongoing threat to self or others. **Having information about these situations enables individuals to think about and plan for eventualities so anxiety can be dealt with in a positive manner. Client may be nonverbal or aware but speaks as though the incident just happened or is related to someone else. Flashbacks may occur with the individual reliving the incident/event. Client may require physical/chemical restraint if perceives others as threatening harm or feels hopeless about situation.**

- Identify social aspects of trauma or incident (e.g., disfigurement, chronic conditions or permanent disabilities, loss of home or community) that affect ability to return to normal involvement in activities and work. **Client may feel embarrassed or guilty of their present situation, causing them to socially isolate from family or friends.**
- Identify ethnic background, cultural and spiritual perceptions, and beliefs about the occurrence. **Client (or SOs) may believe occurrence is retribution from God or result of some indiscretion on client's part; client may in some way also blame self for the incident or occurrence. Individual's view of how they are coping may be influenced by cultural and community background, religious beliefs, and family influence. Note: Some research shows that in certain cultures, people do not voluntarily seek mental help for fear of stigmatization in their communities and will likely be resistant to treatment. One multicultural study (2017) showed that European Americans see mental illness in terms of biomedical illness, whereas Latin and African American cultures focus more on spirituality, moral character, and social rationale for mental illness.**
- Identify how client's experiences may affect current situation. **Individual who has had previous experiences with traumatic events (e.g., victim of violence, natural/man-made disasters; first responder, individual who deals with trauma on a regular basis) may be more susceptible to post-trauma syndrome and ineffective coping abilities.**
- Determine degree of disorganization (e.g., task-oriented activity is not goal directed, organized, or effective; individual is overwhelmed by emotion much of the time). **Presence of persistent frightening thoughts and memories, reliving**

Information that appears in brackets has been added by the authors to clarify and enhance the use of nursing diagnoses.

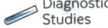 Diagnostic Studies 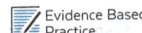 Evidence Based Practice 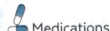 Medications 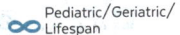 Pediatric/Geriatric/Lifespan

the event, feeling emotionally numb and unable to be close to friends and family members, and suffering from sleep and eating problems that interfere with ability to manage daily living, work, and relationships with others.

- Note verbal and nonverbal expressions of guilt or self-blame. Listen for comments of humiliation, shame, or taking on responsibility, especially when client has survived trauma in which others died (e.g., "I should have been more careful/gone back to get her"; "Don't call me a hero; I should have done more"). **Sense of own responsibility (blame) and guilt about not having been "good enough" to deserve surviving are strong beliefs, especially in individuals who are influenced by family background, religious, and cultural factors. Expressing guilt for actions that individual might have taken can lead to ruminations about lack of responsible behavior, leading to anxiety and post-trauma syndrome.**
- Identify whether incident has reactivated preexisting or coexisting situations (physical or psychological). **Cumulative effects of multiple events can put the individual at higher risk for developing post-trauma syndrome and indicate need for preventive measures to be taken. Traumas or difficulties in client's life and how they were dealt with will affect how the client views the current trauma.**
- Identify client's past coping mechanisms and compare with those currently used. **Resolution of the effects of the trauma is largely dependent on the coping skills the client has developed throughout own life and is able to bring to bear on current situation. Additionally, resilience factors (e.g., having a way of getting through the bad event and learning from it or being able to act and respond effectively despite feeling fear) can facilitate recovery.**
- Note withdrawn behavior, use of denial, and use of chemical substances or impulsive behaviors (e.g., chain smoking, overeating, gambling, aggression). **Indicators of the severity of anxiety and client's difficulty coping with PTS and need for interventions to address behaviors.**
- Be aware of signs of increasing anxiety (e.g., silence, stuttering, inability to sit still). **Increasing anxiety may indicate risk for violence or need for medication or other measures to decrease anxiety and help client manage feelings.**
- Assess signs and stage of client's grieving for self and others. **Identification and understanding of stages of grief**

Information that appears in brackets has been added by the authors to clarify and enhance the use of nursing diagnoses.

assist with choice of interventions, plan of care, and movement toward resolution.
- Determine disruptions in relationships (e.g., family, friends, coworkers, SOs). **Support persons may not know how to deal with client/situation and may be oversolicitous or withdraw; either of these actions will be counterproductive to client's ability to cope with situation.**
- Identify support persons (e.g., loved ones, spiritual advisor/priest or pastor/rabbi/imam). **Having unconditional support from loving and caring others can help the client cope with the situation and move on to live more fully.**
- Determine availability and helpfulness of client's support systems, family, social, community, etc., being aware that family members themselves or community in general may also be at risk. **Having an effective available support system and talking with them about what is happening can help client and family members resolve feelings and move on with life in a positive manner.**
- Identify development of phobic reactions to ordinary articles (e.g., knives) and situations (e.g., walking in groups of people, strangers ringing doorbell). **These may trigger feelings from original trauma and need to be dealt with sensitively, accepting reality of feelings and stressing ability of client to deal with them.**
- Assess client's level of trauma response using screening tool (e.g., SPAN [evaluating responses of startle, physically upset by reminders, anger, and numbness], Trauma Screening Questionnaire [TSQ]). **Short self-report questionnaire or other screening tool suggests presence of post-trauma response requiring a structured interview by a mental health professional.**

Chronic (in addition to previous assessment)

- Evaluate continued somatic symptoms and reports of new or changes in symptoms. **Reports of physical symptoms, such as gastric irritation, anorexia, insomnia, muscle tension, and headache may accompany disorganization and need further evaluation and interventions.**
- Note manifestations of chronic pain or pain symptoms in excess of degree of physical injury. **Psychological responses may magnify or exacerbate physical symptoms, indicating need for interventions to help client deal with pain.**
- Be aware of signs of severe or prolonged depression and note presence of flashbacks, intrusive memories, nightmares,

---

Information that appears in brackets has been added by the authors to clarify and enhance the use of nursing diagnoses.

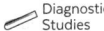 Diagnostic Studies 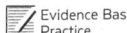 Evidence Based Practice 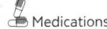 Medications 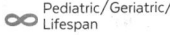 Pediatric/Geriatric/Lifespan

panic attacks, and poor impulse control; problems with memory or concentration; thoughts and perceptions; and conflict, aggression, or rage. **Symptoms are not uncommon following a trauma of such magnitude, although client may feel that they are "going crazy."**

- Assess degree of dysfunctional coping (including substance use or abuse, suicidal ideation) and consequences of their actions. **Identifies needs and depth of interventions required. Individuals display different levels of dysfunctional behavior in response to stress, and often the choice of chemical substances or substance abuse is a way of deadening the psychic pain.** Refer to ND risk for Suicide.
- Identify client's readiness to change dysfunctional behaviors for a healthier approach to PTS. **Attempting to apply interventions prior to the client's readiness (e.g., precontemplation, contemplation, preparation, action, or maintenance) is met with resistance.**

Nursing Priority No. 2.

To assist client to cope with situation that exists post-trauma:

Acute

- Develop nurse/client therapeutic relationship. **Nurse–client relationships are built on honesty, trust, and respect by the nurse, thus allowing the client to feel comfortable and confident sharing their thoughts and feelings so the nurse can assist them with recovery.**
- Provide a calm and safe environment. **Client can cope with disruption of life more effectively when surrounded by quiet and by knowing they are safe.**
- Stay with the client of sexual assault while police collect their data and during the exams by the Sexual Assault Nurse Examiner (SANE). **Being available to support and comfort the client can help maintain a calm and safe environment for the client.**
- Listen to and investigate physical complaints. **Initially, client may not verbalize physical injuries that may have occurred during the event/accident, which may be masked by emotional reactions and limit client's ability to recognize pain or discomfort. These need to be addressed and differentiated from anxiety symptoms for appropriate treatment to begin.**
- Discuss client's thoughts, feelings, behaviors, and currently or recently occurring stressors client is contending with, such as displacement from home due to catastrophic event or individual who suffered abuse as a child or whose own

---

Information that appears in brackets has been added by the authors to clarify and enhance the use of nursing diagnoses.

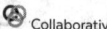 Acute Care 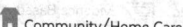 Collaborative Community/Home Care 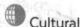 Cultural

child is dying of cancer. **Client's cumulative effects of multiple events may indicate a need for medications (e.g., antidepressants, antianxiety, or antipsychotic), as well as psychological interventions (e.g., mindfulness, medication, counseling/therapy) to help with coping.**

- Allow the client to work through adjustment based on their needs. If the client is withdrawn or unwilling to talk, do not force the issue. **Each person is an individual and has own ways of coping. Being there and allowing client to choose own path conveys sense of confidence in ability to cope with situation.**
- Listen for expressions of fear of crowds or people. **May indicate continuing anxiety and difficulty reentering normal activities.**
- Determine or monitor sleep pattern of children as well as adults. **Sleep disturbances or nightmares may develop, delaying resolution, impairing coping abilities, and interfering with return to desired lifestyle.**
- Be aware of and assist client to use their strengths in a positive way by acknowledging ability to handle what has happened or is happening. **Enhances self-esteem and reduces sense of helplessness and powerlessness, thus enabling client to move on with life.**
- Encourage client to learn stress-management techniques, such as mindfulness, deep breathing, meditation, relaxation, and exercise. **Reduces stress, enhancing coping skills and helping to resolve situation.**
- Assist client in coping with practical concerns and effects of the incident, such as court appearances, altered relationships with SO(s), and employment problems. **In the period immediately following the traumatic incident, individual is in a state of numbness and shock. Thinking becomes difficult, and assistance with practical matters will help manage necessary activities for the person to move through this time.**
- Administer antianxiety or sedative and hypnotic medications with caution. **Client with a history of substance misuse/abuse may relapse, resulting in overuse. Selective serotonin reuptake inhibitors (SSRIs) may help with PTS symptoms such as fear, worry, anger and may help with sleep problems and nightmares.**

Chronic

- Provide emotional and physical presence to strengthen client's coping abilities. **Client with a history of substance**

Information that appears in brackets has been added by the authors to clarify and enhance the use of nursing diagnoses.

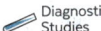 Diagnostic Studies 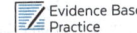 Evidence Based Practice 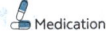 Medications 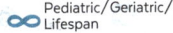 Pediatric/Geriatric/Lifespan

misuse/abuse may relapse, resulting in overuse. **Selective serotonin reuptake inhibitors (SSRIs) may help with PTS symptoms such as fear, worry, anger and may help with sleep problems and nightmares.**

- Continue listening to expressions of concern. **May have recurring symptoms, thus necessitating the need to continue talking about the incident.**
- Permit free expression of feelings (may continue from the crisis phase). Do not rush client through expressions of feelings too quickly and refrain from providing false reassurances (e.g., everything will be fine). **May have recurring symptoms, thus necessitating the need to continue talking about the incident.**
- Encourage client to talk out experience when ready, expressing feelings of fear, anger, loss, or grief. (Refer to ND Grief or dysfunctional Grieving.) **Client may need to repeat story over and over and needs to be accepted and assured that feelings are normal for the unusual event experienced.**
- Determine if feelings expressed appear congruent with events the client experienced. **Expressing feelings helps client recognize and identify them to enhance coping. Incongruency may indicate deeper conflict that can impede resolution.**
- Encourage client to become aware and accepting of own feelings and reactions as being normal reactions in an abnormal situation. **There are no "bad" feelings, and awareness and acceptance enable client to cope with feelings once identified and move forward in recovery from traumatic event.**
- Acknowledge reality of loss of self that existed before the trauma. Assist client to move toward an acceptance of the potential for growth that exists within client. **Recognition that individual can never go back to being the person they were before the incident allows progress toward life as a different person.**
- Continue to allow client to progress at own pace. **Taking own time to talk about what has happened and allowing feelings to be fully expressed aids in the healing process. If rushed, client may believe they are not accepted or understood.**
- Encourage expression of feelings and reinforce that feelings and reactions to trauma are common and not indicators of weakness or failure. Note whether feelings expressed appear congruent with events the client experienced. Give

---

Information that appears in brackets has been added by the authors to clarify and enhance the use of nursing diagnoses.

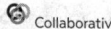 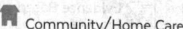

"permission" to express and cope with anger at the assailant or situation in acceptable ways. **Being free to express anger appropriately allows it to be dissipated so underlying feelings can be identified and dealt with, thus strengthening coping skills.**
- Avoid making value judgments. **Client may be judging self, and care provider needs to convey nonjudgmental stance to allow individual to deal with feelings of guilt and recrimination, accepting fact that client did the best client was capable of in the circumstances.**
- Avoid prompting discussion of issues that cannot be resolved (e.g., "if only I had done . . . this would not have happened"). Keep discussion on practical and emotional level rather than intellectualizing the experience. **When feelings (the experience) are intellectualized, uncomfortable insights and/or awareness are avoided by the use of rationalization, blocking resolution of feelings and impairing coping abilities.**
- Provide for sensitive, trained counselors/therapists and engage in therapies, such as psychotherapy in conjunction with medications, implosive therapy (flooding), hypnosis, relaxation, Rolfing therapy, memory work, cognitive behavioral therapy (CBT), eye movement desensitization and reprocessing (EMDR), and physical and occupational therapies. **Treatment approaches are highly individual and thus not universal. Efforts are currently made to attempt to prevent PTS from occurring, or at least to reduce severity of symptoms when they occur. While no definitive studies exist, it is commonly believed that Psychological First Aid (PFA), when applied early in an acute situation, may decrease rates of PTS following a natural disaster or mass casualty situation. PFA includes high levels of emotional support and help with basic needs for shelter, food, clothing, and economic issues. Many studies have shown that brief, trauma-focused CBT started within a few weeks of a traumatic event has been shown to decrease the rate of subsequent PTS, and EMDR has been shown to be most effective in treating clients with PTS.**
- Discuss use of medications. **Treatment will be variable and individualized. Medications to reduce pain and anxiety and promote rest may be components of acute medical intervention. Long term, medications may be used to lift mood and aid in management of behavior until client regains control of own self. Low-dose**

Information that appears in brackets has been added by the authors to clarify and enhance the use of nursing diagnoses.

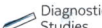 Diagnostic Studies 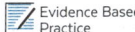 Evidence Based Practice 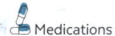 Medications 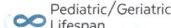 Pediatric/Geriatric/Lifespan

psychotropics may be used when loss of contact with reality is a problem. Recent studies promote use of selective serotonin reuptake inhibitor (SSRI) and serotonin-norepinephrine reuptake inhibitor (SNRI) antidepressants as they appear to be the most effective psychopharmacological interventions for the symptoms of PTS in adults.

Nursing Priority No. 3.

To promote ongoing coping (Teaching/Discharge Considerations) and enhance well-being (long-term goals):

- Review signs/symptoms of a trauma response occurring during daily living. **Promotes awareness and helps client know that control of feelings as they arise will help move beyond traumatic episode.**
- Encourage client to identify and monitor feelings on an ongoing basis. **Promotes awareness of changes in ability to deal with stressors, allowing prompt intervention when necessary.**
- Discuss client's strengths (e.g., supportive family, usually copes well with stress) as well as vulnerabilities (e.g., client tends toward alcohol or other drugs for coping; client has witnessed a murder). **Knowing one's strengths and weaknesses helps client know what actions to take to cope with and prevent anxiety from becoming overwhelming.**
- Discuss coping strategies/stress-management techniques, such as deep breathing, meditation, relaxation, and exercise. **Reduces stress, enhancing coping skills and helping to resolve situation.**
- Encourage routine meetings with supportive persons (e.g., loved ones, spiritual advisor, pastor, rabbi, imam). **Having unconditional support from loving and caring others can help the client cope with the situation and move on to live more fully.**
- Recommend participation in debriefing sessions that may be provided following major events. **Addressing the stressor promptly may facilitate recovery from event and prevent exacerbation. Debriefing is being used by many schools and organizations proactively to cope with traumatic events and lessen development of maladaptive response, although issues about best timing of debriefing continue to be debated.**
- Review what reactions client may expect during each phase. Let client know these are common reactions, and

---

Information that appears in brackets has been added by the authors to clarify and enhance the use of nursing diagnoses.

 Acute Care   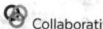 Collaborative   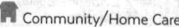 Community/Home Care   Cultural

phrase in neutral terms of "You may or may not . . ." **Knowledge of what may be experienced helps reduce fear of the unknown, thereby enabling client to manage reactions if they occur. Use of neutral terms lets client understand that not all reactions may occur in own situation.**

- Assist client to identify factors that may have created a vulnerable situation and that client may have power to change to protect self in the future. **While client is not responsible for event, they may have unknowingly contributed to occurrence by their actions. Identifying those actions that are within client's power to change provides sense of control over seemingly uncontrollable situations.**
- Discuss lifestyle changes client is contemplating and how they may contribute to recovery. **Client needs to evaluate appropriateness of plans and look at long-range consequences (e.g., moving away from effective support group) to make the best choice for the future.**
- Review stress-management techniques. **Deep breathing, counting to 10 before reacting negatively or with violence, reviewing the situation, and reframing skills assist client in developing constructive ways to cope with feelings of powerlessness and to regain control of self. Reframing stressors or situation in other words or positive ideas can help client recognize and consider alternatives.**
- Review drug regimen, potential side effects of prescribed medications, and necessity of prompt reporting of untoward effects. **Understanding the benefits and potential side effects develops an awareness of medication's effects on the body.**
- Discuss recognition of and ways to manage "anniversary reactions," reinforcing normalcy of recurrence of thoughts and feelings at this time. **Understanding that these feelings are to be expected and planning for them help client get through the anniversary of the event with the least difficulty.**
- Suggest support groups for client/family/SO(s) and employment and community resource groups (e.g., Assistance Support and Self-Help in Surviving Trauma, employee peer assistance programs, Red Cross or other survivor support services, Compassionate Friends). **Family members may not understand client's reactions and need help with accepting them and learning how to cope with client**

POST-TRAUMA SYNDROME

Information that appears in brackets has been added by the authors to clarify and enhance the use of nursing diagnoses.

 Diagnostic Studies 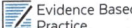 Evidence Based Practice 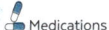 Medications 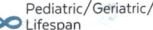 Pediatric/Geriatric/Lifespan

- Encourage psychiatric consultation. **Family members may not understand client's reactions and need help with accepting them and learning how to cope with client in the most helpful manner. Provides opportunity for ongoing support to cope with recurrent stressors as individual moves on with life.**
- Encourage psychiatric consultation. **Family members may not understand client's reactions and need help with accepting them and learning how to cope with client in the most helpful manner. Provides opportunity for ongoing support to cope with recurrent stressors as individual moves on with life.**
- Refer for long-term individual/family/marital counseling, if indicated. **May need additional assistance to prevent continuation of anxiety and the onset or continuation of post-trauma syndrome. Note: While no definitive studies exist, it is commonly believed that PFA, when applied early in an acute situation, may decrease rates of PTS following a natural disaster or mass casualty situation. PFA includes high levels of emotional support and help with basic needs for shelter, food, clothing, and economic issues. Many studies have shown that brief trauma-focused CBT started within a few weeks of a traumatic event has been shown to decrease the rate of subsequent PTS, and EMDR has been shown to be most effective in treating clients with PTS. Additional, ongoing support or therapy may be needed to help family resolve crisis and look at potential for growth. Client problems affect family members and other relationships, and further counseling may help resolve issues of enabling behavior and communication problems.**
- Refer to NDs difficulty Coping, dysfunctional Grief

Documentation Focus

Assessment/Reassessment
- Identified risk factors noting internal and external concerns
- Client's perception of event and personal significance
- Individual findings, noting current dysfunction and behavioral and emotional responses to the incident
- Specifics of traumatic event
- Reactions of family/SO(s)
- Cultural or spiritual beliefs and expectations
- Availability and use of resources

Planning
- Plan of care and who is involved in the planning
- Teaching plan

Information that appears in brackets has been added by the authors to clarify and enhance the use of nursing diagnoses.

 Acute Care  Collaborative 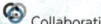 Community/Home Care Cultural

Implementation/Evaluation
- Responses to interventions, teaching, and actions performed
- Emotional changes
- Attainment of or progress toward desired outcome(s)
- Modifications to plan of care

Discharge Planning
- Long-term needs and who is responsible for actions to be taken
- Specific referrals made

Sample Nursing Outcomes & Interventions Classifications NOC/NIC

NOC—Comfort Status: Psychospiritual
NIC—Crisis Intervention
NIC—Support System Enhancement

---

adult PRESSURE INJURY — NANDA-I

[Diagnostic Division: Safety]

Definition: Localized damage to the skin and/or underlying tissue of an individual >18 years of age, as a result of pressure, or pressure in combination with shear (European Pressure Ulcer Advisory Panel, 2019).

Recognizing Cues

Related/Risk Factors
External Factors:
Altered microclimate between skin and supporting surface; inappropriate skin moisture level; use of linen with insufficient moisture wicking property
Inadequate access to appropriate equipment, or health services
Inadequate availability of equipment for individuals with obesity
Inadequate caregiver knowledge of pressure injury prevention strategies
Increased magnitude of mechanical load; sustained mechanical load
Pressure over bony prominence; shearing forces; surface friction

---

Information that appears in brackets has been added by the authors to clarify and enhance the use of nursing diagnoses.

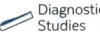 Diagnostic Studies 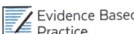 Evidence Based Practice Medications 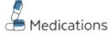 Pediatric/Geriatric/Lifespan

Internal Factors:
Decreased physical activity; impaired physical mobility
Inadequate fluid volume; dry skin
Hyperthermia
Inadequate adherence to incontinence treatment regimen, or to pressure injury prevention plan; inadequate knowledge of pressure injury prevention strategies
Protein-energy malnutrition
Tobacco use; substance misuse
Other Factors:
Factors identified by standardized validated screening tool

Defining Characteristics

Subjective
Pain at pressure points

Objective
Blood-filled blister
Erythemia; purple localized area of discolored intact skin; localized heat in relation to surrounding tissue
Full-thickness tissue loss, loss with exposed bone, muscle, or tendon; partial-thickness loss of dermis
Ulcer is covered by eschar, or slough

Clinical Connections
Para-/quadriplegia; hip fractures; diabetes mellitus; overweight; cerebrovascular accident (CVA), coma, dementia; amputation; burns; peripheral vascular disease, thrombophlebitis

Generate Solutions

Plan Desired Outcomes

Client Will (Include Specific Time Frame)
- Display healthy skin in injured/high-risk areas (e.g., bony prominences, skinfolds) during time in care facility.

Client/Caregiver Will (Include Specific Time Frame)
- Participate in prevention measures.
- Demonstrate behaviors or lifestyle changes to improve circulation (e.g., engage in regular exercise, cessation of smoking, weight reduction, disease management).
- Verbalize understanding when to contact healthcare provider

---

Information that appears in brackets has been added by the authors to clarify and enhance the use of nursing diagnoses.

 Acute Care 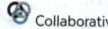 Collaborative 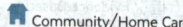 Community/Home Care Cultural

Interventions/Take Action

Nursing Priority No. 1.
To assess contributing factors:

- Note the presence of pressure injury upon admission to care, using National Pressure Injury Advisory Panel (NPIAP) Pressure Injury Stages, Braden risk scale, or similar scale per facility policy. **Using susceptibility factors of sensory perception, skin moisture, activity, mobility, nutritional status, friction, and shear potential, the client's risk can be quickly determined. Note: The term "pressure ulcer" continues to be used widely in clinical areas; however, "pressure injury" better describes the variety of injuries that may demonstrate injury yet intact skin. NPIAP recommends using the term "pressure injury," given that open ulceration does not always occur.**
- Identify/investigate the cause(s) of injury (e.g., pressure, friction, shear, moisture) and implement pressure reduction measures. **Nursing measures include multiple components (e.g., cleansing and drying of skin, repositioning client regularly with sufficient equipment and personnel to reduce friction or shear, and using appropriate padding and support surfaces).**
- Identify/investigate underlying condition(s) that increase(s) the risk of pressure injury. **Skin integrity problems can be the result of (1)** *disease processes that affect circulation and perfusion of tissues* **(e.g., arteriosclerosis, venous insufficiency, hypertension, obesity, diabetes, malignant neoplasms, shock); (2)** *immobility and level of independence* **affecting ability to change own position; (3)** *incontinence* **(fecal and urinary); (4)** *surgical or other trauma, burns, or radiation* **that can break down internal tissues as well as skin; (5)** *nutrition and hydration* **(e.g., malnutrition deprives the body of protein and calories required for cell growth and repair, and dehydration impairs transport of oxygen and nutrients); and (6)** *medications (e.g., vasopressors, corticosteroids, immunosuppressives, antineoplastics)* **that adversely affect or impair healing.**
- Consider client's age, developmental factors (e.g., overall physical and mental health, lifestyle factors [e.g., obesity, sedentary lifestyle, tobacco, alcohol, and recreational drug use] as well as life expectancy), and ability to care for self regarding effect on skin/tissue health. **Skin is affected by both intrinsic and extrinsic factors. Intrinsic factors may**

Information that appears in brackets has been added by the authors to clarify and enhance the use of nursing diagnoses.

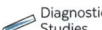 Diagnostic Studies 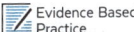 Evidence Based Practice 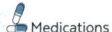 Medications 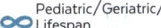 Pediatric/Geriatric/Lifespan

include aging/developmental factors, altered nutritional status, vascular disease issues, and diabetes. Extrinsic factors include falls, accidents, pressure, immobility, and surgical procedures. Older adults experience decreased epidermal regeneration, less subcutaneous fat, elastin, and collagen, causing the skin to become thinner and drier and with generally less tensile strength. The negative effect of immobility and physiological instability on a person's skin does not discriminate by age or developmental level.

- Identify/investigate for compromised skin sensation, vision, hearing, or speech **that may impact the client's self-care regarding skin and pressure area care.**
- Evaluate skin for discoloration (e.g., nonblanchable erythema; persistent red, blue, or purple hues) in pressure areas **suggestive of impaired tissue health. Note: For clients with dark skin, it may be necessary to focus on other evidence of pressure injury development (e.g., induration, coolness, or increased warmth as well as signs of skin discoloration).**
- Evaluate current medication regimen. **Client may be on medications that contribute to the development of pressure injuries or affect wound healing (e.g., vasopressors, corticosteroids, immunosuppressives, antineoplastics) and that can adversely affect the skin.**
- Review laboratory results (e.g., hemoglobin/hematocrit [Hb/Hct], white blood cell count, blood glucose, blood and/or wound culture and sensitivities for infectious agents [viral, bacterial, fungal], albumin, prealbumin, transferrin, hemoglobin A_{1C}, and lipid studies [as needed]) **to evaluate for potential risk factors or ability to heal. Note: Evidence suggests serum albumin less than 3.5 correlates to decreased wound healing and increased incidence of pressure injury. However, albumin levels may be impacted by inflammation and other factors dependent upon the client's condition. For this reason, additional laboratory values and assessments, such as serum prealbumin (i.e., less than 10 mg/dL may be associated with malnutrition) should be used to evaluate the client's nutritional status.**
- Assist with preparation for testing, and review results of imaging studies. **Tissue injury may be visualized via x-rays, computed tomography, bone scans, MRI, tissue or bone biopsy.**

Information that appears in brackets has been added by the authors to clarify and enhance the use of nursing diagnoses.

 Acute Care  Collaborative 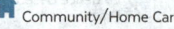 Community/Home Care 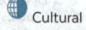 Cultural

Nursing Priority No. 2.

To restore optimal skin/tissue integrity:

- Document/trend progression or failure of wound healing. **The most common method of monitoring utilizes photography and diagrams. Additionally, consistent utilization of an evidence-based skin integrity risk assessment tool (e.g., Braden, etc.) may improve continuity of care through caregiver communication.**
- Determine anatomical location and depth of skin or tissue injury (e.g., wound stage 1 to 4) and describe **to provide baseline and document changes.**
- Note consistency, volume, odor, and color of drainage, when present. **Wound drainage may indicate infection and cause or exacerbate skin injury.**
- Determine, document, and regularly reassess wound (1) dimensions (i.e., length, width, and depth) in centimeters; (2) wound margins (i.e., are wound edges flush with wound base/flat, or are wound walls present/floor of wound is deeper than the edge); (3) presence of tunneling or tracts; and (4) evidence of necrosis (e.g., color gray to black, dry, leathery), or healing (e.g., pink or red granulation tissue, moist) **to establish a comparative baseline and evaluate the effectiveness of interventions.**
- Practice and instruct client/caregiver(s) in scrupulous hand hygiene and clean or sterile technique **to reduce the incidence of contamination or infection.**
- Collaborate in wound care, referring to specialist(s) for further evaluation, and treatments. **Interventions depend on several factors (e.g., whether the lesion is acute or chronic; stage of lesion, client's general health status) and can include reduction of pressure, debridement of necrotic and devitalized tissue (e.g., via cleansing with various solutions and types of dressings), and control of exudate and infection.**
- Participate in treatment of underlying conditions. **Management of conditions such as cardiovascular or neurological impairments, infections, and so on, can improve skin condition and promote healing.**
- Provide optimum nutrition (including adequate protein, lipids, calories, trace minerals, and multivitamins [e.g., A, C, D, E, and zinc]) **to promote skin and tissue health, and to maintain general good health.** Refer to dietitian as indicated.

Information that appears in brackets has been added by the authors to clarify and enhance the use of nursing diagnoses.

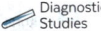 Diagnostic Studies 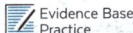 Evidence Based Practice 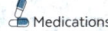 Medications 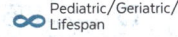 Pediatric/Geriatric/Lifespan

- Provide adequate hydration (e.g., oral, enteral feeding, parenteral fluids, ambient room humidity) **to reduce and replenish transepidermal water loss.**
- Administer medications as indicated. **Medications may include those for management of pain, infections, anemia, or malnutrition.**
- Monitor client for incontinence and promptly remove wet, dirty, or wrinkled linens. Change briefs, pads, padding, and bedding as soon as damp/soiled. Cleanse the affected area and apply barrier ointment. Use appropriate incontinence disposables; however, avoid or limit the use of plastic material (e.g., rubber sheets, plastic-backed linen savers). **Prolonged skin exposure to moisture causes maceration, which causes softening of the skin and predisposes the skin to injury.**
- Develop regularly timed repositioning/turning schedule for clients with mobility and sensation impairments, using a turn sheet/device as needed; encourage or assist with periodic weight shifts for the client in a chair **to reduce stress on pressure points and to promote circulation to tissues.**
- Use proper turning and transfer techniques. Utilize sufficient personnel when repositioning client **to avoid movements that cause friction or shearing (e.g., pulling client with parallel force, or dragging movements).**
- Use appropriate padding or pressure-reducing devices (e.g., heel rolls, foam boots, egg crate, gel pads) or pressure-relieving devices (e.g., air or water mattress) when indicated **to reduce pressure on sensitive areas and enhance circulation to compromised tissues.**
- Special skin/tissue considerations for the critically ill clients placed in the prone position (i.e., coronavirus, acute respiratory distress syndrome [ARDS]):
  (1) Head: Apply soft prophylactic padding to pressure points on the face (e.g., forehead when facing down; around medical devices [e.g., endotracheal tubes, feeding tubes]; cheeks, chin, lips). Ensure face padding is adjusted to avoid direct pressure on eyes and use appropriate measures **to prevent dry eyes with risk of developing corneal abrasions.**
  (2) Torso: Apply ECG leads to back; ensure all central lines and appliances (e.g., ostomies) are secured, padded, and not prone to leaking; ascertain that elbows and shoulders are supported and padded.

Information that appears in brackets has been added by the authors to clarify and enhance the use of nursing diagnoses.

(3) Legs: Apply soft prophylactic padding to pressure points (e.g., kneecaps, dorsal foot, toes).
(4) Breasts and genitalia: Utilize positioning and devices **to relieve pressure points.**

- Utilize practices that prevent medical device–related pressure injury, using guidelines **to guide practice and documentation:**
  (1) Choose the correct size of medical device(s) (e.g., tubing, anti-embolism stocking, splints) to fit the client.
  (2) Remove or adjust the device periodically to assess skin.
  (3) Avoid placement of device(s) over sites of prior or existing pressure injury.
  (4) Cushion and protect skin with cushioning in high-risk areas (e.g., nasal bridge, ears, elbows, sacrum, heels, toes).
  (5) Provide education to other care providers about client's devices and interventions for prevention of skin breakdown.
- Refer to other providers, as indicated. **Neurosurgery, urology, plastic, orthopedic, general surgery, and others (rehabilitation medicine specialists, social workers, home care providers, and mental health workers) may be indicated to improve the patient's health, attitude, support structure, and living environment.**

Nursing Priority No. 3.

To promote healthy, intact skin (Teaching/Discharge Considerations) and enhance well-being (long-term goals):

- Encourage regular inspection and monitoring of skin for changes or failure to heal. **Early detection and reporting to healthcare providers promotes timely evaluation and intervention.**
- Ascertain that client/caregivers understand the client's particular pressure prevention needs and are able and willing to carry out prevention measures.
- Encourage good nutrition, adequate hydration, early and ongoing mobility, and range-of-motion and strengthening exercises **to enhance circulation and promote health of skin and other organs.**
- Discuss proper and safe use of medical equipment or appliances (e.g., appliances, padding for all pressure points when in bed or wheelchair, straps of braces).
- Encourage abstinence from smoking, **which causes vasoconstriction, impairing circulation.**
- Advise client/caregiver of the importance for long-term monitoring of healing and follow-up with medical providers.

Information that appears in brackets has been added by the authors to clarify and enhance the use of nursing diagnoses.

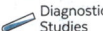 Diagnostic Studies 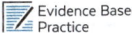 Evidence Based Practice 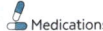 Medications 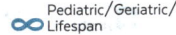 Pediatric/Geriatric/Lifespan

- Refer client to community services, as indicated. **The client may benefit from visits from home health, rehabilitation services, social services, and medical equipment providers to ensure that pressure avoidance strategies are adapted to the home and continued over the long term.**

Documentation Focus

Assessment/Reassessment
- Individual findings, including specific risk factors, condition of skin, ability to manage/direct own care
- Characteristics of pressure injury if present

Planning
- Plan of care and who is involved in planning
- Teaching plan

Implementation/Evaluation
- Responses to interventions, teaching, and actions performed
- Attainment of or progress toward desired outcome(s)
- Modifications to plan of care

Discharge Planning
- Long-term needs and who is responsible for actions to be taken
- Specific referrals made

Sample Nursing Outcomes & Interventions Classifications NOC/NIC

NOC—Wound Healing: Secondary Intention
NIC—Pressure Injury Care

child PRESSURE INJURY NANDA-I

[Diagnostic Division: Safety]

Definition: Localized damage to the skin and/or underlying tissue of an individual 29 days to ≤18 years of age, as a result of pressure, or pressure in combination with shear (European Pressure Ulcer Advisory Panel, 2019).

Information that appears in brackets has been added by the authors to clarify and enhance the use of nursing diagnoses.

Recognizing Cues
Related/Risk Factors
External Factors:

Altered microclimate between skin and supporting surface; inappropriate skin moisture level; use of linen with insufficient moisture wicking property

Difficulty for caregiver to lift patient completely off bed

Inadequate access to appropriate equipment, health services, or supplies

Inadequate access to equipment for overweight child

Inadequate caregiver knowledge of appropriate methods for removing adhesive materials, or for stabilizing devices

Inadequate caregiver knowledge of modifiable factors, or of pressure injury prevention strategies

Increased magnitude of mechanical load; sustained mechanical load

Pressure over bony prominence; shearing forces; surface friction

Internal Factors:

Decreased physical activity; impaired physical mobility; difficulty assisting caregiver with moving self

Inadequate fluid volume; dry skin

Difficulty maintaining position in bed or chair

Hyperthermia

Inadequate adherence to incontinence treatment regimen or pressure injury prevention plan

Inadequate knowledge of appropriate methods for removing adhesive materials, or for stabilizing devices

Protein-energy malnutrition; water-electrolyte imbalance

Other Factors:

Factors identified by standardized validated screening tool

Defining Characteristics

Objective

Blood-filled blister; erythema; purple localized area of discolored intact skin

Full-thickness tissue loss; loss with exposed bone, muscle, or tendon; partial-thickness loss of dermis

Localized heat in relation to surrounding tissue

Pain at pressure points

Ulcer covered with eschar, or slough

Information that appears in brackets has been added by the authors to clarify and enhance the use of nursing diagnoses.

Clinical Connections
Hospitalized child, para-/quadriplegia; diabetes mellitus; overweight; traumatic brain injury (TBI), coma; fractures, amputation; burns; thrombophlebitis, developmental delay

Generate Solutions

Plan Desired Outcomes

Client Will (Include Specific Time Frame)
- Display and maintain healthy skin (e.g., bony prominences, skinfolds) during time in care facility.
- Participate in treatment program (if developmentally able to do so).
- Demonstrate behaviors or lifestyle changes (e.g., engage in regular exercise, weight reduction, disease management) to improve circulation (if developmentally able to do so).

Caregiver Will (Include Specific Time Frame)
- Participate in treatment program.

Interventions/Take Action

Nursing Priority No. 1.
To assess for contributing factors:

- Assess and monitor skin surfaces: (1) back of the head and ears (especially in infants and toddlers); (2) sacrum, hips, buttocks, heels, elbows, spine, and shoulder blades (especially if immobilized in supine position); (3) under edges of plasters, casts, splints, or braces; (4) around medical equipment (e.g., tubes, masks, drains) regularly when in care, noting and documenting changes, or failure to heal. **Early detection and reporting to healthcare providers promotes timely intervention.**
- Consider client's age, developmental level/cognition, body size, coordination, and mobility. **Many skin issues in children, including pressure injuries, can be attributed to skin immaturity and body size. Older gestational age equates to thicker skin and a more robust skin barrier. These factors also impact the client's ability to participate in preventive strategies. Note: Children living with long-term/lifelong special needs (disabilities) are an especially high-risk population for pressure injuries due to compromise in several areas (e.g., acute and/or chronic illnesses; genetic malformations; physical and intellectual disabilities;**

Information that appears in brackets has been added by the authors to clarify and enhance the use of nursing diagnoses.

 Acute Care 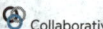 Collaborative 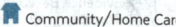 Community/Home Care Cultural

sensation disorders; nonverbal and/or nonambulatory traits; immobility; and reliance on medical device[s] to extend or improve life).
- Identify/investigate underlying condition(s) that increase the risk of pressure injury. **Skin integrity problems can be the result of (1)** *disease processes* **that affect circulation and perfusion of tissues (e.g., heart disease, diabetes, malignant neoplasms, shock); (2)** *medical devices* **(e.g., tracheostomy tube, nasal cannula, ill-fitting devices, etc.); (3)** *medications* **(e.g., vasopressors, corticosteroids, immunosuppressives, antineoplastics) that adversely affect or impair healing; (4)** *trauma, burns, radiation* **that break down internal tissues as well as skin; (5)** *nutrition and hydration* **that affect transport of nutrients and perfusion of tissues and organs.**
- Assess skin/tissue using a standardized validated screening tool (e.g., Braden Q Scale, Braden QD Scale, or similar tool), noting:

  Mobility: **Determines whether child is active on own, has difficulty repositioning self, or is completely dependent.**

  Sensory perception: **Determines whether child is able to respond to stimuli in a meaningful, developmentally appropriate manner; alterations may be related to neurological conditions causing paralysis or loss of pain sensation (e.g., spinal cord injury, brain injury, burns).**

  Moisture and dryness: **Avoiding excess moisture is critical because a child's skin is susceptible to injury not only from moisture but also from the chemicals found in moisture sources (e.g., stool, urine, respiratory devices, and caustic gastrointestinal effluent [e.g., tube leakage]). Conversely, dehydration and a heated environment can cause dry skin, which is fragile and prone to abrasion.**

  Nutrition: **Note whether the child is receiving adequate calories and protein for growth, development, cell repair.**

  Tissue perfusion: **Note overall skin color, oxygen saturation, hemodynamic stability, and urine output.**

  Friction (how skin moves against support surfaces) and shear forces (the skin and bony surfaces slide across one another): **Determined by child's ability to change or maintain position in bed/chair, or requires repositioning by others without sliding or dragging the child across the bed.**

Information that appears in brackets has been added by the authors to clarify and enhance the use of nursing diagnoses.

- Medical devices (e.g., oxygen delivery and measurement devices, feeding tubes).
- Evaluate skin for discoloration (e.g., nonblanchable erythema; persistent red, blue, or purple hues) in pressure areas suggestive of impaired tissue health. **Note: For clients with dark skin, it may be necessary to focus on other evidence of pressure injury development, such as bogginess, induration, coolness, or increased warmth, as well as signs of skin discoloration.**
- Ascertain recent, current, and long-term medication regimens, noting medications that may impact skin health and fragility. **Hospitalized children and those with chronic conditions may be on multiple medications, including some that can impact skin (e.g., corticosteroids, vasopressors, immunosuppressives, antineoplastics, etc.). These effects may have long-term implications even after the medication is discontinued. Physiological differences of immature skin also predispose pediatric skin to higher absorption rates of topical medications (i.e., iodine; isopropyl, ethyl, and methyl alcohol; chlorhexidine; and hydrocortisone).**
- Review laboratory results (e.g., hemoglobin/hematocrit, white blood cell count, blood glucose, albumin, prealbumin, transferrin) **to evaluate for factors affecting ability to protect skin/tissue or heal. Note: Evidence suggests serum albumin less than 3.5 has been correlated with decreased wound healing and increased incidence of pressure injuries. However, albumin levels may be impacted by inflammation and other factors dependent on the client's condition. For this reason, additional laboratory values and assessments, such as serum prealbumin (i.e., less than 10 mg/dL may be associated with malnutrition) should be used to evaluate client's nutritional status.**

Nursing Priority No. 2.
To restore optimal skin/tissue integrity:
- Assist in treatment of underlying conditions, including administration of oxygen, fluids, and medications **to bring about healing to tissues and normalize body functions.**
- Determine anatomical location and depth of skin or tissue injury (e.g., wound stage 1 to 4) and describe **to provide baseline and document changes.**

Information that appears in brackets has been added by the authors to clarify and enhance the use of nursing diagnoses.

- Note consistency, volume, odor, and color of drainage, when present. **Wound drainage may indicate infection and cause or exacerbate skin injury.**
- Regularly reassess wound per protocol: (1) dimensions (i.e., length, width, and depth) in centimeters; (2) wound margins (i.e., are wound edges flush with wound base/flat, or are wound walls present/floor of wound is deeper than the edge); (3) presence of tunneling or tracts; and (4) evidence of necrosis (e.g., color gray to black, dry, leathery) or healing (e.g., pink or red granulation tissue, moist) **to establish a comparative baseline and evaluate the effectiveness of interventions.**
- Document/trend progression or failure of wound healing. **Consistent utilization of an evidence-based skin integrity risk assessment tool (e.g., Braden QD, etc.) may improve continuity of care through caregiver communication.**
- Practice and instruct client/caregiver(s) in scrupulous hand hygiene and clean or sterile technique **to reduce the incidence of contamination or infection.**
- Collaborate with wound care specialist for a complete assessment of needs and initiation of treatment plan, as indicated. **Interventions depend on several factors (e.g., whether the lesion is acute or chronic; stage of lesion, client's general health status). Treatment can include reduction of pressure, debridement of necrotic and devitalized tissue (e.g., via cleansing with various solutions), control of exudate and infection, use of special dressings/devices (e.g., hydrocolloids, hydrogels, polyurethane foams, and transparent films).**
- Determine client's level of discomfort and implement pain relief strategies (e.g., topical, oral, parenteral medication; distraction, etc.). **Pain in children is often underestimated and undertreated; effective pain management may be compromised due to communication difficulties and the lack of effective scales to measure pain. Family members/caregivers may give valuable insight regarding the child's demeanor and response to gauge the client's comfort level.**
- Provide positioning and padding:
  Evaluate mattress/support surfaces (e.g., foam, air cell mattress, pressure reduction mattress overlay) **to provide adequate support and pressure relief. Pediatric clients have softer subcutaneous and muscle tissue. Support surfaces should envelop the client to facilitate the redistribution of pressure.**

Information that appears in brackets has been added by the authors to clarify and enhance the use of nursing diagnoses.

Inspect bed, crib, and chairs to ensure that no tubing, cables, leads, hard toys, or syringe caps are inadvertently left under the child.

Develop regularly timed repositioning/turning schedule for clients according to need. Encourage/assist with periodic weight shifts for the client in a chair **to reduce stress on pressure points and promote circulation to tissues. Note: How often a child needs to move or be moved in bed or chair depends on the child's age, body size, and current disease condition.**

Cushion bony prominences with pillows or gel cushions.

Use needed pillows, padding, strapping to maintain good posture.

- Prevent friction and shear:

Use a draw sheet, transfer aid, or mechanical lift to reposition **to avoid dragging the client patient across the support surface.**

Lift child using enough people **to prevent dragging client across the support surface.**

- Maintain nutrition and hydration:

Evaluate child's food and weight history, current nutrition status, and adequacy of nutritional intake. **Evidence indicates malnutrition, or poor nutritional status, and variables that indicate potential malnutrition (e.g., low body weight and poor oral food intake) are independent risk factors for developing pressure injuries. While much discussion centers on overweight children, underweight children are at equal, or even greater, risk.**

Collaborate with a dietician for specialist screening and dietary management to provide energy and protein needs of the child experiencing metabolic stress of healing wounds. **Nutrition needs should be assessed frequently to avoid over- or underfeeding. Note: When oral intake is inadequate to support healing, enteral feeding may be initiated.**

Evaluate child's hydration status, noting the presence of factors that cause fluid losses. **High temperature, vomiting, profuse sweating, diarrhea, and/or heavily exuding wounds increase the need for water intake to replace losses.**

- Manage secretions, excretions:

Remove urine/stool as soon as present, cleaning with appropriate cleanser and carefully drying area.

Prevent child from sitting or lying in one place for too long, or sitting in wet clothing, a wet bed, or diaper/continence brief.

Information that appears in brackets has been added by the authors to clarify and enhance the use of nursing diagnoses.

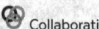

Apply appropriate moisturizers to dry skin areas as indicated **to reduce skin fragility caused by rubbing on linens.**

- Prevent medical device and equipment injury:

Provide the correct type and size of medical device/equipment considering the child's weight, size, development, and mobility. **Approximately 50% of pressure injuries are related to pressure from equipment and devices, a significant source in the pediatric client.**

Avoid device placement over sites of prior or existing pressure injury.

Cushion and protect skin with dressings in high-risk areas (e.g., nasal bridge, rim of cast) and provide sufficient padding under arm boards, orthotics/casts, and traction boots.

Provide device/skin interface monitoring, especially in children with long-term conditions (e.g., critically ill, or in casts/other immobilizers, or receiving fluid resuscitation, or who have unresolved soft-tissue inflammation).

Rotate blood pressure cuffs and transcutaneous oxygen tension ($tcPO_2$) probes regularly.

Collaborate with respiratory therapy to assess/reposition, and provide sufficient padding for endotracheal (ET) tube/tracheostomy, and noninvasive ventilation devices. **Helps identify early concerns of skin/tissue of the nose, lips, cheeks, or mucosal injuries of the tongue and buccal mucosa.**

Nursing Priority No. 3.

To promote healthy, intact skin (Teaching/Discharge Considerations) and enhance well-being (long-term goals):

- Stress importance of evaluating child cries/change in behavior that may reveal change in skin integrity and need for further evaluation/treatment.

- Encourage regular inspection and monitoring of skin and report changes in skin/wound characteristics. **Early detection and reporting to healthcare providers promote timely evaluation and intervention.**

- Instruct care provider in ongoing treatments (if child discharged with a pressure injury), and determine that the caregiver is prepared and able to care for child at home. **Provides for continuity of care.**

- Identify community resources for dressing supplies/equipment, home-care services if needed. **Client discharged with wound will require ongoing treatment and support.**

Information that appears in brackets has been added by the authors to clarify and enhance the use of nursing diagnoses.

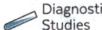 Diagnostic Studies 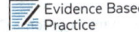 Evidence Based Practice 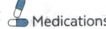 Medications 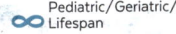 Pediatric/Geriatric/Lifespan

- Encourage good nutrition by discussing individual needs and addressing child's feeding habits and food security issues (if applicable).
- Promote adequate hydration, discussing ways to help child meet this need, **to enhance circulation and promote health of skin and other organs.**
- Discuss proper and safe use of equipment or appliances (e.g., oxygen equipment, sleeping surfaces, padding, wheelchairs).
- Encourage abstinence from smoking (if child/teenager is smoking or using tobacco in another way), **which causes vasoconstriction, impairing circulation.**

Documentation Focus

Assessment/Reassessment
- Individual findings, including specific cause or risk factors, status of skin/tissues
- Ability of child to participate in own care/pressure prevention actions
- Availability and willingness of caregiver to provide pressure prevention measures

Planning
- Plan of care and who is involved in planning
- Teaching plan

Implementation/Evaluation
- Responses to interventions, teaching, and actions performed
- Attainment of or progress toward desired outcome(s)
- Modifications to plan of care

Discharge Planning
- Long-term needs and who is responsible for actions to be taken
- Specific referrals made

Sample Nursing Outcomes & Interventions Classifications NOC/NIC

NOC—Tissue Integrity: Skin and Mucous Membranes
NIC—Pressure Injury Care

Information that appears in brackets has been added by the authors to clarify and enhance the use of nursing diagnoses.

neonatal PRESSURE INJURY NANDA-I

[Diagnostic Division: Safety]

Definition: Localized damage to the skin and/or underlying tissue of an individual up to 28 days of age, as a result of pressure, or pressure in combination with shear (European Pressure Ulcer Advisory Panel, 2019).

Recognizing Cues

Related/Risk Factors

External Factors:

Altered microclimate between skin and supporting surface; inappropriate skin moisture level; use of linen with insufficient moisture wicking property

Inadequate access to appropriate equipment, supplies, or health services

Inadequate caregiver knowledge of pressure injury prevention strategies, modifiable factors, appropriate methods for stabilizing devices, or removing adhesive materials

Increased magnitude of mechanical load; sustained mechanical load

Pressure over bony prominence; shearing forces; surface friction

Internal Factors:

Impaired physical mobility

Inadequate fluid volume; dry skin

Hyperthermia

Water-electrolyte imbalance

Impaired circulation

Other Factors:

Factors identified by standardized validated screening tool

Defining Characteristics

Objective

Blood-filled blister

Erythema; localized heat in relation to surrounding tissue

Full-thickness tissue loss; full tissue loss with exposed bone, muscle, or tendon; partial-thickness loss of dermis

Maroon or purple localized area of discolored intact skin

Skin ulceration; ulcer is covered by eschar, or slough

Clinical Connections

Newborn; premature infant; low-birth-weight infant

Information that appears in brackets has been added by the authors to clarify and enhance the use of nursing diagnoses.

 Diagnostic Studies 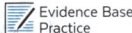 Evidence Based Practice 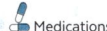 Medications 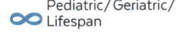 Pediatric/Geriatric/Lifespan

Generate Solutions

Plan Desired Outcomes

Client Will (Include Specific Time Frame)
- Regain and/or maintain healthy skin, especially in risk areas (e.g., bony prominences, skinfolds, skin under medical devices).

Caregiver/Parent Will (Include Specific Time Frame)
- Participate in prevention measures and treatment program.
- Verbalize understanding of risk factors and when to contact healthcare provider.

Interventions/Take Action

Nursing Priority No. 1.
To assess extent of skin/tissue injury and contributing factors:

- Determine neonate's gestational age (less than 37 weeks) and postnatal age, weight at birth (grams), skin maturity, developmental factors affecting skin/tissue health, and period of hospitalization (days). **The skin of a term newborn is not considered mature until 3 weeks have passed, and a preterm newborn requires even more time to mature. The rate of tissue injury is about 57% at gestational ages of 24 to 27 weeks compared with 3% at term. Infants are predisposed to dry, flaky skin, and preterm/ill neonates are further impacted by the negative effect of immobility and physiological instability.**
- Identify presence of underlying condition(s) that contributed to or increase risk of pressure injury. **Low birth weight (less than 2,500 g), hypotension and hypoxemia, edema, anemia/nutritional deficiencies, sepsis, use of therapeutic and diagnostic devices (accounts for 50% to 90% of pressure injuries in the neonate), and prolonged stay in the neonatal intensive care unit (associated with 9.25% to 43.1% of pressure injuries) have a cumulative effect on skin/tissue integrity. Note: Edema reflects compromised circulation and poor nutrition leading to accumulation of interstitial fluid and decrease in tissue oxygenation.**
- Assess skin and continually evaluate high-risk locations. **The most frequent locations of hospital-acquired pressure injuries (HAPIs) in neonates are the (1) back of the head (occipital region) and ears; (2) anatomical areas where therapeutic or diagnostic systems are at risk**

Information that appears in brackets has been added by the authors to clarify and enhance the use of nursing diagnoses.

 Acute Care    Collaborative   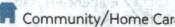 Community/Home Care   Cultural

(e.g., fingers and feet [pulse oximetry sensor]); and (3) skin support areas (vascular catheters), thorax (electrodes), nasal septum, back of the neck, nostrils and cheeks (continuous positive airway pressure [CPAP] interface, both binaural cannulae and face mask). HAPI leads to significant morbidity and increased costs due to prolonged illness, immobilization, increased device utilization.

- Use a standardized risk assessment tool, as indicated. **It is vital that skin risk assessments are routinely performed. Predicting injuries and their progression or healing is complex and often multifactorial in neonates. The three skin assessment tools that have been largely tested and validated are the Braden Q Scale, Glamorgan Q Scale, and the Neonatal Skin Risk Assessment Scale (NSRAS). Similar to the Braden Q Scale, the NSRAS reflects the physical and developmental needs of a neonate and consists of six subscales, with a low score indicating high risk.**

- Ascertain current medication regimen. **Neonate may be receiving medications that can contribute to development of pressure injuries or affect wound healing (e.g., steroids, analgesics [e.g., morphine, fentanyl], sedatives [e.g., midazolam, lorazepam], vasopressors) and can adversely affect the skin.**

- Review laboratory results (e.g., hemoglobin/hematocrit, blood glucose, blood and/or wound culture and sensitivities for infectious agents [viral, bacterial, fungal], albumin, prealbumin, transferrin, protein) **to evaluate for factors affecting ability to heal. Note: Plasma albumin levels are typically low in neonates (between 2.8 and 4.4 g/dL). The primary problem of decreasing plasma albumin concentration in sick hospitalized neonates is transcapillary escape into the interstitial fluid. The edema produced by this process increases tissue fragility and risk of breakdown. In addition, low hemoglobin levels affect oxygen carrying capacity of blood and tissue oxygenation increasing risk of tissue necrosis and ulceration.**

Nursing Priority No. 2.
To promote healing and prevent further injury:

- Coordinate with interdisciplinary team including respiratory therapist, wound care specialist, and nutritionist. **Research demonstrates that an interdisciplinary team is more effective at reducing pressure injuries than a single discipline.**

Information that appears in brackets has been added by the authors to clarify and enhance the use of nursing diagnoses.

 Diagnostic Studies 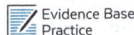 Evidence Based Practice 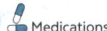 Medications 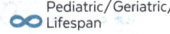 Pediatric/Geriatric/Lifespan

- Assist with medical treatments of underlying conditions. **There are a few goals fundamental to all wound treatment regardless of client age. These include (1) infection identification, control, and treatment; (2) the establishment and maintenance of a clean and hydrated wound bed; (3) debridement or removal of necrotic or devitalized tissue if present; and (4) wound protection or barrier formation to prevent secondary infection, skin breakdown, or dehydration.**
- Assist in early treatment of skin breakdown in pressure areas. Initiate coverage of wound. Refer to wound care specialist for ongoing assessment and treatment concerns. **Goals fundamental to all wound treatment, regardless of age, include (1) infection identification, control, and treatment; (2) the establishment and maintenance of a clean and hydrated wound bed; (3) debridement or removal of necrotic or devitalized tissue if present; and (4) wound protection or barrier formation to prevent secondary infection, skin breakdown, or dehydration. Early wounds should be covered using a safe and effective dressing, such as silicone-bordered foam. Other treatments can include debridement by surgery, enzymatic debriding dressings, medical-grade honey.**
- Provide optimum nutrition (including adequate protein, lipids, calories, trace minerals, and multivitamins [e.g., A, C, D, E]) **to promote skin and tissue health and to maintain general well-being. Note: Parenteral or enteral nutrition may be initiated early for neonates at risk of malnutrition. However, breastfeeding should always be promoted through suckling, feeding bottle, or enteral catheter.**
- Provide adequate hydration (e.g., oral, tube feeding, IV, ambient room humidity) **to reduce and replenish transepidermal water loss.**

Nursing Priority No. 3.

To maintain optimal skin health/prevent breakdown:

- Inspect skin with each repositioning. Note skin color/discoloration (e.g., nonblanchable erythema; persistent red, blue, or purple hues) in pressure areas **suggestive of impaired tissue health. Note: It may be necessary in a darker-skinned individual to focus more on other evidence of pressure injury development, such as bogginess, induration, coolness, or increased warmth.**
- Develop regularly timed repositioning schedule. **Reduces stress on pressure points and promotes circulation to tissues.**

Information that appears in brackets has been added by the authors to clarify and enhance the use of nursing diagnoses.

- Reposition the neonate to relieve or redistribute pressure using appropriate manual handling techniques and equipment. **Avoids movements that cause friction or shearing (e.g., pulling with parallel force, dragging movements).**
- Use appropriate padding or pressure-reducing devices (e.g., gel pads, heel rolls, or foam booties) or pressure-relieving devices (e.g., air or water mattress) as indicated. **Reduces pressure on sensitive areas and enhances circulation.**
- Cleanse/bathe and moisturize skin as needed/or per facility policy. **During the first 2 weeks, skin hygiene is not recommended on a daily basis. Skin cleaning should be done only with warm water and cotton compresses or a soft material. It is advisable to hydrate the skin of newborns at risk for pressure injury (at term, after the first 48 hr) using emollients (oils, emulsion, milk). In preterm infants, no ointment or topical cream or mineral oils should be used as a usual form of skin moisturizing due to the risk of infection (e.g., contamination by bacteria, fungus, or virus).**
- Exercise gentleness when removing adhesives (e.g., probes, film and hydrocolloid dressings, ostomy bag) **to avoid accidental injury. Note: Leaking ostomy sites can lead to severe excoriation and possible secondary infection.**
- Participate in practices that prevent medical device–related pressure injuries:
  Choose the correct size of medical device(s) (e.g., endotracheal tube [ET], CPAP, other tubings, splints) to fit the neonate.
  Remove or move the device periodically to assess skin.
  Avoid placement of device(s) over sites of prior or existing pressure injury.
  Protect skin with cushioning in high-risk areas (e.g., nasal bridge, ears, sacrum, heels, occipital area of head).
  Educate other care providers about client's devices and interventions for prevention of skin breakdown.

Nursing Priority No. 4.

To maintain tissue integrity (Teaching/Discharge Considerations) and enhance well-being (long-term goals):

- Instruct parent/caregivers to regularly inspect skin and report changes or failure to heal. **Early detection and reporting to healthcare providers promote timely evaluation and intervention.**
- Review client's nutrition (calories and nutrients) and hydration needs and ways to meet these needs, as well as ongoing age-appropriate range-of-motion and strengthening exercises

---

Information that appears in brackets has been added by the authors to clarify and enhance the use of nursing diagnoses.

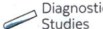 Diagnostic Studies 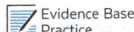 Evidence Based Practice 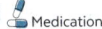 Medications 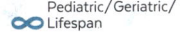 Pediatric/Geriatric/Lifespan

to enhance circulation and promote health of skin and other organs.
- Stress importance of changing diapers after each episode of incontinence, cleaning and drying the area and applying approved barrier product (e.g., creams, lotions, pastes, and/or emollients enriched with zinc oxide, polyurethane spreads). Change ostomy appliances as needed. **Both urine and feces can macerate the skin.**
- Discuss proper and safe use of equipment or appliances. Have caregiver(s) demonstrate knowledge of equipment management and involved safety issues.
- Ascertain that caregiver(s) can provide safe environment for neonate.
- Identify community resources such as home care, respite, support groups.
- Refer for medical and skin/tissue follow-up care.

Documentation Focus

Assessment/Reassessment
- Individual findings, including specific related factors, status of skin
- Parent/caregiver understanding of neonatal care needs and risk factors
- Parent/caregiver ability to participate in treatment regimen

Planning
- Plan of care and who is involved in planning
- Teaching plan

Implementation/Evaluation
- Responses to interventions, teaching, and actions performed
- Attainment of or progress toward desired outcome(s)
- Modifications to plan of care

Discharge Planning
- Long-term needs and who is responsible for actions to be taken
- Specific referrals made

Sample Nursing Outcomes & Interventions Classifications NOC/NIC

NOC—Wound Healing: Secondary Intention [or] Risk Control: Pressure Injury
NIC—Pressure Injury Care [or] Prevention

Information that appears in brackets has been added by the authors to clarify and enhance the use of nursing diagnoses.

ineffective intimate partner RELATIONSHIP NANDA-I

[Diagnostic Division: Roles/Relationships]

Definition: Pattern of mutuality that is insufficient, or that may affect the course, prognosis, or treatment of a health condition of one or both partners.

Recognizing Cues

Related/Risk Factors
Excessive anxiety; excessive stress; depressive symptoms
Inadequate communication skills; inadequate emotional support
Imbalance in autonomy between partners; overinvolvement of one partner
Unaddressed anger, chronic sadness, or apathy about partner
Difficulty accessing support; dissatisfaction with social support
Negative attribution of partner's intentions; unrealistic expectations
Unaddressed conflict between partners
Intimate partner aggression; unaddressed intimate partner violence

Defining Characteristics

Subjective
Dissatisfaction with complementary interpersonal relations between partners
Dissatisfaction with physical or emotional need fulfillment between partners
Dissatisfaction with information, or idea sharing between partners

Objective
Inadequate mutual respect between partners; does not identify partner as support person
Unsatisfactory communication with partner; imbalance in collaboration between partners
Inadequate understanding of partner's functional impairment
Inadequate mutual support in daily activities between partners
Delayed attainment of developmental goals appropriate for partner life-cycle stage

---

Information that appears in brackets has been added by the authors to clarify and enhance the use of nursing diagnoses.

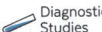 Diagnostic Studies 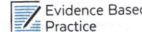 Evidence Based Practice 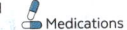 Medications 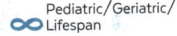 Pediatric/Geriatric/Lifespan

Clinical Connections
Chronic health/debilitating conditions, chronic pain, substance misuse, depression, borderline personality, schizophrenia

Generate Solutions

Plan Desired Outcomes

Client Will (Include Specific Time Frame)
- Verbalize desire to make changes to meet each other's needs as appropriate.
- Express a desire to improve communication skills.
- Develop realistic plans to improve relationship.

Interventions/Take Action

Nursing Priority No. 1.
To access current situation and determine needs:

- Determine makeup of family (e.g., family members, heterosexual/homosexual relationship, roles of each member), length of relationship, and specific stresses. **Stressors of family—developmental issues, elderly parents needing assistance, financial difficulties, and domestic violence—strain relationships between partners. Homosexual partners have similar yet different stressors based on family or society perception, cultural and spiritual expectations.**
- Identify how each partner sees self-image and locus of control. **Do partners view self as a positive or negative person who is in control or controlled by others' influences and how each relates to the other.**
- Discuss needs of each partner and how each views the other's needs. **Identifies misperceptions and areas of disagreement to provide a basis of planning for change.**
- Identify style of communication and understanding of nonverbal cues used by family members. **Poor communication and lack of understanding of what the other is saying, or inferring, leads to conflicts and lack of problem-solving.**
- Determine how partners cope with conflict. **Many individuals try to avoid conflict instead of working to resolve it.**
- Identify cultural beliefs that affect how each person copes with daily activities in family. **Family of origin influences how individuals think roles are to be dealt with, and conflict arises if partners are not willing to discuss and accept or merge beliefs.**
- Identify medical problems/sexual concerns that may affect relationship. **Conditions such as prostate problems,**

Information that appears in brackets has been added by the authors to clarify and enhance the use of nursing diagnoses.

breast cancer, hysterectomy, vaginismus, and erectile dysfunction can affect interactions between partners. **Medical treatment and therapy may be necessary.**
- Assess how the couple cope with sexual aspects of their relationship. **When anger and conflict interfere with intimacy, couple may distance themselves from one another.**
- Identify patterns of intimate partner violence. **Understanding what instigates the problem and what starts the level of aggression between partners is vital for helping to correct the physical and emotional abuse.**
- Determine how partners resolve conflict. **Past coping strategies used can be enhanced, help the partners recognize the use of defense mechanisms, or if the police have been involved in the past or present conflicts.**
- Note how partners as a whole function. **Interactions among partners and situational dynamics provide information about need to improve relationships. Is there a history of dominance or controlling behaviors?**
- Identify partners' readiness to change. **Attempting to present interventions prior to both parties identifying their stage of readiness to resolve the conflict will be met with resistance. Negotiating with partners may help to identify a stage of readiness that both agree on as a starting point.**

Nursing Priority No. 2.

To assist couple to improve relationship:

- Develop a therapeutic nurse/partner relationship. **Listening respectfully to the partners' concerns demonstrates a willingness and caring to help with their issues.**
- Maintain a positive attitude in interactions with individuals. **Provides an environment in which clients feel comfortable and safe discussing problems openly.**
- Promote discussions with partners to foster awareness of each other's thoughts, feelings, and beliefs that may strain relationship. **Enables individuals to begin to discuss potential problem areas and understand other points of view.**
- Have partners identify thoughts and feelings when starting a conversation. **Individuals have a system of thinking that forms the basis for reality, determines how they see the world, and exists below the level of our consciousness.**
- Discuss the skills of emotional intelligence. **The ability to recognize and control own emotions and recognize emotions of others is important to maintain healthy relationships. Recognizing others' emotions is being aware of their body language.**

Information that appears in brackets has been added by the authors to clarify and enhance the use of nursing diagnoses.

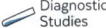 Diagnostic Studies 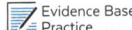 Evidence Based Practice 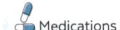 Medications 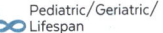 Pediatric/Geriatric/Lifespan

- Assist partners to understand effects of nonverbal language. **Lack of awareness of body language, tone of voice, and subtle movements can be misinterpreted and need to be discussed and clarified.**
- Explore each person's physical, sexual, and emotional needs. **Understanding that unconscious needs underlie desire to gain acceptance, recognition, and sense of being cared about or valued, helps client to deal more openly with these issues.**
- Encourage couple to learn effective conflict-resolution skills. **Family may have used ineffective ways to cope with conflict, resulting in fighting and a lose-lose situation.**
- Role-play a specific problem couple argues about, using the win-win method of resolution. **Practicing how to defuse arguments and repair hurt feelings helps to identify other's feelings and use new skills for resolution.**
- Encourage partners to practice remaining calm and focused regardless of circumstances. **When issue has previously resulted in violence, remaining calm can help individuals think more clearly and be more rational in solving the situation, and avoiding further conflict.**
- Have each person verify what they think they heard the other person say. **Provides the opportunity for the speaker to correct or acknowledge what was said.**
- Discuss issues and provide information about intimate relationships. **Conflict inevitably affects intimacy, and couple may need to resolve issues around this part of their life. Include a sex therapist/counselor to participate in helping the couple.**
- Discuss use of nonblameful self-disclosure during discussions with partner. **Promotes an atmosphere of respect and mutual consideration in which individuals can talk about their feelings and resolve problems.**

Nursing Priority No. 3.

To promote optimal relationship between partners (Teaching/Discharge Considerations) and enhance well-being (long-term goals):

- Review what partners have learned about intimate relationships. **Encourages input from each member so each feels heard and views self as part of the solution.**
- Encourage partners to use active-listening technique. **Allows the partner to share their concerns without fear of judgment. Active-listener does not provide solutions, however, allows the partner to find their own solution that enhances self-esteem and builds confidence.**

Information that appears in brackets has been added by the authors to clarify and enhance the use of nursing diagnoses.

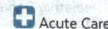 Acute Care 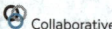 Collaborative 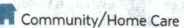 Community/Home Care Cultural

- Discuss appropriate use of humor and playfulness in daily interactions. **Helps partners to identify humor and playfulness, not at the other's expense, to enjoy life and laughter. Humor and laughter makes difficult issues easier to cope with.**
- Encourage use of relaxation and mindfulness techniques. **Promotes calm manner and ability to cope with difficult issues more effectively.**
- Recommend information sources, books, and websites, as appropriate. **Provides additional resources to access information to assist couple in learning to cope with intimate relationships/partner issues.**
- Identify community resources/support groups as appropriate. **Individuals who have successfully resolved similar issues can provide role modeling for change and effective use of problem-solving skills.**
- Refer to therapy as indicated. **May need further in-depth care to cope with individual physical/psychological/sexual issues.**

Documentation Focus

Assessment/Reassessment
- Individual's perception of situation and self.
- Partner's views and expectations.
- How partners communicate and deal with conflict.

Planning
- Plan of care and who is involved in planning.
- Teaching plan.

Implementation/Evaluation
- Response of partners to plan, interventions, and actions performed.
- Attainment or progress toward desired outcomes.
- Modifications to plan of care.

Discharge Planning
- Long-range plan and who is responsible for actions to be taken.
- Any referrals made.

Sample Nursing Outcomes & Interventions Classifications NOC/NIC

NOC—Social Interaction Skills
NIC—Conflict Mediation

Information that appears in brackets has been added by the authors to clarify and enhance the use of nursing diagnoses.

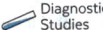 Diagnostic Studies 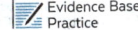 Evidence Based Practice 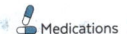 Medications 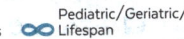 Pediatric/Geriatric/Lifespan

RELATIONSHIP PROBLEM

ICNP

[Diagnostic Division: Roles/Relationships]

Definition: An evolving pattern between individuals with increasing stress, unresolved conflict, and diverging goals for the future.

Recognizing Cues

Related/Risk Factors
Inadequate communication skills; lack of trust
Multiple stressors; unresolved conflict
Different goals; unrealistic expectations
Substance misuse

Defining Characteristics

Subjective
Unhappy with emotional support/responses from family and friends,
Dissatisfied with communications, interactions, and quality time together

Objective
Inability to collaborate or define goals; defined goals not obtained
Lack of mutual respect between family and friends
Inability to trust, support, or respect family and friends, misunderstands compromise functioning of others

Clinical Connections
Chronic conditions (e.g., multiple sclerosis, spinal cord injury, gastric bypass surgery, mental health problems, depression, anxiety, bipolar disorder, personality disorders, substance abuse, dementia), domestic violence

Generate Solutions

Plan Desired Outcomes

Client Will (Include Specific Time Frame)
- Verbalize a desire to improve relationship with family and friends.
- Acknowledge worth and value of family and friends as a person.
- Seek information regarding physical and emotional needs of others.

Information that appears in brackets has been added by the authors to clarify and enhance the use of nursing diagnoses.

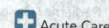 Acute Care 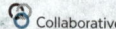 Collaborative 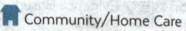 Community/Home Care  Cultural

- Engage in effective communication skills.
- Participate in therapy sessions to learn ways to develop satisfactory relationships.

Interventions/Take Action

Nursing Priority No. 1.
To assess current situation and determine needs:

- Determine makeup of family, length of relationship, and financial situation—parents/children, older/younger, and other members of household. **Stressors of family relationships within a household, difficulties with child-rearing, older adult needing care, and financial difficulties can strain the relationship between partners.**
- Discuss individual's perception of own and other's needs and how family sees own needs. **Identifies how each person sees situation and areas of agreement and disagreement, providing a basis for beginning plan of care.**
- Determine person's self-image and locus of control. **View of self as a positive or negative individual who is in control or controlled by others influences behavior and how family and friends respond.**
- Assess emotional intelligence skills. **This is the ability to recognize and control one's own emotions and recognize the emotions of other.**
- Investigate cultural factors that may be affecting relationship and contributing to conflict. **Roles from family of origin for each person may promote conflict when beliefs clash and neither is willing to change or even discuss thinking.**
- Determine style of communication used (passive, aggressive, passive-aggressive, assertive). **Poor communication is unclear and indirect leading to conflict, ineffective problem-solving, and poor emotional bonding in families with problems.**
- Determine how family as a whole functions (structure, roles, developmental stage, culture, spiritually). **Personal and family history affects relationships between family members, and situational dynamics can create conflict as individuals take sides in disagreements, escalating the situation.**
- Identify ways in which family members cope with conflict. **Conflict is inevitable in relationships, and family need to identify how they cope when it is effective or ineffective.**
- Note medical problems that may be affecting the relationship. **Conditions such as heart disease, diabetes,**

Information that appears in brackets has been added by the authors to clarify and enhance the use of nursing diagnoses.

 Diagnostic Studies 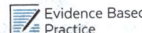 Evidence Based Practice Medications Pediatric/Geriatric/Lifespan

and cancer may cause family and friends to feel overwhelmed with stress and withdraw from one another.
- Identify digital addiction (e.g., social media or games via cell phone or computer). **Digital addiction has become a health concern globally that influences interpersonal relationships.**

Nursing Priority No. 2.
To assist family and friends to resolve existing conflict:

- Maintain positive attitude toward family members and others. **A safe environment allows individuals to speak freely, knowing they will not be judged for comments and opinions, so family or others can get to the deeper roots of current situation.**
- Discuss surface symptoms of dysfunctional relationships and the fact that these are not the problems that need to be dealt with. **Individuals are often not aware of underlying emotions that are influencing their behavior and continue to focus on surface issues.**
- Explore family/friends and others emotional needs. **Unconscious desires to gain acceptance, recognition, and a sense of being cared about or valued are often motivators for relationships.**
- Discuss and clarify nonverbal communication. **Client, family/friends, and others need to be aware of and ask about the meaning of body language, tone of voice, and subtle movements that convey positive or negative messages. When these cues are misinterpreted, they can lead to misunderstandings.**

- Assist client/family/friends and others to learn effective conflict-resolution skills such as the win-win method. **Individuals have traditionally used ineffective means of solving conflict or avoided it altogether. Resolving to listen to each other's needs and agree on a mutually acceptable solution provides new ways to resolve problems and enhances relationship.**
- Provide information about the active-listening technique. **Avoids giving advice and encourages other person to find own solution, enhancing self-esteem.**
- Have clients identify thoughts and feelings when starting a discussion with each other. **A system of thinking (a paradigm), existing below our level of consciousness, forms the basis for how we look at and experience life and determines how we perceive our world, forming the basis for our reality.**

Information that appears in brackets has been added by the authors to clarify and enhance the use of nursing diagnoses.

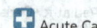 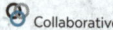 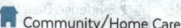

- Discuss the skills of emotional intelligence. **The ability to recognize and control own emotions and recognize emotions of others is important to maintain healthy relationships.**
- Explore each person's emotional needs. **Understanding that unconscious needs underlie desire to gain acceptance, recognition, and sense of being cared about or valued help client to deal more openly with these issues.**
- Assist partners to understand effects of nonverbal language. **Lack of awareness of body language, tone of voice, and subtle movements can be misinterpreted and need to be discussed and clarified.**
- Encourage couple to learn effective conflict-resolution skills. **Family may have used ineffective ways to deal with conflict, resulting in fighting and a lose-lose situation.**
- Recommend individuals verify what they believe they heard. **Allows speaker to correct misperception and respond more effectively.**
- Role-play a specific conflict that is a frequent issue using the win-win method of resolution. **Practicing how to defuse arguments and repair hurt feelings helps to identify other's feelings and use new skills for resolution.**
- Encourage clients to maintain a calm demeanor and focus, regardless of circumstances. **Regardless of circumstances, staying focused enables individuals to think more rationally and come to a desired solution.**
- Promote nonblameful self-disclosure when having a discussion. **Not placing blame results in a more considerate and respectful resolution.**

Nursing Priority No. 3.

To promote optimal relationship between family, friends, and others (Teaching/Discharge Considerations) and enhance well-being (long-term goals):

- Include all family members in discussions, as indicated. **Promotes involvement, provides opportunities for communication and clarification of family dynamics, and enhances commitment to achieving goals.**
- Have individuals acknowledge beliefs they have become aware of during therapy. **Unconscious thinking influences each person's view of the world in negative or positive ways.**

Information that appears in brackets has been added by the authors to clarify and enhance the use of nursing diagnoses.

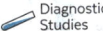 Diagnostic Studies 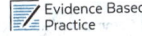 Evidence Based Practice 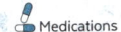 Medications ∞ Pediatric/Geriatric/Lifespan

- Encourage use of relaxation and mindfulness techniques. **Helps individuals to ease anxiety and learn to relate to each other in a calm manner.**
- Encourage family members to use active-listening. **Avoid giving advice and allow others to find their own solution, enhancing self-esteem.**
- Discuss the use of humor and laughter (not at other's expense) in daily lives. **Helps to lighten difficult moments and provide opportunities to share fun moments.**
- Recommend books and websites to provide additional information. **Encourages partners to seek and learn new ways to improve relationship.**
- Refer to support groups and classes as indicated. **Parenting, assertiveness, and financial assistance will help partners learn new skills as needed.**
- Refer to other physical/psychological resources, as needed. **May need further treatment to address pathology and help partners understand other's needs.**

Documentation Focus

Assessment/Reassessment
- Individual's perception of situation and self
- Individuals views and expectations
- How individuals communicate and cope with conflict

Planning
- Plan of care and who is involved in planning
- Teaching plan

Implementation/Evaluation
- Response of individuals to plan, interventions, and actions performed
- Attainment or progress toward desired outcomes

Discharge Planning
- Long-range plan and who is responsible for actions to be taken
- Referrals made

Sample Nursing Outcomes & Interventions Classifications NOC/NIC

NOC—Social Interaction Skills
NIC—Role Enhancement

Information that appears in brackets has been added by the authors to clarify and enhance the use of nursing diagnoses.

impaired RELIGIOSITY NANDA-I

[Diagnostic Division: Values/Beliefs]

Definition: Diminished commitment of oneself to faith-based beliefs, principles, and activities.

Recognizing Cues

Related/Risk Factors
Anxiety; depressive symptoms
Cultural barrier to practicing religion; spiritual distress
Fear of death; insecurity
Inadequate social support, or sociocultural interaction
Unaddressed environmental constraints
Inadequate transportation
Ineffective use of coping strategies; ineffective caregiving
Pain

Defining Characteristics

Subjective
Difficulty reconnecting with previous belief patterns, or religious rituals
Difficulty adhering to religious doctrines, or rituals (e.g., ceremonies, regulations, clothing, prayer, services, holiday observances)
Discomfort with separation from faith community
Questions religious doctrines, or rituals

Clinical Connections
Any acute or chronic condition, palliative care, end-of-life situation, depression, long-term care residents

Generate Solutions

Plan Desired Outcomes

Client Will (Include Specific Time Frame)
- Express understanding of relation of situation/health status to thoughts and feelings of concern about ability to participate in desired religious activities.
- Seek solutions to individual factors that may interfere with reliance on religious beliefs/participation in religious rituals.
- Express ability to once again participate in beliefs and rituals of desired religion.

Information that appears in brackets has been added by the authors to clarify and enhance the use of nursing diagnoses.

- Discuss beliefs and values about spiritual or religious issues.
- Attend religious or worship services of choice as desired.
- Verbalize concerns about end-of-life issues and fear of death.

Interventions/Take Action

Nursing Priority No. 1.
To assess causative/contributing factors:
- Determine client's usual religious and spiritual beliefs, values, and past spiritual commitment. **Provides a baseline for understanding current problem.**
- Identify current situation (e.g., illness, hospitalization, prognosis of death, depression, lack of support systems, financial concerns). **Identifies problems client is dealing with in the moment that may be affecting desire to be involved with spiritual activities.**
- Determine client's usual religious or spiritual beliefs and past or current involvement in specific spiritual activities. **Provides an understanding of how client sees religion in own life before current disruption.**
- Note client's/significant other's (SO's) reports and expressions of anger/concern, alienation from God, and sense of guilt or retribution. **Perception of guilt may cause spiritual crisis and suffering, resulting in rejection of religious beliefs or anger toward God.**
- Identify barriers and beliefs that may hinder growth or self-discovery. **Provides opportunity for self-reflection such as own worthiness and ability to forgive self for past decisions or life choices. Previous practices and beliefs may need to be considered, and then accepted or discarded when new search for religious beliefs is begun. That process may be long.**
- Determine sense of futility, feelings of hopelessness, and lack of motivation to help self. **Indicators that client may see no, or only limited, options or personal choices, and treatment needs to be directed at finding what happened in client's life to bring about these feelings.**
- Assess extent of depression client may be experiencing. **Some studies suggest that a focus on religion may protect against depression.**
- Note recent changes in negative behaviors (e.g., withdrawal from others or religious activities, dependence on alcohol or medications). **Lack of connectedness with self and others impairs ability to trust others or feel worthy of trust from others or God.**

Information that appears in brackets has been added by the authors to clarify and enhance the use of nursing diagnoses.

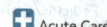 Acute Care 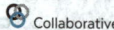 Collaborative 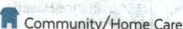 Community/Home Care Cultural

- Identify cultural values and expectations regarding religious beliefs or practices. **Individuals grow up in a family that instills a value system within them. As the person grows up, ideas, values, and expectations may change or be strengthened by new information, different questioning, and alternative viewpoints, which may affect current situation.**
- Note quality of relationships with significant others and friends. **Individual may withdraw from others in relation to the stress of illness, pain, and suffering. Others may be encouraging client to rely on religious beliefs at a time when individual is questioning own beliefs in the current situation.**
- Note socioeconomic status of individual/family. **Women who are poor may have high levels of personal religiosity yet participate less in organized religion because they may feel stigmatized by their situation (e.g., single mothers, those receiving public assistance, those engaging in a lifestyle that conflicts with church norms).**
- Assess lack of transportation or environmental barriers to participation in desired religious activities. **These barriers can be realistic in the face of such issues as poor bus systems, inability of individual to get to bus stop (physical problems of walking or distance to the bus stop), or inability to drive a car.**
- Identify substance use or abuse. **Individuals often turn to use of various substances in distress, and this can affect the ability to deal with problems in a positive manner.**
- Determine client's current thinking about and expressed desire to learn more about religious beliefs and actions. **Provides guidance of client's wishes.**
- Identify religious beliefs or cultural values of family of origin and climate in which client grew up. **Early religious training deeply affects children and is carried on into adulthood. Conflict between family's beliefs and client's current learning may need to be addressed.**

Nursing Priority No. 2.

To assist client/SOs to deal with feelings/situation:

- Use therapeutic communication skills of reflection and active-listening. **Communicates acceptance and enables client to find own solutions to concerns as situation is discussed and deeper meanings are discovered.**
- Have client identify and prioritize current and immediate needs. **Coping with current needs is easier than trying to predict the future. Also, it is important to take care of basic needs before moving on to higher needs.**

Information that appears in brackets has been added by the authors to clarify and enhance the use of nursing diagnoses.

- Encourage expression of feelings about illness, condition, or death. **As people age, they become more concerned about their own mortality, and others often see them as in poor health and as spiritual and religious. If they have been diagnosed with a long-term chronic or terminal illness, they may be feeling more angry and rejecting of God than seeking God's help.**
- Review with client past difficulties in life and coping skills that were used at that time. **Recalling problems with family, peers, and colleagues or individuals in position of authority can help client to remember how those were handled and how those skills could be used in current situation.**
- Provide time for nonjudgmental discussion of individual's spiritual beliefs and fears about impact of current illness and/or treatment regimen. **Helps to clarify thoughts and promote ability to deal with stresses of what is happening.**
- Discuss how cultural beliefs of family of origin have influenced client's religious practices. **As client expands options for learning new or other religious beliefs and practices, these influences will provide information for comparing and contrasting new information.**
- Discuss personal beliefs that may hinder participation in religious activities. **Provides opportunity for self-reflection, such as own worthiness and ability to forgive self for past decisions/life choices.**
- Discuss differences between grief and guilt, and help client to identify and deal with each. Point out consequences of actions based on guilt. **Individuals often feel guilty about the "what-ifs" of life. "If only I had done this!" "If only I had paid more attention!" "If only I had made him go to the doctor!" Most of these guilty feelings are not based on reality, and when they are acted on, the individual does not get the release they seek.**
- Explore connection of desire to strengthen belief patterns and customs to daily life. **Becoming aware of how these issues affect the individual's daily life can enhance ability to incorporate them.**
- Suggest use of journaling and reminiscence. **Promotes life review and can assist in clarifying values and ideas, recognizing and resolving feelings and situation.**
- Review client's religious affiliation, associated rituals, and beliefs. **Helps client examine what was important in the**

Information that appears in brackets has been added by the authors to clarify and enhance the use of nursing diagnoses.

past and may trigger some desire to reconnect with these previous beliefs.
- Provide opportunity for nonjudgmental discussion of philosophical issues related to religious belief patterns and customs. **Open communication can assist client to check reality of perceptions and identify personal options and willingness to resume desired activities.**
- Discuss desire to continue or reconnect with previous belief patterns and customs and perceived barriers. **As client begins to think about current feelings of alienation from religious connections, these discussions can help to clarify and allow client to think about how beliefs can be restored or modified.**
- Identify ways to strengthen spiritual or religious expression. **There are multiple options for enhancing participation in faith community (e.g., joining prayer or study group, volunteering time to community projects, singing in the choir, reading spiritual writings).**
- Take the lead from the client in initiating participation in religious activities, prayer, and/or other activities. **Client may be vulnerable in current situation and needs to be allowed to decide own participation in these actions. Living and participating in desired religious activities will help client to understand the tenets of their choice.**
- Explore alternatives or modifications of ritual based on setting and individual needs and limitations. **Individual may not be able to attend community place of worship, so another location—chapel in the facility or quiet room with appropriate religious artifacts or material—can provide the setting desired.**
- Provide privacy for meditation or prayer and performance of rituals, as appropriate. **Many individuals prefer to pray or meditate in private so they can concentrate without interruption or questions from others.**
- Involve client in refining healthcare goals and therapeutic regimen, as appropriate. **Identifies role that client's illness or condition is playing in current ability to participate and appropriateness of participating in desired religious activities.**
- Help client learn relaxation techniques, meditation, guided imagery, and mindfulness (living in the moment and enjoying it). **Learning to relax can help client to process information and make decisions in a more positive manner.**

Information that appears in brackets has been added by the authors to clarify and enhance the use of nursing diagnoses.

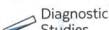 Diagnostic Studies
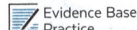 Evidence Based Practice
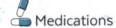 Medications
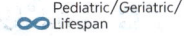 Pediatric/Geriatric/Lifespan

Nursing Priority No. 3.

To promote spiritual growth (Teaching/Discharge Considerations) and enhance well-being (long-term goals):

- Assist client to identify spiritual counselor who could be helpful (e.g., minister, priest, spiritual advisor who has qualifications or experience) in dealing with specific concerns of client. **Provides answers to spiritual questions, assists in the journey of self-discovery, and can help client learn to accept and forgive self.**
- Encourage client to continue stress-reducing activities, such as meditation, relaxation exercises, or mindfulness (method of being in the moment). **Promotes general well-being and sense of control over self and ability to choose desired religious activities.**
- Encourage participation in religious activities and services, as desired. **Enhances client's knowledge and promotes connectedness with self, others, and/or higher power.**
- Refer to community religious leaders (e.g., pastor, rabbi, imam, parish nurse, religion classes, other support groups). **Guides client to leaders in the community.**
- Provide bibliotherapy, including list of relevant resources and websites. **Allows client to use for later reference, promoting self-paced learning and ongoing support.**
- Refer to appropriate resources such as crisis counselor, governmental agencies, spiritual advisor (who has qualifications or experience dealing with specific problems such as death or dying process, relationship problems, substance abuse, suicide), hospice, psychotherapy, and Alcoholics or Narcotics Anonymous. **May require additional help to cope with current situation.**

Documentation Focus

Assessment/Reassessment
- Individual findings, including risk factors or nature of spiritual conflict, effects of participation in treatment regimen
- Physical and emotional responses to conflict
- Availability and use of resources

Planning
- Plan of care and who is involved in planning
- Teaching plan

Information that appears in brackets has been added by the authors to clarify and enhance the use of nursing diagnoses.

Implementation/Evaluation
- Responses to interventions, teaching, and actions performed
- Attainment of or progress toward desired outcome(s)
- Modifications to plan of care

Discharge Planning
- Long-term needs and who is responsible for actions to be taken
- Available resources, specific referrals made

Sample Nursing Outcomes & Interventions Classifications NOC/NIC

NOC—Spiritual Health
NIC—Spiritual Support

---

risk for RELOCATION STRESS ICNP

[Diagnostic Division: Stress Management]

Definition: Susceptible to negative psychological and physical effects associated with moving from one environment to another.

Recognizing Cues

Risk Factors
Limited or no preparation for change; forced change/relocation (e.g., decline in health/cognitive function; house fire, natural disaster)

Lack of control; disruption of situation/daily routines; resistance to change

Unfamiliarity with new environment; lack of resources, social support

Potential loss of independence, friends, possessions, neighborhood/community, and/or school/employment

Depressive symptoms; substance misuse

Individuals facing unpredictability of experience or who move from one environment to another; or who have history of loss

Clinical Connections
Chronic conditions (e.g., multiple sclerosis, asthma, cystic fibrosis), brain injury, stroke, dementia, schizophrenia, developmental delay

---

Information that appears in brackets has been added by the authors to clarify and enhance the use of nursing diagnoses.

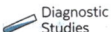 Diagnostic Studies 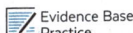 Evidence Based Practice 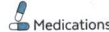 Medications 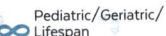 Pediatric/Geriatric/Lifespan

Generate Solutions

Plan Desired Outcomes

Client Will (Include Specific Time Frame)
- Verbalize understanding of reason(s) for change.
- Demonstrate appropriate range of feelings and reduced anxiety.
- Participate in routine and special or social events as able.
- Verbalize acceptance of situation.

Interventions/Take Action

Nursing Priority No. 1.
To assess causative/contributing or risk factors:

- Determine situation or cause for relocation (e.g., planned move for new job; deployment or returning from military duty; loss of home or community due to natural or man-made disaster; older adult unable to care for self, caregiver burnout; change in marital or health status; child in foster care, adolescent leaving for college, death of significant other). **The greatest incidence of relocation stress occurs just before and during a 3-mo period following relocation and increases if there is (1) little or no time to prepare for a move; (2) a lack of predictability about the new environment; and (3) little or no time between notification to move and the move itself.** (Refer to ND risk for disrupted Immigration Transition for interventions appropriate to this population.)
- Determine physical and emotional health status. **Stress associated with a move, even if desired, can cause or exacerbate health problems.**
- Note client's age, developmental level, role in family. **Age and position in life cycle make a difference in the impact of issues involved in relocating. For example, a child can be traumatized by transfer to new school/loss of peers; elderly persons may be affected by loss of long-term home, neighborhood setting, and support persons.**
- Ascertain if client participated in the decision to relocate and perceptions about change(s) and expectations for the future. **Decision may have been made without client's input or understanding of event or consequences, which can impact adjustment.**
- Note whether relocation will be temporary (e.g., extended care for rehabilitation therapies, moving in with family while house is being repaired after fire) or long term or

---

Information that appears in brackets has been added by the authors to clarify and enhance the use of nursing diagnoses.

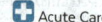 Acute Care 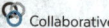 Collaborative 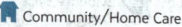 Community/Home Care   Cultural

permanent (e.g., move from home of many years; placement in retirement center or long-term care facility). **Client may be willing to relocate on temporary basis, seeing it as step to health and independence, but may view long-term placement as unbearable loss.**

- Identify cultural and/or spiritual concerns or conflicts **that may affect client's coping or impact social interactions and expectations. For example, client's cultural norm may be that elders are cared for by family—not placed in a facility—causing client to feel abandoned; or individual may be required to defer to family decision-maker and feel powerless in determining own destiny.**
- Note ethnic ties and primary language spoken and read. Obtain interpreter where appropriate. **Affects client, significant other(s) (SO[s]), and healthcare providers who must try to reduce the client's feelings of alienation while communicating with client of another primary language or client who is displaced from cultural attachments.**
- Monitor behavior, noting presence of anxiety, suspiciousness or paranoia, irritability, defensiveness. Compare with SO's/staff's description of customary responses. **Move may temporarily exacerbate mental deterioration (cognitive inaccessibility) and impair communication (social inaccessibility).**
- Determine involvement of family/SO(s). Note availability and use of support systems and resources. Ascertain presence or absence of comprehensive information and planning (e.g., when and how move will take place, if the environment for the client will be similar or greatly changed). **These factors can greatly affect client's ability to cope with change.**
- Identify issues of safety that may be involved, **such as difficulty adjusting to new environment (e.g., navigating streets or choosing correct bus; locating dining hall or bathroom in facility), concerns of elopement or running away.**

Nursing Priority No. 2.
To prevent/minimize adverse response to change:

- Collaborate in treatment of underlying conditions (e.g., chronic confusional states, brain injury, post-trauma rehabilitation) and physical stress symptoms **that are potentially exacerbating relocation stress or that may affect the length of time that relocation is required.**

Information that appears in brackets has been added by the authors to clarify and enhance the use of nursing diagnoses.

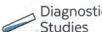 Diagnostic Studies 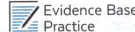 Evidence Based Practice 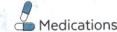 Medications 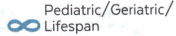 Pediatric/Geriatric/Lifespan

- Anticipate and address feelings of distress and grieving in family/caregivers when placing loved one in a different environment (e.g., nursing home, foster care). **Support and referrals may be needed to help SOs in practical issues and adjustment.**
- Begin relocation planning with client and SO(s) as early as possible. Provide support and advocate for client who is unable to participate in decisions. **Having a well-organized plan for move with support and advocacy may reduce anxiety.**
- Allow as much time as possible for move preparation and provide information and support in planning.
- ∞ Discuss relocation or move with child, providing information aimed at level of understanding and interest. **Child lacks ability to put problem into perspective, so minor mishap may seem catastrophic, and child is more vulnerable to stress because they have less control over environment than most adults.**
- ∞ Encourage age-appropriate decisions for child (e.g., choice of bedroom/paint colors, designated play area) or older adult (e.g., move to nursing home or adult foster care). **Inclusion in decision allows individual to be part of the process, increasing their sense of control.**
- ∞ Avoid moving adolescent in middle of school year when possible. **Adolescent is vulnerable to emotional, social, and cognitive dysfunction because of the great importance of peer group and loss of friends and social standing caused by relocation.**
- Support self-responsibility and coping strategies **to foster sense of control and self-worth.**
- Suggest contact with someone (friend, family, business associate) who has been to or lived in new area where move is being planned **to absorb some of that person's experience and knowledge.**
- Encourage free expression of feelings about reason for relocation, including venting of anger; grief; loss of personal space, belongings, or friends; financial strains; powerlessness; and so forth. Acknowledge reality of situation and maintain hopeful attitude regarding move/change. Refer to NDs relating to client's particular situation (e.g., Grief; difficulty Coping) for additional interventions. **Provides opportunity to shift negative perceptions and identify positive aspects of relocation. Note: Children are particularly sensitive to change when divorce is involved, resulting in new home, environment, and family structure, triggering sense of insecurity, isolation, and/or anger.**

Information that appears in brackets has been added by the authors to clarify and enhance the use of nursing diagnoses.

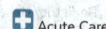 Acute Care 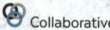 Collaborative 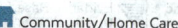 Community/Home Care 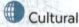 Cultural

- Identify strengths and successful coping behaviors the individual has used previously. **Incorporating them into problem-solving builds on past successes.**
- Encourage client to maintain contact with friends (e.g., telephone, email, video calls, arranged visits) **to reduce sense of isolation.**
- Orient to surroundings and schedules. Introduce to neighbors, staff members, roommate, or residents. Provide clear, honest information about actions and events.
- Encourage individual/family to personalize area with pictures, own belongings, as possible and appropriate. **Enhances sense of belonging and creates personal space.**
- Determine client's usual schedule of activities and incorporate into routine as possible. **Reinforces sense of importance of individual.**
- ∞ Take practical steps to alleviate stress for child. Encourage parents to walk with child to school or rehearse boarding the school bus, visit new classroom, contact friends child left behind, drive past places of interest to child, find a safe play place, unpack child's favorite toys, invite neighborhood children to a get-acquainted party, and so forth. **Helps child to maintain ties and develop new ones, thus reducing sense of loss and shifting focus to the future.**
- Introduce planned diversional activities, such as movies, meals with new acquaintances, art therapy, music, spiritual activities. **Involvement increases opportunity to interact with others, decreasing isolation.**
- Long-Term Placement:

Place client with dementia in private room in facility, if appropriate, and include SO(s)/family in care activities, mealtimes, especially early in transition stage. **Keeping client secluded may be needed under some circumstances (e.g., advanced Alzheimer disease with fear or aggressive reactions) to decrease the client's stress reactions to new environment.**

Encourage physical contact, use of touch unless client prefers to abstain, is paranoid, or is agitated at the moment. **Human connection reaffirms acceptance of individual.**

Deal with aggressive behavior by imposing calm, firm limits. Control environment and protect others from client's disruptive behavior. **Promotes safety for client and others.**

Remain composed, place in a quiet environment, providing time out, as indicated, **to prevent escalation into panic state and violent behavior.**

Information that appears in brackets has been added by the authors to clarify and enhance the use of nursing diagnoses.

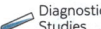 Diagnostic Studies 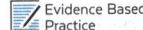 Evidence Based Practice 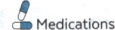 Medications 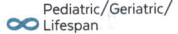 Pediatric/Geriatric/Lifespan

Nursing Priority No. 3.

To promote acceptance (Teaching/Discharge Considerations) and enhance well-being (long-term goals):

- Involve client/family in formulating goals and plan of care when possible. **Supports independence and commitment to achieving outcomes.**
- ∞ Contact facility staff for suggestions to facility relocation of older adult. **Strategies used may include assigning a staff person or knowledgeable resident to act as guide to new facility, accompanying to an activity, having a family meal together in dining room.**
- Encourage communication between client/family/SO **to provide mutual support and problem-solving opportunities.**
- Discuss benefits of adequate nutrition, rest, and exercise **to maintain physical well-being.**
- Involve in anxiety- and stress-reduction activities (e.g., meditation, progressive muscle relaxation, group socialization), as able, **to enhance psychological well-being and coping abilities.**
- Encourage participation in activities, hobbies, and personal interactions as appropriate. **Promotes creative endeavors, stimulating the mind.**
- Provide client with information and list of local social groups, assistance organizations, or community services (e.g., Welcome Wagon, senior citizen or teen clubs, churches, singles' groups, sports leagues) **to provide contacts for client to develop new relationships and learn more about the new setting.**
- Discuss safety issues regarding new environment (e.g., how to navigate streets or choose correct bus; locate dining hall or bathroom in facility), concerns of elopement or running away.
- ∞ Anticipate variety of emotions and reactions that may not occur immediately but be delayed for weeks or months. **May vary from insomnia and loss of appetite to becoming involved with alcohol or other drugs or exacerbation of health problems, onset of serious illness, or behavioral problems. Awareness provides opportunity for timely intervention. Note: Children show signs of stress differently at different ages or school levels, and their reaction is affected by the emotional reactions of parents/adults around them.**

Information that appears in brackets has been added by the authors to clarify and enhance the use of nursing diagnoses.

- Identify resources for professional counseling as indicated. **Inability to express or experience own feelings, behavioral changes, increasing anxiety, depressive symptoms requires mental health support for safety and well-being of individual.**
- Refer to NDs lack of Resilience; Post-Trauma Syndrome for additional interventions.

Documentation Focus

Assessment/Reassessment
- Assessment findings, individual's perception of the situation and changes, sense of loss, specific behaviors
- Cultural, socioeconomic, or spiritual concerns
- Safety issues

Planning
- Note plan of care, who is involved in planning, and who is responsible for proposed actions
- Teaching plan

Implementation/Evaluation
- Response to interventions (especially time out or seclusion), teaching, and actions performed
- Sentinel events
- Attainment of or progress toward desired outcome(s)
- Modifications to plan of care

Discharge Planning
- Long-term needs and who is responsible for actions to be taken
- Specific referrals made

Sample Nursing Outcomes & Interventions Classifications NOC/NIC

NOC—Psychosocial Adjustment: Life Change
NIC—Relocation Stress Reduction

lack of RESILIENCE ICNP

[Diagnostic Division: Self-Perception/Concept]

Definition: Inability to recover psychologically from a stressful, adverse, or traumatic event.

Information that appears in brackets has been added by the authors to clarify and enhance the use of nursing diagnoses.

Recognizing Cues

Related/Risk Factors
Natural, man-made disasters; community discord
Dysfunctional family relationships, communication, roles
Illness; lack of health resources; lack of support
Financial decline; loss of employment
Partner discord; separation, divorce
Substance misuse; overeating

Defining Characteristics (impaired Resilience)

Subjective
Stress; anxiety; depressive symptoms; feels shame, guilt
Recurrent illness; increased somatic complaints
Feels out of control, powerless, vulnerable; lacks confidence
Lack of interest in usual activities, work/academic endeavors

Objective
Ineffective problem-solving skills
Poor self-esteem; lacks self-compassion
Withdrawn; isolation from family/friends
Restless; tearful; angry

Clinical Connections
Substance abuse, mental health issues—depression, phobia, bipolar disorder, schizophrenia; chronic illness—renal failure, heart failure, cancer; debilitating conditions—multiple sclerosis, Parkinson disease, obesity; eating disorders; domestic abuse or violence, human trafficking

Generate Solutions

Plan Desired Outcomes

Client Will (Include Specific Time Frame)
- Verbalize that life is challenging, requiring a reframing of negative events.
- Discuss positive attributes of self and positive thoughts regarding the situation.
- Use community resources for growth and development. express empathy, help others, and express gratitude.
- Express a willingness to help others and express empathy and gratitude toward others.
- Participate in programs based on specific needs, such as promoting mental health, substance abstinence, or learning to manage finances.

Information that appears in brackets has been added by the authors to clarify and enhance the use of nursing diagnoses.

 Acute Care 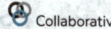 Collaborative 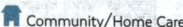 Community/Home Care Cultural

Interventions/Take Action

Nursing Priority No. 1.
To assess causative/contributing factors:

- Identify internal stressors (e.g., acute/chronic health concerns, debilitating conditions, or mental health issues), and external stressors (e.g., substance abuse, unemployment, food/shelter insecurity, discrimination/bullying, exposure to violence/disasters, human trafficking, previously incarcerated populations). Have client complete the General Health Questionnaire (GHQ). **Individuals overwhelmed with stress may lack psychological strength and physical energy, and their immune system may be impaired. The GHQ score reflects the average burden of psychological strain/mental distress. Promotes understanding the depth of distress client is experiencing, effect on health and well-being, to promote client-centered care.**
- Assess functional capacity and how it affects client's ability to cope and manage daily needs. **Stress influences people differently. Presence of physical impairments may bring additional stress, and current adversity or trauma can alter the immune system causing loss of physical and mental endurance to keep up with activities of daily living.**
- Evaluate client's ability to verbalize and comprehend current situation and influence on coping. **Client's psychological growth and developmental level and the number of stressors can impact client, affecting ability to communicate thoughts, feelings, and beliefs congruently.**
- Note speech and communication patterns, comparing with nonverbal behavior. **Communicates thoughts and ideas with others; however, verbal and nonverbal communication must be congruent, or clarified, to understand the client's intentions.**
- Determine client's locus of control. **Ability to control life depends on client's perception of vulnerability to internal and external stressors impacting life. Individuals with external locus of control are less likely to feel in control or rely on their own abilities or judgment to manage a situation.**
- Evaluate client's psychological developmental level and current decision-making ability. **Crises affect individual's ability to think clearly and trust own ability to deal with situation. Recognizing client's developmental stage and willingness and confidence to change guides decision-making capabilities.**

Information that appears in brackets has been added by the authors to clarify and enhance the use of nursing diagnoses.

- Determine timing of stressor(s) and gender of client. **Susceptibility and resilience to stress can depend on several factors including the timing of the exposure across the life span with respect to development as well as genetic sex of the individual (e.g., stress during early postnatal period is more likely to negatively affect males than females, childhood adversity impacts hormonal effects on neural function, stress exposures during puberty tend to have stronger immediate effects on females).**
- Identify coping skills and use of defense mechanisms by individual and in the family. **The use of food or drugs to deal with feelings, acting-out behaviors/poor impulse control or violence, devaluing education or importance of learning new skills, and focusing on the negative in situations lead to members learning these methods of dealing with problems and difficulties that arise, resulting in lack of ability to adjust positively and learn attributes of resiliency.**
- Note parental status (including age and maturity) and parenting style. **Young parents may lack ability to deal with family responsibilities, financial concerns, and low socioeconomic factors.**
- Determine stability of client's relationships with spouse/significant others (e.g., separation or divorce, deteriorating health, or recent death of family member). **Globally, family is the most significant social support for members throughout the life span. Parents role model how to cope with stress and adversity as well as help each other to be resilient.**
- Determine health literacy and availability and use of resources that can foster resilience, including family, support groups, and financial. **Identifies needs and potential supports to strengthen coping strategies.**
- Discuss spiritual/cultural beliefs and ethnic origin of client/family. **Knowing the role of culture and ethnicity in shaping and defining health behavior helps the individual understand how this is important to them. Note: Information is also important to reduce bias in healthcare and empower disadvantaged client/family.**
- Knowing the role of culture and ethnicity in shaping and defining health behavior helps the individual understand how this is important to them. Note: Information is also important to reduce bias in healthcare and empower disadvantaged client/family. **Improving the future is based on**

Information that appears in brackets has been added by the authors to clarify and enhance the use of nursing diagnoses.

 Acute Care 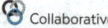 Collaborative 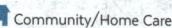 Community/Home Care Cultural developing the client's capacity to cope successfully with obstacles in life.

- Determine presence of suicidal ideation/plan/means. **A client in crisis is unpredictable; however, timely recognition and intervention can lessen stress and promote safety.** (Refer to ND risk for Suicide.)
- Determine client readiness/willingness to change behaviors. **Client's readiness to change stage will guide the level of interventions used to promote change. Interventions applied prior to the readiness of the client may be met with resistance.**

Nursing Priority No. 2.

To assist client to improve skills to deal with adverse situations or crises:

- Discuss primary concern (e.g., obesity, substance use, poor impulse control, violent behavior/abuse), providing information about the risks. Suggest habits client/family members can develop that promote physical and mental well-being. **For example, studies suggest that encouraging children to reduce sedentary behavior (e.g., screen time, aggressive video games) and choose activities/enjoyable exercise promoting movement can result in weight loss and improve feelings of satisfaction and sense of control.**
- Encourage free expressions of thoughts and feelings, including anger and hostility, setting limits on unacceptable/harmful behavior. **When feelings are verbalized, client begins to identify them and recognize how they affect personal behavior. Unacceptable behavior leads to feelings of shame and guilt if not controlled. Note: Reluctance to disclose feelings can be related to past experiences with disapproval or punishment.**
- Active-listen client's concerns and observe body language for congruency when interacting with family or providers. **Being listened to provides opportunity for client to feel valued, capable, and like a survivor rather than a victim. Nonverbal actions, especially facial expressions, eye contact, body posture, contribute 93% of the message to the receiver and may contradict the words spoken.**
- Acknowledge client's adversity and difficulty making changes in situation. **Often, individuals who are feeling that life is difficult begin to doubt their ability to deal with circumstances and are not able to anticipate positive outcomes.**

Information that appears in brackets has been added by the authors to clarify and enhance the use of nursing diagnoses.

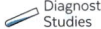 Diagnostic Studies 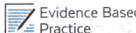 Evidence Based Practice 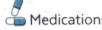 Medications 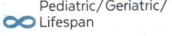 Pediatric/Geriatric/Lifespan

- Determine coping strategies used to cope with problems in the past. **Client's history of coping with previous stressors and awareness of self and others can indicate how much help and coaching is needed to help the client develop resiliency.**
- Help client to assume responsibility for own life, to look at situation as a challenge rather than an obstacle, and to refrain from viewing crisis as insurmountable. **Resilience is not something that people have or do not have; it is learned and developed in people as they deal with adversities of life. Taking care of oneself keeps the mind ready to deal with adverse situations.**
- Determine availability and use of resources, family, support groups, and financial. **Family, friends, and community support agencies are important resources to help the client continue on the path of personal growth and recovery.**
- Encourage client to collaborate with provider/treatment team when developing or revising therapy plan. **Exploring multiple approaches to take control of own thoughts and behaviors with interprofessional providers promotes sense of control and is associated with improving physical and mental well-being.**
- Explore multiple approaches to take control of own thoughts and behaviors with interprofessional providers. Promotes sense of control and is associated with improving physical and mental well-being. **Provides data to assist in decision-making process and enhances client's cooperation in change process. Nurses play a primary role in enhancing health literacy, which is the basis for successful outcomes.**
- Have client paraphrase information provided during teaching sessions. **Teaching sessions include communication, emotional intelligence, managing emotions, positive view of self and abilities, self view as a fighter rather than a victim, and setting realistic goals. Assures client's understanding, provides opportunity to correct misunderstandings, enhancing health literacy, which is the basis of successful outcomes.**
- Encourage spouse, parents, children involved with client to develop a positive mindset that fosters resilience within the family unit. **Family structure and parental presence demonstrate the influence family members gain when coping with distress and building resilience.**

Information that appears in brackets has been added by the authors to clarify and enhance the use of nursing diagnoses.

800 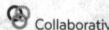 Acute Care 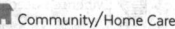 Collaborative Community/Home Care Cultural

- Facilitate communication skills between client and family encouraging open discussion about stressors. **Family relationships and effective communication are important components of socialization and developing coping skills to build resilience.**

Nursing Priority No. 3.

To promote successful adaptation to stressors (Teaching/Discharge Considerations) and enhance well-being (long-term goals):

- Reinforce that client is responsible for self, for choices made, and for actions taken and that resilience is within client's control. **Resiliency is a learned behavior of thinking, feeling, and believing promoted by learned skills/interventions, including cognitive behavioral therapy and mindfulness meditation.**
- Review client's strengths that assisted with emotional growth and development. **Client reinforced about progress toward autonomy and self-reliance may be able to progress with higher levels of change.**
- Identify learning opportunities/resources specific to individual needs, further promoting growth and development of coping strategies. **Activities such as coaching and training of assertiveness, journaling, regular physical exercise, socialization, hobbies, personal/family counseling, or parenting classes can enhance knowledge, promote healthy lifestyle, and help develop a resilience mindset.**
- Discuss use of the problem-solving method to set mutually agreed-on goals. **As family accepts solutions that are acceptable to each member, their self-esteem is enhanced, and individuals are more apt to follow through on decisions.**
- Provide anticipatory guidance relevant to current situation and long-term expectations. **Client may have many issues to resolve, and planning ahead can help client make changes, have hope for the future, and have a sense of control over their life.**
- Encourage client/parents to take time to care for themselves. **Provides opportunity for personal growth; respite allows individuals to pursue own interests and return to tasks of life/parenting with renewed vigor, which is vital to prevent relapse to ineffective behaviors.**
- Refer to community resources, as appropriate, such as social services; financial, domestic violence/elder abuse program;

Information that appears in brackets has been added by the authors to clarify and enhance the use of nursing diagnoses.

family therapy; divorce counseling; special needs support services. **Appropriate support enhances ability to develop resilience in challenges client is dealing with.**

Documentation Focus

Assessment/Reassessment
- Findings, including specifics of individual situations, parental concerns, perceptions, expectations
- Locus of control and cultural beliefs

Planning
- Plan of care and who is involved in the planning
- Teaching plan

Implementation/Evaluation
- Response to interventions, teaching, and actions performed
- Attainment of or progress toward desired outcome(s)
- Modifications to plan of care

Discharge Planning
- Long-term needs and who is responsible for actions to be taken
- Specific referrals made

Sample Nursing Outcomes & Interventions Classifications NOC/NIC

NOC—Personal Resiliency
NIC—Resilience Promotion

---

risk for urinary RETENTION NANDA-I

[Diagnostic Division: Elimination]

Definition: Susceptible to incomplete emptying of the bladder.

Recognizing Cues

Risk/Related Factors
Unaddressed environmental constraints; inadequate privacy
Fecal impaction
Improper toileting posture
Inadequate relaxation of pelvic floor; weakened pelvic floor

Information that appears in brackets has been added by the authors to clarify and enhance the use of nursing diagnoses.

 Acute Care 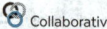 Collaborative 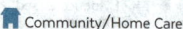 Community/Home Care   Cultural

Clinical Connections
Benign prostatic hyperplasia (BPH); prostatitis, cancer, perineal surgery, birth trauma, urethral calculi, diabetes mellitus, multiple sclerosis (MS), spinal cord compression, urinary tract infection (UTI)

Generate Solutions

Plan Desired Outcomes

Client Will (Include Specific Time Frame)
- Verbalize understanding of causative factors and appropriate interventions for individual situation.
- Demonstrate techniques or behaviors to alleviate or prevent retention.
- Void in sufficient amounts with no palpable bladder distention, experience no postvoid residuals greater than 50 mL, and have no dribbling or overflow.

Interventions/Take Action

Acute Retention

Nursing Priority No. 1.
To assess risk/contributing factors:

- Note client's gender and age. **Retention is most common among men (young men due to renal calculi) and older men (where prostate abnormalities or urethral strictures cause outlet obstruction). Postpartal women are at risk following delivery, and postmenopausal women are at risk because of changes in pelvic floor muscle strength. In either gender, retention may be due to medications; neurogenic bladder such as occurs with spinal cord injury (SCI); diabetes, MS, Parkinson disease; pelvic surgery; or any other condition resulting in bladder denervation.**
- Review client's history for (1) bladder outlet obstruction (e.g., prostatic hypertrophy, urethral stricture, urinary stones or tumors), (2) nonfunctioning detrusor muscle (i.e., sensory or motor paralytic bladder due to underlying neurological disease), or (3) atonic bladder that has lost its muscular tone (i.e., chronic overdistention), **resulting in ineffective emptying of the bladder and urine retention.**
- Ascertain if client can empty bladder completely, partially, or not at all, despite urge to urinate. **These are signs of urinary retention caused by (1) blockage of the urethra or**

Information that appears in brackets has been added by the authors to clarify and enhance the use of nursing diagnoses.

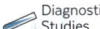 Diagnostic Studies 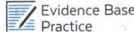 Evidence Based Practice 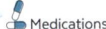 Medications 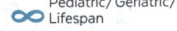 Pediatric/Geriatric/Lifespan

(2) **disruption of complex system of nerves that connects the urinary tract with the brain.**
- Investigate reports of sudden loss of ability to pass urine, great difficulty passing urine, sudden strong urges to urinate but difficulty starting urine stream; pain with urination, or blood in urine. **May indicate acute urinary retention due to UTI or outlet obstruction.**
- Review results of laboratory tests, such as urinalysis for presence of red and white blood cells, nitrates, glucose, bacteria, and cultures, as indicated. Blood may be tested for infection, electrolyte imbalance, and (in men) prostate-specific antigen **to determine presence of treatable conditions.**
- Review results of diagnostic tests. **Urine flow rate, bladder capacity, and postvoid residual scanning may be done to evaluate bladder muscle function and sphincter control; pelvic ultrasound, computed tomography (CT) scan, IV pyelogram, and cystoscopy can help locate the source of obstruction (e.g., lower or upper tract). Lumbar spine radiographs, CT scan, or MRI may be done when retention is thought to be due to an acute spinal problem (e.g., herniated disk, spinal cord disruption, infection) or presence of a chronic neurological conditions such as MS.**
- Review medication regimen **for drugs that can cause or exacerbate retention (e.g., psychotropics, opiates, sedatives, alpha and beta blockers, anticholinergics, antihistamines, neuroleptics, anesthesia).**
- Determine anxiety level. **Client may be too embarrassed to void in presence of others or talk about problem with care providers.**
- Examine for fecal impaction, pelvic or perineal surgical site swelling, postpartal edema, vaginal or rectal packing, enlarged prostate, or other "mechanical" factors **that may produce a blockage of the urethra.**
- Strain urine, if appropriate, **for presence of stones or calculi that may produce a blockage of the urethra, causing outlet obstruction.**

Nursing Priority No. 2.
To determine degree of risk **(risk for urinary Retention):**
- Determine if there has been any significant urine output in the previous 6 to 8 hr. **Small amount of urine may leak out of bladder refelecting overflow and is not enough to relieve symptoms.**
- Note recent amount and type of fluid intake. **Adequate fluid intake is necessary for production of healthy**

Information that appears in brackets has been added by the authors to clarify and enhance the use of nursing diagnoses.

output. If client is not voiding despite adequate fluid intake, fluids may be restricted temporarily to prevent bladder overdistention until adequate urine flow is established.

- Palpate height of the bladder. Ascertain whether client has sensation of bladder fullness and level of discomfort. **Sensation and discomfort can vary depending on underlying cause of retention. Most people with acute retention also feel pain in lower abdomen (pelvis).**
- Catheterize, or perform a bladder scan or ultrasound for bladder residual after voiding **to determine presence of urine retention.**

Nursing Priority No. 3.
To assist in preventing retention/optimizing urinary output:

- Assist in treatment to relieve mechanical obstruction (e.g., removal of local blockage—vaginal packing, bowel impaction) or apply ice **to reduce perineal swelling.**
- Administer medications, as indicated. **Anticholinergics (e.g., oxybutinin [Ditropan]) or beta-3 blockers (e.g., mirabegron [Myrbetriq]) are often used to reduce bladder spasms impeding urine outflow. For some men with an enlarged prostate, treatment with an alpha-adrenergic blocker (e.g., finasteride [Proscar], tamsulosin [Flomax]) can help relax the muscle at the base of the urethra and allow urine to pass from the bladder.**
- Administer additional/supportive medications, as indicated (e.g., antibiotics, stool softeners, pain relievers), **to promote comfort while treating underlying cause.**
- Provide privacy **to reduce retention caused by embarrassment or anxiety.**
- Assist client to sit upright on toilet or commode or stand **to provide functional position of voiding.**
- Encourage warm sitz bath or shower, voiding in tub or shower if need be. **Warm water stimulates bladder to relax and may facilitate voiding.**
- Drain bladder (using the appropriate catheter material and size) intermittently or catheterize with indwelling catheter **to completely decompress bladder and resolve *acute* retention. Typically, the catheter will remain indwelling until the etiology of the obstruction is treated appropriately.**
- Prepare for more intensive interventions (e.g., reconstructive surgery, lithotripsy, prostatectomy), as indicated, **to remove source of obstruction, reconstruct sphincter, or provide for urinary diversion.**

Information that appears in brackets has been added by the authors to clarify and enhance the use of nursing diagnoses.

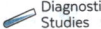 Diagnostic Studies   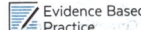 Evidence Based Practice   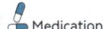 Medications   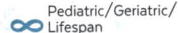 Pediatric/Geriatric/Lifespan

Nursing Priority No. 4.
To promote optimal elimination (Teaching/Discharge Considerations) and enhanced well-being:

- Emphasize good voiding habits (e.g., four to six times/day). **Postponing or holding urination for prolonged periods can, over time, overstretch and weaken bladder muscles.**
- Encourage client to report problems immediately **so treatment can be instituted promptly.**
- Adjust fluid intake and timing, if indicated, **to prevent bladder distention.**

Chronic Retention

Nursing Priority No. 1.
To assess contributing/risk factors:

- Ask client about symptoms common to overflow incontinence and often associated with urinary retention:
  Feeling no need to urinate, while simultaneously losing urine; frequent leaking or dribbling
  Feeling the urge to urinate but not being able to
  Feeling as though the bladder is never completely empty
  Passing a dribbling stream of urine, even after spending a long time at the toilet
  Frequently getting up at night to urinate
- Review medical history for diagnoses, such as congenital defects, neurological disorders (e.g., MS, polio), prostatic hypertrophy or surgery, birth canal injury or scarring, and SCI with lower motor neuron injury or bladder stones, **that may cause detrusor-sphincter dyssynergia (loss of coordination between bladder contraction and external urinary sphincter relaxation), detrusor muscle atrophy, or chronic overdistention because of outlet obstruction.**
- Assess client's medication regimen (e.g., psychotropic, antihistamines, atropine, belladonna) **to consult with primary care provider regarding client's continued use of drugs that are known to potentiate urinary retention.**

Nursing Priority No. 2.
To determine degree of impairment:

- Ascertain effect of condition on functioning and lifestyle. **Chronic urinary retention can limit client's desired lifestyle (e.g., daily activities, social functioning) and can lead to chronic incontinence and life-threatening complications (e.g., intractable UTIs, kidney failure).**

Information that appears in brackets has been added by the authors to clarify and enhance the use of nursing diagnoses.

Nursing Priority No. 3.

To assist in preventing retention/optimizing urinary output:

- Collaborate in treatment of underlying conditions (e.g., medications to treat BPH, reducing or eliminating medications responsible for retention, repairing perineal scarring or outlet obstruction), **which may correct or reduce severity of retention and associated overflow or total incontinence.**
- Encourage continued performance of physical therapy exercises **to stretch tight, and/or strengthen, pelvic floor muscles.**
- Instruct client/SO in management of voiding problems as indicated:

    Emphasize good voiding habits (e.g., four to six times/day) on a timed schedule, whether voiding or using catheter. **Postponing or holding urination for prolonged periods can, over time, overstretch and weaken bladder muscles.**

    Maintain consistent fluid intake **to wash out bacteria, avoid infections, and limit bladder stone formation.**

    Adjust fluid amount and timing, if indicated, **to prevent bladder distention.**
- Administer medications as indicated. **Medications such as 5–alpha reductase inhibitors may be used to shrink prostate, and/or alpha blockers used to relax muscles of the bladder neck and prostate.**
- Consult with urologist and prepare for more intensive interventions, as indicated.

Nursing Priority No. 4.

To promote optimum elimination (Teaching/Discharge Considerations) and enhanced well-being:

- Instruct SO/caregiver(s) in clean intermittent catheterization techniques, whether voiding or using catheter, **so that more than one individual is able to assist the client in care of elimination needs.**
- Emphasize need for adequate fluid intake, including use of acidifying fruit juices or ingestion of vitamin C or methenamine (Mandelamine). **Maintains renal function, prevents infection and formation of bladder stones, and reduces risk of encrustation around indwelling catheter when present.**
- Discuss appropriate use of herbal products, **such as saw palmetto, to improve symptoms of BPH.**

Information that appears in brackets has been added by the authors to clarify and enhance the use of nursing diagnoses.

- Review signs/symptoms of complications **to promote timely contact with healthcare provider for evaluation and intervention.**

Documentation Focus

Assessment/Reassessment
- Individual findings, including nature of problem, degree of impairment, and whether client is incontinent

Planning
- Plan of care and who is involved in planning
- Teaching plan

Implementation/Evaluation
- Response to interventions
- Attainment of or progress toward desired outcome(s)
- Modifications to plan of care

Discharge Planning
- Long-term needs and who is responsible for actions to be taken
- Specific referrals made

Sample Nursing Outcomes & Interventions Classifications NOC/NIC

NOC—Urinary Elimination
NIC—Urinary Elimination Management
NIC—Urinary Retention Care

---

impaired ROLE PERFORMANCE ICNP

[Diagnostic Division: Roles/Relationships]

Definition: Inability to achieve expected sociopersonal or professional roles.

Recognizing Cues

AUTHOR NOTE: There is a typology of roles (e.g., sociopersonal [friendship, family, marital, parenting, community], self-management, socialization [developmental transitions], and spiritual) that can help in understanding impaired Role Performance.

Related/Risk Factors
Altered physical/body image; low self-esteem
Multiple stressors; conflict; violence

Information that appears in brackets has been added by the authors to clarify and enhance the use of nursing diagnoses.

Role confusion/conflict; unrealistic expectations
Substance misuse/abuse
Cognitive impairments (e.g., dementia, psychosis); depression; developmental delay
Inadequate family preparation, socialization, role models; ineffective/lack of support

Defining Characteristics

Subjective
Misperception of role
Lacks confidence, clarity of expectations; feels powerless
Perceives to be unwanted, unliked; reports discrimination
Reports doubt about/dissatisfaction with role

Objective
Inability to fulfill responsibilities
Anxiety; anger; aggression; sarcasm; depressive symptoms
Lacks knowledge of role expectations, motivation, support from others
Inability to adapt to change; inadequate coping strategies; lack of self-management skills

Clinical Connections
Chronic conditions (e.g., multiple sclerosis, pain, chronic fatigue syndrome), cancer, substance abuse, brain or spinal cord injury, major surgery, major depression, bipolar disorder, borderline personality disorder, schizophrenia

Generate Solutions

Plan Desired Outcomes

Client Will (Include Specific Time Frame)
- Verbalize understanding of role expectations and obligations.
- Verbalize realistic perception and acceptance of self in changed role.
- Talk with family/significant other(s) (SO[s]) about situation, changes that have occurred, and limitations imposed.
- Develop realistic plans for adapting to new role or role changes.

Interventions/Take Action

Nursing Priority No. 1.
To assess causative/contributing factors:
- Identify type of role dysfunction—for example, developmental (adolescent, adult, geriatric); situational (husband to father, gender identity); transitions from health to illness.

Information that appears in brackets has been added by the authors to clarify and enhance the use of nursing diagnoses.

- Determine client role in family constellation. **Provides a point of reference for understanding changes due to health alterations (mental or physical) or lack of knowledge about role or appropriate role skills.**
- Identify how client sees self as a man or woman, adult/child in usual lifestyle or role functioning. **Each person has a perception of self that is important to know to understand changes that may be occurring. Low self-esteem, anxiety, and depression can cause an internal struggle with role performance.**
- Establish client's view of sexual functioning (e.g., loss of childbearing ability following hysterectomy), **which can affect how client views self in role as male or female, and may need specific interventions to resolve feelings of loss.**
- Identify cultural factors relating to individual's sexual roles. **Cultures define male and female roles differently (e.g., Muslim culture demands that the woman adopt a subservient role, whereas the man is seen as the powerful one in the relationship).**
- Determine client's perceptions or concerns about current situation. **May believe current role is more appropriate for the opposite sex (e.g., passive role of the client may be somewhat less threatening for women). Life transitions such as divorce, illness, or loss of job can alter or disrupt role performance.**
- Interview SO(s) regarding their perceptions and expectations. **The beliefs of individuals directly involved with the client and the situation (e.g., parents bringing a new baby home from the hospital, adult child assuming responsibility for elder parent) are important to understanding the new roles individuals are undertaking.**
- Evaluate for misuse/abuse of substances. **Substance users are at risk for ineffective role performance causing a loss of financial resources, employment, family/personal relationships, and loss of time and energy to manage life.**
- Identify availability and use of resources. **Individual may be unaware of or have difficulty accessing community support or assistance programs.**
- Investigate history of incidents of domestic violence in the family. Refer to appropriate psychiatric, support, and legal services, as indicated. **The roles of perpetrator and survivor are difficult to alter without intensive therapy as well as support for other family members/children. Neither individual in this situation sees self as worthy, and both have poor self-esteem. Perpetrators do not get what they**

Information that appears in brackets has been added by the authors to clarify and enhance the use of nursing diagnoses.

want through the use of violence, and survivors (the battered persons) often believe they deserve this treatment.

Nursing Priority No. 2.

To assist client to deal with existing situation:

- Discuss perceptions and significance of the situation as seen by client. **Provides opportunity to clarify any misperceptions and discuss changes client may have to make in regard to what has happened (e.g., loss of a limb, disfiguring surgery).**
- Maintain positive attitude toward the client. **Promotes safe relationship in which client feels safe to discuss changes that are occurring and plan for a positive future.**
- Provide opportunities for client to exercise control over as many decisions as possible. **Enhances self-concept and promotes commitment to goals.**
- Offer realistic assessment of situation while communicating sense of hope.
- Discuss and assist client/SO(s) to develop strategies for dealing with changes in role related to past transitions, cultural expectations, and value or belief challenges. **Helps those involved deal with differences between individuals (e.g., adolescent task of separation in which parents clash with child's choices; individual's decision to change religious affiliation).**
- Acknowledge reality of situation related to role change and help client express feelings of anger, sadness, and grief. Encourage celebration of positive aspects of change and expressions of feelings. **Changes in role necessitated by illness, trauma, changes in family structure (new baby, child leaving home for college, elderly parent needing care), or any other circumstance, may result in a sense of loss and the need to deal with the feelings that accompany change.**
- Provide open environment for client to discuss concerns about sexuality. **Embarrassment can block discussion of sensitive subject.** (Refer to NDs impaired Sexual Functioning; ineffective intimate partner Relationship, as appropriate.)
- Educate about role expectations using written and audiovisual materials. **Using different modalities enables client to review material at leisure and begin to incorporate information into own thinking.**
- Assist client to identify role model. **Offers opportunity for client to observe how someone else functions in a role that is new to client.**
- Use techniques of role rehearsal to practice new role. **Provides opportunity for the client to try and develop new skills to cope with anticipated changes.**

Information that appears in brackets has been added by the authors to clarify and enhance the use of nursing diagnoses.

 Diagnostic Studies 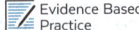 Evidence Based Practice 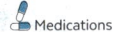 Medications 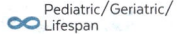 Pediatric/Geriatric/Lifespan

- Discuss use of medication, and refer as appropriate. **Client may benefit from antidepressants to combat depression, or psychotropic medications may be required to address other mental health issues.**

Nursing Priority No. 3.

To strengthen role behaviors (Teaching/Discharge Considerations) and enhance well-being (long-term goals):

- Make information available (including bibliotherapy, appropriate websites) for client to learn about role expectations or demands that may occur. **Provides opportunity to be proactive in dealing with changes, such as classes to help new parent(s) learn about new roles and credible websites for additional information regarding individual's specific concerns.**
- Accept client in changed role. Encourage and give positive feedback for changes and goals achieved. **Provides reinforcement and facilitates continuation of efforts.**
- Refer to support groups, employment counselors, parent effectiveness classes, counseling/psychotherapy, as indicated by individual need(s). **Provides ongoing support to sustain progress.**
- Refer to NDs chronic inadequate Self-Esteem; situational inadequate Self-Esteem; impaired Parenting.

Documentation Focus

Assessment/Reassessment

- Individual findings, including specifics of predisposing crises or situation, perception of role change
- Expectations of SO(s)

Planning

- Plan of care and who is involved in planning
- Teaching plan

Implementation/Evaluation

- Responses to interventions, teaching, and actions performed
- Attainment of or progress toward desired outcome(s)
- Modifications to plan of care

Discharge Planning

- Long-term needs and who is responsible for actions to be taken
- Specific referrals made

Sample Nursing Outcomes & Interventions Classifications NOC/NIC

NOC—Role Performance
NIC—Role Enhancement

Information that appears in brackets has been added by the authors to clarify and enhance the use of nursing diagnoses.

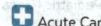 Acute Care 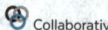 Collaborative 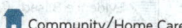 Community/Home Care   Cultural

excessive SEDENTARY BEHAVIORS   NANDA-I

[Diagnostic Division: Activity/Rest]

Definition: Unsatisfactory activity pattern during waking hours that has low energy expenditure.

Recognizing Cues

Related/Risk Factors
Conflict between cultural beliefs and health practices
Inadequate physical endurance; impaired physical mobility; pain
Difficulty adapting areas for physical activity
Exceeds screen time recommendations for age; parenting practices that inhibit child's physical activity
Inadequate interest in physical activity; inadequate motivation for physical activity; negative affect toward physical activity
Inadequate knowledge of consequences of sedentarism, or health benefits associated with physical activities; inadequate training for physical exercise
Inadequate resources for physical activity; inadequate role models, or social support
Inadequate time management skills
Inadequate self-efficacy; low self-esteem
Perceived physical disability, or safety risk

Defining Characteristics

Subjective
Prefers low physical activity

Objective
Average daily physical activity is less than recommended for age and gender
Chooses a daily routine lacking physical exercise; does not exercise during leisure time
Performs majority of tasks in a sitting or reclining posture
Prolonged inactivity

Clinical Connections
Chronic or debilitating conditions (e.g., arthritis, multiple sclerosis [MS], chronic obstructive pulmonary disease, heart failure, paralysis), chronic pain, overweight, depression, long-term care residents

---

Information that appears in brackets has been added by the authors to clarify and enhance the use of nursing diagnoses.

 Diagnostic Studies 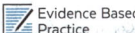 Evidence Based Practice 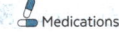 Medications 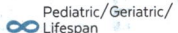 Pediatric/Geriatric/Lifespan

Generate Solutions

Plan Desired Outcomes

Client Will (Include Specific Time Frame)
- Verbalize understanding of importance of regular exercise to general well-being.
- Identify necessary precautions or safety concerns and self-monitoring techniques.
- Formulate realistic exercise program with gradual increase in activity.

Interventions/Take Action

Nursing Priority No. 1.
To assess precipitating/etiological factors:

- Identify conditions that may contribute to immobility or the onset and continuation of inactivity or sedentary lifestyle (e.g., aging, obesity, cardiac and pulmonary conditions, depression, MS, arthritis, Parkinson disease, surgery, hemiplegia or paraplegia, chronic pain, brain injury) **that may contribute to immobility or the onset and continuation of inactivity or sedentary lifestyle.**
- ∞ Assess the client's age, developmental level, motor skills, ease and capability of movement, posture, and gait. **These determine the type and intensity of needed interventions related to activity. Children/adolescents are at risk due to physical inactivity and lengthy screen time.**
- Determine client's current weight and body mass index (BMI); note dietary habits. **If client is overweight and BMI is not in healthy range, a weight-loss program should be suggested along with exercise.**
- Assess physical capabilities to participate in exercise/activities, noting attention span, physical limitations and tolerance, level of interest or desire, and safety needs. **Identifies barriers that need to be addressed.**
- ∞ Review usual activities and work requirements/environment. **Absence of regular exercise and the presence of a stressful job with little physical exercise increases likelihood of deconditioning.**
- Note emotional and behavioral responses to problems associated with self- or condition-imposed sedentary lifestyle. **Feelings of frustration and powerlessness may impede the attainment of goals.**
- Determine family dynamics and support provided by family/friends. **Major lifestyle change may require support of**

Information that appears in brackets has been added by the authors to clarify and enhance the use of nursing diagnoses.

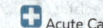 Acute Care 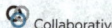 Collaborative 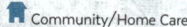 Community/Home Care   Cultural

others to achieve and maintain goals or client may be at increased risk of slipping back into "old" ways.
- Ascertain availability of resources (e.g., finances for gym membership, transportation, exercise facility or gym at work site, proximity of walking trail or bike path, safety of neighborhood for outdoor activity).

Nursing Priority No. 2.
To motivate and stimulate client involvement:
- Establish therapeutic relationship acknowledging reality of situation and client's feelings. **Changing a lifelong habit can be difficult, and the client may be feeling discouragement with body and hopelessness (i.e., unable to turn situation around into a positive experience).**
- Ascertain the client's perception of current activity/exercise patterns, impact on life, and cultural expectations of client/others.
- Discuss motivation for change. **Concerns of significant other(s) (SO[s]) regarding threats to personal health and longevity or acceptance by teen peers may be sufficient to cause the client to initiate change; to sustain change, however, the client must want to change for self.**
- Review necessity for, and benefits of, regular exercise. **Research confirms that exercise has benefits for the whole body (e.g., can boost energy, enhance coordination, reduce muscle deterioration, improve circulation, lower blood pressure, produce healthier skin and a toned body, and prolong youthful appearance). Regular exercise has also been found to boost cardiac fitness in both conditioned and out-of-shape individuals.**
- Counsel client regarding individual health risks. **Focuses attention on own situation and helps prioritize needs, making change more manageable.**
- Involve client, SO, parent, or caregiver in developing exercise plan and goals to meet individual needs, desires, and available resources.
- Introduce activities at the client's current level of functioning, progressing to more complex activities, as tolerated. **Reduces likelihood of overwhelming client at the beginning and maintains interest over time.**
- Recommend a mix of age- and gender-appropriate activities or stimuli (e.g., movement classes, walking, hiking, jazzercise or other dancing, swimming, biking, skating, bowling, golf, or weight training). **Activities need to be personally meaningful for the client to derive the most enjoyment and to sustain motivation to continue with the program.**

Information that appears in brackets has been added by the authors to clarify and enhance the use of nursing diagnoses.

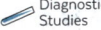 Diagnostic Studies 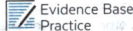 Evidence Based Practice 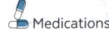 Medications 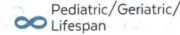 Pediatric/Geriatric/Lifespan

- Encourage a change of scenery (indoors and out, where possible) and periodic changes in the personal environment when the client is confined inside.

Nursing Priority No. 3.

To promote optimal level of function and prevent exercise failure:

- Assist with the treatment of any underlying conditions impacting participation in activities **to maximize function within limitations of the situation.**
- Collaborate with physical medicine specialist or occupational/physical therapist in providing active or passive range-of-motion exercises and isotonic muscle contractions. **Techniques such as gait training, strength training, and exercise to improve balance and coordination can be helpful in rehabilitating the client.**
- Schedule ample time to perform exercise activities balanced with adequate rest periods.
- Review the importance of adequate intake of fluids, especially during hot weather/strenuous activity.
- Provide for safety measures as indicated by individual situation, including environmental management/fall prevention. (Refer to risk for NDs [adult/child] Fall.)
- Reevaluate ability/commitment periodically. **Changes in strength/endurance signal readiness for progression of activities or possibly decrease in exercise if overly fatigued. Wavering commitment may require change in types of activities or the addition of a workout buddy to reenergize involvement.**
- Discuss discrepancies in planned and performed activities with the client aware and unaware of observation. Suggest methods for dealing with identified problems. **May be necessary when the client is using avoidance or controlling behavior or is not aware of own abilities due to anxiety/fear.**

Nursing Priority No. 4.

To sustain increased activity (Teaching/Discharge Considerations) and enhance well-being (long-term goals):

- Educate the client/SO about the benefits of physical activity as related to the client's particular situation. **Many studies have shown the health benefits of physical activity in the setting of chronic illness; for example, it increases function in arthritis, improves glycemic control in type 2 diabetes, and can enhance quality of life.**

Information that appears in brackets has been added by the authors to clarify and enhance the use of nursing diagnoses.

- Review components of physical fitness: (1) **cardiovascular endurance** (ability of heart and lungs to work together to provide the needed oxygen and fuel to the body during sustained workload), (2) **muscular strength** (correlates to ability to move and lift things), (3) **muscular endurance** (capacity of muscles to perform continuously without fatigue), (4) **flexibility** (ability to move easily through expected range of motion), and (5) **body composition** (muscle mass, percentage of body fat). **Fitness routines need to include all elements to attain maximum benefits and prevent deconditioning.**
- Instruct in safety measures as individually indicated (e.g., warm-up and cooldown activities; taking pulse before, during, and after activity; wearing reflective clothing when jogging, placing reflectors on bicycle; locking wheelchair before transfers; judiciously using medications; having supervision as indicated).
- Recommend keeping an activity or exercise log, including physical and psychological responses, changes in weight, endurance, and body mass. **Provides visual evidence of progress or goal attainment and encouragement to continue with program.**
- Encourage the client to involve self in exercise as part of wellness management for the whole person.
- 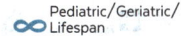 Encourage parents to set a positive example for children by participating in exercise and engaging in an active lifestyle.
- Identify community resources, charity activities, and support groups. **Community walking or hiking trails, sports leagues, and so on, provide free or low-cost options. Activities such as 5K walks for charity, participation in Special Olympics, or age-related competitive games provide goals to work toward.**
- Discuss alternatives for exercise program in changing circumstances (e.g., walking the mall during inclement weather, using exercise facilities at a hotel when traveling, participating in water aerobics at a local swimming pool, joining a gym).
- Promote individual participation in community awareness of problem and discussion of solutions. **Physical inactivity (and associated diseases) is a major public health problem that affects huge numbers of people in all regions of the world. Recognizing the problem and future consequences may empower the global community to develop effective measures to promote physical activity and improve public health.**

Information that appears in brackets has been added by the authors to clarify and enhance the use of nursing diagnoses.

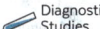 Diagnostic Studies
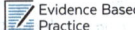 Evidence Based Practice
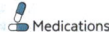 Medications
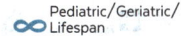 Pediatric/Geriatric/Lifespan

- Promote community goals for increasing physical activity, such as Sports, Play, and Active Recreation for Kids (SPARK) and Physician-Based Assessment and Counseling for Exercise (PACE), **to address national concerns about obesity and major barriers to physical activity, such as time constraints, lack of training in physical activity or behavioral change methods, and lack of standard protocols.**

Documentation Focus

Assessment/Reassessment
- Individual findings, including level of function and ability to participate in specific or desired activities
- Access to individual/community resources
- Motivation for change

Planning
- Plan of care and who is involved in the planning
- Teaching plan

Implementation/Evaluation
- Responses to interventions, teaching, and actions performed
- Attainment of or progress toward desired outcome(s)
- Modifications to plan of care

Discharge Planning
- Discharge and long-range needs, noting who is responsible for each action to be taken
- Specific referrals made
- Sources of and maintenance for assistive devices

Sample Nursing Outcomes & Interventions Classifications NOC/NIC

NOC—Knowledge: Prescribed Activity
NIC—Exercise Promotion

---

bathing, dressing, grooming, feeding, toileting
SELF-CARE DEFICIT [specify] `ICNP`

[Diagnostic Division: Self-Care]

Definition: Inability to independently perform and address personal needs, including eating, personal hygiene, elimination needs, and clothing oneself.

Information that appears in brackets has been added by the authors to clarify and enhance the use of nursing diagnoses.

 Acute Care   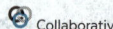 Collaborative   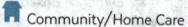 Community/Home Care   Cultural

Recognizing Cues

[**Note:** Self-Care also may be expanded to include the practices used by the client to promote health, the individual responsibility for self, and a way of thinking. Refer to NDs ineffective Health Maintenance Behaviors and ineffective Home Maintenance Behaviors.]

Related/Risk Factors

Inadequate internal motivation, mental impairment, confusion; anxiety

Physical weakness, musculoskeletal impairment; neuromuscular impairment

Pain

Lack of adaptive equipment; inadequate resources

Environmental constraints (e.g., cast, splint, traction, ventilator)

Defining Characteristics

Bathing Difficulty:
- Obtaining bathing supplies
  Accessing bathroom, or water source; difficulty regulating water flow/temperature
  Washing/drying body

Dressing Difficulty:
- Gathering, selecting, putting clothing on lower/upper body, or fastening clothing
  Obtaining clothing (e.g., insufficient choices, inappropriate attire for climate/environment)
- Maintaining clothing (e.g., clothing dirty, in disrepair, excessive odor)

Grooming Difficulty:
- Maintaining personal appearance—combing hair, shaving, applying makeup
  Performing oral hygiene—flossing, brushing teeth; care for dentures
- Caring for finger/toenails

Feeding Difficulty:
- Obtaining food; storing food safely; opening containers; preparing sufficient amount of food
  Getting food onto utensil; bringing food to mouth; manipulating food in mouth; chewing or swallowing food
  Handling utensils; picking up cup; or using assistive device
  Self-feeding in an acceptable manner
- Maintaining acceptable weight; meeting nutritional needs

Information that appears in brackets has been added by the authors to clarify and enhance the use of nursing diagnoses.

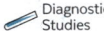 Diagnostic Studies 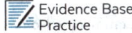 Evidence Based Practice 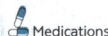 Medications 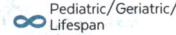 Pediatric/Geriatric/Lifespan

Toileting Difficulty:
- Accessing toilet; sitting on toilet; rising from toilet
  Manipulating clothing for toileting; incontinence
  Performing toileting hygiene—cleaning self, perineal care
- Inability to flush toilet, use a urinal

Clinical Connections

Arthritis, neuromuscular impairment (e.g., multiple sclerosis [MS], brain injury, stroke, Parkinson disease, spinal cord injury [SCI]), chronic pain, chronic fatigue syndrome, depression, dementia, autism, developmental delay, end-of-life/hospice care

Generate Solutions

Plan Desired Outcomes

Client Will (Include Specific Time Frame)
- Identify individual areas of weakness or needs.
- Demonstrate techniques and lifestyle changes to meet self-care needs.
- Perform self-care activities within level of own ability.
- Identify personal and community resources that can provide assistance.

Interventions/Take Action

Nursing Priority No. 1.
To identify causative/contributing factors:

- Determine client's age, developmental issues, and existing conditions (e.g., heart or renal failure, SCI, malnutrition, pain, trauma, surgery) and cognitive or psychological factors (e.g., mental illness, brain injury, cerebrovascular accident, MS, Alzheimer disease) **affecting ability of client to care for own needs. Assists in setting realistic goals and creating a baseline for evaluating the effectiveness of interventions.**
- Identify other etiological factors present, including language barriers, speech impairment, visual acuity or hearing problems, and emotional instability or lability. (Refer to NDs impaired verbal Communication; Sensory Deficit [specify: visual, auditory, kinesthetic, gustatory, tactile, olfactory], for related interventions.)
- Review medication regimen **for possible effects on alertness/mentation, energy level, balance, perception.**
- Assess barriers to client's participation in treatment regimen **that can limit availability of resources or choice of**

Information that appears in brackets has been added by the authors to clarify and enhance the use of nursing diagnoses.

 Acute Care 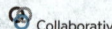 Collaborative 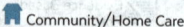 Community/Home Care   Cultural

options (e.g., lack of information, insufficient time for discussion, psychological or intimate family problems that may be difficult to share, fear of appearing stupid or ignorant, social or economic limitations, work or home environment problems).

Nursing Priority No. 2.

To assess degree of disability:

- Identify degree of individual impairment and functional level according to scale as listed in ND impaired physical Mobility.
- Note anticipated duration of self-care disruption and intensity of care required. **A wide variety of factors can impact self-care, some of which may be (1) invariable or permanent (e.g., quadriplegia or advanced dementia); (2) temporary (e.g., fractures requiring immobilization, mild stroke with potential for good recovery); (3) variable (e.g., person having episode of severe depression or episodes of relapsing-remitting MS).**
- Assess cognitive functioning (e.g., memory, intelligence, concentration, ability to attend to task) **to determine client's ability to participate in care and potential to return to normal functioning or to learn/relearn tasks.**
- Determine individual strengths and skills of the client **to incorporate into plan of care enhancing likelihood of achieving outcomes.**

Nursing Priority No. 3.

To assist in correcting/dealing with deficits **in general**:

- Collaborate in treatment of underlying conditions **to enhance client's capabilities, maximize rehabilitation potential.**
- Provide accurate and relevant information regarding current and future needs **so that client can incorporate this into self-care plans while minimizing problems (e.g., heightened anxiety, depression, resistance) often associated with change.**
- Perform or assist with meeting client's needs. **Personal care assistance is part of nursing care and should not be neglected, while self-care independence is promoted and integrated.**
- Promote client's/significant other's (SO's) participation in problem identification and desired goals and decision making. **Enhances commitment to plan, optimizing outcomes, and supporting recovery and/or health promotion.**

Information that appears in brackets has been added by the authors to clarify and enhance the use of nursing diagnoses.

- Develop plan of care appropriate to individual situation, scheduling activities to conform to client's usual or desired schedule.
- Active-listen client's/SO's concerns. **Exhibits regard for client's values and beliefs, clarifies barriers to participation in self-care, provides opportunity to work on problem-solving solutions and to provide encouragement and support.**
- Practice and promote short-term goal setting and achievement **to recognize that today's success is as important as any long-term goal, accepting ability to do one thing at a time and conceptualization of self-care in a broader sense.**
- Provide for communication among those who are involved in caring for or assisting the client. **Enhances coordination and continuity of care.**
- Instruct in or review appropriate skills necessary for self-care, using terms understandable to client (e.g., child, adult, cognitively impaired person) and with sensitivity to developmental needs for practice, repetition, or reluctance. **Individualized teaching best affords reinforcement of learning. Sensitivity to special needs attaches value to the client's needs.**
- Establish "contractual" partnership with client/SO(s), if appropriate, **for motivation or behavioral modification.**
- Encourage client to use vision and hearing aids as appropriate. **Improves reception and interpretation of sensory input to facilitate self-care.**
- Perform or assist with meeting client's needs when client is unable to meet own needs.
- Avoid doing things for client that the client can do for self, but provide assistance as needed. **Client may be fearful or dependent, and although assistance is helpful in preventing frustration (and sometimes easier for the caregivers in terms of their time), it is important for client to do as much as possible for self to regain or maintain self-esteem, reduce helplessness, and promote optimal recovery.**
- Cue client, as indicated. **A cognitively impaired or forgetful client can often successfully participate in many activities with cueing, which can enhance self-esteem and potentiate learning or relearning of self-care tasks.**
- Schedule activities **to conform to client's preferred schedule as much as possible (e.g., bathing at a relaxing time for client rather than on a set routine).**

Information that appears in brackets has been added by the authors to clarify and enhance the use of nursing diagnoses.

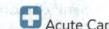 Acute Care 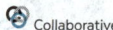 Collaborative 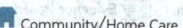 Community/Home Care Cultural

- Plan activities to prevent or accommodate fatigue and/or exacerbation of pain.
- Allow sufficient time for client to accomplish tasks to fullest extent of ability. Avoid unnecessary conversation or interruptions **that divert focus from the task at hand and can contribute to client's level of frustration.**
- Assist with necessary adaptations to accomplish activities of daily living. Begin with familiar, easily accomplished tasks **to encourage client and build on successes.**
- Identify energy-saving behaviors (e.g., sitting instead of standing when possible). (Refer to NDs decreased Activity Tolerance; Fatigue for additional interventions.)
- Assist with medication regimen as necessary, encouraging timely use of medications (e.g., taking diuretics in morning when client is more awake and able to manage toileting, using pain relievers prior to activity to facilitate movement, postponing intake of medications that cause sedation until self-care activities completed).
- Collaborate with rehabilitation professionals to identify and obtain assistive devices, mobility aids, and home modification, as necessary (e.g., adequate lighting, visual aids; bedside commode; raised toilet seat and grab bars for bathroom; modified clothing; modified eating utensils) **to enhance client's capabilities and promote independence.**
- Arrange for a home visit, as indicated, to assess environmental concerns that can impact client's abilities to care for self in the home. **If necessary modifications are not feasible or cannot be made, client may require temporary or long-term relocation or regular home-care assistance.**
- Note availability and use of resources and supportive person(s), access to social support and approval (e.g., support group participants, family members, professionals). **Important for client to have means for sharing common concerns, needs, and wishes.**

Nursing Priority No. 4.
To meet specific self-care needs:

Bathing Deficit
- Ask client/SO for input on bathing habits or cultural bathing preferences. **Creates opportunities for client to (1) keep long-standing routines (e.g., bathing at bedtime to improve sleep) and (2) exercise control over situation. Enhances self-esteem, while respecting personal and cultural preferences.**

Information that appears in brackets has been added by the authors to clarify and enhance the use of nursing diagnoses.

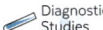 Diagnostic Studies 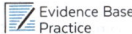 Evidence Based Practice 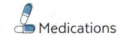 Medications 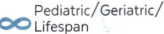 Pediatric/Geriatric/Lifespan

- Bathe or assist client in bathing, providing for any or all hygiene needs as indicated. **The type of bath (e.g., bed bath, towel bath, tub bath, shower) and purpose (e.g., cleansing, removing odor, simply soothing agitation) are determined by the client's need. Note: Bathing is a healing rite and should be a comforting experience that focuses on the client's needs, rather than being a routinely scheduled task.**
- Obtain hygiene supplies (e.g., soap, toothpaste, toothbrush, mouthwash, lotion, shampoo, razor, towels) for specific activity to be performed and place in client's easy reach **to provide visual cues and facilitate completion of activity.**
- Ascertain that all safety equipment is in place and properly installed (e.g., grab bars, antislip strips, shower chair, hydraulic lift) and that client/caregiver(s) can safely operate equipment.
- Instruct client to request assistance when needed and place call device within easy reach, or stay with client as dictated by safety needs.
- Provide privacy during personal care activities. **Maintains client's dignity.**
- Provide for adequate warmth (e.g., covering client during bed bath or warming bathroom). **Certain individuals (especially infants, the elderly, and very thin or debilitated persons) are prone to hypothermia and can experience evaporative cooling during and after bathing.**
- Determine that client can perceive water temperature, adjust water temperature safely, or that water is correct temperature for client's bath or shower **to prevent chilling or burns. This step requires that client is cognitively and physically able to perceive hot and cold and to adjust faucets safely.**
- Assist client in and out of shower or tub, as indicated. Bathe or assist client in bathing, providing for any or all hygiene needs, as indicated. **Needs are variable (e.g., client may need to get into the tub before running water, may require a shower chair, may be independent with one fixture and not another), requiring assessment of the client and of individual situations**
- Assist with or cue client to complete hygiene steps (e.g., oral care, lotion application, applying deodorant, washing and styling hair). **These steps may be completed at the same or different time as bathing but are usually part of a regular routine that is necessary for client's physical well-being and emotional or social comfort.**

Information that appears in brackets has been added by the authors to clarify and enhance the use of nursing diagnoses.

 Acute Care 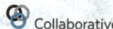 Collaborative 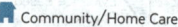 Community/Home Care Cultural

Experiencing the normal process of a task through established routine and guided practice facilitates optimal learning.

Dressing Deficit

- Ascertain that appropriate client clothing is available. **Client may not have sufficient clothing, clothing may be inadequate for the situation or weather conditions, or clothing may need to be modified for client's particular medical condition or physical limitations.**
- Assist client in choosing clothing or lay out clothing, as indicated. **May be needed when client has cognitive, physical, or psychiatric conditions affecting the client's ability to choose appropriate pieces of clothing or to maintain a satisfactory appearance.**
- Dress client or assist with dressing, as indicated. **Client may need assistance in putting on or taking off items of clothing (e.g., shoes and socks, or over-the-head shirt) or may require partial or complete assistance with fasteners (e.g., buttons, snaps, zippers, shoelaces).**
- Allow sufficient time for dressing and undressing **because tasks may be tiring, painful, and difficult to complete. Dressing may be done from a seated position if balance is impaired.**
- Use adaptive clothing as indicated (e.g., clothing with front closure, wide sleeves and pant legs, Velcro or zipper closures). **These may be helpful for client with limited arm or leg movement or impaired fine motor skills or cognitively impaired person who desires to dress self but cannot do so with regular clothing fasteners.**
- Teach client to dress affected side first, then unaffected side (when client has paralysis or injury to one side of body) **to allow for easier manipulation of clothing.**

Grooming Deficit

- Ask client/SO for input on cultural preferences and grooming habits to align care to client's individual needs and desires. **Provides an opportunity for client to (1) keep long-standing routines and (2) exercise control over their situation. This enhances self-esteem while respecting personal and cultural preferences.**
- Inspect client's oral cavity and lips (i.e., mucosal irritation/dryness; chipped, missing, or sharp-edged teeth; excessive plaque, etc.) to evaluate general oral health and address specific client needs. A referral for additional dental care may be needed.

Information that appears in brackets has been added by the authors to clarify and enhance the use of nursing diagnoses.

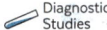 Diagnostic Studies 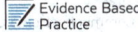 Evidence Based Practice 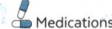 Medications 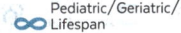 Pediatric/Geriatric/Lifespan

- Assist client with/or provide oral care (e.g., flossing, brush teeth, mouthwash/oral rinse, denture care, etc.) to ensure and maintain oral health.
- Assess client's scalp, hair, and skin for dryness, dandruff, infestations, hair loss, etc., to evaluate skin and hair health and address client's specific needs.
- Assist client with activities to maintain personal appearance (e.g., combing/brushing hair, shaving/beard care, makeup application, etc.). **Maintenance of personal appearance promotes client engagement in daily activities and social presence.**

Feeding Deficit

- Assess client's need and ability to prepare food, as indicated (including shopping, cooking, cutting food, opening containers, and managing the environment, etc.). **Identifies specific assistance required.**
- Ascertain that client can swallow safely, checking gag and swallow reflexes, as indicated. (Refer to ND impaired Swallowing for related interventions.)
- Assess for and alleviate pain where possible **to improve client's desire for food, and ability to eat/manage necessary tasks for food preparation and eating.**
- Have client sitting upright (out of bed at table) as much as possible. **Improves posture for eating and better digestion, and promotes the idea that eating is a social activity.**
- Arrange tray/table place setting to facilitate self-feeding (e.g., rearrange items for easy access; remove plate and cup covers; unwrap utensils; open packets; cut up food; butter bread) **to reduce client's frustration or apathy, and to promote ease of accessing food.**
- Encourage food and fluid choices reflecting individual likes and abilities and that meet nutritional needs **to maximize food intake. (Refer to ND impaired Swallowing for related interventions.)**
- Ascertain that client can swallow safely, checking gag and swallow reflexes, as indicated. Refer to ND impaired Swallowing for related interventions.
- Provide food and fluid of appropriate consistency to facilitate swallowing. **Cut food into bite-size pieces to prevent overfilling mouth and reduce risk of choking.**
- Assist client to handle utensils or in guiding utensils to mouth. **May require specialized equipment (e.g., rocker knife, plate guard, built-up handles) to increase**

Information that appears in brackets has been added by the authors to clarify and enhance the use of nursing diagnoses.

 Acute Care 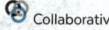 Collaborative 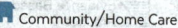 Community/Home Care Cultural

independence or assistance with movement of arms and hands. Provide nutritious finger foods where possible, if the client wants to feed self but experiences difficulty managing utensils.
- Assist client with small cup, glass, or bottle for liquids, using straw or adaptive lids as indicated **to enhance fluid intake while reducing spills.**
- Allow client time for intake of sufficient food **for feeling satisfied or completing a meal.**
- Use verbal cueing and prompting (e.g., "pick up your spoon," "take a bite," "chew," "swallow"), where indicated. **May improve client's efforts when distraction, depression, or cognitive issues are interfering.**
- Remove distractions (e.g., turn off TV to improve client's efforts and facilitate client focus in eating).
- Assist client with social graces when eating with others; provide privacy when manners might be offensive to others or client could be embarrassed.
- Collaborate with nutritionist, speech-language pathologist, occupational therapist, or physician **for special diets or feeding methods necessary to provide adequate nutrition.**
- Feed client, encouraging adequate chewing and swallowing, when client is not able to obtain nutrition by self-feeding. Avoid providing fluids until client has swallowed food and mouth is clear. **Prevents "washing down" foods, reducing risk of choking.**

Toileting Deficit
- Provide mobility assistance to bathroom or commode or place on bedpan or offer urinal, as indicated.
- Direct or accompany cognitively impaired client to bathroom, as needed.
- Provide privacy **to enhance self-esteem and improve ability to urinate or defecate.**
- Assist with manipulation of clothing, if needed, **to decrease incidence of functional incontinence caused by difficulty removing clothing/underwear.**
- Observe need for and assist in obtaining modified clothing or fasteners **to assist client in manipulation of clothing, fostering independence in self-toileting.**
- Provide or assist with use of assistive equipment (e.g., raised toilet seat, support rails, spill-proof urinals, fracture pans, bedside commode) **to promote independence and safety in sitting down or arising from toilet or for aiding elimination when client is unable to go to bathroom.**

Information that appears in brackets has been added by the authors to clarify and enhance the use of nursing diagnoses.

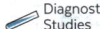 Diagnostic Studies 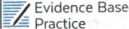 Evidence Based Practice 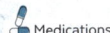 Medications 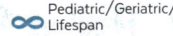 Pediatric/Geriatric/Lifespan

- Keep toilet paper or wipes and handwashing items within client's easy reach.
- Implement bowel or bladder training program, as indicated. **This may include developing a schedule for toileting and other interventions as seen in NDs impaired fecal Continence, chronic functional Constipation, urinary Incontinence [specify], and impaired urinary Elimination.**
- Observe for behaviors such as pacing, fidgeting, or holding crotch **that may be indicative of need for prompt toileting.**

Nursing Priority No. 5.

To promote wellness (Teaching/Discharge Considerations):

- Assist the client to become aware of rights and responsibilities in health and healthcare and to assess own health strengths—physical, emotional, and intellectual.
- Support client in making health-related decisions and assist in developing self-care practices and goals that promote health.
- Instruct client/SO/caregiver in relaxation techniques (e.g., deep breathing, meditation, music, yoga) **to reduce frustration and enhance coping.**
- Provide for ongoing evaluation of self-care program **to note progress and identify changes in needs.**
- Review and modify program periodically to accommodate changes in client's abilities. **Assists client to adhere to plan of care to fullest extent.**
- Encourage keeping a journal of progress and practicing of independent living skills. **Assists client to adhere to plan of care to fullest extent.**
- Review client's/SO's/caregiver's safety concerns. Modify activities or environment **to reduce risk of injury and promote successful community functioning.**
- Refer client/SO to a home-care provider, social services, physical or occupational therapy, rehabilitation, and counseling resources, as indicated.
- Arrange a consult with community resources (e.g., senior services, Meals on Wheels).
- Review client care instructions from other members of healthcare team and provide written copy. **Provides clarification, reinforcement; allows periodic review by client/caregivers.**
- Discuss respite or other care options with family. **Allows them free time away from the care situation to renew**

Information that appears in brackets has been added by the authors to clarify and enhance the use of nursing diagnoses.

 Acute Care 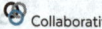 Collaborative 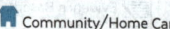 Community/Home Care Cultural

themselves. (Refer to ND excessive Caregiving Burden for additional interventions.)
- Assist and support family with alternative placements as necessary. **Enhances the likelihood of finding individually appropriate environment to meet client's needs.**
- Be available for discussion of feelings about situation (e.g., grieving, anger). **Provides opportunity for client/family to get feelings out in the open and begin to problem-solve solutions as indicated.**
- Refer to NDs difficulty Coping; impaired family Coping; situational Self-Esteem; impaired physical Mobility; as appropriate.

Documentation Focus

Assessment/Reassessment
- Individual findings, functional level, and specifics of limitation(s)
- Needed resources and adaptive devices
- Availability and use of community resources
- Who is involved in care or provides assistance

Planning
- Plan of care and who is involved in planning
- Teaching plan

Implementation/Evaluation
- Response to interventions, teaching, and actions performed
- Attainment of or progress toward desired outcome(s)
- Modifications of plan of care

Discharge Planning
- Long-term needs and who is responsible for actions to be taken
- Type of and source for assistive devices
- Specific referrals made

Sample Nursing Outcomes & Interventions Classifications NOC/NIC

Bathing Deficit
NOC—Self-Care Behavior: Bathing
NIC—Bathing

Dressing Deficit
NOC—Self-Care Behavior: Dressing
NIC—Dressing

Information that appears in brackets has been added by the authors to clarify and enhance the use of nursing diagnoses.

Grooming
NOC—Self-Care Behavior: Hygiene
NIC—Self-Care Assistance

Feeding Deficit
NOC—Self-Care Behavior: Eating
NIC—Feeding

Toileting Deficit
NOC—Self-Care Behavior: Toileting
NIC—Self-Care Assistance: Toileting

---

inadequate SELF-COMPASSION   NANDA-I

[Diagnostic Division: Self Perception/Concept]

Definition: Insufficient ability to extend self-kindness and understanding, acknowledge one's connection to the larger human experience, be mindful and self-aware of one's thoughts and feelings during times of failures, limitations, or suffering.

Recognizing Cues

Related/Risk Factors
Excessive stress; fatigue
Individualism; narcissism
Parental overprotection; impaired family processes
Difficulty independently performing activities of daily living, or instrumental activities of daily living
Ineffective denial; rumination
Perception of weakness, pattern of failure; perfectionism
Overidentification with other's emotions, or thoughts
Avoidance behaviors; social behavior incongruent with social norms; disconnected from society
Conflict between health behaviors and social norms

Defining Characteristics

Subjective
Anxiety; excessive guilt; harsh self-judgment
Loneliness; self-harming thoughts
Exacerbation of signs, or symptoms
Overidentification of feelings, or thoughts

Information that appears in brackets has been added by the authors to clarify and enhance the use of nursing diagnoses.

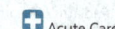 Acute Care 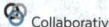 Collaborative 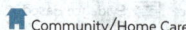 Community/Home Care   Cultural

Objective
Psychological distress, or repression
Cognitive repression; complacent behaviors
Decreased social interaction; hetero-aggressive behavior
Abnormal eating pattern; self-neglect
Risk-taking behaviors; substance misuse

Clinical Connections
Abuse/neglect, borderline personality disorder, schizophrenia, anxiety disorder, phobias, depression

Generate Solutions

Plan Desired Outcomes

Client Will (Include Specific Time Frame)
- Verbalize acceptance of psychical and emotional self.
- Demonstrate self-care, improvement with eating habits, and increased energy.
- Report decreased distress, increased socialization.

Interventions/Take Action

Nursing Priority No. 1.
To identify causative factors:

- Identify thoughts, feelings, and behaviors potentiating self-pity, ruminating, or reliving a negative event. **Feeling sorry for self or self-pity potentiates low-self-esteem, depression, or anxiety.**
- Discuss client's feelings of being a weak person. **Client not admitting to the emotional pain experienced can develop physical and mental illness if not addressed.**
- Identify client's thoughts of feeling defeated. **Self-criticism is defeating, resulting in never being good enough to measure up to family/friends or society.**
- Determine client's reaction to a loss of self-compassion. **A lack of forgiveness and self-compassion increases the risk for poor coping, low self-esteem, depression, anxiety, substance misuse or abuse, and a perception of a lack of social support.**
- Identify thoughts of self-harm or harm to others. **Anxiety and depression due to a lack of self-esteem and compassion can lead to thoughts of harming self or others, necessitating further evaluation/intervention.**

Information that appears in brackets has been added by the authors to clarify and enhance the use of nursing diagnoses.

 Diagnostic Studies 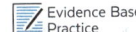 Evidence Based Practice 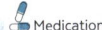 Medications 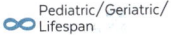 Pediatric/Geriatric/Lifespan

- Determine cultural/spiritual background. **Cultural/spiritual beliefs and values differ; therefore, understanding the client's background defines attitudes and behaviors toward self-compassion in their own community.**
- Identity work or professional background (e.g., first responders such as police, rescue teams, and healthcare professionals) are exposed to a variety of stressful episodes or disasters. **Exposure to disasters or trauma hardens the emotional response, creating a lack of an emotional response and self-compassion. For those who practice self-compassion, they have a reduced risk for anxiety, depression, and fewer accounts of secondary trauma stress, burnout, or compassion fatigue.**
- Assess client's readiness to change behaviors to accept self-compassion. **Attempting to implement strategies prior to the client's readiness to change will be met with resistance. Stages of change are precontemplation, contemplation, preparation, action, maintenance, and relapse. Applying interventions based on the stage is more likely for change to take place.**

Nursing Priority No. 2.

To assist client to cope with current situation:

- Assist client to focus on accepting, experiencing, and acknowledging negative experiences with kindness as a human making a mistake. **Practicing self-forgiveness enhances mental health and overall well-being.**
- Encourage client to see beyond self-judgment, self-pity, and find the ability to forgive self and other that can encourage to try to do better in the future. **Humans make mistakes, and committing to daily self-improvement to do our best is a daily challenge.**
- Direct discussion on self-forgiveness, mindfulness, self-compassion training. **Self-compassion training is learning to have an internal discussion promoting loving, kindness, and acknowledging the imperfection of being human. Mindfulness develops self-awareness, limits negative self-talk, and develops self-acceptance. Self-forgiveness instills resilience.**
- Assist client to develop personally effective coping strategies. **Coping strategies can include exercise, journaling, reading, listening to music, creative arts, or social interactions. Moreover, coping skills help to reduce**

Information that appears in brackets has been added by the authors to clarify and enhance the use of nursing diagnoses.

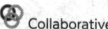 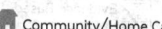

stress, improve overall health conditions, and allow for self-expression.
- Encourage client to connect with family, friends, and community resources for support and guidance. **Support and guidance from others can be a reminder to be kind to self, remembering positive attributes; humans make errors, but this does equate to being worthless or inept.**

Nursing Priority No. 3.

To promote self-compassion (Teaching/Discharge Considerations) and enhance well-being (long-term goals):

- Review coping skills learned. **Helps client remember skills learned during treatment.**
- Discuss client's improvement accomplished during treatment. **Fosters a sense of accomplishment and self-worth.**
- Review community resources available to help the client continue self growth. **Support is available via counselors, therapists, self-help resources, or community support groups.**

Documentation Focus

Assessment/Reassessment
- Individual findings, emotional and behavioral responses to situation
- Physical stress responses such as abnormal eating patterns, fatigue, or substance misuse/abuse
- Cultural/spiritual beliefs
- History of abuse, neglect, substance abuse, social isolation

Planning
- Plan of care and who is involved in the planning
- Teaching plan

Implementation/Evaluation
- Responses to interventions, teaching, and actions performed
- Emotional changes
- Goal attainment or progress toward desired outcomes
- Modifications to plan of care

Discharge Planning
- Long-term goals and who is responsible for actions to be taken
- Specific referrals made

Information that appears in brackets has been added by the authors to clarify and enhance the use of nursing diagnoses.

 Diagnostic Studies 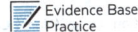 Evidence Based Practice 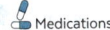 Medications 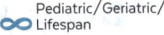 Pediatric/Geriatric/Lifespan

Sample Nursing Outcomes & Interventions Classifications NOC/NIC

NOC—Self-Esteem
NIC—Self-Esteem Enhancement

readiness for enhanced SELF-CONCEPT NANDA-I

[Diagnostic Division: Self-Perception/Concept]

Definition: Pattern of perceptions or ideas about the self, which can be strengthened.

Recognizing Cues

Defining Characteristics

Subjective
Desires to enhance:
 Acceptance of limitations, or strengths
 Body image satisfaction; confidence in abilities
 Congruence between actions and words
 Role performance; satisfaction with personal identity
 Self-esteem; satisfaction with sense of worth

Clinical Connections
Health-seeking behaviors, the client may be healthy or this diagnosis can occur in any clinical condition or life process

Generate Solutions

Plan Desired Outcomes

Client Will (Include Specific Time Frame)
- Verbalize understanding of own sense of self-concept.
- Participate in programs and activities to enhance self-esteem.
- Demonstrate behaviors and lifestyle changes to promote positive self-esteem.
- Participate in family, group, or community activities to enhance self-concept.

Interventions/Take Action

Nursing Priority No. 1.
To assess current situation and desire for improvement:
- Determine client's current belief about self. **Knowing oneself is the basis for personality development such as a**

Information that appears in brackets has been added by the authors to clarify and enhance the use of nursing diagnoses.

 Acute Care 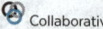 Collaborative 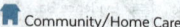 Community/Home Care   Cultural

clarity of self-concept, self-esteem, and dedication to goal attainment. Listening to client's self-report of positive and negative life events allows client to be aware of own thoughts and helps the client to understand the unity of self or self-perception. Information about client's current thinking about self provides a beginning for making changes to improve self.

- Determine client's concept of self in relation to cultural or religious ideals and beliefs. **Cultural characteristics are learned in the family of origin and shape how the individual views self.**
- Assess client's readiness, motivation to change, and willingness to accept assistance. **Identifying client's commitment and willingness to change allows for choosing interventions based on readiness, potentially enhancing outcomes.**
- Observe nonverbal behaviors and note congruence with verbal expressions. Discuss cultural meanings of nonverbal communication. **Incongruences between verbal and nonverbal communication require clarification. Interpretation of nonverbal expressions is culturally determined and needs to be clarified to avoid misinterpretation.**
- Identify family dynamics—present and past. **Provides information about family functioning that will help to develop plan of care for enhancing client's self-concept. Self-esteem begins in early childhood and is influenced by perceptions of how the individual is viewed by significant other(s) (SO[s]).**
- Determine availability and quality of family/SO(s) support. **Presence of supportive people who reflect positive attitudes regarding the individual promotes a positive sense of self.**

Nursing Priority No. 2.
To promote client sense of self-concept:

- Develop therapeutic relationship. Be attentive, validate client's communication, maintain open communication using techniques such as motivational interviewing (MI) and "I" messages. **MI is a goal-oriented, collaborative approach to empower clients to think about their own reasons for changing thinking or behaviors. Asking open-ended questions will help to identify/clarify the client's present thinking and perceptions of current events. The desire to make changes may come over time, depending on client's/SO's need, abilities, and readiness to change.**

Information that appears in brackets has been added by the authors to clarify and enhance the use of nursing diagnoses.

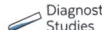 Diagnostic Studies 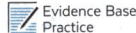 Evidence Based Practice Medications Pediatric/Geriatric/Lifespan

- Collaborate in identifying and developing a list of realistic short- and long-term goals for improvement. **Shared decision making with the client and an interprofessional team promote client-centered care, improving outcomes for the client.**
- Help client recognize their use of defense mechanisms to protect their image. **Defense mechanisms and eight stages of psychosocial development are widely used to project a positive self-image to others.**
- Discuss client's perception of self, confronting misconceptions and identifying negative self-talk. Address distortions in thinking, such as self-referencing (beliefs that others are focusing on individual's weaknesses or limitations), filtering (focusing on negative and ignoring positive), and catastrophizing (expecting the worst outcomes). **Empowered clients can progress with stages of change at their selected pace with better outcomes.**
- Encourage client to review and list current and past successes and strengths. **Listing strengths helps develop self-awareness and mindfulness that can be used to reduce stress in daily living.**
- Acknowledge client's positive behaviors, how they benefit client, and ask if they would like to try other options available that could help client. Provide positive reinforcement to allow for progress at client's own pace. **Developing resilience and finding happiness is a process that is developed or cultivated with intention. Daily cultivation requires reframing thoughts and beliefs about self.**
- Involve in activities or exercise program of choice, and promote socialization. **Client's pursuing or participating in activities that bring enjoyment will not fall into mindless behaviors or activities that can limit their ability to develop optimism, joy, and contentment in daily living.**

Nursing Priority No. 3.

To promote enhanced sense of personal worth (Teaching/Discharge Considerations):

- Assist client to review and add to their personally achievable short- and long-term goals. Provide positive feedback for verbal and behavioral changes reflecting improvement of self-view. **Increases likelihood of success and commitment to change. Functional family and social support are important for individual's overall mental health and emotional well-being.**

Information that appears in brackets has been added by the authors to clarify and enhance the use of nursing diagnoses.

- Reinforce that current decision to improve self-concept is an ongoing process throughout life, requiring strategies to further hope and confidence. **Self-awareness can help and trigger positive coping strategies with daily stressors. Providing the client and family with resources helps with ongoing support strengthening resilience.**
- Recommend client/SO/family enroll in assertiveness training classes. **Promotes expression of feelings in an assertive, rather than aggressive or passive, manner to promote self-esteem.**
- Suggest vocational/emotional counseling as well as activities or hobbies that the client enjoys or would like to experience. **Provide opportunities for learning new skills that can enhance feeling of success and self-worth.**
- Emphasize that self-concept growth includes recognizing confidence in verbal and social presentation, as well as grooming and personal hygiene. **Mindfulness is a strategy of developing both self-awareness and awareness of responses from others. Learning to be mindful helps with personal growth and peace of mind.**
- Provide positive feedback for verbal and behavioral changes reflecting self-view. **Positive reinforcement encourages continued successful behaviors.**

Documentation Focus

Assessment/Reassessment
- Individual findings, including evaluations of self and others, current and past successes
- Interactions with others, lifestyle
- Motivation for and willingness to change

Planning
- Plan of care and who is involved in planning
- Educational plan

Implementation/Evaluation
- Responses to interventions, teaching, and actions performed
- Attainment of or progress toward desired outcome(s)
- Modifications to plan of care

Discharge Planning
- Long-term needs and who is responsible for actions to be taken
- Specific referrals made

Information that appears in brackets has been added by the authors to clarify and enhance the use of nursing diagnoses.

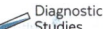 Diagnostic Studies 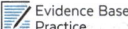 Evidence Based Practice 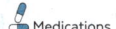 Medications 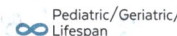 Pediatric/Geriatric/Lifespan

Sample Nursing Outcomes & Interventions Classifications NOC/NIC

NOC—Self-Esteem
NIC—Self-Modification Assistance

chronic inadequate SELF-ESTEEM — NANDA-I

[Diagnostic Division: Self-Perception/Self-Concept]

Definition: Long-standing negative perception of self-worth, self-acceptance, self-respect, competence, and attitude toward self.

Recognizing Cues

Related/Risk Factors

Decreased mindful acceptance; impaired resilience
Difficulty managing finances
Disrupted body image
Fatigue, excessive stress
Fear of rejection; negative resignation orientation; unaddressed repeated negative reinforcement; stigmatization
Impaired religiosity; spiritual incongruence; values incongruent with cultural norms
Inadequate:
  Affection received; respect from others; approval from others
  Attachment behavior, or family cohesiveness
  Group membership, or sense of belonging
  Social support
  Self-efficacy
Ineffective communication skills
Maladaptive grieving

Defining Characteristics (chronic low Self-Esteem)

Subjective
Excessive guilt; shame
Hopelessness; loneliness
Rejects positive feedback; repeated failures
Underestimates ability to deal with situation
Insomnia

Information that appears in brackets has been added by the authors to clarify and enhance the use of nursing diagnoses.

 Acute Care 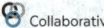 Collaborative 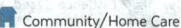 Community/Home Care   Cultural

Objective
Dependent on other's opinions; excessive seeking of reassurance; overly conforming, or obedient behaviors
Depressive symptoms
Decreased eye contact
Rumination, self-negating verbalizations
Suicidal ideation
Hesitant to try new experiences

Clinical Connections
Chronic health conditions, epilepsy, degenerative diseases, eating disorders, substance misuse, anxiety, post-traumatic stress disorder, depressive disorders, personality disorders, bipolar disorder, schizophrenia, pervasive developmental disorders

Generate Solutions

Plan Desired Outcomes

Client Will (Include Specific Time Frame)
- Verbalize understanding of negative evaluation of self and reasons for this problem.
- Participate in treatment program to promote change in self-evaluation.
- Demonstrate behaviors and lifestyle changes to promote positive self-image.
- Verbalize increased sense of self-worth in relation to current situation.
- Participate in family, group, or community activities to enhance change.

Interventions/Take Action

Nursing Priority No. 1.
To assess causative/contributing **or risk** factors:

- Note age and developmental level of client and circumstances surrounding current situation. **Younger people, or those with developmental lag, may not have learned skills to deal with negative occurrences and/or rejection from others.**
- Elicit client's perceptions of current situation (e.g., family crisis, loss of employment, academic failure, physical disfigurement from an accident or illness, relationship problems/divorce with feelings of abandonment by significant other [SO] resulting in social isolation). **Provides insight into**

Information that appears in brackets has been added by the authors to clarify and enhance the use of nursing diagnoses.

 Diagnostic Studies   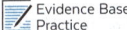 Evidence Based Practice   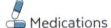 Medications   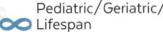 Pediatric/Geriatric/Lifespan

client's view of reality and use of defense mechanisms, which is necessary for choosing interventions appropriate to assist client to address feelings and develop realistic sense of self-worth.
- Assess client's sense of control over self and current situation. **Client's locus of control (or the degree of perceived control) may be a critical factor in ability to cope. Individuals with external locus of control tend to blame others for their problems rather than taking responsibility for their actions using defense mechanisms to protect self-esteem and reduce sense of shame.**
- Determine factors of promoting low self-esteem related to current situation (e.g., family crises, physical disfigurement, social isolation). **Current crises may exacerbate long-standing feelings and perception of self as not being worthwhile.**
- Determine client's awareness of self-destructive behavior, acting out, aggression, or suicidal thoughts. **Detrimental choices may cause feelings of embarrassment or humiliation and lead to feelings of worthlessness. Additionally, client may not be able to accept responsibility for behavior.** Refer to NDs non-suicidal Self-Injurious Behavior; risk for Suicide as indicated for additional interventions.
- Observe nonverbal behavior (e.g., nervous movements, lack of eye contact) and incongruences of verbal expressions. **Important for nurse to be aware of client's culture and healthy communication styles. Incongruences between verbal and nonverbal need to be clarified to be sure perceived meaning of communication is accurate.**
- Note content of negative self-talk and client's perceptions of how others see them. **As negative thoughts are repeated in one's head, they become the basis for believing that the individual is indeed worthless and that others must agree with that conclusion.**
- Determine past and current factors (e.g., negative self-talk or negative perceptions regarding what others think of client) or aggravating occurrences (e.g., family crises, physical disfigurement from an accident or illness, feelings of abandonment by SO[s] resulting in social isolation) that can exacerbate low self-esteem. **Constant repetition of negative words and thoughts reinforces idea that individual is worthless.**
- Note spiritual and cultural factors that influence client's thinking, feelings, and behaviors. **Family of origin affects how one views self in relation to family members and**

Information that appears in brackets has been added by the authors to clarify and enhance the use of nursing diagnoses.

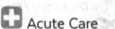 Acute Care 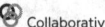 Collaborative 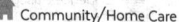 Community/Home Care 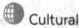 Cultural

others in society. Understanding these factors is necessary to provide appropriate care for client.

- Identify family members, dynamics of interactions present and past,— and cultural influences. **Family communication, parenting styles, ethnicity, cultural beliefs, socioeconomic status, or presence of medical, physical, or mental health issues may result in use of demeaning language, creating embarrassment or shame for client. Inflated praise to children and adolescents can lead to narcissistic traits or lower self-esteem, just as lack of praise damages self-concept.**
- Determine family members/SO(s), relationships, availability, willingness, and quality of support provided to client. **Recognizing family hierarchy and communication patterns helps to understand client's position in the family and potential for support. Resolution for the individual or family can be a lifelong process requiring continuing involvement to promote change and growth.**
- Evaluate current medication regimen, noting client adherence or rationale for nonadherence, as well as use of over-the-counter drugs, herbals, alcohol, and illicit substances. **Important to identify and prevent adverse side effects. Maintaining scheduled medications (e.g., antidepressants, antipsychotics) requires ongoing evaluation and possible changes in regimen. The use of other medications/substances increases the risk of interactions and side effects. Clients experiencing side effects or financial difficulties may stop taking medications as prescribed.**
- Identify client's level of readiness to change and willingness or ability to participate in shared decision making for treatment planning. **Client who acknowledges a need or desire to change is more likely to engage in therapeutic treatment. Motivational interviewing can encourage client to start thinking about changing lifestyle.**

Nursing Priority No. 2.

To promote client sense of self-esteem in coping with situation and life changes:

- Develop therapeutic nurse/client relationship. Use open, honest, and respectful communication using skills of active-listening, and validate client's communication, provide encouragement for efforts, maintaining open communication. **The process of healing begins with a trusting relationship promoting and motivating client to take an active role to change unhealthy thinking and behaviors.**

Information that appears in brackets has been added by the authors to clarify and enhance the use of nursing diagnoses.

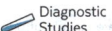 Diagnostic Studies 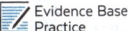 Evidence Based Practice 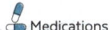 Medications 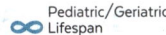 Pediatric/Geriatric/Lifespan

- 🤝 Collaborate with interprofessional treatment team to address presenting medical and safety concerns with the client. **Medical situation/chronic illness may lead to physical changes, such as weight loss or gain, deformity, or amputation, affecting how client sees self as a person. Attitude may contribute to feelings of depression and lack of attention to personal safety requiring evaluation and assistance.**
- Review situations client is currently experiencing and note client's primary concern to be addressed. **Recognizing client's priorities and stage of readiness to change aids the interprofessional team in collaborating with client using shared decision making to develop an effective plan of care.**
- Accept client's perceptions or view of situation while presenting your perception of reality. Avoid threatening existing self-esteem. **Client may not be thinking rationally (e.g., focusing on negative aspects of self, catastrophizing, or expecting the worst outcome, believing others focus on client's weakness) and use defense mechanisms to protect their self-esteem. Promotes trust and allows client to begin to look at options for improving self-esteem. Understanding client's distress and view of situation provides opportunity to be empathetic.**
- Discuss client perceptions of self related to what is happening; confront misconceptions and negative self-talk. **Address distortions in thinking, such as self-referencing (belief that others are focusing on individual's weakness/limitations), filtering (focusing on negative and ignoring positive), catastrophizing (expecting the worst outcomes). Addressing these issues openly provides opportunity for change.**
- Assist client to identify negative thinking and behaviors as they relate to low self-esteem and contribute to feelings of powerlessness. **Self-awareness provides opportunity to reframe thinking toward positive self-esteem and attainment of life goals. Clients who cannot differentiate between what they can and cannot control (or change) may feel defeated and increase negative behaviors (e.g., aggression toward self or others, sabotage treatment plan).**
- Emphasize need to avoid comparing self with others. Encourage client to focus on aspects of self that can be valued. **Important to only compare self (then) to self (now). Changing negative thinking can be effective in developing positive self-talk to enhance self-esteem.**

Information that appears in brackets has been added by the authors to clarify and enhance the use of nursing diagnoses.

- Provide positive reinforcement for progress accomplished. Emphasize importance of progressing at own rate. **Promotes continuation of positive thinking and behaviors that help client regain self-esteem and acceptance of client's progress toward self-improvement at own pace. Note: While praise may be helpful, excessive praise may be heard as manipulative, being rejected as insincere, and actually diminish self-esteem.**
- Assist client to recognize thoughts and feelings leading to a sense of loss of control, aggressive or self-destructive behaviors harming self or others. Set limits on problem behaviors such as acting out, suicide preoccupation, or rumination (unable to stop repetitive thoughts). **Negative thoughts and feelings are a precursor to acting-out behaviors. Helping client to develop self-awareness is a starting point to control negative behaviors. Self-awareness/mindfulness techniques help individuals to find peace of mind in daily living.** Refer to NDs risk for other-directed Violence; risk for Suicide as appropriate
- Encourage involvement in activities/exercise program that client enjoys or would like to experience. **Social interactions with group therapy or activities help client to improve self-esteem. Exercise enhances sense of well-being and can help energize client.**
- Teach client to manage milieu in their home environment (e.g., structure in daily routine and care activities, balance, limit-setting, safety). Prepare client for events or changes that are expected, when possible. **Helping client understand how a behavioral health facility functions and the similarity to healthy home environments can better position client to live a healthy lifestyle. Being prepared for various situations promotes a sense of control and ability to deal with activities as they occur.**
- Emphasize importance of grooming and personal hygiene. Assist in developing skills as indicated (e.g., makeup classes, dressing for success). **Clients with low self-esteem may have overlooked their personal hygiene and need support to improve their personal presentation at home or in social settings.**
- Help client understand that self-worth improves with identifying positive attributes, learning to project confidence, and presenting an appropriate appearance. **Others may judge an individual by outward appearance as well as the positive self-appraisal and sense of confidence one presents.**

Information that appears in brackets has been added by the authors to clarify and enhance the use of nursing diagnoses.

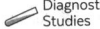 Diagnostic Studies 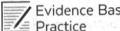 Evidence Based Practice Medications 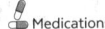 Pediatric/Geriatric/Lifespan

- Promote socialization and participation in recreation and activity programs. **Involvement with others can enhance positive feelings about self. Teaching client self-awareness, approaches to develop resilience and improve self-esteem is a process that takes effort and time.**
- Give reinforcement for progress noted. **Positive words of encouragement promote continuation of efforts, supporting development of coping behaviors.**
- Encourage client to progress at own pace. **Adaptation to a change in self-esteem depends on its significance to individual, disruption to lifestyle, and length of illness/debilitation.**

Nursing Priority No. 3.

To promote thinking and feeling worthy (Teaching/Discharge Considerations) and enhance well-being (long-term goals):

- Review new skills learned and progress made recovering self-esteem. **Client's acknowledgment of improvement develops awareness, confidence, and self-worth.**
- Assist client to identify goals that are personally realistic and achievable. Reinforce that present treatment is a brief encounter in the overall life of client with continued work and ongoing support being necessary to sustain behavior changes and personal growth. **Newly learned approaches to change behaviors require continued work and ongoing support to maintain and sustain improvement in self-esteem/self-worth.**
- Encourage client to structure daily activities by developing a time-management plan. **Successful people self-manage daily living to meet goals.**
- Refer to vocational or employment counselor, educational resources for new skills (e.g., assertiveness training, positive self-image, communication skills), as appropriate. **Assists with development of social or vocational skills, enhancing sense of self-concept and inner locus of control.**
- Encourage participation in class, activities, or hobbies that client enjoys or would like to experience. **Meaningful accomplishment, assuming self-responsibility, and participating in new activities engenders one's sense of competence and self-worth. Successful people self-manage daily living to meet goals.**
- Refer to counseling, therapy, mental health, or special needs/community support groups (e.g., domestic violence, alcohol/substance recovery, grief recovery), as indicated. **Behavioral changes require ongoing effort, and support groups/socialization help sustain life changes.**

Information that appears in brackets has been added by the authors to clarify and enhance the use of nursing diagnoses.

Documentation Focus

Assessment/Reassessment
- Individual findings, including early memories of negative evaluations (self and others), subsequent or precipitating failure events
- Effects on interactions with others, lifestyle
- Specific medical and safety issues
- Motivation for and willingness to change

Planning
- Plan of care and who is involved in planning
- Teaching plan

Implementation/Evaluation
- Responses to interventions, teaching, and actions performed
- Attainment of or progress toward desired outcome(s)
- Modifications to plan of care

Discharge Planning
- Long-term needs and who is responsible for actions to be taken
- Specific referrals made

Sample Nursing Outcomes & Interventions Classifications NOC/NIC

NOC—Self-Esteem
NIC—Self-Esteem Enhancement

---

situational inadequate SELF-ESTEEM — NANDA-I

[Diagnostic Division: Self-Perception/Self-Concept]

Definition: Change from positive to negative perception of self-worth, self-acceptance, self-respect, competence, and attitude toward self in response to a current situation.

Recognizing Cues

Related/Risk Factors
Behavior incongruent with values; values incongruent with cultural norms; impaired religiosity

Decreased mindful acceptance; negative resignation orientation; maladaptive perfectionism; inadequate respect from others; unrealistic self-expectations

---

Information that appears in brackets has been added by the authors to clarify and enhance the use of nursing diagnoses.

 Diagnostic Studies 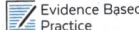 Evidence Based Practice 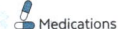 Medications 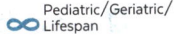 Pediatric/Geriatric/Lifespan

Difficulty accepting alteration in social role; inadequate social support
Difficulty managing finances
Disrupted body image; fear of rejection; stigmatization
Fatigue; excessive stress; powerlessness
Inadequate attachment behavior, or family cohesiveness
Ineffective communication skills; inadequate self-efficacy

Defining Characteristics

Subjective
Loneliness; helplessness; purposelessness
Underestimates ability to deal with situation
Insomnia

Objective
Depressive symptoms
Indecisive behavior; overly obedient behavior
Rumination; self-negating verbalizations

Clinical Connections
Traumatic injuries, surgery, pregnancy, newly diagnosed conditions (e.g., diabetes mellitus), adjustment disorders, substance misuse, stroke, depression, dementia

Generate Solutions

Plan Desired Outcomes

Client Will (Include Specific Time Frame)
- Verbalize understanding of individual factors that precipitated current situation.
- Identify feelings and underlying dynamics for negative perception of self.
- Express positive self-appraisal.
- Demonstrate behaviors to restore positive self-image.
- Participate in treatment regimen or activities to correct factors that precipitated crisis.

Interventions/Take Action

Nursing Priority No. 1.
To assess causative/contributing **or risk** factors:
- Determine individual situation/factors (e.g., family crisis, termination of a relationship, loss of employment, physical disfigurement) related to lowered self-esteem in the present circumstances. **Many factors are involved in a person's**

Information that appears in brackets has been added by the authors to clarify and enhance the use of nursing diagnoses.

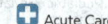 Acute Care   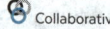 Collaborative   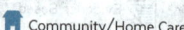 Community/Home Care   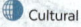 Cultural

self-esteem, and this information is essential for planning accurate care. Refer to appropriate underlying NDs such as disturbed Body Image, Post-Trauma Syndrome, disturbed Personal Identity, risk for disrupted Immigration Transition, impaired Family Process, ineffective intimate partner Relationship.

- Identify client's basic sense of self-esteem and image client has of self: existential, physical, psychological. **The components of self-esteem are (1) how you see yourself/identity, (2) self-confidence, (3) sense of belonging, (4) feeling of competence, and (5) a feeling of security. Each aspect plays a role in the client's ability to cope with current situation/crisis.**
- Assess client's expressions or demonstrations of degree of threat/perception of crisis. **How individuals perceive themselves is based on the self-judgments they make. How the client sees the current situation in relation to ability to cope will affect sense of self-worth and needs to be acknowledged and planned for to help client deal with feelings of low self-esteem.**
- Assess degree of threat and perception of client in regard to crisis. **One individual views a serious situation as manageable, while another individual may be overly concerned about a minor problem.**
- Identify a sense of control client perceives self to have over self and situation. Note client's locus of control (internal or external). **Client's locus of control (degree of control client believes or perceives they have) may be a critical factor in ability to cope with current situation or crisis. Individuals with internal locus of control tend to be more optimistic about their ability to cope with adversity even in the face of current difficulties. Individuals with external locus of control will look to others to solve problems and take care of them.**
- Determine client's awareness of own responsibility for coping with situation, and personal growth. **These factors enhance the ability of the client to effectively manage situation in a positive manner.**
- Evaluate conversations, noting a negative attitude self-talk. **Contributes to view of situation as hopeless and/or too difficult to cope with.**
- Listen for client who makes self-depreciating comments or expresses suicidal thoughts or verbalizes intention to harm self with a plan. **Indicates a high level of stress and urgent need for further evaluation and/or referral to**

Information that appears in brackets has been added by the authors to clarify and enhance the use of nursing diagnoses.

acute or emergent mental health services. Refer to ND risk for Suicide as appropriate.

- Assess family/significant other (SO) dynamics and support of client. **How family members interact affects an individual's development and sense of self-esteem. Effective interactions among family members usually lead to positive support for the client in current situation. Dysfunctional interactions may be detrimental to client's ability to deal with what is happening.**
- Observe nonverbal behaviors, body language. **Clarify with client incongruences between verbal and nonverbal communication to ensure accuracy of interpretation.**
- Verify client's concept of self in relation to cultural/religious ideals. **Cultural and religious influences during the individual's life affect beliefs about self, measure of worth, and ability to deal with current situation or crisis. Note: Recent studies support that self-esteem functions similarly across cultures.**
- Determine past coping skills in relation to current episode. **Past experiences with failure or success will affect client's expectations regarding the eventual outcome of coping with current illness or crisis.**
- Note availability and use of resources to address specific need (e.g., rehabilitation services, home-care support, job placement). **Individual may be unaware or have difficulty accessing community supports or assistance programs.**
- Identify client's desires, abilities, reasons to change, and need to change thinking and feeling about self-worth. **Client seeking help is willing to progress through the stages of change (e.g., precontemplation, contemplation, preparation, action, and maintenance). Client who is not ready to change will resist working through the intervention. Apply interventions based on the client's identified stage of readiness.**

Nursing Priority No. 2.

To assist client to cope with loss/change and recapture sense of positive self-esteem:

- Encourage expression of thoughts, feelings, or anxieties related to the situation. **Hearing client's emotions, loss, or grieving sends a message of accepting the client without judgment and as a human with needs.** Refer to ND Grief or dysfunctional Grief as indicated.

Information that appears in brackets has been added by the authors to clarify and enhance the use of nursing diagnoses.

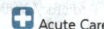 Acute Care 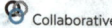 Collaborative 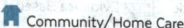 Community/Home Care Cultural

- Assist with treatment of underlying condition as appropriate. **For example, cognitive restructuring and improved concentration in mild brain injury often result in restoration of positive self-esteem.**
- Identify individual strengths and assets and aspects of self that remain intact and can be valued. Reinforce positive traits, abilities, self-view. **Client may not see these in the anxiety and hopelessness of the immediate situation, and reminding client of own positive attributes can help client recover hope and develop a positive attitude about situation.**
- Help client identify own responsibility and control or lack of control in situation. **When able to acknowledge what is out of own control, client can focus attention on area of own responsibility.**
- Assist client to problem-solve situation, developing plan of action and setting goals to achieve desired outcome. **Enhances commitment to plan, optimizing outcomes.**
- Convey confidence in client's ability to cope with current situation. **Validation helps client accept own ability to deal with what is happening.**
- Mobilize support systems. **Feeling hopeless and alone lowers client's ability to manage care and concentrate on healing. Support systems can provide role modeling and the help needed to engender hope and enhance self-esteem.**
- Provide opportunity for client to practice alternative coping strategies, including progressive socialization opportunities. **Involvement with others provides client with situation in which new actions can be tried out and validated or discarded to enhance feelings of self-worth.**
- Encourage use of visualization, guided imagery, and relaxation. **These strategies promote a positive sense of self and general well-being, enhancing client's coping ability.**
- Provide feedback about client's self-negating remarks or behavior, using I-messages. **Allows client to experience a different view. "I" messages are a nonjudgmental way to let individual understand how behavior is perceived by or affecting others and self.**
- Encourage involvement in decisions about care, as appropriate. **Promotes sense of control over what is happening, enhancing feelings of self-worth.**
- Give positive reinforcement for progress. **Positive words of encouragement promote continuation of efforts, supporting development of coping behaviors.**

Information that appears in brackets has been added by the authors to clarify and enhance the use of nursing diagnoses.

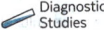 Diagnostic Studies
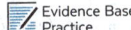 Evidence Based Practice
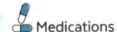 Medications
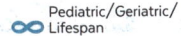 Pediatric/Geriatric/Lifespan

Nursing Priority No. 3.

To promote positive aspects of the individual (Teaching/ Discharge Considerations) and enhance well-being (long-term goals):

- Review progress made during treatment. **Reminds the client of their abilities to change their thinking and feeling about themselves and confidence in their abilities to cope.**
- Assist client to identify personally achievable goals. **Increases likelihood of client's success and commitment to change.**
- Encourage client to look to the future and set long-range goals for achieving necessary lifestyle changes. **Supports view that this is an ongoing process, providing client with hope for the future.**
- Support independence in activities of daily living and mastery of therapeutic regimen. **Individuals who are confident are more secure and positive in self-appraisal.**
- Promote attendance in therapy or support group as indicated. **Provides opportunity to discuss own situation and hear how others are dealing with similar problems, promoting new ideas about own ability to deal with issues.**
- Involve extended family/SO(s) in treatment plan as appropriate. **Enhances their understanding of what client wishes to accomplish, increasing likelihood they will provide appropriate support to client.**
- Provide information and bibliotherapy, including reliable websites as appropriate. **Reinforces learning, allowing client to progress at own pace. Promotes opportunity for making informed decisions and improving ability to deal with situation.**
- Refer to vocational or employment counselor and educational resources, as appropriate. **Assists with development of social or vocational skills, promoting sense of competence and self-responsibility.**
- Suggest participation in group or community activities (e.g., assertiveness classes, volunteer work, support groups). **Provides opportunities for learning new information and being appreciated for contributions, enhancing sense of self-worth.**
- Refer to counseling or therapy, mental health, or other special-needs support groups, as indicated. **May need additional support to deal with crisis.**

Information that appears in brackets has been added by the authors to clarify and enhance the use of nursing diagnoses.

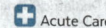 Acute Care 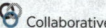 Collaborative 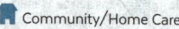 Community/Home Care 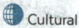 Cultural

Documentation Focus

Assessment/Reassessment
- Individual findings, noting precipitating crisis, client's perceptions, effects on desired lifestyle/interaction with others
- Underlying dynamics and duration of current situation
- Past history of self-esteem issues
- Cultural values or religious beliefs, locus of control
- Family support, availability and use of resources

Planning
- Plan of care and who is involved in planning
- Teaching plan

Implementation/Evaluation
- Responses to interventions, teaching, actions performed, and changes that may be indicated
- Attainment of or progress toward desired outcome(s)
- Modifications to plan of care

Discharge Planning
- Long-term needs and goals and who is responsible for actions to be taken
- Specific referrals made

Sample Nursing Outcomes & Interventions Classifications NOC/NIC

NOC—Self-Esteem
NIC—Self-Esteem Enhancement

---

non-suicidal SELF-INJURIOUS BEHAVIOR NANDA-I

[Diagnostic Division: Stress Management]

Definition: Deliberate self-inflicted harm to oneself without the motive of suicide or sexual deviation, and for purposes that are not socially sanctioned.

Recognizing Cues

Related/Risk Factors
Behavioral factors:
Addictive behaviors; problematic internet use; intentional misuse of prescription medications; substance misuse
Inadequate health literacy

Information that appears in brackets has been added by the authors to clarify and enhance the use of nursing diagnoses.

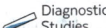 Diagnostic Studies 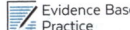 Evidence Based Practice 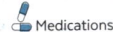 Medications 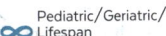 Pediatric/Geriatric/Lifespan

Low level of moderate-to-vigorous physical activity; high level of screen-based sedentary behavior

High frequency score on standardized, validated self-injury instrument

Implicit identification with cutting on standardized, validated self-injury instruments

Psychological factors:

Excessive stress, or anxiety; hopelessness; depressive symptoms

High level of alexithymia; difficulty expressing, or regulating emotions

Emotional dysregulation; difficulty relieving negative emotions

Inability to maintain proper interpersonal-regulation; inadequate self-control; ineffective impulse control

Inadequate self-esteem; loneliness

Hypersensitivity; intolerant of uncertainty; ineffective use of coping strategies

Strong urge to avoid elevated emotional arousal

Elevated severity score using standardized, validated self-injury instrument

Eating disorder

Physiological factors:

Ineffective sleep pattern; insomnia

Ineffective overweight self-management

Situational factors:

Difficulty accessing mental health care

Exposure to peer nonsuicidal self-injury behaviors

Difficulty with immigration transition

Social factors:

Difficulty establishing social interaction; disturbed interpersonal relations

Bullying; peer-related rejection

Ineffective communication between parent and adolescent; harsh parenting; inadequate parental monitoring

Inadequate social support; inadequate parental social support

Defining Characteristics

Subjective
Increased anxiety symptoms

Objective
Abrading skin; scratching, or burning skin; cutting with a sharp object
Biting; hitting
Pulling hair; head banging
Anger behaviors

Information that appears in brackets has been added by the authors to clarify and enhance the use of nursing diagnoses.

Clinical Connections
Borderline personality, dissociative disorders, bipolar disorder, developmental delay, autism spectrum, eating disorders, substance misuse, physical or psychological abuse, gender identity crisis

Generate Solutions

Plan Desired Outcomes

Client Will (Include Specific Time Frame)
- Verbalize understanding of reasons for wanting to cut or harm self, or occurrence of behavior.
- Identify precipitating factors or awareness of arousal state that occurs prior to incident.
- Express increased self-concept or self-esteem.
- Demonstrate self-control, as evidenced by lessened (or absence of) episodes of self-injury.
- Engage in use of alternative methods for managing feelings and individuality.
- Seek help when feeling anxious and having thoughts of harming self.

Interventions/Take Action

Nursing Priority No. 1.
To assess causative/contributing factors:
- Determine underlying dynamics of individual situation (e.g., behavioral, psychological, physiological, situational, or social factors as listed in Related/Risk Factors). Note presence of inflexible, maladaptive personality traits (e.g., impulsive, unpredictable, inappropriate behaviors, intense anger, lack of control of anger) **reflecting personality or character disorder, mental illness. Note: Clients diagnosed as borderline personality disorder are often unstable and prone to self-injury and need a specific treatment plan to diminish these behaviors.**
- Evaluate history of mental illness (e.g., borderline personality, identity disorder, bipolar disorder). **These conditions may be the underlying cause of the self-injurious behavior.**
- Identify previous episodes of self-injurious behavior. **Some body piercing (e.g., ears) is generally accepted as decorative; piercing of multiple sites often is an attempt to establish individuality, addressing issues of separation and belonging, but is not considered self-injury behavior.**

Information that appears in brackets has been added by the authors to clarify and enhance the use of nursing diagnoses.

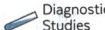 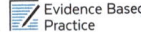 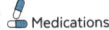 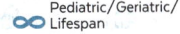

- Note beliefs, cultural and spiritual practices that may be involved in choice of behavior. **Growing up in a family that did not allow feelings to be expressed, individuals learn that feelings are bad or wrong. Family dynamics may come out of spiritual or cultural expectations that believe in strict punishment for transgressions. Individuals may believe mental illness is the result of unacceptable actions, and feelings of guilt may lead to anxiety and subsequent self-injurious behaviors.**
- Determine use or abuse of addicting substances. **Client may be trying to resist impulse to self-injure by turning to drugs.**
- Review laboratory findings (e.g., blood alcohol, polydrug screen, glucose, and electrolyte levels). **Drug use may affect self-injury behavior.**
- Note degree of impairment in social and occupational functioning. **May dictate treatment setting (e.g., specific outpatient program, short-stay inpatient).**
- Identify client's stage of readiness to change. **Attempting to implement interventions prior to the client's stage of readiness will be met with resistance.**

Nursing Priority No. 2.
To structure environment to maintain client safety:

- Assist client to identify feelings leading up to desire for self-harm. **Early recognition of recurring feelings provides opportunity to seek and learn other ways of coping.**
- Provide external controls/limit setting. **May decrease the opportunity for client to engage in self-harm.**
- Include client in development of plan of care. **Commitment to plan increases likelihood of adherence.**
- Encourage appropriate expression of feelings. **Identifies feelings and promotes understanding of what leads to development of tension/harmful behavior.**
- Keep client in continuous staff view and provide special observation checks during inpatient therapy. **Promotes safety by recognizing escalating behaviors and providing timely intervention**
- Structure inpatient milieu to maintain positive, clear, open communication among staff and clients, with an understanding that "secrets are not tolerated" and failure to maintain openness will be addressed. **Prevents manipulative behavior, so client does not pit one staff member against another to fulfill own desires.**

Information that appears in brackets has been added by the authors to clarify and enhance the use of nursing diagnoses.

- Develop schedule of alternative, healthy, success-oriented activities, including involvement in such groups as Self-Harm Support Group, Cutters Awareness & Support Group (or similar program) based on individual needs; self-esteem activities including positive affirmations, connecting with friends and like-minded peers, and exercise.
- Note feelings of healthcare providers and family, such as frustration, anger, defensiveness, need to rescue. **Client may be manipulative, evoking defensiveness and conflict among staff/family. These feelings need to be identified, recognized, and dealt with openly with staff/family and client.**
- Discuss the role neurotransmitters in the brain play in predisposing individual to beginning this behavior. **It is believed that problems in the serotonin system may make the person more aggressive and impulsive, and when combined with a home where they have learned that feelings are bad or wrong, this leads to turning aggression on self.**
- Discuss use of medication, such as clozapine. **This medication has been shown to reduce acts of self-injurious behavior and help client maintain a more stable mood.**
- Provide care for client's self-inflicted wounds in a matter-of-fact manner **conveying empathy and concern.** Refrain from offering sympathy or additional attention **that could provide reinforcement for maladaptive behavior and may encourage its repetition.**

Nursing Priority No. 3.

To promote movement toward positive behaviors:

- Develop a therapeutic relationship between client, nurse, and counselor to enable the client to stay physically safe, pledging: "I will not cut or harm myself for the next 24 hours." Renew commitment daily with client. **Making a commitment helps client to think before acting and can prevent new incidents of self-injury.**
- Encourage client involvement in formulating plan of care and developing goals for preventing undesired behavior. **Being involved in own decisions can help to reestablish ego boundaries and enhance commitment to goals, optimizing outcomes and enhancing self-esteem.**
- Discuss with client/family normalcy of adolescent task of separation and ways of achieving. **Helps individual members understand these actions and begin to recognize normal actions and those that are of concern and need intervention.**

Information that appears in brackets has been added by the authors to clarify and enhance the use of nursing diagnoses.

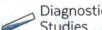 Diagnostic Studies 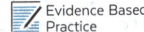 Evidence Based Practice 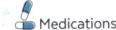 Medications 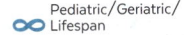 Pediatric/Geriatric/Lifespan

- Identify the consequences and outcomes of current actions (e.g., ask "Does this get you what you want?" or "How does this behavior help you achieve your goals?"). **Provides client with opportunity to look at own behaviors in a different way and begin to understand how they are harmful rather than helpful. Contrasting healthy behaviors versus current actions can help client decide to change them. Dialectic behavior therapy is effective in reducing injurious behavior, along with the use of medication.**
- Assist client to learn assertive behavior. Include the use of effective communication skills, focusing on developing self-esteem by replacing negative self-talk with positive comments. **Low self-esteem is a factor in this behavior, and by learning new ways of expressing self, client can begin to feel better and deal with anxieties in a more positive manner.**
- Provide avenues of communication **for times when client needs to talk to avoid cutting or damaging self.**
- Choose interventions that help the client to reclaim power in own life (e.g., experiential and cognitive). **Beginning to think in a positive manner and then translating that into action provides reinforcement for using power to stop injurious behaviors and develop a more productive lifestyle.**
- Involve client/family in group therapies as appropriate. **Group setting aids in promoting diffusion of anger and provides insight as to how negative, aggressive behavior affects others, making feedback easier to digest and understand.**

Nursing Priority No. 4.

To promote long-term safety (Teaching/Discharge Considerations) and enhance well-being (long-term goals):

- Discuss coping skills, progress made, and commitment to safety and ways in which client will cope with precursors to undesired behavior. **Identifies specific precursors for individual and provides a plan for client to follow when anxiety becomes overwhelming, creating opportunity for client to assume responsibility for self.**
- Identify and mobilize support systems. **Knowing who client can turn to when anxiety becomes a problem can help client avoid injurious behavior.**
- Promote the use of healthy behaviors, identifying consequences and outcomes of current actions. **As client**

Information that appears in brackets has been added by the authors to clarify and enhance the use of nursing diagnoses.

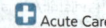 Acute Care 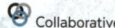 Collaborative 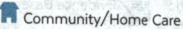 Community/Home Care   Cultural

develops a more positive attitude and accepts the idea that current actions are being destructive to desired lifestyle, new behaviors can help make needed changes.
- Discuss living arrangements when client is discharged/relocated. **May need assistance and support with transition to minimize stressors to avoid recurrence of self-harm.**
- Arrange for continued involvement in group therapy after discharge from program. **Remaining in this supportive environment can help client maintain new behaviors as client begins to increase responsibility for self and own action.**
- Involve family/significant other in planning for discharge and in group therapies, as appropriate. **Promotes coordination and continuation of plan, commitment to goals.**
- Discuss and provide information and discuss the use of medication, as appropriate. **Antidepressant medications may be useful, but they need to be weighed against the potential for overdosing. Note: Medication may be tried for co-occurring disorders like depression or bipolar disorder. However, if the person has no co-occurring disorder, medications may be discouraged, as they can work to cover up feelings that a person has to work through in order to stop the self-harm behavior. Medications that stabilize moods, ease depression, and calm anxiety may be tried to reduce the urge to self-harm.**
- Refer to NDs Anxiety; impaired Social Connectedness; chronic inadequate Self-Esteem; situational inadequate Self-Esteem.

Documentation Focus

Assessment/Reassessment
- Individual findings, including risk factors present, underlying dynamics, prior episodes
- Cultural or spiritual practices
- Laboratory test results
- Substance use or abuse

Planning
- Plan of care and who is involved in planning
- Teaching plan

Implementation/Evaluation
- Response to interventions, teaching, and actions performed
- Attainment of or progress toward desired outcome(s)
- Modifications to plan of care

Information that appears in brackets has been added by the authors to clarify and enhance the use of nursing diagnoses.

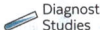 Diagnostic Studies 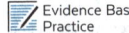 Evidence Based Practice 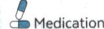 Medications 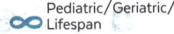 Pediatric/Geriatric/Lifespan

Discharge Planning
- Long-term needs and who is responsible for actions to be taken
- Community resources, referrals made

Sample Nursing Outcomes & Interventions Classifications NOC/NIC

NOC—Self-Harm Restraint
NIC—Behavior Management: Self-Harm

SENSORY DEFICIT [Specify: visual, auditory, kinesthetic, gustatory, tactile, olfactory] ICNP

[Diagnostic Division: Neurosensory]

Definition: Change(s) in actual or perceived sensory data resulting in a compromised or dysfunctional human response.

Recognizing Cues

Related/Risk Factors
Inadequate/excessive environmental stimuli: therapeutically restricted environments (e.g., isolation, bedrest, confining illnesses, incubator); socially restricted environment (e.g., institutionalization, homebound, aging, chronic or terminal illness, infant deprivation), stigmatized (e.g., mental illness, developmentally delayed, disabled); excessive environmental stimulation (e.g., intensive care, work setting, competitive video gaming)

Altered sensory reception, transmission, or integration (e.g., neurological injury due to traumatic brain injury/stroke, facial nerve damage, damage to the olfactory nerve [responsible for smell], neoplasm, multiple sclerosis, etc.)

Biochemical imbalances (e.g., acid-base imbalance, elevated blood urea nitrogen, ammonia; hypoxia); electrolyte imbalance; drugs (e.g., stimulants or depressants, mind-altering drugs)

Psychological stress; sleep deprivation

Defining Characteristics

Subjective
Sensory acuity change (e.g., photosensitivity, hypoesthesias or hyperesthesias, diminished or altered sense of taste, inability to tell position of body parts [proprioception])
Sensory distortions

Information that appears in brackets has been added by the authors to clarify and enhance the use of nursing diagnoses.

 Acute Care  Collaborative 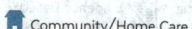 Community/Home Care 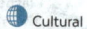 Cultural

Objective

Change in sensory acuity or visual response to stimuli
Behavioral/personality change; restlessness; irritability
Impaired problem-solving abilities; poor concentration
Change in mentation; hallucinations; illusions
Impaired communication
Motor incoordination, syncope/dizziness, falls (e.g., Ménière syndrome)

Generate Solutions

Plan Desired Outcomes

Client Will (Include Specific Time Frame)

- Regain or maintain usual level of cognition.
- Recognize and correct or compensate for sensory impairments.
- Verbalize awareness of sensory needs and presence of overload and/or deprivation.
- Identify and modify external factors that contribute to alterations in sensory or perceptual abilities.
- Use resources effectively and appropriately.
- Be free of injury.

Interventions/Take Action

Nursing Priority No. 1.

To assess causative/contributing factors and degree of impairment:

- Identify client with condition that can affect sensing, interpreting, and communicating stimuli. **Specific clinical concerns (e.g., neurological disease or trauma, intensive care unit confinement, surgery, pain, biochemical imbalances, psychosis, substance abuse, toxemia) have the potential for altering one or more of the senses, with resultant change in the reception, sensitivity, or interpretation of sensory input.**
- Note age and developmental stage. **Problems with sensory perception may be known to client/caregiver (e.g., child wearing hearing aid, elderly adult with known macular degeneration), where compensatory interventions are in place. Screening or evaluation may be required if sensory impairments are suspected but not obvious.**
- Review results of sensory and motor neurological testing and laboratory studies (e.g., cognitive testing or laboratory values, such as electrolytes, chemical profile, arterial blood

---

Information that appears in brackets has been added by the authors to clarify and enhance the use of nursing diagnoses.

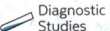 Diagnostic Studies   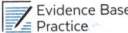 Evidence Based Practice   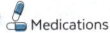 Medications   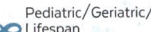 Pediatric/Geriatric/Lifespan

gases, serum drug levels) **to note presence or possible cause of changes in response to sensory stimuli.**

- Evaluate medication regimen and determine possible use or misuse of drugs (prescription, over-the-counter [OTC], illicit) **to identify effects, side effects, or drug interactions that may cause or exacerbate sensory or perceptual problems.**
- Assess ability to speak, hear, interpret, and respond to simple commands **to obtain an overview of client's mental and cognitive status and ability to interpret stimuli.**
- Evaluate sensory awareness (e.g., recognition of hot and cold, dull or sharp; smell, and taste), visual acuity and hearing; and proprioception (e.g., location and movement of body parts).
- Note inattention to body parts, segments of environment; lack of recognition of familiar objects or persons. **Various sensory disturbances can occur with stroke (e.g., loss of ability to feel touch, pain, temperature or to sense how the body is positioned.**
- Determine response to painful stimuli **to note whether response is appropriate to stimulus and is immediate or delayed.**
- Observe for behavioral responses (e.g., illusions, hallucinations, delusions, withdrawal, hostility, crying, inappropriate affect, confusion or disorientation) **that may indicate mental or emotional problems or chemical toxicity (as might occur with digoxin or other drug overdose or reaction) or be associated with brain or neurological trauma or infection.**
- Ascertain client's/significant other's (SO's) perception of problem/changes in activities of daily living. **Client may or may not be aware of changes (e.g., diabetic with neuropathy may not realize they have lost discrimination for pain in feet; or parents may notice child's problem with coordination or difficulty with words).** Listen to and respect client's expressions of deprivation and take these into consideration in planning care.

Nursing Priority No. 2.
To promote normalization of response to stimuli:

- Address client by name and have personnel wear name tags and reintroduce self, as needed, **to preserve client's sense of identity and orientation.**
- Approach from visually intact side, position objects to take advantage of intact visual field, and use eye patch, if

---

Information that appears in brackets has been added by the authors to clarify and enhance the use of nursing diagnoses.

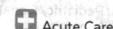 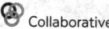 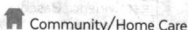 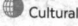

indicated, **to decrease sensory confusion when client has acute loss of vision or field of vision in one eye.**
- Reorient to person, place, time, and events, as necessary, **to reduce confusion and provide sense of normalcy to client's daily life.**
- Explain procedures and activities, expected sensations, and outcomes.
- Provide means of communication, as indicated by client's current situation.
- Determine if client reads lips and turn toward/face client, making sure to have client's attention, and enunciating words clearly.
- Encourage use of hearing devices (e.g., hearing aid, audio-visual amplifier, closed-caption TV, signing interpreter) **to assist in managing auditory impairment.**
- Pay attention to background noise and reduce it to a minimum when attempting conversation. **Background noise is often amplified, causing misinterpretation of conversation or inability to hear words, and often results in overstimulation of senses.**
- Place glasses or contacts where they can be easily found, and encourage client to wear corrective lenses during waking hours.
- Interpret stimuli and offer feedback **to assist client to separate reality from fantasy or altered perception.**
- Avoid isolating client, physically or emotionally, **to prevent sensory deprivation and limit confusion.**
- Promote a stable environment with continuity of care by same personnel as much as possible.
- Eliminate extraneous noise and stimuli, including nonessential equipment, alarms, or audible monitor signals when possible.
- Provide undisturbed rest and sleep periods.
- Speak to visually impaired or unresponsive client during care **to provide auditory stimulation and prevent startle reflex.**
- Provide tactile stimulation as care is given if approved by client. **Touching is an important part of caring and a deep psychological need communicating presence and connection with another human being.**
- Provide sensory stimulation, including familiar smells and sounds, tactile stimulation with a variety of objects, changing of light intensity, and other cues (e.g., clocks, calendars).

Information that appears in brackets has been added by the authors to clarify and enhance the use of nursing diagnoses.

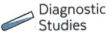 Diagnostic Studies
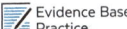 Evidence Based Practice
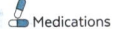 Medications
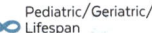 Pediatric/Geriatric/Lifespan

- Investigate reports of changes in tastes of foods (foods taste or smell odd), ability to salivate, or loss of appetite. **May reflect loss or distortion of smell and taste functions or side effects or interactions with medications.**
- Remove offensive odors from client's presence, especially **when client is immobile, debilitated, and/or suffering from oversensitivity to odors, nausea, or vomiting.**
- Encourage SO(s) to bring in familiar objects, talk to, and touch the client frequently.
- Minimize discussion of negatives (e.g., client and personnel problems) within client's hearing. **Client may misinterpret and believe references are to self.**
- Provide diversional activities, as able (e.g., TV, radio, conversation, large-print or audiobooks). (Refer to ND decreased Diversional Activity Engagement.)
- Promote meaningful socialization. (Refer to ND inadequate Social Connectedness.)
- Collaborate with other health team members in providing rehabilitative therapies and stimulating modalities (e.g., music therapy, sensory training, remotivation therapy) **to achieve maximal gains in function and psychosocial well-being.**
- Identify and encourage use of resources and prosthetic devices (e.g., hearing aids, computerized visual aid, glasses with a level plumbline for balance). **Useful for augmenting senses.**

Nursing Priority No. 3.

To prevent injury/complications:

- Record perceptual deficit on chart **so that caregivers are aware.**
- Place call bell or other communication device within reach and be sure client knows where it is and how to use it.
- Provide safety measures, as needed (e.g., siderails, bed in low position, adequate lighting; assistance with walking; use of vision or hearing devices).
- Review basic and specific safety information (e.g., "I am on your right side"; "This water is hot"; "Swallow now"; "Stand up"; "You cannot drive").
- Position doors and furniture so they are out of travel path for client with impaired vision or strategically place items or grab bars **to aid in maintaining balance.**
- Ambulate with assistance and devices **to enhance balance.**
- Describe where affected areas of body are when moving client.

Information that appears in brackets has been added by the authors to clarify and enhance the use of nursing diagnoses.

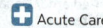 Acute Care 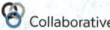 Collaborative 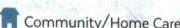 Community/Home Care 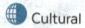 Cultural

- Limit and carefully monitor use of sedation, especially in the elderly, **who are more sensitive to side effects and drug interactions affecting sensory perception and interpretation.**
- Monitor use of heating pads or ice packs; use thermometer to measure temperature of bath water **to protect from thermal injury.**
- Refer to NDs risk for [adult or child] Fall; risk for burn Injury; risk for physical Injury.

Nursing Priority No. 4.

To promote optimal sensory functioning (Teaching/Discharge Considerations) and enhance well-being (long-term goals):

- Review ways to prevent or limit exposure to conditions affecting sensory functions (e.g., how exposure to loud noise and toxins can impair hearing; early childhood screening for speech and language disorders; vaccines to prevent measles, mumps, meningitis, **once known to be major causes of hearing loss**).
- Assist client/SO(s) to learn effective ways of coping with and managing sensory disturbances, anticipating safety needs according to client's sensory deficits and developmental level.
- Identify alternative ways of dealing with perceptual deficits (e.g., vision and hearing aids; augmentative communication devices; computer technologies; specific deficit-compensation techniques).
- Provide explanations of and plan care with client, involving SO(s) as much as possible. **Enhances commitment to and continuation of plan, optimizing outcomes.**
- Review home safety measures pertinent to deficits.
- Discuss drug regimen, noting possible toxic side effects of both prescription and OTC drugs. **Prompt recognition of side effects allows for timely intervention/change in drug regimen.**
- Demonstrate use and care of sensory prosthetic devices (e.g., assistive vision or listening devices, etc.).
- Identify resources and community programs for acquiring and maintaining assistive devices.
- Refer to appropriate helping resources, such as Society for the Blind, Self-Help for the Hard of Hearing (SHHH), or local support groups, screening programs, as indicated.
- Refer to additional NDs Anxiety; acute Confusion; chronic Confusion as appropriate.

Information that appears in brackets has been added by the authors to clarify and enhance the use of nursing diagnoses.

Documentation Focus

Assessment/Reassessment
- Individual findings, noting specific deficit and associated symptoms, perceptions of client/SO(s)
- Assistive device needs

Planning
- Plan of care, including who is involved in planning
- Teaching plan

Implementation/Evaluation
- Responses to interventions, teaching, and actions performed
- Attainment of or progress toward desired outcome(s)
- Modifications to plan of care

Discharge Planning
- Long-term needs and who is responsible for actions to be taken
- Available resources; specific referrals made

Sample Nursing Outcomes & Interventions Classifications NOC/NIC

Auditory
NOC—Sensory Function: Hearing
NIC—Communication Enhancement: Hearing Deficit

Visual
NOC—Sensory Function: Vision
NIC—Communication Enhancement: Visual Deficit

Gustatory/Olfactory
NOC—Sensory Function: Taste & Smell
NIC—Nutrition Management

Kinesthetic
NOC—Sensory Function: Proprioception
NIC—Body Mechanics Promotion

Tactile
NOC—Sensory Function
NIC—Peripheral Sensation Management

Information that appears in brackets has been added by the authors to clarify and enhance the use of nursing diagnoses.

impaired SEXUAL FUNCTIONING ICNP

[Diagnostic Division: Sexuality/Reproduction]

Definition: Interactions between mind and body affecting sexual expression and performance (i.e., desire, arousal, physical pleasure, and orgasm) resulting in a response that is unsatisfying or unrewarding.

Recognizing Cues

Related/Risk Factors
Lack of knowledge regarding sexual functions and the reproductive system
Insufficient sexual role model; lack of partner/significant other (SO)
Insufficient environment lacks privacy, safety
Fear of sexual vulnerability
History of sexual abuse/trauma
Cultural expectations, restrictions

Defining Characteristics

Subjective
Lack of/decreased interest or desire to participate in sexual activities
Unable to maintain physical arousal, sexual activity
Difficulty obtaining or achieving orgasm
Physical, emotional distress; discomfort or pain during intercourse
Thoughts, feelings of shame, embarrassment, guilt; concerns about own desirability

Objective
Erectile dysfunction (ED)
Vaginal photoplethysmography
Decreased hormone levels (e.g., testosterone, estrogen, and prolactin)

Clinical Connections
Sexual pain disorder (e.g., dyspareunia, vaginismus, noncoital sexual pain), urological infections, arthritis, cancer, major surgery, heart disease, hypertension, diabetes mellitus, spinal cord injury, hormonal imbalances, multiple sclerosis (MS), traumatic injury, pregnancy, childbirth, abuse, depression, alcoholism/drug abuse, obesity

---

Information that appears in brackets has been added by the authors to clarify and enhance the use of nursing diagnoses.

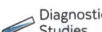 Diagnostic Studies   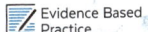 Evidence Based Practice   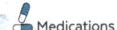 Medications   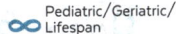 Pediatric/Geriatric/Lifespan

Generate Solutions

Plan Desired Outcomes

Client Will (Include Specific Time Frame)
- Verbalize understanding of sexual anatomy, functions, and processes influencing sexual functioning.
- Verbalize awareness of biological/biochemical/emotional reason for sexual issues.
- Acknowledge lifestyle stressors contributing/causing sexual difficulties.
- Define acceptable, satisfying or alternative approaches to obtain sexual pleasure.
- Share thoughts and feelings with partner/SO regarding their body image, sex role, desirability, and ideas of sexual expression as a sexual partner.

Interventions/Take Action

Nursing Priority No. 1.
To assess causative/contributing factors:

- Perform a complete history and physical, including a sexual history, which would include usual pattern of functioning, level of desire, and problems, such as rape or abuse. **Establishes a database from which an individualized plan of care can be formulated. Note: Obtaining a sexual history from a client may be challenging for the client with a history of sexual abuse/trauma.**
- Allow client adequate time to share their experiences and observe vocabulary and style of communication used by the individual/SO. **Sexual practices are considered personal and private, and clients may feel hesitant or embarrassed to discuss with others. Be aware of incongruences, shame, or guilt. Male/female expressions or thoughts of sexual behaviors are viewed differently, requiring an appreciation of both styles of communication.**
- Have client describe problem in own words. **Sexual dysfunction is divided into four categories—sexual desire (decreased libido), arousal (ED or aversion or avoidance of sex), orgasm (delay, absence), and sexual pain disorders (dyspareunia, vaginismus). Client's perception of the problem may differ from the SO's, and plan of care needs to be based on client's perceptions for maximum effectiveness. Note: Family members may object to elder client's lawful sexual behavior,**

Information that appears in brackets has been added by the authors to clarify and enhance the use of nursing diagnoses.

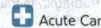 Acute Care 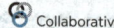 Collaborative 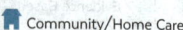 Community/Home Care Cultural

indicating need for family to express concerns and obtain information regarding client's rights.
- Determine importance of sex to individual/partner and client's motivation for change. **Both individuals may have differing levels of desire and expectations that may create conflict in relationship.**
- Be alert to comments/innuendos of client, **as sexual concerns are often disguised as humor, sarcasm, and/or off-hand remarks. It is important for the nurse to recognize and acknowledge client's concern.**
- Assess client's/SO's knowledge regarding sexual anatomy and function and effects of current situation or condition. **Individuals may be ignorant of anatomy of sexual system and how it works, impacting client's understanding of situation and expectations.**
- Determine preexisting problems or conditions that may be factors in current situation (e.g., illness, surgery, trauma). **Physical conditions (e.g., arthritis, MS, hypertension, diabetes mellitus, fatigue, presence of a colostomy, urinary incontinence) can directly affect sexual functioning, or individual can believe that condition precludes sexual activity, such as recent myocardial infarction or heart surgery.**
- Identify current stress factors in individual situation (e.g., marital or job stress, role conflicts). **May be producing enough anxiety to cause depression or other psychological reaction(s) leading to physiological symptoms.**
- Discuss cultural values, spiritual beliefs, or conflicts present. **Client may have anxiety and guilt as a result of family beliefs about sex and genital area of the body because of how sexuality was communicated to the client as they were growing up.**
- Determine pathophysiology, surgery, or trauma involving sexual organs and impact on (perception of) individual/SO. **The client may be more concerned about these issues when the sexual parts of the body are involved (e.g., mastectomy, hysterectomy, prostatectomy).**
- Explore with client the meaning of client's sexual behavior. **Masturbation, for instance, may have many meanings or purposes, such as for relief of anxiety, sexual deprivation, pleasure, a nonverbal expression of need to talk, way of alienating. Or, client's inhibitions may be diminished by changes in cognition increasing risk of inappropriate behavior.** (*Note:* Nurse needs to be aware of and be

---

Information that appears in brackets has been added by the authors to clarify and enhance the use of nursing diagnoses.

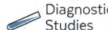 Diagnostic Studies 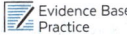 Evidence Based Practice 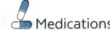 Medications 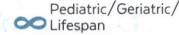 Pediatric/Geriatric/Lifespan

in control of own feelings and response to client expressions or self-revelation.)
- Avoid making value judgments, **as they do not promote client health or assist the client to cope with the situation. Client needs to be free to express concerns in whatever way is comfortable to individual. All clients, even those with limited cognition, have a right to engage in intimate behaviors.**
- Review medication regimen and drug use (prescriptions, over the counter, illegal, alcohol) and cigarette use. **Antihypertensives may cause ED; monoamine oxidase inhibitors and tricyclics can cause erection or ejaculation problems and anorgasmia in women; selective serotonin reuptake inhibitor antidepressants can cause decreased libido or orgasm disorders; antihistamines may cause temporary vaginal dryness (dyspareunia); narcotics and alcohol can produce impotence and inhibit orgasm; smoking creates vasoconstriction and may be a factor in ED. Evaluation of drug and individual response is important to determine accurate intervention.**
- Observe behavior and stage of grieving when related to body changes or loss of a body part (e.g., pregnancy, obesity, amputation, mastectomy). **A change in body image can affect how individual views body in many aspects, but particularly in the sensitive area of sexual functioning, and indicates need for information and additional support.**
- Discuss client's view of body, if indicated (e.g., concern about penis size, failure with performance; loss of desirability).
- Review laboratory results (e.g., hormone levels, serum glucose, red blood cell count, drug levels). **Testing may reveal undiagnosed conditions, such as diabetes resulting in ED in men or anemia affecting arousal. Inappropriate drug levels or hormone deficiencies—decreased estrogen in women and decreased testosterone in men and women—may result in decreased libido; and hypothyroidism may impair sexual arousal.**
- Assist with diagnostic studies to determine cause of ED. **More than half of the cases have a physical cause such as diabetes, vascular problems, etc.** Monitor penile tumescence during rapid eye movement sleep **to determine physical ability. Men are embarrassed to bring up the subject with their healthcare provider even when they are seeing**

Information that appears in brackets has been added by the authors to clarify and enhance the use of nursing diagnoses.

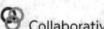 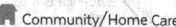 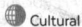

provider for other conditions; unless the provider specifically asks, the subject is not addressed.
- Assist with or review diagnostic studies for female sexual disorders (e.g., vaginal photoplethysmography **to assess vaginal blood flow and engorgement,** vaginal pH **to identify infection or diminished secretions,** and biothesiometer **to test sensitivity of clitoris and labia**).

Nursing Priority No. 2.
To assist client/SO to deal with individual situation:

- Establish therapeutic nurse-client relationship **to promote treatment and facilitate sharing of sensitive information and feelings.**
- Assist with treatment of underlying medical conditions, including changes in medication regimen, weight management, and cessation of smoking. **Successful treatment/management of many conditions (e.g., cardiovascular, diabetes, arthritis) can improve sexual functioning. However, some treatments and medications also have deleterious affects on sexual abilities/desire.**
- Collaborate with physical therapist/other specialist to identify mechanical aides that may be useful for clients with physical conditions/disabilities. **New or different approaches may be needed to promote or enhance sexual satisfaction.**
- Provide factual information about individual condition involved (e.g., premature ejaculation, female problems of dyspareunia; low sexual desire). **Accurate information promotes informed decision making.**
- Determine what client wants to know **to tailor information to client needs.** *Note:* **Information affecting client safety or consequences of actions may need to be reviewed and reinforced.**
- Encourage and accept expressions of concern, anger, grief, fear. **Client needs to feel free to talk about these feelings to begin resolution.**
- Assist client to be aware of and deal with stages of grieving for loss or change. **Sexual dysfunction is often a result of losses such as breast cancer treatment or prostate surgery and need to be addressed in the context of the whole. Healthcare providers need to be willing to help client understand grieving issues.**
- Encourage client to share thoughts and concerns with partner and to clarify values and impact of condition on relationship.

Information that appears in brackets has been added by the authors to clarify and enhance the use of nursing diagnoses.

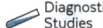 Diagnostic Studies
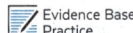 Evidence Based Practice
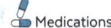 Medications
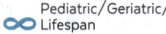 Pediatric/Geriatric/Lifespan

- Provide for or identify ways to obtain privacy **to allow for sexual expression for individual and/or between partners without embarrassment and/or objections of others, especially in communal living situations.**
- Discuss client's rights regarding intimacy in residential or extended care settings with SO/family. Review appropriateness of home visits or provision for privacy for intimate contact. **Family members may not realize that the need for sexual expression is not limited by advancing age, declining cognition, or marital status, and they may be unaware that client has a right to engage in appropriate intimate behaviors.**
- Assist client/SO to problem-solve alternative ways of sexual expression. **When client is unable to perform in usual manner, there are many ways the couple can learn to satisfy sexual needs.**
- Provide information about availability of corrective measures such as medication (e.g., papaverine or sildenafil [Viagra] for ED), lubricating gels, hormone creams, or possibly hormonal replacement therapy for vaginal dryness and dyspareunia, as appropriate, or reconstructive surgery (e.g., penile/breast implants), Eros Therapy (handheld device used to improve blood flow to clitoris and external labia to increase sensitivity of tissues), or behavioral therapies (e.g., self-stimulation, sensate focus exercises, Masters & Johnson treatment strategies), when indicated.
- Refer to appropriate resources, as needed (e.g., healthcare coworker with greater comfort level and/or knowledgeable clinical nurse specialist or professional sex therapist, family counseling). **Not all professionals are knowledgeable about or comfortable dealing with sexual issues, and referrals to more appropriate resources can provide client/couple with accurate assistance.**

Nursing Priority No. 3.

To promote sustained sexual satisfaction (Teaching/Discharge Considerations) and enhance well-being (long-term goals):

- Review sex education, explanation of normal sexual functioning when necessary. **Reinforcing accurate information can help assuage anxiety about unknowns, such as normal changes of aging, or provide an accurate basis for understanding problems being experienced.**
- Provide written material appropriate to individual needs (include bibliotherapy and reliable internet resources related

---

Information that appears in brackets has been added by the authors to clarify and enhance the use of nursing diagnoses.

to client's concerns) **for reinforcement at client's leisure and readiness to deal with sensitive materials.**
- Encourage ongoing dialogue and take advantage of teachable moments. **Within a therapeutic relationship, comfort is achieved and individual is encouraged to ask questions and be receptive to continuing conversation about sexual issues.**
- Demonstrate and assist client to learn relaxation and/or visualization techniques. **Stress is often a component of sexual dysfunction, and using these skills can help with resolution of problems.**
- Emphasize importance of engaging in regular self-examination, as indicated (e.g., breast/testicular examinations). **Encourages client to participate in own health prevention activities, become more aware of potential problems, and become more comfortable with sexual self.**
- Identify community resources for further assistance (e.g., Reach for Recovery, CanSurmount, Ostomy Association, family or sex therapist).
- Refer for further professional assistance concerning relationship difficulties, low sexual desire, and other sexual concerns (e.g., premature ejaculation, vaginismus, painful intercourse). Note: Referral to counselor expert in trauma may be preferred to assist sexual abuse survivors to overcome sexual difficulties.
- Identify resources for assistive devices or sexual aids.

Documentation Focus

Assessment/Reassessment
- Individual findings including nature of dysfunction, predisposing factors, perceived effect on sexuality and relationships
- Cultural or spiritual factors, conflicts
- Response of SO
- Motivation for change

Planning
- Plan of care and who is involved in planning
- Teaching plan

Implementation/Evaluation
- Response to interventions, teaching, and actions performed
- Attainment of or progress toward desired outcome(s)
- Modifications to plan of care

Information that appears in brackets has been added by the authors to clarify and enhance the use of nursing diagnoses.

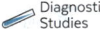 Diagnostic Studies
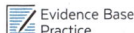 Evidence Based Practice
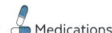 Medications
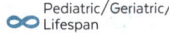 Pediatric/Geriatric/Lifespan

Discharge Planning
- Long-term needs, referrals made, and who is responsible for actions to be taken
- Community resources, specific referrals made

Sample Nursing Outcomes & Interventions Classifications NOC/NIC

NOC—Sexual Functioning
NIC—Sexual Counseling

---

risk for SHOCK · NANDA-I

[Diagnostic Division: Circulation]

Definition: Susceptible to a condition manifested by failure to perfuse or oxygenate vital organs.

Recognizing Cues

Risk Factors
Excessive bleeding; nonhemorrhagic fluid losses; inadequate fluid volume; unstable blood pressure
Hyperthermia, hypothermia; hypoxemia; hypoxia
Inadequate knowledge of bleeding, or infection management strategies; or of modifiable factors
Ineffective medication self-management
Factors identified by standardized, validated screening tool

Clinical Connections
Gastrointestinal (GI) bleed, multiple trauma, burns, disseminated intravascular coagulation; myocardial infarction, cardiomyopathy, malignant hypertension; pulmonary embolus, pneumothorax; spinal cord injury (SCI), anaphylaxis, sepsis

Generate Solutions

Plan Desired Outcomes

Client Will (Include Specific Time Frame)
- Display hemodynamic stability as evidenced by vital signs within normal range for client; prompt capillary refill; adequate urinary output with normal specific gravity; usual level of mentation.

Information that appears in brackets has been added by the authors to clarify and enhance the use of nursing diagnoses.

 Acute Care 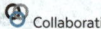 Collaborative 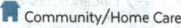 Community/Home Care 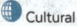 Cultural

- Be afebrile and free of other signs of infection, achieve timely wound healing.
- Verbalize understanding of disease process, risk factors, and treatment plan.

Interventions/Take Action

Nursing Priority No. 1.
To assess causative/contributing factors:

- Note possible medical diagnoses or disease processes that can result in one or more types of shock, such as major trauma with heavy internal or external bleeding; heart failure; head injury or SCI; allergic reactions; pregnancy-related complications; intra-abdominal infections, open wounds, or other conditions associated with sepsis.
- Assess for history or presence of conditions leading to **hypovolemic shock,** such as trauma, surgery, inadequate clotting function, anticoagulant therapy; GI or other organ hemorrhage; prolonged vomiting and diarrhea; diabetes insipidus; misuse of diuretics. **These conditions deplete the body's circulating blood volume and ability to maintain organ perfusion and function.**
- Assess for conditions associated with **cardiogenic shock,** including myocardial infarction, cardiac arrest, lethal ventricular dysrhythmias, severe valvular dysfunction, cardiomyopathies, malignant hypertension. **These conditions directly impair the heart muscle and ability to pump.**
- Assess for conditions associated with **obstructive shock,** including pulmonary embolus, aortic stenosis, cardiac tamponade, tension pneumothorax. **In these conditions, the heart itself may be healthy but cannot pump because of conditions outside the heart that prevent normal filling or adequate outflow.**
- Assess for conditions associated with **distributive shock— neural induced,** including pain, anesthesia, SCI or head injury; or **chemical induced,** including peritonitis, sepsis, burns, anaphylaxis, hyperglycemia. **These situations result in loss of sympathetic tone, blood vessel dilation, pooling of venous blood, and increased capillary permeability with shifting of fluids.**
- Monitor for persistent or heavy fluid loss, including wounds, drains, vomiting, GI tube, chest tube. Check all secretions and excretions for occult blood. Refer to NDs risk for excessive Bleeding; inadequate Fluid Volume, risk for imbalanced Fluid Volume Balance, for additional interventions.

Information that appears in brackets has been added by the authors to clarify and enhance the use of nursing diagnoses.

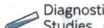 Diagnostic Studies 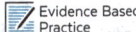 Evidence Based Practice 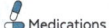 Medications 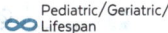 Pediatric/Geriatric/Lifespan

- Inspect skin, noting presence of traumatic or surgical wounds, erythema, edema, tenderness, petechiae; rashes or hives **for evidence of hemorrhage, localized infections, or hypersensitivity reaction.**
- Investigate reports of increased or sudden pain in wounds or body parts, **which could indicate ischemia or infection.**
- Be aware of invasive devices, such as urinary and intravascular catheters, endotracheal tube, implanted prosthetic devices **that potentiate risk for localized and systemic infections.**
- Assess vital signs and tissue and organ perfusion **for changes associated with shock states:**

Heart rate and rhythm—noting progressive changes in heart rate **(reflecting an attempt to increase cardiac output)** and development of dysrhythmias, **suggesting electrolyte imbalances, hypoxia.**

Respirations—noting rapid, shallow breathing, use of accessory muscles **(in an attempt to increase vital capacity and compensate for metabolic acidosis associated with poor tissue perfusion and anaerobic metabolism),** which can progress to respiratory failure.

Blood pressure—noting hypotension, postural hypotension, and narrowed pulse pressure. **May indicate hypovolemia and/or failure of cardiac pumping or compensatory mechanisms.**

Pulses and neck veins—noting rapid, weak, thready peripheral pulses; congested or flat neck veins. **Signs associated with changes in circulating volume, cardiac ouput, and progressive changes in vascular tone and/or capillary permeability.**

Temperature—higher than 100.4°F (38°C) or lower than 96.8°F (36°C) may indicate infectious process. **Temperature changes in presence of elevated heart and respiratory rate, along with mildly elevated white blood cell (WBC) count in absence of documented infection, are suggestive of systemic inflammatory response.**

State of consciousness and mentation—noting anxiety, restlessness, confusion, lethargy, or unresponsiveness. **Can occur because of changes in oxygenation, acid-base imbalances, and toxins associated with hypoperfusion.**

Skin color and moisture—noting overall flushing or pallor; bluish lips and fingernails, slow capillary refill; or cool, clammy skin.

Information that appears in brackets has been added by the authors to clarify and enhance the use of nursing diagnoses.

 Acute Care  Collaborative 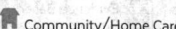 Community/Home Care 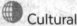 Cultural

Urine output—noting substantially decreased ouput. **One of the most sensitive indicators of change in circulating volume or poor perfusion.**

Urine characteristics—noting color and odor **suggestive of infection source.**

Bowel sounds—noting diminished or absent bowel sounds; other changes in GI function such as vomiting; or change in color, amount, or frequency of stools, **reflecting hypoperfusion of GI tract.**

- Measure invasive hemodynamic parameters when available—central venous pressure, mean arterial pressure, cardiac output—**to determine if intravascular fluid deficit or cardiac dysfunction exists.**
- Obtain specimens of wounds, drains, central lines, blood for culture and sensitivity.
- Review laboratory data such as complete blood count with WBCs and differential; platelet numbers and function; other coagulation factors; tests for cardiac, renal, and hepatic function; pulse oximetry/arterial blood gas; serum lactate, blood urine cultures **to identify potential sources of shock and degree of organ involvement.**
- Review diagnostic studies such as x-rays, electrocardiogram, echocardiogram, angiography with ejection fraction, computed tomography scans or MRI, ultrasound **to determine presence of injuries or disorders that could cause or lead to shock conditions.**
- Refer to NDs ineffective peripheral Tissue Perfusion, risk for impaired Cardiovascular Function, risk for ineffective cerebral Tissue Perfusion as indicated.

Nursing Priority No. 2.
To prevent/correct potential causes of shock:

- Collaborate in prompt treatment of underlying conditions such as trauma, heart failure, infections, and prepare for/assist with medical and surgical interventions **to maximize systemic circulation and tissue and organ perfusion.**
- Administer oxygen by appropriate route (e.g., nasal prongs, mask, ventilator) **to maximize oxygenation of tissues.**
- Administer fluids, electrolytes, colloids, blood or blood products, as indicated, **to rapidly restore or sustain circulating volume, electrolyte balance, and prevent shock state.**
- Administer medications as indicated (e.g., vasoactive drugs, cardiac glycosides, thrombolytics, anticoagulants, antimicrobials, analgesics).

Information that appears in brackets has been added by the authors to clarify and enhance the use of nursing diagnoses.

 Diagnostic Studies 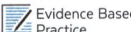 Evidence Based Practice 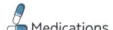 Medications ∞ Pediatric/Geriatric/Lifespan

- Provide client care with infection prevention interventions, such as diligent attention to hand hygiene, aseptic wound care or dressing changes, isolation precautions, early intervention in potential infectious condition **to reduce incidence or progression of infection.**
- Provide nutrition by best means—oral, enteral, or parenteral feeding. Refer to nutritionist or dietitian **to provide foods rich in nutrients, vitamins, and minerals needed to promote healing and support immune system health.**
- Refer to NDs ineffective peripheral Tissue Perfusion; risk for impaired Cardiovascular Function; risk for ineffective cerebral Tissue Perfusion, for additional interventions and rationales.

Nursing Priority No. 3.

Promote cellular perfusion and oxygenation (Teaching/Discharge Considerations) and enhance well-being (long-term goals):

- Instruct client/significant other in ways to prevent and/or manage underlying conditions that cause shock, including heart disease, injuries, dehydration, infection.
- Identify reportable signs and symptoms, including unrelieved pain, unresolved bleeding, excessive fluid loss, persistent fever and chills, change in skin color accompanied by chest pain **for timely evaluation and intervention.**
- Emphasize need for recognition of substances that cause hypersensitivity or allergic reactions (e.g., insects, medicines, foods, latex) **to reduce risk of anaphylactic shock state.**
- Teach client purpose, dosage, schedule, precautions, and potential side effects of medications given to treat underlying conditions. **Enhances compliance with drug regimen, reducing individual risk.**
- Instruct in wound and skin care as indicated **to prevent infection and promote healing.**
- Teach client/caregivers importance of good hand hygiene, clean environment, and avoiding crowds when ill, especially if client is immunocompromised.
- Reinforce importance of immunization against infections such as influenza and pneumonia, especially in client with chronic conditions.
- Encourage consumption of healthy diet, participation in regular exercise, and adequate rest **for healing and immune system support.**

Information that appears in brackets has been added by the authors to clarify and enhance the use of nursing diagnoses.

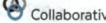 Acute Care 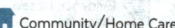 Collaborative  Community/Home Care Cultural

• Recommend that client at risk for hypersensitivity reactions wear medical alert bracelet, maintain readily accessible emergency medication (e.g., Benadryl and/or EpiPen).

Documentation Focus

Assessment/Reassessment
- Individual risk factors such as blood loss, presence of infection
- Assessment findings, including respiratory rate, character of breath sounds; heart rate and rhythm; temperature; frequency, amount, and appearance of secretions; presence of cyanosis; and mentation level
- Results of laboratory tests and diagnostic studies

Planning
- Plan of care, specific interventions, and who is involved in the planning
- Teaching plan

Implementation/Evaluation
- Client's responses to treatment, teaching, and actions performed
- Attainment of or progress toward desired outcome(s)
- Modifications to plan of care

Discharge Planning
- Long-term needs, identifying who is responsible for actions to be taken
- Community resources for equipment and supplies postdischarge
- Specific referrals made

Sample Nursing Outcomes & Interventions Classifications NOC/NIC

NOC—Circulation Status
NIC—Shock Prevention

---

impaired SITTING ABILITY NANDA-I

[Diagnostic Division: Safety]

Definition: Limitation of independent and purposeful attainment and/or maintenance of a rest position that is supported by the buttocks and thighs, in which the torso is upright.

Information that appears in brackets has been added by the authors to clarify and enhance the use of nursing diagnoses.

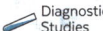 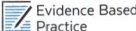 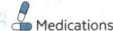 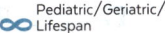

Recognizing Cues

Related/Risk Factors
Inadequate physical endurance; inadequate muscle strength
Inappropriate relief posture
Malnutrition
Pain

Defining Characteristics

Objective
Difficulty:
  Adjusting position of one or both lower limbs on uneven surface
  Attaining, or maintaining postural balance
  Flexing or moving both hips, or both knees
  Difficulty performing bodyweight exercises

Clinical Connections
Neuromuscular disorders (e.g., multiple sclerosis [MS], amyotrophic lateral sclerosis, Parkinson disease), traumatic injuries (e.g., fractures, spinal cord or brain injuries), rheumatoid arthritis, severe depression, dementia

Generate Solutions

Plan Desired Outcomes

Client Will (Include Specific Time Frame)
- Verbalize understanding of individual treatment regimen and safety measures.
- Attain and maintain sitting position that enables activities.
- Participate in activities of daily living (ADLs) and desired activities and prevent complications.

Interventions/Take Action

Nursing Priority No. 1.
To identify causative/contributing factors:
- Determine diagnosis that contributes to sitting balance problems (e.g., MS, arthritis, Parkinson disease, cardiopulmonary disorders, back pain conditions with client use of compensatory positions to reduce pain; traumatic brain injury, spinal cord injury with hemi-/paraplegia; lower-limb injuries or amputations; psychiatric conditions including severe depression, dementias). **These conditions can cause postural and balance impairments, muscular weakness, and inadequate range of motion. Sensory deficits may**

Information that appears in brackets has been added by the authors to clarify and enhance the use of nursing diagnoses.

 Acute Care 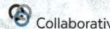 Collaborative 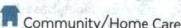 Community/Home Care Cultural

also be involved (e.g., impaired proprioception and/or visual processing, cognitive impairments).
- Note factors affecting current situation (e.g., surgery, fractures, amputation, tubings [chest tube, indwelling catheter, IVs, pumps] and potential time involved [e.g., few hours in bed after surgery versus serious trauma requiring long-term bedrest or debilitating disease or pain limiting movement]). **Identifies potential impairments and determines type of interventions needed to provide for client's safety. Note: Sitting and standing balance are of major concern when assessing amputee's ability to maintain the center of gravity over the base of support. Both balance and coordination are required for weight shifting from one limb to another, thus improving the potential for an optimal gait.**
- Note older client's general health status. **Several aging-related changes can impact sitting ability (e.g., sarcopenia with diminished endurance and core strength, impaired vision, loss of balance, reduced ability to quickly and adequately correct movements affecting center of gravity).**
- Assess nutritional and hydration status and client's report of energy level. **Deficiencies in nutrients and water, electrolytes, and minerals can negatively affect energy and activity tolerance. Note: Research supports that obese individuals show reduced seated functional reach abilities when compared to normal and overweight subjects.**

Nursing Priority No. 2.
To assess functional ability:
- Determine functional status using a 0 to 4 (or other validated) scale, noting muscle strength and tone, joint mobility, cardiovascular status, balance, and endurance. **Identifies strengths and deficits (e.g., inability to sit upright, reach forward, or transfer safely from bed to wheelchair) and may provide information regarding potential for recovery.**
- Determine degree of perceptual or cognitive impairment and ability to follow directions. **Impairments related to age, chronic or acute disease condition, trauma, surgery, or medications require alternative interventions or changes in plan of care.**
- Refer to physician, physical therapy specialists, for special testing, as indicated. **May include many different functional tests to determine potential for improvement and direction for therapies.**

Information that appears in brackets has been added by the authors to clarify and enhance the use of nursing diagnoses.

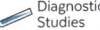 Diagnostic Studies 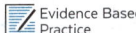 Evidence Based Practice 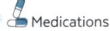 Medications 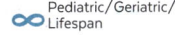 Pediatric/Geriatric/Lifespan

Nursing Priority No. 3.

To promote optimal level of function and prevent complications:

- Assist with treatment of underlying condition(s) **to maximize potential for optimal function.**
- Encourage client's participation in self-care activities and in physical or occupational therapies. **Improves body strength and function; enhances self-concept and sense of independence. Note: Sitting balance affects ADLs, including feeding, dressing, bathing, transfers, and mobility.** Refer to ND Self-Care Deficit, [specify].
- Note changes in client's abilities to perform self-care and participate in therapies **to promote psychological and physical benefits of self-care and to adjust level of assistance as indicated.**
- Support trunk and extremities when in seated position, using pillows or rolls, braces, shoes, gel pads, and so forth, **to maintain upright position and optimal internal organ function and to reduce risk of pressure injury.**
- Demonstrate and assist with use of assistive devices (e.g., siderails, overhead trapeze, roller pads, safety belt, hydraulic lifts, chairs) **for position changes and safe transfers.**
- Avoid routinely doing for client those activities that client can do for self. **Caregivers can contribute to deficits by being overprotective or helping too much.**
- Provide for safety measures as indicated by individual situation, including environmental management and fall prevention. (Refer to NDs risk for [adult or child] Falls.)
- Collaborate with physical medicine specialist and occupational or physical therapists in providing range-of-motion exercise (active or passive), isotonic muscle contractions (e.g., sitting reach, push, and pull exercises), assistive devices, and activities.
- Administer pain medications before activity as needed **to promote maximal effort and involvement in activity.**
- Collaborate with nutritionist in providing nutritious foods and needed feeding assistance, **to optimize available energy for activities.**
- Refer to NDs Activity Intolerance; impaired bed Mobility; impaired physical Mobility; impaired Transferring Ability; impaired Standing Ability; impaired wheelchair Mobility; and impaired Walking Ability for related interventions.

Information that appears in brackets has been added by the authors to clarify and enhance the use of nursing diagnoses.

Nursing Priority No. 4.

To maintain function (Teaching/Discharge Considerations) and enhance well-being (long-term goals):

- Encourage client's/significant other's (SO's) involvement in decision making as much as possible. **Enhances commitment to plan, optimizing outcomes.**
- Demonstrate use of mobility devices (e.g., walkers, strollers, scooters, braces, prosthetics) and have client/care provider demonstrate knowledge about and safe use of device. Identify appropriate resources for obtaining and maintaining appliances or equipment. **Safe use of mobility aids promotes client's independence and enhances quality of life and safety for client and caregiver.**
- Discuss ways that client can exercise safely. **Options may be limited, but attending regular rehabilitation sessions may provide best opportunity for improvement in function, including self-care, social independence, and recreation.**
- Involve client and SO(s) in care, assisting them to learn ways of managing problems of immobility and imbalanced sitting, especially when impairment is expected to be long term. Refer to support and community services as indicated **to provide care, supervision, companionship, respite services, nutritional and ADL assistance, adaptive devices or changes to living environment, financial assistance, and so forth.**

Documentation Focus

Assessment/Reassessment
- Individual findings, including level of function and ability to participate in specific or desired activities

Planning
- Plan of care and who is involved in the planning
- Teaching plan

Implementation/Evaluation
- Responses to interventions, teaching, and actions performed
- Attainment of or progress toward desired outcome(s)
- Modifications to plan of care

Discharge Planning
- Discharge and long-term needs, noting who is responsible for actions to be taken
- Specific referrals made
- Sources of and maintenance for assistive devices

Information that appears in brackets has been added by the authors to clarify and enhance the use of nursing diagnoses.

Sample Nursing Outcomes & Interventions Classifications NOC/NIC

NOC—Body Mechanics Performance
NIC—Body Mechanics Promotion

---

impaired SKIN INTEGRITY NANDA-I

[Diagnostic Division: Safety]

Definition: Damage to epidermis and/or dermis.

Recognizing Cues

Related/Risk Factors

External factors

Inappropriate skin moisture level; excretions; secretions; use of linen with inadequate moisture wicking property

Exposure to environmental temperature extremes

Inadequate caregiver knowledge about maintaining, or protecting tissue integrity

Inadequate caregiver knowledge of appropriate use of adhesive materials

Inappropriate use of chemical agent

Pressure over bony prominences; shearing forces; surface friction

Internal factors

Underweight for age and gender; ineffective overweight self-management

Decreased physical activity; impaired physical mobility

Edema; water-electrolyte imbalance

Inadequate adherence to incontinence treatment program

Inadequate knowledge about maintaining, or protecting tissue integrity

Inadequate knowledge of appropriate use of adhesive materials; unaddressed adhesive allergy

Malnutrition

Psychogenic factor (e.g., obsessive-compulsive disorder); self-directed violence; tobacco use; substance misuse

Defining Characteristics

Subjective

Acute [discomfort]/pain; pruritus

Information that appears in brackets has been added by the authors to clarify and enhance the use of nursing diagnoses.

 Acute Care 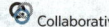 Collaborative 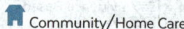 Community/Home Care   Cultural

Objective
Abscess; blister; desquamation; disrupted skin surface; abraded skin; macerated skin; excoriation
Altered skin color, or turgor; dry skin; localized area hot to touch
Hyperkeratosis
Bleeding; hematoma
Foreign matter piercing skin

Clinical Connections
Anemias; arthritis; end-of-life conditions; long-term care residents, contagious diseases, coronary artery disease; dementias; burns; cancer, diabetes mellitus, obesity; peripheral vascular disease

Generate Solutions

Plan Desired Outcomes

Client Will (Include Specific Time Frame)
- Identify individual risk factors.
- Display timely healing of skin lesions or wounds without complication.
- Participate in prevention measures and treatment program.

Interventions/Take Action

Nursing Priority No. 1.
To assess causative/contributing factors:
- Identify/investigate underlying conditions or pathology involved. **The etiology of skin breakdown is multifactorial. Often the combination of environment and client condition(s) results in compromised skin integrity. Only recognition of the appropriate etiology and selection of a relevant treatment plan will produce good client outcomes. Skin integrity problems can be the result of**
  (1) Disease processes that affect circulation and perfusion of tissues (e.g., arteriosclerosis, venous insufficiency, hypertension, obesity, diabetes, malignant neoplasms)
  (2) Conditions that can be associated with skin irritation/rashes (e.g., measles, chickenpox, fungal infection, incontinence)
  (3) Skin disorders such as eczema; contact dermatitis (e.g., latex, poison ivy)
  (4) Disorders caused by parasites/insects (e.g., Lyme disease, lice, bedbugs)
  (5) Autoimmune disorders (e.g., lupus)

Information that appears in brackets has been added by the authors to clarify and enhance the use of nursing diagnoses.

 Diagnostic Studies 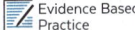 Evidence Based Practice 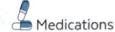 Medications 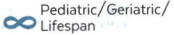 Pediatric/Geriatric/Lifespan

- *(6) Organ dysfunction/metabolic dyscrasia* (e.g., liver disease, celiac disease, kidney failure, iron deficiency anemia, thyroid problems, and cancers [e.g., leukemia and lymphoma])
- *(7) Medications that adversely affect skin or impair healing* (e.g., anticoagulants, antibiotics, corticosteroids, immunosuppressives, antineoplastics)
- *(8) Burns or radiation*
- *(9) Nutrition and hydration* (e.g., malnutrition deprives the body of protein and calories required for cell growth and repair; dehydration impairs transport of oxygen and nutrients)

- Consider client's age, developmental factors, and ability to care for self. **Impacts the client's ability to assess for a problem as well as the ability to prevent harm. Infants and children are prone to skin rashes associated with incontinence; viral, bacterial, fungal infections; and allergic reactions. Infant skin has a higher rate of absorption (i.e., relevant for weight to body surface area and topical medications) and an increased rate of fluid loss as compared to an adult's skin (i.e., increased insensible losses and dry, flaky, impaired skin). Additionally, pediatric clients have a reduced ability to thermoregulate and less mature immune responses than adolescents and adults. In older adults, there is decreased epidermal regeneration, fewer sweat glands, less subcutaneous fat, elastin, and collagen, causing skin to become thinner, drier, and less responsive to pain sensations. In general, the skin of older adults has less tensile strength.** Refer to NDs risk for impaired Fluid Volume Balance, and risk for adult, child, or neonatal Pressure Injury for related assessments and interventions.

- Evaluate client's health status in general terms. **Many factors (e.g., debilitation, immobility, extremes of age, mental status, dehydration or malnutrition, presence of seasonal or substance allergies, chronic disease, occupational, treatment, and environmental hazards) can affect the ability of the skin to perform its functions (e.g., protection, sensation, movement and growth, chemical synthesis, immunity, thermoregulation, and excretion).**

- Perform complete body skin assessment **paying attention to *vulnerable areas* (e.g., skin beneath and around devices, dressings/adhesive, compression hose, splints, or casts); *bony prominences* (e.g., heels, sacrum, occiput); *skin-to-skin areas* (e.g., under breast tissue, inner thighs,**

Information that appears in brackets has been added by the authors to clarify and enhance the use of nursing diagnoses.

neck folds, buttocks); *areas where client lacks sensation* (affects ability to feel discomfort); *area(s) of previous skin breakdown* or prone to breakdown. (Note: In pediatric patients, the most common sites are ears, occiput, and heels).

- Determine the type of skin disruption, as indicated. **Disruption in skin integrity can be** *intentional* (e.g., surgical incision) or *unintentional* (e.g., accidental trauma, drug effect, allergic reaction, rashes); and *open* (e.g., laceration, skin tears, penetrating wound, ulcerations) or *closed* (e.g., contusion, abrasion, rash). Additionally, compromised skin integrity can be further categorized by etiology, such as pressure injury (i.e., injury seen over bony prominences), skin failure (i.e., skin loss associated with a variety of etiologic agents, including mechanical injury), acute skin failure (i.e., disruption in skin integrity related to hemodynamic instability), and end-of-life integument failure (i.e., loss of skin integrity not associated with other injurious factors occurring 1 day to 6 wk prior to death).
- Evaluate hydration status; note presence and degree of edema (1+ to 4+), urine characteristics, and output. **May reveal the presence of circulatory or metabolic imbalances resulting in fluid deficit or overload that can adversely affect skin and tissue health and organ function. Note: Edematous tissues are prone to breakdown.**
- Determine nutritional status and impact of malnutrition on client (e.g., pressure points on emaciated or elderly client, obesity, lack of activity, slow healing or failure to heal). **Clients who are malnourished (i.e., BMI less than 19, or greater than/equal to 40) have an increased risk for skin injury and reduced healing ability. Inadequate intake of dietary protein, vitamin C, and zinc may delay and impair wound healing.**
- Evaluate client's skin care practices noting cultural preferences. **The client's skin may be oily, dry, scaly, or sensitive and affected by bathing frequency (or lack of bathing), temperature of water, types of soap, and other cleansing agents. Note presence/type of body piercing/ punctures, other skin adornments. Ineffective hygiene can result in skin impairment and discomfort.**
- Evaluate for incontinence (urinary or bowel) or consistent skin exposure to urine or fecal material. Evaluate the proximity of dressings to an ostomy/fistula opening. **Moisture-associated skin damage is inflammation and subsequent**

Information that appears in brackets has been added by the authors to clarify and enhance the use of nursing diagnoses.

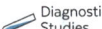 Diagnostic Studies   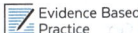 Evidence Based Practice   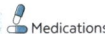 Medications   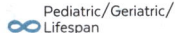 Pediatric/Geriatric/Lifespan

erosion of the skin after prolonged exposure to moisture (e.g., **body fluids like feces, urine, sweat, saliva, wound exudate, mucus, perspiration, digestive secretions).**

- Note presence of compromised mental health, or mobility, sensation, vision, hearing, or speech **that may impact the client's self-care as it relates to skin care. Clients with anxiety or psychiatric disorders may inadvertently pick/scratch at the skin creating injury and irritation. Psychological stress may increase endogenous glucocorticoid production and promote an environment that destabilizes skin barriers. The client with dementia or depression may not have interest in self-care.**

- Ascertain allergy history. **Individuals may be sensitive or allergic to substances (e.g., insects, grasses, medications, adhesives, lotions, soaps, foods) that can adversely affect the skin.**

- Assess blood supply (e.g., capillary refill time, color, and warmth, pulses), skin sensation, pressure points, and broken or abraded skin regularly **to provide a comparative baseline and opportunity for timely intervention when problems are noted. Blood supply to the skin may be compromised by application of a device (i.e., tight splint, cast, or dressing) or by physiological changes caused by chronic disease (e.g., diabetes, hypertension).**

- Determine treatment-related skin or tissue conditions (e.g., surgical incision, IV/invasive line insertion site, presence of casts/braces, use of restraints). Assess surgical sites **for signs of infection (e.g., swelling, redness, pain),** assess IV site **for infiltration (e.g., swelling, erythema, coolness, pain, or failure of infusion), or evidence of extravasation (e.g., blistering, blanching, skin sloughing).** Evaluate skin surrounding casts/braces, and restraints if used, noting abrasions, contusions, skin breaks, or skin color and temperature changes, **suggesting impaired circulation.**

- Review laboratory results (e.g., hemoglobin/hematocrit, white blood cell count with differential, blood glucose, blood and/or wound culture, infectious agents [viral, bacterial, fungal], albumin, hemoglobin A_{1C}, and lipid studies [as needed]) **to evaluate causative factors or ability to heal. Note: Evidence suggests serum albumin less than 3.5 g/dL correlates to decreased wound healing and increased frequency of pressure injury. However, albumin levels may be impacted by inflammation and other factors dependent on the client's condition. For this reason, additional laboratory values and assessments, such**

Information that appears in brackets has been added by the authors to clarify and enhance the use of nursing diagnoses.

as serum prealbumin (i.e., less than 10 mg/dL may be associated with malnutrition) should be used to evaluate the client's nutritional status.

Nursing Priority No. 2.
To assess extent of involvement/injury:

- Obtain a complete history of current skin condition(s) (especially in children where recurrent rash or lesions are common), including age at onset, date of first episode, duration, original site, characteristics of lesions, subjective assessments (e.g., pain, itching, numbness, etc.), and any changes that have occurred. **Common skin manifestations of sensitivity or allergies are hives, eczema, and contact dermatitis. Contagious rashes include measles, rubella, roseola, chickenpox, and scarlet fever. Bacterial, viral, and fungal infections can also cause skin problems (e.g., impetigo, cellulitis, cold sores, shingles, athlete's foot, candidiasis, and diaper rashes).**
- Document and trend results of routine skin inspections, describing observed changes. Note skin color, texture, and turgor. Assess areas of least pigmentation for color changes (e.g., sclera, conjunctiva, nailbeds, buccal mucosa, tongue, palms, and soles of feet). **Systematic inspection can identify improvement or changes for timely intervention.**

General wounds/lesions
- Describe rash or lesion, noting color, and significant characteristics (e.g., flat or raised, weeping blisters, wheal, etc.) and relevant corresponding events (e.g., exposure to contagious disease, medication reaction, recent insect bite, ingrown toenail, sexually transmitted infection) **to assist in diagnosing problem and needed interventions.**
- Determine anatomical location and depth of skin or tissue injury or damage (e.g., epidermis, dermis, underlying issues) and describe (e.g., skin tear, partial or full-thickness burn, abrasion, ulceration, etc.) **to provide baseline and document changes.**
- Utilize a skin integrity assessment tool (e.g., International Skin Tear Advisory Panel [ISTAP] classification or the Payne-Martin classification system, and risk assessment tools, such as Braden, Norton, or Waterlow scales) **to classify skin tears or the risk for skin breakdown according to evidence-based practice guidelines.** Refer to NDs adult, child, or neonate Pressure Injury as indicated for appropriate interventions.

Information that appears in brackets has been added by the authors to clarify and enhance the use of nursing diagnoses.

- Photograph lesion(s) as appropriate **to document status and provide a visual baseline for future comparisons.**
- Note consistency, volume, odor, and color of drainage, when present (e.g., blood, bile, pus, stoma effluent), **which can cause or exacerbate skin irritation.**
- Determine, document, and reassess periodically (1) dimensions and depth in centimeters; (2) margins (i.e., wound edges are flush with wound base/flat, or wound walls are present/floor of wound is deeper than the edge); (3) tunneling or tracts; and (4) evidence of necrosis (e.g., color gray to black, dry, leathery) or healing (e.g., pink or red granulation tissue, moist) **to establish comparative baseline and evaluate effectiveness of interventions.** Refer to NDs adult/child/neonate Pressure Injury; for related assessments and interventions.

Nursing Priority No. 3.
To determine impact of condition:

- Determine client's level of discomfort (e.g., can vary widely from minor itching or aching, to deep pain with burns, or excoriation associated with drainage) **to clarify intervention needs and priorities.**
- Ascertain attitudes of individual/SO(s) about client's condition (e.g., cultural values, stigma). Obtain or review psychological assessment of the client's emotional status, noting the potential for social and relationship problems arising from the presence of the skin condition. **The wholeness and beauty of skin impacts the client's body image and self-esteem. Lesions or wounds that disfigure can be especially devastating.**
- Note sensory deficits of vision, hearing, or speech. **Touch is a particularly important avenue of communication for this population that may be compromised by a major skin condition.**

Nursing Priority No. 4.
To assist/promote healing:

- Practice and instruct client/caregiver(s) in scrupulous hand hygiene and clean or sterile technique **to reduce the incidence of contamination or infection.**
- Provide optimum nutrition (including adequate protein, lipids, calories, trace minerals, and multivitamins [e.g., A, C, D, E]) **to promote skin health and healing and to maintain general good health.**

Information that appears in brackets has been added by the authors to clarify and enhance the use of nursing diagnoses.

- Provide adequate hydration (e.g., oral, enteral feeding, parenteral fluid, ambient room humidity) **to reduce and replenish transepidermal water loss.**
- Manage itching conditions:
  Cover itchy area, trim nails, and wear gloves at night.
  Apply cool, wet compresses.
  Recommend a lukewarm bath with baking soda, colloidal oatmeal (e.g., Aveeno).
  Choose mild soaps without dyes or perfumes. Rinse the soap completely off the body.
  Use a mild, unscented laundry detergent when washing clothes, towels, and bedding.
  Avoid substances that irritate skin or that cause an allergic reaction (e.g., nickel, jewelry, perfume or skin products containing fragrance).
  Encourage use of stress-management techniques (e.g., biofeedback, meditation, yoga).
- Apply high-quality moisturizing cream (e.g., Eucerin) or anti-itch creams (e.g., hydrocortisone cream, menthol, camphor, calamine) or topical anesthetics (e.g., lidocaine or benzocaine), concentrating on the areas where itching is most severe.
- Encourage client to verbalize feelings and discuss how or if condition affects self-concept. (Refer to NDs disturbed Body Image and situational inadequate Self-Esteem.)
- Assist client to work through stages of grief and feelings associated with individual condition.
- Use touch, facial expressions, and tone of voice **to lend psychological support and acceptance of client.**
- Refer for counseling and/or behavior modification therapy, if indicated.
- Prevent skin impairment:
  Maintain or instruct in overall skin hygiene (e.g., shower instead of bath, wash thoroughly, pat dry, gently apply lotion or appropriate cream) **to provide barrier to infection, reduce risk of dermal trauma, and enhance comfort.**
  Cleanse skin after toileting, incontinence, or diaphoretic episodes **to restore normal skin pH and flora, and limit potential for infection.**
  Provide preventative skin care to incontinent client. Change continence pads or diapers frequently, cleanse perineal skin daily and after each incontinence episode, and apply skin protectant **to minimize contact with irritants (urine, stool, excessive moisture).**

Information that appears in brackets has been added by the authors to clarify and enhance the use of nursing diagnoses.

- Handle client gently (particularly infants, young children, elderly frail). **The epidermis of infants and very young children is thin and lacks the subcutaneous depth that will develop with age. The skin of the older client is also thin, less elastic, and prone to injury, such as bruising and skin tears.**
- Use proper turning and transfer techniques. Avoid movements **(e.g., pulling client with parallel force, dragging) that cause friction or shearing.**
- Encourage early ambulation or mobilization. **Reduces risks associated with immobility.**
- Provide safety measures during ambulation (e.g., use of properly fitting hose and footwear).
- Develop regularly timed repositioning/turn schedule for clients with mobility and sensation impairments, using a turn sheet/device as needed; encourage or assist with periodic weight shifts for the client in a chair **to reduce stress on pressure points and to promote circulation to tissues.**
- Use appropriate padding or pressure-reducing devices (e.g., heel rolls, foam boots, egg crate, gel pads) or pressure-relieving devices (e.g., air or water mattress) when indicated **to reduce pressure on sensitive areas and enhance circulation to compromised tissues.**
- Provide adequate clothing or covers **to protect from drafts and prevent vasoconstriction and reduction of circulation to the skin.**
- Avoid or limit the use of plastic material (e.g., rubber sheets, plastic-backed linen savers) and keep bedclothes dry. Remove wet, dirty, or wrinkled linens promptly. **Moisture potentiates skin breakdown and increases the risk for infection.**
- Keep surgical area clean and dry, carefully dress wounds (e.g., use of Steri-Strips, splinting when coughing), prevent infection, and stimulate circulation to surrounding areas **to assist body's natural process of repair.**
- Assist with debridement or enzymatic therapy, as indicated (e.g., burns, wounds with slough/necrotic debris), **to remove nonviable, contaminated, or infected tissue.**
- Use appropriate barrier dressings, wound coverings, drainage appliances, vacuum-assisted closure device (wound vac), and skin-protective agents for open, draining wounds and stomas **to protect the wound and/or surrounding tissues.**

Information that appears in brackets has been added by the authors to clarify and enhance the use of nursing diagnoses.

Apply appropriate dressing (e.g., adhesive or nonadhesive film, hydrofiber or gel, acrylics, hydropolymers) **for wound healing and to best meet needs of client and caregiver or care setting.**

Maintain appropriate moisture environment for client wound (e.g., expose lesion or ulcer to air and light **if excess moisture is impeding healing**, or use occlusive dressings **to maintain a moist environment for autolytic debridement of wound**), as indicated.

Remove adhesive products with care, removing on a horizontal plane while simultaneously supporting the skin. Mineral oil, Vaseline, or alcohol may be used to loosen or soften the adhesive, if needed, **to prevent abrasions or tearing of skin.**

Secure dressings with tape (e.g., elastic, paper tape, etc.) or an abdominal binder. Alternatively, nonadhesive options, such as stockinette, gauze wrap, cohesive bandage (i.e., Coban), or similar products may be used instead of tape to secure dressings and drains **to limit dermal injury.**

Apply hot and cold applications judiciously **to reduce risk of dermal injury in persons with circulatory and neurosensory impairments.**

Elevate lower extremities (as needed) when sitting **to enhance venous return and reduce edema formation.**

Avoid latex products **when client has a known or suspected sensitivity.** Refer to ND risk for Latex Allergy.

- Consult with wound or stoma specialist, as indicated, **to assist with developing plan of care for problematic or potentially serious wounds.**

Nursing Priority No. 5.

To promote healthy, intact skin (Teaching/Discharge Considerations) and enhance well-being (long-term goals):

- Discuss the importance of health, intact skin, as well as measures to maintain proper skin functioning. **The integumentary system is the largest multifunctional organ of the body and thus merits special care.**
- Counsel clients with diabetes and/or neurological impairment regarding the necessity of meticulous skin care, especially the feet and legs. **Healing of lower-extremity injuries tends to be more problematic in this population, resulting in an increased incidence of amputation.**
- Review benefits of medical regimen with the client/SO(s). **Enhances commitment to the plan, optimizing outcomes.**

Information that appears in brackets has been added by the authors to clarify and enhance the use of nursing diagnoses.

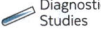 Diagnostic Studies 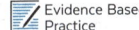 Evidence Based Practice 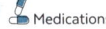 Medications 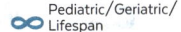 Pediatric/Geriatric/Lifespan

- Encourage regular inspection and monitoring of skin for changes or failure to heal. **Early detection and reporting to healthcare providers promotes timely evaluation and intervention.**
- Identify safety measures for clients with persistent sensation impairments. **Proper care of skin and extremities during cold or hot weather (e.g., wearing gloves; clean, dry socks; properly fitting shoes or boots; and face protection) reduces the risk of injury.**
- Encourage continued mobility, activity, and range of motion (active or assistive) **to enhance circulation and promote overall client health.**
- Discuss avoidance of products containing perfumes, dyes, preservatives (**may cause dermatitis reactions**), alcohol, povidone-iodine, and hydrogen peroxide (**may hinder wound healing**).
- Encourage restriction or abstinence from smoking/tobaccco products, **which causes vasoconstriction and impairs wound healing.**
- Review measures **to avoid infection or reinfection of communicable conditions.**
- Discuss proper and safe use of equipment or appliances (e.g., ostomy appliances, padding straps of braces, splints).
- Discuss importance of limiting lengthy or unnecessary sun exposure, using high sun protection factor (SPF) sunblock, and avoiding tanning beds.
- Assist client to learn stress reduction and alternative therapy techniques **to control feelings of helplessness and enhance coping ability.**
- Refer to dietitian or certified diabetes educator, as appropriate, **to enhance healing, reduce risk of recurrence of diabetic ulcers.**

Documentation Focus

Assessment/Reassessment
- Individual findings, including individual risk factors
- Characteristics of lesion(s) or condition
- Causative and contributing factors
- Impact of condition on personal image and lifestyle

Planning
- Plan of care and who is involved in planning
- Teaching plan

Information that appears in brackets has been added by the authors to clarify and enhance the use of nursing diagnoses.

Implementation/Evaluation
- Responses to interventions, teaching, and actions performed
- Attainment of or progress toward desired outcome(s)
- Modifications to plan of care

Discharge Planning
- Long-term needs and who is responsible for actions to be taken
- Specific referrals made

Sample Nursing Outcomes & Interventions Classifications NOC/NIC

NOC—Tissue Integrity: Skin & Mucous Membranes
NIC—Wound Care

---

ineffective SLEEP PATTERN NANDA-I

[Diagnostic Division: Activity/Rest]

Definition: Difficulty experiencing natural, periodic suspension of relative consciousness, which negatively impairs function.

Recognizing Cues

Related/Risk Factors
Excessive stress; anxiety; fear; loneliness; depressive symptoms; impaired resilience

Decreased sleep efficacy; unaddressed sleep deprivation; pain

Average daily physical activity less than recommended for age and gender; sedentary behaviors

Ineffective sleep hygiene behaviors; sustained inadequate sleep hygiene; inadequate knowledge of importance of sleep hygiene behaviors

Caffeine consumption within 6 hr of sleep; excessive processed food, or sugar intake; inadequate glycemic control

Ineffective overweight self-management

Inadequate knowledge of age-related sleep shifts; unaddressed age-related sleep stage shifts

Excessive caregiving burden; inadequate privacy

Ineffective stoma self-management

Unaddressed environmental disturbances; excessive use of interactive electronic devices

---

Information that appears in brackets has been added by the authors to clarify and enhance the use of nursing diagnoses.

Substance misuse
Sleep hygiene score outside desired range on standardized, validated instrument

Defining Characteristics

Subjective
Feels unrested; dissatisfaction with sleep
Daytime sleepiness; fatigue; decreased attention
Nonrestorative sleep-wake cycle; superficial sleep; insomnia
Difficulty initiating sleep, or maintaining sleep state; unintentional awakening

Objective
Inadequate physical endurance
Decreased functional psychomotor abilities; psychomotor agitation
Decreased efficiency of rapid eye movement (REM) sleep
Evidence of symptoms in standardized diagnostic criteria

Clinical Connections
Hospitalized individuals, long-term care residents, chronic condition of client or family member, sleep apnea, depression, bipolar disorder, schizophrenia, dementia

Generate Solutions

Plan Desired Outcomes

Client Will (Include Specific Time Frame)
- Identify individually appropriate interventions to promote sleep.
- Report improved sleep.
- Report increased sense of well-being and feeling rested.

Interventions/Take Action

Nursing Priority No. 1.
To assess causative/contributing factors:
- Identify presence of factors known to interfere with sleep, including current illness, hospitalization; new baby or sick family member in home. **Sleep problems can arise from internal and external factors and may require assessment over time to differentiate specific cause(s).**
- Ascertain presence of short-term alteration in sleep patterns, such as can occur with travel (jet lag), sharing bed with new sleep partner, fighting with family member, crisis at work, loss of job, death in family. **Helps identify circumstances**

Information that appears in brackets has been added by the authors to clarify and enhance the use of nursing diagnoses.

 Acute Care 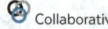 Collaborative 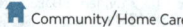 Community/Home Care Cultural

that are known to interrupt sleep acutely, but not necessarily long term.
- Note environmental factors, such as unfamiliar or uncomfortable room; excessive noise and light, uncomfortable temperature; frequent medical and monitoring interventions; and roommate actions—snoring, watching television late at night, wanting to talk. **These factors can reduce client's ability to rest and sleep at a time when more rest is needed.** *Note:* **Clients in critical care units are known to experience lack of sleep or frequent disruptions, often compounding their illness.**

Nursing Priority No. 2.
To evaluate sleep and degree of dysfunction:
- Assess client's usual sleep patterns and compare with current sleep disturbance, relying on client/significant other (SO) report of problem **to ascertain intensity and duration of problems. Understanding client's sleep patterns guides interventions for helping to correct the problem.**
- Listen to reports of sleep quality (e.g., "short," "interrupted") and response from lack of good sleep (feeling foggy, sleepy, and woozy; fighting sleep; fatigue). **Helps clarify client's perception of sleep quantity and quality and response to inadequate sleep.**
- Determine client's sleep expectations. **Individual may have faulty beliefs or attitudes about sleep and/or unrealistic sleep expectations (e.g., "I must get 8 hr of sleep every night or I can't accomplish anything").**
- Observe for physical signs of fatigue (e.g., restlessness, hand tremors, thick speech, drooping eyes, inattention, lack of interest in activities). **Information collected from a comprehensive assessment may be needed to evaluate the type and etiology of sleep disturbance and identify useful treatment options.**
- Incorporate screening information into in-depth sleep diary or testing if needed **to evaluate the type and etiology of sleep disturbance and to identify useful treatment options.**

Nursing Priority No. 3.
To assist client to establish optimal sleep/rest pattern:
- Manage environment for hospitalized client:
  Adjust ambient lighting **to maintain daytime light and nighttime dark.**
  Request visitors to leave, close room door, post "Quiet, patient sleeping" sign, as indicated, **to provide privacy.**

Information that appears in brackets has been added by the authors to clarify and enhance the use of nursing diagnoses.

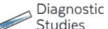 Diagnostic Studies 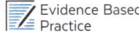 Evidence Based Practice 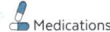 Medications 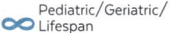 Pediatric/Geriatric/Lifespan

Encourage usual bedtime routines, such as washing face and hands and brushing teeth.

Provide bedtime care, such as straightening bed sheets, changing damp linens or gown, back massage, **to promote physical comfort.**

Turn on soft music, calm TV program, or quiet environment, as client prefers, offer/provide sleep aids such as earplugs, eyemasks, if desired, **to enhance relaxation.**

Minimize sleep-disrupting factors (e.g., shut room door, adjust room temperature as needed, reduce talking and other disturbing noises such as phones, beepers, alarms) **to promote readiness for sleep and improve sleep duration and quality.**

Perform monitoring and care activities without waking client whenever possible. **Allows for longer periods of uninterrupted sleep, especially during night.**

Avoid or limit use of physical restraints in accordance with client's needs and facility policy.

- Refer to provider or sleep specialist as indicated **for specific interventions and/or therapies, including medications, biofeedback.**

Nursing Priority No. 4.

To maintain restorative sleep (Teaching/Discharge Considerations) and enhance well-being (long-term goals):

- Assure client that occasional sleeplessness should not threaten health and that resolving time-limited situation can restore healthful sleep. **Knowledge that occasional insomnia is universal and usually not harmful may promote relaxation and relief from worry, which can perpetuate the problem.**
- Problem-solve immediate needs. **Short-term solutions (e.g., sleeping in different rooms if partner's illness is keeping client awake, acquiring a fan if sleeping quarters too warm or lack ventilation) may be needed until client adjusts to situation or crisis is resolved, with resulting return to more usual sleep pattern.**
- Encourage appropriate indoor light settings during day and night, especially exposure to bright light or sunlight in the morning, avoidance of daytime napping as appropriate for age and situation, being active during day and more passive in evening. **Helps in promotion of normal sleep-wake patterns.**
- Investigate use of aids to block out light and sound, such as sleep mask, room-darkening shades, earplugs, "white noise."

Information that appears in brackets has been added by the authors to clarify and enhance the use of nursing diagnoses.

 Acute Care 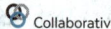 Collaborative 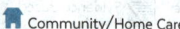 Community/Home Care Cultural

- Discuss use and appropriateness of over-the-counter sleep medications or herbal supplements **to provide assistance in falling and staying asleep.**

Documentation Focus

Assessment/Reassessment
- Assessment findings, including specifics of current and past sleep pattern, and effects on lifestyle and level of functioning
- Specific interventions, medications, or previously tried therapies

Planning
- Plan of care and who is involved in planning
- Teaching plan

Implementation/Evaluation
- Response to interventions, teaching, and actions performed
- Attainment of or progress toward desired outcome(s)
- Modifications to plan of care

Discharge Planning
- Long-term needs and who is responsible for actions to be taken
- Available resources, specific referrals made

Sample Nursing Outcomes & Interventions Classifications NOC/NIC

NOC—Sleep
NIC—Sleep Enhancement

---

inadequate SOCIAL CONNECTEDNESS   NANDA-I

[Diagnostic Division: Roles/Relationships]

Definition: Feeling of not belonging, being cared for, or empowered within a given context.

Recognizing Cues

Related/Risk Factors
Difficulty establishing social interaction, or sharing personal life expectations; inadequate self-esteem; negative opinion of support system

---

Information that appears in brackets has been added by the authors to clarify and enhance the use of nursing diagnoses.

Difficulty independently performing activities of daily living; impaired memory; confusion

Paralyzing fear of crime, or traffic

Impaired physical mobility; inadequate transportation

Inadequate social skills or social support; values incongruent with cultural norms

Defining Characteristics

Subjective

Dissatisfaction with respect from others, with social connection, or social support; impaired ability to meet expectations of others

Preoccupation with own thoughts; purposelessness

Feels different from others; feels insecure in public; loneliness

Objective

Flat affect; hostility; decreased eye contact

Inadequate levels of social activities; minimal interaction with others

Self-neglect

Social behavior incongruent with cultural norms; alienation

Clinical Connections

Any condition that is associated with isolating disorders or treatments such as traumatic injuries, facial scarring/acne, chemotherapy, AIDS, dementia, major depression, conduct disorder, developmental delay, paranoid disorders, schizophrenia

Generate Solutions

Plan Desired Outcomes

Client Will (Include Specific Time Frame)

- Identify causes and actions to correct isolation.
- Verbalize willingness to be involved with others.
- Participate in activities or programs at level of ability and desire.
- Express increased sense of self-worth.

Interventions/Take Action

Nursing Priority No. 1.

To assess causative/contributing factors:

 • Review history and elicit information about traumatic events that may have occurred. (Refer to ND Post-Trauma Syndrome.) **While little is known about the origins of**

Information that appears in brackets has been added by the authors to clarify and enhance the use of nursing diagnoses.

social anxiety disorders, clients who have experienced a traumatic event may withdraw from contact and suffer from anxiety when faced with deciding to participate in social situations. Note: Commonly overlooked causes of emotional trauma include surgery (especially in the first 3 years of life), the sudden death of someone close, the breakup of a significant relationship, or a humiliating or deeply disappointing experience, especially if someone was deliberately cruel.

- Assess factors in client's life that may contribute to desire for isolation. **Causes may be multifactorial and ongoing for months (or years) (e.g., phobias, obsessive-compulsive disorder, chronic pain, facial or body disfigurement, depression, anxiety, or other disabling conditions), resulting in the individual withdrawing, expressing desire to be alone, and refusing to participate in therapeutic activities.**
- Identify client thoughts and feelings of loneliness or disconnection from family/friends or lack of relationships, e.g., (1) immigrants—language barriers, cultural and economic challenges, and limited social ties can contribute to social isolation; (2) marginalized groups—e.g., LGBTQIA individuals, people of color, and others who routinely face discrimination and stigma; (3) older adults—often live alone or separated from families, and have one or more medical conditions, dementia, hearing or vision loss; (4) single or widowed adults. **Lacking social connectedness is a global trend and epidemic crossing demographics and regions. In the United States, nearly half of adults report a lack of social connectedness and loneliness. People with lower income, work excessive hours or work remotely are at greater risk. Many Americans are remaining single, living alone, reducing family size, or not attending faith-based organizations, or participating in community activities. Clients might be housebound due to incontinence, physical immobility, sensory deficits, financial constraints, transportation difficulties, or homeless and fear bullying).**
- Identify behavioral responses of isolation. **Individual may display behaviors such as excessive sleeping, daydreaming, or substance misuse/abuse, which also may potentiate isolation.**
- Assess client for presence of distress (e.g., sad affect, limited social interactions, feelings of loneliness, hopeless, or powerless). **Understanding the client's onset of isolation,**

Information that appears in brackets has been added by the authors to clarify and enhance the use of nursing diagnoses.

 Diagnostic Studies   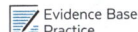 Evidence Based Practice   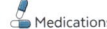 Medications   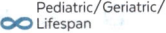 Pediatric/Geriatric/Lifespan and impact on daily living helps reveal the depth of the isolation. Prior to the COVID-19 pandemic, loneliness and social isolation were so prevalent across Europe, the United States, and China that it was described as a behavioral epidemic. The COVID-19 pandemic spawned a global experience of social isolation, impacting every facet of human life from birth to death. Globally, social isolation trends continue, causing physical and mental health concerns. In addition, children of all ages have been socially isolated in many countries due to poverty, oppression, crime/human trafficking, and with few resources.

- Assess client's feelings about self, sense of ability to control situation, sense of hope, and coping skills. **If client is isolating self because of negative feelings, lack of hope, etc., measures to promote self-esteem will need to be taken.**
- Evaluate general health, noting acute illnesses and chronic conditions (e.g., pain, cirrhosis, exacerbation of heart failure, anxiety, and depression). **Isolated individuals appear to be susceptible to acute as well as chronic health problems although little is understood regarding this health issue. The risk for early death for clients can be related to smoking, excessive alcohol and drug use, lack of exercise, obesity, and depression. Adolescents and young adults experiencing loneliness tend to drop out of high school or out of college which influences the productivity of a nation.**
- Identify client's cultural beliefs regarding social connections. **Clients living in societies that value individualism, and self-sufficiency find community, family and religion less essential in their life resulting in less social engagement. Individuals may be reluctant to engage in, or may withdraw from activities because of concern regarding how others view differences in the individual due to cultural dress or physical appearance.**
- Identify support systems available to the client, including presence of/relationship with extended family. **People with social anxiety often lack support systems because of their withdrawal from contact or social awkwardness with others. Often the family of origin is anxious and does not provide the encouragement and support needed by a temperamentally inhibited child (one who is fearful, distressed, withdrawn from new situations, environments, or individuals); alternately, family may be too helpful, enabling client to withdraw further. It is**

Information that appears in brackets has been added by the authors to clarify and enhance the use of nursing diagnoses.

difficult for these individuals to ask for help because they are afraid to meet new people and often find support only when they seek help for other conditions, such as depression.

- Note drug use (prescription and illicit). **Individual may be using substances (e.g., alcohol/other drugs) to control anxiety in social situations.**

Nursing Priority No. 2

To alleviate conditions that contribute to client's sense of isolation:

- Establish therapeutic nurse–client relationship. **Promotes trust and acceptance, allowing client to feel safe and free to discuss sensitive matters without being judged.**
- Identify client's readiness to change/accept developing strategies to interact with others. **Due to client's concerns and fears of interacting one-on-one or in groups, may be taking small steps to gain confidence to socialize in groups or crowds. Patience is needed to establish or reestablish relationships with family or friends. Understanding the client's concerns regarding socialization is the start of getting the client to participate in social activities of interest to the individual.**
- Develop plan of action with client, using a team approach (e.g., psychiatrists, psychologists, and other mental health professionals). Look at available resources; support risk-taking behaviors, financial planning, appropriate medical and self-care, etc. **The interventions, based on client's level of readiness, may include frequent interactions with the healthcare team, developing coping skills to use prior to interactions, role-playing that addresses specific concerns/fears, and how to be assertive rather than aggressive or passive with communication. Helping client to learn how to manage these issues of daily living can increase self-confidence and assist individual to feel more comfortable in social settings.**
- Encourage participation in support groups; introduce client to those with similar or shared interests. **Provides role models and encourages getting to know others who share feelings of anxiety, providing an opportunity to develop social skills and learn some ways of problem-solving to deal with anxiety.**
- Promote participation in recreational or special interest activities in setting that client views as safe. **These activities have the advantage of providing physical and mental**

Information that appears in brackets has been added by the authors to clarify and enhance the use of nursing diagnoses.

 Diagnostic Studies 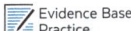 Evidence Based Practice 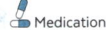 Medications 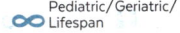 Pediatric/Geriatric/Lifespan

stimulation for client who feels isolated and anxious in social settings.
- Provide positive reinforcement when client makes move(s) toward other(s). **Acknowledges and encourages continuation of efforts, helping client toward independence.**
- Engage medical interpreter as needed during assessment and planning for treatments. Identify language resources for client who speaks another language. Utilize technology as indicated for age and developmentally appropriate interventions. **A professional interpreter is important to ensure accuracy of interpretation and maintain the Health Insurance Portability and Accountability Act; newspapers and radio programming in appropriate foreign language help client feel connected with own community.**
- Assist client to problem-solve solutions to short-term or prescribed isolation. **Condition may require individual to be isolated from others for their and/or others' protection, and working together to decide how to manage loneliness can promote successful outcome.**
- Encourage open visitation when possible and/or telephone or computer contacts for clients homebound or in facilities. **Maintains involvement with others, promoting social involvement, especially when client is unable to go out to activities.**
- Provide/encourage environmental stimuli when client is confined. **Open curtains in room, display pictures of family or views of nature, promote television and radio listening, and encourage groups that provide education related to socialization and recreational activities.**
- Provide for placement in sheltered community when necessary. **The individual who is mentally impaired may be unable to learn to participate in society and display socially acceptable behaviors and will benefit from an environment that offers structure and assistance. Clients are placed in the least restrictive environments based on their illness or behaviors.**

Nursing Priority No. 3.

To promote socialization with family, friends, and the community (Teaching/Discharge Considerations) and enhance well-being (long-term goals):

- Review coping skills learned to improve social skills. **Reinforcing successful coping skills such as problem-solving,**

Information that appears in brackets has been added by the authors to clarify and enhance the use of nursing diagnoses.

communication, social skills, and learning to manage activities of daily living will improve sense of self-esteem.

- Encourage and assist client to enroll in classes pertinent for growth and development. **Continued education such as assertiveness; vocational, cultural, and spiritual organizations; special interests groups (e.g., arts, recreation, cooking, and money management classes) may provide skills to improve ability to engage more effectively in social situations.**
- Involve children and adolescents in age-appropriate programs or activities, as indicated. **Promotes socialization skills and peer contact to enable a young person to learn by interacting with others. For example, after-school activities, the Boys and Girls Club.**
- Help client differentiate between isolation and loneliness or aloneness and discuss how to avoid slipping into an undesired state. **Time for the individual to be alone is important to the maintenance of mental health, but the sadness created by isolation and loneliness needs different interventions.**
- Provide resources that prevent relapse and support client interactions with family, friends, and community. **Activities such as senior citizen services, daily telephone contact, house sharing, pets, day-care centers, and church resources can help individual move out of isolation and become involved in life.**
- Discuss use of medications, as indicated. **Prescribed medications, such as selective serotonin reuptake inhibitors, can be very effective in treating social disorders.**
- Refer to counselor or therapist, as appropriate. **Facilitates grief work, promotes relationship building, and provides opportunity to work toward improvement of individual issues affecting social interactions.**

Documentation Focus

Assessment/Reassessment
- Individual findings, including precipitating factors, effect on lifestyle and relationships, and functioning
- Client's perception of situation
- Cultural or spiritual factors
- Availability and use of resources and support systems

Planning
- Plan of care and who is involved in planning
- Teaching plan

Information that appears in brackets has been added by the authors to clarify and enhance the use of nursing diagnoses.

 Diagnostic Studies 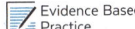 Evidence Based Practice 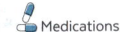 Medications 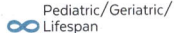 Pediatric/Geriatric/Lifespan

Implementation/Evaluation
- Responses to interventions, teaching, and actions performed
- Attainment of or progress toward desired outcome(s)
- Modifications to plan of care

Discharge Planning
- Long-term needs, referrals made, and who is responsible for actions to be taken
- Available resources, specific referrals made

Sample Nursing Outcomes & Interventions Classifications NOC/NIC

NOC—Social Involvement
NIC—Socialization Enhancement

---

readiness for enhanced transgender SOCIAL IDENTITY NANDA-I

[Diagnostic Division: Self Perception/Concept]

Definition: Pattern of developing gender self-image, including modification of body characteristics, that produce feelings of belonging to a social or cultural group, which can be strengthened.

Recognizing Cues

Defining Characteristics

Subjective

Desires to enhance:
 Autonomy; feelings of recognition, respect for being oneself
 Feelings of being loved, accepted
 Recognition of transgender identity; proximity to the trans community

Desires body transformation

Clinical Connections
Any individual seeking to change gender identity from that assigned at birth.

Information that appears in brackets has been added by the authors to clarify and enhance the use of nursing diagnoses.

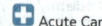 Acute Care 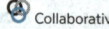 Collaborative 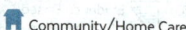 Community/Home Care Cultural

Generate Solutions

Plan Desired Outcomes

Client Will (Include Specific Time Frame)
- Verbalize acceptance and respect of self.
- Accept the affirmation process for gender transition, if desired.
- Verbalize the need for ongoing support from family/significant other (SO)/LGBTQ+ community as a transgender individual.

Interventions/Take Action

Nursing Priority No. 1.
To assess contributing factors and individual responses:

- Establish a therapeutic nurse–client/family/SO relationship. **Conveys an attitude of caring and develops a sense of trust in which client can discuss concerns and find answers to issues confronting the client in new situation.**
- Determine client's demographic information and when client began to think about gender-nonconformity. **Gender assigned at birth does not match the identity or expression of the client. Childhood may be the first sign of a mismatch of gender. Incongruence with assigned gender becomes more apparent in puberty (10 to 13 years of age), sexual desire, and peer support for gender role.**
- Identify how the client/family/SO contend with stigma and stress. **Supportive relationships help the client with coming out and managing their gender identity, transiting into a social life, and support from the LGBTQ+ community.**
- Ask client if they hide their transgender identity. **Some clients want to avoid the psychological distress of discrimination, microaggression, or being marginalized.**
- Determine if client has contacted legal, social, psychological, and medical services for help. **Transgender clients need a wide range of support services from identification, transition, affirmation, and seeking healthcare support.**
- Identify client's level of stress, anxiety, and depression. **Transgender clients have poor self-esteem, discrimination, lack social support, and have relationship problems that can lead to thoughts of suicide if not treated.**
- Ask client about spiritual/cultural thoughts and beliefs and how they want to be identified (e.g., LGBTQ, or other).

Information that appears in brackets has been added by the authors to clarify and enhance the use of nursing diagnoses.

 Diagnostic Studies 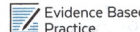 Evidence Based Practice 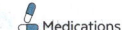 Medications 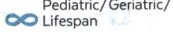 Pediatric/Geriatric/Lifespan

Understanding the client's spiritual/cultural background can guide the nurse to understand conflict or acceptance of the transgender role by the client.

- Determine client's readiness to accept the transgender social identity. **Attempting to implement interventions prior to the client's stage of readiness to change will be met with ambivalence and resistance.**

Nursing Priority No. 2.

To assist client to cope with the situation:

- Provide psychosexual education to client/family/significant others (SOs) to help with decision making. **Client/family/SOs need to understand that legal, educational, and mental health affirmations are important in promoting mental health. During the affirmation process, the client is given the opportunity to make an informed decision to proceed or stop the hormonal or surgical transition process. A lack of family support for gender affirmation is met with stress, anxiety, depression, and even suicide.**
- Allow client and family/SOs time and space to express thoughts, concerns, and feelings regarding client's gender identify. **Client and family need time and space to process the complexity of affirming the transgender process (e.g., legal, educational, mental health), the evaluations prior to transition or in some situations detransition. The detransition process is the reason and need for a full affirming of the transgender process before proceeding with any changes.**
- Help client/family/SO to recognize the importance of the protective power provided by the family/SO for the client. **Clients who have supportive families experience less anxiety, depression, psychosocial issues, and fewer thoughts of suicide.**
- Assist client to make a list of positive attributes of self. Review the list when negative thoughts enter the mind. **Clients keeping a list of attributes, updating the list, and referring to the list frequently helps with self-confidence and self-esteem.**
- Provide client/family/SO with assertiveness training, coping skills, emotional intelligence, mindfulness, and problem-solving skills. **Global misunderstanding of LGBTQ+ individuals has created discrimination even in healthcare, stigma, social isolation, acts of violence, and death to the client. It is vital LGBTQ+ individuals have the**

Information that appears in brackets has been added by the authors to clarify and enhance the use of nursing diagnoses.

communication and coping skills to protect themselves emotionally from verbal abuse.
- Guide client/family/SO to community resources specific to transgender issues, including services that are not available in the present facility. **Family therapy (transgender practice) reduces depression, substance misuse/abuse, suicidal thoughts and attempts by adolescent clients.**
- Provide opportunities for client/family/SO to role-play and practice assertiveness communication. **Role-playing how to respond to negativism from others, builds self-esteem, confidence, and enhances the social identity. In addition, it may enlighten those who are disrespectful to others who are vulnerable.**

Nursing Priority No. 3.

To promote a readiness for transgender social identity (Teaching/Discharge Considerations) and enhance well-being (long-term goals):

- Recap lessons learned with assertiveness, emotional intelligence, and mindfulness.
- Discuss progress made while in treatment. **Recognizing where they were at the beginning of treatment and the progress made encourages the client to continue with their emotional growth and presentation.**
- Provide a list of resources available to the transgender client/family/SO. **Not all community resources are trained to help the LGBTQ+ community; therefore, finding resources for this population is important to get the assistance required.**
- Encourage client/family/SO to follow-up with therapy and community support groups. **Transgender identity is an ongoing process due to the complexity of the affirmation process, transitional period, and affirmation of new gender.**

Documentation Focus

Assessment/Reassessment
- Identify risk factors, emotional/behavioral factors, and support of family/SO
- Client's perception and personal significance of the situation
- Client's cultural/spiritual values, beliefs, and expectations
- Availability and use of resources

Planning
- Plan of care and who is involved in the planning
- Teaching plan

Information that appears in brackets has been added by the authors to clarify and enhance the use of nursing diagnoses.

 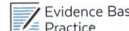 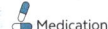 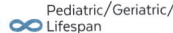

Implementation/Evaluation
- Response to interventions, teaching, and actions performed
- Attainment or progress toward desired outcomes
- Modifications to plan of care

Discharge Planning
- Long-term goals and who is responsible for actions to be taken
- Specific referrals made

Sample Nursing Outcomes & Interventions Classifications NOC/NIC

NOC—Gender Identity
NIC—Self-Awareness

---

inadequate SOCIAL SUPPORT NETWORK NANDA-I

[Diagnostic Division: Roles/Relationships]

Definition: Interpersonal and organizational interactions that are perceived to be unsatisfactory to meet health needs.

Recognizing Cues

Related/Risk Factors
Difficulty trusting that information will remain confidential
Inadequate appreciation of available social support; inadequate trust in other's competence to provide adequate support
Inadequate knowledge, or skill to mobilize support
Inadequate social skills; limited social network; sociocultural dissonance

Defining Characteristics

Subjective
Mistrust of others; decreased perceived emotional support, or positive social interaction
Decreased perceived informational, or instrumental support
Negative opinion of support system; frustration with unmet support expectations; perceived neglect of support demands
Perceived blaming for problems by others; perceived prejudice

Objective
Decreased self-efficacy

Information that appears in brackets has been added by the authors to clarify and enhance the use of nursing diagnoses.

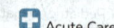 Acute Care 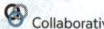 Collaborative 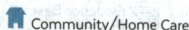 Community/Home Care   Cultural

Clinical Connections

Abuse/neglect, postpartum, depression, substance misuse, dementia, schizophrenia, paranoid personality disorder

Generate Solutions

Plan Desired Outcomes

Client Will (Include Specific Time Frame)

- Express desire to or be involved in achieving positive changes in social behaviors and interpersonal relationships.
- Verbalize awareness of factors causing a lack of a supportive network.
- Identify thoughts, feelings, and behaviors that lead to a lack of social support.
- Self-reinforcement for changes that are achieved.
- Develop effective social support system; use available resources appropriately.

Interventions/Take Action

Nursing Priority No. 1.

To assess causative or contributing factors:

- Review social history with client/significant others (SOs) and go back far enough in time to note when changes in social behavior or patterns of the support network occurred or began to change. **For example, loss or long-term illness of loved one; failed relationships; loss of occupation, financial, or political (power) position; change in status in family hierarchy (job loss, aging, illness); and poor coping or adjustment to developmental stage of life, as with marriage, birth or adoption of child, or children leaving home, are situations that may affect quality of social exchange.**
- Identify client's perception of what they think happened that their needs are not being meet. **Client's support network may be small in numbers, fragile or broken relationships with members no longer wanting to participate or have issues of their own. Or, is the client not reaching out for support.**
- Review medical history, noting stressors of physical or long-term illness/chronic conditions (e.g., stroke, cancer, multiple sclerosis, head injury, Alzheimer disease), mental illness (e.g., schizophrenia), medications, substance use, debilitating accidents, learning disabilities (e.g., sensory integration difficulties, autism spectrum disorder), and emotional

---

Information that appears in brackets has been added by the authors to clarify and enhance the use of nursing diagnoses.

 Diagnostic Studies 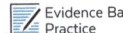 Evidence Based Practice 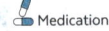 Medications 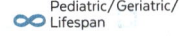 Pediatric/Geriatric/Lifespan

disabilities. **Conditions such as these can isolate individual who feels disconnected from others, resulting in difficulty relating in social situations. Note: Evidence indicates that loneliness heightens sensitivity to social threats and can impair executive functioning, sleep, and mental and physical well-being.**
- Identify presence of visual or hearing impairments. **Individuals with these conditions may find communication barriers are increased, social interaction is affected, and interventions need to be designed to promote involvement with others in positive ways.**
- Observe patterns of communication, relating, social behaviors, and expectations from others while interacting with family/SO. **Individuals may find expressed unrealistic expectations have created barriers, social interactions are affected, and interventions need to be designed to promote involvement with others in positive ways.**
- Encourage client to verbalize feelings of discomfort about social situations. Note any causative factors, recurring precipitating patterns, and barriers to using support systems. **Identifies areas of concern and suggests possible ways to learn new skills.**
- Assess for depression using the Patient Health Questionnaire (PQH-9) tool. **The PHQ-9 is an assessment tool developed to identify depression from mild to severe and intended to be used in a variety of healthcare settings, not just in mental health.**
- Determine client's stage of readiness to change. **Attempting to help client prior to their stage of readiness to change will be met with ambivalence or resistance.**

Nursing Priority No. 2.

To assist client to cope with impaired social and interpersonal interactions:

- Establish therapeutic relationship using positive regard for the person, active-listening, and providing safe environment for self-disclosure. **Client who is having difficulty interacting in social situations needs to feel comfortable and accepted before being willing to talk about self and concerns.**
- Encourage client to verbalize perceptions of reasons for problems. Active-listen, noting indications of hopelessness, powerlessness, fear, anxiety, grief, anger, feeling unloved or unlovable, issues with gender identity, and hate (directed or not). **These feelings arise from the anxiety that comes**

Information that appears in brackets has been added by the authors to clarify and enhance the use of nursing diagnoses.

with the need to participate with others in social situations and can interfere with work, friendships, and the support network.

- Promote social and interpersonal behaviors in objective terms, noting speech patterns and body language with family/SO. **Provides client with an understanding of their approach, patterns of communication, respect, honesty, and expectations from others.**
- Identify client's use of defense mechanisms when communicating with others. **Use of defense mechanisms is a self-protective approach defending their self-esteem and self-concept. Others may find the defensiveness off putting.**
- Help client to use assertiveness communication, emotional intelligence, mindfulness, and coping skills to promote social interactions. **Problems of poor communication lead to frustration/anger that results in not being mindful of what is being said, an inability to read others' body language, and a lack of coping skills may result in destructive behaviors limiting social interactions/support.**
- Role-play social interactions with client using variety of scenarios that client may encounter when interacting with family/friends/SO support network. **Engaging the client in practicing assertive communication while recognizing the recipients' body language is good practice for learning the skills.**
- Debrief and coach the client following the role-play. **Helps client to analyze their approach, message sent, what they think the respondent's response is to the message, and how they may consider a different approach.**
- Help client identify positive approaches to the role-play. **Builds self-esteem, confidence with communication skills, social skills, and interactions.**
- Encourage client to keep a daily journal in which social interactions of each day can be reviewed and the comfort or discomfort experienced noted with possible causes or precipitating factors. **Helps client to identify specific problem areas and begin to choose to take responsibility for own behavior(s).**
- Discuss with client the benefits of self-talk and/or self-talking to a mirror, or to practice a specific message they want to present. **Self-talk or talking to the mirror is helpful to remind self of the positive changes made with communication and positive attributes of self because it reinforces self-esteem and confidence.**

Information that appears in brackets has been added by the authors to clarify and enhance the use of nursing diagnoses.

 Diagnostic Studies 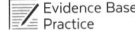 Evidence Based Practice 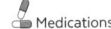 Medications 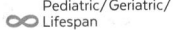 Pediatric/Geriatric/Lifespan

- Discuss use of medications to help with depression. **Clients identified as depressed may benefit with the introduction of an antidepressant. Several kinds of drugs have been found to be effective in the treatment of social anxiety problems; selective serotonin reuptake inhibitors (SSRIs), such as paroxetine (Paxil) and sertraline (Zoloft), are often the first choice. Antianxiety drugs, such as clonazepam (Klonopin), buspirone (BuSpar), and alprazolam (Xanax), can reduce anxiety and may be used alone or in conjunction with SSRIs. Propranolol (Inderal) has been found to be useful for performance anxiety, and when taken an hour before the scheduled event, may suppress the physical symptoms of anxiety.**

Nursing Priority No. 3.

To enhance client's social support network (Teaching/Discharge Considerations) and enhance well-being (long-term goals):

- Review with client the lessons learned and progress made during treatment. **Client's progress builds self-esteem and confidence to continue using the new skills to build a support network.**
- Encourage ongoing family or individual therapy as long as it is promoting growth and positive change. Be alert to possibility of therapy being used as a crutch. **While therapy groups can be useful, individuals can become dependent on the process and not move on to managing on their own.**
- Recommend community resources for client involvement that promote positive behaviors the client desires to achieve. **Encouraging reading materials, attending classes, community support groups, and lectures for self-help can help to alleviate negative self-concepts that lead to impaired social interactions.**
- Encourage follow-up appointments to reinforce positive behaviors. **Change is difficult, and identifying problems that may arise during these contacts can enhance maintenance and enable client/family to continue to progress.**

Documentation Focus

Assessment/Reassessment

- Individual findings, including factors affecting interactions, nature of social exchanges, specifics of individual behaviors.

Information that appears in brackets has been added by the authors to clarify and enhance the use of nursing diagnoses.

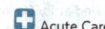 Acute Care 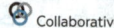 Collaborative 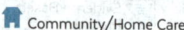 Community/Home Care Cultural

- Cultural or religious beliefs and expectations.
- Perceptions and response of others.

Planning
- Plan of care and who is involved in the planning.
- Teaching plan.

Implementation/Evaluation
- Responses to interventions, teaching, and actions performed.
- Attainment or progress toward desired outcome(s).
- Modifications to plan of care.

Discharge Planning
- Long-term needs and who is responsible for actions to be taken.
- Community resources, specific referrals made.

Sample Nursing Outcomes & Interventions Classifications (NOC/NIC)

NOC—Social Interaction Skills
NIC—Behavior Modification: Social skills

---

impaired SPIRITUAL WELL-BEING — NANDA-I

[Diagnostic Division: Values/Beliefs]

Definition: Diminished integration of meaning and purpose in life through connections with self, others, the world, and/or a power greater than oneself.

Recognizing Cues

Related/Risk Factors
Altered religious ritual, or spiritual practice; cultural conflict
Anxiety; depressive symptoms; loneliness; difficulty accepting the aging process
Barrier to experiencing love; inadequate interpersonal relations; awareness of having unfinished business
Inadequate social support; social alienation; sociocultural deprivation
Loss of independence; inadequate self-esteem; self-alienation
Pain; excessive stress; substance misuse
Anxiety; depression

Information that appears in brackets has been added by the authors to clarify and enhance the use of nursing diagnoses.

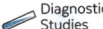 Diagnostic Studies 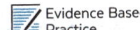 Evidence Based Practice 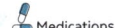 Medications 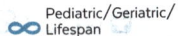 Pediatric/Geriatric/Lifespan

Defining Characteristics

Subjective
Disinterested in nature
Dysomnias [difficulty sleeping]; fatigue
Anger; anger toward power greater than self; alienation, excessive guilt; hopelessness
Concern about beliefs, values system, or the future; insufficient courage
Concerns about family
Feeling abandoned by power greater than self
Feeling of emptiness; feels unloved; feeling worthless; questions own dignity; loss of meaning in life; need for forgiveness; regret
Loss of confidence, control, hope, or serenity; fear
Impaired ability for introspection; inability to experience transcendence
Questions identity, meaning of life, or meaning of suffering

Objective
Anger behaviors; crying
Decreased creativity
Difficulty grieving
Refuses to interact with others
Inadequate sleep quality

Clinical Connections
Chronic conditions (e.g., cancer, AIDS, traumatic brain injury vegetative state, infertility); terminal illness, depression, fetal demise, sudden infant death syndrome (SIDS); death of child; traumatic event with fatal outcome or severe disabilities

Generate Solutions

Plan Desired Outcomes

Client Will (Include Specific Time Frame)
- Identify meaning and purpose in own life that reinforces hope, peace, and contentment.
- Verbalize increased sense of connectedness and hope for future.
- Demonstrate ability to help self and participate in care.
- Participate in activities with others, actively seek relationships.
- Discuss beliefs and values about spiritual issues.
- Verbalize acceptance of self as being worthy, not deserving of illness or situation, and so forth.

Information that appears in brackets has been added by the authors to clarify and enhance the use of nursing diagnoses.

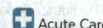 Acute Care 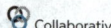 Collaborative 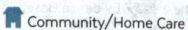 Community/Home Care Cultural

Interventions/Take Action

Nursing Priority No. 1.
To assess causative/contributing factors:

- Identify current situation (e.g., natural disaster, death of a spouse, personal injustice). **Identification of circumstances that puts the individual at risk for loss of connectedness with spiritual beliefs is essential to plan for appropriate interventions.**
- Determine client's cultural beliefs, religious or spiritual orientation, current involvement, presence of conflicts. **Individual cultural/spiritual practices or restrictions may affect client care or create conflict between beliefs and treatment.**
- Note client's reason for living and whether it is directly related to situation (e.g., home and business washed away in a flood, parent whose only child is terminally ill). **Tragic occurrences can cause individual to question previous beliefs or purpose of life.**
- Listen to client's/significant other's (SO's) reports or expressions of concern, anger, alienation from God/higher power, belief that illness or situation is a punishment for wrongdoing, and so forth. **Suggests need for spiritual advisor to address client's belief system, if desired.**
- Assess sense of self-concept, worth, ability to enter into loving relationships. **Lack of connectedness with self and others impairs client's ability to trust others or feel worthy of trust from others. Feelings of abandonment may accompany sense of "not being good enough" in face of illness, disaster.**
- Determine sense of futility, feelings of hopelessness and helplessness, lack of motivation to help self. **Indicators that client may see no, or only limited, options, alternatives, or personal choices available and lacks energy to deal with situation.**
- Note expressions of inability to find meaning in life, reason for living. Evaluate suicidal ideation. **Crisis of the spirit or loss of will to live places client at increased risk for inattention to personal well-being or harm to self requiring further evaluation.**
- Note recent changes in behavior (e.g., withdrawal from others and creative or religious activities, dependence on alcohol or medications). **Helpful in determining severity and duration of situation and possible need for additional referrals, such as substance withdrawal.**

Information that appears in brackets has been added by the authors to clarify and enhance the use of nursing diagnoses.

 Diagnostic Studies 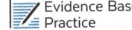 Evidence Based Practice 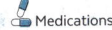 Medications 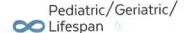 Pediatric/Geriatric/Lifespan

- Observe behavior indicative of poor relationships with others (e.g., manipulative, nontrusting, demanding). **Manipulation is used for management of client's sense of powerlessness because of distrust of others.**
- Ascertain substance use or abuse. **Affects ability to deal with problems in a positive manner.**
- Determine support systems available to client/SO(s) and how they are used. **Provides insight to client's willingness to pursue outside resources.**
- Determine motivation and expectations for change. **Motivation to improve and high expectations can encourage client to make changes that will improve their life. However, unrealistic expectations may hamper efforts.**
- Be aware of influence of care provider's belief system. **It is still possible to be helpful to client while remaining neutral and refraining from promoting own beliefs.**

Nursing Priority No. 2.

To assist client/SO(s) to cope with feelings/situation:

- Develop therapeutic nurse–client relationship. Ascertain client's views as to how care provider(s) can be most helpful. Convey acceptance of client's spiritual beliefs and concerns. **Promotes trust and comfort, encouraging client to be open about sensitive matters and free to express feelings and concerns.**
- Provide calm, peaceful setting when possible. **Promotes relaxation and enhances opportunity for reflection on situation, discussions with others, meditation.**
- Encourage life-review by client. Help client find a reason for living. **Promotes sense of hope and willingness to continue efforts to improve situation.**
- Have client identify and prioritize current or immediate needs. **Helps client focus on what needs to be done and identify manageable steps to take.**
- Encourage client/family to ask questions. **Demonstrates support for individual's willingness to learn.**
- Make time for nonjudgmental discussion of philosophical issues or questions about spiritual impact of illness or situation and/or treatment regimen. **Open communication can assist client in reality checks of perceptions and identifying personal options.**
- Review coping skills used and their effectiveness in current situation. **Identifies strengths to incorporate into plan and techniques needing revision.**

Information that appears in brackets has been added by the authors to clarify and enhance the use of nursing diagnoses.

- Identify use of defense mechanisms currently being used and associated consequences and discuss with client. **Recognizing negative consequences of actions may enhance desire to change.**
- Ascertain past successes and coping behaviors **to determine approaches used previously that may be more effective in dealing with current situation.**
- Problem-solve solutions and identify areas for compromise **that may be useful in resolving possible conflicts.**
- Set limits on acting-out behavior that is inappropriate or destructive. **Promotes safety for client/others and helps prevent loss of self-esteem.**

Nursing Priority No. 3.

To facilitate setting goals and moving forward:

- Involve client in refining healthcare goals and therapeutic regimen, as appropriate. **Enhances commitment to plan, optimizing outcomes.**
- Discuss difference between grief and guilt and help client to identify and deal with each. Point out consequences of actions based on guilt. **Aids client in assuming responsibility for own actions and avoiding acting out of false guilt.**
- Explore ways beliefs give meaning and value to daily living. **As client develops understanding of these issues, client will provide support for dealing with current and future concerns.**
- Use therapeutic communication skills of reflection and active-listening. **Helps client find own solutions to concerns.**
- Clarify reality and appropriateness of client's self-perceptions and expectations. **Necessary to provide firm foundation for growth. Unrealistic ideas can impede desired improvement.**
- Assist client to learn use of meditation, or prayer, and forgiveness **to heal past hurts.**
- Provide information that anger with God/higher power is a normal part of the grieving process. **Realizing these feelings are not unusual can reduce sense of guilt, encourage open expression, and facilitate resolution of conflict.**
- Provide time and privacy to engage in spiritual growth and religious activities (e.g., prayer, meditation, scripture reading, listening to music). **Allows client to focus on self and seek connectedness.**

Information that appears in brackets has been added by the authors to clarify and enhance the use of nursing diagnoses.

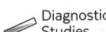 Diagnostic Studies 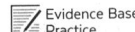 Evidence Based Practice 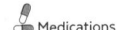 Medications 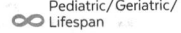 Pediatric/Geriatric/Lifespan

- Encourage and facilitate outings to neighborhood park, nature walks, or similar outings when able. **Sunshine, fresh air, and activity can stimulate release of endorphins, promoting sense of well-being.**
- ∞ Provide play therapy for child that encompasses spiritual data. **Interactive pleasurable activity promotes open discussion and enhances retention of information. Also provides opportunity for child to practice what has been learned.**
- ∞ Abide by parents' wishes in discussing and implementing child's spiritual support. **Limits confusion for child and prevents conflict of values or beliefs.**
- ⊕ Refer to appropriate resources (e.g., pastoral or parish nurse, spiritual counselor, crisis counselor, hospice; psychotherapy; Alcoholics or Narcotics Anonymous). **Useful in dealing with immediate situation and identifying long-term resources for support to help foster sense of connectedness.**
- Refer to NDs difficulty Coping; lack of Resilience; chronic or situational inadequate Self-Esteem; inadequate Social Connectedness; risk for Suicide for additional interventions as indicated.

Nursing Priority No. 4.

To promote sense of connectedness with a higher power (Teaching/Discharge Considerations) and enhance well-being (long-term goals):

- 🏠 Assist client to develop goals for dealing with life/illness situation. **Enhances commitment to goal, optimizing outcomes.**
- Suggest use of journaling. **Can assist in clarifying values and ideas or recognizing and resolving feelings or situation.**
- Review use of relaxation or meditative activities (e.g., yoga, tai chi, prayer). **Helpful in promoting general well-being and sense of connectedness with self, nature, and/or spiritual power.**
- Role-play new coping techniques **to enhance integration of new skills or necessary changes in lifestyle.**
- Assist client to identify SO(s) and people who could provide support as needed. **Ongoing support is required to enhance sense of connectedness and continue progress toward goals. Role models provide opportunities for sharing of experiences, finding hope, and identifying options to deal with situation.**

Information that appears in brackets has been added by the authors to clarify and enhance the use of nursing diagnoses.

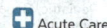 Acute Care 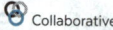 Collaborative 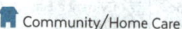 Community/Home Care Cultural

- Encourage family to provide a quiet, calm atmosphere. Be willing to just "be" there and not have a need to "do" something. **Helps client to think about self in the context of current situation.**
- Encourage individual to become involved in cultural activities of their choosing. **Art, music, plays, and other cultural activities provide a means of connecting with self and others.**
- Suggest attendance or involvement in dream-sharing group. **Enhance learning of the characteristics of spiritual awareness and facilitate the individual's growth.**
- Discuss benefit of family counseling, as appropriate. **Issues of this nature (e.g., situational losses, natural disasters, difficult relationships) affect family dynamics.**
- Remind client they are in control of their thinking, feeling, and believing and can make decisions that are best for them. **Gives client the power to determine how the present and future life will heal.**
- Assist client to identify spiritual resources that could be helpful (e.g., contact spiritual advisor who has qualifications or experience in coping with specific problems, such as death and dying, relationship problems, substance abuse, suicide). **Can be helpful in finding answers to spiritual questions, assisting in the journey of self-discovery, and helping client learn to accept and forgive self.**

Documentation Focus

Assessment/Reassessment
- Individual findings, including nature of spiritual conflict, effects on SO/family
- Physical and emotional responses to conflict

Planning
- Plan of care and who is involved in planning
- Teaching plan

Implementation/Evaluation
- Responses to interventions, teaching, and actions performed
- Attainment of or progress toward desired outcome(s)
- Modifications to plan of care

Discharge Planning
- Long-term needs and who is responsible for actions to be taken
- Available resources, specific referrals made

Information that appears in brackets has been added by the authors to clarify and enhance the use of nursing diagnoses.

 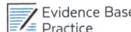 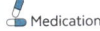 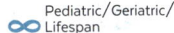

Sample Nursing Outcomes & Interventions Classifications NOC/NIC

NOC—Spiritual Health
NIC—Spiritual Support

---

impaired STANDING ABILITY   NANDA-I

[Diagnostic Division: Activity/Rest]

Definition: Limitation of independent and purposeful attainment and/or maintenance of the body in an upright position from feet to head.

Recognizing Cues

Related/Risk Factors
Excessive emotional disturbance
Inadequate physical endurance; inadequate muscle strength
Malnutrition; ineffective overweight self-management
Pain
Inappropriate relief posture

Defining Characteristics

Objective
Difficulty:
  Adjusting position of one or both lower limbs on uneven surface
  Attaining, or maintaining postural balance
  Extending one or both hips or knees; flexing one or both hips, or knees
  Moving one or both hips, or knees
  Performing bodyweight exercises

Clinical Connections
Neuromuscular disorders (e.g., multiple sclerosis [MS], amyotrophic lateral sclerosis, Parkinson disease), traumatic injuries (e.g., lower extremity fractures, spinal cord or brain injuries), osteoarthritis, rheumatoid arthritis, hip or knee joint replacement; severe depression, dementia

---

Information that appears in brackets has been added by the authors to clarify and enhance the use of nursing diagnoses.

Generate Solutions

Plan Desired Outcomes

Client Will (Include Specific Time Frame)
- Verbalize understanding of individual treatment regimen and safety measures.
- Attain and maintain position of standing function that enables activities and prevents complications.
- Participate in activities of daily living (ADLs) and desired activities.

Interventions/Take Action

Nursing Priority No. 1.
To identify causative/contributing factors:

- Determine diagnosis that contributes to difficulty with standing balance (e.g., stroke, other neurological disorders [e.g., MS, Parkinson disease; traumatic brain injury, spinal cord injury with hemi-/paraplegia]; vestibular disorders/vertigo; osteoarthritis, rheumatoid arthritis, degenerative joint disease; back pain conditions; lower-limb amputations; psychiatric conditions including severe depression, dementias). **These conditions can cause postural and balance impairments, muscular weakness, and inadequate range of motion. Impaired standing balance has a detrimental effect on a person's functional ability and increases the risk of falling. For example, sitting and standing balance are major concerns in an amputee's ability to maintain the center of gravity over the base of support. In persons with chronic neck pain, increased neck muscle activity and increased postural sway during simple balance tasks indicate disturbed sensory feedback patterns, which may have negative consequences when performing daily activities.**
- Assess client's mental status, noting age, developmental stage, and presence of or potential for cognitive dysfunction (e.g., traumatic brain injury, stroke, dementia, extremes of age). **Several studies have suggested that seemingly automatic postural tasks (e.g., standing balance and walking) require some attention and cognitive processing.**
- Determine fall risk, noting factors that may be present. **Fall risk is high in clients with certain conditions (e.g., advanced age or debilitating disease; vision and hearing loss, diminished depth perception; decreased sensation**

Information that appears in brackets has been added by the authors to clarify and enhance the use of nursing diagnoses.

 Diagnostic Studies   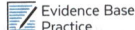 Evidence Based Practice   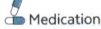 Medications   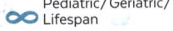 Pediatric/Geriatric/Lifespan

in feet, artificial joints; trauma to lower extremity; amputation, or other surgery or immobilizer; presence of severe vertigo with postural sway; generalized or specific leg weakness; reaching upward, forward, or laterally outside of standing balance position).
- Encourage sitting before attempting standing, when indicated (e.g., supine client with low blood pressure or dehydration, vertigo, or first attempting to get up after long period on bedrest). **Longer sitting pause times may improve postural stability after rising from a supine position.**

Nursing Priority No. 2.

To assess functional ability:

- Determine functional status in relation to 0 to 4 scale, and note muscle strength and tone, joint mobility, cardiovascular status, balance, and endurance. **Identifies strengths and deficits and may provide information regarding potential for recovery.**
- Determine degree of perceptual or cognitive impairment and ability to follow directions. **Impairments (which may be related to age, chronic or acute disease condition, trauma, surgery, or medications) can necessitate alternative interventions or changes in plan of care.**
- Refer to physician, physical therapy specialists, as indicated, **to determine need for additional evaluations, potential for improvement and direction for therapies.**

Nursing Priority No. 3.

To promote optimal level of function and prevent complications:

- Assist with treatment of underlying condition(s) **to maximize potential for optimal function.**
- Assist with/refer for rehabilitation therapies and techniques for implementing standing activities. **Various modalities may be used to gain physiological benefits from standing or modified standing therapy to help preserve joint range of motion, improve muscle flexibility, weight-bearing ability, and bowel and bladder function, even when person is not upright.**
- Provide for safety measures as indicated by individual situation, including environmental management and fall prevention. (Refer to NDs risk for [adult or child] Falls.)
- Encourage client's participation in self-care activities and in physical or occupational therapies. **Improves body**

Information that appears in brackets has been added by the authors to clarify and enhance the use of nursing diagnoses.

strength and function, enhances self-concept and sense of independence.
- Administer pain medications before activity, as needed, **to permit maximal effort and involvement in activity.**
- Collaborate with nutritionist in providing nutritious foods and needed feeding assistance, maximizing client's abilities in ingesting and swallowing (upright position) **to optimize available energy for activities.**
- Demonstrate and assist with use of assistive devices (e.g., siderails, overhead trapeze, roller pads, safety belt, hydraulic lifts, or chairs) **for position changes and transfers. Assists client/caregiver to use device correctly, enhancing safety.**
- Refer to NDs Activity Intolerance; impaired bed Mobility; impaired physical Mobility; impaired wheelchair Mobility; impaired Transferring Ability; impaired Sitting Ability; and impaired Walking Ability for additional interventions.

Nursing Priority No. 4.

To maintain function (Teaching/Discharge Considerations) and enhance well-being (long-term goals):

- Encourage client's/significant other's involvement in decision making as much as possible. **Enhances commitment to plan, optimizing outcomes.**
- Demonstrate use of mobility devices (e.g., walkers, strollers, scooters, braces, prosthetics) and have client/care provider demonstrate knowledge about and safe use of device. Identify appropriate resources for obtaining and maintaining appliances or equipment. **Safe use of mobility aids promotes client's independence and enhances quality of life and safety for client and caregiver.**
- Refer to support and community services, as indicated, **to provide care, supervision, companionship, respite services, nutritional and ADL assistance, adaptive devices or changes to living environment, financial assistance, and so forth.**

Documentation Focus

Assessment/Reassessment
- Individual findings, including level of function and ability to participate in specific or desired activities

Planning
- Plan of care and who is involved in the planning
- Teaching plan

Information that appears in brackets has been added by the authors to clarify and enhance the use of nursing diagnoses.

Implementation/Evaluation
- Responses to interventions, teaching, and actions performed
- Attainment of or progress toward desired outcome(s)
- Modifications to plan of care

Discharge Planning
- Discharge and long-term needs, noting who is responsible for each action to be taken
- Specific referrals made
- Sources of and maintenance for assistive devices

Sample Nursing Outcomes & Interventions Classifications NOC/NIC

NOC—Body Mechanics Performance
NIC—Exercise Therapy: Muscle Control

---

ineffective infant SUCK-SWALLOW RESPONSE NANDA-I

[Diagnostic Division: Food/Fluid]

Definition: Impaired ability to coordinate breathing while safely consuming oral feeding in an individual ≤1 year of age.

Recognizing Cues

Related/Risk Factors
Unaddressed hypoglycemia
Hypothermia
Muscle hypotonia
Inappropriate positioning; unsatisfactory sucking behavior

Defining Characteristics

Subjective
[Caregiver reports infant's inability to achieve effective suck]

Objective
Cardiac arrhythmia; bradycardic events
Choking; excessive coughing; gagging, hiccuping; subcostal retraction; excessive use of accessory respiratory muscles
Finger splaying; hyperextension of extremities; irritable crying
Flaccidity; impaired motor tone
Inability to initiate, or sustain an effective suck

Information that appears in brackets has been added by the authors to clarify and enhance the use of nursing diagnoses.

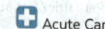 Acute Care 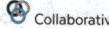 Collaborative 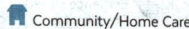 Community/Home Care   Cultural

Inability to coordinate sucking, swallowing, and breathing
Nasal flaring; circumoral cyanosis; pallor; oxygen desaturation
Time-out signals

Clinical Connections
Prematurity, cleft lip/palate, thrush, hydrocephalus, cerebral palsy, fetal alcohol syndrome, respiratory distress syndrome, enteral feeding, severe developmental delay

Generate Solutions

Plan Desired Outcomes

Client Will (Include Specific Time Frame)
- Display adequate output as measured by sufficient number of wet diapers daily.
- Demonstrate appropriate weight gain.
- Be free of aspiration.

Interventions/Take Action

Nursing Priority No. 1.
To identify contributing factors/degree of impaired function:

- Assess infant's suck, swallow, and gag reflexes. Note physiological signs (e.g., cough, apnea, desaturation; bradycardia, pallor; lethargy). **Swallowing requires more than 30 muscles, and the coordination of suckling, swallowing, and breathing is the most complex sensorimotor process the newborn infant undertakes. Information provides a comparative baseline and is useful in determining an appropriate feeding method, including amount and duration of feeds.**

- Note developmental age/neuromuscular coordination (e.g., prematurity, low birth weight), structural abnormalities (e.g., cleft lip/palate), and mechanical barriers (e.g., endotracheal tube and ventilator). **Feeding problems are seen in approximately 40% of premature infants, up to 64% to 78% of infants with developmental disorders and up to 99% of infants with cerebral palsy. Infant maturity and presence of structural/mechanical barriers will require an interdisciplinary team approach and specialized interventions.**

- Determine level of consciousness, neurological impairment, seizure activity, cardiac or respiratory issues, and presence of pain. **Identifies areas of special need to treat comorbidities.**

Information that appears in brackets has been added by the authors to clarify and enhance the use of nursing diagnoses.

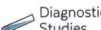 Diagnostic Studies 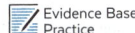 Evidence Based Practice 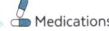 Medications 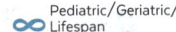 Pediatric/Geriatric/Lifespan

- Observe parent-infant interactions **to determine level of bonding and comfort that could impact stress level during feeding activity.**
- Note type and scheduling of medications, **which could cause sedative effect and impair feeding activity.**
- Note frequency/amount of voiding. Compare birth and current weight and length measurements. **Monitors effectiveness of infant feeding technique.**
- Note the presence of behaviors indicating continued hunger after feeding.

Nursing Priority No. 2.

To promote adequate infant intake:

- Coordinate interdisciplinary approach to determine appropriate method for feeding (e.g., special nipple or feeding device, gavage or enteral tube feeding) and choice of breast milk or formula to meet infant needs.
- Review early infant feeding cues (e.g., rooting, lip smacking, sucking fingers or hand) versus late cue of crying. **Early recognition of infant hunger promotes timely/more rewarding feeding experience for infant and mother.**
- Demonstrate techniques and procedures for feeding. Note proper positioning of infant, latching-on techniques, rate of delivery of feeding, and frequency of burping. **Models appropriate feeding methods and increases parental knowledge base and confidence.** (Refer to ND difficulty performing Breastfeeding, as appropriate.)
- Limit duration of feeding to maximum of 30 min based on infant's response (e.g., signs of fatigue) **to balance energy expenditure with nutrient intake.**
- Monitor caregiver's efforts. Provide feedback and assistance, as indicated. **Enhances learning and encourages the continuation of efforts.**
- Refer nursing mother to lactation specialist for assistance and support in dealing with unresolved issues (e.g., teaching infant to suck). **Provides resource for future needs and problem-solving. Begins pattern of resource utilization.**
- Emphasize the importance of a calm, relaxed environment during feeding **to reduce detrimental stimuli and enhance mother's and infant's focus on feeding activity.**
- Adjust frequency and amount of feeding according to infant's response. **Prevents stress associated with under- or overfeeding.**
- Advance diet, adding solids or thickening agent, as appropriate for age and infant needs.

Information that appears in brackets has been added by the authors to clarify and enhance the use of nursing diagnoses.

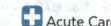 Acute Care 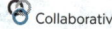 Collaborative 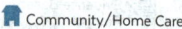 Community/Home Care Cultural

- Alternate feeding techniques (e.g., nipple and gavage) according to infant's ability and level of fatigue.
- Alter medication/feeding schedules, as indicated, **to minimize sedative effects and have infant in alert state.**

Nursing Priority No. 3.

To continue effective feeding (Teaching/Discharge Considerations) and enhance well-being (long-term goals):

- Encourage kangaroo care, placing infant skin-to-skin upright, tummy down, on mother's or father's chest. **Skin-to-skin care increases bonding and may promote stable heart rate, temperature, and respiration in infant.**
- Instruct caregiver in techniques to prevent or alleviate aspiration.
- Discuss anticipated growth and development goals for infant, as well as corresponding caloric needs. **Accommodating infant maturity and development helps to individualize and update plan of care.**
- Suggest monitoring infant's weight and nutrient intake periodically.
- Recommend participation in classes, as indicated (e.g., first aid, infant CPR). **Increases knowledge base for infant safety and caregiver confidence.**
- Refer to support groups (e.g., La Leche League, parenting support groups, stress reduction, or other community resources, as indicated).
- Provide bibliotherapy and appropriate websites for further information.

Documentation Focus

Assessment/Reassessment
- Type and route of feeding, interferences to feeding and infant response
- Frequency/amount of voids
- Infant's measurements
- Parent-infant interactions

Planning
- Plan of care, specific interventions, and who is involved in planning
- Teaching plan

Implementation/Evaluation
- Infant's response to interventions (e.g., amount of intake, weight gain, response to feeding) and actions performed

---

Information that appears in brackets has been added by the authors to clarify and enhance the use of nursing diagnoses.

 Diagnostic Studies 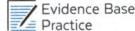 Evidence Based Practice 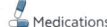 Medications 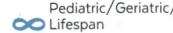 Pediatric/Geriatric/Lifespan

- Caregiver's involvement in infant care, participation in activities, response to teaching
- Attainment of or progress toward desired outcome(s)
- Modifications to plan of care

Discharge Planning
- Long-term needs, referrals made, and who is responsible for follow-up actions

Sample Nursing Outcomes & Interventions Classifications NOC/NIC

NOC—Swallowing Status: Oral Phase
NIC—Swallowing Therapy

---

risk for SUDDEN INFANT DEATH — NANDA-I

[Diagnostic Division: Safety]

Definition: Susceptible to an abrupt and unexplained death in apparently healthy child under one year of age.

Recognizing Cues

Risk Factors
Parents inattentive to secondhand smoke
Infant less than 4 months placed in sitting devices for routine sleep
Infant overheating, or overwrapping
Infant placed in the prone, or side-lying position to sleep
Soft sleep surface; soft, loose objects placed near infant

Clinical Connections
Any child during first year of life

Generate Solutions

Plan Desired Outcomes

Client Will (Include Specific Time Frame)
- Verbalize understanding of modifiable factors.
- Make changes in environment to reduce risk of death occurring from other factors.
- Follow medically recommended prenatal and postnatal care.

Information that appears in brackets has been added by the authors to clarify and enhance the use of nursing diagnoses.

Interventions/Take Action

Nursing Priority No. 1.
To assess causative/contributing factors:
- Identify individual risk factors pertaining to situation, noting presence of Risk Factors, as listed above. **Determines modifiable or potentially modifiable factors that can be addressed.**
- Determine ethnic/cultural background of family. **Although the overall rate of sudden unexpected infant deaths (SUIDs) in the United States declined between 1990 and 2018, statistical reports reveal that disparities in risk factors and SUID rates remain. The Centers for Disease Control and Prevention/National Vital statistics system reports (2024) that SUID rates for American Indian/Alaska Native and non-Hispanic Black infants were more than twice those of non-Hispanic White infants. Rates were lowest for Hispanic and non-Hispanic Asian infants.**
- Note whether mother smoked during pregnancy or is currently smoking. **Many risk factors for sudden infant death syndrome (SIDS) also apply to non-SIDS deaths, and smoking is known to negatively affect the fetus prenatally as well as the infant after birth. It has been reported (2019) that SUID risk more than doubled with any maternal smoking during pregnancy**
- Assess extent of prenatal care and extent to which mother followed recommended care measures. **Prenatal care is important for all pregnancies to afford the optimal opportunity for all infants to have a healthy start to life.**
- Note use of alcohol or other drugs/medications during and after pregnancy. **Research shows that use of tobacco, alcohol, or illicit drugs or misuse of prescription drugs by pregnant women can have severe health consequences for fetus and newborns because many substances pass easily through the placenta. Note: The risk of SIDS was found to be increased 12-fold in infants whose mothers both used alcohol and smoked beyond the first trimester of pregnancy.**

Nursing Priority No. 2.
To promote use of activities to minimize risk of SIDS:
- Emphasize placing infant on back to sleep, both at nighttime and naptime. **Research confirms that fewer infants die of SIDS when they sleep on their backs, not on tummy or side.**

Information that appears in brackets has been added by the authors to clarify and enhance the use of nursing diagnoses.

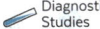 Diagnostic Studies 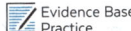 Evidence Based Practice 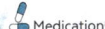 Medications 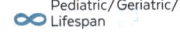 Pediatric/Geriatric/Lifespan

- Advise all caregivers of the infant regarding the importance of maintaining safe sleeping position in own sleeping place with head and face uncovered. **Anyone who will have responsibility for the care of the child during sleep needs to be reminded of the importance of the back to sleep position.**
- Encourage parents to schedule "tummy time" only while infant is awake. **This activity promotes strengthening of back and neck muscles while parents are close and baby is not sleeping.**
- Encourage well-baby checkups and immunizations. **Keeping babies healthy prevents problems that could put the infant at risk for SIDS. Immunizing infants prevents many illnesses that can also be life threatening.** *Note:* **Numerous studies about relationship between SIDS and adverse reactions to vaccines have found no association between SIDS and vaccine receipt.**
- Review benefits of continued breastfeeding, if possible. Recommend sitting up in chair when nursing at night. **Breastfeeding has many advantages (e.g., immunological, nutritional, and psychosocial), promoting a healthy infant. Although this does not preclude the occurrence of SIDS, healthy babies are less prone to many illnesses/problems.** *Note:* **The risk of the mother falling asleep while feeding infant in bed with resultant accidental suffocation could be of concern.**
- Suggest providing pacifier at naptime and bedtime, refraining from placing around neck or attaching to clothing **due to risk of strangulation. Specific mechanism of action is unclear, but studies demonstrate decreased incidence of SIDS with pacifier use.**
- Discuss issues of bed-sharing. **Some of the many concerns include accidental entrapment under a sleeping adult or suffocation by becoming wedged in a couch or cushioned chair. Studies show bed-sharing can increase the risk of SIDS by five times among babies younger than 3 months old. For older babies aged between 3 and 12 months, the risk of dying due to SIDS is three times higher when they share a bed with a parent compared to when they sleep separately in the same room.**
- Note cultural beliefs about bed-sharing. **Bed-sharing is more common among breastfed infants, young**

Information that appears in brackets has been added by the authors to clarify and enhance the use of nursing diagnoses.

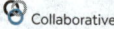 Acute Care 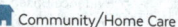 Collaborative Community/Home Care  Cultural

unmarried mothers, low-income families where multiple people share a bed, and those from a minority group.

Nursing Priority No. 3.

To promote positive outcome (Teaching/Discharge Considerations) and enhance well-being (long-term goals):

- Discuss known facts about SIDS with parents. **Corrects misconceptions and helps reduce level of anxiety. SIDS is not preventable, although research indicates that SIDS deaths have reduced since back-sleeping position policy was implemented.**
- Encourage consultation with primary care provider if baby shows any signs of illness or behaviors that concern parent. **Promotes timely evaluation and intervention for treatable problems.**
- Recommend attention to factors below that may help in reducing risk:

    Avoid overdressing or overheating infants during sleep. **Baby should be kept warm, but not too warm. Note: Studies have reported that infants dressed in two or more layers of clothes as they slept had six times the risk of SIDS as those dressed in fewer layers.**

    Place infant on a firm mattress in an approved crib. **Avoiding soft mattresses, sofas, cushions, waterbeds, and other soft surfaces, while not known to prevent SIDS, will minimize chance of suffocation.**

    Remove crib bumper pads, stuffed toys, and fluffy and loose bedding from sleep area, making sure baby's head and face are not covered during sleep. **Minimizes possibility of entrapment and suffocation.**

    Provide pacifier at nap time and bedtime, refraining from placing around neck or attaching to clothing. **Specific mechanism of action is unclear, but studies demonstrate decreased incidence of SIDS with use.**

    Refrain from placing infant under 4 months of age in a sitting position to sleep in commercial devices inconsistent with safe sleep recommendations. **Infant swings with incline angle greater than 10 degrees and/or soft support materials are associated with increased risk of suffocation.**

Information that appears in brackets has been added by the authors to clarify and enhance the use of nursing diagnoses.

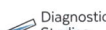 Diagnostic Studies 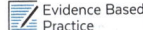 Evidence Based Practice Medications 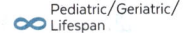 Pediatric/Geriatric/Lifespan

Verify that day-care center/provider(s) are trained in observation and modifying risk factors (e.g., sleeping position) **to reduce risk of death while infant in their care.**

Protect infant and immediate environment from secondhand smoke. **SIDS occurs four times more often in smoke-exposed infants than in those who have a smoke-free environment.**

- Discuss the use of apnea monitors. **Apnea monitors have not proved helpful in preventing SIDS but may be used to monitor other medical problems.**
- Recommend public health nurse or similar resource visit new mothers at least once or twice following discharge. **These early visit programs have demonstrated an improvement in infant safety outcomes.**
- Refer parents to local SIDS programs/other resources for learning (e.g., National SIDS/Infant Death Resource Center and similar websites) and encourage consultation with healthcare provider if baby shows any signs of illness or behaviors that concern them. **Can provide information and support for risk reduction and correction of treatable problems.**
- Recommend monitoring Consumer Product Safety Commission **for commercial products/devices recalled for infant safety.**

Documentation Focus

Assessment/Reassessment
- Baseline findings, degree of parental anxiety/concern
- Individual risk factors

Planning
- Plan of care, interventions, and who is involved in planning
- Teaching plan

Implementation/Evaluation
- Parent's responses to interventions, teaching, and actions performed
- Attainment of or progress toward desired outcome(s)
- Modifications to plan of care

Discharge Planning
- Long-term needs and actions to be taken
- Support systems available, specific referrals made, and who is responsible for actions to be taken

---

Information that appears in brackets has been added by the authors to clarify and enhance the use of nursing diagnoses.

Sample Nursing Outcomes & Interventions Classifications NOC/NIC

NOC—Risk Control
NIC—Risk Identification

risk for accidental SUFFOCATION — NANDA-I

[Diagnostic Division: Safety]

Definition: Susceptible to inadequate oxygen availability.

Recognizing Cues

Risk Factors

Airway Factors:
Inhaling, or swallowing foreign object
Ineffective airway clearance; inadequate airway humidification
Inadequate caregiver knowledge of airway suctioning, or mucous plug prevention
Breathing in excess smoke

Feeding and Eating Factors:
Inadequate chewing before swallowing; swallowing large mouthfuls of food; inappropriate food for age
Does not concentrate on eating; inappropriate posture while eating
Hands-free bottle feeding; inattentive to side-lying chestfeeding
Pacifier attached around neck with string
Inattentive to enteral tube feeding

Sleep Factors:
Sharing sleep surface with others
Sleeping on soft surface; sleeping with soft, or low airflow bedding materials

Play Factors:
Playing with balloon, or plastic bag
Playing in water without adult attendance
Playing near low-hanging clothesline, or in airtight appliance

General Factors:
Inadequate knowledge of, or action to address safety precautions
Inadequate supervision of child [or at-risk individuals]

Information that appears in brackets has been added by the authors to clarify and enhance the use of nursing diagnoses.

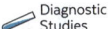 Diagnostic Studies 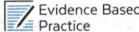 Evidence Based Practice 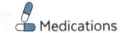 Medications 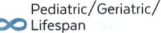 Pediatric/Geriatric/Lifespan

Clinical Connections
Traumatic brain injury, stroke, head/neck trauma, laryngectomy, spinal cord injury, epilepsy, Parkinson disease, depression, substance misuse, overweight, sleep apnea

Generate Solutions

Plan Desired Outcomes

Client Will (Include Specific Time Frame)
- Verbalize knowledge of hazards in the environment.
- Identify interventions appropriate to situation.
- Correct hazardous situations to prevent or reduce risk of suffocation.
- Demonstrate cardiopulmonary resuscitation (CPR) skills and how to access emergency assistance.

Interventions/Take Action

Nursing Priority No. 1.
To assess causative/contributing factors:

- Determine age, developmental level, and mentation (e.g., infant/young child, frail elder, person with developmental delay, altered level of consciousness, or cognitive impairments or dementia) **to identify individuals unable to be responsible for or protect self.**
- Determine client's/significant other's (SO's) knowledge of safety factors or hazards present in the environment **to identify misconceptions and educational needs. Note: Suffocation can be caused by (1) spasm of airway (e.g., food or water going down wrong way, irritant gases, asthma); (2) airway obstruction (e.g., foreign body, tongue falling back in unconscious person, swelling of tissues from burn injury or allergic reaction); (3) airway compression (e.g., tying rope or band tightly around neck, hanging, throttling, smothering); (4) conditions affecting the respiratory mechanism (e.g., epilepsy, tetanus, rabies, nerve diseases causing paralysis of chest wall or diaphragm); (5) conditions affecting respiratory center in brain (e.g., electric shock; stroke or other brain trauma; medications such as morphine, barbiturates); and (6) compression of the chest (e.g., crushing as might occur with cave-in, motor vehicle crash, pressure in a massive crowd).**
- Identify level of concern or awareness and motivation of client/SO(s) to correct safety hazards and improve individual situation. **Lack of knowledge of safety concerns,**

Information that appears in brackets has been added by the authors to clarify and enhance the use of nursing diagnoses.

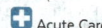 Acute Care 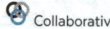 Collaborative 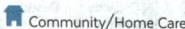 Community/Home Care   Cultural

lack of interest or commitment, unwillingness to make changes, places dependent individuals at risk.
- Assess neurological status and note history/presence of conditions (e.g., stroke, cerebral palsy, multiple sclerosis, amyotrophic lateral sclerosis) **that have potential to compromise airway or affect ability to swallow.**
- Determine use of antiepileptics and how well epilepsy is controlled. **Seizure activity (and especially status epilepticus) is a major risk factor for respiratory inhibition or arrest, particularly when consciousness is impaired.**
- Review medication regimen **to note potential for oversedation and respiratory failure (e.g., central nervous system depressants, analgesics, sedatives, antidepressants).**
- Note reports of sleep disturbance and fatigue; **may be indicative of sleep apnea (airway obstruction).** Refer to NDs Insomnia and Sleep Deprivation.
- Assess for allergies (e.g., medications, foods, environmental) **to which individual could have severe/anaphylactic reaction resulting in respiratory arrest.**
- Be alert to and carefully monitor those individuals who are severely depressed, mentally ill, or aggressive. **These individuals could be at risk for suicide by suffocation (e.g., inhaled carbon monoxide or death by strangling or hanging).** Refer to ND risk for Suicidal Behavior.
- Note signs of respiratory distress (e.g., cough, stridor, wheezing, increased work of breathing) **that could indicate swelling or obstruction of airways.** Refer to NDs ineffective Airway Clearance; risk for Aspiration; ineffective Breathing Pattern; impaired spontaneous Ventilation, as appropriate, for additional interventions.

Nursing Priority No. 2.

To reverse/correct contributing factors:

- Discuss with client/SO(s) identified environmental or work-related safety hazards and problem-solve methods for resolution (e.g., need for smoke and carbon monoxide alarms, vents for household heater, clean chimney, properly strung clothesline, proper venting of machinery exhaust, monitoring of stored chemicals, bracing trench walls when digging).
- Protect airway at all times, especially if client unable to protect self:
  Use proper positioning, suctioning, use of airway adjuncts, as indicated, **for comatose or cognitively impaired individual or client with swallowing impairment or obstructive sleep apnea.**

Information that appears in brackets has been added by the authors to clarify and enhance the use of nursing diagnoses.

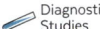 Diagnostic Studies 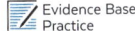 Evidence Based Practice 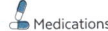 Medications 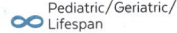 Pediatric/Geriatric/Lifespan

Provide seizure precautions and antiseizure medication, as indicated.

Administer medications when client is sitting or standing upright and can swallow without difficulty.

Emphasize importance of chewing carefully, taking small amounts of food, and using caution **to prevent aspiration when talking or drinking while eating.**

Provide diet modifications as indicated by specific needs (e.g., developmental level; presence/degree of swallowing disability, impaired cognition) **to reduce risk of aspiration or choking.**

Avoid physical and mechanical restraints, including vest or waist restraint, siderails, choke hold. **Can increase client agitation causing struggle to escape, resulting in entrapment of head and hanging.**

- Emphasize with client/SO the importance of getting help when beginning to choke or feel respiratory distress (e.g., staying with people instead of leaving table, make gestures across throat; making sure someone recognizes the emergency) **in order to provide timely intervention, such as abdominal thrusts and calling 911.**
- Refrain from smoking in bed; supervise smoking materials (use, disposal, and storage) for impaired individuals. Keep smoking materials out of reach of children.
- Avoid idling automobile (or using fuel-burning heaters) in closed or unvented spaces.
- Emphasize importance of periodic evaluation and repair of gas appliances and furnace, automobile exhaust system **to prevent exposure to carbon monoxide.**
- Review child protective measures. Refer to ND risk for Sudden Infant Death for interventions relating to infant sleeping safety:

Provide constant supervision of young children in bathtub, swimming pool, other bodies of water.

Make certain that blind and curtain cords, drawstrings on clothing, and so forth, are out of reach of small children **to prevent accidental hanging.**

Prevent young child/impaired individual from putting objects in mouth (e.g., food such as chunks of raw vegetables, nuts and seeds, popcorn, hot dogs; toy parts; buttons; balloons; small balls/marbles; button-type batteries; refrigerator magnets; coins) **that can get lodged in airway and cause choking.**

Lock or remove lid or door of chests, trunks, old refrigerators or freezers **to prevent child from being trapped in airless environment.**

Information that appears in brackets has been added by the authors to clarify and enhance the use of nursing diagnoses.

Nursing Priority No. 3.

To maintain clear airway/adequate air exchange (Teaching/Discharge Considerations) and enhance well-being (long-term goals):

- Review safety factors identified in individual situation and methods for remediation.
- Develop plan with client/caregiver for long-range management of situation to avoid injuries. **Enhances commitment to plan, optimizing outcomes.**
- Review importance of chewing carefully, taking small amounts of food, using caution when talking or drinking while eating. Discuss possibility of choking **because of impaired swallowing or throat muscle relaxation and impaired judgment when drinking alcohol and eating.**
- Promote public education in techniques for clearing blocked airways, back blows, abdominal thrusts (Heimlich maneuver), CPR.
- Discuss fire safety and concerns regarding use of heaters; household gas appliances; and old, discarded appliances. Encourage home fire safety drills yearly.
- Collaborate in community public health education regarding hazards for children (e.g., appropriate toy size for young child); discussing dangers of "huffing" (inhalants) and playing choking or hanging games with preteens; fire safety drills; bathtub rules; how to spot potential for depression and risk of suicidal gestures in adolescents **to reduce potential for accidental or intentional suffocation.**
- Assist individuals to learn to read package labels and identify safety hazards.
- Promote pool safety, use of approved flotation devices, proper fencing enclosure or alarm system for home pools.
- Refer to NDs ineffective Airway Clearance; risk for Aspiration; ineffective Breathing Pattern; impaired Parenting.

Documentation Focus

Assessment/Reassessment
- Individual risk factors, including individual's cognitive status and level of knowledge
- Level of concern and motivation for change
- Equipment or airway adjunct needs

Planning
- Plan of care and who is involved in planning
- Teaching plan

Information that appears in brackets has been added by the authors to clarify and enhance the use of nursing diagnoses.

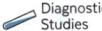 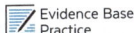 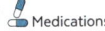 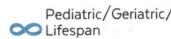

Implementation/Evaluation
- Responses to interventions, teaching, and actions performed
- Attainment of or progress toward desired outcome(s)
- Modifications to plan of care

Discharge Planning
- Long-term needs, appropriate preventive measures, and who is responsible for actions to be taken
- Specific referrals made

Sample Nursing Outcomes & Interventions Classifications NOC/NIC

NOC—Risk Control
NIC—Airway Management

---

risk for **SUICIDE** ICNP

[Diagnostic Division: Safety]

Definition: Susceptible to harming self with intent to die in reaction to excessive stressors or tragic event.

Recognizing Cues

Risk Factors

Behavioral Factors
Mood swings; self-destructive behaviors; using alcohol/drugs; social withdrawal
Inability to ask for help; giving away personal belongings; saying goodbye to people
Preoccupied with death and dying
Change in daily routine; dietary changes; altered sleep pattern; poor personal hygiene
Previous suicide attempts or family members who have suicided
Begun antidepressant medication

Psychological Factors
Anxiety; depressive symptoms; feeling hopeless, worthless, unhappy, trapped, a failure
Angry; frustrated; stressed; personality changes
Wishing had never been born; wanting to be dead; suicidal ideation

---

Information that appears in brackets has been added by the authors to clarify and enhance the use of nursing diagnoses.

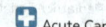 Acute Care 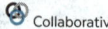 Collaborative 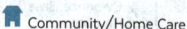 Community/Home Care Cultural

Previous attempts may have residual effects such as permanent or severe injuries causing grief, anger, or guilt

Situational Factors
Access to weapon, or drugs/medications for an overdose
Pressure from peers/family; inability to cope with loss or pressure
Loss of employment; financial problems; loss of housing, transportation, healthcare
Chronic health condition; chronic pain; terminal illness
Conflict with spouse or partner

Social Factors
Family dysfunction; death of a loved one; divorce
Lack of social support, respect; social isolation
Social conflict; legal issues
History of neglect, abuse, or violence

Clinical Connections
Acute or chronic brain syndrome, hormonal imbalances (e.g., premenstrual syndrome [PMS], postpartum psychosis), substance use or abuse, chronic or terminal illness (e.g., amyotrophic lateral sclerosis, cancer), major depression, post-traumatic stress, schizophrenia, bipolar disorder, panic state

Generate Solutions

Plan Desired Outcomes

Client Will (Include Specific Time Frame)
- Verbalize conflict, challenges, and hopelessness perceived with current situation.
- Identify strengths/attributes that can help cope with stressful events.
- Participate in developing plans to cope with concerns and problems.
- Acknowledge suicidal thoughts and feelings are temporary and do not solve the perceived or actual problem.
- Verbalize hope for the future.

Interventions/Take Action

Nursing Priority No. 1.
To assess causative/contributing factors and degree of risk:

- Identify degree of risk or potential for suicide and seriousness of threat. **Information may be obtained from client or significant other (SO) interviews, or over time in the course of care. Note: Most people who are contemplating**

Information that appears in brackets has been added by the authors to clarify and enhance the use of nursing diagnoses.

 Diagnostic Studies   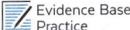 Evidence Based Practice   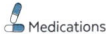 Medications   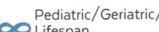 Pediatric/Geriatric/Lifespan

suicide send a variety of signals indicating their intent, and recognizing these warning signs allows for immediate intervention.
- Use a risk scale (where available) to prioritize client risk according to severity of threat and availability of means. **Several risk scales may be used (e.g., Beck's Scale for Suicide Ideation, Linehan's Reasons for Living Inventory, Cole's self-administered adaptation of Linehan's structured interview called the Suicidal Behaviors Questionnaire) to assist in evaluating the severity of risk. Note: In recent years, there have been "several significant changes in how mental health professionals think about, and work with clients who are suicidal. Major modifications include (not a complete listing) (1) acknowledgment that 'traditional' suicide risk factors contribute little to clinicians' suicide prediction and prevention efforts; (2) ongoing clinical encounters and monitoring, including use of comprehensive suicide assessment interviewing protocols; and (3) asking client direct questions about suicide ideation when interviewing." (Sommers-Flannigan, 2017).**
- Note behaviors indicative of intent (e.g., gestures; withdrawal from usual activities or family/friends; presence of means, such as guns; threats; giving away possessions; previous attempts; and presence of hallucinations or delusions). **These are classic behaviors of the individual who is feeling depressed and sad and may be having negative thoughts of worthlessness.**
- Ask directly if person is thinking of acting on thoughts or feelings. **Determines intent. Most people will answer honestly because they actually want help.**
- Note age and gender. **Risk of suicide is greater in males, teens, and the elderly, but there is a rising awareness of risk in early childhood.**
- Determine cultural or spiritual beliefs that may be affecting client's thinking about life and death. **Family of origin and culture in which individual grew up influence attitudes toward taking one's own life. Note: A recent study showed that after other factors were controlled, greater moral objections to suicide and lower aggression level in religiously affiliated subjects seemed to function as protective factors against suicide attempts.**
- Review family history for suicidal behavior. **Individual risk is increased, especially when the person who committed suicide was close to the client.**

Information that appears in brackets has been added by the authors to clarify and enhance the use of nursing diagnoses.

 Acute Care 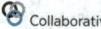 Collaborative 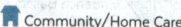 Community/Home Care Cultural

- Identify conditions, such as acute or chronic brain syndrome, panic state, gender identity disorders, post-traumatic stress, hormonal imbalance (e.g., PMS, postpartum psychosis, drug induced) **that may interfere with ability to control own behavior and will require specific interventions to promote safety.**
- Discuss losses client has experienced and meaning of those losses. **Unresolved issues may be contributing to thoughts of hopelessness.**
- Assess physical complaints (e.g., sleeping difficulties, lack of appetite). **Sleeping difficulties, lack of appetite can be indicators of depression and suicidal ideation requiring further evaluation.**
- Determine drug use or "self" medication. **The use of drugs and alcohol, especially the combination of alcohol and barbiturates, increases the risk of suicide.**
- Note history of disciplinary problems or involvement with judicial system. **Feelings of despair over problems with the legal system and lack of hope about outcome can lead to belief that the only solution is suicide.**
- Assess coping behaviors and defense mechanisms presently used. **Client's current negative thinking or the use of defense mechanisms may preclude looking at positive behaviors used in the past that would help in the current situation.**
- Identify presence of SO(s)/friends who are available for support. **Individuals who have positive support systems on whom they can rely during a crisis situation are less likely to commit suicide and are more apt to return to a successful life.**
- Review laboratory findings (e.g., blood alcohol, blood glucose, arterial blood gas, electrolytes, renal function tests) **to identify factors that may affect reasoning ability.**

Nursing Priority No. 2.

To assist clients to accept responsibility for own behavior and prevent suicide:

- Develop therapeutic nurse–client relationship, providing consistent caregiver. **Promotes sense of trust, allowing individual to discuss feelings openly. Collaborating with the client to better understand the problem affirms the client's ability to solve the current situation.**
- Maintain straightforward communication regarding thinking, feeling, and behaviors with depression and suicidal ideation. **By being direct and honest and acknowledging**

Information that appears in brackets has been added by the authors to clarify and enhance the use of nursing diagnoses.

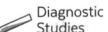 Diagnostic Studies 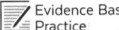 Evidence Based Practice 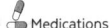 Medications 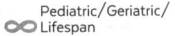 Pediatric/Geriatric/Lifespan

- need for attention, the care provider can avoid reinforcing manipulative behavior.
- Explain concern for safety and willingness to help client stay safe. **Clients often believe their concerns will not be taken seriously, and stating clearly that they will be listened to sends a clear message of support and caring.**
- Encourage expression of feelings and make time to listen to concerns. **Acknowledges reality of feelings and that they are okay. Helps individual sort out thinking and begin to develop understanding of situation and look at other alternatives.**
- Give permission to express angry feelings in acceptable ways and let client know someone will be available to assist in maintaining control. **Promotes acceptance and sense of safety while client is regaining own control.**
- Acknowledge reality of suicide as an option. Discuss consequences of actions if they follow through on intent. Ask how it will help individual to resolve problems. **Helps to focus on consequences of actions and possibility of other options.**
- Maintain observation of client and check environment for, and remove hazards that could be used to commit suicide. Do not leave client alone if expressing "I'm going to kill myself." Do not promise to keep client's suicidal thoughts a secret. **Close observation (e.g., every 15 min or one-to-one with client) increases client safety and may reduce risk of impulsive behavior. Removing potentially harmful objects (e.g., belts, shoelaces, any glass or sharp objects, medications, or any items that could be used to hang self) helps reduce immediate threat.**
- Help client identify more appropriate solutions/behaviors (e.g., motor activities/exercise). **Alternative activities, such as exercise, can lessen sense of anxiety and associated physical manifestations.**
- Provide directions for actions client can take, avoiding negative statements, such as "Do Nots." **Promotes a positive attitude.**
- Discuss use of psychotropic medication, positive and negative aspects. **While the use of medications is often helpful, there are some drawbacks, including the length of time it takes for most medications to take effect and the potential for providing the client a means of suicide.**
- Reevaluate potential for suicide periodically at key times (e.g., mood changes, increasing withdrawal), as well

---

Information that appears in brackets has been added by the authors to clarify and enhance the use of nursing diagnoses.

 Acute Care 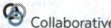 Collaborative 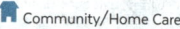 Community/Home Care Cultural as when client is feeling better and discharge planning becomes active. **The highest risk exists when the client has both suicidal ideation and sufficient energy with which to act.**

Nursing Priority No. 3.

To assist client to plan course of action to correct/cope with existing situation:

- Gear interventions to individual needs (e.g., age, relationship, current situation). **Age, relationships, and current situation determine what is needed to help client deal with feelings of despair and hopelessness.**
- Advise client to talk with staff immediately when thoughts of self harm come to mind. **Client's awareness of staffs' concern for client's safety brings an awareness of their concern for the client's well-being and willingness to hear client's thoughts and feelings.**
- Provide directions for client to reframe their negative self-talk into positive attributes of self and make a list to keep available for review if self-talk is not helping. **Providing opportunity for client to have control over circumstances can promote a positive attitude and give client some hope for the future.**
- Assist client to identify a reason to live and to look to the future. **Provides foundation to set meaningful goals and strengthens belief in self.**
- Promote development of internal control. **Helping the client look at new ways to cope with problems can provide a sense of own ability to solve problems, improve situation, and hope for the future.**
- Assist with learning problem-solving, assertiveness training, and social skills. **By learning these new skills, client can begin to feel more confidence in own ability to handle problems that arise and deal with the current situation.**
- Engage in physical activity programs. **Promotes release of endorphins and feelings of self-worth, improving sense of well-being and giving client hope.**
- Determine nutritional needs and help client to plan for meeting them. **Enhances general well-being and energy level.**
- Review use of antidepressants, noting that it takes 4 to 8 weeks for effects of medication to be observed, and different medications may need to be tried to obtain maximum benefit. Stress importance of continuing medication after symptoms of depression resolve to reduce risk of relapse.

Information that appears in brackets has been added by the authors to clarify and enhance the use of nursing diagnoses.

Antidepressants can be effective in quick relief of suffering in severe cases of depression. Studies have shown that cognitive behavior therapy has prevented relapse in 70% more cases than have drugs. In a sample of older adults with depression, the combination of medication and interpersonal psychotherapy was more effective than either alone.
- Involve family/SO in planning. **Improves understanding and support when family knows the facts and has a part in planning for rehabilitation efforts for the client.**

Nursing Priority No. 4.

To promote continued safety and strengthen resilience (Teaching/Discharge Considerations) and enhance well-being (long-term goals):

- Review progress accomplished during treatment. **Client's acknowledgment of accomplishments builds self-esteem and confidence.**
- Encourage continued physical activity programs. **Maintains feelings of self-worth and improving sense of well-being.**
- Include family/SO(s) in discharge planning. **Improve understanding and support when family knows the facts and has a part in planning for rehabilitation efforts for the client.**
- Review use of antidepressants, when prescribed, noting benefits, side effects, and not abruptly stopping the medication due to side effects or when symptoms subside without consulting provider. **Antidepressants can be effective in quick relief of suffering in severe cases of depression, especially in combination with interpersonal psychotherapy; however, abruptly discontinuing medication may result in unpleasant side effects or relapse.**
- Refer to classes/learning opportunities specific to individual needs. **Activities such as assertiveness training, anger management, interpersonal communication classes, developing interpersonal relationships and social skills help client to develop self-esteem, self-confidence, and resilience.**
- Refer to community resources as indicated. **May need referrals to individual, group, or marital psychotherapy, substance abuse treatment program, or social services when situation involves mental illness, family disorganization.**

Information that appears in brackets has been added by the authors to clarify and enhance the use of nursing diagnoses.

 Acute Care 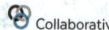 Collaborative 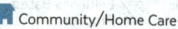 Community/Home Care Cultural

Documentation Focus

Assessment/Reassessment
- Individual findings, including nature of concern (e.g., suicidal/behavioral risk factors and level of impulse control, plan of action and means to carry out plan)
- Client's perception of situation, motivation for change

Planning
- Plan of care and who is involved in the planning
- Details of contract regarding suicidal ideation or plans
- Teaching plan

Implementation/Evaluation
- Actions taken to promote safety
- Response to interventions, teaching, and actions performed
- Attainment of or progress toward desired outcome(s)
- Modifications to plan of care

Discharge Planning
- Long-term needs and who is responsible for actions to be taken
- Available resources, specific referrals made

Sample Nursing Outcomes & Interventions Classifications NOC/NIC

NOC—Suicide Self-Restraint
NIC—Suicide Prevention

---

impaired SURGICAL RECOVERY — NANDA-I

[Diagnostic Division: Health Management]

Definition: Perioperative physiological or psychological alterations extending the recuperation period to achieve and/or enhance preoperative functional health status.

Recognizing Cues

Related/Risk Factors
Excessive anxiety; ineffective health knowledge acquisition
Delirium; negative emotional response to surgical outcome; presumption of unfavorable outcomes

---

Information that appears in brackets has been added by the authors to clarify and enhance the use of nursing diagnoses.

 Diagnostic Studies 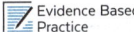 Evidence Based Practice 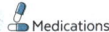 Medications 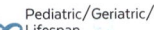 Pediatric/Geriatric/Lifespan

Impaired physical mobility; fear of moving
Increased blood glucose level; malnutrition
Ineffective overweight self-management
Persistent nausea, vomiting, or pain; passive strategies to cope with pain
Tobacco use

Defining Characteristics

Subjective
Difficulty with movement
Physical discomfort; fatigue
Perceives need for more time to recover

Objective
Extended length of hospital stay
Excessive time required for recuperation; requires assistance for self-care
Difficulty resuming activities; postpones resumption of work
Interrupted surgical area healing

Clinical Connections
Major surgical procedures, traumatic injuries with surgical intervention, chronic comorbidity (e.g., diabetes mellitus, cancer, HIV/AIDS, chronic obstructive pulmonary disease [COPD]), postoperative psychosis

Generate Solutions

Plan Desired Outcomes

Client Will (Include Specific Time Frame)
- Display complete healing of surgical area.
- Be able to perform desired self-care activities.
- Report increased energy, able to participate in usual (work or employment) activities.

Interventions/Take Action

Nursing Priority No. 1.
To assess causative/contributing factors:
- Identify vulnerable client (e.g., challenges related to poverty, lack of insurance, or transportation; severe trauma or prolonged hospitalization with multiple complicating factors; client who smokes, is malnourished; or is on steroids or immunotherapy) **who is at higher risk for adverse outcomes.**

Information that appears in brackets has been added by the authors to clarify and enhance the use of nursing diagnoses.

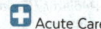 Acute Care   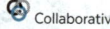 Collaborative   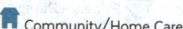 Community/Home Care   Cultural

- Determine extent of surgical involvement of organs or tissues, noting age, developmental level, and general state of health **to help determine time that may be required for client to resume activities of daily living (ADLs) and other activities or expectation of time needed for healing.**
- Note underlying condition or pathology (e.g., cancer, burns, diabetes, hypothyroidism, obesity, steroid therapy, major trauma, infections, radiation therapy, cardiopulmonary disorders, debilitating illness) **that can adversely affect healing and prolong recuperation time. In this population, impaired pulmonary function, hyperglycemia, immobility, and nutritional deficits can compromise wound healing.**
- Determine (1) the length of operative procedure or time under anesthesia (e.g., typical or lengthy); (2) type and severity of perioperative complications (e.g., trauma or other conditions requiring multiple surgeries; heavy bleeding during procedure); (3) type of surgical wound (e.g., clean, clean-contaminated, or grossly contaminated, acutely infected); and (4) development of postoperative complications (e.g., surgical site infection, suture reactions, dehiscence, ventilator-associated pneumonia, deep vein thrombosis) **that can affect the pace of healing or prolong recovery.**
- Evaluate circulation and sensation in surgical area, noting location of incision. **Lack of blood supply at the wound site can slow healing. Note: Areas of the body such as the face and neck receive the most blood supply and heal the fastest, whereas areas such as extremities take longer to heal.**
- Determine nutritional status and current intake **to ascertain if nutrition is adequate to support healing. Client may have preexisting nutritional concerns or may have been fasting perioperatively or have experienced nausea, vomiting, and loss of appetite postoperatively.**
- Review client's preoperative medications/other drug regimen **to ascertain that none could impede healing processes (e.g., aspirin and NSAIDs, chemotherapy agents) or increase bleeding time (e.g., alcohol and some herbals such as garlic and ginkgo biloba can also be associated with bleeding complications).**
- Perform pain assessment **to ascertain whether pain management is adequate to meet client's needs during recovery.**

Information that appears in brackets has been added by the authors to clarify and enhance the use of nursing diagnoses.

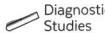 Diagnostic Studies 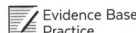 Evidence Based Practice 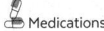 Medications 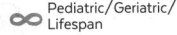 Pediatric/Geriatric/Lifespan

- Evaluate client's cognitive and emotional state, noting presence of postoperative changes, including confusion, depression, apathy, expressions of helplessness **to determine need for further assessment of possible physical or psychological interferences.**
- Ascertain attitudes and cultural values of individual about condition. **Family beliefs and cultural values impact rate and expectations for sick role and recovery.**
- Review results of laboratory tests (e.g., complete blood count [CBC], blood/wound cultures, serum glucose; hormones [e.g., cortisol, glucocorticoid, and other hormones associated with inflammation and immune system dysfunction]) **to assess for presence and type of infections, immunosuppression, metabolic or endocrine dysfunction, or other conditions affecting body's ability to heal.**
- Note allergies or history of skin reactions. Evaluate use of plastics (e.g., incontinence pads or moisture barriers), tape/adhesives, or latex materials. **Client sensitivity to adhesives and/or latex can cause skin or tissue reactions that delay primary wound healing and cause additional skin/tissue damage.** Refer to NDs impaired Skin Integrity, risk for Latex Allergy.
- Note lifestyle factors (e.g., obesity, cigarette smoking, alcohol abuse, lack of exercise/sedentary lifestyle) **that influence circulation and wound healing and can impede recovery.**

Nursing Priority No. 2.
To determine risks or impact of delayed recovery:
- Note length of hospitalization and progress in recovery to date **to compare with expectations for procedure and situation.**
- Determine client's/significant other's (SO's) expectations for recovery and specific stressors related to delay (e.g., return to work or school, home responsibilities, child care, financial difficulties, limited support system).
- Determine energy level and current participation in ADLs. Compare with usual level of function.
- Ascertain whether client usually requires assistance in home setting and who provides it, current availability, and capability.
- Obtain psychological assessment of client's emotional status, noting potential problems arising from current situation.

Information that appears in brackets has been added by the authors to clarify and enhance the use of nursing diagnoses.

 Acute Care 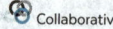 Collaborative 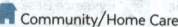 Community/Home Care Cultural

Nursing Priority No. 3.

To promote optimal recovery and reduce risk of complications:

- Inspect incisions or wounds routinely, describing changes (e.g., deepening or healing, wound measurements, presence and type of drainage, development of necrosis).
- Practice and instruct client/caregiver(s) in proper hand hygiene and aseptic technique for incisional care **to reduce incidence of contamination and infection.**
- Administer antibiotics, as appropriate, and medications to manage postoperative discomforts (e.g., pain, nausea, vomiting) and other concurrent or underlying conditions, such as diabetes, osteoporosis, heart failure, COPD. **Several types of medications may be needed. For example, client may require antibiotics perioperatively, insulin to support tissue repair, or management of chronic pain to improve mobility and tissue recovery.**
- Instruct client/SO in necessary self-care of incisions and specific symptom management. **With short hospital stays, client/SO(s) are usually expected to provide a great deal of postoperative care and monitoring at home.**
- Provide wound care expectations and instructions in verbal and written forms **to facilitate self-care and reduce likelihood of misinterpretation of information when client/SO is providing care at home.**
- Instruct client/SO in routine inspection of incision or wound and to report changes in wound indicative of failure to heal (e.g., deepening wound, local or systemic fever, exudates [noting color, amount, and odor], loss of approximation of wound edges) **to establish comparative baseline and allow for early intervention (e.g., antimicrobial therapy, wound irrigation or packing).**
- Avoid or limit use of plastics or latex materials in wound care, as appropriate. **Can delay healing and cause skin breakdown.**
- Collaborate in treatment and assist with wound care, as indicated. **May require barrier dressings, skin-protective agents, wound vac for open or draining wounds, or surgical debridement.** Refer to/include wound care specialist or stomal therapist, as appropriate, **to address treatment interventions to deal with healing difficulties.**
- Provide optimal nutrition with adequate protein **to provide a positive nitrogen balance, which aids in healing and contributes to general good health.**

Information that appears in brackets has been added by the authors to clarify and enhance the use of nursing diagnoses.

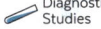 Diagnostic Studies 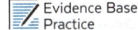 Evidence Based Practice 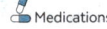 Medications 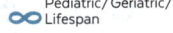 Pediatric/Geriatric/Lifespan

- Encourage adequate fluid and electrolyte intake **to avoid dehydration of tissues and to promote optimal cellular and organ function.**
- Encourage early ambulation and regular exercise **to promote circulation, improve muscle strength and overall endurance, and reduce risks associated with immobility.**
- Recommend pacing activities (alternating activity with adequate rest periods) **to reduce fatigue and allow weakened muscles and tissues to recuperate.**
- Employ nonpharmacological healing measures, as indicated (e.g., breathing exercises, listening to music, relaxation tapes, biofeedback, hot or cold applications) **to promote relaxation of muscles and tissue healing as well as improve coping and outlook for positive healing experience.**
- Refer for follow-up care, as indicated (e.g., telephone monitoring, home visit, wound care clinic, pain management program).

Nursing Priority No. 4.

To promote steady improvement (Teaching/Discharge Considerations) and enhance well-being (long-term goals):

- Demonstrate self-care skills, provide client/SO(s) with health-related information and psychosocial support **to manage symptoms and pain, enhancing well-being.**
- Discuss reality of recovery process in comparison with client's/SO's expectations. **Individuals are often unrealistic regarding energy and time required for healing and own abilities and responsibilities to facilitate process.**
- Involve client/SO(s) in setting incremental goals. **Enhances commitment to plan and reduces likelihood of frustration blocking progress.**
- Refer to physical or occupational therapists, as indicated, **to address exercise program and home-care needs or to identify assistive devices to facilitate independence in ADLs.**
- Identify suppliers for dressings or wound care items and assistive devices as needed.
- Consult dietitian for individual dietary plan **to meet increased nutritional needs that reflect personal situation and resources.**
- Evaluate home situation (e.g., lives alone, bedroom or bathroom on second floor, availability of assistance), where appropriate, **to evaluate for beneficial adjustments, such**

Information that appears in brackets has been added by the authors to clarify and enhance the use of nursing diagnoses.

as moving bedroom to first floor, arranging for commode during recovery, obtaining an in-home emergency call system.
- Discuss alternative placement (e.g., convalescent or rehabilitation center, as appropriate).
- Identify community resources, as indicated (e.g., visiting nurse, home healthcare agency, Meals on Wheels, respite care). **Facilitates adjustment to home setting.**
- Recommend support group or self-help program for smoking cessation.
- Refer for counseling or support. **May need additional help to overcome feelings of discouragement, deal with changes in life, weight management, and/or smoking cessation.**

Documentation Focus

Assessment/Reassessment
- Assessment findings, including wound healing, individual concerns, family involvement, and support factors and availability of resources
- Cultural expectations

Planning
- Plan of care and who is involved in planning
- Teaching plan

Implementation/Evaluation
- Responses of client/SO(s) to plan, interventions, teaching, and actions performed
- Attainment of or progress toward desired outcome(s)
- Modifications to plan of care

Discharge Planning
- Long-range needs and who is responsible for actions to be taken
- Specific referrals made

Sample Nursing Outcomes & Interventions Classifications NOC/NIC

NOC—Self-Care Behavior: Activities of Daily Living (ADLs)/Instrumental Activities of Daily Living (IADL)
NIC—Self-Care Assistance

Information that appears in brackets has been added by the authors to clarify and enhance the use of nursing diagnoses.

risk for SURGICAL WOUND INFECTION NANDA-I

[Diagnostic Division: Safety]

Definition: Susceptible to invasion of pathogenic organisms at location of incision.

Recognizing Cues

Risk Factors
Alcoholism; tobacco use
Ineffective overweight self-management; malnutrition; perioperative hyperglycemia
Perioperative hypothermia, or hypoxia
Unaddressed nasal colonization

Clinical Connections
Surgical procedures, traumatic injuries with surgical intervention, fractures with surgical reduction, joint replacement, comorbidities (e.g., diabetes, hypertension, immunosuppression conditions), amputation

Generate Solutions

Plan Desired Outcomes

Client Will (Include Specific Time Frame)
- Be afebrile and free of signs/symptoms of infection, (e.g., purulent drainage).
- Complete antibiotic therapy as directed.
- Engage in proper wound care techniques.
- Display complete healing of surgical incision.

Interventions/Take Action

Nursing Priority No. 1.
To assess causative/contributing factors:
- Identify client at risk for development of postoperative infections. **Client-related factors are classified as modifiable or nonmodifiable. Modifiable risk factors include alcohol use, smoking, glycemic control (in people with diabetes), obesity, preoperative hypoalbuminemia, and use of immunosuppressive medications.**
- Determine reason for surgical intervention (e.g., trauma, elective joint replacement, traumatic amputation, colon

---

Information that appears in brackets has been added by the authors to clarify and enhance the use of nursing diagnoses.

 Acute Care 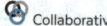 Collaborative 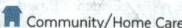 Community/Home Care   Cultural

resection) as well as comorbid conditions (e.g., obesity, current smoking, uncontrolled diabetes/hyperglycemia, advanced age, use of immunosuppressive drugs, poor nutritional status [especially low-protein and albumin levels], renal failure, client being carrier of methicillin-resistant *Staphylococcus aureus* [MRSA] or other antibiotic-resistant bacterium), **that could be a factor in development of postoperative site infections and identify needed interventions.**

Nursing Priority No. 2.
To reduce risk of infection (**perioperatively**):

- Prepare operative site according to specific procedure per agency protocol (e.g., scrubbing with liquid antibacterial soap, swabbing with Betadine or other appropriate prep). **Minimizes bacterial count at operative site.**
- Be aware of the type(s) of surgical wound(s). **Helps in predicting client's risk of surgical site infection (SSI). Note: (1) Superficial incisional SSI: Infection involves only skin and subcutaneous tissue of incision. (2) Deep incisional SSI: Infection involves deep tissues, such as fascial and muscle layers; also includes infection involving both superficial and deep incision sites and organ/space SSI draining through incision. (3) Organ/space SSI: Infection involves any part of the anatomy in organs and spaces other than the incision, which was opened or manipulated during operation.**
- Adhere to all surgical care policies and procedures **to prevent or reduce risks of infections. Note: The Surgical Care Improvement Project (SCIP) measures focus on reduction of surgically related infections through (1) use and timing of prophylactic antibiotics for selected procedures; (2) appropriate hair removal and skin preparation; (3) serum glucose management; (4) perioperative temperature management; and (5) timely removal of urinary catheters.**
- Review laboratory studies **for systemic infections or possible localized infections.**
- Maintain normal client temperature range as much as possible during surgery. **The Centers for Disease Control and Prevention recommends maintaining normothermia in all clients. One study found that patients who experienced mild hypothermia during surgery were three times more likely to have positive cultures from the surgical site.**

Information that appears in brackets has been added by the authors to clarify and enhance the use of nursing diagnoses.

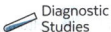 Diagnostic Studies 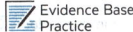 Evidence Based Practice 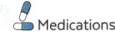 Medications 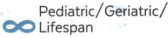 Pediatric/Geriatric/Lifespan

- Identify breaks in aseptic technique and resolve immediately upon occurrence. **Contamination by environmental or personnel contact renders the operative field unsterile, thereby increasing the risk of infection.**
- Insert drain, to evacuate wound bed as necessary, via separate incision distant from the wound; remove the drain as soon as possible.
- Apply sterile dressings and maintain dressings according to facility protocol.
- Administer appropriate antibiotics in timely manner, as indicated. **Antibiotics may be given prophylactically (1) for selected elective surgical procedures; (2) planned in client at high risk for infection; or (3) when procedures need to be performed in the setting of known or suspected wound contamination. SCIP guidelines require the antibiotic to be administered within 1 hr of cut time (any time skin integrity is disrupted, such as in laparoscopic procedures).**

Nursing Priority No. 3.
To reduce risk of surgical site infections (**postoperatively**):

- Obtain information from operating room staff regarding type of procedure performed (clean, contaminated, etc.).
- Determine presence and severity of comorbid conditions that may increase the incidence of SSIs.
- Practice and promote handwashing before and after contact with any client. **Hand hygiene is the single most important factor in the reduction of SSIs. Skin contaminants on the client may be transferred to the caregiver and then passed on to another client if strict adherence to handwashing is not maintained.**
- Perform ongoing assessments: (1) surgical dressing and surrounding areas immediately postoperatively; (2) surgical incision when dressings are removed; (3) assessment of skin surrounding the incision **to evaluate any changes and/or to monitor trends in healing.**
- Protect primary closed incisions with a sterile dressing for 24 to 48 hr (or per surgeon instruction). Use sterile technique for wound dressing change.
- Monitor client's vital signs, and skin color and warmth. **Provides information about systemic tissue perfusion that impacts tissue healing.**
- Monitor laboratory values, such as hematocrit, white blood cell count, serum glucose, serum albumin. **Provides**

Information that appears in brackets has been added by the authors to clarify and enhance the use of nursing diagnoses.

 Acute Care 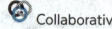 Collaborative 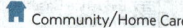 Community/Home Care Cultural

information about fluid and circulatory status, immune and endocrine systems functioning and nutrition needs.
- Administer blood products and fluids, as indicated.
- Administer antibiotics as indicated. **Use of postoperative antibiotics is variable and may be continued (1) if surgical wound was contaminated (either preoperatively or perioperatively); (2) a high risk of infection is associated with the procedure (e.g., colon resection); or (3) consequences of infection are unusually severe (e.g., total joint replacement).**
- Maintain adequate control of serum blood glucose levels in all diabetic clients based on age and situation, and avoid hyperglycemia perioperatively. **Hyperglycemia reduces the body's natural resistance to infection.**
- Provide nutrition by appropriate route (e.g., oral, enteral, parenteral).
- Encourage early ambulation and resumption of activities **to reduce risks associated with immobility and stasis of body fluids.**

Nursing Priority No. 4.
To promote optimal healing (Teaching/Discharge Considerations) and enhance well-being (long-term goals):

- Review client's specific surgical intervention and associated care needs **to promote client's informed self-care and reduce incidence of preventable complications.**
- Instruct client/caregiver in incision care and receive return demonstration, as indicated. **Confirms client/care provider can perform the incision care properly.**
- Review reportable symptoms (postdischarge) such as fever (especially if trending upward), increased pain in surgical site, hardness/redness/warmth of incision, development of drainage or change in character of drainage (e.g., from serosanguinous to blood-tinged pus). **Early intervention may prevent development of serious infectious complications.**
- Advise client to eat nutritious foods and snacks and have adequate fluid intake.
- Instruct client to get adequate rest and to increase activities gradually but steadily as tolerated.
- Ask client about home environment, support, and resources. **May reveal areas of concern (e.g., client unable to provide own incision care; has no access to nutritious food; cannot afford antibiotics).**

Information that appears in brackets has been added by the authors to clarify and enhance the use of nursing diagnoses.

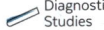 Diagnostic Studies 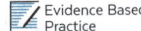 Evidence Based Practice 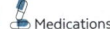 Medications 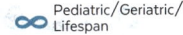 Pediatric/Geriatric/Lifespan

Documentation Focus

Assessment/Reassessment
- Assessment findings, including vital signs, pain level, laboratory results/serum glucose levels
- Character of wound and status of healing
- Self-care ability, family support
- Availability of resources

Planning
- Plan of care and who is involved in planning
- Teaching plan

Implementation/Evaluation
- Responses of client/significant other(s) to plan, interventions, teaching, and actions performed
- Attainment of or progress toward desired outcome(s)
- Modifications to plan of care

Discharge Planning
- Long-term needs and who is responsible for actions to be taken
- Specific referrals made

Sample Nursing Outcomes & Interventions Classifications NOC/NIC

NOC—Self-Management: Wound
NIC—Wound Care

impaired SWALLOWING   NANDA-I

[Diagnostic Division: Food/Fluid]

Definition: Weakened or damaged process of moving substances from the mouth to the stomach.

Recognizing Cues

Related/Risk Factors
Decreased attention
Behavioral feeding problem
Protein-energy malnutrition
Self-injurious behavior

Information that appears in brackets has been added by the authors to clarify and enhance the use of nursing diagnoses.

 Acute Care 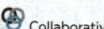 Collaborative 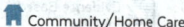 Community/Home Care   Cultural

Defining Characteristics

Subjective

Second Stage: Pharyngeal
Gagging sensation
Food refusal

Third Stage: Esophageal
Volume limiting
Nighttime coughing, or awakening
Feels "something stuck"; odynophagia [pain in esophagus on swallowing]; epigastric pain; heartburn

Objective

First Stage: Oral
Abnormal oral phase of swallow study
Bruxism; inadequate mastication
Choking, coughing, or gagging prior to swallowing; choking when swallowing cold water
Sialorrhea [drooling]; inadequate lip closure
Food falls from, or is pushed out of mouth; impaired ability to clear oral cavity; piecemeal deglutition; nasal reflux
Inadequate consumption during prolonged meal time
Incidence of wet hoarseness twice within 30 sec
Inefficient nippling or suck
Pooling of bolus in lateral sulci; premature entry of bolus; prolonged bolus formation; tongue action ineffective in forming bolus

Second Stage: Pharyngeal
Abnormal pharyngeal phase of swallow study
Altered head position; inadequate laryngeal elevation
Choking; coughing; gurgly voice quality
Delayed, or repetitive swallowing
Fevers of unknown etiology; recurrent pulmonary infection

Third Stage: Esophageal
Abnormal esophageal phase of swallow study
Acidic-smelling breath; regurgitation; vomiting; hematemesis
Hyperextension of head (e.g., arching during or after meals)
Unexplained irritability surrounding mealtimes

Clinical Connections

Brain injury/stroke, neuromuscular conditions (e.g., muscular dystrophy, cerebral palsy, Parkinson disease, amyotrophic lateral sclerosis, Guillain-Barré syndrome), facial trauma, head/neck cancer, radical neck surgery/laryngectomy, cleft

---

Information that appears in brackets has been added by the authors to clarify and enhance the use of nursing diagnoses.

lip/palate, tracheoesophageal fistula, premature infant, gastroesophageal reflux disease, esophageal achalasia, dementia, developmental delays

Generate Solutions

Plan Desired Outcomes

Client Will (Include Specific Time Frame)
- Move food and fluid from mouth to stomach safely.
- Maintain adequate hydration as evidenced by good skin turgor, moist mucous membranes, and individually appropriate urine output.
- Achieve and/or maintain desired body weight.

Client/Caregiver Will (Include Specific Time Frame)
- Verbalize understanding of causative or contributing factors.
- Identify individually appropriate interventions or actions to promote intake and prevent aspiration.
- Demonstrate feeding methods appropriate to the individual situation.
- Demonstrate emergency measures in the event of choking.

Interventions/Take Action

Nursing Priority No. 1.
To assess causative/contributing factors and degree of impairment:

- Evaluate client's potential for swallowing problems, noting age and medical conditions (e.g., Parkinson disease, multiple sclerosis, myasthenia gravis, or other neuromuscular conditions). **Swallowing disorders are especially common in the elderly, possibly due to coexistence of variety of neurological, neuromuscular, or other conditions. Infants at risk include those born prematurely or with tracheoesophageal fistula or lip and palate malformation. Persons with traumatic brain injuries often exhibit swallowing impairments, regardless of age.**
- Determine current situation (e.g., intubation, surgery of head, neck, or jaw; cervical spine injury, vocal cord paralysis, problems with saliva production or management; pain with swallowing; neurological, developmental, cognitive, or psychiatric disorders) **that can affect swallowing. Consequences include problems with oral secretions, nutrition, hydration, quality of life, and social issues.**
- Assess client's cognitive and sensory-perceptual status. **Cognition, sensory awareness, orientation,**

Information that appears in brackets has been added by the authors to clarify and enhance the use of nursing diagnoses.

 Acute Care   Collaborative 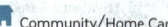 Community/Home Care 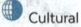 Cultural

concentration, and motor coordination all affect desire and ability to swallow safely and effectively. Also, the muscles of the mouth, pharynx, and upper esophageal sphincter are directly connected to the brain through the cranial nerves and can be weakened in people with neurological disorders.

- Ascertain presence and strength of cough and gag reflex. **Although absence of gag reflex is not necessarily predictive of client's eventual ability to swallow safely, it does increase client's potential for aspiration (overt or silent). Coughing, drooling, double swallowing, decreased ability to move food in mouth, and throat clearing with or after swallowing are indicative of swallowing dysfunction and increase risk for aspiration.**
- Note symmetry of facial structures and muscle tone. Assess strength and excursion of muscles involved in chewing and swallowing.
- Note voice quality and speech. **Abnormal voice (dysphonia) and abnormal speech patterns (dysarthria) are signs of motor dysfunction of structures involved in oral and pharyngeal swallowing.**
- Note hyperextension of head or arching of neck during or after meals or repetitive swallowing, **which suggests inability to complete swallowing process.**
- Determine infant's ability to initiate and sustain effective suck. **Weak suck results in inefficient nippling, suggesting ineffective movement of tongue and mouth muscles, impairing ability to swallow. This problem affects not only the infant's ability to feed but also oral secretion management, increasing risk of overt or silent aspiration.** Refer to ND ineffective infant Suck-Swallow Response.
- Review medications. **Certain drugs can trigger dysphagia or amplify preexisting dysphagia, especially if multiple medications increase the number of side effects on swallowing function. In general, these medications may include (1) drugs that act in the brain (e.g., benzodiazepines, neuroleptics, anticonvulsants, certain sedatives); (2) drugs that act to reduce saliva flow (including but not limited to tricyclic antidepressants and serotonin reuptake inhibitor agents); (3) drugs that affect esophageal and lower sphincter function (including but not limited to glucocorticosteroids, nitrates, neuroleptics, and statins); and (4) drugs that affect esophageal transport ("it gets stuck"; may involve size or coating of pill as well as the active ingredient).**

Information that appears in brackets has been added by the authors to clarify and enhance the use of nursing diagnoses.

- Auscultate breath sounds **to evaluate the presence of aspiration.**
- Inspect oropharyngeal cavity for edema, inflammation, and altered integrity of oral mucosa or structures (e.g., lesions or tumors of the mouth or oral cavity and throat).
- Evaluate state of dentition (e.g., poor or missing teeth, ill-fitting dentures) and adequacy of oral hygiene.
- Review laboratory test results for underlying problems (e.g., complete blood count) **to screen for infectious or inflammatory conditions** or thyroid or other metabolic and nutritional studies **that can affect swallowing.**
- Prepare for or assist with diagnostic testing of swallowing activity (e.g., reflex cough test, swallowing electromyography, transnasal or esophageal endoscopy, videofluorographic swallow studies; fiberoptic endoscopic examination of swallowing) **to identify the pathophysiology of swallowing disorder.**

Nursing Priority No. 2.

To prevent aspiration and maintain airway patency:

- Identify individual factors that can precipitate aspiration or compromise airway.
- Withhold oral feedings until appropriate diagnostic workup is completed to determine client's individual factors causing impaired swallowing and identify specific needs. **Limits complications due to the inability to swallow correctly.**
- Consult with physician or dietitian regarding meeting current nutritional needs. **May need enteral (preferably by peripheral endoscopic gastrostomy tube) or parenteral feedings in order to obtain nutrition, while reducing risk of aspiration that could accompany nasogastric feedings.**
- Move client to chair for meals, snacks, and drinks when possible; if client must be in bed, raise head of bed as upright as possible with head in anatomical alignment and slightly flexed forward during feeding. Keep client seated upright or head of bed elevated for 30 to 45 min after feeding, if possible, **to reduce risk of regurgitation or aspiration.**
- Instruct client to cough and expectorate **when secretion management is of concern.**
- Have suction equipment available during initial feeding attempts and as indicated. Suction oral cavity if client cannot clear secretions **to prevent aspiration.**
- Teach client self-suction when appropriate (e.g., drooling, frequent choking, structural changes in mouth or pharynx). **Promotes airway safety and independence and sense of control with managing secretions.**

Information that appears in brackets has been added by the authors to clarify and enhance the use of nursing diagnoses.

Nursing Priority No. 3.

To enhance swallowing ability to meet fluid and caloric body requirements:

- Consult with physician, speech/language pathologist, dysphagia specialist, gastroenterologist, or rehabilitation team, as indicated. **Various interventions may be implemented for the treatment of dysphagia. For example, disorders of *oral and pharyngeal swallowing* are usually amenable to dietary modification and training in swallowing techniques and maneuvers. Therapies may also include medications, surgery or other procedures.**
- Provide cognitive cues (e.g., remind client to chew and swallow as indicated) **to enhance concentration and performance of swallowing sequence.** Focus attention on feeding and swallowing activity by decreasing environmental stimuli, **which may be distracting during feeding. Also, if client is talking or laughing while eating, risk of aspiration is increased.**
- Encourage a rest period before meals. **Prevents fatigue interfering with efforts.**
- Implement dietary modifications as indicated by type and phase of dysphagia.
- Remain with client during meal **to reduce anxiety and provide assistance as needed.**
- Allow ample time for eating (feeding). Incorporate client's eating style and pace when feeding **to avoid fatigue and frustration with process.**
- Implement dietary modifications as indicated by type and phase of dysphagia:
  Position client on the unaffected side when appropriate, placing food in this side of mouth and having client use the tongue **to assist with managing the food when one side of the mouth is affected (e.g., hemiplegia).**
  Provide proper consistency of food and fluids if oral feedings are determined to be appropriate. **Clients vary in ability to swallow thin and thick substances. Thickened liquids (addition of thickening agent or yogurt, cream soups prepared with less water); thinned purees (hot cereal with water added) or thick drinks, such as nectars or fruit juices that have been frozen into "slush" consistency; and medium to soft boiled or scrambled eggs, canned fruit, and soft-cooked vegetables are most easily swallowed.**
  Feed one consistency or texture of food at a time. **Single-textured foods should be tolerated well before advancing to soft table foods.**

Information that appears in brackets has been added by the authors to clarify and enhance the use of nursing diagnoses.

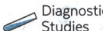 Diagnostic Studies 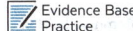 Evidence Based Practice 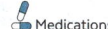 Medications 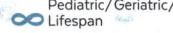 Pediatric/Geriatric/Lifespan

Manage size of bites—use a small spoon or cut all solid foods into small pieces (**e.g., small bites, 1/2 tsp or less, are usually easier to swallow**).

Ensure temperature (hot or cold versus tepid) of foods and fluids, **which will stimulate sensory receptors.**

Feed smaller, more frequent meals **to limit fatigue associated with eating efforts and to promote adequate nutritional intake.**

Avoid pouring liquid into the mouth or "washing food down" with liquid. **May cause client to lose control of food bolus, increasing risk of aspiration.**

Avoid milk products and chocolate, **which may thicken oral secretions and impair swallowing,** and sticky foods (e.g., peanut butter, white bread) **that are difficult to swallow or need fluids to completely swallow.**

Observe oral cavity after each bite, and have client check around cheeks with tongue for remaining or unswallowed food **to prevent overloading mouth with food and reduce risk of aspiration.**

Determine food preferences of client and present foods in an appealing, attractive manner. **Client may make effort to overcome swallowing problems when food is appealing and desired.**

- Provide oral hygiene following each feeding. **Clears mouth of retained food particles and reduces risk of infection and dental caries.**
- Monitor intake, output, and body weight **to evaluate adequacy of fluid and caloric intake and need for changes to therapeutic regimen.**
- Discuss use of enteral or parenteral feedings as indicated, **for the client unable to achieve adequate nutritional intake.**
- Refer to lactation counselor or support group (e.g., La Leche League) **for breastfeeding guidance and problem-solving in infant.**
- Refer to NDs difficulty performing Breastfeeding; ineffective infant Suck-Swallow Response for additional interventions for infants.

Nursing Priority No. 4.

To sustain safe swallowing (Teaching/Discharge Considerations) and enhance well-being (long-term goals):

- Consult with nutritionist/other appropriate practitioners **to establish optimum dietary plan considering specific pathology, nutritional needs, and available resources.**

Information that appears in brackets has been added by the authors to clarify and enhance the use of nursing diagnoses.

- Place medication in gelatin, jelly, or puddings. Consult with pharmacist **to determine if pills may be crushed or if liquids or capsules are available.**
- Refer to ND inadequate Nutritional Intake for related and teaching considerations.
- Assist client and/or significant other(s) (SO[s]) in learning specific feeding techniques and swallowing exercises.
- Encourage continuation of facial exercise program **to maintain or improve muscle strength.**
- Instruct client and/or SO(s) in emergency measures in event of choking **to prevent aspiration or more serious complications.**
- Recommend avoiding food intake within 3 hr of bedtime, eliminating alcohol and caffeine intake, reducing weight if needed, using stress-reduction techniques, and elevating head of bed during sleep **to limit potential for gastric reflux and aspiration.**
- Establish routine schedule for monitoring weight (same time of day and same clothes) and specific weight loss or gain to be reported to primary care provider.

Documentation Focus

Assessment/Reassessment
- Individual findings, including degree and characteristics of impairment, current weight and recent changes
- Nutritional status
- Effects on lifestyle and socialization

Planning
- Plan of care and who is involved in planning
- Teaching plan

Implementation/Evaluation
- Response to interventions, teaching, and actions performed
- Attainment of or progress toward desired outcome(s)
- Modifications to plan of care

Discharge Planning
- Long-term needs and who is responsible for actions to be taken
- Available resources and specific referrals made

Sample Nursing Outcomes & Interventions Classifications NOC/NIC

NOC—Swallowing Status
NIC—Swallowing Therapy

Information that appears in brackets has been added by the authors to clarify and enhance the use of nursing diagnoses.

ineffective THERMOREGULATION   NANDA-I

[Diagnostic Division: Safety]

Definition: Inability to maintain or regulate body temperature within a normal range.

Recognizing Cues

Related/Risk Factors
Inadequate fluid volume
Inappropriate environmental temperature control; inappropriate clothing for environmental temperature
Inactivity; vigorous activity
Increased oxygen demand

Defining Characteristics

Objective
Cyanotic nailbeds; moderate pallor; slow capillary refill
Flushed skin; skin warm, or cool to touch; piloerection; mild shivering
Hypertension; tachycardia; tachypnea seizure
Increased body temperature above normal range; reduction in body temperature below normal range
Seizure

Clinical Connections
Prematurity, central nervous system (CNS) trauma or diseases (e.g., stroke, brain or spinal cord injury, intracranial bleeding or surgery, Parkinson disease, multiple sclerosis); lengthy anesthesia or sedation; prolonged cardiac arrest; infection or sepsis, major surgical procedures; major burns/open wounds

Generate Solutions

Plan Desired Outcomes

Client Will (Include Specific Time Frame)
- Verbalize understanding of individual factors and appropriate interventions.
- Demonstrate techniques and behaviors to correct underlying condition or situation.
- Maintain body temperature within normal limits.

Information that appears in brackets has been added by the authors to clarify and enhance the use of nursing diagnoses.

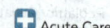 Acute Care 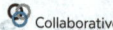 Collaborative 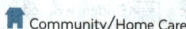 Community/Home Care   Cultural

Interventions/Take Action

Nursing Priority No. 1.
To identify causative/contributing factors:

- Note client's age and developmental level (e.g., premature or very low weight neonate, young child, or aging adult). **Can directly impact ability to maintain or regulate body temperature.**
- Obtain history concerning present symptoms, correlate with previous episodes or family history, and diagnostic studies. **Thermoregulation is a controlled process that maintains the body's core temperature in the range at which most biochemical processes work best (97.7°F to 99.5°F [36.5°C to 37.5°C]).**
- Determine specific factors involved in current temperature fluctuation (e.g., environmental factors [e.g., extreme heat or cold], surgery, infectious process, effects of drugs or toxins, brain or spinal cord injury; behaviors that can increase risk of exposure such as alcoholism, illicit drug use; homelessness). **Thermoregulation is affected in two ways: (1) endogenous factors (via diseases or conditions of body/organ systems that affect temperature homeostasis) and (2) exogenous factors (via environmental exposures, medications, and nutrition).**
- Review client's medications for possible thermoregulatory side effects (e.g., diuretics, certain sedatives and antipsychotic agents, anticholinergics, anticonvulsants, some heart and blood pressure medications, anesthesia).
- Monitor laboratory studies (e.g., tests indicative of infection, thyroid or other endocrine tests, organ damage, drug screens) **to identify potential internal causes of temperature imbalances.**

Nursing Priority No. 2.
To assist with measures to correct/treat underlying cause:

- Monitor temperature by appropriate route (e.g., tympanic, temporal, oral, core), using the same site and device over time and noting variation from client's usual or normal temperature. **Traditionally, temperature measurements have been taken orally (good in alert, oriented adults), rectally (accurate, but not always easy to obtain), or axillary (readings may be lower than core temperature), with each site offering advantages and disadvantages in terms of accuracy and safety. Current technologies allow temperatures to be instantly measured. Tympanic**

Information that appears in brackets has been added by the authors to clarify and enhance the use of nursing diagnoses.

temperature measurement is a noninvasive way to measure core temperature, as blood is supplied to the tympanic membrane by the carotid artery. Abdominal temperature monitoring may be done in the premature neonate.

- Collaborate in treatment of underlying conditions (e.g., sepsis, spinal cord injury, hormonal imbalances, severe malnourishment, dehydration) **that can cause or contribute to body temperature disturbances.**
- Have cooling and warming equipment and supplies readily available during childbirth and following procedures or surgery.
- Initiate emergent and/or immediate interventions, such as cooling or warming measures, fluids, electrolytes, supplemental oral or enteral nutrition, medications (e.g., antipyretics, antibiotics), as indicated, **to restore body temperature within client's usual range, and to optimize organ function.**
- Place newborn infant under radiant warmer, cover infant's head with cap, and use layers of lightweight blankets or occlusive wrap. Provide for skin-to-skin contact with mother as appropriate. **Newborns/infants have temperature instability, especially premature or very low-birth-weight infants. Heat loss is greatest through the head and by evaporation and convection. Skin-to-skin contact helps regulate newborn's temperature and heart rate.**
- Limit clothing or remove blanket from premature infant placed in incubator **to prevent overheating in climate-controlled environment.**
- Instruct care providers to maintain ambient temperature in comfortable range **to prevent or compensate for client's heat production or heat loss (e.g., may need to add or remove clothing or blankets, avoid drafts, reduce or increase room temperature and humidity).**
- Maintain adequate fluid intake. Offer cool or warm liquids, as appropriate. **Hydration assists in maintaining normal body temperature. Note: Ambient temperature affects how much heat is lost through the skin and airways.**
- Ensure that elderly or fragile, high-risk, and debilitated client is evaluated for nutritional deficits, environmental safety, need for social or psychiatric interventions (e.g., need for home health assistance, referral for social services or substance abuse treatment). **Client needs may extend beyond what can be immediately met and require referral for long-term interventions and follow-up.**

Information that appears in brackets has been added by the authors to clarify and enhance the use of nursing diagnoses.

- Review home management of temperature fluctuations especially in risk populations (e.g., newborn infant, person with spinal cord injury, frail elder). **Identifies safety concerns in use of measures such as heating pads, ice bag, radiant heaters or fans; adding or removing clothing or blankets; cool or warm liquids and bath water.**
- Administer fluids, electrolytes, and medications, as appropriate, **to restore or maintain body and organ function.**

Nursing Priority No. 3.

To promote optimal body temperature (Teaching/Discharge Considerations) and enhance well-being (long-term goals):

- Review causative or related factors with client/significant other/caregiver. **Provides information about what, if any, measures can be implemented to protect client from harm or limit potential for problems associated with ineffective thermoregulation.**
- Recommend lifestyle changes, such as cessation of substance use, normalization of body weight, nutritious meals, or regular exercise as indicated **to maximize metabolism and general health.**
- Review home management of temperature fluctuations in special populations (e.g., newborn infant, person with spinal cord injury, frail elder) and possible heating/cooling options. **Older or debilitated persons, infants, and young children typically feel more comfortable in higher ambient temperatures. Women notice feeling cool quicker than men, which may be related to body size or to differences in metabolism and the rate that blood flows to extremities to regulate body temperature. Note: Use of heating pads or ice bags, radiant heaters or fans, cool or warm liquids orally, and bath water, etc., requires close supervision for client safety.**
- Discuss appropriate dressing with client/caregivers, such as:
  Wearing layers of clothing that can be removed or added as needed
  Donning hat and gloves in cold weather
  Using water-resistant outer gear to protect from wet weather chill
  Dressing in light, loose, protective clothing in hot weather
- Review and provide written information concerning client's disease processes, current therapies, and postdischarge precautions regarding hypothermia or hyperthermia, as appropriate to situation. **Allows for review of instructions for**

Information that appears in brackets has been added by the authors to clarify and enhance the use of nursing diagnoses.

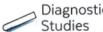 Diagnostic Studies 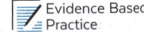 Evidence Based Practice 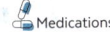 Medications 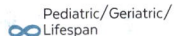 Pediatric/Geriatric/Lifespan

early intervention and implementation of preventive or corrective measures.

- Refer at-risk persons to appropriate community resources (e.g., home care, social services, Foster Adult Care, housing agencies, emergency shelter) **to provide assistance to meet individual needs.**
- Refer to Teaching/Discharge Considerations in NDs decreased Body Temperature, decreased neonatal Body Temperature, or Hyperthermia for related interventions as appropriate.

Documentation Focus

Assessment/Reassessment
- Individual findings, including nature of problem, degree of impairment, or fluctuations in temperature

Planning
- Plan of care and who is involved in planning
- Teaching plan

Implementation/Evaluation
- Responses to interventions, teaching, and actions performed
- Attainment of or progress toward desired outcome(s)
- Modifications to plan of care

Discharge Planning
- Long-term needs and who is responsible for actions to be taken
- Specific referrals made

Sample Nursing Outcomes & Interventions Classifications NOC/NIC

NOC—Thermoregulation
NIC—Temperature Regulation

---

disrupted THOUGHT PROCESS   NANDA-I

[Diagnostic Division: Neurosensory]

Definition: Disturbance in mental processes involved in developing concepts and categories, reasoning, and problem solving.

Information that appears in brackets has been added by the authors to clarify and enhance the use of nursing diagnoses.

NOTE: For clarification, this diagnosis addresses a disruption of thought process and content resulting in disorientation and is not a symptom of a specific disorder. Content includes hallucinations and delusions as may be seen in individuals with schizophrenia, bipolar disorder, anxiety, major depression, etc. Disrupted thought processes may also occur in medical conditions resulting in acute/chronic confusion with treatment focused on the specific cause.

Recognizing Cues

Related/Risk Factors
Acute confusion; disorientation
Excessive anxiety; excessive fear; nonpsychotic depressive symptoms; excessive stress
Maladaptive grieving
Pain; unaddressed trauma
Substance misuse

Defining Characteristics

Subjective
Unreal thoughts; impaired judgment or interpretation of events

Objective
Difficulty communicating verbally
Difficulty independently performing instrumental activities of daily living
Disorganized thought sequences
Inadequate emotional response to situations; difficulty with impulse control
Difficulty finding solutions to everyday situations, or to make decisions
Difficulty planning activities, or performing expected social roles
Obsessions; suspicions

Clinical Connections
Brain injury, cerebrovascular accident, central nervous system (CNS) infections, anorexia nervosa, substance misuse, septicemia, cirrhosis of liver, post surgery, delirium, dementia, schizophrenia, dissociative disorders, paranoid disorder, obsessive-compulsive disorder

---

Information that appears in brackets has been added by the authors to clarify and enhance the use of nursing diagnoses.

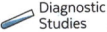 Diagnostic Studies 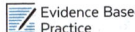 Evidence Based Practice 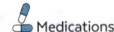 Medications 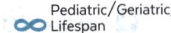 Pediatric/Geriatric/Lifespan

Generate Solutions

Plan Desired Outcomes

Client Will (Include Specific Time Frame)
- Recognize changes in thinking or behavior.
- Identify interventions to deal effectively with situation.
- Maintain usual reality orientation.

Client/Caregiver Will (Include Specific Time Frame)
- Verbalize understanding of causative factors when known.
- Identify interventions to deal effectively with situation.
- Demonstrate behaviors and lifestyle changes to prevent or minimize changes in mentation.

Interventions/Take Action

Nursing Priority No. 1.
To assess causative/contributing factors:

- Identify underlying condition. **Disturbances in thinking can be the result of a wide variety of conditions (e.g., recent stroke, CNS infections; dementias, intellectual disabilities; traumatic brain injury with increased intracranial pressure, anoxic event; acute urinary infections [especially in elderly]; malnutrition, metabolic problems [e.g., acid-base imbalances, diabetes, renal or hepatic failure]; sensory deprivation or overstimulation; toxins, including drug interactions/reactions, drug overdose, accidental exposures; emotional or psychiatric illness [e.g., schizophrenia, bipolar, major depression]).**

- Interview significant other(s) (SO[s])/caregiver(s) to determine client's usual cognitive ability, changes in behavior, length of time problem has existed, and other pertinent information. **Vital to compare present thinking and behaviors with client's history of previous disturbances or if this is the first episode.**

- Identify all prescribed medications, alcohol abuse, illicit or psychoactive drugs, over-the-counter [OTC] medications, use of herbs (e.g., St. John's wort, KavaKava, and Valerian interfere with antidepressants); or elderly client taking three or more medications at one time. **Drugs can have direct effects on the brain, or side effects, dose-related effects, and/or cumulative effects that alter thought patterns and sensory perception, and can create adverse reactions that can be life-threatening.**

Information that appears in brackets has been added by the authors to clarify and enhance the use of nursing diagnoses.

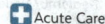 Acute Care 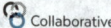 Collaborative 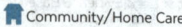 Community/Home Care Cultural

- Note schedule of medication administration. **Evaluating cumulative effects, interactions, or adverse reactions of medications may be indicative of the problem.**
- Assess for presence and severity of pain, as well as use of or need for analgesics. **Both pain and the treatments for pain can diminish the acuity of client's thinking processes. Untreated pain can increase confusion and agitation.**
- Assess dietary intake and nutritional status. **Good nutrition is essential for optimal brain functioning. Persons with anorexia, major depression, substance use, and chronic debilitating conditions may have problems with thinking related to deficits in nutrients, vitamins, electrolytes, and minerals.**
- Evaluate impact of environment. **Excessive noise, multiple people in client's surroundings, chaotic lifestyle, rapid changes in routines, and limited lighting can result in overstimulation/confusion, clouding client's thinking and impairing coping abilities.**
- Monitor laboratory results (e.g., complete metabolic panel, urinalysis/urine drug screen, CBC with differential, thyroid panel, lithium levels). **Abnormalities such as metabolic alkalosis, hypokalemia, hyponatremia, anemia, elevated ammonia levels, infections, drug toxicity for specific medications, illicit drugs, and vitamin B12 and thiamine may be affecting thought processes.**

Nursing Priority No. 2.

To assess degree of impairment:

- Assess baseline for cognitive impairment. **The Mini Mental State Exam (MMSE) is a brief assessment of orientation to person, place and time, immediate recall, short-term verbal memory, calculation, language, and construct ability. Scoring the exam will identify the level of impairment. The MMSE is the tool of choice for a quick assessment in a variety of settings.**
- Complete a more thorough evaluation using Mental Status Exam (MSE) tool as indicated. **The MSE is a comprehensive tool requiring more time to complete and may require a psychiatrist, psychiatric nurse, or trained therapist. If available, compare a previous MSE with the current exam to determine any changes.** Components of the MSE include:

General appearance (e.g., hygiene, speech, eye contact, behaviors, and affect)—**Overall appearance provides an**

Information that appears in brackets has been added by the authors to clarify and enhance the use of nursing diagnoses.

 Diagnostic Studies   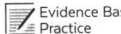 Evidence Based Practice   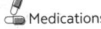 Medications   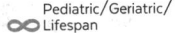 Pediatric/Geriatric/Lifespan impression of whether client is able to attend to activities of daily living. Or is the client's presentation based on their cultural norms? Affect refers to the client's observable emotional reactions and may include lack of emotional response to an event or an overreaction.

Mood—The client's description of how they are feeling (e.g., anxious, angry, irritable) varies depending on how the client is thinking related to the interaction. **Recognizing client's mood guides evaluators' interactions.** Refer to NDs Anxiety; difficulty Coping.

Cognition—**Assesses client's orientation regarding time, place, and personal identity, as well as long- and short-term memory, general intellectual level, ability to think abstractly, and ability to understand and perform a requested task. Note: With a client who is not oriented or has a memory impairment, it will be challenging to determine what concerns them about their health or other issues.** (Refer to NDs acute/chronic Confusion.)

Perception—Confused thoughts may not be based on reality. The perception of something in the absence of external stimuli is a hallucination. On occasion, an auditory or visual hallucination might be considered within the realm of normal depending on cultural and spiritual beliefs (e.g., hearing or seeing a recently deceased loved one). A false or mistaken belief despite evidence to the contrary is a delusion.

Thoughts—**Thought content may reveal hallucination, delusions, obsessions, symptoms of dissociation, or thoughts of self-harm/suicide or harm to others. Thought processes are the logical connection between thinking and their relevance to the main thread of conversation and may be signs of a thought disorder. Depending on the level of thinking to harm self or others, staff may be required to monitor the client every 15 min or provide one-on-one supervision.**

Behaviors—**Context is essential for behavioral evaluation, and the reason for testing may directly affect client's response. Client's behaviors can potentially be harmful and may require close supervision. Also determining client's behavior around and away from caregivers is essential and could indicate issues related to interpersonal relationships.**

Insight and judgment—**Insight refers to a client's ability to recognize a problem and understand its nature and severity. Judgment reveals how a client would respond**

Information that appears in brackets has been added by the authors to clarify and enhance the use of nursing diagnoses.

to a normal event. The client may/may not be aware of changes in these areas and act on their disturbed way of thinking.

- Assist with/prepare client for in-depth diagnostic testing (e.g., MRI, computed tomography [CT] scan, EEG, arterial blood gas, lumbar puncture, ECG). **Disturbed thinking versus confusion can be from issues related to the CNS, metabolic disorders, adverse reaction to medications, infections, cardiogenic shock, overdose/withdrawal, schizophrenia/mood disorders, or traumatic brain injury. Review results to help identify etiology of thinking impairment.**

Nursing Priority No. 3.

To prevent further deterioration, maximize level of function:

- Perform periodic neurological and behavioral assessments, as indicated, and compare with baseline. Note changes in level of consciousness and cognition (e.g., increased lethargy, confusion, drowsiness, irritability; changes in ability to communicate or appropriateness of thinking and behavior). **Early recognition of changes promotes proactive modifications to plan of care.**
- Assist with treatment for underlying problems, such as anorexia; brain injury, increased intracranial pressure; sleep disorders; biochemical imbalances. **Cognition or thinking often improves with treatment and correction of medical or psychiatric problems.**
- Establish alternate means for self-expression (e.g., paper and pencil, or cards showing a variety of emotions or commonly asked questions) if unable to communicate verbally. **Provides way of determining thinking ability.** (Refer to ND impaired verbal Communication for related interventions.)
- Reorient to time, place, and person, as needed. **Inability to maintain orientation is a sign of deterioration.**
- Encourage family/SO(s) to participate in reorientation and provide ongoing input (e.g., current news and family happenings). **Promotes sense of normalcy, maintains contact with family.**
- Stay with client when agitated, frightened. **Support may provide calming effect, reducing anxiety and risk of injury.**
- Identify behavior indicative of potential for violence and take appropriate actions to prevent harm to client/others. **Clients with brain injuries often have lowered impulse**

Information that appears in brackets has been added by the authors to clarify and enhance the use of nursing diagnoses.

 Diagnostic Studies 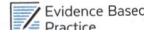 Evidence Based Practice Medications Pediatric/Geriatric/Lifespan

control, problems with anger management, and the potential for violent outbursts, requiring specific interventions designed to help the client learn to control these behaviors. Refer to ND for risk Suicide, or risk for other-directed Violence.

- Provide safety measures appropriate to setting (e.g., door locks, medication safe, side rails, as necessary; close supervision, seizure precautions), as indicated. **May help to prevent accidents and injury to client.**
- Schedule structured activity and rest periods. **Provides stimulation while reducing fatigue.**
- Encourage or provide opportunities for adequate sleep. **Sleep deprivation can increase confusion. Regular sleep routine reinforces the idea of bedtime, and adequate rest can enhance clarity of thinking.** Refer to ND ineffective Sleep Pattern.
- Monitor medication regimen, limit use of sedatives and drugs affecting the nervous system. **Research has shown correlation with episodes of confusion.**
- Refer to appropriate rehabilitation providers (e.g., cognitive retraining program, speech therapist, psychosocial resources, biofeedback, counselor). **May help client to enhance degree of functioning.**

Nursing Priority No. 4.

To create therapeutic milieu and assist client/SO(s) to develop coping strategies—especially when condition is irreversible:

- Manage the milieu (e.g., structure, strategies, support, involvement). **A therapeutic milieu is important in any healthcare setting, promoting and guiding clients/families to understand the specific program/unit purpose, programming, and how to help clients to heal. Communicating with the client/family is critical for understanding what to expect with treatment and safety issues.**
- Provide opportunities for SO(s)/caregivers(s) to ask questions and obtain information. **SOs frequently have difficulty accepting and dealing with client's aberrant behavior and may require assistance in understanding and coping with the situation.**
- Listen with regard to client's verbalizations in spite of speech pattern and content. **Conveys interest and worth to individual, enhancing self-esteem and encouraging continued efforts. Restating and clarifying what you think you heard can help with understanding the client's needs.**

Information that appears in brackets has been added by the authors to clarify and enhance the use of nursing diagnoses.

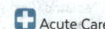 Acute Care 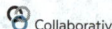 Collaborative 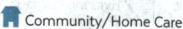 Community/Home Care   Cultural

disrupted THOUGHT PROCESS

- Maintain a calm, quiet environment and approach client in a slow, calm manner. **Client may respond with anxious or aggressive behaviors if startled or overstimulated.**
- Maintain reality-oriented relationship and environment. **Using aids such as clocks, calendars, personal items, and seasonal decorations helps individual maintain current reality.**
- Present reality concisely and briefly and do not challenge illogical thinking. **Helps client stay focused on the present. Client may react defensively if thinking is challenged.**
- Give simple directions, using short words and simple sentences. **Provides for processing of basic communication when thinking is impaired.**
- Reduce provocative stimuli, negative criticism, arguments, and confrontations. **Television programs that are sexual or violent need to be avoided, redirect disrespectful, vulgar, hateful interactions that can result in confrontations, arguments, or violence.**
- Refrain from forcing activities and communications. **Client may feel threatened and may withdraw or rebel.**
- Respect individuality and personal space. **Conveys concern for the person regardless of the circumstances.**
- Use touch judiciously, respecting personal needs and cultural beliefs, but keeping in mind physical and psychological importance of touch. **Touch is a powerful communication tool that can elicit positive or negative reactions. Appropriate touch is defined by family practices, societal expectations, and cultural environment. Always ask permission before touching a client.**
- Provide for nutritionally well-balanced diet, incorporating client's preferences as able. Encourage client to eat. Provide pleasant environment and allow sufficient time to eat. **Enhances intake and general well-being.**
- Provide ample time for client to respond to questions or comments and make simple decisions. **Processing information takes more time when thinking is impaired, and allowing more time promotes communication and client's sense of self-esteem.**
- Inform family/caregiver of the meaning of and reasons for common behaviors observed in client with disturbed thought processes, as well as the probable course of disease process and plan of care. **Helps them to understand and cope with situation and assists them in providing a safe environment for the client.**

Information that appears in brackets has been added by the authors to clarify and enhance the use of nursing diagnoses.

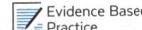 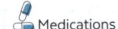

- Support client/SO(s) with grieving process for loss of self or abilities, as in Alzheimer disease. **Progressive loss of mental abilities is difficult for family members to deal with as they grieve the loss of the person they knew. Providing opportunity for individuals to talk about feelings of grief will promote coping abilities.** Refer to NDs Grief or dysfunctional Grief as appropriate for additional interventions.
- Encourage participation in resocialization activities and groups when available. **Can help the individual maintain or regain some degree of social skills. Even in conditions of dementia, client can benefit from these activities.**

Nursing Priority No. 5.

To promote and maintain physical and mental stability (Teaching/Discharge Considerations) and enhance well-being (long-term goals):

- Assist in identifying ongoing treatment needs or rehabilitation program for the individual. **Important to maintain gains and continue progress if able.**
- Promote socialization with individual limitations. **Client may have difficulty tolerating large (or even small) groups of people and unfamiliar or noisy surroundings.** Refer to ND Sensory Deficit [specify: visual, auditory, kinesthetic, gustatory, tactile, olfactory].
- Identify problems related to aging that are remediable, and assist client/SO(s) to seek appropriate assistance and access resources. **Encourages problem-solving to improve condition when possible rather than accept the status quo.**
- Help client/SO(s) develop plan of care when problem is progressive or long term. **Advance planning addressing home care, transportation, assistance with care activities, support and respite for caregivers enhances management of client in home setting.** Refer to ND excessive Caregiving Burden; Self-Care Deficit [specify] for related interventions.
- Refer to community resources (e.g., day-care programs, support groups, drug or alcohol rehabilitation, mental health treatment programs). **Client/caregivers will need assistance and support that maintains a healthy and stable home environment.**
- Refer to NDs acute Confusion; chronic Confusion; impaired Memory; Self-Care Deficit; dysfunctional Grief; Sensory Deficit [specify: visual, auditory, kinesthetic, gustatory, tactile, olfactory], as appropriate, for additional interventions.

Information that appears in brackets has been added by the authors to clarify and enhance the use of nursing diagnoses.

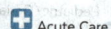 Acute Care 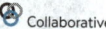 Collaborative 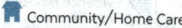 Community/Home Care   Cultural

Documentation Focus

Assessment/Reassessment
- Individual findings, including nature of problem, current and previous level of function, effect on independence and lifestyle
- Results of laboratory tests, diagnostic studies, and mental status or cognitive evaluations
- SO/family support and participation
- Availability and use of resources

Planning
- Plan of care and who is involved in planning
- Teaching plan

Implementation/Evaluation
- Response to interventions, teaching, and actions performed
- Attainment of or progress toward desired outcome(s)
- Modifications to plan of care

Discharge Planning
- Long-term needs and who is responsible for actions to be taken
- Available resources, specific referrals made

Sample Nursing Outcomes & Interventions Classifications NOC/NIC

NOC—Distorted Thought Self-Control
NIC—Dementia Management

---

risk for THROMBOSIS   NANDA-I

[Diagnostic Division: Circulation]

Definition: Susceptible to obstruction of a blood vessel by a blood clot that can break off and lodge in another vessel.

Recognizing Cues

Risk/Related Factors
Atherogenic diet; inadequate fluid volume
Inadequate knowledge of modifiable factors; ineffective management of preventive measures; ineffective medication self-management

---

Information that appears in brackets has been added by the authors to clarify and enhance the use of nursing diagnoses.

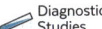 Diagnostic Studies 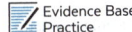 Evidence Based Practice 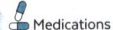 Medications 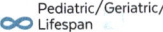 Pediatric/Geriatric/Lifespan

Ineffective overweight self-management; sedentary behaviors; impaired physical mobility; tobacco use

Excessive stress

Clinical Connections

Cerebrovascular accident, cancer, pelvic trauma, upper or lower extremity fracture or crush injuries, orthopedic surgery, varicose veins, infection, sickle cell crisis

Generate Solutions

Plan Desired Outcomes

Client Will (Include Specific Time Frame)

- Identify individual risk factors.
- Develop plan to reduce risk factors.
- Engage in activities/lifestyle changes to prevent thrombus/thromboembolism.
- Be free of signs/symptoms of thrombosis (e.g., extremity pulses/capillary refill equal bilaterally, free of erythema, edema, pain).

Interventions/Take Action

Nursing Priority No. 1.

To identify causative/risk factors:

- Identify predisposing factors including past history of venous thromboembolism (VTE) or cessation of recent anticoagulant therapy; or (2) predisposing factors (e.g., major surgery [especially orthopedic], trauma, extended travel; prolonged immobilization for any cause; spinal cord injury; pregnancy [especially when pregnant client has gestational hypertension, preeclampsia or eclampsia, amniotic fluid embolism]; use of oral contraceptives; valvular heart disease, heart failure, stroke; certain cancers or ongoing cancer treatments; clients requiring critical care for extended periods, indwelling central venous catheter use [especially in children]). **Studies have revealed that while the mechanisms for the development of venous or arterial thrombi are different, the development of venous thrombi is mainly attributable to venous stasis.**
- Evaluate client reports of calf pain or chest pain or shortness of breath. **Symptoms that can be associated with VTE event.**

Information that appears in brackets has been added by the authors to clarify and enhance the use of nursing diagnoses.

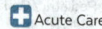 Acute Care 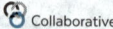 Collaborative 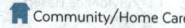 Community/Home Care   Cultural

- Assess and identify client's cardiac rhythm **to assess for thrombogenic dysrhythmias (e.g., atrial fibrillation).**
- Examine all extremities in at-risk client **for signs potentially associated with development of deep vein thrombosis (DVT), such as asymmetry, edema, changes in skin color, pain, obvious tissue injury, prominent veins.**
- Assess client's pulmonary function (i.e., respiratory rate, pulse oximetry, dyspnea/reports of shortness of breath, accessory muscle use, cough, and sputum characteristics) **to evaluate potential pulmonary embolus.**
- Review results of laboratory studies (D-dimer assay [most frequently used screening test]; coagulation profiles, platelet function studies). **Abnormalities in these tests (and others) point toward conditions associated with VTE, such as dehydration or clotting defects or other thrombotic processes.**

Nursing Priority No. 2.
To reduce risk/prevent VTE:

- Initiate active or passive exercises while in bed or chair; for example, flex, extend, and rotate ankles periodically.
- Promote early ambulation after any acute illness, surgery, or trauma.
- Elevate legs when in bed or chair as indicated **to reduce edema and promote venous return.**
- Caution client to avoid crossing legs or hyperflexing knee, such as when in seated position with legs dangling or lying in jackknife position.
- Increase fluid intake to at least 1,500 to 2,000 mL/day, within cardiac tolerance.
- Apply elastic support hose, compression stockings, or sequential compression devices, if indicated.
- Collaborate in treatment of underlying conditions **to manage/treat conditions that can cause or exacerbate risk of thromboembolism.**
- Provide DVT prophylaxis protocol, if indicated, and progressive mobility protocol where available. **The use of chemoprophylaxis (e.g., heparin, enoxaparin, etc.) is associated with a significant reduction in the risk of VTE. Initiation early during hospitalization in patients at high risk for the development of VTE is considered standard of care.**

Information that appears in brackets has been added by the authors to clarify and enhance the use of nursing diagnoses.

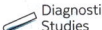 Diagnostic Studies 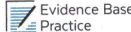 Evidence Based Practice 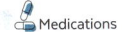 Medications 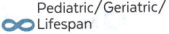 Pediatric/Geriatric/Lifespan

Nursing Priority No. 3.

To promote circulation/venous return (Teaching/Discharge Considerations) and enhance well-being (long-term goals):

- Instruct client/significant other (SO) about client's particular condition and risk factors.
- Recommend continuation of prescribed treatments, exercises, and other measures to prevent immobility and stasis of body fluids.
- Review position recommendations, such as sitting with feet touching the floor and avoiding crossing of legs. **Prevents excess pressure on the popliteal space and enhances venous return.**
- Problem-solve solutions to predisposing factors that may be present, such as employment that requires prolonged standing or sitting, wearing restrictive clothing, use of oral contraceptives, obesity, prolonged immobility, smoking, and dehydration. **Actively involves client in identifying and initiating lifestyle and behavior changes to promote health and prevent occurrence/recurrence of condition or development of complications.**

Documentation Focus

Assessment/Reassessment
- Individual risk factors identified, physical findings
- Client/SO knowledge of modifiable risk factors and concerns

Planning
- Plan of care and who is involved in planning
- Teaching plan

Implementation/Evaluation
- Response to interventions, teaching, and actions performed
- Attainment of or progress toward outcome(s)
- Modifications to plan

Discharge Planning
- Referrals to other resources
- Long-term need and who is responsible for actions

Sample Nursing Outcomes & Interventions Classifications NOC/NIC

NOC—Knowledge: Thrombus Threat Reduction
NIC—Embolus Precautions

Information that appears in brackets has been added by the authors to clarify and enhance the use of nursing diagnoses.

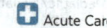 Acute Care 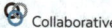 Collaborative 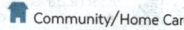 Community/Home Care 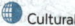 Cultural

impaired TISSUE INTEGRITY NANDA-I

[Diagnostic Division: Safety]

Definition: Damage to the mucous membrane, cornea, integumentary system, muscular fascia, muscle, tendon, blood vessels, lymphatic tissue, bone, cartilage, joint capsule, and/or ligament.

Recognizing Cues

Related/Risk Factors

External Factors
Excretions; secretions
Exposure to environmental temperature extremes
Inadequate caregiver knowledge about maintaining or protecting tissue integrity
Inappropriate use of chemical agent
Pressure over bony prominence; shearing forces; surface friction
Use of linen with insufficient moisture-wicking property

Internal Factors
Underweight for age and gender; ineffective overweight self-management
Decreased blinking frequency
Decreased physical activity
Impaired physical mobility or postural balance
Fluid imbalance; malnutrition
Inadequate adherence to incontinence treatment regimen; inadequate ostomy care
Inadequate blood glucose level management
Inadequate knowledge about maintaining or restoring tissue integrity
Psychogenic factor; psychomotor agitation; self-directed violence
Tobacco use; substance misuse

Defining Characteristics

Subjective
Acute pain; stiffness
Localized numbness; tingling sensation

Information that appears in brackets has been added by the authors to clarify and enhance the use of nursing diagnoses.

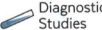 Diagnostic Studies 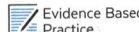 Evidence Based Practice 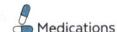 Medications 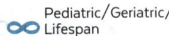 Pediatric/Geriatric/Lifespan

Objective
Abscess; excessive exudate; localized area hot to touch; persistent erythema

Bleeding; hematoma; localized swelling

Muscle weakness, or spasm; decreased range of motion; inadequate balance; difficulty bearing weight

Dry eye

Altered skin color; impaired skin integrity; nonviable tissue

Localized deformity, or loss of hair

Tissue exposure below epidermis; pressure injury; abnormal tissue growth

> [NOTE: In reviewing this ND, it is apparent there is much overlap with other diagnoses. We have chosen to present generalized interventions. Although there are commonalities to injury situations, we suggest that the reader refer to other primary diagnoses as indicated, such as Contamination Exposure; risk for corneal Injury; risk for Dry Eye; risk for [adult/child] Fall; ineffective Health Maintenance Behaviors; impaired physical Mobility; impaired oral Mucous Membrane; impaired Skin Integrity; adult/child/neonate Pressure Injury; ineffective peripheral Tissue Perfusion for additional interventions.

Clinical Connections
Abscess, abuse (physical); traumatic injuries, stroke, paralysis, amputation, anemias, burns, cataracts, deep vein thrombosis; diabetes; falls, frostbite; glaucoma, Parkinson disease, poisoning, substance misuse, malnutrition, vascular occlusive disease, shock, premature infant, hospice

Generate Solutions

Plan Desired Outcomes

Client Will (Include Specific Time Frame)
- Verbalize understanding of condition and causative **or risk** factors.
- Identify interventions appropriate for specific condition.
- Demonstrate behaviors and lifestyle changes to promote healing and prevent complications or recurrence.
- Display progressive improvement in wound or lesion healing if present.

Information that appears in brackets has been added by the authors to clarify and enhance the use of nursing diagnoses.

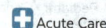 Acute Care 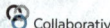 Collaborative 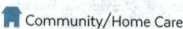 Community/Home Care Cultural

Interventions/Take Action

Nursing Priority No. 1.
To identify causative/contributing factors:

- Identify/investigate underlying conditions to assess for individual factors **that may result in tissue damage or can impede healing, such as:**
  Trauma that causes internal tissue damage (e.g., burns, high-velocity and penetrating trauma) and fractures (especially long-bone fractures) with bleeding
  External pressures (e.g., from tight dressings, splints or casting, burn eschar)
  Immobility (e.g., long-term bedrest)
  Conditions affecting peripheral circulation and sensation (e.g., atherosclerosis, diabetes, venous insufficiency, spinal cord injury)
  Lifestyle factors (e.g., smoking, obesity, sedentary lifestyle)
  Use of medications (e.g., anticoagulants, corticosteroids, immunosuppressives, antineoplastics, vasopressors) that may adversely affect healing
  Malnutrition (deprives the body of protein, calories, and/or nutrients required for cell growth and repair)
  Dehydration (impairs transport of oxygen and nutrients)
- ∞ Consider age, developmental stage, and ability to care for self. **The skin and underlying structures (i.e., subcutaneous fat, muscle) of the very young or older client are thinner and more fragile than the tissues of an adult. Infants, children, young adults, and elderly persons are at greater risk for injury. These factors may impact the client's ability to assess for a problem or prevent self-harm and influence the choice of interventions and teaching.**
- Determine the mechanism of injury where indicated (e.g., chemical burn, electrical/high-voltage injury, motor vehicle accident, gunshot wound, environmental exposure to toxins, or extreme temperatures). **Suggests initial treatment options and potential for tissue damage. Note: Information should include the type, route, and length of exposure to offending agent and possibility of coexisting injuries.**
- Evaluate tissue perfusion by (1) assessing skin and mucous membranes for color (i.e., appropriate for race versus pale or cyanotic); (2) temperature (i.e., warm versus cool);

impaired TISSUE INTEGRITY

Information that appears in brackets has been added by the authors to clarify and enhance the use of nursing diagnoses.

 Diagnostic Studies   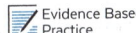 Evidence Based Practice   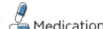 Medications   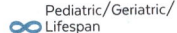 Pediatric/Geriatric/Lifespan

983

(3) skin sensation (e.g., presence of numbness, lack of vibratory sense, etc.); (4) pulses; and (5) calculating ankle-brachial index (ABI) **to evaluate actual or potential for impairment of circulation to lower extremities. An ABI less than 0.9 indicates the need for close monitoring or more aggressive interventions (e.g., tighter blood glucose, weight control, exercise plan, smoking cessation, dietary modifications [low-fat, low-sodium, low-cholesterol diet]). Regular evaluation of an extremity following a fracture is particularly relevant to assess for signs of acute compartment syndrome (e.g., pain [particularly with passive stretch], feeling of tightness/swelling, numbness/tingling, etc.).** Refer to NDs risk for peripheral Neurovascular Dysfunction and ineffective peripheral Tissue Perfusion.

- Evaluate hydration status including skin and mucous membranes (e.g., moist versus dry); note the presence and degree of edema, as needed (nonpitting, or pitting 1+ to 4+); and urine characteristics (e.g., volume of urine, color, clarity). **Determines the presence of circulatory or metabolic imbalances resulting in fluid deficit or overload that can adversely affect cell or tissue health and organ function. Recent evidence strongly suggests the correlation between inadequate fluid intake and kidney disease (e.g., urolithiasis, nephropathy, and chronic kidney disease). Note: Edematous tissues are prone to breakdown.** Refer to ND risk for impaired Fluid Volume Balance.

- Assess client's eyes for conjunctivitis, hemorrhage, burns, abrasions, or lacerations as indicated. Note reports of dry, scratchy eye(s), light sensitivity, vision impairment, or pain. **May indicate injury requiring more intensive evaluation and interventions.**

- Consider race, ethnicity, and family history for genetic factors **that may make the client vulnerable to particular conditions (e.g., sickle cell disease, systemic lupus erythematosus, Marfan syndrome)** and cultural or religious beliefs (e.g., use of folk remedies) or customs **that may damage tissues or impact the client's choice of treatment options.**

- Consider nutritional status and impact of malnutrition on the client's condition (e.g., pressure points on an emaciated client, obesity, lack of activity, slow healing or failure to heal).

- Evaluate client's health and safety practices, noting lack of personal hygiene (e.g., body odor, poor oral care, lack of foot and toenail care), unsafe sexual practices, failure to use

---

Information that appears in brackets has been added by the authors to clarify and enhance the use of nursing diagnoses.

safety equipment (i.e., for occupational or sports-related activities), unprotected excessive sun exposure or self-exposure to toxic substances **that can place the client at risk for tissue injury or impaired function.**
- Note use of prosthetic or external devices (e.g., artificial limbs, contacts, dentures, endotracheal airways, indwelling catheters, esophageal dilators, etc.), **which can cause injury to delicate tissues and provide a point of entry for infection.**

Nursing Priority No. 2.
To assess degree of impairment:

- Obtain a history of client's condition (e.g., pressure injury, venous ulcer, diabetic wound, eye, oral lesions, abscess, etc.), including whether the condition is acute or chronic, original site, wound characteristics, duration of problem, impact on activities of daily living, and changes that have occurred over time.
- Determine psychological effects of the condition on the client and family. **Wounds/tissue injury can be devastating for the client's self-image and esteem—especially if the condition is severe, disfiguring, or chronic—as well as costly and burdensome for the significant other/caregiver.**
- Assess skin and tissues for areas at risk for injury or wound progression (e.g., bony prominences, pressure areas) by noting color, texture, and turgor changes **for comparative baseline:**

  Assess areas of least pigmentation for color changes (e.g., sclera, conjunctiva, nailbeds, buccal mucosa, tongue, palms, and soles of feet).

  Assess wound/lesion, documenting (1) location; (2) dimensions and depth in centimeters; (3) exudates—color, odor, consistency, and amount; (4) margins (i.e., wound edges are flush with wound base/flat, or wound walls are present/floor of wound is deeper than the edge); (5) tunneling/tracts **(full extent of lesions may not be visually discernible)**; and (6) evidence of necrosis (e.g., color gray to black, dry, leathery) or healing (e.g., pink or red granulation tissue, moist) **to establish a comparative baseline and evaluate effectiveness of interventions.**

  Identify and stage pressure injuries using a classification system (e.g., National Pressure Injury Advisory Panel [NPIAP] Pressure Injury Stages, Braden risk scale, Braden Q, Braden QD, or similar scale). (See NDs risk

---

Information that appears in brackets has been added by the authors to clarify and enhance the use of nursing diagnoses.

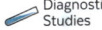 Diagnostic Studies 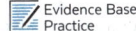 Evidence Based Practice 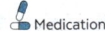 Medications 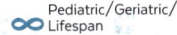 Pediatric/Geriatric/Lifespan

for adult, child, neonatal Pressure Injury.) **Using the susceptibility factors of sensory perception, skin moisture, activity, mobility, nutritional status, friction, and shear potential, the client's risk can be quickly determined. Note: The term "pressure ulcer" continues to be used widely in clinical areas, however, "pressure injury" better describes the variety of injuries that may demonstrate injury yet intact skin. NPIAP recommends the term "pressure injury" given that open ulceration does not always occur.**

Document progression or failure of wound healing. **The most common method of monitoring utilizes photography and diagrams. Additionally, consistent utilization of an evidence-based skin integrity risk assessment tool (e.g., Braden, etc.) may improve continuity of care through caregiver communication.**

- Review diagnostic studies (e.g., x-rays, computed tomography, bone scans, biopsies, MRI) **to visualize tissue injury. May be necessary to determine extent of impairment.**

- Obtain specimens of exudate and lesions for Gram stain, culture and sensitivity, when appropriate **to identify effective antimicrobial therapies.**

- Review and monitor laboratory studies (e.g., hemoglobin/hematocrit, white blood cell count with differential, electrolytes, glucose, blood and/or wound cultures, albumin, prealbumin, hemoglobin A_{1C}, and lipid studies [as needed]) **to evaluate causative factors or ability to heal. May demonstrate systemic changes indicative of infection or other systemic complications. Note: Evidence suggests serum albumin less than 3.5 correlates to decreased wound healing and increased incidence of pressure ulcers. However, albumin levels may be impacted by inflammation and other factors dependent on the client's condition. For this reason, additional laboratory values and assessments, such as serum prealbumin (i.e., less than 10 mg/dL may be associated with malnutrition) should be used to evaluate the client's nutritional status.**

Nursing Priority No. 3.

To facilitate healing:

- Modify or eliminate factors contributing to client's condition, if possible. Assist with treatment of underlying condition(s), as appropriate.

- Provide or encourage optimum nutrition (including adequate protein, lipids, calories, trace minerals, and multivitamins

---

Information that appears in brackets has been added by the authors to clarify and enhance the use of nursing diagnoses.

[vitamin C, zinc, B-complex vitamins, vitamin E, copper]) **to promote tissue health/healing. Nutrients should include adequate protein for tissue/organ maintenance, growth and repair, good immune function, and hormone production. High-quality fats improve energy production and reduce inflammation. Good-quality carbohydrates provide immediate energy, stable blood sugar and insulin levels. Note: Adequate calories and protein are a primary focus for each phase of wound healing.**

- Provide/encourage adequate hydration **to reduce cellular water loss and replenish fluid to enhance circulation. Note: Dehydration can impair tissue perfusion to a wound site by reducing the blood volume, thus limiting the supply of oxygen and nutrients.**
- Provide or assist with oral care (e.g., teaching oral and dental hygiene, changing position of nasogastric tubes, lubricating lips, etc.) **to prevent damage to mucous membranes.** Refer to ND impaired oral Mucous Membrane for related interventions.
- Encourage adequate periods of rest and sleep **to promote healing and meet comfort needs.**
- Promote early and ongoing mobility. Assist with/encourage position changes, active, passive, and assistive exercises in immobile client **to promote circulation and prevent excessive tissue pressure.**
- Incisions/wounds
- Inspect wounds daily for signs of infection (e.g., erythema, edema, pain, odorous drainage, warmth) **to promote timely intervention and revision of the plan of care.**
- Practice and instruct client/caregiver(s) in scrupulous hand hygiene and clean or sterile technique **to reduce the incidence of contamination or infection.**
- Keep surgical area(s) clean and dry, carefully dress wounds, and support incision (e.g., use of Steri-Strips, splinting when coughing) **to prevent wound dehiscence or further injury.**
- Use body temperature physiological solutions (e.g., isotonic saline) **to clean or irrigate wounds and prevent washout of electrolytes.**
- Cleanse wound with irrigation syringe or gauze squares, avoiding cotton balls or other products **that shed fibers.**
- Maintain appropriate moisture environment according to wound needs (e.g., leave wound open to air and light if excess moisture is impeding healing, use occlusive dressings to maintain a moist environment) as indicated.

Information that appears in brackets has been added by the authors to clarify and enhance the use of nursing diagnoses.

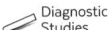 Diagnostic Studies 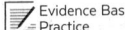 Evidence Based Practice 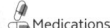 Medications 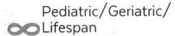 Pediatric/Geriatric/Lifespan

Moisture-associated skin damage (MASD) is multifactorial; too much moisture causes erosion of skin layers, promotes bacterial proliferation, and impairs the skin's compensatory and healing mechanisms. However, appropriate wound moisture is necessary for cell growth and health.

- Use appropriate dressings (e.g., semipermeable, occlusive, wet-to-moist, DuoDERM, Tegaderm, hydrocolloid, hydrofiber or gel, hydropolymers, etc.), drainage appliances, and skin-protective agents for open or draining wounds and stomas **to protect the wound and surrounding tissues from excoriating, drainage, and to promote wound healing. Note: Recent studies report wet-to-dry dressings are beneficial only for mechanical debridement of wounds, yet can damage healthy granulation tissue, and can increase the risk of infection.**
- Administer topical or systemic drugs as indicated **for condition.**
- Collaborate with other healthcare providers (e.g., physician, nurse practitioner, burn specialist, ophthalmologist, infection or wound specialist, ostomy nurse), as indicated, **to assist with developing plan of care for problematic or potentially serious wounds. Note: A general surgeon or burn specialist/burn center may be needed for burns (especially burns to hands, face, or perineum). Ophthalmological consultation is recommended for clients with ocular burns from acids or bases if there is any significant degree of corneal or scleral injury. Caustic ingestions may require multiple specialties, including gastroenterology, gastrointestinal surgery, ear, nose, and throat.**
- Assist with debridement (e.g., mechanical or sharp, as indicated) or enzymatic therapy as indicated (e.g., burns, skin tears, severe pressure sores) **to remove nonviable, contaminated, or infected tissue.**
- Provide appropriate protective and healing devices (e.g., eye pads or goggles, heel protectors, padding, cushions, gel pads, therapeutic beds and mattresses, splints, chronic wound dressings, compression wrap, etc.).
- Refer to NDs dependent on client's situation (e.g., risk for impaired peripheral Neurovascular Function; risk for perioperative positioning Injury; adult, child, or neonatal Pressure Injury; impaired physical/bed Mobility; impaired Skin Integrity; delayed Surgical Recovery; ineffective peripheral Tissue Perfusion) **for related interventions.**

Information that appears in brackets has been added by the authors to clarify and enhance the use of nursing diagnoses.

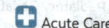 Acute Care 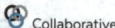 Collaborative 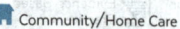 Community/Home Care   Cultural

Nursing Priority No. 4.

To correct hazards/minimize impairment:

- Assess IV catheter sites regularly for erythema, edema, tenderness, burning, etc., **which indicate infiltration or phlebitis, requiring immediate discontinuation of site use or interventions to heal the area.**
- Use appropriate catheter (e.g., peripheral or central venous catheter) when infusing medications at high risk for localized tissue injury (e.g., chemotherapy drugs, vancomycin, phenytoin, calcium chloride, potassium chloride, concentrated dextrose solutions, etc.) and ascertain that IV device is patent and infusing well **to prevent extravasation with resulting tissue damage.**
- Inspect skin and tissues routinely around incisions, cast edges, splints, and traction devices **to ensure proper application and function; the development of pressure, friction, and shear with medical devices is a common source of inpatient injury.**
- Remove adhesive products with care, removing on the horizontal plane, using mineral oil or Vaseline for softening, if needed, **to prevent abrasions or tearing of skin and damage to underlying tissues.**
- Monitor skin surrounding tubes and drains **to ensure correct placement and assess for effects of adhesive, closure devices, injury from device dislocation, and injury as a result of pressure, friction, or shear forces.**
- Develop regularly timed repositioning/turning schedule for clients with mobility and sensation impairments, using adequate personnel and assistive devices (i.e., turn sheet, etc.), as needed. **Small shifts in position and weight reduce stress on pressure points and prevent injury to skin and subcutaneous structures.**
- Use/demonstrate proper turning and transfer techniques **to avoid movements that cause friction or shearing (e.g., pulling client with parallel force, dragging movements).**
- Provide appropriate mattress (e.g., foam, flotation, alternating-pressure or air mattress) and appropriate padding devices (e.g., foam boots, heel protectors, ankle rolls), when indicated, **to reduce tissue pressure and prevent injury.**
- Limit use of plastic material (e.g., rubber sheets, plastic-backed linen savers, etc.) and remove wet or wrinkled linens promptly. **MASD is caused by exposure of skin layers to excessive moisture and the physiological changes to the skin associated with too much moisture (i.e., wound drainage, digestive secretions, urine or stool,**

Information that appears in brackets has been added by the authors to clarify and enhance the use of nursing diagnoses.

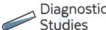 Diagnostic Studies   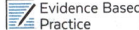 Evidence Based Practice   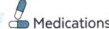 Medications   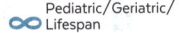 Pediatric/Geriatric/Lifespan

diaphoresis, etc.). **Excessive moisture causes erosion of skin layers, promotes bacterial proliferation, and impairs the skin's compensatory and healing mechanisms.**

- Avoid or restrict use of restraints; use adequate padding and evaluate circulation, movement, and sensation of extremities frequently when restraints are required. **Reduces the risk of impaired circulation and tissue ischemia.**
- Elevate linens over affected extremity with bed cradle **to reduce pressure on and irritation of compromised tissues.**
- Encourage physical activity and exercise **to promote circulation and prevent/limit potential complications of immobility.**
- Provide or assist with oral care (e.g., oral and dental hygiene, change position of nasogastric tubes, lubricate lips) **to prevent damage to oral mucous membranes.** Refer to NDs impaired oral Mucous Membrane and risk for adult, child, or neonatal Pressure Injury for additional interventions.
- Encourage use of adequate clothing or covers; protect from drafts and cold environment **to prevent vasoconstriction that can compromise circulation.**
- Provide or instruct in proper care of extremities during cold or hot weather. **Individuals with impaired sensation or young children/individuals unable to verbalize discomfort require special attention to deal with extremes in weather (e.g., dressing in layers and wearing gloves, clean dry socks, properly fitting shoes or boots, and a face mask in winter; using sunscreen and wearing light clothing to protect from dermal injury in summer).**
- Advise smoking/tobacco cessation and refer for resources, if indicated. **Smoking causes vasoconstriction/interferes with healing.**

Nursing Priority No. 5.

To promote healthy tissue (Teaching/Discharge Considerations) and enhance well-being (long-term goals):

- Encourage verbalizations of feelings and expectations regarding client's condition and potential for recovery of structure and function.
- Help client and family to identify and implement successful coping skills **to reduce pain or discomfort and to improve quality of life.**
- Discuss the importance of follow-up care (e.g., diabetic foot care clinic, wound care specialist, enterostomal

---

Information that appears in brackets has been added by the authors to clarify and enhance the use of nursing diagnoses.

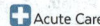 Acute Care   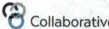 Collaborative   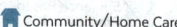 Community/Home Care   Cultural

therapist) as appropriate, self-monitoring, and reporting of changes in condition or pain characteristics. **Promotes early intervention and reduces the potential for complications.**

- Educate client/caregivers on proper safety precautions regarding hazardous materials, as indicated:

  Inform client/caregivers of various substances in the home that are potentially dangerous.

  Counsel parents on how to keep chemicals out of the reach of children and cognitively impaired clients.

- Consult with local social services agency to evaluate the client's/child's home situation if indicated.
- Refer client to appropriate agencies for adequate training and protective equipment to protect against hazardous materials/agents in the community or employment setting.
- Review medical regimen (e.g., proper use of topical sprays, creams, ointments, soaks, or irrigations) with client/caregiver **to facilitate tissue healing and prevent complications associated with lack of knowledge about maintaining tissue integrity.**
- Identify and discuss required changes in lifestyle, occupation, or environment **necessitated by limitations imposed by condition or to avoid causative factors.**
- Refer to community or governmental resources as indicated (e.g., Public Health Department, Occupational Safety and Health Administration) **for information regarding specific conditions and to report hazards.**

Documentation Focus

Assessment/Reassessment
- Individual findings, including history of condition, characteristics of wound or lesion, and evidence of other organ or tissue involvement
- Impact on functioning and lifestyle
- Availability and use of resources

Planning
- Plan of care and who is involved in planning
- Teaching plan

Implementation/Evaluation
- Responses to interventions, teaching, and actions performed
- Attainment of or progress toward desired outcome(s)
- Modifications to plan of care

Information that appears in brackets has been added by the authors to clarify and enhance the use of nursing diagnoses.

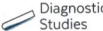 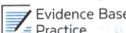 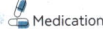 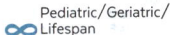

Discharge Planning
- Long-term needs and who is responsible for actions to be taken
- Specific referrals made

Sample Nursing Outcomes & Interventions Classifications NOC/NIC

NOC—Tissue Integrity: Skin & Mucous Membranes
NIC—Wound Care

---

ineffective peripheral TISSUE PERFUSION NANDA-I

[Diagnostic Division: Circulation]

Definition: Decrease in blood circulation to the extremities.

Recognizing Cues

Related/Risk Factors
Ineffective health self-management
Excessive sodium intake
Inadequate knowledge of disease process, or modifiable factors; inadequate action to address modifiable factors
Sedentary behaviors; tobacco use

Defining Characteristics

Subjective
Extremity pain; intermittent claudication
Paresthesia

Objective
Absence of or decreased peripheral pulses; ankle-brachial index less than 0.90; decreased blood pressure in extremities; femoral bruit
Altered motor function
Cold extremity; decreased, or absence of extremity sweating; dystrophic nails; extremity cyanosis; delayed peripheral wound healing; edema
Capillary refill time greater than 3 sec; color does not return to lowered limb after 1-min leg elevation; extremity color pales with limb elevation
Decreased pain-free distances during a 6-min walk test; distance in the 6-min walk test below normal range

---

Information that appears in brackets has been added by the authors to clarify and enhance the use of nursing diagnoses.

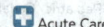 Acute Care 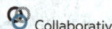 Collaborative 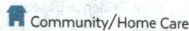 Community/Home Care Cultural

Clinical Connections

Atherosclerosis, anemias, arthritis, coronary artery disease, amputation, Buerger disease, trauma, burns, cerebrovascular accident, chronic obstructive pulmonary disease, congestive heart failure, diabetes mellitus, overweight, peripheral vascular disease, Raynaud disease, thrombophlebitis

Generate Solutions

Plan Desired Outcomes

Client Will (Include Specific Time Frame)

- Demonstrate increased perfusion as individually appropriate (e.g., skin warm and dry, peripheral pulses present and strong, absence of edema, free of pain or discomfort).
- Verbalize understanding of risk factors or condition, therapy regimen, side effects of medications, and when to contact healthcare provider.
- Demonstrate behaviors and lifestyle changes to improve circulation (e.g., engage in regular exercise, cessation of smoking, weight reduction, disease management).

Interventions/Take Action

Nursing Priority No. 1.

To assess causative/contributing **or risk** factors:

- Identify the presence of high-risk factors or conditions (e.g., smoking, cardiovascular disease, dyslipidemia, hypertension, diabetes, sickle cell disease [SCD], circumferential burn, compartment syndrome [CS]). **Places the client at greater risk of developing arterial insufficiency/occlusion. Recent studies have linked depression as an indicator of the presence and progression of peripheral arterial disease (PAD). Furthermore, exposure to toxins (e.g., air pollution, lead) has also been shown to increase the incidence of cardiovascular disease, including PAD.**
- Note current situation or presence of conditions that may affect perfusion to all body systems (e.g., heart failure exacerbation, major trauma, distributive or hypovolemic shock, coagulopathies, sickle cell crisis, heparin-induced thrombocytopenia [HIT]).
- Note location of restrictive clothing, pressure dressings, circular wraps, and cast or traction device **that may restrict circulation to limb. Development of acute CS is associated with the application of external forces that result in compression and impaired perfusion to distal tissues.**

Information that appears in brackets has been added by the authors to clarify and enhance the use of nursing diagnoses.

- Note client's age, gender, and ethnicity. **The risk for PAD increases with age. Current evidence suggests that women are at a slightly increased risk of PAD, possibly due to smaller arterial diameter. Furthermore, African American clients are at a significantly higher risk for PAD and more severe disease than non-Hispanic White clients. Conversely, studies have found young males to be at the highest risk for acute CS.**
- Review client's medications. **Administration of vasoactive medications (e.g., norepinephrine, phenylephrine, epinephrine, and dopamine) may cause vasoconstriction, impairing perfusion of smaller vessels. Additionally, administration via peripheral IV can lead to extravasation of these substances known to cause tissue ischemia and necrosis.**
- Review laboratory tests (e.g., cholesterol, high-density lipoprotein, CRP [C-reactive protein], IL-6 [interleukin-6]). **Recent studies have suggested abnormal cholesterol studies and inflammatory markers may be strong predictors of PAD and more severe disease.**

Nursing Priority No. 2.

To evaluate degree of impairment (ineffective peripheral Tissue Perfusion):

- Palpate arterial pulses (bilateral femoral, popliteal, dorsalis pedis, posterior tibial), using a handheld Doppler if indicated. **For example, client with intermittent claudication may have palpable pulses that disappear after ambulation and using a handheld Doppler to verify peripheral pulses provides a more objective and reliable method to confirm perfusion rather than palpation of peripheral pulses. Note: In 5% to 8% of healthy clients, the dorsalis pedis pulse is absent; however, the posterior tibial pulse is usually palpable.**
- Determine pulse equality as well as intensity (e.g., bounding, normal, diminished, absent) and compare with unaffected extremity **to evaluate distribution and quality of blood flow and success or failure of therapy.**
- Measure ankle-brachial index (ABI) or toe-brachial index (TBI) in clients demonstrating symptoms of PAD. **ABI is obtained by dividing the blood pressure in the ankle by the systolic brachial pressure. Normal ABI is higher than 1; ABI is a first-line noninvasive test to diagnose PAD. In clients with chronic kidney disease and/or diabetes, stiffening of larger arteries may cause falsely elevated ABI**

Information that appears in brackets has been added by the authors to clarify and enhance the use of nursing diagnoses.

values; for this reason, TBI values may be more reliable in these clients.
- Perform a neurovascular assessment of the affected extremity. **Acute impairment of arterial blood flow results in a common presentation of pain, pulselessness, paresthesia, paralysis, and pallor.**
- Compare skin temperature and color with other limbs when assessing extremity circulation. **Helps differentiate type of problem. Severe PAD may present as mottling of the lower extremities in a "fishnet pattern" (livedo reticularis).**
- Measure capillary refill **to determine adequacy of systemic circulation.**
- Inspect lower extremities for skin and nail texture changes (e.g., brittle nails; atrophic, shiny appearance, lack of hair; or dry/scaly, reddened skin; skin breaks or ulcerations) **that often accompany diminished peripheral circulation. Positional changes of the lower extremities may also cause changes in skin color in more severe PAD (e.g., dependent rubor, elevated pallor). Evaluation of wounds/ulcers of the lower extremities warrants close consideration of etiology to discern the appropriate plan of care.**
- Evaluate extremity pain reports, noting location, quality (e.g., cramping, heaviness, burning) and duration. Determine time (day or night) that symptoms are worse, precipitating or aggravating events (e.g., walking), and relieving factors (e.g., rest, sitting down with legs in dependent position, oral analgesics). **Helps isolate and differentiate problems such as intermittent chronic claudication versus loss of function and pain due to acute sustained ischemia related to loss of arterial blood flow. In PAD, the location of the client's pain can be dependent on the vessels affected. Intermittent claudication occurs in only 10% to 30% of clients with PAD; the presentation of pain in PAD may be atypical (e.g., weakness, pain attributed to arthritis) leading to potential misdiagnosis. Evaluation via a 6-min walk test may help the clinician appreciate exertional discomfort or discern a reduction in walking speed. Pain out of proportion to injury or condition of an extremity may be an indication of acute CS. In a sickle cell crisis, severe pain may be accompanied by swelling of the hands and feet.**
- Assess motor function. **Problems with ambulation, hypersensitivity or loss of sensation, numbness and tingling are changes that can indicate neurovascular dysfunction**

Information that appears in brackets has been added by the authors to clarify and enhance the use of nursing diagnoses.

 Diagnostic Studies 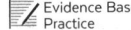 Evidence Based Practice 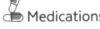 Medications 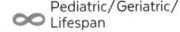 Pediatric/Geriatric/Lifespan or limb ischemia, requiring more evaluation for differentiation of problem. **Pain aggravated by elevation of the lower extremities and alleviated by a dependent position is suggestive of disease progression, as is pain experienced at rest.**

- Ascertain impact on functioning and lifestyle (e.g., leg pain may restrict ambulation or impair activities of daily living). **Reduction in mobility may contribute to the development of skin ulceration and healing problems that seriously impact quality of life.**
- Note client's nutritional and fluid status. **Protein-energy malnutrition and weight loss make ischemic tissues more prone to breakdown. Dehydration reduces blood volume and compromises peripheral circulation.**
- Review laboratory studies (e.g., lipid profile, coagulation studies, hemoglobin/hematocrit, renal/cardiac function tests, inflammatory markers [e.g., CRP, IL6]), and diagnostic studies (e.g., Doppler ultrasound, magnetic resonance angiography, contrast angiography) **to determine probability, location, and degree of impairment. Evaluation of PAD by Doppler ultrasound is a valuable noninvasive strategy but is dependent on the skill of the technician. Utilization of contrasted computed tomographic angiography and magnetic resonance angiography provides higher-resolution images but has more client risk.**

Nursing Priority No. 3.
To maximize tissue perfusion:

- Collaborate in treatment of underlying conditions, such as diabetes, hypertension, cardiovascular conditions, SCD, blood disorders, traumatic injury, hypovolemia, and sepsis **to maximize systemic circulation and organ perfusion.**
- Administer medications such as antiplatelet agents, antithrombotics, and antibiotics **to improve tissue perfusion and organ function. The American Heart Association (AHA) and American College of Cardiology (ACC) guidelines recommend cilostazol to alleviate leg pain and increase walking distance in PAD. However, treatment guidelines include the use of antiplatelets (e.g., aspirin and/or clopidogrel), cholesterol-lowering medications (i.e., statins), antihypertensives (e.g., angiotensin-converting enzyme inhibitors or angiotensin-receptor blockers), and oral anticoagulants.**

Information that appears in brackets has been added by the authors to clarify and enhance the use of nursing diagnoses.

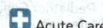 Acute Care 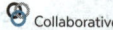 Collaborative 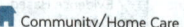 Community/Home Care   Cultural

- Administer fluids, electrolytes, and oxygen as indicated **to promote optimal blood flow, organ perfusion, and function.**
- Assist with or prepare for medical procedures such as endovascular stent placement, surgical revascularization procedures, and thrombectomy **to improve peripheral circulation.**
- Collaborate with wound care specialist if arterial ulcerations are present. **Wound care may include debridement, topical medications, antibiotics, hyperbaric oxygen therapy, and various specialized dressings that facilitate an optimal environment for healing, prevention of infection, and further injury.**
- Provide interventions to promote peripheral circulation and limit complications:
  - Encourage early ambulation when possible and recommend regular exercise. **Supervised exercise therapy (SET) is an important intervention to improve walking functionality in clients with PAD and is part of the recommended guidelines by the ACC, AHA, and Wound, Ostomy, and Continence Nurses Society. Exercise training is an effective treatment to promote collateral circulation and may provide some symptom alleviation via multiple mechanisms, including reduced limb symptoms, improved functional capacity, and reduced systemic cardiovascular risk. Although clinical guidelines support SET, strong evidence exists for community and home-based exercise to achieve similar outcomes when SET is not available or preferred.**
  - Provide pressure-relieving devices for immobilized client (e.g., heel floating, air mattress, foam or sheepskin padding) **to reduce excessive tissue pressure that could lead to skin breakdown.**
  - Assist with or cue client to change position at timed intervals rather than using presence of pain as signal to change positions **because sensation may be impaired.**
  - Avoid or carefully monitor use of heat or cold, such as hot water bottle/heating pad or cold pack. **Decreased tissue sensitivity due to ischemia increases risk of dermal injury.**
- Administer a diet and recommend dietary choices that promote wound healing and support treatment of underlying conditions (e.g., diabetes, hypertension, cardiovascular disease, renal insufficiency, SCD).

Information that appears in brackets has been added by the authors to clarify and enhance the use of nursing diagnoses.

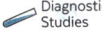 Diagnostic Studies 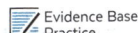 Evidence Based Practice 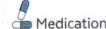 Medications 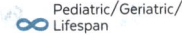 Pediatric/Geriatric/Lifespan

- Refer to NDs risk for Thrombosis; risk for impaired peripheral Neurovascular Function; impaired Skin Integrity; impaired Tissue Integrity; and Sensory Deficit [specify: visual, auditory, kinesthetic, gustatory, tactile, olfactory] for related interventions, as appropriate.

Nursing Priority No. 4.

To maintain optimal tissue perfusion (Teaching/Discharge Considerations) and enhance well-being (long-term goals):

- Discuss relevant risk factors (e.g., family history, overweight, age, smoking, hypertension, diabetes, clotting disorders) and potential outcomes of atherosclerosis (e.g., systemic atherosclerotic conditions, PAD). **Information necessary for client to make informed decisions concerning risk factors and to commit to lifestyle changes necessary to prevent onset of complications or manage symptoms when condition present.**
- Identify necessary changes in lifestyle and assist client to incorporate disease management into activities of daily living. **Promotes independence and enhances self-concept regarding ability to deal with change and manage own needs.**
- Emphasize need for regular exercise program. **Enhances circulation and promotes general well-being. Clinical practice guidelines recommend SET approximately 30 to 45 min, three times per week for at least 2 wk to enhance lower extremity collateral circulation, improved functional capacity, and reduced systemic cardiovascular risk. Alternatively, a similar home-based schedule may be equally as effective in the client with PAD.**
- Refer client/caregiver to nutritionist for nutritional needs and dietary modifications as indicated. **Developing dietary plan with client to address specific risk factors/disease process increases likelihood of achieving desired outcomes.**
- Encourage weight reduction if indicated in overweight client.
- Encourage client to refrain from alcohol consumption or limit use to moderate consumption.
- Discuss care of dependent limbs and foot care as appropriate. **Special attention should be paid to avoid injury or tissue loss on the toes, feet, or lower extremities. Shoes, socks, and hosiery should be properly fitted.**

Information that appears in brackets has been added by the authors to clarify and enhance the use of nursing diagnoses.

- Educate client to avoid leg elevation. **Legs should be maintained in a dependent position (unless medically prescribed otherwise).**
- Teach client/caregivers to examine toes, feet, and legs daily **for injury, ulceration, and/or infection.**
- Encourage client to regularly evaluate peripheral sensation using the Ipswich Touch Test (light touch test) on the tips of the first, third, and fifth toes. **The Ipswich Touch Test is a useful alternative to the monofilament test to evaluate loss of sensation.**
- Review relationship between smoking and peripheral vascular circulation, as indicated. **Smoking contributes to development and progression of PAD and is associated with higher rate of amputation in presence of Buerger disease.**
- Discuss reportable symptoms, including any changes in pain level, difficulty walking, and nonhealing wounds, **to provide opportunity for timely evaluation and intervention.**
- Encourage client to obtain an annual flu vaccination.
- Emphasize need for regular medical and laboratory follow-up **to evaluate disease progression and response to therapies, including medications for desired and untoward effects.**
- Review medication regimen with client/SO. **Client may be on various medications (e.g., antiplatelets, antihypertensives, blood viscosity–reducing agents, anticoagulants, cholesterol-lowering agents, antibiotics). Any of these medications have harmful side effects and require client teaching and medical monitoring.**
- Refer to community resources such as smoking-cessation assistance, weight control program, and exercise group **to provide support for lifestyle changes.**

Documentation Focus

Assessment/Reassessment
- Individual risk factors identified
- Individual findings, noting nature, extent, and duration of problem, effect on independence and lifestyle
- Characteristics of pain, precipitators, and what relieves pain
- Pulse and blood pressure, including above and below suspected lesion as appropriate

Planning
- Plan of care and who is involved in planning
- Teaching plan

Information that appears in brackets has been added by the authors to clarify and enhance the use of nursing diagnoses.

 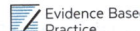 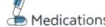 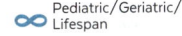

Implementation/Evaluation
- Response to interventions, teaching, and actions performed
- Attainment of or progress toward desired outcome(s)
- Client concerns or difficulty making and following through with plan
- Modifications to plan of care

Discharge Planning
- Long-term needs and who is responsible for actions to be taken
- Available resources, specific referrals made

Sample Nursing Outcomes & Interventions Classifications NOC/NIC

NOC—Tissue Perfusion: Peripheral
NIC—Circulatory Care: Arterial [or] Venous Insufficiency

---

risk for ineffective cerebral
TISSUE PERFUSION   NANDA-I

[Diagnostic Division: Circulation]

Definition: Susceptible to a decrease in blood circulation to the brain.

Recognizing Cues

Risk Factors
Inadequate knowledge of disease process, or modifiable factors
Inadequate action to address modifiable factors
Inadequate blood pressure, or arrhythmia treatment self-management
Ineffective overweight self-management
Sedentary behaviors
Excessive stress; tobacco use; excessive alcohol consumption; substance misuse

Clinical Connections
Traumatic brain injury (TBI), transient ischemic attack, cerebrovascular accident (CVA)/stroke; atherosclerosis, hypertension, atrial fibrillation, mitral valve stenosis or replacement, cardiomyopathy, endocarditis, sleep apnea, sickle cell disease (SCD), cocaine use

---

Information that appears in brackets has been added by the authors to clarify and enhance the use of nursing diagnoses.

 Acute Care 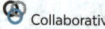 Collaborative 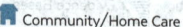 Community/Home Care Cultural

Generate Solutions

Plan Desired Outcomes

Client Will (Include Specific Time Frame)
- Display neurological signs within client's normal range.
- Verbalize understanding of condition, therapy regimen, side effects of medications, and when to contact healthcare provider.
- Demonstrate behaviors and lifestyle changes to improve circulation (e.g., cessation of smoking, relaxation techniques, exercise and dietary program).

Interventions/Take Action

Nursing Priority No. 1.
To assess causative/contributing factors:

- Determine history of conditions associated with thrombus or emboli such as stroke, complicated pregnancy, SCD, fractures (especially long bones and pelvis) **to identify client at higher risk for decreased cerebral perfusion related to vascular occlusion or clot migration.**
- Note current situation or presence of conditions (e.g., acute heart failure, major trauma, sepsis, hypertension) **that can affect multiple body systems and systemic circulation/perfusion.**
- Ascertain potential for the presence of acute neurological conditions, such as TBI, increased cerebrospinal fluid (CSF), tumors, hemorrhage, anoxic brain injury, and toxic or viral encephalopathies. **These conditions alter the relationship between intracranial volume and pressure, potentially increasing intracranial pressure (ICP) and decreasing cerebral perfusion. ICP is dependent on three factors: brain tissue, cerebrospinal fluid (CSF), and blood inside the skull. Brain size is relatively constant; thus, the body will change the amount of CSF and blood in the skull to maintain a consistent ICP. However, additional compensatory mechanisms will cause these mechanisms to be overridden when brain tissue senses hypoxia or hypercapnia, potentially causing an increase in ICP and additional injury to brain tissue.**
- Investigate client reports of headaches; headaches associated with lying down or recurring in the morning and other clinical manifestations such as nausea and vomiting, loss of coordination/motor dysfunction, confusion, visual disturbances (e.g., blurred vision, double vision, loss of

---

Information that appears in brackets has been added by the authors to clarify and enhance the use of nursing diagnoses.

 Diagnostic Studies 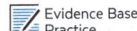 Evidence Based Practice 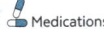 Medications 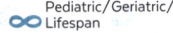 Pediatric/Geriatric/Lifespan vision in one eye, photophobia, optic disc edema), difficulty understanding or using language, or a range of progressive neurological deficits. **These symptoms may accompany cerebral perfusion deficits associated with conditions such as stroke, transient ischemic attack, brain trauma, or cerebral arteriovenous malformations. Note: Bulging of the anterior fontanelle may be noted in infants.**

- Ascertain if client has history of cardiac problems (e.g., recent myocardial infarction, heart failure, heart valve dysfunction or replacement, chronic/paroxysmal atrial fibrillation), **which can impair systemic and cerebral blood flow or cause thromboembolic events to brain.**
- Determine presence of cardiac dysrhythmias (e.g., chronic/paroxysmal atrial fibrillation, bradycardia). **Stroke can be precipitated by dysrhythmias.**
- Assess level of consciousness (LOC), mental status, speech, pupillary changes, and behavior. **Clinical symptoms of decreased cerebral perfusion include fluctuations in consciousness, motor, sensory, and cognitive function. Utilization of the Glasgow Coma Scale (GCS) or the Full Outline of UnResponsiveness (FOUR) score can provide an objective measurement of client LOC that can be easily communicated to other healthcare providers.**
- Evaluate blood pressure. **Chronic or severe hypertension can precipitate cerebrovascular spasm and stroke. Low blood pressure or severe hypotension causes inadequate perfusion of brain. Note: Hypervigilance is necessary for Cushing triad (e.g., hypertension, bradycardia, and irregular respiration), which indicates worsening ICP.**
- Verify proper use of antihypertensive medications. **Individuals may stop medication because of lack of symptoms, presence of undesired side effects, and/or cost of drug, potentiating risk of stroke.**
- Review medication regimen noting use of anticoagulants/antiplatelet agents/other drugs **that could cause intracranial bleeding.**
- Review pulse oximetry or arterial blood gases, noting oxygenation level and saturation. **Hypoxia (Pao_2 level less than 60 mg Hg, or O_2 saturation level less than 94%) is associated with reduced cerebral perfusion and increased morbidity and mortality from severe brain injury.**
- Review laboratory studies (e.g., coagulation profiles, complete blood count, electrolytes, lipids, B-type natriuretic peptide) **to identify disorders that increase risk**

Information that appears in brackets has been added by the authors to clarify and enhance the use of nursing diagnoses.

of clotting or bleeding or conditions contributing to decreased cerebral perfusion.

- Review results of diagnostic studies (e.g., ultrasound or other imaging scans such as echocardiography, computed tomography [CT], or magnetic resonance angiography [MRA]; diffusion and perfusion MRI) **to determine location and severity of disorder that can cause or exacerbate cerebral perfusion problem.**
- Review client's nutritional patterns and use of alcohol. **Increased alcohol consumption and unhealthy eating patterns (i.e., high fat, high sodium, high cholesterol) have been associated with risk factors such as high blood pressure, stroke, atrial fibrillation, and heart disease.**

Nursing Priority No. 2.
To maximize tissue perfusion:

- Assist with the placement and monitoring of invasive monitoring (e.g., extraventricular drain or intraparenchymal monitor) **to assess and track ICP.**
- Collaborate in treatment of underlying conditions as indicated **to improve systemic perfusion and organ function:**
  Restore or maintain fluid balance **to maximize cardiac output and prevent decreased cerebral perfusion associated with hypovolemia.**
  Assist with treatment/management of cardiac dysrhythmias (such as with medication administration, pacemaker insertion, cardioversion). **Reduces risk of diminished cerebral perfusion due to blood clots or low cardiac output.**
  Assist with treatment/management of cardiac dysrhythmias (such as with medication administration, pacemaker insertion, cardioversion). **Reduces risk of diminished cerebral perfusion due to blood clots or low cardiac output.**
  Restrict fluids, administer diuretics, as indicated, **to prevent decreased cerebral perfusion associated with hypertension, and cerebral edema.**
  Keep head in midline position, as indicated, **to promote cerebral venous drainage, preventing or reducing risk of elevated ICP. Note: Caution should be used in clients with suspected (or at risk for) increased ICP to keep hip flexion minimized to prevent compromise of cerebral venous drainage.**
  Maintain optimal head of bed placement (e.g., 0, 15, 30 degrees) as indicated, **to promote cerebral perfusion.**

Information that appears in brackets has been added by the authors to clarify and enhance the use of nursing diagnoses.

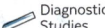 Diagnostic Studies 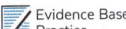 Evidence Based Practice 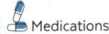 Medications 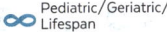 Pediatric/Geriatric/Lifespan

Control fever, monitor hypothermia therapy, as indicated, **to decrease cerebral metabolism and cerebral edema.**

Provide supplemental oxygen to maintain Spo_2 levels at or above 94%; monitor airway, breathing, and circulation. **Increasing ICP may result in changes in LOC and loss of protective airway mechanisms, requiring insertion of an airway adjunct. Note: Hyperventilation is a therapeutic intervention in some clients to reduce ICP.**

Administer vasoactive medications, as indicated, **to increase cardiac output and/or arterial blood pressure to maintain cerebral perfusion. Prevention of hypotension is a priority.**

Administer other medications, as indicated. **Osmotic agents (e.g., mannitol, hypertonic saline solutions) may be used to reduce cerebral edema, antihypertensives may be used to manage high blood pressure, anticoagulants/antiplatelets may be used to prevent cerebral embolus, and thrombolytics may be used to treat cerebral ischemia.**

Minimize noxious stimuli (e.g., client coughing, suctioning, etc.) **to reduce deleterious effects on ICP.**

Prepare client for surgery, as indicated (e.g., carotid endarterectomy, evacuation of hematoma or space-occupying lesion), **to improve cerebral perfusion.**

Refer to NDs impaired Cardiac Output for additional interventions.

Nursing Priority No. 3.

To promote optimal cerebral perfusion (Teaching/Discharge Considerations) and enhance well-being (long-term goals):

- Review modifiable risk factors, as indicated. **Information can help client make informed choices about remedial risk factors and commit to lifestyle changes, as appropriate:**

  Uncontrolled hypertension: **Incidence of stroke increases with systolic blood pressure greater than 140/90 mm Hg. Clients at risk can learn to self-monitor blood pressure, take prescribed antihypertensive agents consistently, and identify symptoms to report to their healthcare provider.**

  Smoking: **Smoking causes vasoconstriction and increased arterial wall stiffness, increasing fibrinogen levels and platelet aggregation, and abnormal blood lipids. Numerous recent studies have confirmed a relationship between active and passive smoking, with the**

Information that appears in brackets has been added by the authors to clarify and enhance the use of nursing diagnoses.

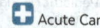 Acute Care 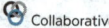 Collaborative 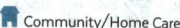 Community/Home Care Cultural

maximum risk period being middle life. Smoking cessation immediately lowers risk of stroke.

- *Overweight and unhealthy diet:* **Abdominal obesity has been associated with increased risk for ischemic stroke. Diet high in cholesterol contributes to development of cerebral atherosclerosis. High intake of sodium can contribute to hypertension.**
- *Physical inactivity:* **Contributes to obesity and hypertension.**
- *Excessive alcohol intake:* **Linked to higher risk of stroke because it can cause hypertension, which is a major risk factor. Note: Alcohol intake consumption at higher amounts is associated with increased risk of atrial fibrillation, ventricular fibrillation, dilated cardiomyopathy, hypertension, dyslipidemia, and a systemic anticoagulant effect, all of which increase the risk of stroke.**
- *Illicit drug use:* **Can significantly boost the risk of a deadly or debilitating stroke. Note: Many illicit drugs have been linked to increased stroke risk (i.e., cocaine, amphetamines, heroin). Additionally, misuse of prescription pain or anxiety medications, such as oxycodone or fentanyl, also increases client risk.**
- Discuss impact of unmodifiable risk factors such as family history, age, race. **Understanding the effects and interrelationship of all risk factors may encourage clients to address what can be changed to improve general well-being and reduce individual risk.**
- Assist client to incorporate disease management into activities of daily living. **Promotes independence; enhances self-concept regarding ability to deal with change and manage own needs.**
- Emphasize necessity of routine follow-up and laboratory monitoring, as indicated, **for effective disease management and possible changes in therapeutic regimen.**
- Refer to educational and community resources, as indicated. **Client/significant other may benefit from instruction and support provided by agencies to engage in healthy activities (e.g., weight loss, smoking cessation, exercise).**

Documentation Focus

Assessment/Reassessment
- Individual findings, noting specific risk factors
- Vital signs, blood pressure, cardiac rhythm
- Medication regimen
- Diagnostic studies, laboratory results

Information that appears in brackets has been added by the authors to clarify and enhance the use of nursing diagnoses.

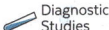 Diagnostic Studies 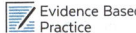 Evidence Based Practice 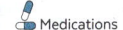 Medications 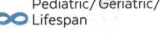 Pediatric/Geriatric/Lifespan

Planning
- Plan of care and who is involved in planning
- Teaching plan

Implementation/Evaluation
- Response to interventions, teaching, and actions performed
- Attainment of or progress toward desired outcome(s)
- Modifications to plan of care

Discharge Planning
- Long-term needs and who is responsible for actions to be taken
- Available resources, specific referrals made

Sample Nursing Outcomes & Interventions Classifications NOC/NIC

NOC—Tissue Perfusion: Cerebral
NIC—Cerebral Perfusion Promotion

---

impaired TRANSFERRING ABILITY NANDA-I

[Diagnostic Division: Activity/Rest]

Definition: Limitation of independent movement between two nearby surfaces.

Recognizing Cues

Related/Risk Factors
Unaddressed environmental constraints (e.g., bed height, inadequate space, wheelchair type, treatment equipment, restraints)
Impaired postural balance; inadequate muscle strength; prolonged immobility
Inadequate knowledge of transfer techniques
Ineffective overweight self-management
Pain

Defining Characteristics

Subjective or Objective
Difficulty moving:
Between bed and chair; between bed or chair or floor and standing position
Between car and chair; between chair and floor
Between uneven levels

Information that appears in brackets has been added by the authors to clarify and enhance the use of nursing diagnoses.

 Acute Care 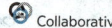 Collaborative 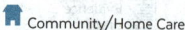 Community/Home Care Cultural

Difficulty transferring:
  In or out of bathtub, or shower stall
  On or off a bedside commode, or a toilet

Clinical Connections

Arthritis, fractures, amputation, neuromuscular diseases (e.g., multiple sclerosis [MS], amyotrophic lateral sclerosis, Guillain-Barré syndrome), paralysis, glaucoma, macular degeneration, dementia

Generate Solutions

Plan Desired Outcomes

Client Will (Include Specific Time Frame)

- Verbalize understanding of situation and appropriate safety measures.
- Master techniques of transfer successfully.
- Make desired transfers safely.

Interventions/Take Action

Nursing Priority No. 1.

To assess causative/contributing factors:

- Determine presence of conditions that contribute to transfer problems. **Neuromuscular and musculoskeletal problems (e.g., MS, fractures with splints or casts, back injuries, knee/hip replacement surgery, amputation, quadriplegia or paraplegia, contractures or spastic muscles); agedness (diminished faculties, multiple medications, painful conditions, decreased balance, muscle mass, tone, or strength), and effects of dementias, brain injury, and so forth, can seriously impact balance and physical and psychological well-being.**
- Evaluate perceptual and cognitive impairments and ability to follow directions. **Plan of care and choice of interventions are dependent on nature of condition—acute, chronic, or progressive.**
- Note factors complicating current situation. **Recent surgery or traction apparatus, debilitating illness or weakness, and mechanical ventilation or multiple IV/indwelling tubings can restrict movement.**
- Review medication regimen and schedule **to determine possible side effects or drug interactions impairing balance and/or muscle tone.**

Information that appears in brackets has been added by the authors to clarify and enhance the use of nursing diagnoses.

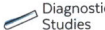 Diagnostic Studies   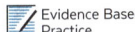 Evidence Based Practice   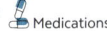 Medications   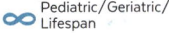 Pediatric/Geriatric/Lifespan

Nursing Priority No. 2.

To assess functional ability:

- Evaluate degree of impairment using functional level classification scale of 0 to 4. **Identifies client's strengths and deficits (e.g., ability to ambulate with assistive devices or problems with balance, inability to bear weight [client is non-weight-bearing or partial weight-bearing]) and determines needs and safety concerns.**
- Note emotional or behavioral responses of client/significant other to problems of immobility. **Restrictions or limitations imposed by immobility can cause physical, social, emotional, and financial difficulties for everyone.**
- Perform the timed up-and-go (TUG) test, as indicated, **to assess client's basic ability to transfer and ambulate safely, and risks of falling. Note: Client may perform this test adequately and still have difficulty with some transfers, such as in or out of a car or bathtub or from floor to chair.**
- Observe movement when client is unaware of observations **to note any incongruence with reported abilities.**

Nursing Priority No. 3.

To promote optimal level of movement:

- Assist with treatment of underlying condition causing dysfunction. **Treatment of condition (e.g., surgery for hip replacement, therapy for unilateral neglect following stroke) can alleviate or improve difficulties with transfer activity.**
- Consult with physical therapist, occupational therapist, or rehabilitation team **to develop general and specific muscle strengthening and range-of-motion exercises, transfer training and techniques, as well as recommendations and provision of balance, gait, and mobility aids or adjunctive devices.**
- Use appropriate number of people to assist with transfers and correct equipment (e.g., mechanical lift/sling, gait belt, transfer pole, sitting or standing disk pivot) **to safely transfer the client in a particular situation (e.g., chair to bed, chair to car, in or out of shower or tub).**
- Demonstrate and assist with use of overhead trapeze, transfer boards, transfer or sit-to-stand hoist, safety grab bars, side rails or stand pole, cane, walker, wheelchair, crutches, as indicated, **to protect client and care providers from injury during transfers and movements.**

Information that appears in brackets has been added by the authors to clarify and enhance the use of nursing diagnoses.

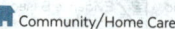

- Position devices (e.g., call light, bed-positioning switch) within easy reach on the bed or chair. **Allows client to obtain assistance for transfer, as needed.**
- Provide instruction or reinforce information for client and caregivers regarding body and equipment positioning **to improve or maintain balance when transferring.**
- Monitor body alignment, posture, and balance and encourage wide base of support when standing to transfer.
- Use full-length mirror, as needed, **to facilitate client's view of own postural alignment.**
- Demonstrate and reinforce safety measures, as indicated, such as transfer board, gait belt, supportive footwear, good lighting, clearing floor of clutter **to avoid possibility of fall and subsequent injury.**

Nursing Priority No. 4.

To maintain safe transfers (Teaching/Discharge Considerations) and enhance well-being (long-term goals):

- Assist client/caregivers to learn safety measures as individually indicated. **Actions (e.g., using correct body mechanics for particular transfer, locking wheelchair before transfer, using properly placed and functioning hoists, ascertaining that floor surface is even and clutter free) are important in facilitating transfers and reducing risk of falls or injury to client and caregiver.**
- Discuss need for and sources of care or supervision. **Homecare agency, before- and after-school programs, senior day care, personal companions, etc., may be required to assist with or monitor activity.**
- Refer to appropriate community resources for evaluation and modification of environment (e.g., shower or tub, uneven floor surfaces, steps, use of ramps, standing tables or lifts). **Guides client and family to resources available to help with handicap services and home remodeling.**
- Refer also to NDs impaired bed/physical/wheelchair Mobility; risk for [adult or child] Fall; impaired Sitting Ability; impaired Standing Ability; impaired Walking Ability, for related interventions.

Documentation Focus

Assessment/Reassessment

- Individual findings, including level of function and ability to participate in desired transfers
- Mobility aids or transfer devices used
- Availability of support person/caregiver

Information that appears in brackets has been added by the authors to clarify and enhance the use of nursing diagnoses.

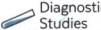 Diagnostic Studies 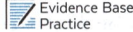 Evidence Based Practice 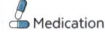 Medications 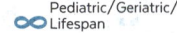 Pediatric/Geriatric/Lifespan

Planning
- Plan of care and who is involved in the planning
- Teaching plan

Implementation/Evaluation
- Responses to interventions, teaching, and actions performed
- Attainment of or progress toward desired outcome(s)
- Modifications to plan of care

Discharge Planning
- Discharge and long-term needs, noting who is responsible for each action to be taken
- Specific referrals made
- Sources for and maintenance of assistive devices

Sample Nursing Outcomes & Interventions Classifications NOC/NIC

NOC—Transfer Performance
NIC—Self-Care Assistance: Transfer

---

ineffective UNDERWEIGHT SELF-MANAGEMENT NANDA-I

[Diagnostic Division: Food/Fluid]

Definition: Unsatisfactory handling of treatment regimen, consequences, and lifestyle changes associated with having a body weight less than standardized norms for age and gender.

Recognizing Cues

Related/Risk Factors
Inadequate knowledge of appropriate nutritional requirements, or weight management strategies; conflicting information sources

Inadequate appetite, eating plan, or meal planning; inappropriate dietary intake; unhealthy family meals

Inadequate nutrient intake to meet increased caloric expenditure

Decreased taste perception, or sense of smell

Inadequate autonomy, self-efficacy, or self-confidence; excessive stress; self-defeating thoughts; inadequate intrinsic motivation; depressive symptoms

---

Information that appears in brackets has been added by the authors to clarify and enhance the use of nursing diagnoses.

 Acute Care 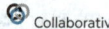 Collaborative 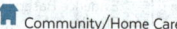 Community/Home Care   Cultural

Food insecurity; decreased awareness of available nutrition services

Inadequate access to accurate weight management information, or programs

Inadequate structured lifestyle support; inadequate social support network

Unaddressed absence of affordable, or local availability of healthy food options

Inadequate caregiver knowledge of appropriate nutritional requirements, or weight management strategies

Decreased access to iron folate, or deworming tablets

Ineffective fatigue self-management; unaddressed sleep deprivation

Defining Characteristics

Subjective

Underweight Symptoms

- Anxiety; fatigue; weakness
- Headache; migraines; increased sensitivity to light
- Diarrhea

Underweight Consequences

- Altered sleep-wake cycle
- Frequent respiratory infections
- Frequent miscarriage; infertility; low sperm count

Objective

Underweight Signs

- Unintended weight loss; 5% reduction in body weight in 6 to 12 mo
- Inadequate muscle mass; low fat-free mass index; mid upper arm circumference below norms for age and gender
- Body mass index less than fifth percentile in individuals 2 to 20 years of age
- Body mass index less than 18.5 kg/m² in individuals 20 to 70 years of age
- Body mass index less than 22 kg/m² in individuals older than 70 years of age

Underweight Symptoms

- Irritable mood; decreased ability to concentrate
- Pallor; excessive hair loss
- Bruises easily; bleeding gums; cold extremities
- Micronutrient deficiencies

Information that appears in brackets has been added by the authors to clarify and enhance the use of nursing diagnoses.

 Diagnostic Studies 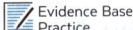 Evidence Based Practice Medications 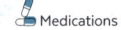 Pediatric/Geriatric/Lifespan

Underweight Consequences
- Decreased blood pressure, or heart rate (greater than 20% reduction from baseline)
- Impaired wound healing; prolonged hospitalization
- Decreased bone density
- Infant growth failure
- Decreased serum glucose, or hemoglobin level
- Decreased serum iron, magnesium, or vitamin B level

Clinical Connections
Chronic health conditions, anorexia/bulimia, cystic fibrosis, celiac disease, facial trauma, oral cancer, abuse/neglect, substance misuse, depression

Generate Solutions

Plan Desired Outcomes

Client Will (Include Specific Time Frame)
- Demonstrate progressive weight gain toward goal.
- Display normalization of laboratory values and be free of signs of malnutrition as reflected in Defining Characteristics.
- Verbalize understanding of causative factors when known and necessary interventions.
- Demonstrate behaviors and lifestyle changes to regain or maintain appropriate weight.

Interventions/Take Action

Nursing Priority No. 1.
To identify contributing factors/health status:

- Assess risk and presence of factors or conditions associated with weight loss (e.g., thyroid dysfunction, gastrointestinal disease, depression, anxiety, cancer, poor dentition, diabetes, HIV/AIDs, tuberculosis, substance abuse, genetic, etc.). **Unintentional weight loss may occur due to the presence of organ dysfunction/disease, or weight loss may be compounded by the presence of physical or psychological illness.**
- Investigate client's dietary history to determine chronic problems and ongoing needs, such as:
  Patterns of food intake, including binge eating, purging, and inadequate, extremely limited food intake,

---

Information that appears in brackets has been added by the authors to clarify and enhance the use of nursing diagnoses.

 Acute Care 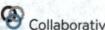 Collaborative 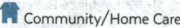 Community/Home Care 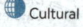 Cultural

experimentation with numerous types of diets and/or repeated dieting efforts ("yo-yo" dieting), preoccupation with weight loss, intense fear of being overweight/fat, rigid rules for food consumption, etc.

Preoccupation with weight loss, intense fear of being overweight/fat, rigid rules for food consumption, etc.

Increased caloric requirements with difficulty ingesting sufficient calories (e.g., cancer, burns).

Maturational or developmental issues (e.g., premature baby with sucking difficulties, child with lack of emotional stimulation or neurodevelopmental conditions, frail elderly living alone, hospitalized, or in nursing home).

Swallowing difficulties (e.g., stroke, Parkinson disease, cerebral palsy, dementia [especially Alzheimer disease]; other neuromuscular/neurodevelopmental disorders).

Decreased absorption (e.g., lactose intolerance, Crohn disease).

Diminished desire or refusal to eat (e.g., anorexia nervosa, cirrhosis, pancreatitis, alcoholism, bipolar disorder, depression, chronic fatigue).

Treatment-related issues (e.g., chemotherapy, radiation, stomatitis, facial surgery, wired jaw).

Personal or situational factors (e.g., inability to procure or prepare food, social isolation, grief, loss).

- Assess pediatric concerns (e.g., changes in nutritional needs related to growth phase; congenital anomalies, including tracheoesophageal fistula, cleft lip/palate; metabolic or malabsorption problems, such as diabetes, phenylketonuria, cerebral palsy; chronic infections).
- Determine lifestyle factors that may affect weight. **Socioeconomic resources, the amount of money available for purchasing food, proximity of grocery stores, and available storage space for food are all factors that may impact food availability and intake.**
- Note client's ability to feed self or the presence of interfering factors. **Difficulties such as paralysis, tremor, or injury to hands or arms with inability to grasp or lift utensils to mouth; cognitive impairments affecting coordination or remembering to eat.**
- Evaluate the impact of cultural, familial, ethnic, and religious influences. **The nutritional balance of a diet is recognized by most cultures, with distinct theories of**

Information that appears in brackets has been added by the authors to clarify and enhance the use of nursing diagnoses.

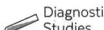 Diagnostic Studies 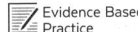 Evidence Based Practice 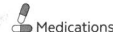 Medications 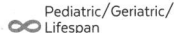 Pediatric/Geriatric/Lifespan

nutritional practices for health promotion and disease prevention. Social media, internet, and American culture promote the concept of thinness as the ideal female form, which may contribute to the development of eating disorders. Negative feedback from significant others (SOs) may impact client motivation for change and promote unhealthy behaviors.

- Assess client's knowledge of nutritional needs and ways client is meeting these needs **to identify teaching needs and/or help guide choice of interventions. Use of a psychosocial assessment tool (e.g., SCOFF questionnaire, Eating Disorder Examination [EDE], Eating Disorder Assessment for *Diagnostic and Statistical Manual of Mental Disorders, Fifth Edition* [EDA-5], Structured Interview for Anorexic and Bulimic Syndromes [SIAB-EX]) or client self-assessment (e.g., Eating Disorder Examination–Questionnaire [EDE-Q], Eating Disorder Inventory [EDI], Eating Attitudes Test [EAT], etc.) facilitates data collection regarding eating behaviors, body image, and client mood. Interview strategies should be empathetic and nonjudgmental to promote open and productive discourse.**
- Obtain client vital signs, including orthostatic values, routinely and as needed, **to evaluate impaired fluid balance and decompensated health associated with malnutrition and inadequate caloric intake.**
- Evaluate client's routine medications. **Some medications can contribute to weight loss (e.g., glucagon-like peptide-1 [GLP-1] receptor agonists, appetite suppressants, central nervous system stimulants, antidepressants, antidiabetic agents, blood pressure medications, chemotherapy, etc.).**
- Evaluate client's routine activity or exercise regimen. **Male clients with eating disorders may focus on muscularity and body leanness rather than severe caloric restriction. Compulsive and excessive exercise may be a contributor to excessive weight loss. Individuals with dementia may pace or be in constant motion, increasing energy needs.**
- Review laboratory test results (e.g., amylase, basic metabolic panel, complete blood count with differential, cholesterol, prealbumin, thyroid function) **that may reveal medical conditions associated with malnutrition/undernutrition, and identify problems that may compromise client health or recovery.**

Information that appears in brackets has been added by the authors to clarify and enhance the use of nursing diagnoses.

 Acute Care 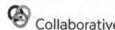 Collaborative 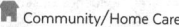 Community/Home Care   Cultural

Nursing Priority No. 2.
To evaluate the degree of compromise:

- Obtain client anthropometric measurements (e.g., height, weight, body mass index [BMI], percentile changes, and growth curves) **to determine the presence and severity of undernutrition/malnutrition. A BMI below 18.5 kg/m^2 is considered underweight and may indicate malnutrition.**
- Perform a focused physical examination evaluating the client for characteristics often seen in clients with protein-energy malnutrition:
  Poor dentition, sore throat, and or inflamed oral mucosa
  Parotid gland enlargement, bleeding gums
  Hair loss (i.e., axilla, pubic), increased body hair (i.e., lanugo), dull hair
  Brittle/fissuring of nails; dry, yellow skin, poor turgor
  Muscle wasting, cachectic appearance
  Edema (i.e., associated with hypoalbuminemia)
  Amenorrhea/menstrual changes, breast atrophy
  Cold intolerance; cold hands and feet
  Delayed healing
- Investigate client's bowel habits, including frequency, stool characteristics, and consistency. **Severe starvation may lead to hepatic steatosis.**
- Monitor pulmonary, cardiovascular, and fluid volume status **to monitor for refeeding complications**:
  Monitor vital signs. **Electrolyte abnormalities may result in cardiac dysrhythmia or myocardial compromise.**
  Auscultate lung sounds and assess pulmonary function. **Fluid and electrolyte shifts seen during refeeding can cause swelling of lung tissue impairing gas exchange.**
  Monitor fluid intake and output. **Initial refeeding may result in considerable renal fluid loss.**
- Perform or review results of nutritional assessment using screening tools such as the Malnutrition Universal Screening Tool, the Veterans Affairs Nutrition Status Classification system, the screening tool developed by Brugler et al. (2005), or the Mini Nutritional Assessment.
- Monitor and trend laboratory test results (e.g., complete blood count with differential, glucose, thyroid, electrolytes [i.e., potassium, magnesium, sodium, phosphate], albumin, arterial blood gas, renal function, etc.) **to evaluate client response to treatment and recovery. Refeeding in the presence of inadequate caloric intake can result in serum electrolyte deficiencies.**

Information that appears in brackets has been added by the authors to clarify and enhance the use of nursing diagnoses.

 Diagnostic Studies   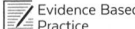 Evidence Based Practice   Medications   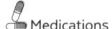 Pediatric/Geriatric/Lifespan

- Assist with and evaluate results of diagnostics (e.g., EKG, chest x-ray, endoscopic evaluation, etc.) **to evaluate client response to treatment and recovery, and assess for potential complications.**

Nursing Priority No. 3.
To correct/improve existing deficiencies:

- Collaborate in the treatment of client conditions to correct, treat, or promote client's recovery. **Counseling and psychological treatment (e.g., enhanced cognitive behavioral therapy (CBT-e), family-based therapy, dialectical behavioral therapy) can improve eating habits to support weight gain, enhance problem-solving, improve mood and client relationships.**
- Administer medication(s), as indicated. Medicate client for pain or nausea and manage drug side effects **to increase physical comfort and appetite. Appetite stimulants, dietary supplements, digestive drugs/enzymes, vitamins and minerals (e.g., iron), antacids, anticholinergics, antiemetics, antidiarrheals, etc., may be used to enhance intake, improve digestion, and correct nutritional deficiencies. Antidepressants may be used for clients with eating disorders to maximize psychological interventions and alleviate anxiety. The Food and Drug Administration (FDA) has approved fluoxetine, a selective serotonin reuptake inhibitor, for the treatment of bulimia.**
- Engage client and family in a structured program of medical supervision, talk therapy, and nutritional interventions. **Eating disorders represent complex client problems that require an interdisciplinary, team approach. The severely underweight client is at risk for significant complications during treatment (e.g., suicide, refeeding syndrome, electrolyte abnormalities, cardiopulmonary dysfunction, etc.).**
- Provide optimum nutrition (including adequate protein, lipids, calories, trace minerals, and multivitamins [e.g., A, C, D, E, and zinc]) **to promote return to a healthy weight and client health.**
- Encourage a pleasant, relaxing eating environment, including socialization when possible. Minimize the presence of unpleasant odors, sights, or cooking odors **to prevent a negative effect on appetite and enhancing food intake.**
- Encourage client/SO/caregiver engagement in food selection without undue emphasis on food consumption.

Information that appears in brackets has been added by the authors to clarify and enhance the use of nursing diagnoses.

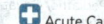 Acute Care 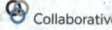 Collaborative 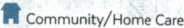 Community/Home Care Cultural

- Educate client/SO/caregiver in strategies to increase client caloric intake, such as add nonfat milk powder to foods with a high liquid content (e.g., gravy, puddings, cooked cereal) and sugar or honey to beverages for carbohydrates.
- Instruct client/SO/caregiver to avoid foods that cause intolerances or increase gastric motility (e.g., gas-forming foods, hot or cold, spicy, caffeinated beverages, milk products, etc.) **to reduce postprandial discomfort that may discourage client from eating.**
- Collaborate with a dietitian **to address meal planning and educate client/SO/caregiver on nutritional strategies.**
- Collaborate with occupational therapist **to identify appropriate assistive devices to facilitate independence in feeding and self-esteem.**
- Consult a speech therapist **to develop specific exercises or activities to address swallowing difficulties related to neurological problems (e.g., stroke, amyotrophic lateral sclerosis).** (Refer to ND impaired Swallowing for additional interventions.)
- Refer for dental care **to correct missing teeth or poorly fitting dentures that affect client's ability to chew food or enjoy the process of eating.**

Nursing Priority No. 4.

To promote client weight gain without complications (Teaching/Discharge Considerations) and enhance well-being (long-term goals):

- Emphasize the importance of client follow-up with the therapeutic program. **Despite treatment, many clients with eating disorders continue to struggle with unhealthy eating behaviors for years to come.**
- Involve client in developing behavior modification program appropriate to specific needs based on consistent, realistic weight gain goal. **Enhances commitment to change and likelihood of accomplishing desired outcomes.**
- Provide positive regard, love, and acknowledgment of "voice within" guiding client with eating disorder. **These efforts encourage the client to recognize maladaptive eating patterns as defense mechanisms to ease the emotional pain and begin to resolve underlying issues and develop more adaptive coping strategies for dealing with stressful situations.**
- Emphasize importance of well-balanced, nutritious intake. Provide nutritional information as indicated, taking into account client's age and developmental stage (e.g., toddler,

---

Information that appears in brackets has been added by the authors to clarify and enhance the use of nursing diagnoses.

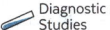 Diagnostic Studies 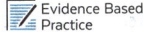 Evidence Based Practice 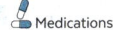 Medications 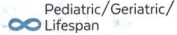 Pediatric/Geriatric/Lifespan

teenager, pregnant woman, elderly person with chronic disease), physical health and activity tolerance, financial and socioeconomic factors, and client's/SO's potential **for management of underlying conditions. For example, older adults need same nutrients as younger adults but in smaller amounts and with attention to certain components, such as calcium, fiber, vitamins, protein, and water. Infants/children require small meals and constant attention to needed nutrients for proper growth and development while dealing with the child's food preferences and eating habits.**

- Assist client/SO(s) to learn how to blenderize food or perform enteral feeding when indicated. **Promotes independence in self-care and sense of some degree of control in a difficult situation.**
- Encourage client to continue routine monitoring of weight. **Client may express anxiety with the weighing-in process, engaging the client's caregiver/SO to record weights and support client may be beneficial.**
- Discuss with client/SO the importance of healthy levels of regular activity and exercise. **Participation in a structured exercise program may provide consistency and accountability to enhance client success.**
- Address financial issues and identify ways to meet dietary needs using nutrient-dense, low-budget foods.
- Refer for dental hygiene and professional care, counseling or psychiatric care, and family therapy as indicated.
- Assist client to identify and access community resources such as nutrition assistance program, budget counseling, Meals on Wheels, community food banks, or other appropriate assistance programs.

Documentation Focus

Assessment/Reassessment
- Baseline and subsequent assessment findings to include signs/symptoms and laboratory diagnostic findings
- Caloric and nutrient intake
- Individual cultural or religious restrictions, personal preferences
- Availability and use of resources
- Personal understanding and perception of problem

Planning
- Plan of care and who is involved in planning
- Teaching plan

Information that appears in brackets has been added by the authors to clarify and enhance the use of nursing diagnoses.

Implementation/Evaluation
- Client's responses to interventions, teaching, and actions performed
- Results of periodic weigh-in
- Attainment or progress toward desired outcome(s)
- Modifications to plan of care

Discharge Planning
- Long-term needs and who is responsible for actions to be taken
- Specific referrals made

Sample Nursing Outcomes & Interventions Classifications NOC/NIC

NOC—Eating Disorder Self-Control
NIC—Eating Disorders Management

---

impaired spontaneous VENTILATION NANDA-I

[Diagnostic Division: Respiration]

Definition: Inability to maintain independent breathing that is adequate to support life.

Recognizing Cues

Related/Risk Factors
Respiratory muscle fatigue
Body position that inhibits lung expansion

Defining Characteristics

Subjective
Dyspnea
Apprehensiveness

Objective
Decreased arterial oxygen saturation, or partial pressure of oxygen; increased partial pressure of carbon dioxide (Pco_2)
Deterioration in arterial blood gases from baseline; hypoxia; increased heart rate
Decreased tidal volume
Decreased cooperation; psychomotor agitation
Increased accessory muscle use; increased metabolic rate

Information that appears in brackets has been added by the authors to clarify and enhance the use of nursing diagnoses.

 Diagnostic Studies 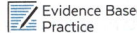 Evidence Based Practice 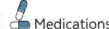 Medications ∞ Pediatric/Geriatric/Lifespan

Clinical Connections

Chronic obstructive pulmonary disease, asthma, pulmonary embolus, acute respiratory distress syndrome, SARS-CoV2, brain injury, chest trauma or surgery, Guillain-Barré syndrome, amyotrophic lateral sclerosis (ALS), shock

Generate Solutions

Plan Desired Outcomes

Client Will (Include Specific Time Frame)
- Reestablish and maintain effective respiratory pattern via ventilator with absence of retractions or use of accessory muscles, cyanosis, or other signs of hypoxia; and with arterial blood gases (ABGs)/Sao$_2$ within acceptable range.
- Participate in efforts to wean within individual ability, as appropriate.

Caregiver/Client Will (Include Specific Time Frame)
- Demonstrate behaviors necessary to maintain respiratory function.

Interventions/Take Action

Nursing Priority No. 1.
To determine degree of impairment:

- 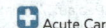 Identify client with impending respiratory failure (e.g., elevated respiratory rate; apnea or slow, shallow breathing; declining mentation or obtunded with the need for airway protection).
- Determine presence of conditions that could be associated with hypoventilation. **Causes include (1) central alveolar hypoventilation as a result of congenital defects, drugs, and central nervous system disorders (e.g., stroke, trauma, and neoplasms); (2) obesity hypoventilation syndrome is another well-known cause of hypoventilation; (3) chest wall deformities (e.g., kyphoscoliosis and changes after thoracic surgery) can be associated with alveolar hypoventilation leading to respiratory insufficiency and failure; (4) neuromuscular diseases that can cause alveolar hypoventilation include myasthenia gravis, ALS, Guillain-Barré, and muscular dystrophy.**
- Assess spontaneous respiratory pattern, noting rate, depth, rhythm, symmetry of chest movement, use of accessory muscles. **Tachypnea, shallow breathing, demonstrated or reported dyspnea (using a numeric or similar scale);**

Information that appears in brackets has been added by the authors to clarify and enhance the use of nursing diagnoses.

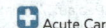 Acute Care 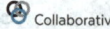 Collaborative 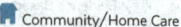 Community/Home Care   Cultural

increased heart rate, dysrhythmia; pallor or cyanosis; and intercostal retractions and use of accessory muscles indicate increased work of breathing or gas exchange impairment.
- Auscultate breath sounds, noting presence or absence and equality of breath sounds, adventitious breath sounds.
- Evaluate ABGs and/or pulse oximetry and capnography **to determine presence and degree of arterial hypoxemia (Pao_2 less than 55 mm Hg) and hypercapnia ($Paco_2$ greater than 45 mm Hg) requiring ventilatory support.**
- Obtain or review results of pulmonary function studies (e.g., lung volumes, **inspiratory and expiratory pressures, and forced vital capacity**), as appropriate, **to assess the presence and degree of respiratory insufficiency.**
- Investigate etiology of current respiratory failure **to determine ventilation needs and most appropriate type of ventilatory support.**
- Review serial chest x-rays and imaging (MRI/computed tomography scan) results **to diagnose underlying disorder and monitor response to treatment. Client may already be receiving treatments to maintain airway patency and enhance gas exchange or may have respiratory failure associated with sudden event (e.g., severe trauma, sudden-onset respiratory illness, surgery with complications).**
- Note response to current measures and respiratory therapy (e.g., bronchodilators, steroids, diuretics, supplemental oxygen, nebulizer or intermittent positive-pressure breathing treatments).
- Ascertain desires of client/significant others (SOs) regarding plan for treatment of respiratory failure, as indicated. **Client may have advance directives and/or prior stated decisions about the level of therapy aggressiveness that client desires if situation is chronic or long term. Family members may help in decision-making processes if the client is a minor or is incapacitated.**

Nursing Priority No. 2.
To provide/maintain ventilatory support:
- Collaborate with physician, respiratory care practitioners regarding effective mode of ventilation (e.g., noninvasive oxygenation via continuous positive airway pressure and biphasic positive airway pressure, prone positioning); or intubation and mechanical ventilation (e.g., continuous mandatory, assist control, intermittent mandatory ventilation

---

Information that appears in brackets has been added by the authors to clarify and enhance the use of nursing diagnoses.

 Diagnostic Studies 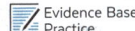 Evidence Based Practice 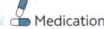 Medications 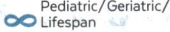 Pediatric/Geriatric/Lifespan

[IMV], pressure support). **Specific mode is determined by client's respiratory requirements, presence of underlying disease process, and the extent to which client can participate in ventilatory efforts.**

- Ensure that ventilator settings and parameters are correct as determined by client situation, including respiratory rate, fraction of inspired oxygen (FIO_2, expressed as a percentage); tidal volume; peak inspiratory pressure.
- Observe overall breathing pattern, distinguishing between spontaneous respirations and ventilator breaths. **The client may be completely dependent on the ventilator or able to take breaths but have poor oxygen saturation without the ventilator. The client on assist-control ventilation mode can still experience hyper-/hypoventilation or "air hunger" and attempt to correct the deficiency by overbreathing.**
- Verify that client's respirations are in phase with the ventilator. **Decreases work of breathing and maximizes O_2 delivery when the client is not fighting the ventilator.**
- Collaborate with respiratory therapy to maintain appropriate tracheal or endotracheal tube cuff pressure. Proper cuff pressure **ensures adequate ventilation and delivery of desired tidal volume without air leak or tracheal tissue injury.**
- Check tubing for obstruction (e.g., kinking or accumulation of water) **that can impede flow of oxygen.** Drain tubing as indicated.
- Check ventilator alarms for proper functioning. Do not turn off alarms, even for suctioning. Remove from ventilator and ventilate manually if source of ventilator alarm cannot be quickly identified and rectified. Verify that alarms can be heard in the nurses' station by care providers.
- Remove from ventilator and ventilate manually **if source of ventilator alarm cannot be quickly identified and rectified.**
- Suction only as needed **to clear secretions (e.g., if client is coughing excessively, has visible secretions, or is tripping high-pressure alarm on ventilator).**
- Verify that oxygen line is in proper outlet/tank; monitor in-line oxygen analyzer or perform periodic oxygen analysis **to deliver an acceptable oxygen percentage and saturation for client's specific needs.**
- Verify client's tidal volume is set to the volume as ordered, and proper functioning of spirometer, bellows, or computer readout of delivered volume. Note alterations from desired volume delivery **to determine alteration in lung**

Information that appears in brackets has been added by the authors to clarify and enhance the use of nursing diagnoses.

 Acute Care 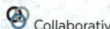 Collaborative 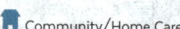 Community/Home Care Cultural

compliance or leakage through machine/around tube cuff (if used).
- Monitor airway pressure **for developing complications or equipment problems (e.g., increased airway resistance, retained secretions, decreased lung compliance, client out of phase or off ventilator).**
- Promote periodic maximal ventilation of alveoli; check sigh rate intervals (usually 1½ to 2 times tidal volume), as needed. **Reduces the risk of atelectasis, helps mobilize secretions.**
- Note inspired humidity and temperature; maintain hydration **to prevent excessive drying of mucosa and secretions.**
- Auscultate breath sounds periodically. Investigate frequent crackles or rhonchi that do not clear with coughing or suctioning, **which are suggestive of developing complications (atelectasis, pneumonia, acute bronchospasm, pulmonary edema).**
- Note changes in chest symmetry. **May indicate improper placement of endotracheal tube or development of barotrauma.**
- Keep resuscitation bag at bedside **to allow for manual ventilation whenever indicated (e.g., if client is removed from ventilator or troubleshooting equipment problems).**
- Administer sedation as required **to synchronize respirations and reduce work of breathing and energy expenditure, as indicated.**
- Administer and monitor response to medications that promote airway patency and gas exchange.
- Refer to NDs impaired Airway Clearance; ineffective Breathing Pattern; impaired Gas Exchange, for related interventions.

Nursing Priority No. 3.
To prepare for/assist with weaning process if appropriate:
- Determine physical and psychological readiness to wean, soon after intubation, whenever possible, **to limit complications associated with long-term mechanical ventilation. Successful weaning is based on parameters such as (1) evidence for some reversal of the underlying cause of respiratory failure, (2) adequate oxygenation and normal pH, (3) hemodynamic stability, (4) capability and willingness to initiate inspiratory effort, (5) absence of excessive secretions, and (6) nutritional status sufficient to maintain work of breathing.**

Information that appears in brackets has been added by the authors to clarify and enhance the use of nursing diagnoses.

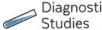 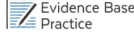 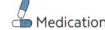 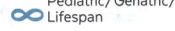

- 🤝 • Determine mode for weaning. **Pressure support mode or multiple daily T-piece trials may be superior to IMV; low-level pressure support may be beneficial for spontaneous breathing trials; and early extubation and institution of noninvasive positive pressure ventilation may have substantial benefits in alert, cooperative client.**
- Explain weaning activities and techniques, individual plan, and expectations. **Reduces fear of the unknown, provides opportunities to deal with concerns, clarifies reality of fears, and helps reduce anxiety to manageable level.**
- 🤝 • Engage client in a specialized exercise program **to enhance respiratory muscle strength and general endurance.**
- Maximize weaning effort:
  Elevate head of bed/place in an orthopedic chair, if possible, or position **to alleviate dyspnea and to facilitate oxygenation.**
  Coach client in "taking control" of breathing during weaning periods (e.g., to take slower, deeper breaths; practice abdominal or pursed-lip breathing; assume a position of comfort) **to maximize respiratory function and reduce anxiety.**
  Instruct in or assist client to perform effective coughing techniques. **Necessary for secretion management after extubation.**
  Provide a quiet environment, a calm approach, and the undivided attention of nurse. **Promotes relaxation, decreasing energy and oxygen requirements.**
  Involve family/SO(s) as appropriate. Provide diversionary activity. **Helps client focus on something other than breathing.**
  Instruct client in use of energy-saving techniques during care activities **to limit oxygen consumption and fatigue associated with work of breathing.**
- Acknowledge and provide ongoing encouragement for client's efforts. Communicate hope for successful weaning response (even partial). **Enhances commitment to continue activity, maximizing outcomes.**

Nursing Priority No. 4.
To prepare for discharge on ventilator when indicated:
- 🏠 • Ascertain plan for discharge placement (e.g., return home, short-term stay in subacute or rehabilitation center, or permanent placement in long-term care facility) **to determine care needs and fiscal impact of home care versus extended-care facility.**
- Review layout of home, noting size of rooms, doorways, placement of furniture, and number and type of

---

Information that appears in brackets has been added by the authors to clarify and enhance the use of nursing diagnoses.

electrical outlets **to identify necessary modifications and safety needs.**
- Determine specific equipment needs. Identify resources for equipment needs and maintenance and arrange for delivery prior to client discharge **to allow SO/caregivers to prepare for transfer.**
- Allow sufficient opportunity for SO(s)/family to practice new skills. Role-play potential crisis situations **to enhance confidence in ability to handle client's needs.**
- Demonstrate airway management techniques and proper equipment cleaning practices **to reduce risk of infection.**
- Instruct SO(s)/caregivers in pulmonary physiotherapy measures, as indicated. Refer for home respiratory therapy support, as needed.
- Provide positive feedback and encouragement for the efforts of SO(s)/caregivers. **Promotes continuation of desired behaviors.**
- List names and phone numbers for identified contact persons and resources **to reduce the sense of isolation and enhance the likelihood of obtaining assistance and support when needed.**
- Review and provide written or audiovisual materials regarding proper ventilator management, maintenance, and safety for reference in home setting. **Provides information to enhance client's/SO's level of comfort with challenging tasks.**
- Identify signs/symptoms requiring prompt medical evaluation or intervention. **Timely treatment may prevent progression of problem or untoward complications.**
- Obtain No Smoking signs to be posted in home. Encourage family members to refrain from smoking.
- Have family/SO(s) notify utility companies and fire department about presence of a ventilator in the home. **Client will be placed on a high-risk list for follow-up in case of a power outage or fire.**
- Develop emergency disaster plan **to address backup electrical needs and possible evacuation if required.**

Nursing Priority No. 5.

To promote spontaneous ventilation (Teaching/Discharge Considerations) and enhance well-being (long-term goals):

- Discuss the impact of specific activities on respiratory status and problem-solve solutions to maximize weaning effort or to reduce the incidence of respiratory distress or failure.
- Monitor the health of visitors and persons involved in care **to protect client from sources of infection.**

Information that appears in brackets has been added by the authors to clarify and enhance the use of nursing diagnoses.

 Diagnostic Studies 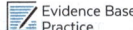 Evidence Based Practice 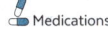 Medications 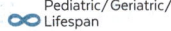 Pediatric/Geriatric/Lifespan

- Recommend involvement in support group; introduce to individuals dealing with similar problems **to provide role models, assistance for problem-solving.**
- Encourage time out for caregivers **so that they may attend to personal needs, wellness, and growth.** Refer to ND risk for caregiver Role Strain.
- Provide opportunities for client/SO(s) to discuss advance directives. **Clarifies parameters for termination of therapy or other end-of-life decisions, as desired.**
- Recommend involvement in a support group; introduce to other ventilator-dependent individuals who are successfully managing home ventilation, if desired, **to answer questions, provide role model, assist with problem-solving, and offer encouragement and hope for the future.**
- Refer to additional resources (e.g., spiritual advisor, counselor).

Documentation Focus

Assessment/Reassessment
- Baseline findings, subsequent alterations in respiratory function
- Results of diagnostic testing
- Individual risk factors and concerns

Planning
- Plan of care and who is involved in planning
- Teaching plan

Implementation/Evaluation
- Client's/SO's responses to interventions, teaching, and actions performed
- Skill level and assistance needs of SO(s)/family
- Attainment of or progress toward desired outcome(s)
- Modifications to plan of care

Discharge Planning
- Discharge plan, including appropriate referrals, action taken, and who is responsible for each action
- Equipment needs and source
- Resources for support persons or home-care providers

Sample Nursing Outcomes & Interventions Classifications NOC/NIC

NOC—Respiratory Function: Ventilation
NIC—Mechanical Ventilation Management: Invasive

Information that appears in brackets has been added by the authors to clarify and enhance the use of nursing diagnoses.

impaired adult VENTILATORY WEANING RESPONSE NANDA-I

[Diagnostic Division: Respiration]

Definition: Inability to successfully transition to spontaneous ventilation of individuals >18 years of age who have required mechanical ventilation at least 24 hours.

Recognizing Cues

Related/Risk Factors
Altered sleep-wake cycle
Excessive airway secretions; ineffective cough
Malnutrition

Defining Characteristics

Subjective
Early Response (30 min)
Apprehensiveness, or fear of machine malfunction, or perceived need for increased oxygen
Feels warm

Objective
Early Response (30 min)
Audible airway secretions; adventitious respiratory sounds
Decreased blood pressure (less than 90 mm Hg or greater than 20% reduction from baseline); increased blood pressure (systolic pressure greater than 180 mm Hg or greater than 20% from baseline)
Decreased heart rate (greater than 20% reduction from baseline); increased heart rate (greater than 140 bpm or greater than 20% from baseline)
Decreased oxygen saturation (less than 90% when fraction of inspired oxygen ratio greater than 40%)
Increased respiratory rate (greater than 35 rpm or greater than 50% over baseline); panting; shallow breathing
Hyperfocused on activities; psychomotor agitation: wide-eyed appearance
Nasal flaring; paradoxical abdominal breathing; uses significant respiratory accessory muscles

---

Information that appears in brackets has been added by the authors to clarify and enhance the use of nursing diagnoses.

 Diagnostic Studies
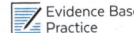 Evidence Based Practice
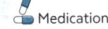 Medications
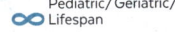 Pediatric/Geriatric/Lifespan

Intermediate Response (30 to 90 min)
Decreased pH (less than 7.32 or greater than 0.07 reduction from baseline); hypercapnia (greater than 50 mm Hg increased in partial pressure of carbon dioxide or greater than 8 mm Hg increased from baseline); hypoxemia (partial pressure of oxygen 50% or oxygen greater than 6 L/min)
Diaphoresis
Difficulty cooperating with instructions
Late Response (Greater Than 90 min)
Fatigue
Cyanosis
Recent-onset arrhythmias; cardiopulmonary arrest

Clinical Connections
Traumatic brain injury, stroke, substance overdose, chronic obstructive pulmonary disease, infections, SARS-CoV2, crushing chest trauma, paralysis, respiratory or cardiac arrest

Generate Solutions

Plan Desired Outcomes

Client Will (Include Specific Time Frame)
- Indicate understanding of weaning process and future needs.
- Reestablish independent respiration with arterial blood gases (ABGs) within client's normal range and be free of signs of respiratory failure.
- Demonstrate increased tolerance for activity and participate in self-care within level of ability.

Interventions/Take Action

Nursing Priority No. 1.
To identify contributing factors/degree of dysfunction:

- Determine the extent and nature of underlying disorders or factors (e.g., respiratory muscles/diaphragmatic dysfunction/weakness, lung/chest wall compliance, or gas exchange, cardiovascular dysfunction, neuromuscular disorders, psychological factors [e.g., depressive disorders or delirium], metabolic/endocrine diseases, alone or combined) **that contribute to client's reliance on mechanical support, thus affecting weaning efforts. Note: Recent studies have reported on various predictors of weaning outcome, which included maximal inspiratory pressure (PImax), rapid shallow breathing index (RSBI), fluid balance,**

Information that appears in brackets has been added by the authors to clarify and enhance the use of nursing diagnoses.

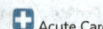 Acute Care 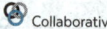 Collaborative 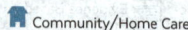 Community/Home Care   Cultural

comorbidity burden, severity of illness, emphysematous changes, and low serum albumin. **Although age was not an independent predictor of weaning failure, the correlation of advanced age and the presence of comorbidities, particularly diabetes, cerebrovascular disorders, heart disease, and chronic pulmonary diseases, demonstrated more common difficulty in ventilatory weaning.**

- Investigate previous unsuccessful weaning attempts to determine the level of response to weaning interventions (as noted in Defining Characteristics) noting the length of time the client has been on the ventilator and previous episodes of extubation and reintubation. **Although most individuals remain on the ventilator for 7 days or less, some require support for several weeks or more. Note: Studies have shown that if client fails to wean from ventilator dependence within 60 days, client will probably not do so later.**

- Complete the modified Burns Weaning Assessment Program (m-BWAP) or similar checklist (e.g., stability of vital signs, factors that increase metabolic rate [e.g., sepsis, fever]; hydration status; need for/recent use of analgesia or sedation; nutritional state; muscle strength; activity level) **to assess systemic parameters that may affect readiness for weaning. Evidence suggests successful spontaneous breathing trials (SBTs), low RSBI, high PImax, stable Pao_2 and $Paco_2$, stable pulmonary infiltrate(s) and/or pleural effusion, adequate body strength and condition, and ability to clear and maintain patent airway correlate with successful extubation and decreased risk for postextubation respiratory failure (PERF).**

- Ascertain client's awareness and understanding of the weaning process, expectations, and concerns. **Unrealistic expectations or unvoiced concerns can impair weaning process or willingness to participate.**

- Determine client's psychological readiness, presence and degree of anxiety. **Weaning provokes anxiety regarding the ability to breathe on one's own and the potential of ventilator dependence, especially if repeated attempts at weaning have been unsuccessful. The client must be highly motivated, be able to actively participate in the weaning process, and be physically comfortable enough to work at weaning.**

- Review client's laboratory studies, such as complete blood count, **to determine the number and quality of red blood cells for oxygen transport,** serum albumin, and electrolyte levels indicating nutritional status **to determine if client**

Information that appears in brackets has been added by the authors to clarify and enhance the use of nursing diagnoses.

 Diagnostic Studies 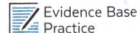 Evidence Based Practice 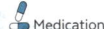 Medications 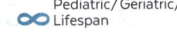 Pediatric/Geriatric/Lifespan

has sufficient nutritional stores to meet demands of spontaneous breathing and weaning.
- Review chest x-ray, pulse oximetry, capnography, and/or ABGs. **Before client's weaning attempts, chest x-ray should show stable processes without advancement of infectious or inflammatory activity. ABGs should demonstrate satisfactory oxygenation. Capnometry measures end-tidal carbon dioxide values and can be used to monitor readiness for weaning.**

Nursing Priority No. 2.
To support weaning process:
- Discuss with client/SO an individual plan and expectations regarding ventilatory weaning. **May reduce client's anxiety about the process and increase willingness to work at SBTs.**
- Consult with dietitian and nutritional support team for adjustments in client's diet (i.e., enteral/parenteral nutrition) prior to weaning **to support respiratory muscle strength and work of breathing and to prevent excessive production of CO_2, which could alter respiratory drive. Individuals on long-term ventilation may require enteral formulas with a high concentration of carbohydrates, protein, and calories to improve respiratory muscle function.**
- Collaborate in implementing weaning protocols and varying ventilator mode (e.g., spontaneous breathing trials, automatic tube compensation, partial client support by means of synchronized intermittent mandatory ventilation, pressure support ventilation during client's spontaneous breathing) **to optimize the work of breathing and to provide support for spontaneous ventilation.**
- Perform a focused physical examination of client **to evaluate weaning tolerance.** The examination may include:
Respiratory rate **to evaluate client's work of breathing.**
Depth of client's respirations (i.e., RSBI). **RSBI is a strong predictor of ventilatory weaning success. Values greater than 105 min/L predict weaning failure.**
Spontaneous tidal volume **to evaluate client's work of breathing.**
Heart rate **to evaluate for signs of hypoxia and client decompensation. Note that elevation of client's heart rate (i.e, greater than 140 or 25% above baseline) may be seen as an early compensatory response; however,**

Information that appears in brackets has been added by the authors to clarify and enhance the use of nursing diagnoses.

 Acute Care 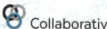 Collaborative 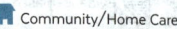 Community/Home Care 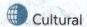 Cultural

bradycardia (i.e., heart rate less than 60) may also be seen but is a more ominous presentation.

Blood pressure **to evaluate for signs of hypoxia and client decompensation (i.e., SBP 40 mm Hg above baseline).**

- Note client's response to activity or client care during weaning, as indicated. Provide undisturbed rest or sleep periods. Avoid stressful procedures or situations and nonessential activities **to prevent excessive oxygen consumption or demand with an increased possibility of weaning failure.**
- Assist the client with secretion management by suctioning client's airway, as needed **to maintain a patent airway and facilitate ventilation.**
- Discuss the impact of specific activities (e.g., muscle-strengthening activities, physiotherapy with positive pressure, cough augmentation, respiratory muscle training, etc.) on respiratory status, and problem-solve solutions **to maximize weaning effort.**
- Time medications during weaning efforts **to minimize sedative effects.**
- Provide quiet room, calm approach, and undivided attention. **Enhances relaxation, thereby conserving energy.**
- Involve SO(s)/family, as appropriate (e.g., sit at bedside, provide encouragement, help monitor client status).
- Provide diversionary activity (e.g., watching TV, listening to audiobooks, music) **to focus attention away from breathing when not actively working at breathing exercises.**
- Acknowledge and provide ongoing encouragement for client's efforts.
- Minimize setbacks and focus client attention on gains and progress to date **to reduce frustration that may further impair progress.**

Nursing Priority No. 3.

To prepare for discharge on ventilator when indicated:

- Prepare client/SO for alternative actions when client is unable to resume spontaneous ventilation (e.g., tracheostomy with long-term ventilation support in alternate care setting or home, palliative care or end-of-life procedures). **Client discharged from intensive care unit may be sent to specialized units (long-term acute care), extended care facilities, or home. Customized discharge planning for people new to home ventilation is essential, and must include assessment of the environment, availability of resources, and capability of caregivers.**

Information that appears in brackets has been added by the authors to clarify and enhance the use of nursing diagnoses.

- Ascertain that all needed equipment is in place, caregivers are trained, and safety concerns have been addressed (e.g., notifying fire department, utility company; alternative power source, backup equipment, client call or alarm system, established means of client/caregiver communication) **to ease the transfer when client is going home on ventilator.**
- Evaluate caregiver capabilities and burden when client requires a long-term ventilator in the home **to determine potential or presence of skill-related problems or emotional issues (e.g., caregiver overload, burnout, or depression). Note: All home caregivers (professionals, family, friends) should receive a comprehensive orientation before caring for someone using a home ventilator. This includes familiarization with the ventilator; alarms and the subsequent actions that must be taken; tracheostomy care; safe transfer of the ventilator user; suctioning techniques; and bag-valve-mask ventilation (use of an Ambu bag) in the case of an emergency, such as accidental disconnection of the ventilator circuit.**
- Discuss with client/SO signs/symptoms requiring prompt medical evaluation or intervention. Timely treatment may prevent progression of a problem or untoward complications.
- Obtain no-smoking signs to be posted in client's home and remind family members/visitors to refrain from smoking to reduce risk of fire.
- Have family/SO(s) notify the utility company and fire department of the presence of a ventilator in client's home. The client will be placed on a high-risk list for follow-up in case of a power outage or fire.
- Refer to ND impaired spontaneous Ventilation for additional interventions.

Nursing Priority No. 4.

To promote optimal ventilation (Teaching/Discharge Considerations) and enhance well-being (long-term goals):

- Encourage client/SO(s) to evaluate the impact of ventilatory dependence on their lifestyle and changes they are willing or unwilling to make when client is discharged on ventilator. **Quality-of-life issues must be examined, including issues of privacy and intimacy, and resolved by client and SO(s). All parties need to understand that ventilatory support is a 24-hr job that ultimately affects everyone. Findings may dictate alternative placement is desirable or needed.**

Information that appears in brackets has been added by the authors to clarify and enhance the use of nursing diagnoses.

- Stress need for caregivers to monitor physical well-being. **Caregivers have reported insufficient sleep, physical exhaustion, back pain, and significantly higher physical burden levels.**
- Discuss importance of time for self and identify appropriate sources for respite care for client and caregiver. **Initially, caregivers may have limited understanding of the magnitude of the demands on their time and energy. Knowing support is available enhances coping abilities.** Refer to ND excessive Caregiving Burden.
- Emphasize to client/SO(s) importance of monitoring health of visitors and persons involved in care, avoiding crowds during flu season, obtaining immunizations, and so forth, **to protect client from sources of infection.**
- Engage in rehabilitation program, if possible, **to enhance respiratory muscle strength and general endurance.**
- Encourage client/SO(s) to discuss advance directives and ascertain that all caregivers and care providers are aware of the plan of care. **Clarifies parameters for emergency situations, termination of therapy, or other end-of-life decisions, as desired.**
- Recommend client/SO(s) involvement in a support group and introduce to other ventilator-dependent individuals who are successfully managing home ventilation, **to answer questions, provide role models, assist with problem-solving, and offer encouragement and hope for the future.**

Documentation Focus

Assessment/Reassessment
- Baseline findings and subsequent changes
- Results of diagnostic testing and procedures
- Home evaluation as indicated

Planning
- Plan of care, specific interventions, and who is involved in the planning
- Teaching plan

Implementation/Evaluation
- Client/SO response to interventions
- Attainment of or progress toward desired outcome(s)
- Modifications to plan of care

Discharge Planning
- Status at discharge, long-term needs and referrals, indicating who is to be responsible for each action
- Equipment needs and supplier

Information that appears in brackets has been added by the authors to clarify and enhance the use of nursing diagnoses.

Sample Nursing Outcomes & Interventions Classifications NOC/NIC

NOC—Mechanical Ventilation Weaning Response: Adult
NIC—Mechanical Ventilatory Weaning

---

impaired child VENTILATORY WEANING RESPONSE — NANDA-I

[Diagnostic Division: Respiration]

Definition: Inability to successfully transition to spontaneous respiration of individuals <18 years of age who have required mechanical ventilation at least 24 hours.

Recognizing Cues

Related/Risk Factors

Physiological Factors:
Altered sleep-wake cycle
Ineffective airway clearance
Malnutrition
Pain

Psychological Factors:
Anxiety; inadequate self-esteem
Decreased motivation; hopelessness; powerlessness
Fear; inadequate trust in health professional
Inadequate knowledge of weaning process; uncertainty about ability to wean

Situational Factors:
Unaddressed environmental disturbances
Inappropriate pace of weaning process
Uncontrolled episodic energy demands

Defining Characteristics
Mild

Subjective
Breathing discomfort
Feels warm
Fatigue
Fear of machine malfunction
Perceived need for increased oxygen

Information that appears in brackets has been added by the authors to clarify and enhance the use of nursing diagnoses.

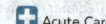 Acute Care 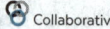 Collaborative 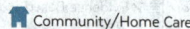 Community/Home Care   Cultural

Objective
Mildly increased respiratory rate over baseline
Increased focus on breathing
Psychomotor agitation

Moderate

Subjective
Apprehensiveness

Objective
Abnormal skin color

Blood pressure increased from baseline (less than 20 mm Hg), heart rate increased from baseline (less than 20 beats/min); moderately increased respiratory rate over baseline

Decreased air entry on auscultation; minimal use of respiratory accessory muscles

Diaphoresis; facial mask of fear

Difficulty cooperating, or responding to coaching; hyperfocused on activities

Severe

Objective
Adventitious breath sounds; asynchronized breathing with the ventilator

Blood pressure increased (≥20 mm Hg) or heart rate increased (≥20 beats/min) from baseline; significantly increased respiratory rate above baseline

Deterioration in arterial blood gases (ABGs) from baseline

Gasping breaths; shallow breathing; paradoxical abdominal breathing; uses significant respiratory accessory muscles

Profuse diaphoresis

Clinical Connections
Traumatic brain injury, paralysis, chest trauma, substance overdose, premature infant, infection, near drowning, stroke, respiratory or cardiac arrest

Generate Solutions

Plan Desired Outcomes

Client Will (Include Specific Time Frame)
- Actively participate in the weaning process depending on age/condition.
- Reestablish independent respiration with ABGs within client's normal range and be free of signs of respiratory failure.

Information that appears in brackets has been added by the authors to clarify and enhance the use of nursing diagnoses.

 Diagnostic Studies   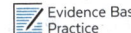 Evidence Based Practice   Medications   Pediatric/Geriatric/Lifespan

- Demonstrate increased tolerance for activity and participate in self-care within level of ability.

Interventions/Take Action

Nursing Priority No. 1.
To identify contributing factors/degree of dysfunction:

- Note client age and developmental factors. **Individuals at any age (from preterm neonates to teenagers) may require ventilatory support. However, interventions and equipment needs are individually determined. For example, pathologies affecting a newborn's lungs are different from others observed later in life. Also, neonates and infants have smaller airway caliber, few collateral airways, poor airway stability, and low functional residual capacity. Infants and children younger than 24 mo who require mechanical ventilation for longer than 48 hr may be at higher risk for extubation failure.**
- Determine extent and nature of underlying disorders or factors (e.g., adequate respiratory drive, respiratory muscles/diaphragmatic dysfunction or weakness, lung/chest wall compliance, gas exchange, cardiovascular dysfunction, neuromuscular disorders, well as metabolic/endocrine diseases, alone or combined) **that contribute to client's reliance on mechanical support and can affect future weaning efforts.**
- Note length of time client has been receiving ventilator support. Review previous episodes of extubation and reintubation noting the level of response to weaning interventions (as noted in Defining Characteristics). **Although most individuals remain on the ventilator for 7 days or less, some require support for several weeks or more. Commonly, if the client fails to wean from ventilator dependence within 60 days, the client will probably not do so later. Upper airway obstruction is the single most common cause of extubation failure in children.**
- Assess systemic parameters that may affect readiness for weaning using the modified Burns Weaning Assessment Program (m-BWAP) or similar checklist (e.g., stability of vital signs, factors that increase metabolic rate [e.g., sepsis, fever]; hydration status; need for/recent use of analgesia or sedation; nutritional state; muscle strength; activity level) **to assess systemic parameters that may affect readiness for weaning.**

Information that appears in brackets has been added by the authors to clarify and enhance the use of nursing diagnoses.

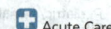 Acute Care 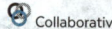 Collaborative 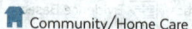 Community/Home Care Cultural

- Ascertain client's and parents' awareness and understanding of weaning process, expectations, and concerns. **Client/parents may need specific and repeated instructions during the weaning process. Unrealistic expectations or unvoiced concerns can impair the weaning process or willingness to participate.**
- Consider client's age/developmental level when determining client's readiness for weaning and presence and degree of anxiety. **Weaning provokes anxiety regarding ability to breathe on own and likelihood of ventilator dependence. The child must be motivated, be able to actively participate in the weaning process, and be physically comfortable enough to work at weaning.**
- Review laboratory studies (e.g., complete blood count reflecting number and quality of red blood cells **[affects oxygen transport]**, serum albumin, and electrolyte levels indicating nutritional status **[to confirm sufficient energy to meet demands of spontaneous breathing and weaning])**.
- Review chest x-ray, pulse oximetry or capnography, and/or ABGs. **Before weaning attempts, chest radiograph should show stable processes without advancement of infectious or inflammatory activity. ABGs should demonstrate satisfactory oxygenation.**

Nursing Priority No. 2.

To support weaning process:

- Discuss with client/parents the client's plan and expectations. Assure client of nurse's presence and assistance during weaning attempts. **Helps to reduce client's anxiety about the weaning process and enhance willingness to work at spontaneous breathing.**
- Consult with dietitian, nutritional support team for adjustments in composition of diet prior to weaning **to support respiratory muscle strength, work of breathing, and to prevent excessive production of CO_2, which could alter respiratory drive. Individuals on long-term ventilation may require gavage/enteral formulas with a high concentration of carbohydrates, protein, and calories to improve respiratory muscle function.**
- Implement weaning protocols and varying ventilator mode as ordered (e.g., spontaneous breathing trials, assist-control and synchronized intermittent mandatory ventilation [SIMV], volume-targeted, and high-frequency ventilation) **to optimize the work of breathing and to provide support for spontaneous ventilation.**

Information that appears in brackets has been added by the authors to clarify and enhance the use of nursing diagnoses.

- Perform a focused physical examination of client **to evaluate weaning tolerance.** The examination may include:
  Respiratory rate **to evaluate the client's work of breathing.**
  Inspiratory pressure and time, flow, and synchronization of the ventilator with the client's spontaneous breaths **to assess lung compliance and the gas volume that reaches the alveoli.**
  Depth of the client's respirations (i.e., RSBI). **RSBI may be a strong predictor of ventilatory weaning success. Values greater than 105 min/L may predict weaning failure.**
  Client's spontaneous tidal volume **to evaluate the client's work of breathing.**
  Pulse oximetry **to determine client's ability to ventilate and exchange gases.**
  Heart rate **to evaluate signs of hypoxia and client decompensation.**
  Blood pressure **to evaluate for signs of hypoxia and client decompensation.**
- Note client's response to activity/client care during weaning and limit, as indicated. Provide undisturbed rest or sleep periods. Avoid stressful procedures or situations and nonessential activities. **Prevents excessive oxygen consumption or demand with an increased possibility of weaning failure.**
- Assist client with secretion management by suctioning airway, as needed **to maintain a patent airway and facilitate ventilation.**
- Discuss/observe impact of specific activities (e.g., muscle-strengthening activities, physiotherapy with positive pressure, cough augmentation, respiratory muscle training, etc.) on respiratory status, and problem-solve solutions to maximize weaning effort.
- Time medications during weaning efforts **to minimize sedative effects.**
- Provide quiet room, calm approach, undivided attention of nurse. **Enhances relaxation, conserving energy.**
- Involve family, as appropriate (e.g., sitting at bedside, providing encouragement, and helping monitor client status).
- Provide client with age-appropriate diversional activity (e.g., watching TV, videos, listening to audiobooks, music) **to focus attention away from breathing when not actively working on breathing exercises.**
- Acknowledge and provide ongoing encouragement for client's efforts.

Information that appears in brackets has been added by the authors to clarify and enhance the use of nursing diagnoses.

- Minimize setbacks, focus client/parent attention on gains and progress to date **to reduce frustration that may further impair progress.**

Nursing Priority No. 3.
To prepare for discharge on ventilator when indicated:

- Prepare client/parent/family for alternative actions when client is unable to resume spontaneous ventilation (e.g., tracheostomy with long-term ventilatory support in alternate care setting or home, palliative care, or end-of-life procedures). **Despite meeting all weaning criteria and succeeding in a weaning trial, failure of planned extubation occurs in about 10% to 20% of cases. Client discharged from intensive care unit may be sent to specialized units (long-term acute care), extended-care facilities, or home.**
- Assess home environment, availability of resources, and capability of caregivers when developing customized discharge plan. **All home caregivers (professionals, family, friends) should receive a comprehensive orientation before caring for someone using a home ventilator. This includes familiarization with the ventilator; alarms and the subsequent actions that must be taken; tracheostomy care; safe transfer of the ventilator user; suctioning techniques; and bag-valve-mask ventilation (use of an Ambu bag) in the case of an emergency.**
- Ascertain that all needed equipment is in place, caregivers are trained, and safety concerns have been addressed (e.g., notify fire department, utility company; availability of alternative power source, backup equipment, client call or alarm system, established means of client/caregiver communication) **to ease the transfer when client is going home on ventilator.**
- Discuss with the client/SO signs/symptoms requiring prompt medical evaluation or intervention. **Timely treatment may prevent the progression of a problem or untoward complications.**
- Obtain no-smoking signs to be posted in the client's home, and remind family members to refrain from smoking **to reduce the risk of fire.**
- Have parents/family notify the utility company and fire department of the presence of a ventilator in the client's home. **Client will be placed on a high-risk list for follow-up in case of a power outage or fire.**
- Refer to ND impaired spontaneous Ventilation for additional interventions.

Information that appears in brackets has been added by the authors to clarify and enhance the use of nursing diagnoses.

 Diagnostic Studies 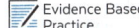 Evidence Based Practice Medications 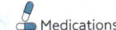 Pediatric/Geriatric/Lifespan

Nursing Priority No. 4.

To promote optimal ventilation (Teaching/Discharge Considerations) and enhance well-being (long-term goals):

- Encourage client/parents to evaluate impact of ventilatory dependence on their lifestyle and changes they are willing or unwilling to make when client is discharged on ventilator. **All parties need to understand that ventilatory support is a 24-hr job that ultimately affects everyone. Quality-of-life issues must be examined, including issues of privacy and intimacy, and resolved by the ventilator-dependent client and SO(s).**
- Discuss importance of time for self and identify appropriate sources for respite care. Stress the need for caregivers to monitor physical well-being. **Caregivers have reported insufficient sleep, physical exhaustion, back pain, and significantly higher physical burden levels.** (Refer to ND excessive Caregiving Burden.)
- Emphasize importance of monitoring health of visitors and people involved in care, avoiding crowds during flu season, obtaining immunizations, and so forth, **to protect client from sources of infection.**
- Engage in rehabilitation program **to enhance respiratory muscle strength and general endurance or to compensate for deficits.**
- Encourage discussion of advanced directives and ascertain that all caregivers and care providers are aware of the plan of care. **Clarifies parameters for emergency situations, termination of therapy, or other end-of-life decisions, as desired.**
- Recommend involvement in support group; introduce to other ventilator-dependent individuals who are successfully managing home ventilation **to answer questions, provide role model, assist with problem-solving, and offer encouragement and hope for the future.**
- Review conditions requiring immediate medical intervention **to treat developing complications and potentially prevent respiratory failure.**

Documentation Focus

Assessment/Reassessment
- Baseline findings and subsequent changes
- Results of diagnostic testing or procedures
- Home evaluation as indicated

Information that appears in brackets has been added by the authors to clarify and enhance the use of nursing diagnoses.

 Acute Care 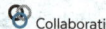 Collaborative 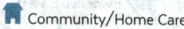 Community/Home Care Cultural

Planning
- Plan of care, specific interventions, and who is involved in the planning
- Teaching plan

Implementation/Evaluation
- Client/parent response to interventions
- Attainment of or progress toward desired outcome(s)
- Modifications to plan of care

Discharge Planning
- Status at discharge, long-term needs and referrals, indicating who is to be responsible for each action
- Equipment needs and supplier

Sample Nursing Outcomes & Interventions Classifications NOC/NIC

NOC—Respiratory Function: Ventilation
NIC—Mechanical Ventilatory Weaning

---

risk for other-directed VIOLENCE NANDA-I

[Diagnostic Division: Stress Management]

Definition: Susceptible to behaving in a physically, emotionally, and/or sexually harmful manner toward another.

Recognizing Cues

Risk/Related Factors
Anger behaviors; ineffective impulse control; psychomotor agitation
Easy access to weapon
Negative body language (e.g., rigid posture, clenching of fists/jaw, pacing, threatening stances); suicidal behaviors
Pattern of aggressive antisocial behavior (disruptive, confrontational)
Pattern of indirect violence (e.g., tearing objects off walls, urinating/defecating on floor, temper tantrum) or other-directed violence (e.g., hitting/kicking/spitting/scratching others, throwing objects, sexual molestation); pattern of threatening violence (e.g., verbal threats against property/people, threatening notes/gestures)

Information that appears in brackets has been added by the authors to clarify and enhance the use of nursing diagnoses.

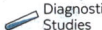 Diagnostic Studies 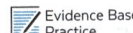 Evidence Based Practice 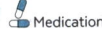 Medications 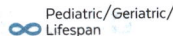 Pediatric/Geriatric/Lifespan

Clinical Connections
Psychotic conditions (e.g., schizophrenia, paranoia), antisocial personality disorder, dementia, substance misuse (e.g., phencyclidine [PCP], delirium tremens), abuse, postpartum psychosis, premenstrual syndrome [PMS], brain injury

Generate Solutions

Plan Desired Outcomes

Client Will (Include Specific Time Frame)
- Acknowledge realities of the situation.
- Verbalize understanding of why behavior occurs.
- Identify precipitating factors in individual situation.
- Express realistic self-evaluation and increased sense of self-esteem.
- Participate in care and meet own needs in an assertive manner.
- Demonstrate self-control as evidenced by relaxed posture, nonviolent behavior or verbalizations.
- Use resources and support systems in an effective manner.

Interventions/Take Action

Nursing Priority No. 1.
To assess causative/contributing factors:
- Assess clients with a history of aggression, violence, or homicide, keeping the door open and advising team of your proximity to client. **Protection for self, others, and client.**
- Determine underlying dynamics such as frustration, anger, mood swings, history of aggression or violence. **Uncontrolled emotions can lead to unacceptable behaviors that harm others.**
- Identify conditions, such as acute or chronic brain syndrome, panic state, hormonal imbalance, PMS, psychosis, drug-induced psychotic states, and postanesthesia or postseizure confusion. **These conditions may interfere with ability to control own behavior and lead to violent episodes.**
- Review laboratory findings (e.g., blood alcohol, drug/toxicology screen, blood glucose, arterial blood gases, electrolytes, renal function tests, and lithium level). **Provides information about possible treatable sources of behavior. For example, lithium is the gold standard for treating bipolar disorders.**
- Determine client's perception of self and situation. Note use of defense mechanisms. **Individuals who are prone to**

Information that appears in brackets has been added by the authors to clarify and enhance the use of nursing diagnoses.

violent behavior may see themselves as victims (denial), may blame others (projection), may not follow social norms, and may be impulsive.

- Observe and listen for early cues of distress or increasing anxiety. **Behaviors, such as irritability, lack of cooperation, and demanding behavior, and body posture or expression may signal escalating potential for violent behavior and need for immediate intervention.**
- Observe for signs of aggression or verbalized homicidal intent. **Perceived morbid or anxious feelings while with the client; warning from the client, "He is going to get what he deserves," or self-destructive behavior; and possession of alcohol or other drug(s) by known substance abuser need to be noted, and access to a weapon must be taken seriously. Various Tarasoff statutes, Duty to Warn, exist in many states requiring therapists/healthcare providers to report specific threats to both the individual named and law enforcement when client expresses homicidal intent overtly or covertly. Follow hospital or agency protocol for duty to warn. In addition, help client realize that the proposed action is not wise or in client's own interest.**
- Note family history of suicidal or homicidal behavior. **Dynamics in family of origin, current family, and parental deprivation or abuse in the early years of an individual's life may contribute to violent behavior in current situation as individual uses violence as a means of solving problems.**
- Ask directly if the person is thinking of acting on thoughts or feelings. **Can determine reality and urgency of violent intent and importance of immediate intervention. Implement duty to warn as needed.**
- Determine availability of violence or homicidal means. **Identifies urgency of situation and need to intervene by removing lethal means, possibly hospitalizing client, or instituting other measures to ensure safety of client and others.**
- Assess client coping behaviors. **Client believes there are no alternatives other than violence and has been dealing with frustration and anger in unacceptable ways (yelling, hitting, other violent behaviors) and needs to learn alternative coping skills.**
- Identify risk factors and assess for indicators of child abuse or neglect (e.g., unexplained or frequent injuries, failure to thrive). **Visible evidence of physical abuse or neglect**

Information that appears in brackets has been added by the authors to clarify and enhance the use of nursing diagnoses.

 Diagnostic Studies 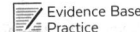 Evidence Based Practice 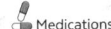 Medications 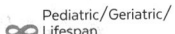 Pediatric/Geriatric/Lifespan makes it more easily recognized; however, behaviors of withdrawal and acting out may also signal the presence of abuse.

- Determine presence, extent, and acceptance of violence in the client's culture. **Youth violence has become a national concern with widely publicized school shootings and an increase in arrests of both boys and girls for violent crimes and weapons violations.**

Nursing Priority No. 2.

To assist client to accept responsibility for impulsive behavior and potential for violence:

- Develop therapeutic nurse-client relationship. Provide consistent caregiver when possible. **Promotes sense of trust, allowing client to discuss feelings openly and to begin to identify sources of anger and more acceptable ways of coping with it.**
- Maintain straightforward communication. **Avoids reinforcing manipulative behavior. Manipulation is used for management of powerlessness because of distrust of others, fear of loss of power or control, fear of intimacy, and search for approval.**
- Discuss motivation for change (e.g., failing relationships, job loss, involvement with judicial system). **Crisis situation can provide impetus for change but requires timely therapeutic intervention to sustain efforts.**
- Make time to listen to expressions of feelings. Acknowledge reality of client's feelings and that feelings are okay, except harm to others. (Refer to ND Self-Esteem, [specify].) **Promotes understanding of how feelings lead to actions and that individual is responsible for controlling behavior in acceptable ways.**
- Help client recognize that client's actions may be in response to client's fear (may be afraid of own behavior, loss of control), dependency, and feeling of powerlessness. **Promotes understanding of self and ability to deal with feelings in acceptable ways.**
- Confront client's tendency to minimize situation or behavior. **Individuals often want to say that things "are not as bad" as portrayed. By confronting this minimization, the reality of the situation can be brought out and discussed, leading to better understanding of the situation and changes in behavior.**
- Identify feelings or events (e.g., individual's view of self, hallucinations, individual/family or peer conflict, aggressive

---

Information that appears in brackets has been added by the authors to clarify and enhance the use of nursing diagnoses.

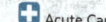 Acute Care 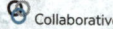 Collaborative 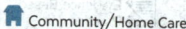 Community/Home Care Cultural

behavior) involved in precipitating violent behavior. **By identifying the factors involved in current situation, an appropriate plan can be made to change actions to prevent future violent behavior.**
- Discuss impact of behavior on others and consequences of actions. **Discussing these issues openly can help client to develop empathy and understand other person's reactions and begin to change behaviors that can lead to violence.**
- Acknowledge reality of homicide as an option. Discuss consequences of actions if they were to follow through on intent. Ask how it will help client to resolve problems. **Acknowledging the reality of individual's thoughts provides opportunity to look at how actions would affect others, ability to control own behavior, and make choices to live and make a better life for self.**
- Accept client's anger without reacting on emotional basis. Give permission to express angry feelings in acceptable ways and let client know that therapist will be available to assist in maintaining control. **Promotes acceptance and sense of safety. Client's anger is usually directed at the situation and not at the caregiver, and by remaining separate, the therapist can be more helpful for resolution of the anger.**
- Help client identify more appropriate solutions/behaviors. **Motor activities or exercise can lessen sense of anxiety and associated physical manifestations, thus diminishing feelings of anger.**
- Provide directions for actions client can take, avoiding negatives, such as "do nots." **Discussing positive ideas to help client begin to look toward a better future can provide hope that violent behaviors can be changed, promoting feelings of self-worth and belief in control of own self.**

Nursing Priority No. 3.
To assist client in controlling behavior:
- Discuss with client regarding safety of self/others. **Encourage client to contact staff when thoughts and feelings of aggression, violence, or homicidal ideations are entering the mind. Early interventions can help to mitigate violent actions.** Note: One recent study of parental intervention in their child's risky behavior over a 10-year time frame suggests that early parenting intervention may reduce association of high-risk females with aggressive peers and partners in adolescence.

Information that appears in brackets has been added by the authors to clarify and enhance the use of nursing diagnoses.

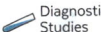 Diagnostic Studies 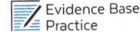 Evidence Based Practice 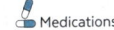 Medications 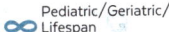 Pediatric/Geriatric/Lifespan

- Give client as much control as possible within constraints of individual situation. **Because control issues are a factor in violent behavior, giving client control in appropriate ways can enhance self-esteem and promote confidence in ability to change behavior.**
- Be truthful when giving information and interacting with individual. **Builds trust, enhancing therapeutic relationship, and prevents manipulative behavior.**
- Identify current and past successes, and strengths. Discuss effectiveness of coping techniques used and possible changes. Refer to ND difficulty Coping. **Client is often not aware of positive aspects of life and once recognized they can be used as a basis for change.**
- Give positive reinforcement for client's efforts. **Encourages continuation of desired behaviors.**
- Assist client to distinguish between reality, hallucinations, or delusions. **Violent behavior in clients with major mental disorders (schizophrenia, mania) may be in response to command hallucinations and may require more aggressive treatment or hospitalization until behavior is under control.**
- Approach in positive manner, acting as if the client has control and is responsible for own behavior. Be aware, though, that the client may not have control, especially if under the influence of drugs (including alcohol). **Individuals will often respond to a positive expectation, reducing threatening actions. Staff needs to be trained in management of this behavior and be prepared to take control of the situation if client is out of control.**
- Maintain distance and do not touch client when situation indicates client does not tolerate such closeness. **Individuals who have experienced traumatic events, such as rape, or suffer from post-trauma response may fear close contact even with trusted persons.**
- Remain calm offering client a quiet place to relax, medications to help calm client, and state limits on inappropriate behavior (including consequences) in a firm manner. **A calm approach helps client to de-escalate anger, and knowing there are alternatives to help become calm or what the consequences will be gives an opportunity to choose to change behavior and cope appropriately with situation. Use a step-by-step approach using the least restrictive and progressing to more restrictive strategies depending on the client's responses to calming interventions. Speak softly, calmly, and clearly, using basic**

Information that appears in brackets has been added by the authors to clarify and enhance the use of nursing diagnoses.

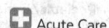 Acute Care 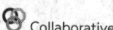 Collaborative 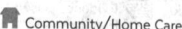 Community/Home Care Cultural

language, to explain what can happen as the situation continues to escalate.

- Advise client as the process of de-escalation is progressing to a higher level of intervention. **Moving to a higher level of more restrictive behaviors may be a reason for client to calm down. Intervention needs to be maintained for the safety of client/staff, and others.** Refer to ND risk for Suicide.
- Administer prescribed medications (e.g., antianxiety or antipsychotic), taking care not to oversedate client. **May be least restrictive way to help client control violent behaviors while learning new coping skills to handle anger and impulsive behavior. The chemistry of the brain is changed by early violence and has been shown to respond to serotonin as well as related neurotransmitter systems, which play a role in restraining aggressive impulses.**
- Monitor for possible drug interactions and cumulative effects of drug regimen (e.g., anticonvulsants, antidepressants). **May be contributing factor in violent behavior.**

Nursing Priority No. 4

To assist client/SO(s) to correct/cope with existing situation:

- Gear interventions to individual(s) involved based on age, relationship, communication, and social interactions. **Conflict-resolution skills can be learned by all age groups when age-appropriate materials are used.**
- Maintain calm, matter-of-fact, nonjudgmental attitude. **Decreases defensive response, allowing individual to think about own responsibility in the conflict and choose positive behaviors instead of usual angry reaction.**
- Notify potential victims in the presence of serious homicidal threat in accordance with legal and ethical guidelines. **Duty to Warn is mandated in many states, healthcare systems, and professional organizations. Not following protocol may result in a variety of legal actions taken against the healthcare system and the healthcare provider.**
- Discuss situation with abused or battered person, providing accurate information about choices and effective actions that can be taken. **Promotes understanding of options, giving hope and support for planning for a violence-free future.**
- Assist individual to understand that angry feelings are appropriate in the situation and need to be expressed but not acted on. (Refer to ND Post-Trauma Syndrome, as psychological responses may be similar.) **Helps client accept**

Information that appears in brackets has been added by the authors to clarify and enhance the use of nursing diagnoses.

 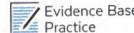 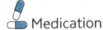 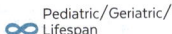

feelings as natural and begin to learn effective coping skills, and promotes sense of control over situation.
- Identify resources available for assistance to family/SO (e.g., battered women's shelter, social services, financial). **Helps client to manage immediate needs such as food, shelter, and safety with a long-range goal of attaining or maintaining independence and violence-free life.**

Nursing Priority No. 5.

To promote safety in event of violent behavior:

- Provide a safe, quiet environment and remove items from the client's environment that could be used to inflict harm to self/others. **Reducing stimuli can help client to calm down, and removing articles provides for safety of client and staff (e.g. sharp objects, belts, shoelaces, mouthwash due to alcohol content).**
- Maintain distance from client who is striking out or hitting and take evasive or controlling actions, as indicated. **Staff safety is of prime importance, and avoiding physical confrontation until client regains control or restraint team is assembled can prevent injury.**
- Call for additional staff/security personnel. **Having sufficient people available to handle the situation may defuse client's anger, allowing situation to calm down without further action. All personnel need to be trained in de-escalation/restraint techniques.**
- Approach an aggressive or attacking client using appropriate restraint approaches. Keep hands at side allowing client to see you are not holding something to harm them. **Safety is a prime concern, and these actions may defuse the situation.**
- Maintain direct and constant eye contact when appropriate. **Assists in identifying client's intentions and conveys sense of caring. Eye contact may be perceived as threatening, so it needs to be used cautiously.**
- Speak in a low, commanding voice. **Tone of voice conveys message of control and concern and can help to calm the client's anger.**
- Provide client with a sense that caregiver is in control of the situation. **Client is feeling out of control, and seeing that staff are in control provides a feeling of safety.**
- Maintain clear route for staff and client and be prepared to move quickly. **Safety for all is of prime importance, and staff may need to leave the room to regroup while**

Information that appears in brackets has been added by the authors to clarify and enhance the use of nursing diagnoses.

continuing to protect the client. Client takedown needs to be done quickly to gain control of the individual.

- Hold client, using restraints or place in seclusion when necessary until client regains self-control. **Brief period of physical restraint may be required until client regains control or other therapeutic interventions take effect. Doctor's orders are required for restraints and seclusion and is the most restrictive care. Client must be monitored 1:1 until calm enough to release restraints.**
- Administer medication, as indicated (e.g., Haldol, Ativan, and Benadryl). **Client may require chemical restraint until control is regained.**
- Discuss event with client after situation is calmed down and control is regained. **Helping client to understand how feelings of anger had gotten out of control and what can be done to prevent a recurrence can provide a learning opportunity for the individual. Also, debrief with staff about the restraint process and their thoughts and feelings.**

Nursing Priority No. 6.

To prevent future violence (Teaching/Discharge Considerations) and enhance well-being (long-term goals):

- Promote client involvement in planning care within limits of situation, allowing for meeting own needs for enjoyment. **Individuals often believe they are not entitled to pleasure and good things in their lives and need to learn how to meet these needs in acceptable ways.**
- Assist client to learn assertive behaviors. **Manipulative, nonassertive, or aggressive behaviors lead to anger, which can result in violence. Learning assertiveness skills can facilitate change, increase self-esteem, and promote interpersonal relationships.**
- Provide information about conflict-resolution skills and help client learn how to use them effectively. **Conflict is always present in human relationships, and learning how to manage conflict is one of the most important tools we can use to solve disagreements and improve relationships.**
- Discuss reasons for client's behavior with SO(s). Determine desire and commitment of involved parties to sustain current relationships. **Family members may believe individual is purposefully behaving in angry ways, and understanding underlying reasons for behavior can defuse**

Information that appears in brackets has been added by the authors to clarify and enhance the use of nursing diagnoses.

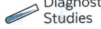 Diagnostic Studies 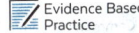 Evidence Based Practice 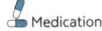 Medications 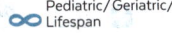 Pediatric/Geriatric/Lifespan

feelings of anger on their part, leading to willingness to resolve problems.
- Develop strategies to help parents learn more effective parenting skills. **Participating in parenting classes and learning appropriate ways of dealing with frustrations can improve family relationships and prevent angry interactions and the possibility of violent behavior.**
- Identify support systems. **Presence of family/friends and clergy who can serve as mentors and listen to individual nonjudgmentally can help client defuse angry feelings and learn appropriate ways of dealing with them. Note: Not just the client needs help; those around them also need to learn how to provide positive role models and display a broader array of skills for resolving problems.**
- Refer to formal resources, as indicated. **May need individual or group psychotherapy, substance-abuse treatment program, anger-management class, social services, and/or safe house to facilitate change.**
- Promote violence prevention and emotional literacy programs in the schools and community. **Young people who are at risk for violence need to be identified, and positive programs aimed at promoting emotional wellness need to be instituted in schools, parent education meetings, churches, and community centers. These programs are based on the premise that intelligent management of emotions is critical to successful living. Aggressive youth lack skills in arousal management and nonviolent problem-solving, which can be learned in programs and reinforced by the adults in their lives.**
- Refer to NDs impaired Parenting, impaired family Coping, and Post-Trauma Syndrome.

Documentation Focus

Assessment/Reassessment
- Individual findings, including nature of concern (e.g., suicidal, homicidal), behavioral risk factors, and level of impulse control, plan of action, and means to carry out plan
- Client's perception of situation, motivation for change
- Family history of violence
- Availability and use of resources

Planning
- Plan of care and who is involved in the planning
- Details of contract regarding violence to self/others
- Teaching plan

Information that appears in brackets has been added by the authors to clarify and enhance the use of nursing diagnoses.

Implementation/Evaluation
- Actions taken to promote safety, including notification of parties at risk
- Response to interventions, teaching, and actions performed
- Attainment or progress toward desired outcome(s)
- Modifications to plan of care

Discharge Planning
- Long-term needs and who is responsible for actions to be taken
- Available resources, specific referrals made

Sample Nursing Outcomes & Interventions Classifications NOC/NIC

NOC—Aggression Self-Restraint
NIC—Behavior Management

---

impaired WALKING ABILITY   NANDA-I

[Diagnostic Division: Activity/Rest]

Definition: Limitation of independent movement within the environment on foot.

Recognizing Cues

Related/Risk Factors
Altered mood
Unaddressed environmental constraints
Fear of falling; inadequate knowledge of mobility techniques
Insufficient muscle strength or physical endurance; prolonged immobility
Ineffective overweight self-management
Pain

Defining Characteristics

Subjective or Objective
Difficulty:
  Ambulating on level, decline, incline, or uneven surface
  Climbing, or descending stairs
  Navigating curbs; ambulating required distance

Information that appears in brackets has been added by the authors to clarify and enhance the use of nursing diagnoses.

 Diagnostic Studies   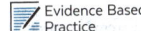 Evidence Based Practice   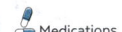 Medications   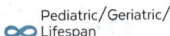 Pediatric/Geriatric/Lifespan

Clinical Connections

Arthritis, overweight, amputation, brain injury, stroke, traumatic injury, fractures, chronic pain, peripheral vascular disease, spinal nerve compression, multiple sclerosis (MS), cerebral palsy, Parkinson disease, macular degeneration, dementia

Generate Solutions

Plan Desired Outcomes

Client Will (Include Specific Time Frame)
- Move about within environment as needed or desired within limits of ability or with appropriate adjuncts.
- Verbalize understanding of situation or risk factors and safety measures.

Interventions/Take Action

Nursing Priority No. 1.
To assess causative/contributing factors:

- Identify conditions or diagnoses (e.g., acute/chronic illness; musculoskeletal injuries or surgery, balance problems—including inner ear conditions; movement disorders [e.g., MS, Parkinson disease, cerebral palsy], spinal abnormalities [e.g., congenital, disease, trauma, degeneration], impaired circulation or neuropathies, degenerative bone or muscle disorders, foot conditions [e.g., plantar warts, bunions, ingrown toenails, pressure injuries]) **that contribute to walking impairment and identify specific needs and appropriate interventions.**
- Note client's particular symptoms related to walking (e.g., unable to bear weight, cannot walk usual distance, limping, staggering, stiff leg, leg pain, shuffling, asymmetric or unsteady gait, can walk on certain surfaces but not on others).
- Determine ability to follow directions and note emotional/behavioral responses **that may be affecting client's ability or desire to engage in activity.**

Nursing Priority No. 2.
To assess functional ability:

 • Perform timed up-and-go (TUG) test, as indicated, **to assess client's basic ability to ambulate safely. Factors**

Information that appears in brackets has been added by the authors to clarify and enhance the use of nursing diagnoses.

assessed include sitting balance, ability to transfer from sitting to standing and back to sitting, the pace and stability of ambulation, and the ability to turn without staggering.

- Evaluate components of walking (e.g., gait, distance covered over time). Determine muscle strength and tone, joint mobility, cardiovascular status, balance, endurance, and use of assistive device. **Identifies strengths and deficits (e.g., ability to ambulate with/without assistive devices) and may provide information regarding potential for recovery.**
- Note whether impairment is temporary or permanent. **Condition may be caused by reversible condition (e.g., weakness associated with acute illness or fractures/surgery with weight-bearing restrictions), or walking impairment can be permanent (e.g., congenital anomalies, amputation, severe rheumatoid arthritis).**
- Determine degree of impairment in relation to suggested functional scale (0 to 4), noting that impairment can be temporary, permanent, or progressive.
- Assist with or review results of mobility testing (e.g., gait, timing of walking over fixed distance, distance walked over set period of time [endurance], limb movement analysis, leg strength and speed of walking, ambulatory activity monitoring) **for differential diagnosis and to guide treatment interventions.**
- Note emotional and behavioral responses of client/significant other(s) (SO[s]) to problems of mobility. **Walking impairments can negatively affect self-concept and self-esteem, autonomy, and independence. Social, occupational, and relationship roles can change, leading to isolation, depression, and economic consequences.**

Nursing Priority No. 3.
To promote safe, optimal level of independence in walking:

- Assist with treatment of underlying condition causing dysfunction, as indicated by individual situation.
- Consult with physical therapist, occupational therapist, or rehabilitation team **for individualized mobility program and to identify and create appropriate devices (e.g., shoe insert, leg brace to maintain proper foot alignment for walking, quad cane, hemiwalker).**
- Instruct in proper application of prostheses, immobilizers (e.g., walking cast or boot), and braces before walking

---

Information that appears in brackets has been added by the authors to clarify and enhance the use of nursing diagnoses.

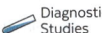 Diagnostic Studies 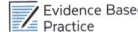 Evidence Based Practice 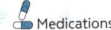 Medications 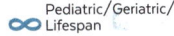 Pediatric/Geriatric/Lifespan

to maintain joint alignment/stability, immobilization, or to maintain alignment or balance during movement. **Prevents harm or further disability.**

- Demonstrate safe use of and help client become comfortable with assistive devices (e.g., cane, crutches, walker) **to maintain stability and balance during movement.**
- Provide assistance when indicated (e.g., walking on uneven surfaces; client is weak or has to walk a distance; or vision, coordination, or posture are impaired).
- Use adequate personnel and safety devices (e.g., gait belt, properly fitted nonslip shoes, handrail) when ambulating **to prevent injury to client or caregivers.**
- Monitor client's cardiopulmonary tolerance for walking. **Increased pulse rate, chest pain, breathlessness, irregular heartbeat are indicative of need to reduce level of activity.** (Refer to ND Activity Intolerance; impaired Cardiac Output, for related interventions.)
- Encourage adequate rest and gradual increase in walking distance **to reduce fatigue or leg pain associated with walking and improve stamina.** (Refer to NDs Fatigue; risk for impaired peripheral Neurovascular Function.)
- Administer medication, as indicated, **to manage pain and maximize level of functioning.** (Refer to NDs acute/chronic Pain; Chronic Pain Syndrome.)
- Implement fall precautions for high-risk clients (e.g., frail or ill elderly, visually or cognitively impaired, person on multiple medications, presence of balance disorders) **to reduce risk of accidental injury.** (Refer to ND risk for [adult/child] Fall for related interventions.)
- Provide cueing as indicated. **Client may need reminders (e.g., lift foot higher, look where going, walk tall) to concentrate on/perform tasks of walking, especially when balance or cognition is impaired.**
- Assist client to obtain needed information, such as handicap placard for close-in parking, sources for mobility scooter, or special public transportation options, when indicated.

Nursing Priority No. 4.

To maintain ambulation abilities (Teaching/Discharge Considerations) and enhance well-being (long-term goals):

- Involve client/SO(s) in problem-solving, assisting them to learn ways of managing deficits **to enhance safety for client and SO(s)/caregivers.**
- Encourage participation in regular active and passive exercise program. Advance levels of exercise, as able

---

Information that appears in brackets has been added by the authors to clarify and enhance the use of nursing diagnoses.

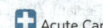 Acute Care 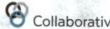 Collaborative 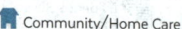 Community/Home Care   Cultural

to improve muscle tone and strength and increase stamina and endurance.
- Identify appropriate resources for obtaining and maintaining appliances, equipment, and environmental modifications **to promote mobility.**
- Evaluate client's home (or work) environment for barriers to walking (e.g., uneven surfaces, many steps, no ramps, long distances between places client needs to walk) **to determine needed changes, make recommendations for client safety.**
- Instruct client/SO in safety measures in home, as individually indicated (e.g., maintaining safe travel pathway, proper lighting, wearing glasses, handrails on stairs, grab bars in bathroom, using walker instead of cane when tired or when walking on uneven surface) **to reduce risk of falls.**
- Discuss appropriate use of electric scooter, if indicated. **Enhances mobility, especially over distances, to maintain independence and socialization.**
- Discuss need for emergency call/support system (e.g., Lifeline, HealthWatch) **to provide immediate assistance for falls or other home emergencies when client lives alone.**

Documentation Focus

Assessment/Reassessment
- Individual findings, including level of function and ability to participate in specific or desired activities
- Equipment and assistive device needs

Planning
- Plan of care and who is involved in the planning
- Teaching plan

Implementation/Evaluation
- Responses to interventions, teaching, and actions performed
- Attainment of or progress toward desired outcome(s)
- Modifications to plan of care

Discharge Planning
- Discharge and long-term needs, noting who is responsible for actions to be taken
- Specific referrals made
- Sources for and maintenance of assistive devices

Sample Nursing Outcomes & Interventions Classifications NOC/NIC

NOC—Ambulation
NIC—Exercise Therapy: Ambulation

Information that appears in brackets has been added by the authors to clarify and enhance the use of nursing diagnoses.

 Diagnostic Studies 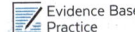 Evidence Based Practice 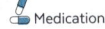 Medications 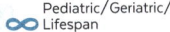 Pediatric/Geriatric/Lifespan

risk for impaired WATER-ELECTROLYTE IMBALANCE

NANDA-I

[Diagnostic Division: Food/Fluid]

Definition: Susceptible to changes in serum electrolyte levels.

Recognizing Cues

Risk Factors
Diarrhea; vomiting
Excessive or insufficient fluid volume
Inadequate knowledge of, or action to address modifiable factors

Clinical Connections
Renal failure, anorexia nervosa, diabetes mellitus, diabetes insipidus, Crohn disease, gastroenteritis, pancreatitis, traumatic brain injury, cancer, multiple trauma, burns, sickle cell disease

Generate Solutions

Plan Desired Outcomes

Client Will (Include Specific Time Frame)
- Display laboratory results within normal range for individual.
- Be free of complications resulting from electrolyte imbalance.
- Identify individual risks and engage in appropriate behaviors or lifestyle changes to prevent or reduce frequency of electrolyte imbalances.

Interventions/Take Action

Nursing Priority No. 1.
To assess causative/contributing factors:
- Identify the client with current or newly diagnosed condition commonly associated with electrolyte imbalances, such as inability to eat or drink, febrile illness, active bleeding, or other fluid loss, including vomiting, diarrhea, gastrointestinal (GI) drainage, or burns.
- Assess specific client risk, noting chronic disease processes that may lead to electrolyte imbalances, including kidney

---

Information that appears in brackets has been added by the authors to clarify and enhance the use of nursing diagnoses.

disease, metabolic or endocrine disorders, chronic alcoholism, cancer or cancer treatments, conditions causing hemolysis such as massive trauma, multiple blood transfusions, and sickle cell disease.

- Note the client's age and developmental level, **which may increase the risk for electrolyte imbalance. Note: This risk group can include the very young or premature infant, the elderly, or individuals unable to meet their own needs or monitor their health status.**
- Review the client's medications **for those associated with electrolyte imbalance. Note: There are many, including (and not limited to) diuretics, laxatives, corticosteroids, barbiturates, certain antidepressants (e.g., selective serotonin reuptake inhibitors [SSRIs]), antihypertensive agents, antiepileptics, some hormones/birth control pills, some antibiotics, and antifungal agents.**

Nursing Priority No. 2.
To identify potential electrolyte deficit:

- Assess mental status, noting client/caregiver report of change—altered attention span, recall of recent events, and other cognitive functions. **Can be associated with electrolyte imbalance; for example, it is the most common sign associated with sodium imbalances.**
- Monitor heart rate and rhythm by palpation and auscultation. **Tachycardia, bradycardia, and other dysrhythmias are associated with potassium, calcium, and magnesium imbalances.**
- Auscultate breath sounds, assess rate and depth of respirations and ease of respiratory effort, observe color of nailbeds and mucous membranes, and note pulse oximetry or blood gas measurement, as indicated. **Certain electrolyte imbalances, such as hypokalemia, can cause or exacerbate respiratory insufficiency.**
- Review the electrocardiogram (ECG). **Because the ECG reflects electrophysiological, anatomical, metabolic, and hemodynamic alterations, it is routinely used for the diagnosis of electrolyte and metabolic disturbances, as well as myocardial ischemia, cardiac dysrhythmias, structural changes of the myocardium, and drug effects.**
- Assess GI symptoms, noting presence, absence, and character of bowel sounds; presence of acute or chronic diarrhea; and persistent vomiting, high nasogastric tube output. **Any disturbance of the GI functioning carries with it the potential for electrolyte imbalances.**

Information that appears in brackets has been added by the authors to clarify and enhance the use of nursing diagnoses.

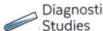 Diagnostic Studies 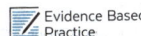 Evidence Based Practice 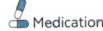 Medications 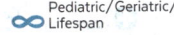 Pediatric/Geriatric/Lifespan

- Review the client's food intake. Note the presence of anorexia, vomiting, recent fad or unusual diet, long-term parenteral nutrition; look for signs of chronic malnutrition. **These conditions can point to potential electrolyte imbalances, either deficiencies or excesses, such as high sodium content.**
- Evaluate motor strength and function, noting steadiness of gait, hand grip strength, and reactivity of reflexes. **These neuromuscular functions can provide clues to electrolyte imbalances, including calcium, magnesium, phosphorus, sodium, and potassium.**
- Assess fluid intake and output. **Many factors, such as inability to drink, diuresis or chronic kidney failure, trauma, and surgery, affect an individual's fluid balance, disrupting electrolyte transport, function, and excretion.**
- Review laboratory results for abnormal findings. **Electrolytes include sodium, potassium, calcium, chloride, bicarbonate (carbon dioxide), and magnesium. These chemicals are essential in many bodily functions, including fluid balance, movement of fluid within and between body compartments, nerve conduction, muscle contraction—including the heart, blood clotting, and pH balance. Excitable cells, such as nerve and muscle, are particularly sensitive to electrolyte imbalances.**
- Assess for specific imbalances:

<u>Sodium (Na^+)</u> **This is a dominant extracellular cation, thus found in higher concentrations in the extracellular fluid.**

Review laboratory results—normal range in adults is 135 to 145 mEq/L. **Elevated sodium (hypernatremia) can occur if the client has an overall deficit of total body water owing to inadequate fluid intake or water loss and can be associated with low potassium, metabolic acidosis, and hypoglycemia.**

Monitor for physical or mental disorders impacting fluid intake. **Impaired thirst sensation or an inability to express thirst or obtain needed fluids may lead to hypernatremia.**

Note the presence of medical conditions that may impact sodium level. **Hyponatremia may be associated with disorders such as congestive heart failure, liver and kidney failure, pneumonia, metabolic acidosis, and intestinal conditions resulting in prolonged GI suction. Hypernatremia can result from simple conditions, such as febrile illness, causing fluid loss and/or**

Information that appears in brackets has been added by the authors to clarify and enhance the use of nursing diagnoses.

 Acute Care 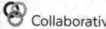 Collaborative 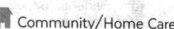 Community/Home Care 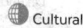 Cultural

restricted fluid intake, or from complicated conditions such as kidney and endocrine diseases, affecting sodium intake or excretion.

Note the presence of cognitive dysfunction such as confusion, restlessness, and abnormal speech, **which may be a cause or effect of sodium imbalance.**

Assess for orthostatic blood pressure changes, tachycardia, low urine output, or other clinical findings, such as generalized weakness, swollen tongue, weight loss, and seizures. **These signs suggest hypernatremia.**

Assess for nausea, abdominal cramping, lethargy, and orthostatic blood pressure changes—if fluid volume is also depleted; confusion, decreased level of consciousness, or headache. **These signs and symptoms are suggestive of hyponatremia, which can lead to seizures and a coma if untreated.**

Review drug regimen. **Drugs such as anabolic steroids, angiotensin, cisplatin, and mannitol may increase sodium level. Diuretics, laxatives, theophylline, and triamterine can decrease sodium level.**

Potassium (K$^+$) **Most abundant intracellular cation, thus found in higher concentrations in the intracellular fluid, and obtained through diet, is excreted via the kidneys.**

Identify at-risk populations. **Extremes of age (premature or elderly); ingestion of unusual diet with high-potassium, low-sodium foods; clients receiving IV potassium boluses or transfusions of whole blood or packed cells; and use of potassium supplements, including over-the-counter (OTC) herbals or salt substitutes, increase possibility of hyperkalemia.**

Review laboratory results—the normal range in adults is 3.5 to 5 mEq/L.

Note current medical conditions that may impact potassium level. **Metabolic acidosis, burn or crush injuries, massive hemolysis, diabetes, kidney disease/renal failure, cancer, and sickle cell trait are associated with hyperkalemia. Fasting, diarrhea or nasogastric suctioning, alkalosis, administration of IV potassium boluses, or transfusions of whole blood or packed red blood cells increase the risk of hypokalemia.**

Identify conditions or situations **that potentiate risk for hyperkalemia, including ingestion of an unusual diet with high-potassium, low-sodium foods or use of potassium supplements, including over-the-counter (OTC) herbals or salt substitutes.**

Information that appears in brackets has been added by the authors to clarify and enhance the use of nursing diagnoses.

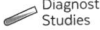 Diagnostic Studies 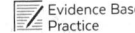 Evidence Based Practice 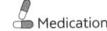 Medications 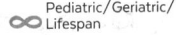 Pediatric/Geriatric/Lifespan

- Monitor ECG, as indicated. **Abnormal potassium levels, both low and high, are associated with changes in the ECG.**
- Evaluate reports of abdominal cramping, hyperactive bowel motility, muscle twitching, and cramps, followed by muscle weakness. Note the presence of depressed reflexes, ascending flaccid paralysis of legs and arms. **These signs/symptoms suggest hyperkalemia.**
- Note the presence of weakness and fatigue (most common), anorexia, abdominal distention, diminished bowel sounds, palpitations, postural hypotension, muscle cramps, and pain (severe hypokalemia); also note flaccid paralysis. **May be manifestations of hypokalemia.**
- Review drug regimen. **Use of potassium-sparing diuretics or other medications, such as NSAIDs, angiotensin-converting enzyme (ACE) inhibitors, angiotensin-receptor blockers (ARBs), heparin, and certain antibiotics such as pentamidine may increase potassium level. Medications such as some chronic obstructive pulmonary disease (COPD) medications (e.g., albuterol, terbutaline), steroids, certain antimicrobials (e.g., penicillins, aminoglycosides), laxatives, and some diuretics may cause hypokalemia.**

<u>Calcium (Ca^{2+})</u> **Most abundant cation in the body, participates in almost all vital processes, working with sodium to regulate depolarization and the generation of action potentials.**

- Review laboratory results—the normal range for adults is 8.5 to 10.5 mg/dL.
- Note the presence of medical conditions impacting calcium level. **Acidosis, Addis disease, cancers (e.g., bone, lymphoma, and leukemias), hyperparathyroidism, lung disease (e.g., tuberculosis [TB], histoplasmosis), thyrotoxicosis, and polycythemia may lead to an increased calcium level. Chronic diarrhea, intestinal disorders such as Crohn disease; pancreatitis, alcoholism, renal failure, or renal tubular disease; recent orthopedic surgery or bone healing, history of thyroid surgery, or irradiation of upper middle chest and neck; and psychosis may result in decreased calcium levels.**
- Monitor for excessive urination (polyuria), constipation, lethargy, muscle weakness, anorexia, headache, and coma, **which can be associated with hypercalcemia.**
- Monitor for cardiac dysrhythmias, hypotension, and heart failure; muscle cramps, facial spasms—positive

---

Information that appears in brackets has been added by the authors to clarify and enhance the use of nursing diagnoses.

Chvostek sign; numbness and tingling sensations, muscle twitching—positive Trousseau sign; seizures, or tetany, **which suggest hypocalcemia.**

Review drug regimen. **Drugs such as anabolic steroids, some antacids, lithium, oral contraceptives, vitamins A and D, and amoxapine, can increase calcium levels. Drugs such as albuterol, glucocorticoids, insulin, phosphates, trazodone, laxative overuse, or long-term anticonvulsant therapy can decrease calcium levels.**

<u>Magnesium (Mg^{2+})</u> **The second most abundant intracellular cation after potassium, magnesium controls absorption or function of sodium, potassium, calcium, and phosphorus.**

Review laboratory results—normal range in adults is 1.5 to 2 mEq/L.

Note the presence of medical conditions impacting magnesium level. **Diabetic acidosis, multiple myeloma, renal insufficiency, eclampsia, asthma, GI hypomotility; adrenal insufficiency, extensive soft tissue injury, severe burns, shock, sepsis, and cardiac arrest are associated with hypermagnesemia. Conditions resulting in decreased intake (starvation, alcoholism, and parenteral feeding), excess GI losses (diarrhea, vomiting, nasogastric suction, and malabsorption), renal losses (inherited renal tubular defects among others), or miscellaneous causes (including calcium abnormalities, chronic metabolic acidosis, and diabetic ketoacidosis) can lead to hypomagnesemia.**

Note GI and renal function. **The main controlling factors of magnesium are GI absorption and renal excretion. Low levels of magnesium, potassium, calcium, and phosphorus may be manifest at the same time if absorption is impaired. High levels of magnesium, calcium, phosphate, and potassium often occur together in the setting of kidney disease.**

Monitor for nausea, vomiting, weakness, and vasodilation, **which suggest a mild to moderate elevation of magnesium level (from 3.5 to 5 mEq/L).**

Monitor ECG, as indicated. **The presence of heart blocks, especially if accompanied by ventilatory failure and stupor, suggests severe hypermagnesemia (greater than 10 mEq/L). Hypomagnesemia can lead to potentially fatal ventricular dysrhythmias, coronary artery vasospasm, and sudden death.**

Information that appears in brackets has been added by the authors to clarify and enhance the use of nursing diagnoses.

 Diagnostic Studies 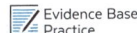 Evidence Based Practice Medications 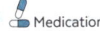 Pediatric/Geriatric/Lifespan

- Review drug regimen. **Drugs such as aspirin and progesterone may increase magnesium level; albuterol, digoxin, diuretics, oral contraceptives, aminoglycosides, proton-pump inhibitors, immunosuppressants, cisplatin, and cyclosporines are some of the medications that may decrease magnesium levels.**

Nursing Priority No. 3.
To prevent imbalances:

- Collaborate in the treatment of underlying conditions **to prevent or limit effects of electrolyte imbalances caused by disease or organ dysfunction.**
- Observe and intervene with elderly hospitalized person on admission and during facility stay. **Elderly are more prone to electrolyte imbalances related to fluid imbalances, use of multiple medications including diuretics, heart and blood pressure medications, lack of appetite or interest in eating or drinking; or lack of appropriate dietary and/or medication supervision.**
- Provide or recommend balanced nutrition, using the best route for feeding. Monitor intake, weight, and bowel function. **Obtaining and utilizing electrolytes and other minerals depends on the client regularly receiving them in a readily available form, including food and supplements via ingestion, enteral, or parenteral routes.**
- Measure and report all fluid losses, including emesis, diarrhea, wound, or fistula drainage. **Loss of fluids rich in electrolytes can lead to imbalances.**
- Maintain fluid balance **to prevent dehydration and shifts of electrolytes.**
- Use pump or controller device when administering IV electrolyte solutions **to provide medication at desired rate and prevent untoward effects of excessive or too rapid delivery.**

Nursing Priority No. 4.
To promote fluid and electrolyte balance (Teaching/Discharge Considerations) and enhance well-being (long-term goals):

- Discuss ongoing concerns for the client with chronic health problems, such as kidney disease, diabetes, or cancer; individuals taking multiple medications; and/or client deciding to take medications or drugs differently than prescribed. **Early intervention can help prevent serious complications.**

Information that appears in brackets has been added by the authors to clarify and enhance the use of nursing diagnoses.

- Consult with dietitian for specific teaching needs. **Learning how to incorporate foods that increase electrolyte intake or identifying food or condiment alternatives increases client's self-sufficiency and likelihood of success.**
- Review the client's medications at each visit **for possible change in dosage or drug choice based on the client's response, change in condition, or development of side effects.**
- Discuss medications with primary care provider **to determine if different pharmaceutical intervention is appropriate. For example, changing to potassium-sparing diuretic or withholding a diuretic may correct imbalance.**
- Teach the client/caregiver to take or administer drugs as prescribed, especially diuretics, antihypertensives, and cardiac drugs, **to reduce the potential of complications associated with medication-induced electrolyte imbalances.**
- Instruct the client/caregiver in reportable symptoms. **For example, a sudden change in mentation or behavior 2 days after starting a new diuretic could indicate hyponatremia, or an elderly person taking digitalis (for atrial fibrillation) and a diuretic may be hypokalemic.**
- Provide information regarding calcium supplements, as indicated. **It is popular wisdom to instruct people, women in particular, to take calcium for prevention of osteoporosis. However, calcium absorption cannot take place without vitamins D and K and magnesium. A client taking calcium may need additional information or resources.**

Documentation Focus

Assessment/Reassessment
- Identified or potential risk factors for individual
- Assessment findings, including vital signs, mentation, muscle strength and reflexes, presence of fatigue, respiratory distress
- Results of laboratory tests and diagnostic studies

Planning
- Plan of care, specific interventions, and who is involved in the planning
- Teaching plan

Information that appears in brackets has been added by the authors to clarify and enhance the use of nursing diagnoses.

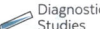 Diagnostic Studies 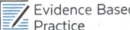 Evidence Based Practice 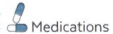 Medications 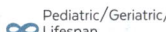 Pediatric/Geriatric/Lifespan

Implementation/Evaluation
- Client's responses to treatment, teaching, and actions performed
- Attainment of or progress toward desired outcome(s)
- Modifications to plan of care

Discharge Planning
- Long-term needs, identifying who is responsible for actions to be taken
- Specific referrals made

Sample Nursing Outcomes & Interventions Classifications NOC/NIC

NOC—Electrolyte & Acid/Base Balance
NIC—Fluid/Electrolyte Management

---

readiness for enhanced WEIGHT SELF-MANAGEMENT NANDA-I

[Diagnostic Division: Food/Fluid]

Definition: Pattern of pursuing and/or maintaining healthy body weight, which can be strengthened.

Recognizing Cues

Defining Characteristics

Subjective
Desires to enhance:
  Healthy lifestyle; ability to set achievable goals; congruency of decisions about goals
  Knowledge about essential nutrients; the need for physical activity; to make appropriate food choices to promote health
  Nutrition; nutrient intake; positive eating behaviors
  Participation in weight management program
  Desires to maintain physical well-being through physical activity

Clinical Connections
Chronic conditions or healthy individuals

Information that appears in brackets has been added by the authors to clarify and enhance the use of nursing diagnoses.

 Acute Care 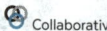 Collaborative 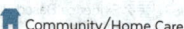 Community/Home Care   Cultural

Generate Solutions

Plan Desired Outcomes

Client Will (Include Specific Time Frame)
- Ingest adequate nutrients/balanced diet to meet individual needs.
- Routinely engage in safe food preparation and storage practices.
- Achieve/maintain optimum personal weight goal.

Interventions/Take Action

Nursing Priority No. 1.
To determine current nutritional status and eating patterns:

- Assess client's knowledge of current nutritional needs and ways client is meeting these needs. **Provides baseline for further teaching or interventions.**
- Assess eating patterns and food and fluid choices in relation to any health-risk factors and health goals. **Helps to identify specific strengths and weaknesses that can be addressed.**
- Verify that age-related and developmental needs are met. **These factors are constantly present throughout the life span, although differing for each age group. For example, older adults need the same nutrients as younger adults, but in smaller amounts and with attention to certain components, such as calcium, fiber, vitamins, protein, and water. Infants/children require small meals and constant attention to needed nutrients for proper growth and development while dealing with child's food preferences and eating habits.**
- Evaluate influence of cultural and religious factors **to determine what client considers to be normal dietary practice as well as to identify food preferences and restrictions and eating patterns that can be strengthened or altered if indicated.**
- Assess how client perceives food, food preparation, and the act of eating **to determine client's feeling and emotions regarding food (including the use of food for celebrations or as a reward) and self-image.**
- Ascertain occurrence of or potential for negative feedback from significant others (SOs). **May reveal control issues that could impact client's motivation for and commitment to change.**

Information that appears in brackets has been added by the authors to clarify and enhance the use of nursing diagnoses.

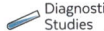 Diagnostic Studies 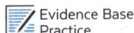 Evidence Based Practice 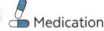 Medications 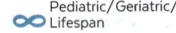 Pediatric/Geriatric/Lifespan

- Determine patterns of hunger and satiety. **Helps identify strengths and weaknesses in eating patterns and potential for change (e.g., person predisposed to weight gain may need a different time for a big meal than evening or may need teaching as to what foods reinforce feelings of satisfaction).**
- Assess client's ability to shop for, safely store, and prepare foods **to determine if health information or financial resources might be needed.**

Nursing Priority No. 2.

To assist client/SO(s) to develop plan to meet individual needs:

- Determine motivation and expectation for change. **Motivation to improve and high expectations can encourage client to make changes that will improve client's life. However, the presence of unrealistic expectations may hamper efforts. Client may be satisfied with current nutritional state and eating behaviors or may be changing some aspect of food intake or preparation in response to new dietary information or a change in health status.**
- Assist in obtaining and reviewing results of individual testing (e.g., weight, height, body fat percentage, lipids, glucose, complete blood count, total protein) **to determine that client is healthy and/or identify dietary changes that may help attain health goals.**
- Encourage client's beneficial eating patterns and habits **to provide reinforcement and support client's efforts to incorporate changes into lifestyle habits and continue with new behaviors, such as:**

  Limit added sugars and sugary drinks
  Drink water
  Eat frequent, smaller meals
  Eat a variety of foods, including grain products, fruits, and vegetables
  Eat only moderate amounts of dairy and meat products
  Be mindful while eating
  Follow specific dietary program, as indicated

- Provide instruction and reinforce information regarding special needs. **Client/SO may benefit from or desire assistance learning new eating habits or following medically prescribed diets (e.g., very low-calorie diet, enteral feedings, diabetic or renal dialysis diet).**
- Encourage the client to carefully read food labels, instructing in the meaning of labeling information, **to assist client/SO in making healthful choices.**

Information that appears in brackets has been added by the authors to clarify and enhance the use of nursing diagnoses.

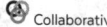 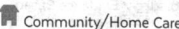

- Consult with or refer to a dietitian/physician, as indicated. **Client/SO may benefit from advice regarding specific nutrition or dietary issues or may require regular follow-up to determine that needs are met when following a medically prescribed program.**
- Encourage client to get enough physical activity at moderate intensity within client's tolerance.
- Encourage client to get enough sleep (e.g., at least 7 hr a night).
- Develop a system for self-monitoring **to provide a sense of control and enable the client to track progress as well as to assist in making informed choices.**

Nursing Priority No. 3.

To promote a healthy weight (Teaching/Discharge Considerations) and enhance well-being (long-term goals):

- Review client risk factors and provide additional information or response to concerns. **Assists the client with motivation and decision making.**
- Provide client/SO(s) with a reference list of local and online resources. **Reinforces learning, allows client to progress at own pace, and encourages client to be responsible for own learning. When referencing the internet, nontraditional, or unproven resources, the client must exercise some restraint and determine the reliability of the source and information before acting on it.**
- Encourage variety and moderation in dietary plans **to decrease boredom and encourage client in efforts to make healthy choices about eating and food.**
- Discuss the use of nutritional supplements and over-the-counter herbal products. **Confusion may exist regarding the need for and use of these products in a balanced dietary regimen.**
- Assist client to identify and access community resources when indicated. **May benefit from assistance, such as nutritional assistance program, budget counseling, Meals on Wheels, community food banks, use of digital applications to track nutrition, and other assistance programs.**

Documentation Focus

Assessment/Reassessment
- Baseline information, client's perception of need
- Nutritional intake and metabolic needs
- Motivation and expectations for change

Information that appears in brackets has been added by the authors to clarify and enhance the use of nursing diagnoses.

 Diagnostic Studies   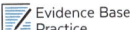 Evidence Based Practice   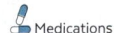 Medications   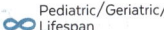 Pediatric/Geriatric/Lifespan

Planning
- Plan of care, specific interventions, and who is involved in planning
- Teaching plan

Implementation/Evaluation
- Client's responses to interventions, teaching, and actions performed
- Attainment or progress toward desired outcome(s)
- Modifications to plan of care

Discharge Planning
- Long-term needs and actions to be taken
- Support systems available, specific referrals made, and who is responsible for actions to be taken

Sample Nursing Outcomes & Interventions Classifications NOC/NIC

NOC—Weight Maintenance Behavior
NIC—Nutritional Counseling

Information that appears in brackets has been added by the authors to clarify and enhance the use of nursing diagnoses.

 Acute Care 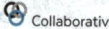 Collaborative 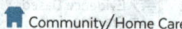 Community/Home Care Cultural

CHAPTER 3

Health Conditions and Client Concerns

This section facilitates and helps validate the assessment and diagnosis steps of the nursing process. Because the nursing process is perpetual and ongoing, other nursing diagnoses may be appropriate based on changing individual situations. Therefore, the nurse must continually assess, identify, and validate new client needs and evaluate subsequent care. To facilitate access to the health conditions/concerns and nursing diagnoses, the conditions are listed alphabetically and coded to identify nursing specialty areas:

- MS: Medical-Surgical
- PED: Pediatric
- OB/GYN: Obstetric/Gynecological
- CH: Community/Home
- PSY: Psychiatric/Behavioral

There is no separate category for geriatrics because concerns and conditions in this population are subsumed under the other specialty areas and because older adults are susceptible to the majority of these problems. To use this tool, cues that could be collected from the assessment of a client with the given condition/concern are provided. Our nursing-focused assessment tool is divided into concepts or Diagnostic Divisions (DDs) that group similar nursing diagnoses together. The cues included here generally reflect a specific DD noted for your review. A Nursing Diagnosis (ND) *concept* within the DD is suggested for you to consider. Refer to the DD page 1205 and locate the ND concept. A page reference is provided to facilitate reviewing the ND definition and cues to determine if the diagnosis reflects your client's specific problem. Some concepts contain more than one ND, for example Fluid, which could include excessive Fluid Volume, inadequate Fluid Volume, or risk for impaired Fluid Volume Balance. Furthermore, the authors believe the majority of NDs can be an actual problem, a risk diagnosis, or an opportunity for enhancing the client's well-being. When considering a problem versus a risk diagnosis, the Related Factors of a problem diagnosis are also the Risk Factors for a risk diagnosis. Clinical judgment is required to choose the appropriate ND to begin generating solutions and taking action to provide effective client care.

Abdominal hysterectomy — MS
Refer to Hysterectomy

Abdominal perineal resection — MS
Also refer to Surgery, general

Verbalizes concern about change in appearance/body function, fear of rejection by significant other(s) (SO[s]) or reaction of others, low self-esteem, anxiety, depressive symptoms
  Review DD Self-Perception/Concept—consider Body image

Fears intimacy, feels vulnerable, questioning ability to engage in sexual activity, concerned about bodily changes (e.g., radical resection or treatment procedures), decreased sexual interest/desire, lacks information about alternate sexual activities
  Review DD Sexuality/Reproduction—consider Sexual functioning

Abortion, elective termination — OB
Conflicting information, misinformation, concern about moral or spiritual consequences of potential decision, young age, unplanned pregnancy, partner not involved, worried about reaction of others, muscle tension, hesitant to choose action
  Review DD Values/Beliefs—consider Decision making

Concerns about perception of moral or ethical implications of therapeutic procedure, young age, single mother, unsure about decision while reporting procedure is her only option
  Review DD Values/Beliefs—consider Moral distress

Questions regarding reproduction, contraception, self-care, and Rh factor; misperceptions, unfamiliar with resources
  Review DD Health Management—consider Health knowledge

Abortion, spontaneous termination — OB
Missed or incomplete abortion, anemia, low platelets, abdominal trauma, disseminated intravascular coagulopathy (DIC)
  Review DD Circulation—consider Bleeding

Perinatal loss, crying, anger, expresses sorrow, distress
  Review DD Stress Management—consider Grief

Abruptio placentae — OB
Also refer to Hemorrhage, prenatal

Frank bleeding from vagina, increased heart/respiration rate, signs of fetal distress
  Review DD Circulation—consider Bleeding

Verbal report of pain, diaphoresis, pupil dilation, protective behaviors/positioning to ease pain
  Review DD Comfort—consider Pain

Alarm, intense dread (related to threat of death to fetus/self)
  Review DD Stress Management—consider Fear

Pregnancy/labor complications, compromised fetal oxygen transport
  Review DD Sexuality/Reproduction—consider Maternal-fetal dyad

Abscess, brain (acute) — MS
Restlessness, irritability, reports headache
  Review DD Comfort—consider Pain

Dehydration, temperature above normal range
    Review DD Safety—consider Thermoregulation
Cerebral edema, hyperthermia, change in level of consciousness, restlessness, agitation, hallucinations
    Review DD Neurosensory—consider Confusion

Abscess, skin/tissue   CH/MS
Redness, swelling, hematoma/bleeding, localized area hot to touch
    Review DD Safety—consider Skin/Tissue integrity
Exposure to toxins, malnutrition, insufficient knowledge to avoid exposure to pathogens
    Review DD Safety—consider Infection

Abuse, physical   CH/PSY
Also refer to Battered child syndrome
History of physical abuse, bruises/scratches/burns/fractures consistent with physical violence
    Review DD Safety—consider Injury
Overwhelming threat to self, personal vulnerability, inability to deal with current situation, chronic worry, anxiety, destructive behavior toward self or others
    Review DD Stress Management—consider Coping
Decreased eye contact, dependent on others' opinions, excessive guilt/seeking of reassurance, overly obedient behaviors
    Review DD Self-Perception/Concept—consider Self-esteem
Perceived vulnerability, powerlessness, dysfunctional family processes, lack of social support, feeling of shame
    Review DD Stress Management—consider Resilience
Decreased sexual desire, pain with sexual activity, excessive anxiety in response to anticipated/attempted sexual activity
    Review DD Sexuality/Reproduction—consider Sexual functioning

Abuse, psychological   CH/PSY
Overwhelming threat to self, personal vulnerability, inability to deal with current situation, chronic worry, anxiety, destructive behavior toward self or others
    Review DD Stress Management—consider Coping
Perceived vulnerability, powerlessness, dysfunctional family processes, lack of social support, feeling of shame
    Review DD Stress Management—consider Resilience
Verbal expressions of lack of control, alienation, shame; repeated negative reinforcement, inadequate self-efficacy, lack of social support, apathy, passivity
    Review DD Self-Perception/Concept—consider Self-esteem

[esophageal] Achalasia (cardiospasm)   MS
Dysphagia, heartburn, regurgitation, inability to ingest food, insufficient dietary intake, recurrent respiratory infections
    Review DD Food/Fluid—consider Swallowing
Inability or reluctance to ingest adequate nutrients to metabolic or nutritional needs, inadequate intake, weight loss, pallor
    Review DD Food/Fluid—consider Nutritional intake

A

Regurgitation, recurrent respiratory infections
   Review DD Respiration—consider Aspiration

Acidosis, metabolic   MS
Refer to underlying cause/condition, e.g., Diabetic ketoacidosis

Acidosis, respiratory   MS
Also refer to underlying cause/condition
Dyspnea with exertion, tachypnea, changes in mentation, irritability, tachycardia, hypoxia, hypercapnia
   Review DD Respiration—consider Gas exchange

Acne   CH/PED
Disruptions of skin surface
   Review DD Safety—consider Skin integrity
Fear of rejection by others, focus on appearance, negative feelings about body change in social involvement
   Review DD Self-Perception/Concept—consider Body image
Self-negating verbal statements, expressions of helplessness, inadequate approval/respect from others
   Review DD Self-Perception/Concept—consider Self-esteem

Acoustic neuroma   MS
Also refer to Surgery, general
Hearing loss, tinnitus
   Review DD Neurosensory—consider Sensory deficit
Hearing difficulties, dizziness, sense of unsteadiness
   Review DD Safety—consider Fall

Acquired immune deficiency syndrome (AIDS)   MS
Also refer to HIV infection
Depressed immune system, use of antimicrobial agents, broken skin, traumatized tissue, malnutrition, environmental exposure, invasive procedures, chronic disease processes
   Review DD Safety—consider Immunologic Impairment
Diarrhea, profuse sweating, vomiting, fever, nonelastic skin turgor, weight loss, dry mucous membranes
   Review DD Food/Fluid—consider Fluid volume
Tissue inflammation, cutaneous lesions, myalgia/arthralgia, verbal report of pain, paresthesias, paralysis, guarding behaviors, changes in vital signs (acute), restlessness
   Review DD Comfort—consider Pain
Respiratory muscle impairment, decreased lung expansion, retained secretions, ineffective cough
   Review DD Respiration—consider Airway clearance

    CH

Weight loss, decreased subcutaneous fat or muscle mass, lack of appetite, nausea, altered taste sensation, abdominal cramping, hyperactive bowel sounds, diarrhea, inflamed oral mucosa, abnormal laboratory results (vitamin, mineral, protein deficiencies or electrolyte imbalance)
   Review DD Food/Fluid—consider Nutritional intake

Lack of energy, inability to maintain usual routines, impaired ability to concentrate, lethargy, listlessness, disinterest in surroundings
Review DD Activity/Rest—consider Fatigue

PSY

Verbalized feelings of aloneness or rejection, absence of supportive significant others, poor self-esteem, withdrawal from usual activities
Review DD Roles/Relationships—consider Social connectedness

Altered attention span, memory deficit, disorientation, delusional thinking, impaired ability to make decisions, altered personality, inability to follow commands/mental tasks
Review DD Neurosensory—consider Confusion

Acromegaly CH

Verbal expressions of pain, impaired ability to participate in usual activities, changes in sleep pattern, fatigue
Review DD Comfort—consider Pain

Verbalizations of feelings or concerns, fear of rejection or reaction of others, negative comments about body, change in appearance, change in social involvement
Review DD Self-Perception/Concept—consider Body image

Altered body structure, changes in libido
Review DD Sexuality/Reproduction—consider Sexual functioning

Acute respiratory distress syndrome MS
Refer to Respiratory distress syndrome, acute

Adams-Stokes syndrome CH
Refer to Dysrhythmia, cardiac

ADD PED
Refer to Attention-deficit disorder

Addiction MS
Refer to specific substance used; Substance dependence/abuse rehabilitation

Addison disease MS

Vomiting, diarrhea, increased renal losses, thirst, delayed capillary refill, poor skin turgor, dry mucous membranes
Review DD Food/Fluid—consider Fluid volume

Low body weight, decreased subcutaneous fat and muscle mass, lack of interest in food, inflamed oral mucosa, laboratory evidence of protein or vitamin deficiencies
Review DD Food/Fluid—consider Nutritional intake

Vomiting, diarrhea, endocrine dysfunction, desires salty foods, thirst, abnormal lab values
Review DD Food/Fluid—consider Water-electrolyte balance

Hypovolemia, electrolyte imbalance, changes in vital signs, irregular pulse, dysrhythmias, change in mentation
Review DD Circulation—consider Cardiac output

Health Conditions and Client Concerns

Overwhelming lack of energy, inability to perform desired activities, lethargy, poor concentration
  Review DD Activity/Rest—consider Fatigue
Body consciousness, unrealistic self-expectations, preoccupation with change, concern about reaction of others
  Review Self Perception/Concept—consider Body image

Adenoidectomy   PED/MS
Sedation, collection of secretions/blood in oropharynx, vomiting
  Review DD Respiration—consider Airway clearance
Crying, apprehension, trembling, sympathetic stimulation (pupil dilation, tachycardia)
  Review DD Stress Management—consider Anxiety
Restlessness, crying, grimacing, verbalization of discomfort
  Review DD Comfort—consider Pain

Adjustment disorder   PED/PSY
Refer to Anxiety disorders

Adoption/loss of child custody   PSY
Loss of child, expectations for future of child/self, emotional distress, altered grieving process, depressive symptoms
  Review DD Stress Management—consider Grief
Lack of control, powerlessness, hopelessness, lack of social support, poor self-esteem, depressive symptoms
  Review DD Stress Management—consider Resilience

Adrenal crisis, acute   MS
Also refer to Addison disease; Shock
Vomiting, diarrhea, endocrine dysfunction, desires salty foods, thirst, abnormal lab values (decreased serum sodium), hypotension, dry mucus membranes, changes in mentation
  Review DD Food/Fluid—consider Water-electrolyte balance
Verbalization of severe pain in abdomen, lower back, or legs
  Review DD Comfort—consider Pain
Generalized weakness, inability to perform activities/movement
  Review DD Activity/Rest—consider Mobility
Low body weight, decreased subcutaneous fat and muscle mass, lack of interest in food, inflamed oral mucosa, laboratory evidence of protein or vitamin deficiencies
  Review DD Food/Fluid—consider Nutritional intake

Adrenalectomy   MS
Diminished pulse, pallor, cyanosis, hypotension, changes in mentation
  Review DD Circulation—consider Tissue perfusion
Inadequate primary defenses (incision, traumatized tissues), suppressed inflammatory response, invasive procedures
  Review DD Safety—consider Infection

Unfamiliarity with long-term therapy needs, statements of concern or misconception, request for information
Review DD Health Management—consider Health knowledge

Adrenal insufficiency — CH
Refer to Addison disease

Affective disorder — PSY
Refer to Bipolar disorder; Depression, major

Affective disorder, seasonal — PSY
Also refer to Depression, major
Verbalizations of inability to cope, changes in sleep pattern, reports lack of energy, fatigue, behavioral changes (irritability, discouragement)
Review DD Stress Management—consider Coping
Change in usual activity level, decreased appetite, lack of energy or interest to prepare food
Review DD Food/Fluid—consider Nutritional intake

Agoraphobia — PSY
Also refer to Phobia
Tachycardia, chest pain, dyspnea, gastrointestinal distress, faintness, sense of impending doom
Review DD Stress Management—consider Anxiety
Sympathetic stimulation, apprehension, panic, withdrawal
Review DD Stress Management—consider Fear
Change in style or pattern of interaction, discomfort in social situations, avoidance of phobic stimuli
Review DD Roles/Relationships—consider Social connectedness

Agranulocytosis — MS
Suppressed inflammatory response, low neutrophil count
Review DD Safety—consider Infection

AIDS — MS/CH
Refer to Acquired immune deficiency syndrome; *also refer to* HIV infection

AIDS dementia — CH
Also refer to Dementia, HIV
Impaired cognition, increased agitation, restlessness, altered response to stimuli, clinical evidence of organic impairment
Review DD Neurosensory—consider Confusion
Reports of feeling scared, shaky, increasing tension, loss of control, apprehension, extraneous movements, tremors, increased somatic complaints
Review DD Stress Management—consider Anxiety
Intolerance, rejection, abandonment, neglectful relationships, distortion of reality of health problems
Review DD Roles/Relationships—consider Coping, family

Alcohol intoxication, acute — MS
Also refer to Delirium tremens

Health Conditions and Client Concerns

A

Hallucinations, exaggerated emotional response, fluctuation in cognition or level of consciousness, increased agitation
Review DD Neurosensory—consider Confusion

Tracheobronchial obstruction, presence of chronic respiratory problems, decreased energy, fatigue
Review DD Respiration—consider Breathing pattern

Reduced level of consciousness, depressed cough or gag reflex, delayed gastric emptying
Review DD Respiration—consider Aspiration

Increased tension, apprehension, feelings of inadequacy, shame, self-disgust, remorse, fear
Review DD Stress Management—consider Anxiety

Disorientation, restlessness, sleep deprivation, exaggerated emotional responses, bizarre thinking, hallucinations
Review DD Neurosensory—consider Sensory deficit

Altered systemic vascular resistance, presence of dysrhythmias
Review DD Circulation—consider Cardiac output

Alteration in balance, reduced muscle coordination, cognitive impairment, involuntary muscle activity
Review DD Safety—consider Injury

Inadequate food intake, altered taste sensation, lack of interest in food, debilitated state, decreased subcutaneous fat or muscle mass, laboratory evidence of mineral or electrolyte deficiency
Review DD Food/Fluid—consider Nutritional intake

Alcoholism CH
Refer to Substance dependence/abuse rehabilitation

Aldosteronism, primary MS
Dry mucous membranes, poor skin turgor, dilute urine, excessive thirst, weight loss
Review DD Food/Fluid—consider Fluid volume

Impaired coordination, decreased muscle strength, paralysis, positive Chvostek's and Trousseau's signs
Review DD Activity/Rest—consider Mobility

Hypovolemia, cardiac dysrhythmias
Review DD Circulation—consider Cardiac output

Alkalosis, metabolic MS
Refer to underlying cause/condition, e.g., Renal failure, Dialysis

Alkalosis, respiratory MS
Also refer to underlying cause/condition

Dyspnea, tachypnea, changes in mentation, tachycardia, hypoxia, hypocapnia
Review DD Respiration—consider Gas exchange

Allergies, seasonal CH
Refer to Hay fever

ALS CH
Refer to Amyotrophic lateral sclerosis

Alzheimer disease CH
Also refer to Dementia, presenile/senile

Inability to recognize danger in environment, disorientation, confusion, impaired judgment, weakness, muscular incoordination, impaired balance, altered perception, seizure activity
  Review DD Safety—consider Injury

Inaccurate or inappropriate response to stimuli, progressive cognitive impairment, short-term memory deficit, impaired socialization, altered personality, clinical evidence of organic impairment
  Review DD Neurosensory—consider Confusion

Changes in usual response to stimuli, change in problem-solving ability, exaggerated emotional response (anxiety, paranoia, hallucinations), inability to tell position of body parts, diminished or altered sense of taste
  Review DD Neurosensory—consider Sensory deficit

Wakefulness, disorientation (day/night reversal), increased aimless wandering, inability to identify need or time for sleeping, changes in behavior, lethargy, dark circles under eyes, frequent yawning
  Review DD Sleep/Rest—consider Sleep pattern

Reported or observed inability to take responsibility for meeting basic health practices, lack of equipment or financial resources, impairment of personal support system
  Review DD Health Management—consider Health maintenance

PSY

Complex/increasing care needs, lack of privacy, respite; ineffective coping skills, lack of support/resources, unstable health of care receiver, problem behaviors
  Review DD Roles/Relationships—consider Caregiving burden

Limited preparation for change, resistance to change, decline in health, decreased cognition; potential loss of independence, possessions, friends; lack of social support
  Review DD Stress Management—consider Relocation stress

Amphetamine abuse PSY
Refer to Stimulant abuse

Amputation MS
Reduced arterial or venous blood flow, tissue edema, hematoma formation, hypovolemia
  Review DD Circulation—consider Cardiovascular function

Reports of incisional or phantom pain, guarding or protective behavior, narrowed focus, changes in vital signs
  Review DD Comfort—consider Pain

Reluctance to attempt movement, impaired coordination, decreased muscle strength, control, and mass
  Review DD Activity/Rest—consider Mobility

Health Conditions and Client Concerns

Loss of body part, tearfulness, poor eye contact, unwillingness to look at or touch residual limb, negative feelings about body, preoccupation about loss
Review DD Stress Management—consider Grief

Amyotrophic lateral sclerosis (ALS) — MS/CH

Impaired coordination, limited range of motion, impaired purposeful movement
Review DD Activity/Rest—consider Mobility

Shortness of breath, fremitus, shallow respirations, reduced vital capacity
Review DD Respiration—consider Breathing pattern

Recurrent coughing shocking, signs of aspiration
Review DD Food/Fluid—consider Swallowing

Impaired articulation, inability to speak in sentences, use of nonverbal cues
Review DD Roles/Relationships—consider Communication

PSY

Expressions of frustration about inability to care for self and depression over physical deterioration, powerlessness
Review DD Self-Perception/Concept—consider Resilience

Sorrow, choked feelings, expression of distress, changes in eating and sleeping patterns, altered communication patterns, changes in libido
Review DD Stress Management—consider Grief

Illness severity of care receiver, complexity and amount of homecare needs, duration of caregiving required, caregiver is spouse, family/caregiver isolation, lack of respite or recreation for caregiver
Review DD Roles/Relationships—consider Caregiving burden

Anaphylaxis — CH/MS

Also refer to Shock

Diminished or adventitious breath sounds, ineffective or absent cough, difficulty vocalizing, anxious
Review DD Respiration—consider Airway clearance

Tachycardia, palpitations, changes in blood pressure, anxiety, restlessness
Review DD Circulation—consider Cardiac output

Anemia — CH

Reports of fatigue, weakness, abnormal heart rate or blood pressure, decreased exercise or activity level, dyspnea on exertion
Review DD Activity/Rest—consider Activity intolerance

Weight loss or weight below normal for age, height, body build; change in oral mucosa; decreased activity tolerance; weakness; loss of muscle tone
Review DD Food/Fluid—consider Nutritional intake

Inadequate dietary intake, request for information, development of preventable complications
Review DD Health Management—consider Health knowledge

Anemia, iron-deficiency   CH
Also refer to Anemia

Reports of tiredness, inability to maintain usual routines or level of physical activity
  Review DD Activity/Rest—consider Fatigue

Active or chronic blood loss, poor skin turgor, dry mucous membranes, low blood pressure, tachycardia
  Review DD Food/Fluid—consider Fluid volume

Dehydration, malnutrition, vitamin deficiency, dry mouth, inflamed tongue
  Review DD Food/Fluid—consider Mucous membrane

Anemia, pernicious   CH
Also refer to Anemia

Paresthesia, impaired proprioception, loss of vibratory sensation, visual changes (yellow-blue color blindness)
  Review DD Neurosensory—consider Sensory deficit

Muscle weakness, changes in gastrointestinal motility, diarrhea/constipation
  Review DD Elimination—consider Elimination, intestinal

Generalized weakness, paresthesia of extremities, loss of proprioception, ataxia
  Review DD Safety—consider Injury

Anemia, sickle cell   MS

Dyspnea, use of accessory muscles, hypoxia (cyanosis, tachycardia, changes in mentation, restlessness)
  Review DD Respiration—consider Gas exchange

Renal impairment (decreased specific gravity, pale urine), cerebral impairment (paralysis, visual disturbances), peripheral impairment (distal ischemia, tissue infarctions, ulcerations, bone pain), cardiac impairments (angina, palpitations)
  Review DD Circulation—consider Cardiovascular function

CH/PED

Reports of localized, generalized, or migratory joint pain or abdominal/back pain; guarding; distracting behaviors (moaning, crying, restlessness); facial grimacing; narrowed focus; autonomic responses
  Review DD Comfort—consider Pain

Questions, statements of concern or misinterpretation of information, exacerbation of condition, inadequate follow-through of therapy instructions, development of preventable complications
  Review DD Health Management—consider Health knowledge

Altered/delayed physical growth, difficulty performing skills typical of age group
  Review DD Health Management—consider Growth, child
  Review DD Health Management—consider Development, child

Significant other displaying protective behavior disproportionate to client's ability or need for autonomy
  Review DD Roles/Relationships—consider Coping, family

Aneurysm, abdominal aortic   MS
Refer to Aortic aneurysm, abdominal

Aneurysm, cerebral   MS
Refer to Cerebrovascular accident

Aneurysm, ventricular   MS
Dyspnea, adventitious breath sounds, S_3/S_4 heart sounds, changes in hemodynamic measurements, dysrhythmias
   Review DD Circulation—consider Cardiac output

Blood pressure changes, diminished pulses, edema, dyspnea, dysrhythmias, altered mental status decreased renal function
   Review DD Circulation—consider Cardiovascular function

Weakness, fatigue, abnormal heart rate/blood pressure response to activity, dysrhythmias
   Review DD Activity/Rest—consider Activity intolerance

Angina pectoris   MS
Verbalization of chest pain, narrowed focus, restlessness, moaning, diaphoresis, changes in vital signs
   Review DD Comfort—consider Pain

Transient or prolonged myocardial ischemia, effects of medications, alterations in cardiac rate, rhythm, and electrical conduction
   Review DD Circulation—consider Cardiac output

Verbalized apprehension, expressed concerns, association of condition with loss of abilities, facial tension, restlessness, narrowed focus
   Review DD Stress Management—consider Anxiety

   CH

Exertional dyspnea, abnormal pulse/blood pressure response to activity, electrocardiogram changes
   Review DD Activity/Rest—consider Activity intolerance

Lack of understanding or training on specific exercise needs, safety concerns, fear of myocardial injury
   Review DD Activity/Rest—consider Sedentary behaviors

Questions, request for information, statements of concern, inaccurate follow-through of instructions
   Review DD Health Management—consider Health knowledge

Long-term therapy requiring lifestyle changes, multiple stressors, assault to self-concept, altered locus of control
   Review DD Health Management—consider Health maintenance

Anorexia nervosa   MS
Weight loss, poor skin turgor and muscle tone, denial of hunger, unusual hoarding or handling of food, amenorrhea, electrolyte imbalance, cardiac irregularities, hypotension
   Review DD Food/Fluid—consider Nutritional intake

Chronic laxative or diuretic use, poor skin turgor, dry mucous membranes
   Review DD Food/Fluid—consider Fluid volume

Impaired ability to make decisions or problem solve, unrealistic verbalizations, altered sleep patterns, ideas of reference, altered attention span, distractibility, perceptual disturbances, failure to recognize hunger cues, fatigue, anxiety, depression
Review DD Neurosensory—consider Thought process

Distorted view of body as fat, severe emaciation, overly conforming, dependence on others' opinion
Review DD Self-Perception/Concept—consider Body image

Enmeshed family, dissonance among family members, enabling behavior of family members; ill-defined family rules, functions, and roles
Review DD Roles/Relationships—consider Parenting

Antisocial personality disorder

Contempt for authority or rights of others, inability to tolerate frustration, need for immediate gratification, easy agitation, vulnerable self-concept, inability to verbalize feelings, use of poor coping mechanisms, substance use
Review DD Stress Management—consider Violence

Use of aggression and manipulation to handle problems or conflicts, inappropriate use of defense mechanisms (denial, projection), chronic worry, anxiety, destructive behaviors, high rate of accidents
Review DD Stress Management—consider Coping

Substance abuse, sexual promiscuity, feelings of inadequacy, nonparticipation in therapy
Review DD Self-Perception/Concept—consider Self-esteem

Expressions of concern or complaints, situational preoccupation, display of protective behaviors disproportionate to client's abilities or need for autonomy
Review DD Roles/Relationships—consider Coping, family

Difficulty meeting expectations of others, lack of belief that rules pertain to self, sense of emptiness or inadequacy covered by expressions of self-conceit, arrogance, contempt, behavior unaccepted by dominant cultural group
Review DD Roles/Relationships—consider Social connectedness

Anxiety disorder, generalized

Sympathetic stimulation (pupil dilation, tachycardia), extraneous movements (pacing, rocking, fidgeting), restlessness, poor eye contact, focus on self, impaired functioning, nonparticipation in decision making
Review DD Stress Management—consider Anxiety
Review DD Stress Management—consider Resilience

Verbalization of inability to cope or problem-solve, compulsive behaviors (smoking, drinking), emotional tension, change in social involvement
Review DD Stress Management—consider Coping

Inadequate or incorrect information or understanding of primary person, temporary family disorganization and role changes, prolonged disability that exhausts resources and support capacity
Review DD Roles/Relationships—consider Coping, family

A

Discomfort in social situations, withdrawal from usual activities or interactions, dysfunctional interactions, sad/flat affect
Review DD Roles/Relationships—consider Social connectedness

Anxiety disorders   PSY/PED

Sympathetic stimulation (pupil dilation, tachycardia), extraneous movements (pacing, rocking, fidgeting), restlessness, poor eye contact, focus on self, impaired functioning, nonparticipation in decision making
Review DD Stress Management—consider Anxiety

Verbalization of inability to cope or problem-solve, compulsive behaviors (smoking, drinking), emotional tension, change in social involvement
Review DD Stress Management—consider Coping

Panic states, dysfunctional family, history of self-destructive behaviors, emotional disturbance, increasing motor activity
Review DD Stress Management—consider Suicide
Review DD Stress Management—consider Self-injurious behavior

Difficulty falling asleep, awakening earlier or later than desired, reports of not feeling rested, dark circles under eyes, frequent yawning
Review DD Activity/Rest—consider Sleep pattern

Inadequate or incorrect information or understanding of primary person, temporary family disorganization and role changes, prolonged disability that exhausts resources and support capacity
Review DD Roles/Relationships—consider Coping, family

Discomfort in social situations, withdrawal from usual activities or interactions, dysfunctional interactions, sad/flat affect
Review DD Roles/Relationships—consider Social connectedness

Anxiolytic abuse   PSY

Refer to Depressant abuse

Aortic aneurysm, abdominal (AAA)   MS

Interruption of arterial blood flow (embolus or spontaneous blockage of aorta); signs and symptoms of shock
Review DD Circulation—consider Tissue perfusion

Turbulent blood flow through arteriosclerotic lesion; abdominal pain, pallor, hyperthermia, leukocytosis
Review DD Safety—consider Infection

Reports of severe pain, guarding behavior, facial mask, change in abdominal muscle tone
Review DD Comfort—consider Pain

Aortic aneurysm repair, abdominal   MS

Also refer to Surgery, general

Verbalization of fear, apprehension, decreased self-assurance, increased tension, changes in vital signs
Review DD Stress Management—consider Fear

Weakening in arterial wall, failure of vascular repair
Review DD Circulation—consider Bleeding

Interruption of arterial blood flow, hypovolemia, signs of poor renal perfusion
   Review DD Circulation—consider Tissue perfusion

Aortic stenosis   MS
Also refer to Valvular heart disease
Fatigue, dyspnea, changes in vital signs and hemodynamic parameters, syncope
   Review DD Circulation—consider Cardiac output
Alveolar-capillary membrane changes, congestion
   Review DD Respiration—consider Gas exchange
Episodic ischemia of myocardial tissue and stretching of left atrium; angina, vital sign changes
   Review DD Comfort—consider Pain

        CH

Exertional dyspnea, reports of fatigue, weakness, abnormal blood pressure or ECG changes, dysrhythmias in response to activity
   Review DD Activity/Rest—consider Activity intolerance

Aplastic anemia   CH
Also refer to Anemia
Abnormal blood profile (leukopenia, thrombocytopenia), drug therapies (antineoplastics, antibiotics, NSAIDs, anticonvulsants)
   Review DD Safety—consider Immunologic impairment
Verbalization of lack of energy, inability to maintain usual routines or level of physical activity, tiredness, decreased libido, lethargy, increase in physical complaints
   Review DD Activity/Rest—consider Fatigue

Appendicitis   MS
Verbal report of pain, guarding behavior, narrow focus, diaphoresis, autonomic responses (changes in vital signs)
   Review DD Comfort—consider Pain
Nausea/vomiting, anorexia, hyperthermia, diaphoresis, dry mucous membranes, dry skin, thirst
   Review DD Food/Fluid—consider Fluid volume
Possible release of pathogens into peritoneal cavity; abdominal pain, guarding, leukocytosis, hyperthermia, diaphoresis, chills
   Review DD Safety—consider Infection

ARDS   MS
Refer to Respiratory distress syndrome, acute

Arrhythmia, cardiac   MS/CH
Refer to Dysrhythmia, cardiac

Arterial occlusive disease, peripheral   CH
Skin discoloration, temperature changes, altered sensation, claudication, delayed healing
   Review DD Circulation—consider Tissue perfusion
Pain with activity/walking, presence of circulatory problems
   Review DD Activity/Rest—consider Walking

Altered circulation and sensation, delayed healing of wounds
  Review DD Safety—consider Skin/Tissue integrity

Arthritis, juvenile rheumatoid PED/CH
Also refer to Arthritis, rheumatoid
Physical disabilities, bone/joint damage, growth/height velocity lower that 30th percentile
  Review DD Health Management—consider Growth, child
Difficulty performing motor skills typical of age group, joint stiffness, decreased range of motion
  Review DD Health Management—consider Development, child
Delay in accomplishing developmental tasks, altered state of wellness, changes in physical appearance, decreased social interaction
  Review DD Roles/Relationships—consider Social connectedness

Arthritis, rheumatoid CH
Verbal reports, narrow focus, guarding or protective behaviors, physical or social withdrawal
  Review DD Comfort—consider Pain
Limited range of motion, impaired coordination, decreased muscle strength, control, and mass
  Review DD Activity/Rest—consider Mobility
Inability to manage activities of daily living, decreased muscle strength, limited range of motion, pain on movement, decreased strength and endurance
  Review DD Self-Care—consider Self-care
Negative self-talk, feelings of helplessness, changes in lifestyle and physical abilities, dependence on others for assistance, decreased social involvement
  Review DD Self-Perception/Concept—consider Body image

Arthritis, septic CH
Joint inflammation, verbalization of pain, guarding behaviors, restlessness, narrow focus
  Review DD Comfort—consider Pain
Limited range of motion, slowed movement, joint stiffness or discomfort, impaired coordination
  Review DD Activity/Rest—consider Mobility
Inability to perform activities of daily living, discomfort, limited range of motion, decreased strength
  Review DD Self-Care—consider Self-care
Presence of infectious process, chronic disease state, invasive procedures, leukocytosis, hyperthermia
  Review DD Safety—consider Infection

Arthroplasty MS
Break in primary defenses, exudate at operative site, altered inflammatory response, leukocytosis, hyperthermia
  Review DD Safety—consider Infection
Surgical procedure, trauma to vasculature
  Review DD Circulation—consider Bleeding

Impaired coordination, reluctance to move, discomfort with movement
  Review DD Activity/Rest—consider Mobility
Verbal reports, narrow focus, guarding behavior, autonomic response (diaphoresis, changes in vital signs)
  Review DD Comfort—consider Pain

Arthroscopy, knee MS
Questions, requests for information, misconceptions
  Review DD Health Management—consider Health knowledge
Joint stiffness, discomfort, prescribed movement restrictions, use of assistive devices for ambulation
  Review DD Activity/Rest—consider Walking

Asperger disorder PED/PSY
Refer to Autism spectrum disorder

Aspiration, foreign body CH
Dyspnea, ineffective cough, diminished or adventitious breath sounds
  Review DD Respiration—consider Airway clearance
Apprehension, fearfulness, pupil dilation, increased tension
  Review DD Stress Management—consider Anxiety
Lack of safety education or precautions, eating large mouthfuls or pieces of food
  Review DD Safety—consider Suffocation

Asthma MS
Also refer to Emphysema
Wheezing, dyspnea, changes in depth and rate of respirations, use of accessory muscles, persistent ineffective cough with or without sputum production
  Review DD Respiration—consider Airway clearance
Dyspnea, restlessness, reduced activity tolerance, cyanosis, change in vital signs, abnormal arterial blood gases
  Review DD Respiration—consider Gas exchange
Restlessness, apprehension, fearful expression, extraneous movements
  Review DD Stress Management—consider Anxiety

CH

Fatigue, exertional dyspnea
  Review DD Activity/Rest—consider Activity intolerance
Presence of atmospheric pollutants, environmental contaminants in the home (smoking or secondhand smoke exposure)
  Review DD Safety—consider Contamination exposure

Athlete's foot CH
Disruption of skin surface, reports of painful itching
  Review DD Safety—consider Skin integrity
Multiple breaks in skin integrity, exposure to warm/moist environment
  Review DD Safety—consider Infection

Atrial fibrillation CH
Also refer to Dysrhythmia, cardiac

A

Dyspnea, dizziness, presyncope or syncopal episodes
  Review DD Activity/Rest—consider Activity intolerance
Interruption of arterial blood flow (microemboli), change in mentation, dizziness, numbness/tingling face or scalp
  Review DD Circulation—consider Tissue perfusion

Atrial flutter CH
Also refer to Dysrhythmia, cardiac
Expressed concerns, apprehension, awareness of physiological symptoms (palpitations, dizziness, syncope), focus on self
  Review DD Stress Management—consider Anxiety

Atrial tachycardia CH
Refer to Dysrhythmia, cardiac

Attention-deficit disorder PED/PSY
Easily distracted by extraneous stimuli, shifting between incomplete activities
  Review DD Stress Management—consider Coping
Poor eye contact, derogatory self-comments, hesitance to try new activities, low level of self-confidence
  Review DD Self-Perception/Concept—consider Self-esteem
Verbalization of misconceptions, poor school performance, unrealistic expectations of medication regimen, lack of resource use
  Review DD Health Management—consider Health knowledge

Autism spectrum disorder PED/PSY
Lack of responsiveness to others, lack of eye contact or facial responsiveness, treating persons as objects, lack of awareness of feelings in others; indifference or aversion to comfort, affection, or physical contact; failure to develop cooperative social play and peer friendships in childhood
  Review DD Roles/Relationships—consider Social connectedness
Lack of interactive communication mode, no use of gestures or spoken language, absent or abnormal nonverbal communication, lack of eye contact or facial expression, peculiar patterns of speech, impaired ability to initiate or sustain conversation despite adequate speech
  Review DD Roles/Relationships—consider Communication
Organic brain dysfunction, inability to trust others, disturbance in self-concept, inadequate sensory stimulation, abnormal response to stimuli (sensory overload); history of physical, emotional, or sexual abuse; realization of severity of condition
  Review DD Safety—consider Nonsuicidal behavior
Lack of awareness of the feeling of existence of others, increased anxiety resulting from physical contact with others, absent or impaired imitation of others, repeating what others say, persistent preoccupation with parts of objects, obsessive attachment to objects, marked distress over changes in environment, autoerotic or ritualistic behaviors, self-touching, rocking, swaying
  Review DD Self-Perception/Concept—consider Personal identity

Denial of existence or severity of disturbed behaviors, preoccupation with personal emotional reaction to situation, rationalization that problem will be outgrown, attempts to intervene with child are achieving increasingly ineffective results, family withdraws from or becomes overly protective of child
Review DD Roles/Relationships—consider Coping, family

Barbiturate abuse CH/PSY
Refer to Depressant abuse

Battered child syndrome PED/CH
Also refer to Abuse, physical

Vulnerability, history of previous abuse or neglect, lack of or nonuse of support systems by caregivers, dependent position in relationship, signs of abuse (multiple healed fractures, unusual bruising patterns)
Review DD Safety—consider Injury

Delay or difficulty in performing age-appropriate skills, loss of previously acquired skills, precocious or accelerated sexual awareness, flat affect, decreased responsiveness
Review DD Health Management—consider Development, child

Verbalization of negative feelings, inappropriate caretaking behaviors, evidence of physical or psychological trauma to child
Review DD Roles/Relationships—consider Family process
Review DD Roles/Relationships—consider Parenting

PSY

Lack of eye contact, withdrawal from social contacts, discounting own needs, nonassertive or passive behavior, indecisive, overly conforming behaviors
Review DD Self-Perception/Concept—consider Self-esteem

Acting-out behavior, development of phobias, poor impulse control, emotional numbness
Review DD Stress Management—consider Post-trauma syndrome

Benign prostatic hyperplasia CH/MS
Urinary frequency, hesitancy, inability to empty bladder completely, incontinence or dribbling, nocturia, bladder distension, residual urine
Review DD Elimination—consider Retention, urinary

Verbal reports of bladder spasms, narrow focus, altered muscle tone, grimacing, distraction behaviors, restlessness, autonomic responses
Review DD Comfort—consider Pain

Active fluid volume loss through post obstructive diuresis, endocrine, or renal dysfunction
Review DD Food/Fluid—consider Fluid volume
Review DD Food/Fluid—consider Water-electrolyte balance

Increased tension, apprehension, worry, expressed concerns
Review DD Stress Management—consider Fear
Review DD Stress Management—consider Anxiety

Bipolar disorder   PSY
Irritability, impulsive behavior, delusional thinking, angry response when ideas or wishes are denied, manic excitement
  Review DD Self-Perception/Concept—consider Impulse control
Threatening body language or verbalizations, increased motor activity, overt and aggressive acts, hostility, statements of worthlessness or hopelessness
  Review DD Stress Management—consider Violence
Body weight 20% or more below IBW, inadequate intake, inattention to mealtimes, distraction during eating, laboratory evidence of nutritional deficits
  Review DD Food/Fluid—consider Nutritional intake
Narrow therapeutic range of drug (lithium), inability to follow medication regimen, denial of need for therapy
  Review DD Safety—consider Poisoning
Denial of need for sleep, interrupted nighttime sleep, one or more nights without sleep, changes in behavior or performance, increasing irritability, restlessness, dark circles under eyes
  Review DD Activity/Rest—consider Sleep pattern
Increased distractibility, agitation, anxiety, disorientation, poor concentration, auditory or visual hallucinations, bizarre thinking, motor incoordination
  Review DD Neurosensory—consider Sensory deficit
Statements of difficulty coping with situation, lack of adaptation to change, ineffective family decision-making process, poor communication, inappropriate boundaries
  Review DD Roles/Relationships—consider Family process/Interaction patterns
Reports of nervousness or fearfulness, feelings of inadequacy, agitation, angry or tearful outbursts, rambling speech, restlessness, hand rubbing or wringing, poor concentration, impaired ability to make decisions, numerous or repetitive physical complaints without organic cause, hallucinations, delusions
  Review DD Stress Management—consider Anxiety
Discomfort in social situations, withdrawal from usual activities, dysfunctional interactions, sad/flat affect, remaining home
  Review DD Roles/Relationships—consider Social connectedness

Bladder cancer   MS
Also refer to Cancer; Urinary diversion
Urinary frequency, dysuria
  Review DD Elimination—consider Elimination, urinary
Sensation of bladder fullness, bladder distension, residual urine, dysuria
  Review DD Elimination—consider Retention

Bone cancer   MS/CH
Also refer to Myeloma, multiple; Amputation
Verbal reports of pain, protective behaviors, autonomic responses
  Review DD Comfort—consider Pain

Bone fragility, generalized weakness, balance difficulties
Review DD Safety—consider Injury

Decreased fine/gross motor skills, decreased range of motion, altered gait, postural instability
Review DD Activity/Rest—consider Mobility

Bone marrow transplantation — MS/CH

Also refer to Transplantation, recipient

Immune dysfunction or suppression, abnormal blood profile, action of donor T cells
Review DD Safety—consider Injury

Expressions of boredom, restlessness, withdrawal, requests for something to do
Review DD Activity/Rest—consider Diversional activity

Increased metabolic needs for healing, altered ability to ingest nutrients due to nausea, vomiting, loss of appetite, taste changes, oral lesions
Review DD Food/Fluid—consider Nutritional intake

Borderline personality disorder — PSY

Mood swings, feel disconnected from body or reality, engage in reckless/dangerous behaviors, sensation seeking
Review DD Self-Perception/Concept—consider Impulse control

Projection as a defense mechanism, negative transference, feelings of guilt or need to "punish" self, distorted sense of self, inability to cope with increased psychological or physiological tension in a healthy manner
Review DD Stress Management—consider Violence
Review DD Stress Management—consider Nonsuicidal behavior

Easy frustration or feelings of hurt, abuse of alcohol or other drugs, transient psychotic symptoms, performance of self-mutilating acts
Review DD Stress Management—consider Anxiety

Poor sense of belonging, seeks reassurance of others, lack of tolerance of rejection or of being alone, unhappiness with self, rejects positive feedback
Review DD Self-Perception/Concept—consider Self-esteem

Difficulty identifying self or defining self-boundaries, feelings of depersonalization, extreme mood changes, poor interpersonal relations, ineffective role performance
Review DD Self-Perception/Concept—consider Personal identity

Alternating clinging and distancing behaviors, difficulty meeting expectation of others, experiencing feelings of difference from others, expressing interests inappropriate for developmental age, exhibiting behavior unacceptable by dominant cultural group
Review DD Roles/Relationships—consider Social connectedness

Botulism (foodborne) — MS/CH

Reports of thirst, dry skin and mucous membranes, hypotension, decreased urine output, change in mental status, increased hematocrit
Review DD Food/Fluid—consider Fluid volume

Limited ability to perform gross or fine motor skills
  Review DD Activity/Rest—consider Mobility
Nervousness, self-focused, expression of concern for well-being, tension, psychomotor agitation, change in vital signs
  Review DD Stress Management—consider Anxiety
Neuromuscular impairment, presence of infectious process
  Review DD Respiration—consider Ventilation, spontaneous

Bowel obstruction — MS
Refer to Ileus

Brain tumor — MS
Also refer to Cancer
Reports of headache, facial expression of pain, narrow focus, autonomic response
  Review DD Comfort—consider Pain
Memory loss, personality changes, impaired ability to make decisions or conceptualize, inaccurate interpretation of environment
  Review DD Neurosensory—consider Thought process
Changes in visual acuity, alterations of sense of balance, gait disturbance, paresthesia
  Review DD Neurosensory—consider Sensory deficit
Recurrent vomiting, decreased intake, poor skin turgor, dry mucous membranes
  Review DD Neurosensory—consider Fluid volume
Unkempt or disheveled appearance, body odor, verbalization or observation of inability to perform activities of daily living
  Review DD Neurosensory—consider Self-care

Breast cancer — MS/CH
Also refer to Cancer
Expressed concerns, apprehension, uncertainty, focus on self, diminished productivity
  Review DD Stress Management—consider Anxiety
Verbalizations, statements of misconception, inappropriate behaviors
  Review DD Health Management—consider Health knowledge
Significance of body part with regard to sexual perceptions
  Review DD Self-Perception/Concept—consider Body image
Health-related changes, medical treatments, concern about relationship with SO
  Review DD Sexuality/Reproduction—consider Sexual functioning

Bronchitis — CH
Rhonchi, tachypnea, ineffective cough
  Review DD Respiration—consider Airway clearance
Reports of fatigue, dyspnea, abnormal vital signs in response to activity
  Review DD Activity/Rest—consider Activity intolerance
Reports of pleuritic chest pain, guarding, distraction behaviors, restlessness
  Review DD Comfort—consider Pain

Bronchopneumonia MS/CH
Also refer to Bronchitis
Changes in rate and depth of respirations, abnormal breath sounds, use of accessory muscles, dyspnea, cyanosis, cough with or without sputum production
  Review DD Respiration—consider Airway clearance
Restlessness, changes in mentation, dyspnea, tachycardia, pallor, cyanosis, abnormal arterial blood gas results, hypoxia
  Review DD Respiration—consider Gas exchange
Decreased ciliary action, stasis of secretions, presence of existing infection, immunosuppression, chronic disease, malnutrition, leukocytosis, hyperthermia
  Review DD Safety—consider Infection

Bulimia nervosa PSY/MS
Also refer to Anorexia nervosa
Erosion of tooth enamel, multiple caries, abraded teeth due to dietary habits, poor oral hygiene, chronic vomiting
  Review DD Health Management—consider Health maintenance
Sore, inflamed buccal mucosa; swollen salivary glands; ulcerations of mucosa; reports of constant sore mouth or throat
  Review DD Food/Fluid—consider Mucous membrane
Self-induced vomiting, excessive laxative or diuretic use, esophageal erosion or tear, poor skin turgor, dry mucous membranes
  Review DD Food/Fluid—consider Fluid volume
Repeated vomiting, laxative use, inadequate fluid intake
  Review DD Food/Fluid—consider Water-electrolyte balance
Verbalization of misconception of current situation related to binging and purging behaviors; distortion of body image; verbalization of the problem
  Review DD Health Management—consider Health knowledge

Burns (dependent on type, degree, and severity of the injury) MS/CH
Loss of fluids through wound drainage, capillary damage, and evaporation; hypermetabolic state; insufficient intake; poor skin turgor; dry mucous membranes; concentrated urine
  Review DD Food/Fluid—consider Fluid volume
Hypermetabolic state, protein catabolism, anorexia, restricted oral intake
  Review DD Food/Fluid—consider Nutritional intake
Tracheobronchial obstruction (edema and loss of ciliary action); circumferential full thickness burns of the chest, neck, and thorax; compression of the airway; limited chest excursion; trauma due to direct upper airway injury; fluid shifts; pulmonary edema; decreased lung compliance
  Review DD Respiration—consider Airway clearance
Loss of protective dermal layer; traumatized tissue; necrosis; decreased hemoglobin; suppressed inflammatory response; environmental exposure; invasive procedures
  Review DD Safety—consider Infection

Impaired healing, deficient immunity, fatigue, anorexia
  Review DD Safety—consider **Immunologic impairment**
Verbal reports of pain, narrow focus, distraction and guarding behaviors, facial grimacing, changes in vital signs
  Review DD Comfort—consider **Pain**
Reexperiencing the event, repetitive dreams or nightmares, psychic or emotional numbness, sleep disturbance
  Review DD Stress Management—consider **Post-trauma syndrome**

PED

Expressions of boredom, restlessness, withdrawal, requests for something to do
  Review DD Activity/Rest—consider **Diversional activity**
Effects of physical disability, separation from SO(s), environmental deficiencies
  Review DD Activity/Rest—consider **Development, child**

Bursitis CH

Verbal reports, guarding behavior, narrow focus
  Review DD Comfort—consider **Pain**
Decreased range of motion, reluctance to attempt movement, activity restrictions by medical treatment
  Review DD Activity/Rest—consider **Mobility**

Calculi, urinary CH/MS

Reports of sudden, severe, colicky pains; guarding and distraction behaviors; self-focus; autonomic response
  Review DD Comfort—consider **Pain**
Urinary urgency or frequency, oliguria, hematuria
  Review DD Elimination—consider **Elimination, urinary**
Nausea, vomiting, diarrhea, changes in urinary output, post obstructive diuresis, poor skin turgor, dry mucous membranes
  Review DD Food/Fluid—consider **Fluid volume**
Stasis of urine, leukocytosis, hyperthermia
  Review DD Safety—consider **Infection**
Requests for information, statements of concern, recurrence or development of preventable complications
  Review DD Health Management—consider **Health knowledge**

Cancer MS

Also refer to Chemotherapy; Radiation therapy
Expressed concerns, feelings of inadequacy/helplessness, insomnia, increased tension, restlessness, focus on self, sympathetic stimulation
  Review DD Stress Management—consider **Fear**
  Review DD Stress Management—consider **Death anxiety**
Anger, sadness, withdrawal, choked feelings; changes in eating or sleep patterns, activity level, libido, communication patterns
  Review DD Stress Management—consider **Grief**

Verbalizations of impact of crisis on own values, priorities, goals, or relationships, desires to enhance positive outlook on life
   Review DD Stress Management—consider Hope

Verbal reports, self-focus, narrow focus, alteration in muscle tone, facial expression of pain, distraction or guarding behaviors, autonomic responses, restlessness
   Review DD Comfort—consider Pain

Relentless or overwhelming lack of energy, inability to maintain usual routines, decreased performance, impaired ability to concentrate, lethargy, listlessness, disinterest in surroundings
   Review DD Activity/Rest—consider Fatigue

Verbalization of problem, request for assistance, lack of necessary equipment or aids
   Review DD Self-Care—consider Home maintenance

PSY/PED

Situational or transitional crisis (long-term illness, change in roles or economic status, developmental); anticipated loss of a family member
   Review DD Roles/Relationships—consider Family process
   Review DD Roles/Relationships—consider Coping, family

Candidiasis   CH
Also refer to Thrush

Infectious lesions disrupting skin surface and mucous membranes
   Review DD Safety—consider Skin/Tissue integrity

Verbal report of pain, guarded behavior, restlessness
   Review DD Comfort—consider Pain
   Review DD Comfort—consider Discomfort

Presence of infectious lesions, vaginal discomfort
   Review DD Sexuality/Reproduction—consider Sexual functioning

Cannabis abuse   CH
Refer to Depressant abuse

Carbon monoxide poisoning   MS

Headache, confusion, somnolence, elevated carbon monoxide levels
   Review DD Respiration—consider Gas exchange

Fatigue, exertional dyspnea
   Review DD Activity/Rest—consider Activity intolerance

Use of therapeutic intervention (hyperbaric oxygen therapy); cognitive impairment
   Review DD Safety—consider Injury

Altered consciousness, loss of large and small muscle coordination, seizure activity
   Review DD Safety—consider Suffocation

Cardiac catheterization (aka heart cath, angiogram, angiography)   MS

Expressed concerns, apprehension, uncertainty, focus on self
   Review DD Stress Management—consider Anxiety

Altered heart rate or rhythm (vasovagal response), decreased myocardial contractility
  Review DD Circulation—consider Cardiac output
Impaired arterial blood flow, local hematoma formation, emboli, allergic dye response
  Review DD Circulation—consider Tissue perfusion

Cardiac surgery   MS/PED
Altered myocardial contractility secondary to temporary factors such as ventricular wall surgery, recent myocardial infarction, response to certain medications or drug interactions, altered preload (hypovolemia) or afterload (vascular resistance), dysrhythmias
  Review DD Circulation—consider Cardiac output
Interoperative bleeding, insufficient heparin reversal, fibrinolysis, platelet destruction, volume depletion, postoperative diuretic therapy
  Review DD Circulation—consider Bleeding
  Review DD Circulation—consider Fluid volume
Atelectasis, inadequate function or premature removal of chest tubes, diminished oxygen-carrying capacity of the blood, abnormal arterial blood gas results, hypoxia
  Review DD Respiration—consider Gas exchange
Reports of incisional pain in chest or donor site; paresthesia or pain in hand, arm, shoulder; anxiety; restlessness; irritability; distraction behaviors; changes in heart rate and blood pressure
  Review DD Comfort—consider Pain
  Review DD Comfort—consider Discomfort
Surgical incision, puncture wounds, disruption of skin surface and tissues
  Review DD Safety—consider Skin/Tissue integrity

Cardiogenic shock   MS
Refer to Shock, cardiogenic

Cardiomyopathy   CH/MS
Dyspnea, fatigue, chest pain, dizziness, syncope
  Review DD Circulation—consider Cardiac output
Weakness, fatigue, dyspnea, abnormal heart rate or blood pressure in response to activity, ECG changes
  Review DD Activity/Rest—consider Activity intolerance
Change in usual patterns of responsibility, role strain, change in capacity to resume role
  Review DD Roles/Relationships—consider Role performance

Carotid endarterectomy   MS
Also refer to Surgery, general
Interruption in arterial blood flow (wound hematoma or emboli, pressure changes, edema formation), change in mentation/level of consciousness
  Review DD Circulation—consider Tissue perfusion

Carpal tunnel syndrome CH/MS
Verbal reports, reluctance to use affected extremity, guarding behaviors, expressed fear of reinjury, altered ability to continue previous activities
  Review DD Comfort—consider Pain
Decreased hand strength, weakness, limited range of motion, reluctance to attempt movement
  Review DD Activity/Rest—consider Mobility
Mechanical compression (brace), repetitive tasks or motions, immobilization
  Review DD Circulation—consider Neurovascular function
Questions, statements of concern, request for information, inaccurate follow-through of instructions, development of preventable complications
  Review DD Health Management—consider Health knowledge

Casts CH/MS
Also refer to Fractures
Presence of fracture(s), mechanical compression (cast), immobilization, vascular obstruction; pallor, paresthesia, diminished or absent pulse, pain/pressure, impaired mobility, coolness in affected extremity
  Review DD Circulation—consider Neurovascular function
Pressure of cast, moisture, debris under cast, objects under cast to relieve itching, altered sensation or circulation
  Review DD Safety—consider Skin integrity
Statements of need for assistance, observed difficulty in performing activities of daily living
  Review DD Self-Care—consider Self-care

Cataract CH
Diminished activity, visual distortions, change in usual response to stimuli
  Review DD Neurosensory—consider Sensory deficit
Poor vision, reduced hand-eye coordination
  Review DD Safety—consider Injury
Expressed concerns, apprehension, feelings of uncertainty
  Review DD Stress Management—consider Anxiety
  Review DD Stress Management—consider Fear
Requests for information, statement of concern, inaccurate follow-through of instructions, development of preventable complications
  Review DD Health Management—consider Health knowledge

Cat scratch disease CH
Verbal reports, guarding behaviors, autonomic response
  Review DD Comfort—consider Pain
Increased body temperature, flushed or warm skin, tachypnea, tachycardia, chills, aches, headache
  Review DD Safety—consider Thermoregulation

Health Conditions and Client Concerns

Celiac disease   CH

Weight loss, abdominal distention, steatorrhea, anemia, vitamin deficiencies
  Review DD Food/Fluid—consider Nutritional intake

Abdominal pain, hyperactive bowel sounds, at least three loose stools per day
  Review DD Elimination—consider Elimination, intestinal

Mild to massive steatorrhea, diarrhea, poor skin turgor, dry mucous membranes
  Review DD Food/Fluid—consider Fluid volume

Cellulitis   CH/MS

Broken skin, chronic disease, presence of pathogens, insufficient knowledge to avoid exposure to pathogens
  Review DD Safety—consider Infection

Reports of localized pain, headache, guarding behaviors, restlessness, autonomic response
  Review DD Comfort—consider Pain
  Review DD Comfort—consider Discomfort

Inflammation, trauma, erythema, warmth, edema, tenderness or pain
  Review DD Safety—consider Skin/Tissue integrity

Cerebrovascular accident (CVA)   MS

Altered level of consciousness, changes in vital signs, changes in motor or sensory responses, restlessness, memory loss; sensory, language, intellectual, and emotional deficits
  Review DD Circulation—consider Tissue perfusion

Inability to purposefully move involved body parts, limited range of motion, impaired coordination, decreased muscle strength or control
  Review DD Activity/Rest—consider Mobility

Impaired articulation, dysarthria, inability to modulate speech, inability to find or name words or identify objects, inability to comprehend spoken/written language, inability to produce written communication
  Review DD Roles/Relationships—consider Communication

Stated or observed inability to perform activities of daily living, requests for assistance, disheveled appearance, incontinence
  Review DD Self-Care—consider Self-care

Muscle paralysis, perceptual impairment, ineffective cough or gag reflex
  Review DD Food/Fluid—consider Swallowing

Sensory loss of part of visual field with perceptual loss of corresponding body segment
  Review DD Health Management—consider Health maintenance

CH

Members expressing difficulty in managing home in a comfortable manner, requesting assistance with home maintenance, disorderly surroundings, overtaxed family members
  Review DD Self-Care—consider Home maintenance

Actual change in structure or function, change in usual patterns of responsibility or physical capacity to resume role, verbal or nonverbal response to actual or perceived change
    Review DD Self-Perception/Concept—consider Self-esteem
    Review DD Self-Perception/Concept—consider Body image
    Review DD Self-Perception/Concept—consider Role performance

Cervix, dysfunctional   OB
Refer to Dilation of Cervix, premature

Cesarean birth   OB
Also refer to Cesarean birth, unplanned/postpartal
Statements of concern, questions, misconceptions
    Review DD Health Management—consider Health knowledge
Restriction of oral intake, blood loss, poor skin turgor, dry mucous membranes
    Review DD Food/Fluid—consider Fluid volume
Separation, existing maternal/child health conditions, lack of privacy
    Review DD Roles/Relationships—consider Caregiver child attachment

Cesarean birth, postpartal   OB
Also refer to Postpartum periods
Developmental transition, situational crisis (surgical intervention), physical complications interfering with initial interaction, negative self-appraisal
    Review DD Roles/Relationships—consider Caregiver child attachment
Verbal reports of incisional pain, cramping, afterpains, spinal headache; guarding or distraction behaviors; irritability; facial mask of pain
    Review DD Comfort—consider Pain
    Review DD Comfort—consider Discomfort
Perception of self as "failing" at life event, maturational transition, perceived loss of control in unplanned delivery
    Review DD Self-Perception/Concept—consider Self-esteem
Orthostatic hypotension, development of pregnancy-induced hypertension or eclampsia, effects of anesthesia, thromboembolism, anemia, excessive blood loss, rubella sensitivity, Rh incompatibility, tissue trauma
    Review DD Safety—consider Injury
Tissue trauma, broken skin, decreased hemoglobin, invasive procedures or increased environmental exposure, prolonged rupture of amniotic membranes, malnutrition
    Review DD Safety—consider Infection
Verbalization of inability to perform desired activities of daily living
    Review DD Self-Care—consider Self-care

Cesarean birth, unplanned   OB
Also refer to Cesarean birth, postpartal
Request for information, verbalization of concerns or misconceptions, inappropriate behavior or response
    Review DD Health Management—consider Health knowledge

Increased tension, apprehension, feelings of inadequacy, sympathetic stimulation, narrow focus, restlessness
   Review DD Stress Management—consider Anxiety
Verbalization of lack of control, lack of participation in care or decision making, passivity
   Review DD Self-Perception/Concept—consider Resilience
Altered blood flow to placenta or through umbilical cord, decreased fetal oxygen transport
   Review DD Sexuality/Reproduction—consider Maternal-fetal dyad
Increased or prolonged contractions, psychological reaction
   Review DD Comfort—consider Pain
Invasive procedures, rupture of amniotic membranes, break in skin, decreased hemoglobin, exposure to pathogens
   Review DD Safety—consider Infection

Chemotherapy MS/CH
Also refer to Cancer
Gastrointestinal loss through vomiting, inadequate oral intake due to stomatitis or anorexia; abnormal fluid loss through indwelling tubes, wounds, fistulas; hypermetabolic state
   Review DD Food/Fluid—consider Fluid volume
Weight loss, muscle wasting, aversion to eating, reported altered sense of taste, sore and inflamed buccal mucosa, diarrhea, constipation
   Review DD Food/Fluid—consider Nutritional intake
Oral mucosa ulcerations, leukoplakia, decreased salivation, reports of pain
   Review DD Food/Fluid—consider Mucous membrane
Verbalization of negative feelings about body, preoccupation with change, feelings of helplessness or hopelessness, change in social environment
   Review DD Self-Perception/Concept—consider Body image
Impaired healing, deficient immunity, anorexia, fatigue
   Review DD Safety—consider Immunologic impairment
Expressed desire to enhance belief in possibilities or sense of meaning of life and positive outlook
   Review DD Self-Perception/Concept—consider Hope

Cholecystectomy MS
Verbal reports, guarding or distraction behaviors, autonomic responses
   Review DD Comfort—consider Pain
Fremitus, tachypnea, decreased respiratory depth and vital capacity, holding breath, reluctance to cough
   Review DD Respiration—consider Breathing pattern
Fluid loss from vomiting or nasogastric suction, medically restricted intake
   Review DD Food/Fluid—consider Fluid volume

Cholelithiasis MS
Verbal reports, guarding or distraction behaviors, focus on self, narrow focus, changes in vital signs
   Review DD Comfort—consider Pain

Dietary restrictions, nausea, vomiting, dyspepsia, abdominal or epigastric pain, loss of nutrients, impaired fat digestion due to obstructed bile flow
  Review DD Food/Fluid—consider Nutritional intake
Verbalization of concerns, questions, recurrence of condition
  Review DD Health Management—consider Health knowledge

Chronic obstructive lung disease   CH/MS

Presence of wheezes, crackles, tachypnea, dyspnea, changes in depth of respirations, use of accessory muscles, persistent cough, chest radiograph findings
  Review DD Respiration—consider Airway clearance
Dyspnea, restlessness, confusion, abnormal arterial blood gas values, hypoxia, hypercapnia, changes in vital signs, reduced activity tolerance
  Review DD Respiration—consider Gas exchange
Verbal reports of fatigue, exertional dyspnea, abnormal vital sign response
  Review DD Activity/Rest—consider Activity intolerance
Weight loss, reported altered taste sensation, decreased muscle mass and subcutaneous fat, poor muscle tone, aversion to eating or lack of interest in food
  Review DD Food/Fluid—consider Nutritional intake
Decreased ciliary action, stasis of secretions, debilitated state, malnutrition
  Review DD Safety—consider Infection

Circumcision   PED

Request for information, verbalization of concern or misconception, inaccurate follow-through of instructions
  Review DD Health Management—consider Health knowledge
Crying, changes in sleep pattern, refusal to eat
  Review DD Comfort—consider Pain
Edema, difficulty voiding
  Review DD Elimination—consider Elimination, urinary
Circumcision procedure, decreased clotting factors immediately after birth, previously undiagnosed bleeding or clotting problems
  Review DD Circulation—consider Bleeding
Immature immune system, invasive procedure, tissue trauma, environmental exposure
  Review DD Safety—consider Infection

Cirrhosis   MS

Also refer to Substance dependence/abuse rehabilitation; Hepatitis, acute viral
Viral infection, alcohol abuse, hepatotoxic agents/chemicals
  Review DD Safety—consider Liver function
Abnormal blood profile, altered clotting factors, impaired vitamin K absorption, release of thromboplastin, portal hypertension, development of esophageal varices
  Review DD Circulation—consider Bleeding

CH

Aversion to eating, observed lack of intake, muscle wasting, weight loss, imbalances in nutritional studies
  Review DD Food/Fluid—consider Nutritional intake

Generalized or abdominal edema, weight gain, dyspnea, blood pressure changes, positive hepatojugular reflex, change in mentation, altered electrolytes, changes in urine specific gravity, pleural effusion
  Review DD Food/Fluid—consider Fluid volume

Altered circulation or metabolic state, poor skin turgor, skeletal prominence, presence of edema, ascites, accumulation of bile salts on skin
  Review DD Safety—consider Skin integrity

Alcohol abuse, increased serum ammonia level, inability of liver to detoxify certain enzymes and drugs, disorientation
  Review DD Neurosensory—consider Confusion

Verbalization of changes in lifestyle, fear of rejection or reaction of others, negative feelings about body or abilities; feelings of helplessness, hopelessness, powerlessness
  Review DD Self-Perception/Concept—consider Self-esteem
  Review DD Self-Perception/Concept—consider Body image

Cleft lip/palate   PED/MS

Also refer to Newborn, special needs

Inability to sustain an effective suck; inability to coordinate sucking, swallowing, and breathing
  Review DD Food/Fluid—consider Suck-swallow response

Impaired swallowing, regurgitation
  Review DD Respiration—consider Aspiration

Anatomic defect, developmental delay, impaired ability to speak
  Review DD Roles/Relationships—consider Communication

Altered appearance, anatomic defect, significance of body part (face)
  Review DD Self-Perception/Concept—consider Body image

Cocaine hydrochloride poisoning, acute   MS

Also refer to Stimulant abuse; Substance dependence/abuse rehabilitation

Tachypnea, altered depth of respiration, shortness of breath, abnormal arterial blood gas values
  Review DD Respiration—consider Breathing pattern

Drug effect on myocardium; alterations in electrical rate, rhythm, or conduction; preexisting myocardiopathy
  Review DD Circulation—consider Cardiac output

CH

Cocaine abuse, abnormal liver enzyme levels, jaundice
  Review DD Safety—consider Liver function

Altered taste, food aversion, anorexia, food insecurity, evidence of vitamin deficiencies
  Review DD Food/Fluid—consider Nutritional intake

Localized tissue trauma, injection techniques, exposure to pathogens, malnutrition, impaired immune system
   Review DD Safety—consider Infection
Ineffective coping skills, substance abuse, inadequate problem-solving skills, insufficient goal-directed behavior
   Review DD Stress Management—consider Coping
Altered sensory reception or integration, anxiety, panic, hallucinations, bizarre thinking, change in sense of taste or smell
   Review DD Neurosensory—consider Sensory deficit

Coccidioidomycosis (San Joaquin Valley/Valley Fever) CH
Verbal reports, distraction behaviors, narrow focus
   Review DD Comfort—consider Pain
Reports of overwhelming lack of energy, inability to maintain usual routine, emotional lability, irritability, impaired ability to concentrate, decreased endurance, decreased libido
   Review DD Activity/Rest—consider Fatigue
Statements of concern or questions
   Review DD Health Management—consider Health knowledge

Colitis, ulcerative MS
Increased bowel sounds and peristalsis; urgency; frequent, watery stools; abdominal pain; cramping
   Review DD Elimination—consider Elimination, intestinal
Verbal reports, guarding or distraction behaviors (restlessness), self-focus
   Review DD Comfort—consider Pain
Severe diarrhea, vomiting, capillary plasma loss, restricted intake, nausea, anorexia, hypermetabolic state (inflammation, fever)
   Review DD Food/Fluid—consider Fluid volume

CH

Weight loss, decreased subcutaneous fat or muscle mass, poor muscle tone, hyperactive bowel sounds, steatorrhea, pale conjunctiva and mucous membranes, aversion to eating
   Review DD Food/Fluid—consider Nutritional intake
Verbalization of inability to cope, discouragement, anxiety, preoccupation with physical self, chronic worry, emotional tension, depression, recurrent exacerbation of symptoms
   Review DD Stress Management—consider Coping
Unresolved dependency conflicts, feelings of insecurity, resentment, repression of anger and aggressive feelings, lacking a sense of control in stressful situations, sacrificing own wishes for others, retreating from aggression or frustration
   Review DD Self-Perception/Concept—consider Resilience

Colostomy MS
Also refer to surgery, general
Absence of sphincter at stoma, character and flow of effluent from stoma, reaction to product or removal of adhesive, improperly fitted appliance
   Review DD Safety—consider Skin integrity

Interruption or alteration of normal bowel function, changes in dietary or fluid intake, effects of medications
  Review DD Elimination—consider Elimination, intestinal

Questions, statements of concern, inaccurate follow-through of instruction or performance of ostomy care, development of preventable complications
  Review DD Health Management—consider Health knowledge

Verbalization of change in perception of self, negative feelings about body, fear of rejection or reaction of others, not touching or looking at stoma, refusal to participate in ostomy care
  Review DD Self-Perception/Concept—consider Body image

Reduced participation in usual activities, verbalized or observed discomfort in social situations
  Review DD Roles/Relationships—consider Social connectedness

Altered body structure and function, radical resection and treatment procedures, vulnerability, psychological concern about response of SO(s) disruption of sexual response pattern (erection difficulty)
  Review DD Sexuality/Reproduction—consider Sexual functioning

Coma   MS

Cognitive impairment, loss of protective reflexes and purposeful movement
  Review DD Safety—consider Suffocation

Inability to ingest food or fluids, hypermetabolic state, poor skin turgor, dry mucous membranes
  Review DD Food/Fluid—consider Fluid volume

Inability to perform activities of daily living
  Review DD Self-Care—consider Self-care

Reduced or interrupted cerebral arterial or venous blood flow, metabolic alterations, effects of drug or alcohol overdose, hypoxia, anoxia
  Review DD Circulation—consider Tissue perfusion

Stasis of body fluids (oral, pulmonary, urinary), invasive procedures, nutritional deficits
  Review DD Safety—consider Infection

Coma, diabetic   MS
Refer to Diabetic ketoacidosis

Compartment syndrome, extremity   MS

Reports of progressing pain distal to injury unrelieved by analgesics
  Review DD Comfort—consider Pain

Absent or diminished distal pulses, pallor, pain, paresthesia, paralysis, coolness of extremity
  Review DD Circulation—consider Tissue perfusion

Reduction or interruption of blood flow, tissue trauma, excessive edema, elevated tissue pressures, hypovolemia
  Review DD Neurosensory—consider Neurovascular function

Complex regional pain syndrome CH
Verbal reports of pain, ineffective pain self-management, impaired physical mobility, changes in sleep pattern, altered ability to continue previous activities, decreased social interactions
  Review DD Comfort—consider Pain
Reports of pain, decreased skin temperature, pallor, diminished arterial pulsations, tissue swelling
  Review DD Circulation—consider Tissue perfusion
Change in usual response to stimuli, abnormal sensitivity to touch, physiological anxiety, irritability
  Review DD Neurosensory—consider Sensory deficit
Situational crisis, chronic disability, debilitating pain
  Review DD Roles/Relationships—consider Role performance
Temporary family disorganization or role changes, prolonged disability that exhausts the supportive capacity of SO(s)
  Review DD Roles/Relationships—consider Coping, family

Concussion, brain CH
Reports of headache, guarding or distraction behaviors, narrow focus
  Review DD Comfort—consider Pain
Vomiting, decreased intake, hypermetabolic state (fever), poor skin turgor, dry mucous membranes, concentrated urine
  Review DD Food/Fluid—consider Fluid volume
Traumatic brain injury, difficulty recalling events/information, decreased motivation, decreased socialization
  Review DD Neurosensory—consider Memory
Questions, statements of concern, development of preventable complications
  Review DD Health Management—consider Health knowledge

Conduct disorder (childhood, adolescence) PSY/PED
Delayed ego development, antisocial character, poor impulse control, dysfunctional family system, loss of significant relationships, history of suicidal or acting-out behaviors
  Review DD Stress Management—consider Nonsuicidal behavior
  Review DD Stress Management—consider Violence
Inappropriate use of defense mechanisms, inability to meet role expectations, poor self-esteem, failure to assume responsibility for own actions, hypersensitivity to criticism; excessive smoking, drinking, or drug use
  Review DD Stress Management—consider Coping
Dangerous behavior, temper outbursts, irritable mood, deficits in problem-solving skills, physical aggression as the solution to problems
  Review DD Self-Perception/Concept—consider Impulse control
Self-negating verbalizations, anger, rejection of positive feedback, frequent lack of success in life events
  Review DD Self-Perception/Concept—consider Self-esteem

Health Conditions and Client Concerns

Unrealistic parental expectations, rejection or overprotection of child; exaggerated expressions of anger, disappointment, or despair regarding child's behavior or ability to improve or change
  Review DD Roles/Relationships—consider Coping, family
Dysfunctional interaction with others (difficulty waiting turn in games or group situations, not seeming to listen to what is being said), difficulty playing quietly and maintaining attention to task or play activity, shifting from one activity to another and interrupting or intruding on others
  Review DD Roles/Relationships—consider Social connectedness

Congestive heart failure   MS
Refer to Heart failure, chronic

Conn syndrome   MS/CH
Refer to Aldosteronism, primary

Constipation   CH
Change in character and frequency of stools, feeling of abdominal or rectal fullness or pressure, changes in bowel sounds, abdominal distention
  Review DD Elimination—consider Elimination, intestinal
Verbal report, reluctance to defecate, distraction behaviors
  Review DD Comfort—consider Pain
Development of preventable problems, verbalization of concerns, questions
  Review DD Health Management—consider Health knowledge

Coronary artery bypass surgery   MS
Decreased myocardial contractility, diminished circulating volume (preload), alterations in electrical conduction, increased systemic vascular resistance (afterload)
  Review DD Circulation—consider Cardiac output
Verbal reports, changes in vital signs, distraction behaviors, restlessness, irritability
  Review DD Comfort—consider Pain

CH
Delay or alteration in physical capacity to resume role, change in usual role or responsibility, change in self/other's perception of role
  Review DD Roles/Relationships—consider Role performance

Coronary artery disease   CH/MS
Exertional discomfort, pain, fatigue, abnormal heart rate response, ECG changes (dysrhythmias)
  Review DD Activity/Rest—consider Activity intolerance
Altered heart rate or rhythm, altered contractility, increased peripheral vascular resistance, dizziness, weakness, pallor
  Review DD Circulation—consider Cardiac output

Craniotomy   MS
Also refer to Surgery, general

Increased intracranial pressure due to brain injury, surgical procedure; change in mentation, pupillary changes
  Review DD Circulation—consider Tissue perfusion
Disorientation to time, place, person; motor incoordination; altered communication patterns; restlessness; irritability; change in behavior pattern
  Review DD Neurosensory—consider Confusion
Traumatized tissues, break in skin integrity, invasive procedures, nutritional deficits, altered integrity of closed system (cerebrospinal fluid leak)
  Review DD Safety—consider Infection

Crohn disease CH/MS
Also refer to Colitis, ulcerative
Weight loss, decreased subcutaneous fat or muscle mass, poor muscle tone, aversion to eating, observed lack of intake
  Review DD Food/Fluid—consider Nutritional intake
Hyperactive bowel sounds, increased peristalsis, cramping, frequent loose liquid stools
  Review DD Elimination—consider Elimination, intestinal
Statements of concern, questions, inaccurate follow-through of instructions, development of preventable complications or exacerbation
  Review DD Health Management—consider Health knowledge

Croup PED/CH
Harsh, brassy cough; tachypnea; use of accessory muscles; presence of wheezes
  Review DD Respiration—consider Airway clearance
Threat to well-being, difficulty breathing, transmitted fears from others, restlessness, crying, tension, irritable mood, change in vital signs
  Review DD Stress Management—consider Anxiety
  Review DD Stress Management—consider Fear
Dry mucous membranes, poor skin turgor, scant/concentrated urine
  Review DD Food/Fluid—consider Fluid volume

Croup, membranous PED/CH
Also refer to Croup
Inflammation of larynx with formation of false membrane
  Review DD Safety—consider Suffocation

C-section OB
Refer to Cesarean birth, unplanned

Cubital tunnel syndrome CH
Verbal reports, reluctance to use affected extremity, guarding behaviors, expressed fear of reinjury, altered ability to continue previous activities
  Review DD Comfort—consider Pain
Decreased pinch or grasp strength, hand fatigue, reluctance to attempt movement
  Review DD Activity/Rest—consider Mobility

Mechanical compression (brace, repetitive tasks/motions), immobilization
  Review DD Neurosensory—consider Neurovascular function

Cushing syndrome CH
Compromised regulatory mechanism (fluid and sodium retention) leading to edema, weight gain
  Review DD Food/Fluid—consider Fluid volume
Immunosuppressed inflammatory response, skin and capillary fragility, negative nitrogen balance
  Review DD Safety—consider Infection
Decreased muscle mass, increased resistance to insulin
  Review DD Food/Fluid—consider Nutritional intake
Statements of or observed inability to complete or perform activities of daily living
  Review DD Self-Care—consider Self-care
Negative feelings about body, feelings of hopelessness, changes in social involvement
  Review DD Self-Perception/Concept—consider Body image
Verbalization of concerns or dissatisfaction/alteration in relationship with SO
  Review DD Sexuality/Reproduction—consider Sexual functioning
Increased protein breakdown, negative protein balance, demineralization of bone
  Review DD Safety—consider Injury

CVA MS/CH
Refer to Cerebrovascular accident

Cystic fibrosis CH/PED
Abnormal breath sounds, ineffective cough, cyanosis, altered respiratory rate/depth
  Review DD Respiration—consider Airway clearance
Stasis of respiratory secretions and development of atelectasis
  Review DD Safety—consider Infection
Weight loss, underweight, muscle wasting, delayed physical growth
  Review DD Food/Fluid—consider Nutritional intake
Statements of concern, questions, inaccurate follow-through of instructions, development of preventable complications
  Review DD Health Management—consider Health knowledge
SO attempting assistive or supportive behaviors with unsatisfactory results, protective behavior disproportionate to client's abilities or need for autonomy
  Review DD Roles/Relationships—consider Coping, family

Cystitis CH
Verbal reports, distraction behaviors, narrow focus
  Review DD Comfort—consider Pain
Inflammation or irritation of bladder; urinary frequency, nocturia, dysuria
  Review DD Elimination—consider Elimination, urinary

Statements of concern, questions, inaccurate follow-through of instructions, development of preventable complications, recurrent infections
   Review DD Health Management—consider Health knowledge

Cytomegalic inclusion disease   CH
Refer to Cytomegalovirus (CMV) infection

Cytomegalovirus (CMV) infection   CH
Transplacental exposure, contact with blood or body fluids
   Review DD Safety—consider Infection, [fetal]
Inflammation of retina
   Review DD Neurosensory—consider Sensory deficit

Deep vein thrombosis   CH/MS
Refer to Thrombophlebitis

Degenerative disc disease   CH/MS
Refer to Herniated nucleus pulposus

Degenerative joint disease   CH
Refer to Arthritis, rheumatoid

Dehiscence, abdominal wound   MS
Poor or delayed wound healing, disruption of skin surface or wound closure; exposure of abdominal contents to external environment
   Review DD Safety—consider Skin/Tissue integrity
Inadequate primary defenses (separation of incision, traumatized intestines, environmental exposure)
   Review DD Safety—consider Infection
Perceived threat of death, fearfulness, restlessness, sympathetic stimulation
   Review DD Stress Management—consider Fear
   Review DD Stress Management—consider Anxiety
Statements of concern, questions, inaccurate follow-through of instructions, development of preventable complications
   Review DD Health Management—consider Health knowledge

Dehydration   PED/CH
Dry mucous membranes, poor skin turgor, decreased pulse volume and pressure, thirst
   Review DD Health Management—consider Fluid volume
Statements of concern, questions, inaccurate follow-through of instructions, development of preventable complications
   Review DD Health Management—consider Health knowledge

Delirium tremens   MS/PSY
Also refer to Alcohol intoxication, acute
Increased tension; apprehension; feelings of inadequacy, shame, self-disgust, remorse; fear of unspecific consequences; identifies object of fear
   Review DD Stress Management—consider Anxiety
   Review DD Stress Management—consider Fear

Disorientation, restlessness, irritability, exaggerated emotional responses, bizarre thinking, visual or auditory distortions or hallucinations
  Review DD Neurosensory—consider Sensory deficit
Direct effect of alcohol on cardiac muscle, altered systemic vascular resistance, dysrhythmias
  Review DD Circulation—consider Cardiac output
Alterations in balance, reduced muscle coordination, cognitive impairments, involuntary clonic/tonic muscle activity
  Review DD Safety—consider Injury
  Review DD Safety—consider Violence
Reports of inadequate food intake, altered taste sensation, lack of interest in food; debilitated state, decreased subcutaneous fat or muscle mass, signs of mineral or electrolyte imbalance, abnormal laboratory findings
  Review DD Food/Fluid—consider Nutritional

Delivery, precipitous/out of hospital   OB
Also refer to Labor, precipitous; Labor stages
Nausea, vomiting, lack of intake
  Review DD Food/Fluid—consider Fluid volume
Excessive blood loss
  Review DD Circulation—consider Bleeding
Broken or traumatized tissue, increased environmental exposure, rupture of amniotic membranes
  Review DD Safety—consider Infection
Rapid descent, pressure changes, compromised circulation, environmental exposure
  Review DD Safety—consider Injury, [fetal]

Delusional disorder   PSY
Perceived threats of danger, increased feelings of anxiety, acting out in an irrational manner
  Review DD Safety—consider Nonsuicidal behavior
  Review DD Safety—consider Violence
Inability to trust, rigid delusional system, fear of other people and own hostility
  Review DD Stress Management—consider Anxiety
Difficulty managing complex treatment regimen or accessing healthcare system, failure to include treatment plan in daily living, ineffective choices for meeting health goals
  Review DD Health Management—consider Health self-management
Verbal expressions of no control or influence over situation, use of paranoid delusions, aggressive behavior to compensate for lack of control
  Review DD Self-Perception/Concept—consider Resilience
Interference with ability to think clearly and logically, fragmentation and autistic thinking, delusions, beliefs and behaviors of suspicion/violence
  Review DD Neurosensory—consider Thought process

Discomfort in social situations, difficulty in establishing relationships with others, expression of feelings of rejection, no sense of belonging
Review DD Roles/Relationships—consider Social connectedness

Dementia, HIV CH/PSY
Also refer to Dementia, presenile/senile
Fluctuation of cognition, progressive cognitive impairment, increased agitation, restlessness, altered interpretation or response to stimuli, clinical evidence of organic impairment
Review DD Neurosensory—consider Confusion

Reports of feeling scared, shaky, increased tension, loss of control, apprehension, extraneous movements, tremors, increased somatic complaints
Review DD Stress Management—consider Anxiety

Intolerance, rejection, abandonment, neglectful relationships with other family members, SO preoccupied with personal reaction, distortion of reality of health problem
Review DD Roles/Relationships—consider Coping, family

Dementia, presenile/senile CH/PSY
Also refer to Alzheimer disease
Observed experiences of forgetting, inability to determine if a behavior was performed, inability to perform previously learned skills, inability to recall factual information or recent/past events
Review DD Neurosensory—consider Memory

Social isolation, apprehension, irritability, defensiveness, suspiciousness, aggressive behavior
Expressions of distress, anger at potential loss, choked feelings, crying; alteration in activity level, communication patterns, eating habits, sleep patterns
Review DD Stress Management—consider Anxiety
Review DD Stress Management—consider Fear
Review DD Stress Management—consider Grief

Impaired ability to perform activities of daily living
Review DD Self-Care—consider Self-care deficit

Impaired muscle coordination and balance, confusion, impaired judgment, psychomotor agitation, seizure activity
Review DD Safety—consider Injury
Review DD Safety—consider Nonsuicidal behavior
Review DD Safety—consider Violence

Illness severity of care receiver, duration of caregiving required, complexity or amount of caregiving tasks, care receiver exhibiting deviant or bizarre behavior, family/caregiver isolation, lack of respite or recreation, spouse is caregiver
Review DD Roles/Relationships—consider Caregiving burden

Depressant abuse CH/PSY
Also refer to Drug overdose, acute (depressants)
Inability to admit impact of condition on life, minimizes symptoms or problem, refuses healthcare attention, abuse of chemical

substances, lack of goal-directed behavior, inadequate problem-solving, destructive behavior toward self
  Review DD Stress Management—consider Coping
Weight loss, pale conjunctiva or mucous membranes, pallor, anemia, electrolyte imbalances
  Review DD Food/Fluid—consider Nutritional intake
Changes in sleep patterns, decreased concentration, loss of inhibitions
  Review DD Safety—consider Injury

Depression, major   PSY/CH

Depressed mood, feelings of worthlessness and hopelessness; risk for injury due to effects of electroconvulsive therapy
  Review DD Safety—consider Injury
  Review DD Safety—consider Nonsuicidal behavior
  Review DD Safety—consider Suicide
Reports of nervousness or fearfulness; feelings of inadequacy; agitation, angry or tearful outbursts, rambling, discoordinated speech; restlessness, poor memory or concentration, decreased ability to grasp ideas, inability to make decisions, ideas of reference, hallucinations, delusions
  Review DD Stress Management—consider Anxiety
  Review DD Stress Management—consider Fear
Difficulty falling or remaining asleep, early morning awakening or waking later than desired, reports of not feeling rested, physical signs (dark circles under eyes, excessive yawning), hypersomnia (using sleep as an escape)
  Review DD Activity/Rest—consider Sleep pattern
Discomfort in social situations, withdrawal from usual activities, dysfunctional interactions with others, sad/flat affect, remaining home or in bed
  Review DD Roles/Relationships—consider Social connectedness
Statements of difficulty coping with situation, family system not meeting needs of its members, difficulty accepting or receiving help appropriately, ineffective family decision-making process, failure to send or receive clear messages
  Review DD Roles/Relationships—consider Family process
Poor memory or concentration, decreased ability to grasp ideas, inability to make decisions, numerous or repetitious physical complaints without organic cause, ideas of reference, hallucinations, delusions
  Review DD Neurosensory—consider Thought process

Depression, postpartum   OB/PSY
Also refer to Depressive disorders
Anxiety associated with parental role, inability to meet personal needs, perceived guilt regarding relationship with infant
  Review DD Roles/Relationships—consider Caregiver child attachment
Stressors, sleep deprivation, depression, insufficient energy, inability to maintain usual routines, increase in physical symptoms
  Review DD Activity/Rest—consider Fatigue

Developmental transition, change in body image, self-negating statements, perceived inability to cope with situation, sense of helplessness
  Review DD Self-Perception/Concept—consider Self-esteem
Hopelessness, increased anxiety, mood swings, despondency, severe depression, psychosis
  Review DD Safety—consider Violence

Dermatitis, contact CH
Verbal reports, irritability, scratching
  Review DD Comfort—consider Pain
  Review DD Comfort—consider Discomfort
Inflammation, epidermal edema, development of vesicles or bullae
  Review DD Safety—consider Skin integrity
Broken skin and tissue trauma
  Review DD Roles/Relationships—consider Infection
Alterations in physical appearance, expressed feelings of rejection, deceased interaction with peers
  Review DD Roles/Relationships—consider Social connectedness

Diabetes, gestational OB
Also refer to Diabetes mellitus
Pregnancy, dietary intake, lack of diabetes management, inadequate blood glucose monitoring
  Review DD Food/Fluid—consider Blood glucose
Impaired glucose metabolism, compromised oxygen transport due to changes in circulation, treatment-related side effects
  Review DD Sexuality/Reproduction—consider Maternal-fetal dyad
Questions, statements of misconception, inaccurate follow-through of instructions, development of preventable complications
  Review DD Health Management—consider Health knowledge

Diabetes insipidus MS/CH
Urinary frequency, thirst, polydipsia, dilute urine, dry skin and mucous membranes, decreased skin turgor, nocturia, increased serum sodium
  Review DD Food/Fluid—consider Fluid volume
Complexity of medication regimen, presence of side effects, economic difficulties, inadequate knowledge, perceived seriousness and benefits
  Review DD Health Management—consider Health self-management

Diabetes, juvenile (Type 1) PED
Also refer to Diabetes mellitus
Failure to take actions that prevent health problems, minimizes health status change, failure to achieve optimal sense of control
  Review DD Health Management—consider Health maintenance
Ineffective control of serum glucose level, changes in mentation, developmental age, risk-taking behaviors
  Review DD Safety—consider Injury

Use of maladaptive coping strategies, inadequate problem-solving, risk-taking/destructive behaviors toward self
  Review DD Stress Management—consider Coping
Family expression of confusion about plan of care, verbalization of difficulty coping with situation, family not meeting physical and emotional needs of its members, feelings of guilt/fear by SO, display of protective behaviors disproportionate to client's abilities or need for autonomy
  Review DD Roles/Relationships—consider Coping, family

Diabetes mellitus CH/PED
Requests for information, statements of concern, misconceptions, inadequate follow-through of instructions, development of preventable complications
  Review DD Health Management—consider Health knowledge
Complexity and duration of treatment, perceived excessive demands on individual, powerlessness, perceived susceptibility to complications
  Review DD Health Management—consider Health self-management
Lack of adherence to diabetes management, medication management; inadequate blood glucose monitoring, physical activity; multiple stressors, rapid growth periods
  Review DD Food/Fluid—consider Blood glucose
Decreased leukocyte function, circulatory changes, delayed healing
  Review DD Safety—consider Infection
Glucose, insulin, and electrolyte imbalances; development of retinopathy/neuropathy
  Review DD Neurosensory—consider Sensory deficit

Diabetic ketoacidosis CH/MS
Increased urinary output, dilute urine, reports of weakness, thirst, nausea/vomiting, sudden weight loss, hypotension, tachycardia, delayed capillary refill, dry mucous membranes, poor skin turgor
  Review DD Food/Fluid—consider Fluid volume
Elevated serum glucose levels, presence of ketones in urine, nausea, weight loss, blurred vision, irritability
  Review DD Food/Fluid—consider Blood glucose
Endocrine regulatory dysfunction, altered fluid intake, vomiting, polyuria
  Review DD Food/Fluid—consider Water-electrolyte
Overwhelming lack of energy, inability to maintain usual routines, decreased performance, impaired ability to concentrate, listlessness
  Review DD Activity/Rest—consider Fatigue
High serum glucose levels, decreased leukocyte function, stasis of body fluids, invasive procedures, alteration in circulation and perfusion
  Review DD Safety—consider Infection

Dialysis, general CH
Also refer to Dialysis, peritoneal; Hemodialysis

Reported inadequate intake, aversion to eating, altered taste sensation, poor muscle tone, weakness, sore and inflamed oral mucosa, pale conjunctiva and mucous membranes
Review DD Food/Fluid—consider Nutritional intake

Verbal expression of distress or unresolved issues, denial of loss; altered eating habits, sleep and dream patterns, activity levels, libido; crying, labile affect; feelings of sorrow, guilt, anger
Review DD Stress Management—consider Grief

Verbalization of changes in lifestyle, focus on past function, negative feelings about body, feelings of helplessness or powerlessness, extension of body boundary to incorporate environmental objects (dialysis setup), change in social interaction, overdependence on others for care, not taking responsibility for self-care, lack of follow-through, self-destructive behaviors
Review DD Self-Perception/Concept—consider Body image

Inability to perform activities of daily living, disheveled, unkempt appearance, strong body odor
Review DD Self-Care—consider Self-care

Verbal expression of having no control, depression over physical deterioration, nonparticipation in care, anger, passivity
Review DD Self-Perception/Concept—consider Resilience

Expressions of concern or reports about response of SO to patient's health problem, preoccupation of SO with own personal reactions, display of intolerance or rejection, protective behaviors disproportionate to client's abilities or need for autonomy
Review DD Roles/Relationships—consider Coping, family

Dialysis, peritoneal MS/CH

Also refer to Dialysis, general

Inadequate osmotic gradient of dialysate, fluid retention due to malpositioned/kinked/clotted PD catheter, bowel distention, peritonitis, scarring of peritoneum, excessive PO/IV intake
Review DD Food/Fluid—consider Fluid volume

Improper placement of PD catheter, catheter manipulation during insertion
Review DD Safety—consider Injury

Contamination of catheter or infusion system, skin contaminants, signs of peritonitis (rigid/painful abdomen, cloudy effluent, hyperthermia, leukocytosis)
Review DD Safety—consider Infection

Verbal reports, guarding or distraction behaviors, self-focus
Review DD Comfort—consider Pain
Review DD Comfort—consider Discomfort

Increased abdominal pressure restricting diaphragmatic movement, rapid infusion of dialysate, pain or discomfort, inflammatory process (atelectasis or pneumonia)
Review DD Respiration—consider Breathing pattern

Diaper rash PED
Refer to Candidiasis

Diarrhea PED/CH
Statements of concern, questions, development of preventable complications
   Review DD Health Management—consider Health knowledge

Losses through gastrointestinal tract, altered intake, poor skin turgor, dry mucous membranes
   Review DD Food/Fluid—consider Fluid volume

Verbal reports, facial grimacing, abdominal guarding, autonomic responses
   Review DD Comfort—consider Pain

Reports of discomfort, disruption of skin surface, destruction of skin layers
   Review DD Safety—consider Skin integrity

Digitalis toxicity MS/CH
Changes in cardiac rate, rhythm, and conduction; dysrhythmias; changes in mentation; worsening of heart failure; elevated serum drug levels
   Review DD Circulation—consider Cardiac output

Excess fluid loss through vomiting or diarrhea, decreased fluid intake, nausea, decreased plasma proteins, malnutrition, continued use of diuretics, excess sodium and fluid retention
   Review DD Food/Fluid—consider Fluid volume

Inaccurate follow-through of instructions, statements of concern, misconceptions, questions, development of complication (toxicity)
   Review DD Health Management—consider Health knowledge

Physiological effects of toxicity, reduced cerebral perfusion—confusion, decreased consciousness
   Review DD Neurosensory—consider Thought process

Dilation and curettage OB/GYN
Also refer to Abortion, elective or spontaneous termination

Requests for information and statements of concern, misconceptions
   Review DD Health Management—consider Health knowledge

Dilation of cervix, premature OB
Also refer to Preterm labor

Increased tension, apprehension, feelings of inadequacy, sympathetic stimulation, repetitive questioning
   Review DD Stress Management—consider Anxiety

Surgical intervention, use of tocolytic drugs
   Review DD Sexuality/Reproduction—consider Maternal-fetal dyad

Perceived potential fetal loss, expressions of distress, anger, guilt, choked feelings
   Review DD Stress Management—consider Grief

Dislocation/subluxation of joint CH
Verbal or coded reports, guarded or protective behaviors, narrow focus, autonomic responses
   Review DD Comfort—consider Pain

Nerve impingement, improper fitting of splint device
   Review DD Safety—consider Injury

Limited range of motion, limited ability to perform motor skills, gait changes
Review DD Activity/Rest—consider Mobility

Disruptive behavior disorder   PED/PSY
Refer to Oppositional defiant disorder

Disseminated intravascular coagulation (DIC)   MS
Failure of regulatory mechanism (coagulation process), hemorrhage
Review DD Circulation—consider Shock
Changes in respiratory rate and depth, changes in mentation, decreased urinary output, development of acral cyanosis and focal gangrene
Review DD Circulation—consider Tissue perfusion
Sympathetic stimulation, restlessness, focus on self, apprehension
Review DD Stress Management—consider Anxiety
Review DD Stress Management—consider Fear
Reduced oxygen-carrying capacity, development of acidosis, fibrin deposits in microcirculation, ischemic damage of lung parenchyma
Review DD Respiration—consider Gas exchange
Verbal reports, narrow focus, alteration in muscle tone, guarding or distraction behaviors, restlessness, autonomic responses
Review DD Comfort—consider Pain

Dissociative disorders   PSY
Maladaptive response to stress (dissociation, fragmentation of the personality), increased tension, feelings of inadequacy, focus on self, projection of personal perceptions onto the environment
Review DD Stress Management—consider Anxiety
Review DD Stress Management—consider Fear
Dissociative state, conflicting personalities, depressed mood, panic states, suicidal or homicidal behaviors
Review DD Safety—consider Nonsuicidal behavior
Review DD Safety—consider Violence
Review DD Safety—consider Suicide
Alteration in perception or experience of the self, loss of one's own sense of reality and the external world, poorly differentiated ego boundaries; confusion about sense of self, purpose, or direction in life; memory loss, presence of more than one personality within the individual
Review DD Self-Perception/Concept—consider Personal identity
Family/SO describing inadequate understanding or knowledge that interferes with assistive or supportive behaviors, relationships and marital conflict
Review DD Roles/Relationships—consider Coping, family

Diverticulitis   CH
Verbal reports, guarding or distraction behaviors, autonomic responses, narrow focus
Review DD Comfort—consider Pain
Increase or decrease in frequency of stools, change in stool consistency and appearance
Review DD Elimination—consider Elimination, intestinal

Statements of concern, request for information, development of preventable complications
 Review DD Health Management—consider Health knowledge
Chronic nature of disease process, recurrent episodes despite cooperation with medical regimen
 Review DD Self-Perception/Concept—consider Resilience

Down syndrome PED/CH
Also refer to Mental delay
Delay or inability to perform skills/activities and self-care appropriate for age
 Review DD Health Management—consider Development, child
 Review DD Health Management—consider Motor development, infant
Cognitive difficulties, poor muscle tone and coordination, weakness
 Review DD Safety—consider Injury
Weak and ineffective sucking or swallowing, observed lack of adequate intake, weight loss, failure to gain
 Review DD Food/Fluid—consider Nutritional intake
Confusion about plan of care, verbalized difficulty coping with situation
 Review DD Roles/Relationships—consider Family process
Infant/child unable to effectively initiate parental contact due to altered behavioral organization, inability of parents to meet the personal needs of the child
 Review DD Roles/Relationships—consider Caregiver child attachment
Withdrawal from usual interactions and activities, assumption of total child care, becoming overindulgent or overprotective
 Review DD Roles/Relationships—consider Social connectedness
Loss of "perfect child," chronic condition requiring long term care, unresolved feelings
 Review DD Stress Management—consider Grief

Drug overdose, acute (depressants) MS/PSY
Also refer to Substance dependence/abuse rehabilitation
Changes in respiratory rate and depth, cyanosis, abnormal arterial blood gases, hypoxia
 Review DD Respiration—consider Breathing pattern
 Review DD Respiration—consider Gas exchange
Central nervous system depression, agitation, hypersensitivity to the drug(s), psychological stress, seizures
 Review DD Safety—consider Injury
 Review DD Safety—consider Suffocation
 Review DD Safety—consider Poisoning
Suicidal behaviors, toxic reactions to drug(s)/unintentional overdose
 Review DD Safety—consider Nonsuicidal behavior
 Review DD Safety—consider Suicide
 Review DD Safety—consider Violence
Nonsterile drug injection techniques, impurities in injected drugs, localized tissue trauma, malnutrition, altered immune state
 Review DD Safety—consider Infection

Drug withdrawal CH/MS
Inaccurate interpretation of environment, inappropriate or nonreality-based thinking, paranoia
  Review DD Neurosensory—consider Thought process
Central nervous system agitation (withdrawal from depressant use)
  Review DD Safety—consider Injury
Alcohol or substance abuse, legal or disciplinary problems, depressed mood (stimulants)
  Review DD Safety—consider Suicide
Reports of muscle aches, fever, diaphoresis, rhinorrhea, lacrimation, malaise
  Review DD Comfort—consider Pain
  Review DD Comfort—consider Discomfort
Perceptual or cognitive impairment, therapeutic management (restraints), inability to meet own physical needs
  Review DD Self-Care—consider Self-care
Reports of insomnia or hypersomnia, decreased ability to function, increased irritability
  Review DD Activity/Rest—consider Sleep pattern
  Review DD Activity/Rest—consider Fatigue

Duchenne muscular dystrophy PED/CH
Refer to Muscular dystrophy (Duchenne)

DVT CH/MS
Refer to Thrombophlebitis

Dysmenorrhea GYN
Verbal reports, guarding or distraction behaviors, narrow focus, changes in vital signs
  Review DD Comfort—consider Pain
Presence of pain and secondary symptoms such as nausea, vomiting, syncope, chills; fatigue, depression
  Review DD Activity/Rest—consider Activity intolerance
Muscle tension, headaches, irritability, depression, verbalization of inability to cope, report of poor self-concept
  Review DD Stress Management—consider Coping

Dysrhythmia, cardiac CH/MS
Altered cardiac conduction, reduced myocardial contractility, abnormal ECG
  Review DD Circulation—consider Cardiac output
Multiple questions, misinterpretation of information, inaccurate statements regarding information, failure to improve on previous regimen, development of preventable complications
  Review DD Health Management—consider Health knowledge
Imbalance between myocardial oxygen supply and demand, cardiac depressant effects of certain drugs (beta-blockers, antidysrhythmics)
  Review DD Activity/Rest—consider Activity intolerance
Use of digitalis, lack of education regarding medication use, reduced vision, cognitive impairments
  Review DD Safety—consider Poisoning

Ebola MS
Also refer to Disseminated intravascular coagulation; Multiple organ dysfunction syndrome

Reports of headache, myalgia, abdominal or chest pain, sore throat, fever
    Review DD Comfort—consider Pain
    Review DD Comfort—consider Discomfort

Inflammatory process leads to increased body temperature, warm skin, headache
    Review DD Safety—consider Thermoregulation

Spread of infection or secondary infection risk based on mode of transmission, invasive monitoring and procedures, debilitated state, malnutrition, insufficient knowledge or resources to avoid exposure to pathogens
    Review DD Safety—consider Infection

Inadequate intake due to nausea, painful swallowing, abdominal pain; increased fluid loss (vomiting, diarrhea, hemorrhage, DIC); hypermetabolic state
    Review DD Food/Fluid—consider Fluid volume

Fluctuations in cognition, agitation, change in level of consciousness (stupor, coma)
    Review DD Neurosensory—consider Confusion

Eclampsia OB
Also refer to Hypertension, intrapartum

Expressed concerns, apprehension, increased tension, decreased self-assurance, difficulty concentrating
    Review DD Stress Management—consider Anxiety
    Review DD Stress Management—consider Fear

Tissue edema, hypoxia, tonic-clonic seizures, abnormal blood profile or clotting factors
    Review DD Safety—consider Injury, [maternal]

Prescribed bedrest, discomfort, difficulty turning, postural instability
    Review DD Activity/Rest—consider Mobility

Weakness, discomfort, physical restrictions
    Review DD Self-Care—consider Self-care

ECT PSY
Refer to Electroconvulsive therapy

Ectopic pregnancy (tubal) OB
Also refer to Abortion, spontaneous termination

Verbal reports, guarding or distraction behaviors, facial grimacing, diaphoresis, changes in vital signs
    Review DD Comfort—consider Pain

Pregnancy-related complications, decreased or restricted intake
    Review DD Food/Fluid—consider Fluid volume

Pregnancy-related complications, hemorrhagic loss
    Review DD Circulation—consider Bleeding

Increased tension, apprehension, sympathetic stimulation, restlessness, self-focus
    Review DD Stress Management—consider Anxiety
    Review DD Stress Management—consider Fear

Edema, pulmonary — MS
Dyspnea, presence of crackles, pulmonary congestion, restlessness, anxiety, increased central venous pressure and pulmonary pressure
  Review DD Food/Fluid—consider Fluid volume
Hypoxia, restlessness, confusion
  Review DD Respiration—consider Gas exchange
Apprehension, panic state, restlessness, self-focus
  Review DD Stress Management—consider Anxiety
  Review DD Stress Management—consider Fear

Electrical injury — MS
Also refer to Burns
Altered heart rate and rhythm (ventricular fibrillation, asystole)
  Review DD Circulation—consider Cardiac output
Reduction of venous or arterial blood flow (venous coagulation, muscle edema), increased tissue pressure (compartment syndrome)
  Review DD Circulation—consider Tissue perfusion
Damaged or destroyed tissue, necrosis
  Review DD Safety—consider Tissue integrity
Muscle paralysis (central nervous system damage), loss of large and small muscle coordination (seizures)
  Review DD Safety—consider Injury
  Review DD Safety—consider Suffocation

Electroconvulsive therapy (ECT) — PSY
Lack of relevant or multiple and divergent sources of information, mistrust of regimen or healthcare personnel, sense of powerlessness, support system deficit
  Review DD Values/Beliefs—consider Decision-making
Effects of therapy on cardiovascular, respiratory, musculoskeletal, and nervous system; pharmacologic effects of anesthesia
  Review DD Safety—consider Injury
Fluctuation in cognition, agitation
  Review DD Neurosensory—consider Confusion
Reported or observed experiences of forgetting, difficulty recalling recent events or factual information
  Review DD Neurosensory—consider Memory

Emphysema — CH/MS
Dyspnea, restlessness, changes in mentation, abnormal arterial blood gas values
  Review DD Respiration—consider Gas exchange
Abnormal breath sounds (rhonchi), ineffective cough, changes in respiratory rate or depth, dyspnea
  Review DD Respiration—consider Airway clearance
Fatigue, weakness, exertional dyspnea, abnormal vital sign response to activity
  Review DD Activity/Rest—consider Activity intolerance
Lack of interest in food, reported altered taste, loss of muscle mass and tone, fatigue, weight loss
  Review DD Food/Fluid—consider Nutritional intake

Inadequate primary defenses (stasis of body fluids, decreased ciliary action), chronic disease process, malnutrition
Review DD Safety—consider Infection

Verbal expression of having no control, depression over physical deterioration, nonparticipation in therapeutic regimen, anger, passivity
Review DD Self-Perception/Concept—consider Resilience

Encephalitis   MS

Cerebral edema altering cerebral arterial or venous blood flow, hypovolemia, cellular exchange problems (acidosis)
Review DD Circulation—consider Tissue perfusion

Increased body temperature, flushed/warm skin, increased pulse and respiratory rates
Review DD Safety—consider Thermoregulation

Restlessness, tonic-clonic activity, altered sensorium, cognitive impairment, generalized weakness, ataxia, vertigo
Review DD Safety—consider Injury
Review DD Safety—consider Suffocation

Verbal reports of headache, photophobia, distraction behaviors, restlessness, changes in vital signs
Review DD Comfort—consider Pain

Encopresis   PSY/PED

Involuntary passage of stool at least once monthly, strong odor of feces on client, hiding soiled clothing
Review DD Elimination—consider Continence, fecal

Anger, oppositional behavior, verbalization of powerlessness, reluctance to engage in social activities
Review DD Self-Perception/Concept—consider Body image

Attempts to intervene with child are increasingly ineffective, SO describes preoccupation with personal reaction (excessive guilt, anger, blame regarding child's condition or behavior), overprotective behavior
Review DD Roles/Relationships—consider Coping, family

Endocarditis   MS

Inflammation of lining of the heart and structural change in valve leaflets
Review DD Circulation—consider Cardiac output

Embolic or valvular vegetative interruption of atrial blood flow
Review DD Circulation—consider Tissue perfusion

Apprehension, expressed concerns, self-focus
Review DD Stress Management—consider Anxiety

Verbal reports, narrow focus, distraction behaviors, autonomic responses (changes in vital signs)
Review DD Comfort—consider Pain

Imbalance between oxygen supply and demand, debilitating condition, dyspnea/weakness with activity
Review DD Activity/Rest—consider Activity intolerance

Endometriosis GYN
Verbal reports of pain between and with menstruation, guarding or distraction behaviors, narrow focus
  Review DD Comfort—consider Pain
Presence of adhesions, verbalization of problem, altered relationship with partner
  Review DD Sexuality/Reproduction—consider Sexual functioning
Lack of information, misinterpretations, statements of concern, misconceptions
  Review DD Health Management—consider Health knowledge

Enteral feeding MS/CH
Body weight 10% or more under ideal, decreased subcutaneous fat or muscle mass, poor muscle tone, changes in gastric motility and stool characteristics
  Review DD Food/Fluid—consider Nutritional intake
Active loss or failure of regulatory mechanisms, inability to obtain or ingest fluids
  Review DD Food/Fluid—consider Fluid volume
Invasive procedure, surgical placement of feeding tube, malnutrition, chronic disease
  Review DD Safety—consider Infection
Presence of feeding tube, bolus tube feedings, increased intragastric pressure, delayed gastric emptying, medication administration
  Review DD Safety—consider Aspiration
Overwhelming lack of energy, inability to maintain usual routines/tasks, lethargy, impaired ability to concentrate
  Review DD Activity/Rest—consider Fatigue

Enteritis MS/CH
Refer to Colitis, ulcerative; Crohn disease

Enuresis PSY/PED
Nocturnal or diurnal enuresis, strong odor of urine on client, hiding soiled clothing
  Review DD Elimination—consider Elimination, urinary
Anger, oppositional behaviors, verbalization of powerlessness, reluctance to engage in social activities
  Review DD Self-Perception/Concept—consider Body image
Attempts to intervene with child are increasingly ineffective, SO describes preoccupation with personal reaction (guilt, anger, blame), overprotective behavior
  Review DD Roles/Relationships—consider Coping, family

Epilepsy CH
Refer to Seizure disorder

Erectile dysfunction CH/PSY
Reports of disruption of sexual response pattern, inability to achieve desired satisfaction
  Review DD Sexuality/Reproduction—consider Sexual functioning

Self-negating verbalizations, expressions of helplessness, powerlessness
   Review DD Self-Perception/Concept—consider Self-esteem

Failure to thrive, adult   CH/MS
Expressed lack of appetite, difficulty performing self-care activities, altered mood state, inadequate intake, weight loss, physical decline
   Review DD Food/Fluid—consider Nutritional intake
   Review DD Food/Fluid—consider Elder frailty syndrome
   Review DD Food/Fluid—consider Underweight self-management
Inadequate nutrition, anemia, extremes of age, fatigue, weakness, deficient immunity, impaired healing, pressure ulcers
   Review DD Self-Perception/Concept—consider Resilience

Failure to thrive, infant/child   PED
Lack of appropriate weight gain or weight loss, poor muscle tone, pale conjunctiva, laboratory results indicating nutritional deficiencies
   Review DD Food/Fluid—consider Nutritional intake
   Review DD Food/Fluid—consider Feeding behavior, infant
   Review DD Food/Fluid—consider Eating dynamics, child
Altered physical growth, flat affect, listlessness, decreased response, delay or difficulty in performing skills appropriate for age
   Review DD Health Management—consider Growth, child
   Review DD Health Management—consider Development, child
Verbalization of concerns, questions, misconceptions, development of preventable complications
   Review DD Health Management—consider Health knowledge
Lack of knowledge, inadequate bonding, unrealistic expectations for self/infant, lack of appropriate response of child to relationship
   Review DD Roles/Relationships—consider Parenting

Fatigue syndrome, chronic   CH
Verbalization of unremitting or overwhelming lack of energy, inability to maintain usual routines, listlessness, compromised concentration
   Review DD Activity/Rest—consider Fatigue
Verbal reports of headache, sore throat, arthralgia, abdominal pain, muscle aches, altered ability to continue previous activities, changes in sleep pattern
   Review DD Comfort—consider Pain
Reports of inability to perform desired activities of daily living
   Review DD Self-Care—consider Self-care
Health alterations, stress, difficulty performing usual activities
   Review DD Roles/Relationships—consider Role performance

Femoral popliteal bypass   MS
Also refer to Surgery, general
Interruption in arterial blood flow, hypovolemia
   Review DD Circulation—consider Tissue perfusion
Vascular obstruction, immobilization, mechanical compression, dressings
   Review DD Neurovascular—consider Neurovascular function

Inability to walk desired distance, climb stairs, negotiate inclines
  Review DD Activity/Rest—consider Walking

Fetal alcohol syndrome   PED
External chemical factors (alcohol intake by mother), placental insufficiency, fetal drug withdrawal in utero or postpartum, prematurity
  Review DD Neurosensory—consider Neurodevelopmental organization
Change from baseline physiological measures, tremors, startles, twitches, hyperextension of arms and legs, deficient self-regulatory behaviors, deficient response to visual or auditory stimuli
  Review DD Activity/Rest—consider Motor development
Mental or physical illness, inability of mother to assume the task of unselfish giving and nurturing, presence of stressors (legal, financial), lack of available or ineffective role models, interruption of bonding process, lack of appropriate response of child to relationship
  Review DD Roles/Relationships—consider Parenting

PSY

Inability to meet basic needs, fulfill role expectations, problem solve; excessive use of drug(s)
  Review DD Stress Management—consider Coping, [maternal]
Abandonment, rejection, neglectful relationships with family members, detrimental decisions and actions by family
  Review DD Roles/Relationships—consider Family process
  Review DD Roles/Relationships—consider Family identity syndrome

Fetal demise   OB
Also refer to Perinatal loss/death of child
Death of fetus, altered delivery process
  Review DD Sexuality/Reproduction—consider Childbearing process
Expresses distress, anger; crying, change in eating habits, sleep pattern
  Review DD Stress Management—consider Grief

Fibromyalgia syndrome, primary   CH
Reports of achy pain in fibrous tissues (muscles, tendons, ligaments), muscle stiffness and spasms, disturbed sleep, guarding behaviors, fear of injury or exacerbation, restlessness, irritability, self-focus, reduced interaction with others
  Review DD Comfort—consider Pain
Verbalization of overwhelming lack of energy, inability to maintain usual routines or level of physical activity, tiredness, feelings of guilt for not keeping up with responsibilities, increase in physical complaints, listlessness
  Review DD Activity/Rest—consider Fatigue
Chronic debilitating physical condition, prolonged activity restriction, isolation, lack of specific therapeutic cure, prolonged stress
  Review DD Self-Perception/Concept—consider Resilience

Fractures MS/CH
Also refer to Casts; Traction

Loss of skeletal integrity, movement of skeletal fragments, use of traction apparatus
  Review DD Safety—consider Injury

Verbal reports, distraction behaviors, self-focus, narrow focus, facial grimacing, guarding or protective behaviors, alteration in muscle tone, changes in vital signs
  Review DD Comfort—consider Pain

Reduction or interruption of blood flow due to direct vascular injury, tissue trauma, excessive edema, thrombus formation, hypovolemia
  Review DD Neurosensory—consider Neurovascular function

Inability to purposefully move within physical environment, imposed restrictions, reluctance to attempt movement, limited range of motion, decreased muscle strength and control
  Review DD Activity/Rest—consider Mobility
  Review DD Activity/Rest—consider Transferring
  Review DD Activity/Rest—consider Standing

Statements of concern, questions, misconceptions
  Review DD Health Management—consider Health knowledge

Frostbite MS/CH

Altered circulation and thermal injury, damaged or destroyed tissue
  Review DD Safety—consider Tissue integrity

Traumatized tissue, tissue destruction, altered circulation, compromised immune system in affected area
  Review DD Safety—consider Infection

Verbal reports, guarding or distraction behaviors, narrow focus, changes in vital signs
  Review DD Comfort—consider Pain

Gallstones CH
Refer to Cholelithiasis

Gas, lung irritant MS/CH

Persistent cough, abnormal breath sounds (wheezes), dyspnea, tachypnea
  Review DD Respiration—consider Airway clearance

Irritation or inflammation of alveolar membrane, altered arterial blood gases, cyanosis
  Review DD Respiration—consider Gas exchange

Verbalizations, increased tension, apprehension, restlessness, sympathetic stimulation
  Review DD Stress Management—consider Anxiety

Gastritis, acute MS

Verbal reports of epigastric pain/indigestion, guarding or distraction behaviors, changes in vital signs
  Review DD Comfort—consider Pain

Excessive fluid loss through vomiting, diarrhea; reluctance to ingest fluid; restrictions of oral intake
  Review DD Food/Fluid—consider Fluid volume

Blood loss, inattention to early signs of complications
  Review DD Circulation—consider Bleeding

Gastritis, chronic CH
Inability to ingest adequate nutrients, nausea, vomiting, anorexia, epigastric pain
   Review DD Food/Fluid—consider Nutritional intake
Verbalization of concerns, questions, continuation of problems, development of preventable complications
   Review DD Health Management—consider Health knowledge

Gastroenteritis CH/MS
At least three liquid stools per day, hyperactive bowel sounds, abdominal pain
   Review DD Elimination—consider Elimination, intestinal
Excessive fluid loss through diarrhea, vomiting; hypermetabolic state (infection); decreased intake, nausea, vomiting; extremes of age or weight
   Review DD Food/Fluid—consider Fluid volume
Lack of knowledge to prevent contamination (inappropriate hand hygiene/food handling)
   Review DD Safety—consider Infection

Gastroesophageal reflux disease (GERD) CH
Reports of heartburn, distraction behaviors
   Review DD Comfort—consider Pain
Reports of heartburn or something "stuck" when swallowing, food refusal, nighttime coughing or awakening
   Review DD Food/Fluid—consider Swallowing
Limited intake, recurrent vomiting
   Review DD Food/Fluid—consider Nutritional intake
Nighttime heartburn, regurgitation of stomach contents upon lying down, interrupted sleep, not feeling well rested
   Review DD Activity/Rest—consider Sleep pattern
Incompetent lower esophageal sphincter, regurgitation of gastric acid
   Review DD Safety—consider Aspiration

Gender dysphoria PSY
Increased tension, helplessness, hopelessness, feelings of inadequacy, uncertainty, insomnia, self-focus, impaired daily functioning
   Review DD Stress Management—consider Anxiety
Confusion about sense of self, purpose, direction in life, sexual identity or preference, desire to be of the opposite sex, change in self-perception of role, conflict in roles
   Review DD Roles/Relationships—consider Role performance
   Review DD Roles/Relationships—consider Social identity, transgender
Inadequate or incorrect information or understanding, SO unable to perceive or to act effectively regarding client's needs, temporary family disorganization and role changes, client providing little support for primary person
   Review DD Roles/Relationships—consider Coping, family
Attempts to describe growth or impact of crisis on own values, priorities, goals, or relationships; moving toward health-promoting and enriching lifestyle; choosing experiences that optimize health
   Review DD Self-Perception/Concept—consider Self-concept

Health Conditions and Client Concerns

Verbalizations of discomfort with sexual orientation or role, lack of information about human sexuality
    Review DD Sexuality/Reproduction—consider Sexual functioning

Genetic disorder (fetal)   CH/OB

Increased tension, apprehension, uncertainty, feelings of inadequacy, expressed concerns
    Review DD Stress Management—consider Anxiety
Suffering, blame, despair, change in usual routines and activities of daily living
    Review DD Stress Management—consider Grief
Verbalization of concerns, statement of misconceptions, request for information
    Review DD Health Management—consider Health knowledge
Situational crisis, individual/family vulnerability, difficulty reaching agreement regarding options
    Review DD Roles/Relationships—consider Family process
Verbalization of inner conflict about beliefs, questioning of the moral and ethical implications of therapeutic choices, viewing situation as punishment, anger, hostility, crying
    Review DD Values/Beliefs—consider Spiritual well-being
    Review DD Values/Beliefs—consider Religiosity

Gigantism   CH
Refer to Acromegaly

Glaucoma   CH

Progressive loss of visual field
    Review DD Neurosensory—consider Sensory deficit
Apprehension, uncertainty, expressed concern regarding changes in life events
    Review DD Stress Management—consider Anxiety

Glomerulonephritis   PED

Weight gain, edema, anasarca, intake greater than output, blood pressure changes
    Review DD Food/Fluid—consider Fluid volume
Aversion to eating, reported alteration in taste, weight loss, decreased intake
    Review DD Food/Fluid—consider Nutritional intake
Verbal reports, guarding or distraction behaviors, changes in vital signs
    Review DD Comfort—consider Pain
Statements of boredom, restlessness, irritability
    Review DD Activity/Rest—consider Diversional activity
Renal damage with fluid retention, malnutrition, chronic illness
    Review DD Health Management—consider Growth, child

Goiter   CH

Verbalization of feelings, fear of rejection by others, actual change in structure, change in social involvement
    Review DD Self-Perception/Concept—consider Body image

Change in health status, progressive growth of mass, perceived threat of death
  Review DD Stress Management—consider Anxiety
Decreased ability to ingest or difficulty swallowing
  Review DD Food/Fluid—consider Nutritional intake
Tracheal compression or obstruction
  Review DD Respiration—consider Airway clearance

Gonorrhea CH
Also refer to Sexually transmitted infection
Presence of infectious process in highly vascular area, lack of recognition of disease process
  Review DD Safety—consider Infection
Verbal reports of genital or pharyngeal irritation, perineal or pelvic pain, guarding, distraction behaviors
  Review DD Comfort—consider Pain
Statements of concern, questions, misconceptions, inaccurate follow-through of instructions, development of preventable complications
  Review DD Health Management—consider Health knowledge

Gout CH
Verbal reports, guarding, distraction behaviors, changes in vital signs
  Review DD Comfort—consider Pain
Reluctance to attempt movement, limited range of motion, therapeutic restriction of movement
  Review DD Activity/Rest—consider Mobility
Statements of concern, questions, misconceptions, inaccurate follow-through of instructions, development of preventable complications
  Review DD Health Management—consider Health knowledge

Guillain-Barré syndrome (acute polyneuritis) MS
Reported or observed change in usual response to stimuli, altered communication patterns, change in sensory acuity and motor coordination
  Review DD Neurosensory—consider Sensory deficit
Impaired coordination, partial or complete paralysis, decreased muscle strength and control
  Review DD Activity/Rest—consider Mobility
Increased tension, apprehension, restlessness, helplessness uncertainty, fearfulness, self-focus, sympathetic stimulation
  Review DD Stress Management—consider Anxiety
  Review DD Stress Management—consider Fear
Weakness or paralysis of respiratory muscles, impaired gag or swallow reflexes, decreased energy, fatigue
  Review DD Respiration—consider Breathing pattern
Inability to perform usual activities of daily living
  Review DD Self-Care—consider Self-care

Gulf War syndrome CH/MS
Overwhelming lack of energy, inability to maintain usual routines or level of physical activity, lethargy, compromised concentration
  Review DD Activity/Rest—consider Fatigue

Expressed concerns, apprehension, uncertainty, fear of unspecific consequences, sleep disturbance, irritability, preoccupation
  Review DD Stress Management—consider Anxiety
  Review DD Stress Management—consider Fear
Reported or observed experiences of forgetting, inability to recall events
  Review DD Neurosensory—consider Memory
Blurred vision, photosensitivity
  Review DD Neurosensory—consider Sensory deficit
Verbal reports of muscle or joint pain, headaches, altered ability to continue previous activities, fatigue, reduced interaction with others
  Review DD Comfort—consider Pain
Exposure to toxins, liquid/loose stools, abdominal pain
  Review DD Elimination—consider Elimination, intestinal

Hallucinogen abuse   CH/PSY
Also refer to Substance dependence/abuse rehabilitation
Acute confusion, inaccurate interpretation of environment, bizarre thinking, disorientation, inability to make decisions, unpredictable behaviors, distractibility, nonreality-based thinking
  Review DD Neurosensory—consider Thought process
Assumptions of "losing mind/control," apprehension, preoccupation with feelings of impending doom, sympathetic stimulation
  Review DD Stress Management—consider Anxiety
  Review DD Stress Management—consider Fear
Inability to meet own physical needs
  Review DD Self-Care—consider Self-care

Hansen disease   CH
Symmetric skin lesions lighter than normal color, nodules, plaques, thickened dermis with loss of sensation, frequent involvement of nasal mucosa (nasal congestion, epistaxis)
  Review DD Safety—consider Skin/Tissue integrity
Inadequate primary and secondary defenses, insufficient knowledge to avoid exposure to/early treatment of infectious bacterial agent
  Review DD Safety—consider Infection
Muscle weakness, numbness, absence of sensation in hands, arms, legs, feet
  Review DD Activity/Rest—consider Mobility
Permanent nerve damage, change in body structure, missing body part, fear of reaction or rejection by others
  Review DD Self-Perception/Concept—consider Body image

Hantavirus pulmonary syndrome   MS
Also refer to Disseminated intravascular coagulation
Reports of headache, myalgia, gastrointestinal distress, fever
  Review DD Comfort—consider Pain
  Review DD Comfort—consider Discomfort
Dyspnea, restlessness, irritability, abnormal respiratory rate and depth, lethargy, confusion
  Review DD Respiration—consider Gas exchange

Respiratory muscle fatigue, impaired secretion management
  Review DD Respiration—consider Ventilation, spontaneous
Expressed concerns, distress, apprehension, extraneous movement
  Review DD Stress Management—consider Anxiety

Hay fever — CH
Inflammation/irritation of mucous membranes, conjunctiva; itching, verbalization of pain; irritability, restlessness
  Review DD Comfort—consider Discomfort
Statements of concern, questions, or misconceptions related to condition and management
  Review DD Health Management—consider Health knowledge

Heart failure, chronic — MS
Tachycardia, dysrhythmias, changes in blood pressure, extra heart sounds, decreased urine output, diminished peripheral pulses, cool and pale skin, orthopnea, crackles, dependent or generalized edema, chest pain
  Review DD Circulation—consider Cardiac output
Orthopnea, abnormal breath sounds, S_3 heart sound jugular vein distention, positive hepatojugular reflex, weight gain, hypertension, oliguria, generalized edema
  Review DD Food/Fluid—consider Fluid volume
Alveolar-capillary membrane changes (fluid collection or shifts into interstitial space and alveoli), dyspnea
  Review DD Respiration—consider Gas exchange

CH
Weakness, fatigue, changes in vital signs, dysrhythmias, dyspnea, pallor, diaphoresis
  Review DD Activity/Rest—consider Activity intolerance
Prolonged chair or bedrest, edema, vascular pooling, decreased tissue perfusion
  Review DD Safety—consider Skin integrity
Statements of concern, questions, or misconceptions; development of preventable complications or exacerbation of condition
  Review DD Health Management—consider Health knowledge

Heatstroke — MS
High body temperature (greater than 105°F [40.6°C]), flushed/hot skin, tachycardia, seizure activity
  Review DD Safety—consider Hyperthermia
Decreased peripheral pulses, dysrhythmias, tachycardia, changes in mentation
  Review DD Circulation—consider Cardiac output

Hematoma, epidural — MS
Fluctuation in cognition or level of consciousness
  Review DD Neurosensory—consider Confusion
Brain injuries, decreased cerebral perfusion pressure, systemic hypotension with intracranial hypertension
  Review DD Circulation—consider Tissue perfusion

Health Conditions and Client Concerns

Neuromuscular dysfunction (injury to respiratory center of brain), perception or cognitive impairment
  Review DD Respiration—consider Breathing pattern
Restricted oral intake, hypermetabolic state, loss of fluid through injuries
  Review DD Food/Fluid—consider Fluid volume

Hematoma, subdural-chronic   CH
Reports of increasing frequency, duration, or severity of headaches
  Review DD Comfort—consider Pain
Fluctuations in cognition, increased agitation, restlessness, misperceptions, inappropriate responses
  Review DD Neurosensory—consider Confusion
Limited ability to perform gross or fine motor skills, gait changes, postural instability
  Review DD Activity/Rest—consider Mobility

Hemodialysis   MS/CH
Also refer to Dialysis, general
Clotting, thrombosis, infection, disconnection, hemorrhage risks
  Review DD Safety—consider Injury
Chronic disease state, drug therapy, abnormal blood profile, inadequate nutrition, altered clotting, altered healing, fatigue, anorexia
  Review DD Safety—consider Immunologic impairment
Excessive fluid losses or shifts via ultrafiltration, fluid restrictions, altered coagulation, disconnection of shunt
  Review DD Food/Fluid—consider Fluid volume
Rapid or excessive fluid intake via IV, blood, plasma expanders, or saline given to support blood pressure during procedure
  Review DD Food/Fluid—consider Fluid volume

Hemophilia   PED
Impaired coagulation, inherent coagulopathies, trauma, hemorrhagic losses
  Review DD Circulation—consider Bleeding
Nerve compression from hematomas, nerve damage, hemorrhage into joint spaces
  Review DD Comfort—consider Pain
Joint hemorrhage, swelling, degenerative changes, muscle atrophy
  Review DD Activity/Rest—consider Mobility
Protective behaviors disproportionate to client's abilities or need for autonomy
  Review DD Roles/Relationships—consider Coping, family

Hemorrhage, postpartum   OB
Postpartum complications, disseminated intravascular coagulation leading to hypovolemia
  Review DD Circulation—consider Shock

Traumatized tissue, stasis of body fluids (lochia), decreased hemoglobin, invasive procedure
    Review DD Circulation—consider Infection

Increased tension, apprehension, feelings of inadequacy, helplessness, sympathetic stimulation
    Review DD Stress Management—consider Anxiety

Interruption in bonding process, physical condition, perceived threat to own survival
    Review DD Roles/Relationships—consider Caregiver child attachment

Hemorrhage, prenatal   OB

Hypovolemia due to ectopic or molar pregnancy, abruptio placentae
    Review DD Circulation—consider Shock

Compromised oxygen transport due to hypovolemia
    Review DD Sexuality/Reproduction—consider Maternal-fetal dyad

Verbalization of specific concerns, increased tension, sympathetic stimulation
    Review DD Stress Management—consider Fear

Verbal report of pain, distraction behaviors, change in blood pressure/pulse
    Review DD Comfort—consider Pain

Excessive or rapid replacement of fluid losses
    Review DD Food/Fluid—consider Fluid volume

Hemorrhoidectomy   MS/CH

Verbal reports, guarding or distraction behaviors, self-focus, changes in vital signs
    Review DD Comfort—consider Pain

Perineal trauma, edema, or swelling; pain
    Review DD Elimination—consider Elimination, urinary

Pain with defecation, reluctance to defecate, hard/formed stools
    Review DD Elimination—consider Elimination, intestinal

Lack of information, misconceptions, statements of concern and questions
    Review DD Health Management—consider Health knowledge

Hemothorax   MS

Also refer to Pneumothorax

Concurrent disease or injury process, dependence on external device (chest drainage system), lack of safety education or precautions
    Review DD Safety—consider Injury
    Review DD Safety—consider Suffocation

Increased tension, restlessness, expressed concern, sympathetic stimulation, self-focus
    Review DD Stress Management—consider Anxiety

Hepatitis, acute viral   MS/CH

Jaundice, hepatic enlargement, abdominal pain, elevation in serum liver function results
    Review DD Safety—consider Liver function

Inadequate secondary defenses, immunosuppression, malnutrition, insufficient knowledge to avoid exposure to pathogens or spread to others
  Review DD Safety—consider Infection
Bile salt accumulation in the tissues, pruritus
  Review DD Safety—consider Tissue integrity
Reports of lack of energy, inability to maintain usual routines, decreased performance, increased physical complaints
  Review DD Activity/Rest—consider Fatigue
Aversion to eating, lack of interest in food, altered taste sensation, observed lack of intake, weight loss
  Review DD Food/Fluid—consider Nutritional intake
Verbal reports, guarding or distraction behaviors, self-focus, changes in vital signs
  Review DD Comfort—consider Pain
  Review DD Comfort—consider Discomfort
Debilitating effects of disease process and inadequate support systems
  Review DD Self-Care—consider Home maintenance
Questions, statements of concern, misconceptions, inaccurate follow-through of instructions, development of preventable complications
  Review DD Health Management—consider Health knowledge

Hernia, hiatal CH

Verbal reports, facial grimacing, self-focus
  Review DD Comfort—consider Pain
Questions, statements of concern, recurrence of condition
  Review DD Health Management—consider Health knowledge

Herniated nucleus pulposus (ruptured intervertebral disc) CH/MS

Verbal reports, guarding or distraction behaviors, preoccupation with pain, self-focus, narrow focus, changes in vital signs (acute), altered muscle tone or function, changes in appetite or sleep pattern, change in libido, physical or social withdrawal
  Review DD Comfort—consider Pain
  Review DD Comfort—consider Pain self-management
Reports of pain with movement, reluctance to attempt or difficulty with purposeful movement, decreased muscle strength, impaired coordination, limited range of motion
  Review DD Activity/Rest—consider Mobility
Statements of boredom, disinterest, restlessness, irritability, withdrawal
  Review DD Activity/Rest—consider Diversional activity

Heroin withdrawal CH/MS

Muscles aches, hot and cold flashes, diaphoresis, lacrimation, rhinorrhea, drug cravings
  Review DD Comfort—consider Pain
  Review DD Comfort—consider Discomfort
Apprehension, pervasive anxious feelings, jittery, restlessness, weakness, insomnia, anorexia
  Review DD Stress Management—consider Anxiety

Prolonged withdrawal, economic difficulties, lack of family or social support, perceived barriers or benefits
 Review DD Health Management—consider Health self-management

Herpes simplex   CH
Verbal reports, distraction behaviors, restlessness
 Review DD Comfort—consider Pain
Risk for secondary infection due to broken or traumatized tissue, altered immune response, untreated infection or treatment failure
 Review DD Safety—consider Infection
Lack of knowledge, values conflict, fear of transmitting disease
 Review DD Sexuality/Reproduction—consider Sexual functioning

Herpes zoster (shingles)   CH
Verbal reports, guarding or distraction behaviors, narrow focus, changes in vital signs
 Review DD Comfort—consider Pain
Statements of concern, questions, misconceptions
 Review DD Health Management—consider Health knowledge

High-altitude pulmonary edema (HAPE)   MS
Also refer to Mountain sickness, acute
Dyspnea, confusion, cyanosis, tachycardia, abnormal blood gases
 Review DD Respiration—consider Gas exchange
Shortness of breath, anxiety, edema, abnormal breath sounds, pulmonary congestion
 Review DD Food/Fluid—consider Fluid volume

High-altitude sickness   MS
Refer to Mountain sickness, acute; High-altitude pulmonary edema

HIV infection   CH
Also refer to Acquired immune deficiency syndrome (AIDS)
Verbalization of nonacceptance or denial of diagnosis, failure to take action that prevents health problem
 Review DD Health Management—consider Health maintenance
Statement of misconception, request for information, inappropriate or exaggerated behaviors (hostile, agitated, apathetic), inaccurate follow-through of instructions, development of preventable complications
 Review DD Health Management—consider Health knowledge
Complexity of healthcare system, access to care, economic difficulties, complexity of therapeutic regimen (confusing dosing schedule, duration of regimen, mistrust of regimen and/or healthcare personnel), health beliefs, cultural influences, perceived seriousness, susceptibility, benefits of therapy, decisional conflicts, powerlessness
 Review DD Health Management—consider Health self-management
Overwhelmed, anger, preloss psychological symptoms, anxiety regarding future, feelings of inadequacy, self-blame
 Review DD Stress Management—consider Grief

Hodgkin disease CH/MS
Also refer to Cancer; Chemotherapy

Apprehension, insomnia, self-focus, increased tension
- Review DD Stress Management—consider Anxiety
- Review DD Stress Management—consider Fear

Statements of concern, questions, misconceptions
- Review DD Health Management—consider Health knowledge

Verbal reports of pain, distraction behaviors, self-focus
- Review DD Comfort—consider Pain
- Review DD Comfort—consider Discomfort

Tracheobronchial obstruction (enlarged mediastinal nodes or airway edema)
- Review DD Respiration—consider Breathing pattern

Hospice/End-of-life care CH

Verbal reports; preoccupation with pain; changes in appetite, sleep pattern; altered ability to continue desired activities; guarded or protective behaviors; restlessness; irritability, narrow focus; altered time perception; impaired thought processes
- Review DD Comfort—consider Pain
- Review DD Comfort—consider Pain self-management
- Review DD Comfort—consider End-of-life comfort

Inability to maintain usual routine, verbalized lack of desire or interest in activity, decreased performance, lethargy
- Review DD Activity/Rest—consider Activity intolerance
- Review DD Activity/Rest—consider Fatigue

Changes in communication pattern, denial of potential loss, choked feelings, anger, fear of loss of physical or mental abilities, negative death images or unpleasant thoughts about any event related to death or dying, anticipated pain related to dying, powerlessness over issues related to dying, worrying about impact of one's own death on SO(s), being the cause of other's grief or suffering, concerns of overworking caregiver as terminal illness progresses
- Review DD Stress Management—consider Grief
- Review DD Stress Management—consider Death anxiety

Client expressing despair about family reactions or lack of involvement, history of poor relationship between caregiver and client, altered caregiver health status, SO attempting assistive or supportive behaviors with unsatisfactory results, apprehension about future ability of caregiver's ability to provide care; SO describing preoccupation about personal reactions, displaying intolerance, abandonment, rejection; family behaviors detrimental to client's well-being
- Review DD Roles/Relationships—consider Coping, family
- Review DD Roles/Relationships—consider Caregiving burden

Physical or psychological stress, energy-consuming anxiety, situational losses, blocks to self-love, low self-esteem, inability to forgive
- Review DD Values/Beliefs—consider Spiritual well-being
- Review DD Values/Beliefs—consider Religiosity

Conflict among decision makers, cultural conflicts, end-of-life decisions, loss of autonomy, physical distance of decision makers
  Review DD Values/Beliefs—consider Moral distress

Hydrocephalus   PED/MS
Changes in mentation, restlessness, irritability, reports of headache, pupillary changes, changes in vital signs
  Review DD Circulation—consider Tissue perfusion
Double vision, development of strabismus, nystagmus, pupillary changes, optic atrophy
  Review DD Neurosensory—consider Sensory deficit
Neuromuscular impairment, decreased muscle strength, impaired coordination
  Review DD Activity/Rest—consider Mobility
Questions, statements of concern, request for information, misperceptions
  Review DD Health Management—consider Health knowledge

                                                                CH
Invasive procedure, presence of shunt
  Review DD Safety—consider Infection

Hyperactivity/Attention-deficit disorder   PED/PSY
Irritable mood, acting without thinking, temper outbursts, dangerous behavior
  Review DD Self-Perception/Concept—consider Impulse control
Denial of problem, projection of blame or responsibility, grandiosity, difficulty in perception of reality
  Review DD Stress Management—consider Coping
Discomfort in social situations, interrupts or intrudes on others, difficulty waiting turn in games or group activities, difficulty maintaining attention to task
  Review DD Roles/Relationships—consider Social connectedness
Unrealistic parental expectations, rejection or overprotection of child, exaggerated response of feelings, despair regarding child's behavior
  Review DD Roles/Relationships—consider Coping, family

Hyperbilirubinemia   PED
Abnormal blood profile (elevated blood urea nitrogen), yellow-orange skin and sclera, clay-colored stool
  Review DD Safety—consider Hyperbilirubinemia
Effects of phototherapy, effects on body regulatory mechanisms, invasive procedure (exchange transfusion), abnormal blood profile, chemical imbalances
  Review DD Safety—consider Injury
Questions, statements of concern, inaccurate follow-through of instructions, development of preventable complications
  Review DD Health Management—consider Health knowledge

Hyperemesis gravidarum   OB

Dry mucous membranes, decreased and concentrated urine, decreased pulse volume and pressure, thirst, hemoconcentration
  Review DD Food/Fluid—consider Fluid volume
Vomiting, dehydration, altered fluid intake
  Review DD Food/Fluid—consider Water-electrolyte balance
Inadequate food intake, lack of interest in food or aversion to eating, weight loss
  Review DD Food/Fluid—consider Nutritional intake
Situational or maturational crisis (pregnancy, change in health status, projected role changes, concern about outcome)
  Review DD Stress Management—consider Coping

Hypertension   CH

Statements of concern, questions, misconceptions, inaccurate follow-through of instructions, lack of blood pressure control, development of preventable complications
  Review DD Health Management—consider Health knowledge
Verbalization of nonacceptance of health status change, lack of movement toward independence
  Review DD Health Management—consider Health maintenance
Generalized weakness, imbalance between oxygen supply and demand
  Review DD Activity/Rest—consider Activity intolerance
Verbal reports of throbbing pain in suboccipital region present upon waking and disappearing spontaneously once moving around; reluctance to move head, avoidance of bright lights or noise, increased muscle tension
  Review DD Comfort—consider Pain
Adverse effects of medications, decreased desire/satisfaction
  Review DD Sexuality/Reproduction—consider Sexual functioning

    MS

Increased afterload (vasoconstriction), fluid shifts, hypovolemia, myocardial ischemia, ventricular hypertrophy and rigidity
  Review DD Circulation—consider Cardiac output
  Review DD Circulation—consider Blood pressure

Hypertension, gestational   OB/CH
Also refer to Eclampsia

Decreased plasma proteins, decreased osmotic pressure; increased hematocrit, decreased urine output, increased urine concentration/specific gravity, edema, sudden weight gain
  Review DD Food/Fluid—consider Fluid volume
Increased blood pressure, weight gain/edema, dyspnea
  Review DD Circulation—consider Cardiac output
Tissue edema, hypoxia, tonic-clonic seizures, abnormal blood profile or clotting factors
  Review DD Safety—consider Injury, [maternal]
Pregnancy complication with compromised oxygen transport—vasospasm of spiral arteries, maternal hypovolemia, hypertension
  Review DD Sexuality/Reproduction—consider Maternal-fetal dyad

Prescribed bedrest, discomfort, difficulty turning, postural instability
  Review DD Activity/Rest—consider Mobility
Weakness, discomfort, physical restrictions
  Review DD Self-Care—consider Self-care

Hypertension, intrapartum   OB
Compromised regulatory mechanisms, fluid shifts, excessive fluid intake, effects of drug therapy (oxytocin infusion)
  Review DD Food/Fluid—consider Fluid volume balance
Altered blood flow, vasospasm, prolonged uterine contractions
  Review DD Respiration—consider Gas exchange, [fetal]
Changes in amount and frequency of voiding, bladder distention, changes in urine specific gravity, presence of albumin
  Review DD Elimination—consider Elimination, urinary
Tonic-clonic convulsions, altered clotting factors (release of thromboplastin from placenta)
  Review DD Safety—consider Injury, [maternal]

Hypertension, pulmonary   CH/MS
Refer to Pulmonary hypertension

Hyperthyroidism   CH
Also refer to Thyrotoxicosis
Verbal report of overwhelming lack of energy, inability to maintain usual routine, decreased performance, emotional lability, irritability, impaired ability to concentrate
  Review DD Activity/Rest—consider Fatigue
Increased feelings of apprehension, overexcitement, distress; emotional lability; shakiness; restlessness; tremors
  Review DD Stress Management—consider Anxiety
Inability to ingest adequate nutrients, hypermetabolic state, constant activity level, impaired absorption of nutrients (diarrhea, vomiting), hyperglycemia, insulin insufficiency
  Review DD Food/Fluid—consider Nutritional intake
Periorbital edema, altered protective mechanisms of eye (reduced ability to blink)
  Review DD Safety—consider Tissue integrity

Hypoglycemia   CH
Irritability, changes in mentation, disorganized thinking, altered attention span, emotional lability
  Review DD Neurosensory—consider Confusion
Inadequate dietary intake, lack of adherence to diabetes management, inadequate blood glucose monitoring, medication management
  Review DD Food/Fluid—consider Blood glucose
Statements of concern, questions, misconceptions, development of hypoglycemia
  Review DD Health Management—consider Health knowledge

Hypoparathyroidism (acute)   MS
Impaired regulatory mechanisms, abnormal heart rhythm, tingling lips, fingers, toes; muscle cramps
  Review DD Food/Fluid—consider Water-electrolyte balance

Neuromuscular excitability (tetany), formation of renal stones
  Review DD Safety—consider Injury
Verbal report of pain, distraction behaviors, narrow focus
  Review DD Comfort—consider Pain
Spasm of the laryngeal muscles
  Review DD Respiration—consider Airway clearance
Change in health status, physiological responses
  Review DD Stress Management—consider Anxiety

Hypothermia (systemic) — CH
Also refer to Frostbite
Reduction in body temperature below normal range, shivering, cool skin, pallor, change in vital signs, slow capillary refill, impaired cognition
  Review DD Safety—consider Injury, cold
  Review DD Safety—consider Body temperature
Statements of concern, misconceptions, questions, development of complications
  Review DD Health Management—consider Health knowledge

Hypothyroidism — CH
Also refer to Myxedema
Verbalization of overwhelming lack of energy, inability to maintain usual routines, impaired ability to concentrate, decreased libido, irritability, listlessness, decreased performance, increase in physical complaints
  Review DD Activity/Rest—consider Fatigue
Decreased muscle strength or control, impaired coordination
  Review DD Activity/Rest—consider Mobility
Bowel movement frequency less than usual pattern, decreased bowel sounds, hard dry stools, development of fecal impaction
  Review DD Elimination—consider Elimination, intestinal
  Review DD Elimination—consider Constipation
Paresthesia of hands and feet, decreased hearing
  Review DD Neurosensory—consider Sensory deficit

Hysterectomy — GYN/MS
Also refer to Surgery, general
Verbal report of pain, guarding or distraction behaviors, facial grimacing, changes in vital signs
  Review DD Comfort—consider Pain
Immobilization, lithotomy position
  Review DD Safety—consider Injury, perioperative
Mechanical trauma, surgical manipulation, localized edema, hematoma, nerve trauma with temporary bladder atony
  Review DD Elimination—consider Elimination, urinary
Altered body function and structure, perceived changes in femininity, changes in hormone levels, loss of libido, changes in sexual response pattern
  Review DD Sexuality/Reproduction—consider Sexual functioning

Ileocolitis — MS/CH
Refer to Crohn disease

Ileostomy MS/CH
Refer to Colostomy

Ileus MS
Verbal report of abdominal pain, guarding or distraction behaviors, narrow focus, changes in vital signs
  Review DD Comfort—consider Pain
Changes in frequency and consistency of stool, absence of stool, alteration in bowel sounds, presence of abdominal pain or distention, cramping
  Review DD Elimination—consider Elimination, intestinal
Increased intestinal losses (vomiting, diarrhea), decreased intake
  Review DD Food/Fluid—consider Fluid volume

Impetigo PED/CH
Open, crusted skin lesions, pruritus
  Review DD Safety—consider Skin integrity
Broken skin, traumatized tissue, altered immune response, virulence or contagious nature of pathogen; lack of knowledge to prevent secondary infection or spread of infection to others
  Review DD Safety—consider Infection
Verbal report of localized pain, distraction behaviors, self-focus
  Review DD Comfort—consider Pain

Infant (at 4 weeks) PED
Questions, expressed concerns or desire to learn more, misconceptions
  Review DD Health Management—consider Health knowledge
Failure to ingest, digest, or absorb adequate nutrients; insufficient intake; malabsorption; congenital problem; neglect, emotional abuse, failure to thrive; obesity in one or both parents; rapid transition across growth percentiles
  Review DD Food/Fluid—consider Nutritional intake
  Review DD Food/Fluid—consider Suck-swallow response
  Review DD Food/Fluid—consider Human milk production
  Review DD Food/Fluid—consider Breastfeeding
Accumulation of gas in abdominal cavity, abdominal cramping
  Review DD Comfort—consider Pain
  Review DD Comfort—consider Discomfort
Immature immunological response, increased environmental exposure
  Review DD Safety—consider Infection
Sleeping position, secondhand smoke exposure, type of bedding
  Review DD Safety—consider Sudden infant death
Immature development of sensory organs, inappropriate or inadequate environmental stimuli, effects of prenatal or intranatal complications, maternal drug use
  Review DD Neurosensory—consider Neurodevelopmental organization

Infection, prenatal OB
Also refer to AIDS

Presence of infection, anemia, inadequate acquired immunity, environmental exposure, rupture of amniotic membranes, treatment-related side effects
  Review DD Roles/Relationships—consider Maternal-fetal dyad

Verbalization of problem, inaccurate follow-through of instructions, development of preventable complications, continuation of infectious process
  Review DD Health Management—consider Health knowledge

Verbal reports, illness-related symptoms, restlessness, withdrawal from usual activities
  Review DD Comfort—consider Discomfort

Infection, puerperal OB/CH

Risk for sepsis or spread of infection, break in skin integrity, traumatized tissues, vascularity of affected area, invasive procedures, increased environmental exposure, anemia, chronic disease
  Review DD Safety—consider Infection

Verbal report of pain, restlessness, guarding or distraction behaviors, self-focus, changes in vital signs
  Review DD Comfort—consider Pain

Aversion to eating, decreased or lack of oral intake, unplanned weight loss
  Review DD Food/Fluid—consider Nutritional intake

Interruption in bonding process, separation, physical barriers, maternal fatigue or apathy
  Review DD Roles/Relationships—consider Caregiver child attachment

Infection, wound MS/CH

Presence of infectious process, break in skin integrity, traumatized tissue, stasis of body fluids, invasive procedures, increased environmental exposure, chronic disease (e.g., diabetes, anemia, malnutrition), altered immune response, adverse effect of medication
  Review DD Safety—consider Infection
  Review DD Safety—consider Surgical wound infection

Delayed healing of wound, damaged tissues, invasive procedures
  Review DD Safety—consider Skin/Tissue integrity

Presence of infection, activity restrictions, nutritional deficiencies
  Review DD Health Management—consider Surgical recovery

Infertility CH

Self-negating statements, expressions of helplessness, perceived inability to deal with situation
  Review DD Self-Perception/Concept—consider Self-esteem

Expressions of anger, disappointment, emptiness, self-blame, helplessness, sadness, feelings interfering with ability to achieve maximum well-being
  Review DD Stress Management—consider Grief

Energy-consuming anxiety, low self-esteem, deteriorating relationship with SO, viewing situation as deserved or punishment for past behaviors
  Review DD Values/Beliefs—consider Spiritual well-being

Inflammatory bowel disease — Ch
Refer to Colitis, ulcerative; Crohn disease

Influenza — Ch
Verbal reports of discomfort, distraction behaviors, narrow focus
  Review DD Values/Beliefs—consider Pain
  Review DD Values/Beliefs—consider Discomfort
Excessive gastric losses through vomiting or diarrhea, hypermetabolic state, altered intake
  Review DD Values/Beliefs—consider Fluid volume
Increased body temperature, warm flushed skin, tachycardia
  Review DD Values/Beliefs—consider Thermoregulation
Infectious process, decreased energy, fatigue, increased respiratory secretions, altered respiratory rate/depth
  Review DD Values/Beliefs—consider Breathing pattern

Insulin shock — MS/CH
Refer to Hypoglycemia

Intestinal obstruction — MS
Refer to Ileus

Irritable bowel syndrome — CH
Verbal reports of abdominal pain or discomfort, guarding or distraction behaviors, restlessness, moaning, irritability
  Review DD Comfort—consider Pain
Frequent, liquid stools upon rising or immediately after eating; rectal pressure or urgency; fecal incontinence; abdominal distention
  Review DD Elimination—consider Elimination, intestinal
  Review DD Elimination—consider Gastrointestinal motility
Change in bowel pattern with decreased frequency, sensation of incomplete evacuation, abdominal pain or pressure, distention
  Review DD Elimination—consider Elimination, intestinal
  Review DD Elimination—consider Constipation

Kawasaki disease — PED
Increased body temperature, flushed skin, tachypnea, tachycardia
  Review DD Safety—consider Thermoregulation
Break in skin integrity (macular rash, desquamation)
  Review DD Safety—consider Skin integrity
Verbal report of pain, restlessness, guarding or distraction behaviors, narrow focus
  Review DD Comfort—consider Pain
Oral pain, hyperemia of tissue, dry/cracked lips
  Review DD Food/Fluid—consider Mucous membrane
Structural changes and inflammation of coronary arteries, alterations in cardiac rate and rhythm, dysrhythmias
  Review DD Circulation—consider Cardiac output

Kidney disease, polycystic CH
Inadequate primary defenses (tissue trauma, stasis of body fluids), inadequate secondary defenses (suppressed inflammatory response), chronic disease state
  Review DD Safety—consider Infection
Verbal reports of back or lower flank pain, severe headache, guarding or protective behaviors, narrow focus, sleep disturbances, distraction behaviors
  Review DD Comfort—consider Pain
Oliguria, edema, abnormal breath sounds, jugular vein distention, hypertension
  Review DD Food/Fluid—consider Fluid volume

Kidney stone(s) CH
Refer to Calculi, urinary

Labor, induced/augmented OB
Questions, statements of concern, misconceptions, preventable complications
  Review DD Health Management—consider Health knowledge
Adverse effects to medications or therapeutic interventions
  Review DD Safety—consider Injury, [maternal]
Altered placental perfusion, umbilical cord prolapse
  Review DD Respiration—consider Gas exchange, [fetal]
Verbal report of pain, muscle tension, guarding or distraction behaviors, narrow focus
  Review DD Comfort—consider Pain

Labor, precipitous OB
Increased tension, apprehension, scared, fearfulness, restlessness, sympathetic stimulation
  Review DD Stress Management—consider Anxiety
Rapid progress of labor, lack of necessary equipment and safe environment
  Review DD Safety—consider Skin/Tissue integrity
Verbal reports of inability to use pain management techniques, sympathetic stimulation, distraction behaviors, moaning, restlessness
  Review DD Comfort—consider Pain

Labor, preterm OB/CH
Continued uterine contractions, irritability, altered placental perfusion, cord prolapse
  Review DD Sexuality/Reproduction—consider Maternal-fetal dyad
Dose-related toxic or adverse effects of tocolytics
  Review DD Safety—consider Poisoning
Delivery of premature infant
  Review DD Safety—consider Injury, [fetal]
Increased tension, apprehension, restlessness, expressions of concern, changes in vital signs
  Review DD Stress Management—consider Anxiety

Questions, statements of concern, misconceptions about risks and treatment plan
Review DD Health Management—consider Health knowledge

Labor, stage I (active phase) — OB
Verbal reports, guarding or distraction behaviors, restlessness, muscle tension, narrow focus
Review DD Comfort—consider Pain
Review DD Comfort—consider Discomfort
Changes in amount and frequency of voiding, urinary retention, slowed progression of labor, reduced sensation to void
Review DD Elimination—consider Elimination, urinary
Situational crisis, personal vulnerability, use of ineffective coping mechanisms, inadequate support systems, pain/discomfort
Review DD Stress Management—consider Coping

Labor, stage II (expulsion) — OB
Verbal reports, guarding or distraction behaviors, restlessness, muscle tension, narrow focus, facial grimacing, diaphoresis
Review DD Comfort—consider Pain
Review DD Comfort—consider Discomfort
Decreased venous return, changes in vital signs (blood pressure, pulse), decreased urinary output, fetal bradycardia
Review DD Circulation—consider Cardiac output
Mechanical compression of head or cord, maternal position or prolonged labor affecting placental perfusion, effects of maternal anesthesia, hyperventilation
Review DD Respiration—consider Gas exchange, [fetal]
Stretching/laceration of delicate tissue due to precipitous labor, hypertonic contractions, adolescence, large fetus; application of forceps
Review DD Safety—consider Skin/Tissue integrity
Pregnancy, stress, anxiety, sleep deprivation, increased physical exertion, anemia, environmental stimuli (temperature, noise, lights)
Review DD Activity/Rest—consider Fatigue

Laminectomy, cervical — MS
Also refer to Laminectomy, lumbar
Immobilization, muscle weakness, obesity, advanced age
Review DD Safety—consider Injury
Pain, retained secretions, muscle weakness
Review DD Respiration—consider Airway clearance
Operative site edema, pain, neuromuscular impairment
Review DD Food/Fluid—consider Swallowing

Laminectomy, lumbar — MS
Also refer to Surgery, general
Diminished or interrupted blood flow due to pressure dressing, edema at operative site, hematoma formation, hypovolemia
Review DD Circulation—consider Tissue perfusion
Spinal trauma due to weakness of spinal column, balance impairment, altered muscle tone, incoordination
Review DD Safety—consider Injury

Veral reports of pain, guarding or distraction behaviors, muscle tension, changes in vital signs, diaphoresis, pallor
  Review DD Comfort—consider Pain
Limited range of motion, decreased muscle strength and control, impaired coordination, reluctance to attempt movement
  Review DD Activity/Rest—consider Mobility
Pain/swelling at operative site, reduced mobility, restriction of position or activity
  Review DD Elimination—consider Elimination, urinary

Laryngectomy   MS/CH
Also refer to Cancer; Chemotherapy
Dyspnea, changes in respiratory rate or depth, use of accessory muscles, weak/ineffective cough, abnormal breath sounds, cyanosis
  Review DD Respiration—consider Airway clearance
Disruption of skin and tissue layers, surgical removal of tissues and grafting, effects of radiation or chemotherapy, altered blood supply, malnutrition, edema of tissues, pooling or continuous drainage of secretions
  Review DD Safety—consider Skin/Tissue integrity
Impaired swallowing, facial and/or neck surgery, presence of tracheostomy or feeding tube
  Review DD Safety—consider Aspiration
Xerostomia, oral discomfort, thick oral secretions, decreased saliva production, dry/crusted/cracked tongue, inflamed lips, absent teeth and gums, poor dental health, halitosis
  Review DD Food/Fluid—consider Mucous membrane

CH

Inability to speak, change in vocal characteristics, impaired articulation
  Review DD Roles/Relationships—consider Communication

Laryngitis   CH/PED
Refer to Croup

Latex allergy   CH
Contact dermatitis (erythema, blisters), delayed hypersensitivity (eczema, irritation), hypersensitivity (generalized edema, wheezing, bronchospasm, hypotension, cardiac arrest)
  Review DD Safety—consider Latex allergy
Expressed concerns, tension, apprehension, hypervigilance, restlessness, self-focus
  Review DD Stress Management—consider Anxiety
  Review DD Stress Management—consider Fear
Health status requiring change in occupation; preventable exposure to latex-containing materials
  Review DD Health Management—consider Health maintenance

Laxative abuse   CH
Faulty health beliefs, expectation of a daily bowel movement, expected passage of stool at same time every day
  Review DD Elimination—consider Constipation

Lead poisoning, acute PED/CH
Also refer to Lead poisoning, chronic

Contamination of food/water, lead-based paint, unprotected occupational exposure, with abdominal cramping, headache, irritability, decreased attentiveness, constipation, tremors
  Review DD Safety—consider Contamination

Loss of coordination, altered level of consciousness, tonic-clonic muscle activity, neurological damage
  Review DD Safety—consider Injury

Excessive vomiting or diarrhea, decreased oral fluid intake
  Review DD Food/Fluid—consider Fluid volume

Statements of concern, questions, misconceptions
  Review DD Health Management—consider Health knowledge

Lead poisoning, chronic CH
Also refer to Lead poisoning, acute

Contamination of food/water, lead-based paint, unprotected occupational exposure, imported herbals/medicinal products, with chronic abdominal cramping, headache, personality changes, cognitive deficits, seizures, neuropathy
  Review DD Safety—consider Contamination

Anorexia, abdominal cramping, reported metallic taste, weight loss
  Review DD Food/Fluid—consider Nutritional intake

Personality changes, learning disabilities, impaired ability to conceptualize and reason, cognitive deficits
  Review DD Neurosensory—consider Thought process

Verbal report of pain, distraction behaviors, self-focus
  Review DD Comfort—consider Pain

Developmental regression, intellectual disability
  Review DD Health Management—consider Development, child

Leukemia, acute MS
Also refer to Chemotherapy

Inadequate secondary defenses (alterations in mature white blood cells, increased number of immature lymphocytes), immunosuppression, bone marrow suppression, invasive procedures, malnutrition
  Review DD Safety—consider Infection

Apprehension, feelings of helplessness, self-focus, insomnia, sympathetic stimulation
  Review DD Stress Management—consider Anxiety
  Review DD Stress Management—consider Fear

Generalized weakness, fatigue, exertional dyspnea, abnormal heart rate or blood pressure in response to activity
  Review DD Activity/Rest—consider Activity intolerance

Verbal reports of abdominal pain, arthralgia, bone pain, headache; distraction or guarding behaviors; narrow focus; autonomic response in vital signs
  Review DD Comfort—consider Pain

Excessive fluid loss (vomiting, diarrhea); decreased intake (nausea, anorexia); hypermetabolic state; predisposition for renal stone formation and tumor lysis syndrome
  Review DD Food/Fluid—consider Fluid volume
Hemorrhage, impaired clotting
  Review DD Circulation—consider Bleeding

Leukemia, chronic   CH
Immune deficiency, impaired healing, altered clotting ability, weakness
  Review DD Safety—consider Immunologic impairment
Verbal report of lack of energy, inability to maintain usual routines, listlessness
  Review DD Activity/Rest—consider Fatigue
Lack of interest in food, anorexia, weight loss, abdominal fullness or pain
  Review DD Food/Fluid—consider Nutritional intake

Long-term care   CH
Apprehension, restlessness, insomnia, repetitive questioning, pacing, purposeless activity, expressed concern regarding changes in life events, self-focus
  Review DD Stress Management—consider Anxiety
  Review DD Stress Management—consider Fear
Denial of feelings, depression, sorrow, guilt; alterations in activity level, sleep patterns, eating habits, libido
  Review DD Stress Management—consider Grief
Voluntary/involuntary, temporary or permanent move; lack of predeparture counseling, multiple losses, feeling of powerlessness, lack of or inappropriate use of support system, decreased psychosocial or physical health status
  Review DD Stress Management—consider Relocation stress
Effects of aging (reduced metabolism, impaired circulation, physiological imbalance, co-morbidities), use of multiple prescribed and over-the-counter drugs
  Review DD Safety—consider Poisoning
Slower reaction times, memory loss, altered attention span, disorientation, inability to concentrate, altered sleep patterns, personality changes
  Review DD Neurosensory—consider Memory
  Review DD Neurosensory—consider Thought process
Reports of difficulty falling asleep, not feeling well rested upon waking, interrupted sleep, waking earlier than desired, change in behavior or performance, increasing irritability, listlessness
  Review DD Activity/Rest—consider Sleep pattern
Physical/psychosocial alteration of sexuality, interference in psychological or physical well-being, self-image, lack of privacy, lack of SO
  Review DD Sexuality/Reproduction—consider Sexual functioning

Life transition, ineffective support system or coping mechanisms, lack of social interaction, depression
  Review DD Values/Beliefs—consider Religiosity

Lupus erythematosus, systemic (SLE)   CH

Reports of overwhelming lack of energy, inability to maintain usual routines, decreased performance, lethargy, decreased libido
  Review DD Activity/Rest—consider Fatigue
Verbal report of pain, guarding or distraction behaviors, self-focus, changes in vital signs
  Review DD Comfort—consider Pain
Presence of skin rash or lesions, ulcerations of mucous membranes, photosensitivity
  Review DD Safety—consider Skin/Tissue integrity
Hiding body/body parts, negative feelings about body, feelings of helplessness, change in social involvement
  Review DD Self-Perception/Concept—consider Body image

Lyme disease   CH/MS

Verbal report of pain, guarding or distraction behaviors, autonomic responses, narrow focus
  Review DD Comfort—consider Pain
Reports of overwhelming lack of energy, inability to maintain usual routines, decreased performance, lethargy, malaise
  Review DD Activity/Rest—consider Fatigue
Alteration in cardiac rate, rhythm, or conduction; pallor, cyanosis, dizziness, change in pulse strength
  Review DD Circulation—consider Cardiac output

Macular degeneration   CH

Verbal report or measured change in visual acuity, changes in usual response to visual stimuli
  Review DD Neurosensory—consider Sensory deficit
Expressed concerns, apprehension, feelings of inadequacy, diminished productivity, impaired attention
  Review DD Stress Management—consider Anxiety
  Review DD Stress Management—consider Fear
Impaired cognitive functioning, inadequate support systems
  Review DD Self-Care—consider Home maintenance
Limited physical mobility, environmental barriers
  Review DD Roles/Relationships—consider Social connectedness

Mallory-Weiss syndrome   MS

Also refer to [esophageal] Achalasia (cardiospasm)
Presence of vomiting, reduced fluid intake; poor skin turgor, dry skin and mucous membranes, thirst
  Review DD Food/Fluid—consider Fluid volume
Excessive vascular losses, changes in vital signs
  Review DD Circulation—consider Bleeding
Statements of concern, questions, recurrence of problem
  Review DD Health Management—consider Health knowledge

Malnutrition CH
Also refer to Anorexia nervosa

Verbal report of lack of appetite, difficulty performing self-care tasks, altered mood, inadequate intake, weight loss, physical decline
  Review DD Food/Fluid—consider Nutritional intake
  Review DD Food/Fluid—consider Underweight self-management

Fatigue, weakness, deficient immunity, impaired healing, pressure injuries, diet deficient in protein, vitamins
  Review DD Safety—consider Immunologic impairment
  Review DD Safety—consider Elder frailty syndrome

Mastectomy MS

Disruption in skin and tissue, altered circulation, destruction of skin and subcutaneous layers
  Review DD Safety—consider Skin/Tissue integrity

Hyperthermia, leukocytosis, purulent drainage, chills
  Review DD Safety—consider Surgical wound infection

Reluctance to attempt movement, limited range of motion, decreased muscle mass and strength
  Review DD Activity/Rest—consider Mobility

Inability to perform self-care tasks due to temporary decreased range of motion of one or both arms
  Review DD Self-Care—consider Self-care

Not looking at or touching surgical site, self-negating statements, preoccupation with loss, change in social involvement or relationships
  Review DD Self-Perception/Concept—consider Body image

Preloss psychological symptoms, predisposition for anxiety, feelings of inadequacy, frequency of major life events
  Review DD Stress Management—consider Grief

Edema in affected arm following mastectomy
  Review DD Circulation—consider Lymphedema self-management

Mastitis OB/GYN

Verbal reports of chest/breast pain, guarding or distraction behaviors, self-focus, changes in vital signs
  Review DD Comfort—consider Pain

Traumatized tissues, stasis of fluids, lack of knowledge of ways to prevent complications
  Review DD Safety—consider Infection

Statements of concern, questions, misconceptions
  Review DD Health Management—consider Health knowledge

Inability to feed on affected side, interruptions in breastfeeding schedule
  Review DD Food/Fluid—consider Breastfeeding

Mastoidectomy PED/MS
Also refer to Surgery, general

Preexisting infection, surgical trauma, stasis of body fluids in close proximity to brain
  Review DD Safety—consider Infection

Verbal report of breast/chest pain, guarding or distraction behaviors, restlessness, self-focus, changes in vital signs
  Review DD Comfort—consider Pain
Reported or tested hearing loss in affected ear
  Review DD Neurosensory—consider Sensory deficit

Measles   CH/PED
Verbal report of discomfort, distraction behaviors, self-focus, changes in vital signs
  Review DD Comfort—consider Pain
  Review DD Comfort—consider Discomfort
Increased body temperature, flushed/warm skin, tachycardia
  Review DD Safety—consider Thermoregulation
Altered immune response, traumatized dermal tissues
  Review DD Safety—consider Infection
Statements of concern, questions, misconceptions, development of preventable complications
  Review DD Health Management—consider Health knowledge

Melanoma, malignant   MS/CH
Refer to Cancer; Chemotherapy

Meningitis, acute meningococcal   MS
Hematologic dissemination of pathogen, stasis of body fluids, suppressed inflammatory response (medication-induced), exposure of others to pathogens
  Review DD Safety—consider Infection
Increased body temperature, warm/flushed skin, tachycardia
  Review DD Safety—consider Thermoregulation
Altered level of consciousness, possible development of tonic-clonic muscle activity, generalized weakness, prostration, ataxia, vertigo
  Review DD Safety—consider Injury
  Review DD Safety—consider Suffocation
Cerebral edema altering or interrupting cerebral arterial or venous blood flow; hypovolemia; gas exchange impairment at cellular level (acidosis)
  Review DD Circulation—consider Tissue perfusion
Verbal report of pain, guarding or distraction behaviors, narrow focus, photophobia, changes in vital signs, restlessness
  Review DD Comfort—consider Pain

Meniscectomy   MS/CH
Impaired ability to move about environment
  Review DD Activity/Rest—consider Walking
Statements of concern, questions, misconceptions, development of preventable complications
  Review DD Health Management—consider Health knowledge

Menopause   GYN
Flushed/warm skin, diaphoresis, night sweats, cold hands and feet
  Review DD Safety—consider Thermoregulation

Reports of overwhelming lack of energy, tiredness, inability to maintain usual routines, decreased performance
  Review DD Activity/Rest—consider Fatigue
Perceived altered body functioning, changes in physical response, misconceptions, impaired relationship with SO
  Review DD Sexuality/Reproduction—consider Sexual functioning
Degenerative changes in pelvic muscles and structural support; urgency, frequency, dribbling
  Review DD Elimination—consider Incontinence
Expressed desire for increased control of health practices, desire for reduction of symptoms
  Review DD Health Management—consider Health self-management

Mental delay   CH
Also refer to Down syndrome
Impaired articulation, difficulty with phonation, inability to modulate speech or find appropriate words (dependent on degree of mental delay)
  Review DD Roles/Relationships—consider Communication
Impaired interaction with peers, family, and/or SO(s); verbalized or observed discomfort in social situations
  Review DD Roles/Relationships—consider Social connectedness
Impaired cognitive ability and motor skills (dependent on degree of mental delay)
  Review DD Self-Care—consider Self-care
Impaired cognition, insufficient finances/planning, lack of support, difficulty maintaining home, disorderly surroundings
  Review DD Self-Care—consider Home maintenance
Decreased metabolic rate, impaired cognitive development, dysfunctional eating patterns, sedentary activity level
  Review DD Food/Fluid—consider Body weight problem
Lack of interest or motivation, lack of resources; lack of training or knowledge of specific exercise needs, safety concerns, fear of injury
  Review DD Activity/Rest—consider Sedentary behaviors
Preoccupation of SO with personal reaction, SO(s) withdraws or has limited interaction with individual, protective behavior disproportionate to client's abilities or need for autonomy/support
  Review DD Roles/Relationships—consider Coping, family

Metabolic syndrome   CH
Inappropriate dietary intake, weight gain, activity level leading to elevated or decreased blood glucose levels
  Review DD Food/Fluid—consider Blood glucose
Verbalized preference for activities low in physical exertion, choosing a daily routine lacking in physical exercise
  Review DD Activity/Rest—consider Sedentary behaviors
Arterial plaque formation, low levels of high-density lipoproteins, high levels of triglycerides, prothrombotic state, proinflammatory state
  Review DD Circulation—consider Tissue perfusion

Miscarriage   OB
Refer to Abortion, spontaneous termination

Mitral stenosis   MS/CH
Reports of fatigue, weakness, exertional dyspnea, tachycardia
    Review DD Activity/Rest—consider Activity intolerance

Restlessness, hypoxia, cyanosis, orthopnea, paroxysmal nocturnal dyspnea
    Review DD Respiration—consider Gas exchange

Jugular vein distention, peripheral or dependent edema, orthopnea, paroxysmal nocturnal dyspnea, weight gain
    Review DD Circulation—consider Cardiac output

Statements of concern, questions, inaccurate follow-through of instructions, development of preventable complications
    Review DD Health Management—consider Health knowledge

Mononucleosis, infectious   CH
Reports of overwhelming lack of energy, inability to maintain usual routines, lethargy, malaise
    Review DD Activity/Rest—consider Fatigue

Verbal reports of pain, guarding or distraction behaviors, self-focus, irritability
    Review DD Comfort—consider Pain
    Review DD Comfort—consider Discomfort

Increased body temperature, warm/flushed skin, tachycardia
    Review DD Safety—consider Thermoregulation

Statements of concern, questions, inaccurate follow-through of instructions, development of preventable complications
    Review DD Health Management—consider Health knowledge

Mood disorders   PSY
Refer to Depressive disorders; Bipolar disorder; Premenstrual dysphoric disorder

Mountain sickness, acute (AMS)   CH/MS
Reports of headache, irritability
    Review DD Comfort—consider Pain

Reports of overwhelming lack of energy, inability to perform usual routines, lack of ability to restore energy after sleep, compromised concentration, decreased performance
    Review DD Activity/Rest—consider Fatigue

Increased water loss (over-breathing dry air), exertion, decreased fluid intake (nausea)
    Review DD Food/Fluid—consider Fluid volume

Multiple personality   PSY
Refer to Dissociative disorders

Multiple sclerosis   CH
Verbal report of overwhelming lack of energy, inability to maintain usual routines, decreased performance, impaired ability to concentrate, increase in physical complaints
Review DD Activity/Rest—consider Fatigue

Limited ability to perform motor skills, limited range of motion, gait changes, postural instability
Review DD Activity/Rest—consider Mobility

Impaired vision, diplopia, disturbance of vibratory or position sense, paresthesia, numbness, blunting of sensation
Review DD Neurosensory—consider Sensory deficit

Verbal expressions of having no control or influence over situation, depression over physical deterioration despite compliance with regimen, nonparticipation in care or decision making, passivity, decreased verbalization, flat affect, isolating behaviors
Review DD Neurosensory—consider Resilience

Reported difficulty managing home management tasks, observed disorderly home environment, poor hygienic conditions of the home
Review DD Self-Perception/Concept—consider Home maintenance

Stated or observed inability to complete activities of daily living
Review DD Self-Care—consider Self-care

Expressions of concern about SO's response to client's illness, SO(s) preoccupation with personal response, intolerance, abandonment, neglectful care, distortion of reality regarding client's illness or prognosis
Review DD Roles/Relationships—consider Coping, family

Mumps   PED/CH

Verbal report of neck/throat pain, body aches, guarding or distraction behaviors, self-focus, autonomic responses in vital signs
Review DD Comfort—consider Pain

Increased body temperature, warm/flushed skin, tachycardia
Review DD Safety—consider Thermoregulation

Hypermetabolic state, painful swallowing, decreased intake; dry skin and mucous membranes, poor skin turgor, thirst
Review DD Food/Fluid—consider Fluid volume

Muscular dystrophy (Duchenne)   PED/CH

Decreased muscle strength, control, and mass; limited range of motion; impaired coordination
Review DD Activity/Rest—consider Mobility
Review DD Activity/Rest—consider Mobility, wheelchair

Learning disability, altered ability to perform self-care/self-control activities appropriate for age
Review DD Health Management—consider Development, child

Sedentary lifestyle, dysfunctional eating patterns, weight gain
Review DD Food/Fluid—consider Overweight

Preoccupation with personal reactions to client's disability, displaying protective behaviors disproportionate to client's abilities and need for autonomy/support
Review DD Roles/Relationships—consider Coping, family

Myasthenia gravis   MS

Dyspnea, changes in respiratory rate or depth, ineffective cough, abnormal breath sounds
Review DD Respiration—consider Breathing pattern
Review DD Respiration—consider Airway clearance

Facial weakness, impaired articulation, hoarseness, inability to speak
  Review DD Roles/Relationships—consider Communication
Reported or observed dysphagia, coughing, choking, evidence of aspiration
  Review DD Food/Fluid—consider Swallowing
Expressed concerns, increasing tension, apprehension, restlessness, sympathetic stimulation, crying, self-focus, uncooperative behavior, withdrawal, anger, noncommunication
  Review DD Stress Management—consider Anxiety
  Review DD Food/Fluid—consider Fear

CH

Statements of concern, questions, misconceptions, development of preventable complications
  Review DD Health Management—consider Health knowledge
Progressive fatigue with repetitive or prolonged muscle use, impaired coordination, decreased muscle strength and control
  Review DD Activity/Rest—consider Mobility
Visual distortions (diplopia), loss of motor coordination
  Review DD Neurosensory—consider Sensory deficit

Myeloma, multiple   MS/CH
Also refer to Cancer
Verbal or coded report of pain; guarding or distraction behaviors; changes in appetite, weight, sleep; reduced social interaction
  Review DD Comfort—consider Pain
Verbalizations, limited range of motion, slowed movement, pain with movement, gait changes
  Review DD Activity/Rest—consider Mobility
Presence of cancer, drug therapies, radiation treatments inadequate nutrition
  Review DD Safety—consider Immunologic impairment
Adverse effects of medical regimen (GI distress), poor appetite/food aversion
  Review DD Food/Fluid—consider Nausea

Myocardial infarction   MS
Also refer to Myocarditis
Verbal report of chest pain/pressure, guarding or distraction behaviors, restlessness, facial grimacing, self-focus, diaphoresis, changes in vital signs
  Review DD Comfort—consider Pain
Increased tension, apprehension, fearfulness, restlessness, expressed concerns, uncertainty, sympathetic stimulation, somatic complaints
  Review DD Stress Management—consider Anxiety
  Review DD Stress Management—consider Fear
Change in cardiac rate and rhythm, reduced preload, increased systemic vascular resistance, altered muscle contractility, infarcted cardiac muscle, structural defects
  Review DD Circulation—consider Cardiac output

Lack of resources, training, or knowledge of specific exercise needs, safety concerns, fear of injury
  Review DD Activity/Rest—consider Sedentary behaviors

Myocarditis MS
Also refer to Myocardial infarction
Fatigue, exertional dyspnea, tachycardia and palpitations in response to activity, dysrhythmias, weakness
  Review DD Activity/Rest—consider Activity intolerance
Degeneration of cardiac muscle; weak peripheral pulse, pallor, cyanosis
  Review DD Circulation—consider Cardiac output
Statements of concern, questions, misconceptions, inaccurate follow-through of instructions, development of preventable complications
  Review DD Health Management—consider Health knowledge

Myringotomy PED/MS
Refer to Mastoidectomy

Myxedema CH
Also refer to Hypothyroidism
Negative feelings about body, feelings of helplessness, change in social involvement
  Review DD Self-Perception/Concept—consider Body image
Weight gain greater than ideal for height and frame
  Review DD Food/Fluid—consider Overweight
Altered electrical conduction and myocardial contractility
  Review DD Circulation—consider Cardiac output

Narcolepsy CH
Hypersomnia, reports of poor nighttime sleep, vivid visual or auditory illusions or hallucinations at the onset of sleep, sleep interrupted by vivid or frightening dreams
  Review DD Activity/Rest—consider Sleep pattern
Sudden loss of muscle tone, momentary paralysis (cataplexy), sudden inappropriate sleep episodes
  Review DD Safety—consider Injury
Negative statements about self, personal vulnerability, chronic physical condition, impaired work or school performance, problems with social relationships, reduced quality of life
  Review DD Self-Perception/Concept—consider Self-esteem

Necrotizing cellulitis/fasciitis PED
Also refer to Cellulitis; Sepsis
Elevated body temperature, flushed/warm skin, tachycardia, lethargy, listlessness
  Review DD Safety—consider Thermoregulation
Inflammation and edema of skin, tissue damage, dermal gangrene
  Review DD Safety—consider Tissue integrity

Necrotizing enterocolitis   PED
Also refer to Sepsis
Abdominal pain and distention, gastric residuals after feedings, failure to gain weight, weight loss
   Review DD Safety—consider Nutritional intake
Vomiting, third-space fluid shifts (bowel inflammation, peritonitis), lack of oral fluid intake
   Review DD Safety—consider Fluid volume

Neglect/abuse   CH/PSY
Refer to Abuse; Battered child syndrome

Nephrectomy   MS
Verbal report of flank or back pain, guarding or distraction behaviors, self-focus, changes in vital signs
   Review DD Comfort—consider Pain
Nausea/vomiting, restricted oral fluid intake
   Review DD Food/Fluid—consider Fluid volume
Excessive vascular losses
   Review DD Circulation—consider Bleeding
Decreased bowel sounds, reduced frequency/amount of stool, hard/formed stool
   Review DD Elimination—consider Elimination, intestinal

Nephrolithiasis   MS/CH
Refer to Calculi, urinary

Nephrotic syndrome   MS/CH
Also refer to Renal failure, acute/chronic
Edema, anasarca, respiratory effusion, ascites, weight gain, intake greater than output, hypertension
   Review DD Food/Fluid—consider Fluid volume
Weight loss, muscle wasting, lack of interest in food, observed inadequate intake
   Review DD Food/Fluid—consider Nutritional intake
Chronic disease process, immunosuppression, malnutrition
   Review DD Safety—consider Infection
Presence of edema and pruritus, activity restrictions
   Review DD Safety—consider Skin integrity

Neuritis   CH
Verbal report of pain, guarding or distraction behaviors, self-focus, changes in vital signs
   Review DD Comfort—consider Pain
Statements of concern, questions, misconceptions
   Review DD Health Management—consider Health knowledge

Newborn, normal   PED
Prenatal or intrapartal stressors, excess production of mucus, cold stress
   Review DD Respiration—consider Gas exchange

Limited amount of subcutaneous fat, thin epidermis with close proximity of blood vessels to skin surface, inability to shiver, movement from warm uterine environment to cooler post-delivery setting
Review DD Safety—consider Body temperature, neonatal

Inadequate secondary defenses (inadequate acquired immunity), inadequate primary defenses (environmental exposure, break in skin integrity, traumatized tissues, decreased ciliary action)
Review DD Safety—consider Infection

Developmental transition or gain of a family member, anxiety related to parental role, lack of privacy in healthcare setting
Review DD Roles/Relationships—consider Caregiver child attachment

Hypermetabolic state, high-calorie requirements, increased insensible water loss, fatigue, potential for inadequate glucose stores
Review DD Food/Fluid—consider Nutritional intake
Review DD Food/Fluid—consider Breastfeeding

Newborn at 1 week   PED
Also refer to Newborn, normal

Risks include physical (hyperbilirubinemia), environmental (inadequate safety precautions), chemical (drugs in breastmilk), psychological (impaired parental interaction)
Review DD Safety—consider Injury

Perineal irritation from urine/stool exposure, chemical irritation from laundry detergent or materials, mechanical irritation (scratches from long fingernails)
Review DD Safety—consider Skin integrity

Alteration in stool consistency and amount, abdominal bloating, irritability with inability to soothe
Review DD Elimination—consider Elimination, intestinal

Newborn, premature   PED

Respiratory difficulties, inadequate oxygenation of tissues, anemia, cyanosis, pallor, poor capillary refill, listlessness
Review DD Respiration—consider Gas exchange

Dyspnea, tachypnea, periods of apnea, nasal flaring, use of accessory muscles, cyanosis, abnormal arterial blood gases, tachycardia
Review DD Respiration—consider Breathing pattern

Immature central nervous system development (temperature regulation center), decreased ratio of body mass to surface area, decreased subcutaneous fat, limited brown fat stores, inability to shiver or sweat, poor metabolic reserves, limited response to hypothermia, frequent medical/nursing interventions/manipulations
Review DD Safety—consider Body temperature

Tissue hypoxia, altered clotting ability, metabolic imbalances (hypoglycemia, electrolyte imbalances, elevated bilirubin)
Review DD Safety—consider Injury

Extremes of age and weight, excessive fluid loss (thin skin, lack of insulating fat, increased environmental temperature, immature kidney function/failure to concentrate urine)
Review DD Food/Fluid—consider Fluid volume

Decreased energy, fatigue, poor positioning, drug-related respiratory depression; inability to coordinate sucking, swallowing, and breathing
Review DD Food/Fluid—consider Suck-swallow response

Immaturity of central nervous system; hypoxia; lack of containment or boundaries; pain, overstimulation; separation from parents
  Review DD Neurosensory—consider Neurodevelopmental organization

Newborn, special needs   PED
Expressions of distress over loss (perfect child), sorrow, guilt, anger, choked feelings, interference with life activities, tearfulness
  Review DD Stress Management—consider Grief [family]
Statements of concern, questions, misconceptions, inadequate performance of caregiver role
  Review DD Health Management—consider Health knowledge
Delay or interruption in bonding process, perceived threat to infant's survival, multiple stressors (financial, needs of family), lack of appropriate response of newborn, lack of support between or from SOs
  Review DD Roles/Relationships—consider Caregiver child attachment
Perceived situational crisis, assumption of full-time responsibility for infant's care, lack of or inappropriate use of resources
  Review DD Roles/Relationships—consider Social connectedness [parental]

Nicotine withdrawal   CH
Expressed concerns or desire to achieve higher level of wellness; lack of support from SO/friends; continued environmental exposure to secondhand smoke or smoking activity
  Review DD Health Management—consider Health maintenance
  Review DD Health Management—consider Health self-management
Return of appetite, normalization of basal metabolic rate, eating in response to internal cues (substitution of food for smoking behaviors)
  Review DD Food/Fluid—consider Overweight

Nonketotic hyperosmolar syndrome   MS
Sudden weight loss, dry skin and mucous membranes, poor skin turgor, hypotension, tachycardia, fever, change in mental status
  Review DD Food/Fluid—consider Fluid volume
Recent weight loss, weakness, hyperglycemia
  Review DD Food/Fluid—consider Nutritional intake
Decreased hemodynamic pressures, electrocardiogram changes, dysrhythmias
  Review DD Circulation—consider Cardiac output
Weakness, cognitive impairments, altered level of consciousness, loss of muscle coordination, risk for seizure activity
  Review DD Safety—consider Injury

Obesity   CH
Weight 20% greater than ideal body weight, sedentary activity level, reported or observed dysfunctional eating pattern, excess body fat by triceps skinfold or other measurement
  Review DD Food/Fluid—consider Overweight
Demonstration of physical deconditioning, daily routine lacking physical exercise or activity
  Review DD Activity/Rest—consider Sedentary behaviors

Fatigue, weakness, exertional discomfort, abnormal heart rate and blood pressure response to activity
    Review DD Activity/Rest—consider Activity intolerance
Sleep apnea; interrupted sleep pattern; daytime drowsiness
    Review DD Activity/Rest—consider Sleep pattern

                                                                                PSY
Negative feelings or statements about body, fear of rejection or reaction of others, feeling of hopelessness or powerlessness, lack of follow-through on treatment plan
    Review DD Self-Perception/Concept—consider Body image
    Review DD Self-Perception/Concept—consider Self-esteem
Reluctance to participate in social gatherings, verbalized or observed discomfort in social situations, dysfunctional interaction with others, feelings of rejection
    Review DD Roles/Relationships—consider Social connectedness

Obsessive-compulsive disorder   PSY

Repetitive actions, recurring thoughts, decreased social and role functioning
    Review DD Stress Management—consider Anxiety
Repetitive behaviors associated with cleaning (e.g., hand hygiene, brushing teeth, showering)
    Review DD Safety—consider Skin/Tissue integrity
Psychological stress, health-illness problems, role dissatisfaction
    Review DD Roles/Relationships—consider Role performance

Opioid abuse   CH/PSY

Refer to Depressant abuse

Oppositional defiant disorder   PED/PSY

Inability to meet age-appropriate expectations, hostility toward others, defiant response to requests or rules, inability to delay gratification
    Review DD Stress Management—consider Coping
Discomfort in social situations, difficulty playing or interacting with others, aggressive behaviors, refusal to comply with requests of others
    Review DD Roles/Relationships—consider Social connectedness
Lack of eye contact, lack of self-confidence, physical risk-taking, distraction of others to cover up own failures, projection of blame
    Review DD Self-Perception/Concept—consider Self-esteem
Unrealistic parental expectations, rejection or overprotection of child; exaggerated expressions of anger, disappointment, despair
    Review DD Roles/Relationships—consider Coping, family

Organic brain syndrome   CH

Refer to Alzheimer's disease

Osteoarthritis (degenerative joint disease)   CH

Refer to Arthritis, rheumatoid

Osteomyelitis   MS/CH

Verbal report of pain, guarding or distraction behaviors, self-focus, autonomic responses, restlessness
    Review DD Comfort—consider Pain

Increased body temperature, warm/flushed skin, chills, tachycardia
  Review DD Safety—consider Thermoregulation
Bone necrosis, extension of infectious process, delayed healing
  Review DD Circulation—consider Tissue perfusion [bone]
Pain upon walking, joint instability
  Review DD Activity/Rest—consider Walking
Statements of concern, questions, misconceptions, inaccurate follow-through of instructions, development of preventable complications
  Review DD Health Management—consider Health knowledge

Osteoporosis   CH
Loss of bone density and integrity increases risk of fracture with minimal to no stress on bone
  Review DD Safety—consider Injury
Verbal report of localized bone pain, guarding or distraction behaviors, self-focus, changes in sleep pattern
  Review DD Comfort—consider Pain
Limited range of motion, reluctance to attempt movement, expressed fear of reinjury, imposed activity restrictions or limitations
  Review DD Activity/Rest—consider Mobility

Palsy, cerebral   PED/CH
Decreased muscle strength, control, mass; limited range of motion; impaired coordination
  Review DD Activity/Rest—consider Mobility
Impaired coordination, limited range of motion
  Review DD Safety—consider Injury
  Review DD Safety—consider Fall, [child]
Verbalized anxiety or guilt regarding client's disability, inadequate understanding and knowledge base, displaying protective behaviors disproportionate to client's abilities or need for autonomy
  Review DD Stress Management—consider Coping, family
Delay or difficulty in performing skills (motor, social, expressive), altered ability to perform self-care or self-control activities appropriate for age
  Review DD Health Management—consider Development, child

Pancreatitis   MS
Verbal report of abdominal or flank pain, guarding or distraction behaviors, self-focus, facial grimacing, changes in vital signs, muscle tension
  Review DD Comfort—consider Pain
Excessive gastric losses (vomiting, nasogastric suction), vasodilation, third-space fluid shifts, ascites; bleeding risk due to alteration in clotting process, hemorrhage
  Review DD Food/Fluid—consider Fluid volume
Decreased insulin production, increased glucagon release, physical health status, stress
  Review DD Food/Fluid—consider Blood glucose
Reported or observed inadequate food intake, aversion to eating, reported altered taste sensation, weight loss, reduced muscle mass and strength
  Review DD Food/Fluid—consider Nutritional intake

Inadequate primary defenses (stasis of body fluids, altered peristalsis, change in pH balance), immunosuppression, nutritional deficiencies, tissue destruction, chronic disease state
Review DD Safety—consider Infection

Panic disorder   PSY

Physiological symptoms, mental or cognitive behaviors indicative of panic, withdrawal from or total avoidance of situations that place client in contact with feared object
Review DD Stress Management—consider Fear

Immobilizing apprehension or physical, mental, or cognitive behaviors indicative of panic; expressed feelings of terror of inability to cope
Review DD Stress Management—consider Anxiety

Paranoid personality disorder   PSY

Perceived threats of danger, paranoid delusions, use of aggressive behavior to compensate, increased feelings of anxiety
Review DD Safety—consider Violence

Rigid delusional system, frightened of other people or own hostility
Review DD Stress Management—consider Anxiety

Family system not meeting physical, emotional, or spiritual needs of its members; inability to express or to accept wide range of feelings; inappropriate boundary maintenance; SO(s) describes preoccupation with personal reactions
Review DD Stress Management—consider Coping, family

Paranoid delusions, lacks sense of control, powerlessness, disrupted family processes, inadequate resources/social support
Review DD Self-Perception/Concept—consider Resilience

Difficulty with the process and character of thoughts, interference with the ability to think clearly and logically, delusions, fragmentation, autistic thinking
Review DD Neurosensory—consider Thought process

Paraplegia   MS/CH

Also refer to Quadriplegia

Loss of muscle function, control, or strength; injury to upper extremity joints due to overuse
Review DD Activity/Rest—consider Transfer ability

Inability to perform usual activities of daily living
Review DD Self-Care—consider Self-care

Reported or observed change in sensory acuity—absence of sensation below level of injury
Review DD Neurosensory—consider Sensory deficit

Limited ability to reposition self in bed/wheelchair; development of skin irritation, breakdown over bony prominences
Review DD Safety—consider Pressure injury

Lack of awareness of bladder distention, retention, incontinence, or overflow; urinary tract infections; renal stone formation; renal dysfunction
Review DD Elimination—consider Elimination, urinary
Review DD Elimination—consider Incontinence, urinary

Negative statements about body or self, feelings of helplessness or powerlessness, delay in taking responsibility for self-care or participation in therapy, change in social involvement
   Review DD Self-Perception/Concept—consider Self-esteem
Negative statements about body, voiced concerns, alteration in relationship with SO, change in interest in self/others
   Review DD Sexuality/Reproduction—consider Sexual functioning

Parathyroidectomy   MS
Verbal report of pain, guarding or distraction behaviors, self-focus, changes in vital signs
   Review DD Comfort—consider Pain
Preoperative renal involvement, stress-induced release of antidiuretic hormone, altered calcium or other electrolyte levels
   Review DD Food/Fluid—consider Fluid volume
Edema in neck region, laryngeal nerve damage
   Review DD Respiration—consider Airway clearance
Statements of concern, questions, misconceptions, development of preventable complications
   Review DD Health Management—consider Health knowledge

Parent-child relational problem   PED/PSY
Lack of effective role model, unrealistic expectations of self/child/partner, verbalization of disappointment in child, inability to care for or discipline child, lack of parental attachment behaviors, child abuse or abandonment
   Review DD Roles/Relationships—consider Parenting
Situational/maturational crisis, family system not meeting needs of its members; difficulty accepting assistance; parents not respecting each other's parenting behaviors
   Review DD Roles/Relationships—consider Family process
   Review DD Roles/Relationships—consider Family interaction
Temporary family disorganization, exhausted supportive capacity of members, detrimental decisions/actions, neglected relationships, intolerance, agitation, depression, hostility, aggression
   Review DD Roles/Relationships—consider Coping, family

Parenteral feeding   MS/CH
Body weight 10% or more under ideal, decreased subcutaneous fat or muscle mass, poor muscle tone
   Review DD Food/Fluid—consider Nutritional intake
Active fluid loss, impaired ability to regulate fluid levels, complications of therapy (hyperglycemia, severe dehydration), inability to obtain or ingest fluids
   Review DD Food/Fluid—consider Fluid volume
Invasive procedure, surgical placement of feeding tube, malnutrition, chronic disease
   Review DD Safety—consider Infection
Catheter-related complications such as air emboli, septic thrombophlebitis
   Review DD Safety—consider Injury

Overwhelming lack of energy, inability to maintain usual routines or tasks, lethargy, impaired ability to concentrate
  Review DD Activity/Rest—consider Fatigue

Parkinson disease   CH
Difficulty moving about the environment, increased occurrence of falls
  Review DD Activity/Rest—consider Walking
Reported or observed dysphagia, drooling, choking, coughing
  Review DD Food/Fluid—consider Swallowing
Neuromuscular impairment affecting ability to swallow effectively; choking, coughing, pocketing food, frequent bouts of pneumonia
  Review DD Safety—consider Aspiration
Impaired articulation, difficulty with phonation, changes in rhythm and tone
  Review DD Roles/Relationships—consider Communication
Feeling stressed, depressed, worried; lack of resources or support; family conflict
  Review DD Roles/Relationships—consider Caregiving burden
Inadequate resources, chronic illness, physical demands
  Review DD Stress Management—consider Anxiety

Pelvic inflammatory disease   OB/GYN/CH
Infectious process in highly vascular pelvic area, delay in seeking treatment
  Review DD Safety—consider Infection
Increased body temperature, warm/flushed skin, tachycardia
  Review DD Safety—consider Thermoregulation
Verbal report of pelvic pain, guarding or distraction behaviors, self-focus, changes in vital signs
  Review DD Comfort—consider Pain
Perceived stigma of physical condition
  Review DD Self-Perception/Concept—consider Self-esteem
Statements of concern, questions, misconceptions, development of preventable complications
  Review DD Health Management—consider Health knowledge

Periarteritis nodosa   MS/CH
Refer to Polyarteritis nodosa

Pericarditis   MS
Verbal report of chest pain increased with movement or certain positions, guarding or distraction behaviors, self-focus, changes in vital signs
  Review DD Comfort—consider Pain
Weakness, fatigue, exertional dyspnea, abnormal heart rate or blood pressure response to activity, signs of heart failure
  Review DD Activity/Rest—consider Activity intolerance
Accumulation of pericardial fluid (effusion), restricted atrial and ventricular filling and contractility
  Review DD Circulation—consider Cardiac output
Increased tension, apprehension, restlessness, expressed concerns
  Review DD Stress Management—consider Anxiety

Perinatal loss/death of child   OB/CH

Verbal expressions of distress, anger, loss, crying, alteration in eating habits or sleep pattern
  Review DD Stress Management—consider Grief

Negative self-appraisal in response to life event in a person with previous positive self-evaluation, verbalization of negative feelings about self (helplessness, uselessness), difficulty making decisions
  Review DD Self-Perception/Concept—consider Self-esteem

Stress, family conflict, inadequate social system
  Review DD Roles/Relationships—consider Role performance

Situational crisis, developmental transition (loss of child), shift in family roles
  Review DD Roles/Relationships—consider Family process

Loss of loved one, blame for loss directed at self/God, alienation from SO/support system, challenged belief and value system, intense suffering
  Review DD Values/Beliefs—consider Spiritual well-being

Peripheral arterial occlusive disease   CH
Refer to Arterial occlusive disease, peripheral

Peripheral vascular disease (atherosclerosis)   CH

Changes in skin temperature and color, lack of hair growth, blood pressure and pulse changes in extremity, presence of bruits, reports of claudication
  Review DD Circulation—consider Tissue perfusion

Reports of muscle fatigue, weakness, exertional discomfort (claudication)
  Review DD Activity/Rest—consider Activity intolerance

Altered circulation with decreased sensation and impaired healing
  Review DD Safety—consider Skin/Tissue integrity

Peritonitis   MS

Inadequate primary defenses (break in skin, traumatized tissue, altered peristalsis), inadequate secondary defenses (immunosuppression), invasive procedures
  Review DD Safety—consider Infection

Dry skin and mucous membranes, poor skin turgor, delayed capillary refill, weak peripheral pulses, diminished urinary output, dark/concentrated urine, hypotension, tachycardia
  Review DD Food/Fluid—consider Fluid volume

Nausea, vomiting, intestinal dysfunction, metabolic abnormalities, increased metabolic needs, increase risk for imbalance
  Review DD Food/Fluid—consider Nutritional intake

Verbal report of abdominal pain, guarding or distraction behaviors, rebound tenderness, facial grimacing, self-focus, changes in vital signs
  Review DD Comfort—consider Pain

Pheochromocytoma   MS

Apprehension, increased tension, shakiness, restlessness, self-focus, fearfulness, diaphoresis, sense of impending doom
  Review DD Stress Management—consider Anxiety

Health Conditions and Client Concerns

Hemoconcentration, dry skin and mucous membranes, poor skin turgor, thirst, weight loss
  Review DD Food/Fluid—consider Fluid volume
Cool/clammy skin, hypertension, postural hypotension, visual disturbances, severe headache, angina
  Review DD Circulation—consider Cardiac output
Statements of concern, questions, misconceptions
  Review DD Health Management—consider Health knowledge

Phlebitis   CH
Refer to Thrombophlebitis

Phobia   PSY
Also refer to Anxiety disorder, generalized
Sympathetic stimulation, apprehension, panic, withdrawal from or total avoidance of situations that place individual in contact with feared object
  Review DD Stress Management—consider Anxiety
  Review DD Stress Management—consider Fear
Reported change in style or pattern of interaction, discomfort in social situations, avoidance of phobic stimulus
  Review DD Roles/Relationships—consider Social connectedness

Placenta previa   OB
Pregnancy-related complication, hypovolemia, hypotension
  Review DD Circulation—consider Bleeding
  Review DD Circulation—consider Shock
Changes in fetal heart rate and rhythm, release of meconium
  Review DD Respiration—consider Gas exchange, [fetal]
Verbalization of specific concerns, increased tension, apprehension, sympathetic stimulation
  Review DD Stress Management—consider Anxiety
  Review DD Stress Management—consider Fear
Imposed activity restrictions, bedrest
  Review DD Activity/Rest—consider Diversional activity

Pleurisy   CH
Verbal report of pleuritic chest pain, guarding or distraction behaviors, self-focus, changes in vital signs
  Review DD Comfort—consider Pain
Decreased respiratory depth, tachypnea, dyspnea
  Review DD Respiration—consider Breathing pattern
Stasis of pulmonary secretions, decreased lung expansion, ineffective cough
  Review DD Safety—consider Infection

Pneumonia   CH/MS
Refer to Bronchitis; Bronchopneumonia

Pneumothorax   MS
Also refer to Hemothorax
Dyspnea, tachypnea, altered chest excursion, respiratory depth changes, use of accessory muscles, nasal flaring, cough, cyanosis, abnormal arterial blood gases
  Review DD Respiration—consider Breathing pattern

Compression or displacement of cardiac structures
  Review DD Circulation—consider Cardiac output
Verbal report of chest pain, guarding or distraction behaviors, self-focus, changes in vital signs
  Review DD Comfort—consider Pain

Polyarteritis nodosa   MS/CH
Organ tissue infarctions, changes in organ function, development of organic psychosis
  Review DD Circulation—consider Tissue perfusion
Increased body temperature, warm/flushed skin, tachycardia
  Review DD Safety—consider Thermoregulation
Verbal report of pain, guarding or distraction behaviors, self-focus, changes in vital signs
  Review DD Comfort—consider Pain
Expressions of sorrow or anger, altered sleep and eating patterns, changes in activity level and libido
  Review DD Stress Management—consider Grief

Polycythemia vera   CH
Reports of fatigue, weakness, decreased ability to perform usual routines
  Review DD Activity/Rest—consider Activity intolerance
Pain in affected area, impaired mental ability, visual disturbances, color changes of skin and mucous membranes
  Review DD Circulation—consider Tissue perfusion

Polyradiculitis, acute inflammatory   MS
Refer to Guillain-Barré syndrome

Postoperative recovery period   MS
Changes in respiratory rate and depth, reduced vital capacity, apnea, bradypnea, cyanosis, sonorous respirations
  Review DD Respiration—consider Breathing pattern
Exposure to cool environment, effect of medications and anesthesia, extremes of age or weight, dehydration
  Review DD Safety—consider Body temperature, perioperative
Disruption of skin and tissues, presence of wound drains
  Review DD Safety—consider Skin/Tissue integrity
Break in skin integrity, tissue trauma, stasis of body fluids, presence of pathogens or contaminants, environmental exposure, invasive procedures
  Review DD Safety—consider Infection
  Review DD Safety—consider Surgical wound
Changes in usual response to stimuli; motor incoordination; impaired ability to concentrate, reason, or make decisions; disorientation to person, place, time
  Review DD Neurosensory—consider Confusion
Verbal report of pain, muscle tension, facial grimacing, guarding or distraction behaviors, narrow focus, self-focus, changes in vital signs
  Review DD Comfort—consider Pain

Restriction of oral fluid intake, loss of fluid through indwelling tubes/ drains, vomiting, blood loss, impaired clotting ability, extremes of age or weight
Review DD Food/Fluid—consider Fluid volume

Postpartum period, 4 to 48 hours　　　　　　　　　　OB/CH

Reports of pelvic cramping (afterpains), self-focus, muscle tension, guarding or distraction behaviors, changes in vital signs, restlessness
Review DD Comfort—consider Pain
Review DD Comfort—consider Discomfort

Maternal verbalization or observations regarding level of satisfaction with breastfeeding process, infant response and weight gain
Review DD Food/Fluid—consider Breastfeeding

Reduced oral intake or inadequate fluid replacement, nausea, vomiting, increased urine output, insensible fluid losses
Review DD Food/Fluid—consider Fluid volume

Excessive blood loss during delivery
Review DD Circulation—consider Bleeding

Lack of support between or from SO(s), ineffective or no role model, anxiety associated with parental role, unrealistic expectations, unmet social or emotional maturation needs of client/partner, presence of stressors (financial, housing, employment)
Review DD Roles/Relationships—consider Caregiver child attachment

Urinary frequency, dysuria, urgency, incontinence, retention
Review DD Elimination—consider Elimination, urinary

Decrease in bowel movement frequency and amount, hard-formed stool, straining with bowel movement, decreased bowel sounds, abdominal distention
Review DD Elimination—consider Elimination, intestinal

Verbal reports of difficulty falling asleep or staying asleep, not feeling well-rested upon waking, interrupted sleep, lack of energy
Review DD Activity/Rest—consider Sleep pattern

Postpartum period, postdischarge to 4 weeks　　　　OB/CH

Physical and emotional demands of infant and other family members, psychological stressors, continued discomfort
Review DD Activity/Rest—consider Fatigue

Maternal verbalization regarding level of satisfaction with breastfeeding process, observation of feeding, infant response and weight gain
Review DD Food/Fluid—consider Breastfeeding

Insufficient intake to meet metabolic demands, lactation, anemia, excessive weight loss, desire to return to prenatal weight
Review DD Food/Fluid—consider Nutritional intake

Tissue trauma, broken skin, decreased hemoglobin, invasive procedures, increased environmental exposure, malnutrition
Review DD Safety—consider Infection

Situational or developmental changes, temporary family disorganization or role changes, minimal support from partner/SO
  Review DD Stress Management—consider Coping
Situational crisis (addition or demands of infant), changes in role, sleep disruption, lack of support from SO/family members, young parental age, life stressors (financial, employment, home environment, lack of resources)
  Review DD Roles/Relationships—consider Parenting
  Review DD Roles/Relationships—consider Coping, family

Postpartum psychosis OB/PSY
Also refer to Depression, postpartum
Anxiety associated with parental role, inability to meet personal needs, perceived guilt regarding relationship with infant
  Review DD Roles/Relationships—consider Caregiver child attachment
Hopelessness, increased anxiety, mood swings, indirect violence, threatening violence, despondency, severe depression, psychosis
  Review DD Safety—consider Violence

Postpolio syndrome CH
Expressed concerns, uncertainty, awareness of physiological symptoms, worry, sleep disturbance, forgetfulness
  Review DD Stress Management—consider Anxiety
  Review DD Stress Management—consider Fear
Overwhelming lack of energy, inability to maintain usual routines or level of physical activity, difficulty concentrating
  Review DD Activity/Rest—consider Fatigue
Impaired gait, joint or postural instability, decreased ability to perform gross motor skills
  Review DD Activity/Rest—consider Walking
  Review DD Activity/Rest—consider Mobility
Daytime drowsiness, decreased ability to function, inability to concentrate
  Review DD Activity/Rest—consider Sleep pattern
Reports of deep aching pain, altered ability to continue previous activities, altered sleep patterns, reduced interaction with others
  Review DD Comfort—consider Pain
Coughing, choking, recurrent pulmonary infections
  Review DD Food/Fluid—consider Swallowing
Diminished or adventitious breath sounds (chronic microatelectasis), poor cough (decreased pulmonary compliance, increased chest wall tightness)
  Review DD Respiration—consider Airway clearance

Post-traumatic stress disorder (PTSD) PSY
Reexperiencing event, somatic reactions, psychological or emotional numbness, altered lifestyle, impaired sleep, self-destructive behaviors, difficulty with interpersonal relationships, development of phobias, poor impulse control, irritability, explosiveness
  Review DD Stress Management—consider Post-trauma syndrome

Verbalization of inability to cope, difficulty asking for help, muscle tension, headaches, chronic worry, emotional tension
  Review DD Stress Management—consider Coping

Verbalization of distress at loss, anger, sadness, labile affect; alteration in eating, sleeping, or dream patterns; difficulty concentrating
  Review DD Stress Management—consider Grief

Startle reaction, intrusive memory causing sudden response of acting out the traumatic event, use of alcohol or other drugs to numb the pain and emotions, intense anxiety, panic state, loss of control
  Review DD Safety—consider Violence

Expressions of confusion about plan of action, impaired family coping; family not meeting physical, emotional, spiritual needs of its members; inability to deal with change or adapt in a constructive manner, ineffective family decision making
  Review DD Roles/Relationships—consider Family process

Pregnancy, 1st trimester OB/CH

Changes in appetite, nausea, vomiting, inadequate financial resources, inadequate nutritional knowledge, insufficient intake, increased metabolic demands
  Review DD Food/Fluid—consider Nutritional intake

Verbal report of breast pain, nausea, leg cramps, hemorrhoids, nasal stuffiness; muscle tension; inability to relax
  Review DD Comfort—consider Discomfort

Situational or environmental changes, hereditary factors, impaired maternal well-being (malnutrition, substance use)
  Review DD Sexuality/Reproduction—consider Maternal-fetal dyad

Variations in blood pressure and pulse, syncopal episodes, pathological edema
  Review DD Circulation—consider Cardiac output

Lack of movement toward health-promoting and enriching lifestyle; choosing activities that negatively impact pregnancy
  Review DD Roles/Relationships—consider Coping, family

Maturational crisis, developmental level, history of maladaptive coping, absence of support systems
  Review DD Roles/Relationships—consider Role performance

Altered food and fluid intake, smooth muscle relaxation, decreased peristalsis, effects of medications (iron)
  Review DD Elimination—consider Elimination, intestinal

Overwhelming lack of energy, inability to maintain usual routines, difficulty falling asleep, dissatisfaction with sleep quality, decreased quality of life
  Review DD Activity/Rest—consider Fatigue
  Review DD Activity/Rest—consider Sleep pattern

Statements of concern, questions, misconceptions, inaccurate follow-through of instructions, development of preventable complications
  Review DD Health Management—consider Health knowledge

Pregnancy, 2nd trimester OB/CH
Also refer to Pregnancy, 1st trimester

Perception of physiological changes, response of others
   Review DD Self-Perception/Concept—consider Body image

Reports of shortness of breath, dyspnea, changes in respiratory depth
   Review DD Respiration—consider Breathing pattern

Decompensated cardiac output due to increased circulatory demand, changes in preload (decreased venous return) and afterload (increased peripheral vascular resistance), ventricular hypertrophy
   Review DD Circulation—consider Cardiac output

Changes in regulatory mechanisms, sodium and water retention
   Review DD Food/Fluid—consider Fluid volume

Reported difficulties, limitations or changes in sexual behaviors or activities
   Review DD Sexuality/Reproduction—consider Sexual functioning

Pregnancy, 3rd trimester OB/CH
Also refer to Pregnancy, 1st and 2nd trimesters

Statements of concern, questions, misconceptions, inaccurate follow-through of instructions, development of preventable complications
   Review DD Health Management—consider Health knowledge

Urinary frequency, urgency, dependent edema
   Review DD Elimination—consider Elimination, urinary

Situational or maturational crisis, personal vulnerability, unrealistic expectations, absent or insufficient support systems
   Review DD Stress Management—consider Coping

Presence of hypertension, infection, substance use or abuse, altered immune system, abnormal blood profile, tissue hypoxia, premature rupture of membranes
   Review DD Sexuality/Reproduction—consider Maternal-fetal dyad

Pregnancy, adolescent OB/CH
Also refer to Pregnancy, 1st, 2nd, and 3rd trimesters

Family expressing confusion about plan; unable to meet physical, emotional, spiritual needs of its members; family inability to adapt to change or deal with traumatic experience in a constructive manner; lack of respect for individuality or autonomy of its members, ineffective family decision-making process, inappropriate boundary maintenance
   Review DD Roles/Relationships—consider Family process

Expressions of feelings of aloneness, rejection, or indifference from others; uncommunicative; withdrawn; lack of eye contact; seeking to be alone; unacceptable behavior; absence of support systems
   Review DD Roles/Relationships—consider Social connectedness

Chronological age, developmental age; unmet social, emotional, or maturational needs; ineffective role model or social support; lack of role identity; presence of stressors (financial, social)
   Review DD Roles/Relationships—consider Parenting

Health Conditions and Client Concerns

Self-negating verbalizations, expressions of shame or guilt, fear of rejection or reaction of others, hypersensitivity to criticism, lack of follow-through or nonparticipation in prenatal care
  Review DD Self-Perception/Concept—consider Self-esteem
Statements of concern, questions, misconceptions, inaccurate follow-through of instructions, development of preventable complications
  Review DD Health Management—consider Health knowledge

Pregnancy, high-risk   OB/CH
Also refer to Pregnancy, 1st, 2nd, and 3rd trimesters
Edema formation, sudden weight gain, hemoconcentration, nausea, vomiting, epigastric pain, headaches, vision changes, decreased urine output
  Review DD Food/Fluid—consider Fluid volume
Variations in blood pressure and hemodynamic readings, edema, shortness of breath, change in mentation
  Review DD Circulation—consider Cardiac output
Compromised oxygen transport (vasospasm of spiral arteries and relative hypovolemia)
  Review DD Sexuality/Reproduction—consider Maternal-fetal dyad
Difficulty managing complex treatment regimen, decisional conflicts, insufficient support, financial challenges
  Review DD Health Management—consider Health self-management

Pregnancy-induced hypertension   OB
Refer to Hypertension, gestational

Premenstrual dysphoric disorder   GYN/PSY
Increased tension, apprehension, restlessness, verbal report of pain, distraction behaviors, somatic complaints, self-focus, physical and social withdrawal
  Review DD Comfort—consider Pain
Feelings of inability to cope or loss of control, depersonalization, increased tension, apprehension, restlessness, somatic complaints, impaired functioning
  Review DD Stress Management—consider Anxiety
Verbalization of difficulty coping or inability to problem solve, inability to meet role expectations, reluctance to ask for help, emotional or muscular tension, chronic fatigue, insomnia, lack of appetite or overeating, frequent illness, decreased social interaction, cyclical irritability
  Review DD Stress Management—consider Coping
Edema, weight gain
  Review DD Food/Fluid—consider Fluid volume
Statements of concern, questions, misconceptions, inaccurate follow-through of instructions, development of preventable complications
  Review DD Health Management—consider Health knowledge

Premenstrual tension syndrome   GYN/PSY
Refer to Premenstrual dysphoric disorder

Pressure Injury   CH

Pressure over bony prominence, shearing forces, surface friction, blisters, tissue loss, discolored intact skin or open wound
    Review DD Safety—consider Pressure injury

Impaired skin integrity, exposure to pathogens, difficulty managing wound care, malnutrition
    Review DD Safety—consider Infection

Statements of concern, questions, misconceptions, inaccurate follow-through of instructions, development of preventable complications
    Review DD Health Management—consider Health knowledge

Preterm labor   OB/CH

Refer to Labor, preterm

Prostatectomy   MS

Also refer to Surgery, general

Dysuria, frequency, dribbling, incontinence, retention, bladder fullness, suprapubic discomfort
    Review DD Elimination—consider Elimination, urinary

Restricted intake, nausea, post-obstructive diuresis
    Review DD Food/Fluid—consider Fluid volume

Vascular-rich tissue trauma, excessive blood loss
    Review DD Circulation—consider Bleeding

Verbal report of suprapubic pain or bladder spasms, distraction behaviors, self-focus, changes in vital signs
    Review DD Comfort—consider Pain

         CH

Preoccupation with change or loss, negative feelings about body, statements of concern about urinary and sexual functioning
    Review DD Self-Perception/Concept—consider Body image

Situational crisis (incontinence, leakage of urine after catheter removal, involvement of genital area), threat to self-concept, change in health status
    Review DD Sexuality/Reproduction—consider Sexual functioning

Pruritus   CH

Verbal report of pain, distraction behaviors, self-focus, restlessness
    Review DD Comfort—consider Pain

Mechanical trauma (scratching), development of vesicles that may rupture
    Review DD Safety—consider Skin integrity

Psoriasis   CH

Loss of protective skin layers, scaling papules and plaques
    Review DD Safety—consider Skin integrity

Hiding affected body part, negative statements about body, feelings of helplessness, change in social involvement
    Review DD Self-Perception/Concept—consider Body image

Pulmonary edema   MS

Dyspnea, restlessness, irritability, abnormal respiratory rate and depth, lethargy, change in mentation
  Review DD Respiration—consider Gas exchange
Respiratory muscle fatigue, impaired secretion management
  Review DD Respiration—consider Ventilation
Expressed concerns, apprehension, increased tension, distress, restlessness
  Review DD Stress Management—consider Anxiety

Pulmonary edema, high altitude   MS
Refer to High-altitude pulmonary edema

Pulmonary embolus   MS

Change in respiratory rate or depth, dyspnea, use of accessory muscles, altered chest excursion, abnormal breath sounds (crackles, wheezes), cough (productive or nonproductive)
  Review DD Respiration—consider Breathing pattern
Profound dyspnea, restlessness apprehension, somnolence, cyanosis, changes in arterial blood gases or pulse oximetry (hypoxemia or hypercapnia)
  Review DD Respiration—consider Gas exchange
Radiologic and laboratory evidence of ventilation-perfusion mismatch, dyspnea, central cyanosis
  Review DD Circulation—consider Tissue perfusion, [pulmonary]
Restlessness, irritability, withdrawal or attack behaviors, tachycardia, pupil dilation, diaphoresis, vomiting, diarrhea, crying, tremulous voice, impending sense of doom
  Review DD Stress Management—consider Fear
  Review DD Stress Management—consider Anxiety

Pulmonary hypertension   CH/MS

Dyspnea, restlessness, irritability, decreased mental acuity, somnolence, abnormal arterial blood gases
  Review DD Respiration—consider Gas exchange
Tachycardia, dyspnea, fatigue, cyanosis
  Review DD Circulation—consider Cardiac output
Weakness, fatigue, abnormal blood pressure and pulse response to activity
  Review DD Activity/Rest—consider Activity intolerance
Expressed concerns, increased tension, apprehension, restlessness, diminished productivity, impaired ability to problem-solve
  Review DD Stress Management—consider Anxiety

Purpura, idiopathic thrombocytopenic   CH

Altered clotting ability
  Review DD Circulation—consider Bleeding
Reports of fatigue, weakness
  Review DD Activity/Rest—consider Activity intolerance
Statements of concern, questions, misconceptions, inaccurate follow-through of instructions, development of preventable complications
  Review DD Health Management—consider Health knowledge

Pyelonephritis   MS

Verbal report of pelvic, back, or flank pain; guarding or distraction behaviors, self-focus, changes in vital signs
  Review DD Comfort—consider Pain
Increased body temperature, warm/flushed skin, chills, tachycardia
  Review DD Safety—consider Thermoregulation
Dysuria, frequency, urgency
  Review DD Elimination—consider Elimination, urinary
Statements of concern, questions, misconceptions, inaccurate follow-through of instructions, development of preventable complications
  Review DD Health Management—consider Health knowledge

Quadriplegia   MS/CH

Also refer to Paraplegia

Decreased respiratory depth, dyspnea, cyanosis, abnormal arterial blood gases
  Review DD Respiration—consider Breathing pattern
Instability of spinal column
  Review DD Safety—consider Injury
Expressions of distress, anger, sorrow; choked feelings; changes in eating habits, sleep pattern, communication pattern; tearfulness
  Review DD Stress Management—consider Grief
Inability to perform self-care tasks
  Review DD Self-Care—consider Self-care
Expressions of difficulties, requests for information or assistance, outstanding debt or financial crisis, lack of necessary aids and equipment
  Review DD Self-Care—consider Home maintenance
Inability to evacuate bowels voluntarily, increased abdominal pressure or distention, dry/hard formed stools, change in bowel sounds
  Review DD Elimination—consider Continence, fecal
  Review DD Elimination—consider Constipation, chronic
Loss of muscle function and control
  Review DD Activity/Rest—consider Mobility
Altered nerve function (spinal cord injury at T6 or above); bladder, bowel, or skin stimulation (tactile, pain, thermal)
  Review DD Neurosensory—consider Autonomic dysreflexia

Rape   CH

Statements of concern, questions, misconceptions, inaccurate follow-through of instructions
  Review DD Health Management—consider Health knowledge
Forceful sexual penetration and trauma to fragile tissues, physical force/battery
  Review DD Safety—consider Tissue integrity

    PSY

Wide range of emotional reactions (anxiety, fear, anger, embarrassment), multisystem physical complaints
  Review DD Stress Management—consider Post-trauma syndrome

Health Conditions and Client Concerns

Verbalization of inability to cope or difficulty asking for help, muscle tension, headaches, emotional tension, chronic worry
  Review DD Stress Management—consider Coping
Alteration in achieving sexual satisfaction, change in interest in self/others, preoccupation with self
  Review DD Sexuality/Reproduction—consider Sexual functioning

Raynaud disease   CH
Verbal report of pain/discomfort, guarding of affected parts, self-focus, restlessness
  Review DD Comfort—consider Pain
Pallor, cyanosis, coolness, numbness, paresthesia, slow healing of lesions
  Review DD Circulation—consider Tissue perfusion
Statements of concern, questions, misconceptions, inaccurate follow-through of instructions, development of preventable complications
  Review DD Health Management—consider Health knowledge

Raynaud phenomenon   CH
Refer to Raynaud disease

Reflex sympathetic dystrophy (RSD)   CH
Refer to Complex regional pain syndrome

Regional enteritis   CH
Refer to Crohn disease

Renal disease, end-stage   CH/MS
Also refer to Renal failure, chronic
Fear of process of dying or loss of abilities, concerns over unfinished business, powerlessness, loss of control, denial of impending death
  Review DD Stress Management—consider Death anxiety

Renal failure, acute (Kidney injury, acute)   MS
Weight gain, edema, anasarca, intake greater than output, venous congestion, changes in blood pressure and central venous pressure, altered electrolyte balance, decreased hemoglobin and hematocrit levels, pulmonary congestion
  Review DD Food/Fluid—consider Fluid volume
Inability to ingest or digest adequate nutrients (anorexia, nausea, vomiting, ulcerations of the oral mucosa, increased metabolic needs), protein catabolism, therapeutic dietary restrictions
  Review DD Food/Fluid—consider Nutritional intake
Depressed immune response, invasive procedures or devices, anemia, malnutrition, changes in dietary intake
  Review DD Safety—consider Infection
Accumulation of toxic waste products and altered cerebral perfusion
  Review DD Neurosensory—consider Confusion

Renal failure, chronic   CH/MS
Also refer to Dialysis, general
Weight gain, edema, anasarca, intake > output, venous congestion, changes in blood pressure and central venous pressure, altered

electrolyte levels, decreased hemoglobin and hematocrit, pulmonary congestion
  Review DD Food/Fluid—consider Fluid volume
Anorexia, nausea, vomiting, ulcerations of oral mucosa, increased metabolic needs, protein catabolism, dietary restrictions
  Review DD Food/Fluid—consider Nutritional intake
Depressed immunological defenses, invasive procedures or devices, malnutrition
  Review DD Safety—consider Infection
Altered metabolic rate, impaired circulation, peripheral neuropathy, decreased skin turgor, reduced activity, immobility, accumulation of toxins in skin
  Review DD Safety—consider Skin integrity
Accumulation of toxic waste products, altered cerebral perfusion, disorientation
  Review DD Neurosensory—consider Thought process
Inability to perform activities of daily living, disheveled, unkempt, strong body odor
  Review DD Self-Care—consider Self-care
Fluid imbalances, myocardial workload, systemic vascular resistance; alterations in cardiac rate/rhythm/conduction (electrolyte imbalances, hypoxia); accumulation of toxins (urea)
  Review DD Circulation—consider Cardiac output
Suppressed erythropoietin production, decreased red blood cell production, altered clotting factors, increased capillary fragility
  Review DD Circulation—consider Bleeding

Renal transplantation   MS
Also refer to Transplantation, recipient
Compromised regulatory mechanisms (new kidney requiring adjustment period for optimal functioning)
  Review DD Food/Fluid—consider Fluid volume
Preoccupation with loss or change, negative feelings about body, focus on past abilities
  Review DD Self-Perception/Concept—consider Body image
Increased tension, apprehension, verbalization of concerns, difficulty concentrating
  Review DD Stress Management—consider Fear
Anxiety, fatigue, difficulty meeting role expectations/basic needs, depression, difficulty problem-solving
  Review DD Stress Management—consider Coping
Break in skin integrity or traumatized tissue, stasis of body fluids, immunosuppression, invasive procedures, nutritional deficits, chronic disease
  Review DD Safety—consider Infection

                                                                CH
Situational crisis, family disorganization, role changes, prolonged disease exhausting support from family members, long-term therapy needs, financial challenges
  Review DD Roles/Responsibilities—consider Coping, family

Repetitive motion injury CH
Refer to Carpal tunnel syndrome

Respiratory distress syndrome, acute MS
Dyspnea, changes in rate and depth of respirations, use of accessory muscles, wheezes, crackles, cough
  Review DD Respiration—consider Airway clearance
Tachypnea, use of accessory muscles, cyanosis, hypoxia, anxiety, changes in mentation, restlessness
  Review DD Respiration—consider Gas exchange
Hypovolemia, vascular pooling, use of diuretics, increased intrathoracic pressure, use of ventilator and positive end-expiratory pressure (PEEP)
  Review DD Circulation—consider Cardiac output
Increased tension, apprehension, restlessness
  Review DD Stress management—consider Anxiety
Active fluid loss through use of diuretics, restricted intake
  Review DD Food/Fluid—consider Fluid volume
Risk for pulmonary injury due to increased airway pressure associated with mechanical ventilation (PEEP)
  Review DD Safety—consider Injury

Respiratory distress syndrome (premature infant) PED
Also refer to Newborn, premature
Tachypnea, use of accessory muscles, retractions, expiratory grunting, pallor or cyanosis, abnormal arterial blood gases, tachycardia
  Review DD Respiration—consider Gas exchange
Dyspnea, increased metabolic rate, restlessness, use of accessory muscles, abnormal arterial blood gases
  Review DD Respiration—consider Ventilation
Inadequate primary defenses (decreased ciliary action, stasis of body fluids, traumatized tissues), inadequate secondary defenses (deficiency of neutrophils and specific immunoglobulins), invasive procedures, malnutrition, increased metabolic demands
  Review DD Safety—consider Infection
Inability to digest/absorb nutrients, altered bowel sounds, abdominal distention, regurgitation/vomiting, abdominal pain
  Review DD Food/Fluid—consider Nutritional intake
Premature/ill infant unable to effectively initiate parental contact, separation, physical barriers, anxiety associated with the parental role and demands of infant
  Review DD Roles/Relationships—consider Caregiver child attachment, impaired

Respiratory syncytial virus (RSV) PED
Dyspnea, abnormal arterial blood gases, hypoxia
  Review DD Respiration—consider Gas exchange
Dyspnea, adventitious breath sounds, cough
  Review DD Respiration—consider Airway clearance
Increased insensible fluid loss (fever, diaphoresis), decreased oral intake
  Review DD Food/Fluid—consider Fluid volume

Retinal detachment   CH
Visual distortions, decreased visual field, changes in visual acuity
   Review DD Neurosensory—consider Sensory deficit
Expressed concerns, apprehension, tension, uncertainty, self-focus
   Review DD Stress Management—consider Anxiety
Statements of concern, questions, misconceptions, inaccurate follow-through of instructions, development of preventable complications
   Review DD Health Management—consider Health knowledge
Visual limitations, activity restrictions
   Review DD Self-Care—consider Home maintenance

Reye syndrome   PED
Increased excretion of dilute urine, sudden weight loss, decreased venous filling, dry skin and mucous membranes, poor skin turgor, hypotension, tachycardia
   Review DD Food/Fluid—consider Fluid volume
Memory loss, altered consciousness, restlessness, agitation
   Review DD Circulation—consider Tissue perfusion, cerebral
Tachypnea, abnormal arterial blood gases, cough, use of accessory muscles
   Review DD Respiration—consider Breathing pattern
Generalized weakness, reduced coordination, agitation, confusion
   Review DD Safety—consider Injury

Rheumatic fever   PED
Verbal report of pain, guarding or distraction behaviors, self-focus, narrow focus, restlessness, changes in vital signs
   Review DD Comfort—consider Pain
Increased body temperature, warm/flushed skin, chills, tachycardia
   Review DD Safety—consider Thermoregulation
Reports of fatigue, exertional discomfort, abnormal heart rate response to activity
   Review DD Activity/Rest—consider Activity intolerance
Cardiac inflammation, enlargement, and altered contractility
   Review DD Circulation—consider Cardiac output

Rickets   PED
Inadequate nutrition, economically disadvantaged, altered physical growth, delay or difficulty in performing motor skills appropriate for age
   Review DD Health Management—consider Growth, child
   Review DD Health Management—consider Development, child
Statements of concern, questions, misconceptions, inaccurate follow-through of instructions, development of preventable complications
   Review DD Health Management—consider Health knowledge

Ringworm, tinea   CH
Also refer to Athlete's foot
Disruption of skin surfaces and presence of lesions
   Review DD Safety—consider Skin integrity

Health Conditions and Client Concerns

Statements of concern, questions, misconceptions, inaccurate follow-through of instructions, development of preventable complications
  Review DD Health Management—consider Health knowledge

Rubella   PED/CH
Verbal report of pain, distraction behaviors, restlessness, changes in vital signs
  Review DD Comfort—consider Pain
  Review DD Comfort—consider Discomfort
Statements of concern, contagious nature of disease, questions, misconceptions, inaccurate follow-through of instructions, development of preventable complications
  Review DD Health Management—consider Health knowledge

Scabies   CH
Disruption of skin surface and inflammation
  Review DD Safety—consider Skin integrity
Statements of concern, communicable nature of disease, questions, misconceptions, inaccurate follow-through of instructions, development of preventable complications
  Review DD Health Management—consider Health knowledge

Scarlet fever   PED
Elevated body temperature, chills, warm/flushed skin, tachycardia
  Review DD Safety—consider Thermoregulation
Verbal report of pain, guarding or distraction behaviors, self-focus, restlessness
  Review DD Comfort—consider Pain
  Review DD Comfort—consider Discomfort
Hypermetabolic state, reduced oral intake
  Review DD Food/Fluid—consider Fluid volume

Schizophrenia (schizophrenic disorders)   PSY
Impaired ability to reason or problem-solve, inappropriate affect, presence of delusional system, command hallucinations, obsessions, ideas of reference, cognitive dissonance
  Review DD Neurosensory—consider Thought process
Difficulty in establishing relationships, dull affect, uncommunicative, withdrawn, seeking to be alone, inadequate or absent significant purpose in life, expressions of rejection
  Review DD Roles/Relationships—consider Social connectedness
Disturbances in thinking and feeling (depression, paranoia, suicidal ideation), lack of development of trust and appropriate interpersonal relationships, catatonic or manic excitement, toxic reactions to drugs (alcohol)
  Review DD Stress Management—consider Self-injurious behavior
  Review DD Stress Management—consider Violence
  Review DD Stress Management—consider Suicide
Impaired judgment, cognition, perception; diminished problem-solving or decision-making ability; poor self-concept; chronic anxiety; depression; inability to perform role expectations; alteration in social participation
  Review DD Stress Management—consider Coping

CH

Deterioration in family functioning, ineffective family decision-making process, difficulty relating to each other, client's expression of despair at family's lack of reaction or involvement, neglectful relationships with client, extreme distortion regarding client's health problem, denial about client's health problem, prolonged overconcern
Review DD Roles/Relationships—consider Family process
Review DD Roles/Relationships—consider Coping, family

Inability to take responsibility for meeting basic health needs in all functional areas, demonstrated lack of adaptive behaviors to internal or external changes, poor hygiene
Review DD Health Management—consider Health maintenance
Review DD Health Management—consider Health self-management
Review DD Health Management—consider Health management, family

Disorderly environment, accumulation of dirt, unwashed clothes
Review DD Self-Care—consider Home maintenance

Sciatica CH

Verbal report of buttock or leg pain, guarding or distraction behaviors, self-focus, changes in vital signs
Review DD Comfort—consider Pain
Review DD Comfort—consider Discomfort

Reluctance to attempt movement, decreased muscle strength and mass
Review DD Activity/Rest—consider Mobility

Scleroderma CH

Also refer to Lupus erythematosus, systemic (SLE)

Decreased strength, decreased range of motion, reluctance to attempt movement
Review DD Activity/Rest—consider Mobility

Changes in skin temperature and color, pressure ulcer formation, organ function changes (cardiopulmonary, gastrointestinal, renal)
Review DD Circulation—consider Tissue perfusion

Weight loss, decreased intake, reported or observed dysphagia
Review DD Food/Fluid—consider Nutritional intake

Verbalization of nonacceptance of health status change, lack of movement toward independence or goal-directed thinking
Review DD Safety—consider Health maintenance

Verbalization of negative feelings about body, focus on past appearance or abilities, fear of rejection or reaction by others, hiding body parts, change in social involvement
Review DD Self-Perception/Concept—consider Body image

Scoliosis PED

Negative feelings about body, change in social involvement, preoccupation with past appearance or abilities
Review DD Self-Perception/Concept—consider Body image

Statements of concern, questions, misconceptions, inaccurate follow-through of instructions, development of preventable complications
Review DD Health Management—consider Health knowledge

Minimizing health status change, failure to take action, evidence of failure to improve
Review DD Health Management—consider Health maintenance

Health Conditions and Client Concerns

Seizure disorder CH

Statements of concern, questions, misconceptions, inaccurate follow-through of instructions, development of preventable complications
  Review DD Health Management—consider Health knowledge

Statements about lifestyle change, fear of rejection, negative feelings about "brain" or self, change in usual pattern of responsibility, denial of problem resulting in lack of follow-through or nonparticipation in therapy
  Review DD Self-Perception/Concept—consider Self-esteem
  Review DD Self-Perception/Concept—consider Personal identity

Decreased self-assurance, statements of concern, discomfort in social situations, ineffective communication with others, withdrawal from social contacts or activities
  Review DD Roles/Relationships—consider Social connectedness

Weakness, balance impairment, cognitive limitations, altered consciousness, loss of large- and small-muscle coordination during seizure
  Review DD Safety—consider Injury
  Review DD Safety—consider Suffocation

Sepsis MS

Also refer to Sepsis, puerperal

Fluid shifts (massive vasodilation, shift into interstitial space), reduced intake
  Review DD Food/Fluid—consider Fluid volume

Decreased preload (venous return, circulating blood volume), altered afterload (increased systemic vascular resistance), negative inotropic effects of hypoxia, complement activation, lysosomal hydrolase
  Review DD Circulation—consider Cardiac output

Infection, hypovolemia, hypotension, hypoxemia
  Review DD Circulation—consider Shock

Sepsis, puerperal OB

Risk of spread due to presence of infection, break in skin integrity, traumatized tissue, rupture of amniotic membranes, high vascularity of involved area, stasis of body fluids, invasive procedures, increased environmental exposure, chronic disease (diabetes mellitus, anemia, malnutrition), altered immune response, adverse effects of medications
  Review DD Safety—consider Infection

Elevated body temperature, warm/flushed skin, tachycardia, chills
  Review DD Safety—consider Thermoregulation

Interruption or reduction in blood flow (infectious thrombi)
  Review DD Circulation—consider Tissue perfusion

Infection, hypovolemia, hypotension, hypoxemia
  Review DD Circulation—consider Shock

Interruption in bonding process, physical illness, perceived threat to own survival
  Review DD Roles/Relationships—consider Caregiver child attachment

Serum sickness   CH
Verbal report of pain, guarding or distraction behaviors, self-focus, changes in vital signs
  Review DD Comfort—consider Pain
Statements of concern, questions, misconceptions, inaccurate follow-through of instructions, development of preventable complications
  Review DD Health Management—consider Health knowledge

Sexually transmitted infection (STI)   GYN/OB
Transmission of infection due to contagious nature of pathogen, insufficient knowledge of ways to avoid exposure or transmit to others
  Review DD Safety—consider Infection
Disruptions of skin surface and tissues, inflammation of mucous membranes
  Review DD Safety—consider Skin/Tissue integrity
Statements of concern, questions, misconceptions, inaccurate follow-through of instructions, development of preventable complications
  Review DD Health Management—consider Health knowledge

Shock   MS
Also refer to Shock, cardiogenic; Shock, hypovolemic/hemorrhagic; Sepsis
Changes in skin color and temperature, altered pulse pressure, hypotension, tachycardia, changes in mentation, decreased urinary output
  Review DD Circulation—consider Tissue perfusion
Apprehension, increased tension, sympathetic stimulation, restlessness, expressions of concern
  Review DD Stress Management—consider Anxiety

Shock, cardiogenic   MS
Also refer to Shock
Electrocardiogram changes, hemodynamic changes, jugular vein distention, cold/clammy skin, diminished peripheral pulses, decreased urinary output
  Review DD Circulation—consider Cardiac output
Ventilation-perfusion imbalance, alveolar-capillary membrane changes
  Review DD Respiration—consider Gas exchange

Shock, hypovolemic/hemorrhagic   MS
Also refer to Shock
Hypotension, tachycardia, decreased pulse volume and pressure, change in mentation, decreased urine concentration
  Review DD Food/Fluid—consider Fluid volume

Shock, septic   MS
Refer to Sepsis

Sick sinus syndrome MS
Also refer to Dysrhythmia, cardiac

Dysrhythmias, reports of palpitations, weakness, changes in mentation or consciousness, syncope
  Review DD Circulation—consider Cardiac output
Changes in cerebral perfusion, altered level of consciousness, loss of balance, syncope
  Review DD Safety—consider Injury

SLE CH
Refer to Lupus erythematosus, systemic

Sleep apnea CH
Daytime drowsiness, tiredness, decreased ability to perform or focus, slowed mentation
  Review DD Activity/Rest—consider Sleep pattern
Morning headache, decreased mental acuity, abnormal arterial blood gases (hypoxemia, hypercapnia), dysrhythmias
  Review DD Respiration—consider Gas exchange
Duration of therapy, associated discomfort, perceived seriousness or benefit
  Review DD Health Management—consider Health self-management

Smallpox MS
Spread of infection due to contagious nature of pathogen, inadequate acquired immunity, presence of chronic disease, immunosuppression
  Review DD Safety—consider Infection
Disruption of skin surface, cornea, or mucous membranes
  Review DD Safety—consider Tissue integrity
Thirst, hypotension, tachycardia, decreased venous filling, decreased urinary output, dry skin or mucous membranes, poor skin turgor, change in mentation, elevated hematocrit
  Review DD Food/Fluid—consider Fluid volume
Expressed concerns, apprehension, increased tension, restlessness, self-focus
  Review DD Stress Management—consider Anxiety
  Review DD Stress Management—consider Fear

CH
Changes in satisfaction with family, stress-reduction behaviors, mutual support; expression of isolation from community resources
  Review DD Roles/Relationships—consider Family process
Deficits of community participation, high illness rate, excessive community conflicts, expressed vulnerability or powerlessness
  Review DD Roles/Relationships—consider Coping, community

Snow blindness CH
Intolerance to light (photophobia), decrease or loss of visual acuity
  Review DD Neurosensory—consider Sensory deficit
Verbal report of eye pain, guarding or distraction behaviors, self-focus
  Review DD Comfort—consider Pain

Increased tension, apprehension, uncertainty, worry, restlessness, self-focus
Review DD Stress Management—consider Anxiety

Somatoform disorders PSY
Verbalized inability to cope or problem-solve, frequent illness rate, multiple somatic complaints, decreased functioning in social or occupational settings, narcissistic tendencies with total focus on self and physical symptoms demanding behaviors, poor adherence to medical regimen and frequent changes in healthcare providers
Review DD Stress Management—consider Coping
Verbal reports of severe or prolonged pain, guarded or protective behaviors, facial masking, fear of reinjury, altered ability to continue previous routines, social withdrawal, demands for therapy and medication
Review DD Comfort—consider Pain
Reported change in voluntary motor or sensory function (paralysis, loss of smell, aphonia, deafness, blindness, loss of tactile or pain sensation), lack of concern over functional loss
Review DD Neurosensory—consider Sensory deficit
Preoccupation with own thoughts, sad/dull affect, absence of supportive SO(s), noncommunicative or withdrawn behavior, lack of eye contact, seeking to be alone
Review DD Roles/Relationships—consider Social connectedness

Spinal cord injury (SCI) MS/CH
Refer to Paraplegia; Quadriplegia

Sprain of ankle or foot CH
Verbal report of ankle pain, guarding or distraction behaviors, self-focus, restlessness, changes in vital signs
Review DD Comfort—consider Pain
Review DD Comfort—consider Discomfort
Reluctance to attempt movement, inability to move about environment as desired
Review DD Activity/Rest—consider Walking

Stapedectomy MS
Increased middle ear pressure with displacement of prosthesis, balance difficulties, dizziness
Review DD Safety—consider Injury
Surgically traumatized tissue, invasive procedures, environmental exposure to upper respiratory infections
Review DD Safety—consider Infection
Verbal report of ear or head pain, guarding or distraction behaviors, self-focus
Review DD Comfort—consider Pain

STI CH
Refer to Sexually transmitted infection

Health Conditions and Client Concerns

Stimulant abuse   CH/PSY
Also refer to Cocaine hydrochloride poisoning, acute; Substance dependence/abuse rehabilitation

Use of harmful substances despite evidence of negative consequences
  Review DD Stress Management—consider Coping
Feelings or belief that others are conspiring against them or ready to attack or kill them
  Review DD Stress Management—consider Fear
  Review DD Stress Management—consider Anxiety
Reported inadequate intake, weight loss or less than normal weight gain, lack of interest in food, poor muscle tone, laboratory evidence of vitamin deficiencies
  Review DD Food/Fluid—consider Nutritional intake
High-risk injection techniques, impurities of drugs, localized tissue trauma, nasal septum tissue damage, malnutrition, altered immune state
  Review DD Safety—consider Infection
Constant state of alertness, racing thoughts, denial of need to sleep, inability to stay awake, initial insomnia then hypersomnia
  Review DD Activity/Rest—consider Sleep pattern
Response to internal stimuli (hallucinations-visual/auditory), bizarre thinking, anxiety, panic, changes in sensory acuity (smell, taste)
  Review DD Neurosensory—consider Sensory deficit

Substance dependence/abuse rehabilitation
(following acute detoxification)   PSY/CH
Lack of acceptance that drug use is causing the present situation, delay in seeking or refusal of healthcare attention to the detriment of health, manipulative behavior, projection of blame or responsibility for problems
  Review DD Stress Management—consider Coping
Ineffective recovery attempts, statements of inability to stop behavior, requests for help, constantly thinking about drug or obtaining drug, alteration in personal, occupational, or social life
  Review DD Self-Perception/Concept—consider Resilience
Inadequate food intake, altered taste sensation, lack of interest in food, debilitated state, decreased subcutaneous fat or muscle mass, laboratory evidence of mineral or electrolyte deficiency
  Review DD Food/Fluid—consider Nutritional intake
Progressive interference with sexual function, testicular atrophy, gynecomastia, impotence, decreased sperm counts, loss of body hair, thin skin, spider angiomas, amenorrhea, increase in miscarriages
  Review DD Sexuality/Reproduction—consider Sexual functioning
Feelings of anger, frustration, responsibility for alcoholic's behavior, suppressed rage, shame, embarrassment, repressed emotions, guilt, vulnerability, closed communication, manipulation, blaming, enabling behavior, inability to accept or receive help
  Review DD Roles/Relationships—consider Family process

Fetal exposure to teratogens, continued use despite risk to fetus
  Review DD Safety—consider Injury, [fetal]
Statements of concern, questions, misconceptions, inaccurate follow-through of instructions, development of preventable complications, continued substance use despite risk of complications
  Review DD Health Management—consider Health knowledge

Sudden infant death   PED
Expressions of distress, guilt, anger; idealization of child, labile affect, crying, prolonged interference with daily functioning, withdrawal
  Review DD Stress Management—consider Grief
Recent crisis, change in family unit, ineffective coping strategies, sleep disruptions, depression
  Review DD Roles/Relationships—consider Parenting
Situational crisis, loss of family, anger, feeling of failure
  Review DD Roles/Relationships—consider Family process

Surgery, general   MS
Also refer to Postoperative recovery period
Statements of concern, questions, misconceptions
  Review DD Health Management—consider Health knowledge
Apprehension, increased tension, decreased self-assurance, fear of unspecific consequences, self-focus, sympathetic stimulation, restlessness
  Review DD Stress Management—consider Anxiety
  Review DD Stress Management—consider Fear
Disorientation, immobilization, muscle weakness, obesity, edema
  Review DD Safety—consider Injury, perioperative positioning
Wrong client, procedure, site, implants, equipment, or materials; external factors (physical design and structure of environment, exposure to equipment, instrumentation, positioning, use of pharmacologic agents); exposure to internal stressors (tissue hypoxia, abnormal blood profile, altered clotting factors, break in skin integrity)
  Review DD Safety—consider Injury
Exposure to cool environment, effects of medications/anesthetic agents, extremes of age/weight, dehydration, open wound
  Review DD Safety—consider Body temperature, perioperative
Preoperative fluid deprivation, blood loss, excessive gastrointestinal fluid loss (vomiting, gastric suction), inappropriate use or rapid replacement of fluids
  Review DD Food/Fluid—consider Fluid volume

Synovitis (knee)   CH
Verbal report of joint pain, guarding or distraction behaviors, self-focus, restlessness, changes in vital signs
  Review DD Comfort—consider Pain

Health Conditions and Client Concerns

Reluctance to attempt movement, inability to move about environment as desired
   Review DD Activity/Rest—consider Walking

Syphilis, congenital   PED
Also refer to Sexually transmitted infection
Irritability, crying, changes in vital signs
   Review DD Comfort—consider Pain
Disruption of skin surface, tissue trauma
   Review DD Safety—consider Skin/Tissue integrity
Altered physical growth, delay or difficulty performing skills appropriate for age
   Review DD Health Management—consider Development, child
Statements of concern, questions, misconceptions, inaccurate follow-through of instructions, development of preventable complications
   Review DD Health Management—consider Health knowledge

Syringomyelia   MS
Change in usual response to stimuli, decreased sensitivity to pain/temperature or touch, motor incoordination
   Review DD Neurosensory—consider Sensory deficit (kinesthetic)
Increased tension, apprehension, uncertainty, self-focus, expressed concerns, restlessness
   Review DD Stress Management—consider Anxiety
   Review DD Stress Management—consider Fear
Decreased muscle strength, control, and mass; impaired coordination
   Review DD Activity/Rest—consider Mobility
Inability to perform self-care tasks
   Review DD Self-Care—consider Self-care

Tay-Sachs disease   PED
Loss of or failure to acquire skills appropriate for age, flat affect, decreased response to stimuli
   Review DD Health Management—consider Development, child
Loss of visual/hearing acuity
   Review DD Neurosensory—consider Sensory deficit

     CH
Expressions of distress, denial, guilt anger, sorrow; choked feelings; changes in sleep or eating habits; altered libido
   Review DD Stress Management—consider Grief
Verbalization of no control over situation or outcome, depression over physical and mental deterioration
   Review DD Stress Management—consider Resilience
Preoccupation with personal reaction, expressed concern about reaction of other family members, inadequate support of one another, altered communication patterns
   Review DD Roles/Relationships—consider Coping, family
Spiritual distress due to challenged belief and value system by presence of fatal condition with racial or religious connotations and intense suffering
   Review DD Values/Beliefs—consider Spiritual well-being

Thrombophlebitis   CH/MS/OB

Changes in skin color and temperature over affected area, edema, pain, diminished peripheral pulses distal to affected area, slow capillary refill
  Review DD Circulation—consider Tissue perfusion
Verbal report of localized pain, guarding or distraction behaviors, restlessness self-focus, changes in vital signs
  Review DD Comfort—consider Pain
  Review DD Comfort—consider Discomfort
Increased tension, apprehension, restlessness, sympathetic stimulation
  Review DD Stress Management—consider Anxiety
  Review DD Stress Management—consider Fear
Pain with walking, restrictive therapies, safety precautions
  Review DD Activity/Rest—consider Mobility
Statements of concern, questions, misconceptions, inaccurate follow-through of instructions, development of preventable complications
  Review DD Health Management—consider Health knowledge

Thrombosis, venous   MS

Refer to Thrombophlebitis

Thrush   CH

White patches or plaques on oral mucosa, oral discomfort, mucosal irritation or bleeding
  Review DD Food/Fluid—consider Mucous membranes
Decreased/inability to ingest adequate nutrients (oral pain, dysphagia)
  Review DD Food/Fluid—consider Nutritional intake

Thyroidectomy   MS

Also refer to Hyperthyroidism; Hypoparathyroidism (acute); Hypothyroidism
Tracheal obstruction, edema, hematoma formation, laryngeal spasm
  Review DD Respiration—consider Airway clearance
Impaired articulation, inability to speak, use of nonverbal cues or gestures
  Review DD Roles/Relationships—consider Communication
Tetany due to chemical imbalance (hypocalcemia, increased release of thyroid hormones), excessive central nervous system stimulation
  Review DD Safety—consider Injury, [tetany]
Loss of muscle control and support, position of suture line
  Review DD Safety—consider Injury
Verbal report of neck pain, guarding or distraction behaviors, narrow focus, changes in vital signs
  Review DD Comfort—consider Pain

Health Conditions and Client Concerns

Thyrotoxicosis **MS**
Also refer to Hyperthyroidism

Uncontrolled hypermetabolic state, increasing cardiac workload, changes in venous return, systemic vascular resistance; alteration in cardiac rate, rhythm, and conduction
  Review DD Circulation—consider Cardiac output

Apprehension, increased tension, restlessness, shakiness, loss of control, panic, changes in cognition, distortion of environmental stimuli, extraneous movements, tremors
  Review DD Stress Management—consider Anxiety

Physiological changes, increased central nervous system stimulation, accelerated mental activity, altered sleep patterns
  Review DD Neurosensory—consider Thought process

Statements of concern, questions, misconceptions, inaccurate follow-through of instructions, development of preventable complications
  Review DD Health Management—consider Health knowledge

TIA **CH**
Refer to Transient ischemic attack

Tic douloureux **CH**
Refer to Neuralgia, trigeminal

Tonsillectomy **PED/MS**
Refer to Adenoidectomy

Tonsillitis **PED**
Verbal report of painful swallowing, guarding or distraction behaviors, reluctance or refusal to swallow, self-focus, changes in vital signs
  Review DD Comfort—consider Pain

Increased body temperature, chills, warm/flushed skin, tachycardia
  Review DD Safety—consider Thermoregulation

Statements of concern, questions, misconceptions, possible transmission, potential complications
  Review DD Health Management—consider Health knowledge

Total joint replacement **MS**
Inadequate primary defenses (broken skin, exposure of joint), inadequate secondary defenses (immunosuppression due to long-term corticosteroid use), invasive procedures, surgical manipulation, implantation of foreign body, decreased mobility
  Review DD Safety—consider Infection

Reluctance to attempt movement, difficulty with purposeful movement, reports of pain with movement, limited range of motion, decreased muscle strength and control
  Review DD Activity/Rest—consider Mobility
  Review DD Activity/Rest—consider Walking

Reduced arterial or venous blood flow, trauma to blood vessels, tissue edema, improper location or dislocation of prosthesis, hypovolemia
  Review DD Circulation—consider Tissue perfusion

Verbal report of joint pain, guarding or distraction behaviors, restlessness, changes in vital signs, self-focus
   Review DD Comfort—consider Pain
Decreased activity level, impaired mobility, weakness, insufficient fiber or fluid intake, dehydration, poor eating habits, decreased gastrointestinal motility, effects of medications (anesthesia, opiate analgesics), environmental changes
   Review DD Elimination—consider Elimination, intestinal

Toxemia of pregnancy · OB
Refer to Hypertension, gestational

Toxic shock syndrome · MS
Also refer to Sepsis
Increased body temperature, warm/flushed skin, tachycardia
   Review DD Safety—consider Thermoregulation
Development of desquamating rash, hyperemia, inflammation of mucous membranes
   Review DD Safety—consider Skin/Tissue integrity
Dry skin and mucous membranes, poor skin turgor, hypotension, tachycardia, delayed venous filling, decreased amount of concentrated urine, hemoconcentration
   Review DD Food/Fluid—consider Fluid volume
Verbal reports of perineal or pelvic pain, guarding or distraction behaviors, self-focus, changes in vital signs
   Review DD Comfort—consider Pain

Traction · MS
Also refer to Casts; Fractures
Verbal report of extremity pain, guarding or distraction behaviors, restlessness, self-focus, muscle tension, changes in vital signs
   Review DD Comfort—consider Pain
Limited range of motion, inability to move purposefully, reluctance to attempt movement, decreased muscle strength and control
   Review DD Activity/Rest—consider Mobility
Statements of boredom, restlessness, irritability
   Review DD Activity/Rest—consider Diversional activity
Invasive procedures (insertion of foreign body through skin and bone), tissue trauma, stasis of body fluids
   Review DD Safety—consider Infection

Transfusion reaction, blood · MS
Also refer to Anaphylaxis
Infusion of cold blood products, systemic response to toxins
   Review DD Safety—consider Thermoregulation
Risk for impairment due to immunologic response, rash
   Review DD Safety—consider Skin integrity
Increased tension, apprehension, sympathetic stimulation, statements of concern
   Review DD Stress Management—consider Anxiety

Transient ischemic attack (TIA) — CH
Altered mentation, behavioral changes, language deficit, change in motor or sensory response
    Review DD Circulation—consider Tissue perfusion

Apprehension, increased tension, expressed concerns, restlessness, irritability
    Review DD Stress Management—consider Anxiety
    Review DD Stress Management—consider Fear

Possible denial of change in health status, required change in lifestyle, fear of consequences, lack of motivation
    Review DD Stress Management—consider Coping

Transplantation, recipient — MS
Also refer to Surgery, general; Cardiac surgery

Expressed concerns, apprehension, increased tension, restlessness, uncertainty, somatic complaints, sympathetic stimulation
    Review DD Stress Management—consider Anxiety
    Review DD Stress Management—consider Fear

Verbalizations, sleep pattern changes, fatigue, poor concentration,
    Review DD Stress Management—consider Coping

CH

Medically-induced immunosuppression, suppressed inflammatory response, antibiotic therapy, invasive procedures, break in skin integrity, tissue trauma, effects of chronic and debilitating disease
    Review DD Safety—consider Infection

Multiple drug therapies, compromised immune system, effects of debilitating disease
    Review DD Safety—consider Immunologic impairment

Role changes, support fatigue, family demonstrating protective behaviors disproportionate to client's needs, SO describes preoccupation with personal reaction
    Review DD Roles/Relationships—consider Coping, family

Complexity of therapeutic regimen, length of therapy, navigating healthcare system, economic difficulties
    Review DD Health Management—consider Health self-management

Traumatic brain injury (TBI) — MS
Altered level of consciousness, memory loss, changes in motor or sensory responses, restlessness, changes in vital signs, systemic hypotension with intracranial hypertension
    Review DD Circulation—consider Tissue perfusion

Neuromuscular dysfunction (injury to respiratory center of brain, perception or cognitive impairment, tracheobronchial obstruction)
    Review DD Respiration—consider Breathing pattern

Altered sensory reception, integration—neurological trauma or deficit, psychological stress, motor incoordination; change in behavior pattern
    Review DD Neurosensory—consider Sensory deficit

Traumatized tissues, break in skin integrity, invasive procedures, decreased ciliary action, stasis of body fluids, malnutrition,

suppressed inflammatory response (steroid use), altered integrity of closed system (cerebrospinal fluid leak)
Review DD Safety—consider Infection

Decreased intake, altered level of consciousness, weakness of muscles used for chewing or swallowing, hypermetabolic state
Review DD Food/Fluid—consider Nutritional intake

CH

Inability to purposefully move, impaired coordination, limited range of motion, decreased muscle strength and motor skills
Review DD Activity/Rest—consider Mobility

Memory deficits, distractibility, altered attention span or concentration, disorientation; impaired ability to make decisions, problem-solve, reason, or conceptualize; personality changes
Review DD Neurosensory—consider Confusion

Difficulty adapting to change, family not meeting needs of its members, difficulty accepting help, inability to express or to accept feelings of its members
Review DD Roles/Relationships—consider Family process

Inability to perform desired activities of daily living
Review DD Self-Care—consider Self-care

Trichinosis   CH

Verbal reports of discomfort, guarding or distraction behaviors, restlessness, changes in vital signs, tissue edema, development of urticaria
Review DD Comfort—consider Pain

Nausea/vomiting, decreased intake, dry skin and mucous membranes, poor skin turgor, concentrated urine, tachycardia, hemoconcentration, decreased venous filling
Review DD Food/Fluid—consider Fluid volume

Changes in respiratory depth, tachypnea, dyspnea, abnormal arterial blood gases
Review DD Respiration—consider Breathing pattern

Statements of concern, questions, misconceptions, prevention of condition
Review DD Health Management—consider Health knowledge

Tuberculosis (pulmonary)   CH

Inadequate primary defenses (decreased ciliary action, stasis of secretions, tissue destruction, extension of infection), lowered resistance or suppressed inflammatory response, malnutrition, inadequate therapeutic interventions
Review DD Safety—consider Infection

Abnormal respiratory rate, depth, and rhythm; adventitious breath sounds (rhonchi, wheezes, stridor); dyspnea
Review DD Respiration—consider Airway clearance

Decrease in effective alveolar surface area, atelectasis, destruction of alveolar-capillary membrane, bronchial edema, thick/viscous secretions
Review DD Respiration—consider Gas exchange

Health Conditions and Client Concerns

Reports of fatigue, weakness, exertional dyspnea
  Review DD Activity/Rest—consider Activity intolerance
Weight loss, lack of interest in food, altered taste sensation, poor muscle tone
  Review DD Food/Fluid—consider Nutritional intake
Complexity of therapeutic regimen, economic difficulties, family patterns of healthcare, perceived seriousness or benefits (especially during remission), side effects of therapy
  Review DD Health Management—consider Health self-management

Typhus   CH/MS
Elevated body temperature, chills, warm/flushed skin, tachycardia
  Review DD Safety—consider Thermoregulation
Verbal reports of pain, guarding or distraction behaviors, self-focus, changes in vital signs
  Review DD Comfort—consider Pain
Reports of headache, changes in mentation, abdominal pain, peripheral ulceration or necrosis
  Review DD Circulation—consider Tissue perfusion

Ulcer, peptic (acute)   MS/CH
Hypovolemia, hypotension, blood loss
  Review DD Circulation—consider Shock
Apprehension, increased tension, restlessness, uncertainty, self-focus, poor eye contact, expressed concerns, withdrawal, panic or attack behavior
  Review DD Stress Management—consider Fear
  Review DD Stress Management—consider Anxiety
Verbal report of abdominal or epigastric pain, guarding or distraction behaviors, self-focus, changes in vital signs
  Review DD Comfort—consider Pain
Statements of concern, questions, misconceptions, inaccurate follow-through of instructions, development of preventable complications
  Review DD Health Management—consider Health knowledge

Ulcer, venous stasis   CH
Destruction of skin layers, open sores
  Review DD Safety—consider Skin/Tissue integrity
Interruption of venous blood flow (small-vessel vasoconstriiction reflex), skin color changes, edema, tingling/itching, delayed wound healing
  Review DD Circulation—consider Tissue perfusion

Unconsciousness   MS
Refer to Coma

Urinary diversion   MS/CH
Absence of stomal sphincter, character and flow of urine from stoma, reaction to stoma products or chemicals, improperly fitted appliance, removal of adhesive
  Review DD Safety—consider Skin integrity
Verbalization of change in body image, fear of rejection or reaction by others, negative feelings about body, not touching or looking at stoma, refusal to participate in care
  Review DD Self-Perception/Concept—consider Body image

Verbal report of stomal pain or discomfort, self-focus, guarding or distraction behaviors, restlessness, self-focus, changes in vital signs
    Review DD Comfort—consider Pain
Loss of continence, changes in amount and character of urine, urinary retention
    Review DD Elimination—consider Elimination, urinary

Urolithiasis   MS/CH
Refer to Calculi, urinary

Uterine bleeding, dysfunctional   GYN
Apprehension, increased tension, worry, uncertainty, restlessness, expressed concerns, self-focus
    Review DD Stress Management—consider Anxiety
Reports of fatigue, weakness
    Review DD Activity/Rest—consider Activity intolerance

Uterine myomas (also called fibroids)   GYN
Also refer to Anemia
Reports of pelvic pain or pressure, cramping, guarding behavior, irritability
    Review DD Comfort—consider Pain
    Review DD Comfort—consider Discomfort
Urinary frequency, urgency
    Review DD Elimination—consider Elimination, urinary
Excessive or chronic blood loss
    Review DD Food/Fluid—consider Fluid volume

Vaginitis   GYN
Damaged or destroyed tissue, presence of lesions
    Review DD Safety—consider Tissue integrity
Verbal reports of vaginal pain, distraction behaviors, self-focus
    Review DD Comfort—consider Pain
Statements of concern, questions, misconceptions, poor hygiene, risk sexual behaviors, transmission of pathogen
    Review DD Health Management—consider Health knowledge

Valvular heart disease   MS
Variations in hemodynamic parameters, dysrhythmias and electrocardiogram changes, dyspnea, adventitious breath sounds, cyanosis or pallor, jugular vein distention, fatigue
    Review DD Circulation—consider Cardiac output
Interruption of arterial-venous flow (systemic emboli), venous thrombosis (venous stasis, decreased activity)
    Review DD Circulation—consider Tissue perfusion
Fatigue, weakness, abnormal heart rate and blood pressure response to activity, exertional discomfort or dyspnea
    Review DD Activity/Rest—consider Activity intolerance
Apprehension, increased tension, expressed concerns, uncertainty, sympathetic stimulation, insomnia
    Review DD Stress Management—consider Anxiety

Increased sodium and water retention, changes in glomerular filtration
    Review DD Food/Fluid—consider Fluid volume

VAP MS/CH
Refer to Ventilator assist/dependence; Bronchopneumonia

Varices, esophageal MS
Also refer to Ulcer, peptic (acute)
Presence of varices, vascular loss, inattentive to early warning signs
    Review DD Circulation—consider Bleeding
Reduced intake, vomiting, thirst, changes in vital signs, decreased urine output
    Review DD Food/Fluid—consider Fluid volume
Apprehension, increased tension, restlessness, sympathetic stimulation, self-focus, expressed concerns
    Review DD Stress Management—consider Anxiety

Varicose veins CH
Verbal report of leg pain, burning
    Review DD Comfort—consider Pain
Hiding affected body part, negative statements about body
    Review DD Self-Perception/Concept—consider Body image
Altered circulation, venous stasis, edema formation
    Review DD Safety—consider Skin/Tissue integrity

Venereal disease CH
Refer to Sexually transmitted infection

Ventilator assist/dependence MS/CH
Dyspnea, increased work of breathing, use of accessory muscles, reduced vital capacity and total lung volume, changes in respiratory rate, decreased Po_2 and Sao_2, increased Pco_2
    Review DD Respiration—consider Breathing pattern
    Review DD Respiration—consider Ventilation, spontaneous
Changes in respiratory rate and depth, abnormal breath sounds, anxiety, restlessness, cyanosis
    Review DD Respiration—consider Airway clearance
Abnormal response due to limited or insufficient energy stores, sleep disturbance, pain or discomfort, perceived inability to wean, decreased motivation, inadequate support system, adverse environment, history of ventilator dependence greater than 1 week or unsuccessful weaning attempts
    Review DD Respiration—consider Ventilatory weaning
Inability to speak
    Review DD Roles/Relationships—consider Communication
Increased muscle and facial tension, hypervigilance, restlessness, fearfulness, apprehension, expressed concerns, insomnia, negative self-talk
    Review DD Stress Management—consider Fear
    Review DD Stress Management—consider Anxiety

Inability to swallow oral fluids, decreased salivation, ineffective oral hygiene, presence of endotracheal tube
  Review DD Food/Fluid—consider Mucous membranes
Risk for imbalance due to inability to ingest nutrients, increased metabolic demands
  Review DD Food/Fluid—consider Nutritional intake

Ventricular fibrillation   MS
Also refer to Dysrhythmia, cardiac
Absence of measurable cardiac output, loss of consciousness, no palpable pulse
  Review DD Circulation—consider Cardiac output

Ventricular tachycardia   MS
Also refer to Dysrhythmia, cardiac
Altered electrical conduction and reduced myocardial contractility
  Review DD Circulation—consider Cardiac output

West Nile Fever   CH/MS
Elevated body temperature, chills, warm/flushed skin, tachycardia, tachypnea
  Review DD Safety—consider Thermoregulation
Hyperthermia, decreased fluid intake, alterations in skin turgor, immobility, circulating toxins
  Review DD Safety—consider Skin integrity
Verbal reports of headache, myalgia, eye pain, abdominal discomfort
  Review DD Comfort—consider Pain
Hypermetabolic state, decreased intake, anorexia, nausea, fluid loss through vomiting or diarrhea
  Review DD Food/Fluid—consider Fluid volume

Wilms tumor   PED
Also refer to Cancer; Chemotherapy
Fearful/scared affect, distress, crying, insomnia, sympathetic stimulation
  Review DD Stress Management—consider Anxiety
  Review DD Stress Management—consider Fear
Nature of tumor (vascular with thin barrier), increased risk of metastasis when manipulated
  Review DD Safety—consider Injury
Family having difficulty meeting physical, emotional, spiritual needs of its members; inability to effectively deal with traumatic experience
  Review DD Roles/Relationships—consider Family process
Restlessness, crying, lethargy, acting-out behavior
  Review DD Activity/Rest—consider Diversional activity

Wound, gunshot   MS/CH
Tissue trauma, vascular losses
  Review DD Circulation—consider Bleeding
Restricted oral intake, hypovolemia
  Review DD Food/Fluid—consider Fluid volume

Verbal report of pain, guarding or distraction behaviors, restlessness, self-focus, changes in vital signs
  Review DD Comfort—consider Pain
Damaged or destroyed tissue
  Review DD Safety—consider Tissue integrity
Tissue destruction, increased environmental exposure, invasive procedures, decreased hemoglobin
  Review DD Safety—consider Infection
Catastrophic nature of incident (accident, assault, suicide attempt), possibly injury or death of others involved
  Review DD Stress Management—consider Post-trauma syndrome

CHAPTER 4

Using Clinical Judgment to Create Client Plan of Care

The client assessment is the foundation on which identification of individual needs, responses, and problems is based. To facilitate the steps of assessment and diagnosis in the nursing process, an assessment tool has been constructed using a nursing focus instead of the medical approach of "review of systems." This has the advantage of identifying and validating nursing diagnoses (NDs) as opposed to medical diagnoses. To achieve this nursing focus, we have grouped the NDs from NANDA International (NANDA-I) and the International Classification for Nursing Practice (ICNP) used in this text into related categories or concepts titled Diagnostic Divisions that reflect a blending of theories, primarily Maslow's Hierarchy of Needs and a self-care philosophy. These divisions or concepts serve as the framework or outline for data collection and clustering that focuses attention on the nurse's phenomena of concern—the human responses to health and illness—facilitating recognition of cues and directing the nurse to the most likely corresponding NDs, thereby guiding the nurse's clinical judgement in generating the best solutions for the client. This tool is a basic screening tool, and additional data/focused assessment may be required on the basis of the client's responses.

Adult Medical/Surgical Assessment Tool

General Information

Name/DOB _____ Race _____ Gender _____
Source of information—self/other _____
Adm date _____ Time _____ From _____
Reason for encounter/admission _____
Vital signs _____

Activity/Rest

Subjective (Reports)
Usual activities/occupation _____
Leisure activities/hobbies _____
Exercise pattern/frequency _____
Sufficient energy for required/desired activities _____
Mobility limitations/aids _____
Motor development milestones achieved _____
Sleep pattern/hours _____
Sleep challenges/barriers _____
Sleep aids _____
Continuous positive airway pressure (CPAP)/oxygen use _____

Objective (Exhibits)
Cardiac/respiratory response to activity _____
Gait/balance _____
Muscle tone/strength _____
Range of motion—joints _____

Circulation

Subjective (Reports)
Chronic conditions _____
Treatment _____
Leg pain with activity _____
History blood clots, bleeding episodes _____
History dysreflexia episodes (spinal cord injury) _____

Objective (Exhibits)
Blood pressure, heart rate/rhythm _____
Heart sounds _____
Carotid pulse/bruits _____
Color: Skin _____ mucus membranes _____ nailbeds _____
Peripheral pulses _____
Capillary refill _____
Edema/jugular vein distension _____

Comfort

Subjective (Reports)
Pain/discomfort characteristics _____
Verbal rating ____; acceptable/manageable level of pain _____
Aggravating/alleviating factors _____
Effect on activities of daily living (ADLs) _____
Labor pattern (refer to obstetrical tool) _____

Objective (Exhibits)
Nonverbal behaviors _____

Elimination

Subjective (Reports)
Describe bowel pattern/changes _____
Describe urinary pattern/changes _____
Continence bowel/bladder _____
Laxative/diuretic use _____

Objective (Exhibits)
Bowel sounds _____
Abdomen soft/nontender _____
Urinary catheter _____
Ostomy _____

Food/Fluid

Subjective (Reports)
Describe diet/daily food intake _____
Use of supplements _____
Diet restrictions/allergies _____
Chewing/swallowing difficulties _____
Nausea/vomiting _____
Usual weight/changes _____
Breastfeeding satisfaction _____

Objective (Exhibits)
Weight/height _____, body mass index (BMI) _____,
   waist circumference _____
Edema _____
Skin turgor _____ oral mucous membranes (moisture) _____
Dentition/dentures _____
Blood glucose level _____

Health Management

Subjective (Reports)
Dominate language _____ English literate _____
Describe general health _____
Developmental milestones achieved _____
Family health history/risks _____

Using Clinical Judgment to Create Client Plan of Care

SAMPLE ASSESSMENT TOOL

Health goals/expectations of care _____
Exercise engagement/plan _____
Cultural/spiritual values impacting health choices/practices
_____

Health literacy/understanding of health, needs, resources ___
Health behaviors/decision making _____
Advance directives/resuscitation status _____
Medical power of attorney _____
Health screenings/frequency _____
Chronic health conditions _____
Effect on life/relationships _____
Prescribed medications _____
Supplements/herbals _____
Recent illness/health concerns _____
Actions taken including home remedies _____
Results _____
_____

Use of substances (including nicotine, alcohol, marijuana, illicit drugs) _____
Plan/needs postdischarge _____
Resources _____

Neurosensory

Subjective (Reports)
Hearing/vision changes _____
Hearing aids/glasses/contacts _____
Sense of taste/smell changes _____
History of headaches, head trauma, stroke (residual effects) ___
Seizures _____ describe _____
Treatment _____
_____

Tingling/numbness _____

Objective (Exhibits)
Consciousness/orientation _____
Behavior _____
Speech clarity _____
Memory _____
Pupils _____
Facial symmetry _____
Hand grasps _____
Weakness/paralysis _____

Respiration

Subjective (Reports)
Difficulty breathing _____
Cough/sputum _____
Chronic conditions _____

Treatment _____
Use of respiratory aids/oxygen _____

Objective (Exhibits)
Respiratory rate/pulse oximetry _____
Lung sounds _____
Work of breathing/distress _____
Skin/mucous membrane color _____

Roles/Relationships

Subjective (Reports)
Relationship status _____
Family structure—nuclear/extended _____
Problems in family/community _____
How managed _____
Communication difficulties/aids _____
Roles in family/community _____
Ability to perform _____
_____
Caregiver for others _____
Member of ethnic/cultural community _____

Objective (Exhibits)
Communication with family/significant others _____
Interaction pattern—family/others _____

Safety

Subjective (Reports)
Allergies/sensitivities—medications, food, environment, latex, contrast media _____
Exposure to infectious disease, environmental pollution, toxins/poisons/pesticides _____
Immunization history _____
Impaired immune system _____
Able to protect self from internal/external threats (illness, injury) _____
Engages in safety behaviors (e.g., uses seat belt, helmet, occupational safety equipment) _____
Feels safe in home/work/community environment _____
History of sensory limitations (specify) _____
History of accidental injuries _____
Substance abuse; exposure (neonatal) _____
Exposure to violence (specify) _____

Objective (Exhibits)
Body temperature _____
Skin/tissue integrity (e.g., bruises/abrasions, rashes, blisters, ulcerations/pressure injury, lacerations, wounds/drainage, burns): record on body diagram

Using Clinical Judgment to Create Client Plan of Care

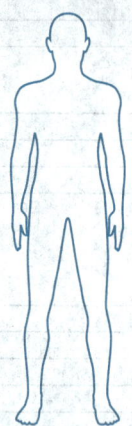
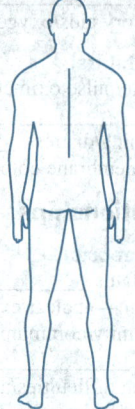

Self-Care

Subjective (Reports)
Perceived ability to perform ADLs _____
Feeding/shopping/cooking _____
_____

Bathing/grooming _____
_____

Dressing _____
_____

Toileting _____
_____

Use of assistive aids/person _____
Management/safety of home environment _____
Discharge plan—needs/changes required _____

Objective (Exhibits)
General appearance _____
Hygiene/body odor _____

Self-Perception/Concept

Subjective (Reports)
Perception of self-worth, competence, personal abilities
_____
Acceptance of self (e.g., body, appearance, gender) ____
Expectations for future, ability to achieve goals; outlook on life _____
Presence of plan/achievable goals _____
Frequently feels annoyed, angry, anxious _____

Feelings of emptiness ___, failure ___, lack of respect ___, rejection ___, shame/guilt ___, discrimination ___, hopelessness ___, powerlessness ___

Engages in harmful activities (e.g., temper outbursts, dangerous behaviors, sensation seeking, gambling, sexual promiscuity) _____

Objective (Exhibits)
Body language, eye contact _____
Self-negative verbalizations _____, rejection of positive feedback
Focused on past appearance, function, successes/failures _____

Sexuality [Component of Roles/Relationships and Self-Perception/Concept]

Subjective (Reports)
Sexually active/contraceptive methods _____
Sexual relationships satisfactory _____
Sexual concerns/changes _____
Practices breast/genital self-examinations _____

Objective (Exhibits)
Sexually transmitted infection (STI) test results _____

Female: Subjective (Reports)
Menstrual history/concerns _____
Breast/vaginal discharge or lesions _____
Pregnancy preparedness/concerns/complications _____
Hormonal therapies _____

Objective (Exhibits)
Labor pattern _____

Male: Subjective (Reports)
Circumcised _____
Sexual performance/erectile difficulties _____
Breast/penile discharge or lesions _____
Last prostate exam _____

Male: Objective (Exhibits)
PSA results _____

Stress Management

Subjective (Reports)
Concerns/stressors _____
How managed (e.g., coping techniques, medications, substance use) _____
Losses (including anticipated) _____
Emotions/feelings (e.g., tension, anxiety, fear) _____

Acceptance/denial of situation _____
Desire to harm self/others _____

Objective (Exhibits)
Emotional status (e.g., calm, anxious, irritable, outbursts, withdrawn) _____
Nonverbal/body language _____
Energy field flow _____

Values/Beliefs

Subjective (Reports)
What gives meaning to client's life _____
Member of a spiritual community _____
Freedom to engage in cultural/spiritual practices _____
Sense of connectedness/harmony with self/others _____
Ability to make decisions/moral choices _____

Diagnostic Divisions: Index of Nursing Diagnoses Included in This Text Organized According to a Nursing Focus

After data are collected and cues are recognized identifying areas of concern or need for the client, the nurse is directed to the Diagnostic Divisions to review the list of NDs used in this text that fall within the individual concepts. The Diagnostic Divisions will assist the nurse in choosing the specific diagnostic label to accurately describe the recognized cues. Then, with the addition of etiology or risk/related factors and signs and symptoms (defining characteristics), when present, the client diagnostic statement emerges.

The authors believe that the majority of NDs approved for use can be either a problem (actual), a risk for, or an opportunity for enhancement, and the interventions for each are similar and overlap. For this reason, where duplicate concepts existed, the ND list has been trimmed to focus primarily on problem diagnoses. When writing a client diagnostic statement, the Related Factors associated with a problem diagnosis also serve as the Risk Factors in a risk diagnosis.

ACTIVITY/REST. *Ability to engage in necessary/desired activities of life (work and leisure) and to obtain adequate sleep/rest*
Activity Intolerance, p. 5–11
Diversional Activity Engagement, decreased, p. 237–242
Fatigue, p. 329–335
Mobility, impaired bed, p. 598–603
Mobility, impaired physical, p. 603–609
Mobility, impaired wheelchair, p. 609–613
Motor Development, delayed infant, p. 622–626
Sedentary Behaviors, excessive, p. 813–818
Sitting Ability, impaired, p. 877–882
Sleep Pattern, ineffective, p. 893–897
Standing Ability, impaired, p. 920–923
Transferring Ability, impaired, p. 1006–1010
Walking Ability, impaired, p. 1051–1055

CIRCULATION. *Ability to transport oxygen and nutrients necessary to meet cellular needs*
Autonomic Dysreflexia, risk for, p. 41–45
Bleeding, risk for excessive, p. 45–50
Blood Pressure, risk for imbalanced, p. 58–63
Cardiac Output, impaired, p. 111–121

Cardiovascular Function, risk for impaired, p. 122–126
Lymphedema Self-Management, ineffective, p. 581–586
Neurovascular Function, risk for impaired peripheral, p. 653–658
Shock, risk for, p. 872–877
Thrombosis, risk for, p. 977–980
Tissue Perfusion, ineffective peripheral, p. 992–1000
Tissue Perfusion, risk for ineffective cerebral, p. 1000–1006

COMFORT. *Ability to control internal/external environment to maintain comfort*

Chronic Pain Syndrome, p. 692–702
Discomfort [specify physical, psychological], p. 229–237
Dry Eye, risk for, p. 242–245
Dry Mouth Self-Management, ineffective, p. 246–250
End-of-Life Comfort Syndrome, impaired, p. 297–300
Pain, acute, p. 684–692
Pain, chronic, p. 692–702
Pain, labor, p. 702–708
Pain Self-Management, ineffective, p. 709–717

ELIMINATION. *Ability to excrete waste products (bowel, bladder)*

Constipation, chronic functional, p. 171–176
Continence, impaired fecal, p. 185–192
Elimination, impaired intestinal, p. 267–275
Elimination, impaired urinary, p. 276–283
Gastrointestinal Motility, impaired, p. 383–391
Incontinence, disability-associated urinary, p. 487–494
Incontinence, mixed urinary, p. 494–503
Incontinence, stress urinary, p. 503–510
Incontinence, urge urinary, p. 510–517
Injury, risk for urinary tract, p. 555–559
Retention, risk for urinary, p. 802–808

FOOD/FLUID. *Ability to maintain intake of and utilize nutrients and liquids to meet physiological needs*

Blood Glucose Within Normal Limits, p. 51–58
Body Weight Problem, p. 83–89
Breastfeeding, difficulty performing, p. 90–98
Breastfeeding, interrupted, p. 98–105
Eating Dynamics, ineffective adolescent, p. 251–255
Eating Dynamics, ineffective child, p. 256–260
Feeding Behavior, impaired infant, p. 342–347
Fluid Volume, excessive, p. 358–365
Fluid Volume, inadequate, p. 365–374
Fluid Volume Balance, risk for impaired, p. 351–358
Liver Function, risk for impaired, p. 570–575
Mucous Membrane, impaired oral, p. 627–634

Nausea, p. 634–640
Nipple-Areolar Complex Integrity, impaired, p. 658–663
Nutritional Intake, inadequate, p. 663–671
Overweight Self-Management, ineffective, p. 675–683
Suck-Swallow Response, ineffective infant, p. 924–928
Swallowing, impaired, p. 956–963
Underweight Self-Management, ineffective, p. 1010–1019
Water-Electrolyte Balance, risk for impaired, p. 1056–1064

HEALTH MANAGEMENT. *Ability to incorporate and act on information to achieve healthy lifestyle/optimal wellness*

Development, impaired child, p. 220–225
Elder Frailty Syndrome, p. 261–267
Emancipated Decision-Making, impaired, p. 289–293
Exercise Engagement, readiness for enhanced, p. 305–308
Growth, delayed child, p. 403–408
Health Knowledge, inadequate, p. 409–415
Health Literacy, inadequate, p. 415–420
Health Maintenance Behaviors, ineffective, p. 420–425
Health Management, ineffective community, p. 425–430
Health Management, ineffective family, p. 430–434
Health Self-Management, ineffective, p. 434–440
Healthy Aging, readiness for enhanced, p. 440–443
Surgical Recovery, impaired, p. 945–951

NEUROSENSORY. *Ability to perceive, integrate, and respond to internal and external cues*

Confusion, acute, p. 160–166
Confusion, chronic, p. 166–170
Memory, impaired, p. 594–598
Sensory Deficit [specify: visual, auditory, kinesthetic, gustatory, tactile, olfactory], p. 858–864
Thought Process, disrupted, p. 968–977

RESPIRATION. *Ability to provide and use oxygen to meet physiological needs*

Airway Clearance, impaired, p. 18–24
Aspiration, risk for, p. 35–40
Breathing Pattern, ineffective, p. 105–111
Gas Exchange, impaired, p. 374–382
Ventilation, impaired spontaneous, p. 1019–1026
Ventilatory Weaning Response, impaired adult, p. 1027–1034
Ventilatory Weaning Response, impaired child, p. 1034–1041

ROLES/RELATIONSHIPS. *Ability to accomplish role development and establish and maintain relationships*

Caregiver Child Attachment, impaired, p. 126–132
Caregiving Burden, excessive, p. 133–140

Communication, impaired verbal, p. 151–160
Coping, impaired community, p. 200–203
Coping, impaired family, p. 203–208
Disrupted Family Identity Syndrome, p. 316–322
Family Process, impaired, p. 322–328
Interaction Patterns, disrupted family, p. 559–566
Loneliness, excessive, p. 575–580
Parenting, impaired, p. 718–725
Relationship, ineffective intimate partner, p. 773–777
Relationship, problem, p. 778–782
Role Performance, impaired, p. 808–812
Social Connectedness, inadequate, p. 897–904
Social Support Network, inadequate, p. 908–913

SAFETY. *Ability to provide safe, growth-promoting environment*

Acute Substance Withdrawal Syndrome, p. 11–18
Allergy Reaction, risk for, p. 24–28
Body Temperature, decreased, p. 70–76
Body Temperature, decreased neonatal, p. 76–80
Body Temperature, risk for decreased perioperative, p. 80–83
Contamination Exposure, p. 176–185
Elopement, risk for, p. 283–288
Falls, risk for [specify adult, child], p. 309–316
Hyperbilirubinemia, neonatal, p. 457–463
Hyperthermia, p. 463–471
Immunologic Impairment, p. 476–482
Infection, risk for, p. 517–524
Injury, risk for burn, p. 525–531
Injury, risk for cold, p. 531–534
Injury, risk for corneal, p. 535–538
Injury, risk for occupational physical, p. 538–544
Injury, risk for perioperative positioning, p. 544–548
Injury, risk for physical, p. 549–555
Latex Allergy, risk for, p. 567–570
Neonatal Abstinence Syndrome, p. 640–645
Occupational Illness, risk for, p. 672–675
Poisoning, risk for, p. 732–737
Pressure Injury, adult, p. 751–758
Pressure Injury, child, p. 758–766
Pressure Injury, neonate, p. 767–772
Skin Integrity, impaired, p. 882–862
Sudden Infant Death, risk for, p. 928–933
Suffocation, risk for accidental, p. 933–938
Surgical Wound Infection, risk for, p. 952–656
Thermoregulation, ineffective, p. 964–968
Tissue Integrity, impaired, p. 981–991

SELF-CARE. *Ability to perform activities of daily living*

Home Maintenance Behaviors, ineffective, p. 443–447
Self-Care Deficit [specify: bathing, dressing, grooming, feeding, toileting], p. 818–830

SELF–PERCEPTION/CONCEPT. *Ability to develop and use skills and behaviors to understand own attitudes and beliefs to integrate and manage life experiences*

Body Image, disrupted, p. 63–70
Dignity, risk for compromised, p. 225–229
Hope, readiness for enhanced, p. 447–451
Impulse Control, ineffective, p. 483–487
Mood Regulation, impaired, p. 613–617
Personal Identity, disturbed, p. 726–731
Resilience, lack of, p. 795–802
Self-Compassion, inadequate, p. 830–834
Self-Concept, readiness for enhanced, p. 834–838
Self-Esteem, chronic inadequate, p. 838–845
Self-Esteem, situational inadequate, p. 845–851
Social Identity, readiness for enhanced transgender, p. 904–908

SEXUALITY/REPRODUCTION. *Ability to meet requirements/characteristics of male/female role [component of Self-Perception/Concept and Roles/Relationships]*

Childbearing Process, ineffective, p. 141–151
Female Genital Mutilation, risk for, p. 347–351
Maternal-Fetal Dyad, risk for impaired, p. 586–593
Sexual Functioning, impaired, p. 865–872

STRESS MANAGEMENT. *Preventing or adapting to life changes, managing individual response to stressors*

Anxiety [mild, moderate, severe, panic level], p. 28–35
Coping, difficulty, p. 192–199
Death Anxiety, p. 209–214
Emotion Regulation, ineffective, p. 293–297
Energy Field, disrupted, p. 301–305
Fear, p. 336–342
Grief, p. 391–396
Grieving, dysfunctional, p. 396–403
Immigration Transition, risk for disrupted, p. 472–476
Post-Trauma Syndrome, p. 738–751
Relocation Stress, p. 789–795
Self-Injurious Behavior, non-suicidal, p. 851–858
Suicide, risk for, p. 935–945
Violence, risk for other-directed, p. 1041–1051

VALUES/BELIEFS. *Ability to use personal values, beliefs (including spiritual), and goals to guide life choices/decisions*

Decision-Making, impaired, p. 215–220
Moral Distress, p. 617–621
Religiosity, impaired, p. 783–789
Spiritual Well-Being, impaired, p. 913–920

---

*Information that appears in brackets in the section has been added by authors to clarify or enhance an ND.

Using Tools and Engaging Clinical Judgment

A sample plan of care formulated using data collected with the nursing model assessment tool along with appropriate pathophysiology and laboratory results is provided. The cues recognized are used to create individualized client diagnostic statements. Then while generating solutions using clinical judgment, desired client outcomes (with timelines added to reflect anticipated length of stay and individual client and nurse expectations) are identified, and interventions/actions were chosen based on problems or needs identified by the client and nurse during data collection, as well as by provider orders. Although not normally included in a written plan of care, rationales are included in this sample for the purpose of explaining or clarifying the choice of interventions to enhance the nurse's learning.

Client Situation and Prototype Plan of Care

Client Situation

Mr. R. S., a client with type 2 diabetes for 10 years, presented to his provider's office with a nonhealing ulcer of 3 weeks' duration on his left foot. Screening studies done in the office revealed blood glucose of 356/fingerstick and urine Chemstix of 2%. Because of distance from medical provider and lack of local community services, he is admitted to the hospital.

Admitting Provider's Orders

Culture/sensitivity of foot ulcer
Random blood glucose on admission and fingerstick BG qid
CBC, electrolytes, serum lipid profile, glycosylated Hb in a.m.
Chest x-ray and ECG in a.m.
Humulin R 10 units SC on admission
DiaBeta 10 mg, PO bid
Glucophage 500 mg, PO daily to start—will increase gradually
Humulin N 10 units SC q a.m. Begin insulin instruction for postdischarge self-care if necessary
Dicloxacillin 500 mg PO q6h, start after culture obtained
Percocet 2.5/325 mg 2 tabs PO q6h prn pain
Diet—2,400 calories, three meals with two snacks
Consult with dietitian
Up in chair ad lib with feet elevated
Foot cradle for bed
Irrigate lesion L foot with NS tid, cover with sterile dressing
Vital signs qid

Client Assessment Database

Name: R. S.   Informant: client
Age: 78   DOB: 5/3/46   Race: Caucasian   Gender: M
Adm. date: 4/28/2024   Time: 7 p.m.   From: home

Activity/Rest

Subjective (Reports)

Occupation: farmer
Usual activities/hobbies: reading, playing cards. "Don't have time to do much. Anyway, I'm too tired."
Limitations imposed by condition: "Can't walk very far, about 1/4 mile."
Sleep: Hours: 6 to 8 hr/night   Naps: no   Aids: no
Insomnia: "Not unless I drink coffee after supper."
Feels somewhat rested when awakens at 4:30 a.m.

Objective (Exhibits)
Observed response to activity: limps, favors L foot when walking
Mental status: alert/active
Muscle mass/tone: bilaterally equal/firm   Posture: slightly stooped
ROM: full   Strength: equal 3 extremities/(favors L foot currently)

Circulation

Subjective (Reports)
History of slow healing: lesion L foot, 3 weeks' duration
Extremities: Numbness/tingling: "My feet feel cold and tingly like sharp pins poking the bottom of my feet when I walk the quarter mile to the mailbox."
Cough/character of sputum: occ./white
Change in frequency/amount of urine: yes/voiding more lately

Objective (Exhibits)
Peripheral pulses: radials 2+; popliteal, dorsalis, post-tibial/pedal, all 1+
BP: R: Lying: 146/90   Sitting: 140/86   Standing: 138/90
    L: Lying: 142/88   Sitting: 138/88   Standing: 138/84
Pulse: Apical: 86   Radial: 86   Strong/regular
Chest auscultation: few wheezes clear with cough, no murmurs/rubs
Jugular vein distention: 0
Extremities:
  Temperature: feet cool bilaterally/legs warm
  Color: Skin: legs pale
  Capillary refill: slow both feet (approx. 4 sec)
  Varicosities: few enlarged superficial veins on both calves
Color:
  General: ruddy face/arms
  Mucous membranes/lips: pink
  Nailbeds: pink

Comfort

Subjective (Reports)
Primary focus: Location: medial aspect, L heel
Intensity (0 to 10): 4 to 5   Quality: dull ache with occ. sharp stabbing sensation
Frequency/duration: "Seems like all the time."
  Radiation: no
Precipitating factors: shoes, walking
  How relieved: ASA, not helping
Other complaints: sometimes has back pain following chores/heavy lifting, relieved by ASA/liniment rubdown

Objective (Exhibits)
Facial grimacing, tense/irritated, pulls foot away when lesion border palpated

Elimination

Subjective (Reports)
Usual bowel pattern: almost every p.m.
Last BM: last night Character of stool: firm/brown
 Constipation: occ.
Laxative use: hot prune juice on occ.
Urinary: no problems Character of urine: pale yellow, no odor/burning

Objective (Exhibits)
Abdomen soft/nontender
Bowel sounds: active all 4 quads

Food/Fluid

Subjective (Reports)

Usual diet 2,400 calorie; 3 meals/1 snack
Dietary pattern:
 B: fruit juice/toast/ham/decaf coffee—1 egg 3 times/wk
 L: meat/potatoes/veg/fruit/milk
 D: ½ meat sandwich/soup/fruit/decaf coffee
Snack: milk/crackers at HS. Usual beverage: skim milk, 2 to 3 cups decaf coffee, drinks "lots of water"—several quarts
Appetite: "I feel hungrier than usual."
Food allergies: none
Heartburn/food intolerance: cabbage causes gas, coffee after supper causes heartburn
Dentures: partial upper plate—fits well
Usual weight: 175 lb Has lost about 5 lb this month

Objective (Exhibits)

Wt: 170 lb Ht: 5 ft 10 in. Build: stocky
Skin turgor: good/leathery Mucous membranes: moist/pink/intact
Condition of teeth/gums: good, no irritation/bleeding noted
Bowel sounds: active all 4 quads
Urine Chemstix: 2% Fingerstick: 356 (provider office) 450 random BG on adm

Health Management

Subjective (Reports)
Dominant language: English Literate: yes
Education level: 2 yr college
Health and illness/beliefs/practices/customs: "I take care of the minor problems and see my provider only when something's broken."

Presence of advance directives: yes—wife to bring in
Durable medical power of attorney: wife
Familial risk factors/relationship:
- Diabetes: maternal uncle
- Tuberculosis: paternal uncle died, age 27
- Heart disease: father died, age 78, heart attack
- Stroke: mother died, age 81
- High BP: mother

Prescribed medications:
- Drug: DiaBeta Dose: 10 mg bid
- Schedule: 8 a.m./6 p.m., last dose 6 p.m. today
- Purpose: control diabetes
- Takes medications regularly? yes

Home urine/glucose monitoring: Only using test strips, stopped some months ago when he ran out. "It was always negative, anyway, and I don't like sticking my finger."
Nonprescription (OTC) drugs: occ. ASA
Use of alcohol (amount/frequency): socially, occ. beer
Tobacco: ½ pk/day
History of current problem: "Three weeks ago, I got a blister on my foot from breaking in my new boots. It got sore, so I lanced it, but it isn't getting any better."
Client's expectations of this hospitalization: "Clear up this infection and control my diabetes."
Evidence of failure to improve: lesion L foot, 3 wk
Last physical examination: complete 1 yr ago, office follow-up 5 mo ago

Neurosensory

Subjective (Reports)

Headache: "Occasionally behind my eyes when I worry too much."
Tingling/numbness: feet, 4 or 5 times/wk (as noted)
Eyes: Vision loss, farsighted, "Seems a little blurry now." Examination: 2 yr ago
Ears: Hearing loss R: "Some." (has not been tested)
Sense of taste/smell: "No problem."

Objective (Exhibits)

Alert, oriented to person, place, time, situation
Affect: concerned   Memory intact
Speech: clear/coherent, appropriate
Pupil: PERRLA/small
Glasses: reading   Hearing aid: no
Handgrip/release: strong/equal
Weakness/paralysis: no

Using Clinical Judgment to Create Client Plan of Care

Respiration

Subjective (Reports)
Cough: occ. morning cough, white sputum
Smoker: filters Pk/day: ½ No. yr: 60+
No CPAP/O_2 required

Objective (Exhibits)
Respiratory rate: 22 Depth: good Symmetry: equal, bilateral
Auscultation: few wheezes, clear with cough
Sputum characteristics: none to observe

Roles/Relationships

Subjective (Reports)
Relationship status: married 49 yr; Living with: wife
Reports no problems/concerns
Family: 1 daughter lives in town (30 miles away); 1 daughter married with a son, living out of state
Other: several couples, he and wife play cards/socialize with 2 to 3 times/mo, church fellowship weekly
Role: works farm alone; husband/father/grandfather; church elder

Objective (Exhibits)
Speech: clear
Verbal/nonverbal communication with family/SO(s): speaks quietly with wife, looking her in the eye; relaxed posture
Family interaction patterns: wife sitting at bedside, relaxed, both reading paper, making occasional comments to each other

Safety

Subjective (Reports)
Allergies: None
Wears seat belt
Fractures/dislocations: L clavicle, 1960s, fell getting off tractor
Arthritis/unstable joints: "Some in my knees."
Back problems: occ. lower back pain
Vision impaired: requires glasses for reading
Hearing impaired: slightly (R), compensates by turning "good ear" toward speaker
Immunizations: Annual COVID/flu last Oct./pneumonia 3 yr ago/tetanus maybe 8 yr ago
Feels safe in home/community

Objective (Exhibits)
Temperature: 99.4°F (37.4°C) Tympanic
Skin integrity: impaired L foot Scars: R inguinal, surgical

Ulcerations: medial aspect L heel, 2.5 cm diameter, approx. 3 mm deep, wound edges inflamed, draining small amount cream-color/pink-tinged matter, slight musty odor noted
Strength (general): equal all extremities   Muscle tone: firm
ROM: good   Gait: favors L foot   Tingling, prickly sensation in feet after walking ¼ mile

Self-Care

Subjective (Reports)
Independent in all ADLs

Objective (Exhibits)
General appearance: clean-shaven, short-cut hair; hands rough and dry; skin on feet dry, cracked, and scaly
No body odor

Self-Perception/Concept

Subjective (Reports)
Feels competent, successful in life
Feels respected by family/community
Denies any harmful activities

Objective (Exhibits)
Body language relaxed, good eye contact
Verbalizations positive, future oriented

Sexuality: Male

Subjective (Reports)
Sexually active: yes Use of condoms: no (monogamous)
Circumcised
Recent changes/concerns: "I've been too tired lately and some erection issues."
No self-examination practices
Last prostate exam: last year

Stress Management

Subjective (Reports)
Concerns/stress factors: "Normal farmer's problems: weather, pests, bankers, etc."
Ways of handling stress: "I get busy with the chores and talk things over with my livestock, and my wife and I have always talked things out."
Financial concerns: Medicare only and might need to hire someone to do chores while here
Lifestyle: middle class/self-sufficient farmer
Recent changes: no

Acceptance/denial of situation: "I'm in control of most things, except the weather and this diabetes now. Tried to avoid dealing with condition—left responsibility to my wife."
Concerned about possible therapy change "from pills to shots."
No desire to harm self/others

Objective (Exhibits)
Emotional status: generally calm, appears frustrated at times
Nonverbal/nonverbal body language: relaxed, congruent
Observed physiological response(s): occasionally sighs deeply/ frowns, throws up hands

Values/Beliefs

Subjective (Reports)
What gives meaning to your life: Successful family man, farmer; church and friends
Cultural factors: rural/agrarian, eastern European descent, "American," no ethnic ties
Member of spiritual community: Protestant/practicing weekly
Comfortable making decisions/moral choices
Feels connected/in harmony w/self/others/nature

Discharge Considerations (as of 4/28)
Anticipated discharge: 5/1/24 (3 days)
Resources: self, wife
Financial: "If this doesn't take too long to heal, we got some savings to cover things."
Community supports: diabetic support group (has not participated)
Anticipated lifestyle changes: "Become more involved in management of condition"
Assistance needed: may require farm help for several days
Teaching: learn new medication regimen and wound care; review diet; encourage smoking cessation
Referral: Supplies: the Downtown Pharmacy or AARP
Equipment: Glucometer—AARP
Follow-up: primary care provider 1 wk after discharge to evaluate wound healing and potential need for additional changes in diabetic regimen

Plan of Care for Mr. R. S. with Diabetes Mellitus

Recognizing Cues:
Nonhealing wound L heel 3 wks duration, 2.5-cm diameter, 3-mm deep, wound edges inflamed, small amount drainage—pinkish/cream color, R/T breaking in new boots; pain 4–5/10, random blood sugar 450 on admission

Client Diagnostic Statement: *adult Pressure Injury* related to surface friction, pressure over bony prominence, lack of knowledge of risk prevention as evidenced by partial thickness loss of dermis, pain 4–5/10 at pressure point, draining wound left heel.

Outcome: Wound Healing: Secondary Intention (NOC) Indicators: Client Will:
Be free of purulent drainage within 48 hr (4/30 1900).
Display signs of beginning healing with wound edges clean/ pink within 60 hr (5/1 0700).

INTERVENTIONS/ TAKE ACTION	RATIONALE
Wound Care (NIC)	
Irrigate wound with room-temperature sterile normal saline (NS) tid.	Cleans wound without harming delicate tissues.
Assess wound with each dressing change. Obtain wound tracing on admission and at discharge.	Provides information about effectiveness of therapy, and identifies additional needs.
Apply sterile dressing. Use paper tape.	Keeps wound clean/minimizes cross contamination. Note: Adhesive tape may be abrasive to fragile tissues.
Infection Control (NIC)	
Follow wound precautions.	Use of gloves and proper handling of contaminated dressings reduces likelihood of spread of infection.
Obtain sterile specimen of wound drainage on admission.	Culture/sensitivity identifies pathogens and therapy of choice.

Using Clinical Judgment to Create Client Plan of Care

INTERVENTIONS/ TAKE ACTION	RATIONALE
Administer dicloxacillin 500 mg per os (PO) q6h, starting 10 p.m.	Treatment of infection and prevention of complications. Note: Food interferes with drug absorption, requiring scheduling around meals.
Observe for signs of hypersensitivity: pruritus, urticaria, rash.	Although no history of penicillin reaction, it may occur at any time.

Recognizing Cues:

T2 diabetes mellitus for 10 yr, random blood sugar 450 on adm, stopped monitoring diabetes some months ago

Client Diagnostic Statement:

Blood Glucose [Not] Within Normal Limits as evidenced by lack of understanding and poor control of blood glucose (fingerstick 450/adm).

Outcome: Blood Glucose Level (NOC)
Indicators: Client Will:

Demonstrate correction of metabolic state as evidenced by fasting blood sugar (FBS) less than 170 mg/dL within 36 hr (4/30 0700).

INTERVENTIONS/ TAKE ACTION	RATIONALE
Hyperglycemia Management (NIC)	
Perform fingerstick blood glucose (BG) qid. Call for BG > 250.	Bedside analysis of blood glucose levels is a more timely method for monitoring effectiveness of therapy and provides direction for alteration of medications such as additional regular insulin.
Administer antidiabetic medications:	Treats underlying metabolic dysfunction, reducing hyperglycemia and promoting healing.

INTERVENTIONS/ TAKE ACTION	RATIONALE
10 Units Humulin N insulin subcutaneous (SC) every a.m. after fingerstick BG	Intermediate-acting preparation with onset of 2 to 4 hr, peaks at 6 to 12 hr, with a duration of 18 to 24 hr. Increases transport of glucose into cells and promotes the conversion of glucose to glycogen.
DiaBeta 10 mg PO bid	Lowers blood glucose by stimulating the release of insulin from the pancreas and increasing the sensitivity to insulin at the receptor sites.
Glucophage 500 mg PO daily; note onset of side effects	Glucophage lowers serum glucose levels by decreasing hepatic glucose production and intestinal glucose absorption and increasing sensitivity to insulin. By using it in conjunction with DiaBeta, client may be able to discontinue insulin once target dosage is achieved (e.g., 2,000 mg/day). An increase of 1 tablet per week is necessary to limit side effects of diarrhea, abdominal cramping, vomiting, possibly leading to dehydration and prerenal azotemia.
Provide diet of 2,400 cals—3 meals/2 snacks.	Proper diet decreases glucose levels/insulin needs, prevents hyperglycemic episodes, can reduce serum cholesterol levels and promote satiation.
Schedule consultation with dietitian to restructure meal plan and evaluate food choices.	Calories are unchanged on new orders but have been redistributed to three meals and two snacks. Dietary choices (e.g., increased vitamin C) may enhance healing.

CLIENT SITUATION AND PROTOTYPE PLAN OF CARE

Using Clinical Judgment to Create Client Plan of Care

Recognizing Cues:
Open wound L heel, pain 4–5/10, constant dull ache with occasional sharp stabbing, limps/favors L foot when walking, grimacing/tense and withdraws foot when lesion palpated

Client Diagnostic Statement:
acute Pain related to physical injury agent (open wound left foot), as evidenced by self-report of pain intensity using standardized pain scale (4 to 5/10), facial expression, and protective behavior.

Outcome: Pain Level (NOC) Indicators:
Client Will:
Report pain is minimized/relieved within 1 hr of analgesic administration (ongoing).
Report absence or control of pain by discharge (5/1).

Outcome: Pain Disruptive Effects (NOC) Indicators: Client Will:
Ambulate with ease, full weight-bearing by discharge (5/1).

INTERVENTIONS/ TAKE ACTION	RATIONALE
Pain Management: Acute (NIC)	
Determine pain characteristics through client's description.	Establishes baseline for assessing improvement/changes.
Place foot cradle on bed; encourage use of loose-fitting slipper when up.	Avoids direct pressure to area of injury, which could result in vasoconstriction/increased pain.
Administer Percocet 2.5/325 mg 2 tabs PO q6h as needed. Document effectiveness.	Provides relief of discomfort when unrelieved by other measures.

Recognizing Cues:
Leg pulses 1+, capillary refill 4 sec, skin pale legs, legs warm/feet cool, tingling/numbness feet walking distance, delayed peripheral wound healing, tobacco use

Client Diagnostic Statement:
ineffective peripheral Tissue Perfusion related to inadequate knowledge of disease process and modifiable factors, as evidenced by decrease in peripheral pulses, alteration in skin characteristics [pale/cool feet]; capillary refill 4 sec; parathesia [feet "when walks ¼ mile."]

Outcome: Knowledge: Diabetes Management (NOC) Indicators: Client Will:

Verbalize understanding of relationship between chronic disease (diabetes mellitus) and circulatory changes within 48 hr (4/30 1900).

Demonstrate awareness of safety factors and proper foot care within 48 hr (4/30 1900).

Maintain adequate level of hydration to maximize perfusion, as evidenced by balanced intake/output, moist skin/mucous membranes, and capillary refill less than 4 sec (daily/ongoing).

INTERVENTIONS/ TAKE ACTION	RATIONALE
Circulatory Care: Arterial Insufficiency (NIC)	
Elevate feet when up in chair. Avoid long periods with feet in a dependent position.	Minimizes interruption of blood flow, reduces venous pooling.
Assess for signs of dehydration. Monitor intake/output. Encourage oral fluids.	Glycosuria may result in dehydration with consequent reduction of circulating volume and further impairment of peripheral circulation.
Instruct client to avoid constricting clothing and socks, and ill-fitting shoes.	Compromised circulation and decreased pain sensation may precipitate or aggravate tissue breakdown.
Reinforce safety precautions regarding use of heating pads, hot water bottles, or soaks.	Heat increases metabolic demands on compromised tissues. Vascular insufficiency alters pain sensation, increasing risk of injury.
Recommend cessation of smoking.	Vascular constriction associated with smoking and diabetes impairs peripheral circulation.

Using Clinical Judgment to Create Client Plan of Care

INTERVENTIONS/ TAKE ACTION	RATIONALE
Discuss complications of disease that result from vascular changes: ulceration, gangrene, muscle or bony structure changes.	Although proper control of diabetes mellitus may not prevent complications, severity of effect may be minimized. Diabetic foot complications are the leading cause of nontraumatic lower extremity amputations. **Note:** Client's dry, cracked, scaly skin; feet cool; and pain when walking a distance suggest mild to moderate vascular disease (peripheral arterial insufficiency) that can limit response to infection, impair wound healing, and increase risk of bony deformities.
Review proper foot care as outlined in teaching plan.	Altered perfusion of lower extremities may lead to serious or persistent complications at the cellular level.

Recognizing Cues:

T2DM 10 yr, random BG 450 on adm, Chemstic 2%, increased thirst/urination, stopped home glucose monitoring, inappropriate foot care—lanced heel blister, smokes ½ pk/day, relies on wife to manage his condition, concerned about changing meds and addition of insulin

Client Diagnostic Statement:

ineffective Health Self-Management related to inadequate knowledge of therapeutic regimen, unaware of seriousness of condition or susceptibility to sequela as evidenced by failure to include treatment regimen in daily living [home glucose monitoring, foot care], inattentive to disease signs/symptoms, and failing to take action that reduces risk factors.

Outcome: Knowledge: Diabetes Management (NOC) Indicators: Client Will:

Perform procedure for home glucose monitoring correctly within 36 hr (4/30 0700).

Verbalize basic understanding of disease process and treatment within 38 hr (4/30 0900).

Explain reasons for actions within 38 hr (4/30 0900).

Perform insulin administration correctly within 60 hr (5/1 0700).

GENERATE SOLUTIONS/ TAKE ACTION	RATIONALE
Teaching: Disease Process (NIC)	
Determine client's level of knowledge, priorities of learning needs, desire/need for including wife in instruction.	Establishes baseline and direction for teaching/planning. Involvement of wife, if desired, will provide additional resource for recall/understanding and may enhance client's follow-through.
Provide teaching guide, "Understanding Your Diabetes," 4/29 a.m. Show film "Living with Diabetes," 4/29 4 p.m., when wife is visiting. Include in group teaching session 4/30 a.m. Review information and obtain feedback from client/wife.	Provides different methods for accessing/reinforcing information and enhances opportunity for learning/understanding.
Discuss factors related to and altering diabetic control such as stress, illness, exercise.	Drug therapy/diet may need to be altered in response to both short-term and long-term stressors and changes in activity level.
Review signs/symptoms of hyperglycemia (e.g., fatigue, nausea, vomiting, polyuria, polydipsia). Discuss how to prevent and evaluate this situation and when to seek medical care. Have client identify appropriate interventions.	Recognition and understanding of these signs/symptoms and timely intervention will aid client in avoiding recurrences and preventing complications.

Using Clinical Judgment to Create Client Plan of Care

GENERATE SOLUTIONS/ TAKE ACTION	RATIONALE
Review and provide information about necessity for routine examination of feet and proper foot care (e.g., daily inspection for injuries, pressure areas, corns, calluses; proper nail care; daily washing and application of good moisturizing lotion such as Eucerin, Nivea bid). Recommend wearing loose-fitting socks and properly fitting shoes (break new shoes in gradually) and avoid going barefoot. If foot injury/skin break occurs, wash with soap/dermal cleanser and water, cover with sterile dressing, and inspect wound and change dressing daily; report redness, swelling, or presence of drainage.	Reduces risk of tissue injury; promotes understanding and prevention of pressure injury formation and wound-healing difficulties.

Teaching: Prescribed Medication (NIC)

Instruct regarding prescribed insulin therapy:	May be a temporary treatment of hyperglycemia with infection or may be permanent addition to/replacement of oral hypoglycemic agent.
Humulin N Insulin, SC.	Intermediate-acting insulin generally lasts 18 to 24 hr, with peak effect between 6 and 12 hr.
Keep vial in current use at room temperature (if used within 30 days).	Cold insulin is poorly absorbed.
Store extra vials in refrigerator.	Refrigeration prevents wide fluctuations in temperature, prolonging the drug shelf life.

GENERATE SOLUTIONS/ TAKE ACTION	RATIONALE
Roll bottle and invert to mix, or shake gently, avoiding bubbles.	Vigorous shaking may create foam, which can interfere with accurate dose withdrawal and may damage the insulin molecule. **Note:** New research suggests that shaking the vial may be more effective in mixing suspension. (Refer to Facility Procedure Manual.)
Choice of injection sites (e.g., across lower abdomen in a Z pattern).	Provides for steady absorption of medication. Site is easily visualized and accessible by client, and a Z pattern minimizes tissue damage.
Demonstrate, then observe client drawing insulin into syringe, reading syringe markings, and administering dose. Assess for accuracy.	May require several instruction sessions and practice before client/wife feel comfortable drawing up and injecting medication.
Instruct in signs/symptoms of insulin reaction or hypoglycemia: fatigue, nausea, headache, hunger, sweating, irritability, shakiness, anxiety, or difficulty concentrating.	Knowing what to watch for and appropriate treatment such as ½ cup of grape juice for immediate response and a snack within ½ hr (e.g., one slice of bread with peanut butter or cheese, or fruit and slice of cheese for sustained effect) may prevent or minimize complications.
Review "Sick Day Rules" (e.g., call the doctor if too sick to eat normally or stay active) and take insulin as ordered. Keep record as noted in Sick Day Guide.	Understanding of necessary actions in the event of mild-to-severe illness promotes competent self-care and reduces risk of hyper-/hypoglycemia.

Using Clinical Judgment to Create Client Plan of Care

GENERATE SOLUTIONS/ TAKE ACTION	RATIONALE
Instruct client/wife in fingerstick glucose monitoring to be done qid until stable, then bid, rotating times such as FBS and before dinner or before lunch and HS. Observe return demonstrations of the procedure.	Fingerstick monitoring provides accurate and timely information regarding diabetic status. Return demonstration verifies correct learning.
Recommend client maintain record/log of fingerstick testing, antidiabetic medication, insulin dosage/site, unusual physiological response, and dietary intake. Outline desired goals of FBS 80–110, premeal 80–130.	Provides accurate record for review by caregivers for assessment of therapy effectiveness/needs.
Discuss other healthcare issues, such as smoking habits, self-monitoring for cancer (breasts/testicles), and reporting changes in general well-being.	Encourages client involvement awareness, and responsibility for own health; promotes wellness. **Note:** Smoking tends to increase client's resistance to insulin.

Another Approach to Planning Client Care—Mind or Concept Mapping

Another way to conceptualize the client's problems/care needs is to create a Mind or Concept Map. This technique was developed to help visualize the linkages between various client symptoms, problems, or interventions, as they impact each other. The parts that are great about traditional care plans (problem-solving and categorizing) are retained, but the linear or columnar nature of the plan is changed to a design that uses the whole brain—a design that brings left-brain, linear problem-solving thinking together with the freewheeling, interconnected, creative right brain. Joining mind mapping and care planning enables the nurse to create a holistic view of the client, strengthening critical-thinking skills and facilitating the creative process of planning client care.

Mind mapping starts in the center of the page with a representation of the main concept—the client. (This helps keep in mind that the client is the focus of the plan, not the medical diagnosis or condition.) From that central thought, other main ideas that relate to the client are added. Different concepts can be grouped together by geometric shapes, color coding, or placement on the page. Connections and interconnections between groups of ideas are represented by the use of arrows or lines with defining phrases added that explain how the interconnected thoughts relate to one another. In this manner, many different pieces of information/cues *about* the client can be connected directly *to* the client.

Whichever piece is chosen becomes the first layer of connections—clustered assessment data, NDs, or outcomes. For example, a map could start with NDs featured as the first "branches," each one being listed separately in some way on the map. Next, the signs and symptoms or cues supporting the diagnoses could be added, or the plan could begin with the client outcomes to be achieved with connections then to NDs. When the plan is completed, there should be an ND (supported by cues from the assessment data and the nurse's general knowledge), solutions generated using clinical judgment–nursing interventions/actions, desired client outcomes, and any evaluation data, all connected in a manner that shows there is a relationship between them. It is critical to understand that there is no preset order for the pieces because one cluster is not more or less important than another (or one is not "subsumed" under another). It is important, however, that those pieces within a branch be in the same order in each branch.

Using Clinical Judgment to Create Client Plan of Care

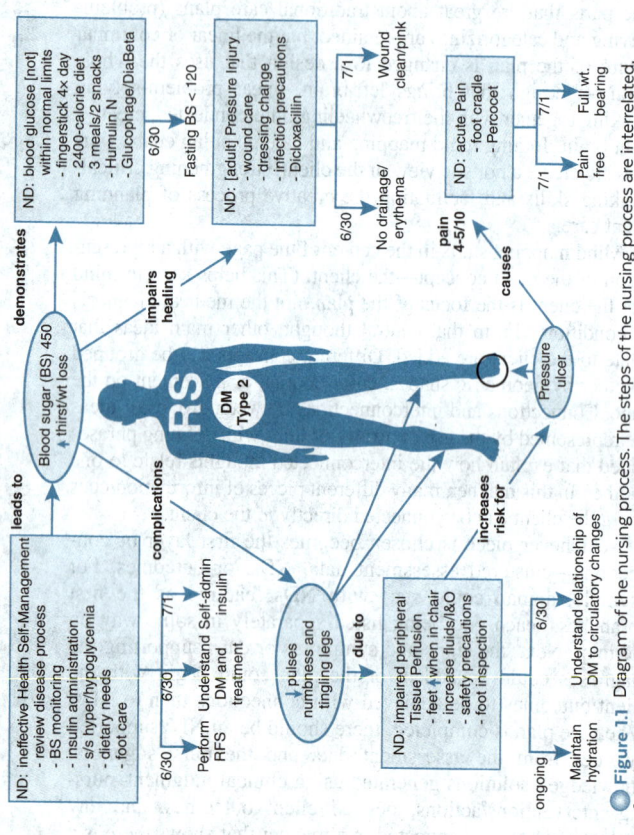

Figure 1.1 Diagram of the nursing process. The steps of the nursing process are interrelated, forming a continuous circle of thought and action that is both dynamic and cyclic.

Index

A

Abdominal aortic aneurysm. *See* Aortic aneurysm, abdominal (AAA)
Abdominal hysterectomy, 1070
Abdominal perineal resection, 1070
Abdominal wound dehiscence, 1107
Abortion
  elective termination, 1070
  spontaneous termination, 1070
Abruptio placentae, 1070
Abscess
  brain, 1070–1071
  skin/tissue, 1071
Abuse
  depressant, 1109–1110
  hallucinogen, 1128
  laxative, 1144
  neglect and, 1155
  opioid, 1158
  physical, 1071
  psychological, 1071
  rehabilitation, 1184–1185
  stimulant, 1184
Achalasia, 1071–1072
Acidosis
  metabolic, 1072
  respiratory, 1072
Acne, 1072
Acoustic neuroma, 1072
Acquired immune deficiency syndrome (AIDS), 1072–1073
  dementia, 1075
Acromegaly, 1073
Activity intolerance, 5–11
Activity/rest diagnostic division
  activity intolerance, 5–11
  in adult medical/surgical assessment tool, 1198
  diversional activity engagement, decreased, 237–242
  fatigue, 329–335
  mobility, impaired bed, 598–603
  mobility, impaired physical, 603–609
  mobility, impaired wheelchair, 609–613
  motor development, delayed infant, 622–626
  nursing diagnoses related to, 1205
  in prototype plan of care, 1212–1213
  sedentary behaviors, excessive, 813–818
  sitting ability, impaired, 877–882
  sleep pattern, ineffective, 893–897
  standing ability, impaired, 920–923
  transferring ability, impaired, 1006–1010
  walking ability, impaired, 1051–1055
Acute mountain sickness (AMS), 1151
Acute polyneuritis, 1127
Acute respiratory distress syndrome, 1073
Acute substance withdrawal syndrome, 11–18
Adams-Stokes syndrome, 1073
Addiction, 1073
Addison disease, 1073–1074

Adenoidectomy, 1074
Adjustment disorder, 1074
Adolescent pregnancy, 1169–1170
Adoption/loss of child custody, 1074
Adrenal crisis, acute, 1074
Adrenalectomy, 1074–1075
Adrenal insufficiency, 1075
Affective disorder, 1075
    seasonal, 1075
Agoraphobia, 1075
Agranulocytosis, 1075
Airway clearance, impaired, 18–24
Alcohol intoxication, acute, 1075–1076
Alcohol use disorder, 1076
Aldosteronism, primary, 1076
Alkalosis
    metabolic, 1076
    respiratory, 1076
Allergies, seasonal, 1076
Allergy reaction, risk for, 24–28
Alzheimer disease, 1077
American College of Cardiology/American Heart Association (ACC/AHA) heart failure guidelines, 112
American Nurses Association (ANA), 1
Amphetamine abuse, 1077
Amputation, 1077–1078
Amyotrophic lateral sclerosis (ALS), 1078
Anaphylaxis, 1078
Anemia, 1078
    aplastic, 1083
    iron-deficiency, 1079
    pernicious, 1079
    sickle cell, 1079
Aneurysm
    abdominal aortic, 1080
    cerebral, 1080
    ventricular, 1080
Angina pectoris, 1080
Ankle sprain, 1183
Anorexia nervosa, 1080–1081
Antisocial personality disorder, 1081
Anxiety, 28–35
    death, 209–214
Anxiety disorder, generalized, 1081–1082
Anxiety disorders, 1082
Anxiolytic abuse, 1082
Aortic aneurysm, abdominal (AAA), 1082
    repair, 1082–1083
Aortic stenosis, 1083
Aplastic anemia, 1083
Appendicitis, 1083
Arrhythmia, cardiac, 1083
Arterial occlusive disease, peripheral, 1083–1084
Arthritis
    juvenile rheumatoid, 1084
    rheumatoid, 1084
    septic, 1084
Arthroplasty, 1084–1085
Arthroscopy, knee, 1085
Asperger disorder, 1085

Aspiration
 foreign body, 1085
 risk for, 35–40
Assessment tools, adult medical/surgical, 1198–1204
Asthma, 1085
Atherosclerosis, 1163
Athlete's foot, 1085
Atrial fibrillation, 1085–1086
Atrial flutter, 1086
Atrial tachycardia, 1086
Attention-deficit disorder, 1086
Autism spectrum disorder, 1086–1087
Autonomic dysreflexia, risk for, 41–45

B

Barbiturate abuse, 1087
Battered child syndrome, 1087
Benign prostatic hyperplasia, 1087
Bipolar disorder, 1088
Bladder cancer, 1088
Bleeding, risk for excessive, 45–50
Blood glucose within normal limits, 51–58
 in sample plan of care for diabetes mellitus, 1220–1222
Blood pressure, risk for imbalanced, 58–63
Blood transfusion reaction, 1189
Body image, disturbed, 63–70
Body temperature
 decreased, 70–76
 decreased neonatal, 76–80
 risk for decreased perioperative, 80–83
Body weight problem, 83–89
Bone cancer, 1088–1089
Bone marrow transplantation, 1089
Borderline personality disorder, 1089
Botulism, 1089–1090
Bowel obstruction, 1090
Brain abscess, 1070–1071
Brain concussion, 1103
Brain injury, traumatic, 1190–1191
Brain tumor, 1090
Breast cancer, 1090
Breastfeeding
 difficulty performing, 90–98
 interrupted, 98–105
Breathing pattern, ineffective, 105–111
Bronchitis, 1090
Bronchopneumonia, 1091
Bulimia nervosa, 1091
Burns, 1091–1092
Bursitis, 1092

C

Calculi, urinary, 1092
Cancer, 1092–1093
 bladder, 1088
 bone, 1088–1089
 brain tumor, 1090
 breast, 1090
 chemotherapy, 1098

Cancer, (*continued*)
   leukemia, acute, 1145–1146
   leukemia, chronic, 1146
   malignant melanoma, 1149
   multiple myeloma, 1153
   Wilms tumor, 1195
Candidiasis, 1093
Cannabis abuse, 1093
Carbon monoxide poisoning, 1093
Cardiac arrhythmia, 1083
Cardiac catheterization, 1093–1094
Cardiac dysrhythmia, 1117–1118
Cardiac output, impaired, 111–121
Cardiac surgery, 1094
Cardiogenic shock, 1094, 1181
Cardiomyopathy, 1094
Cardiovascular function, risk for impaired, 122–126
Caregiver child attachment, impaired, 126–132
Caregiving burden, excessive, 133–140
Carotid endarterectomy, 1094
Carpal tunnel syndrome, 1095
Casts, 1095
Cataract, 1095
Cat scratch disease, 1095
Celiac disease, 1096
Cellulitis, 1096
Cerebral aneurysm, 1080
Cerebral palsy, 1159
Cerebrovascular accident (CVA), 1096–1097
Cervical laminectomy, 1143
Cervix, dysfunctional, 1097
Cesarean birth
   postpartal, 1097
   unplanned, 1097–1098
Chemotherapy, 1098
Childbearing process, ineffective, 141–151
Cholecystectomy, 1098
Cholelithiasis, 1098–1099
Chronic fatigue syndrome, 1122
Chronic obstructive lung disease, 1099
Circulation diagnostic division
   in adult medical/surgical assessment tool, 1198
   autonomic dysreflexia, risk for, 41–45
   bleeding, risk for excessive, 45–50
   blood pressure, risk for imbalanced, 58–63
   cardiac output, impaired, 111–121
   cardiovascular function, risk for impaired, 122–126
   lymphedema self-management, ineffective, 581–586
   neurovascular function, risk for impaired peripheral, 653–658
   nursing diagnoses related to, 1205–1206
   in prototype plan of care, 1213
   shock, risk for, 872–877
   thrombosis, risk for, 977–980
   tissue perfusion, ineffective peripheral, 992–1000
   tissue perfusion, risk for ineffective cerebral, 1000–1006
Circumcision, 1099
Cirrhosis, 1099–1100
Cleft lip/palate, 1100
Client assessment database, 1212
Clinical judgment, 2–4, 1197, 1211
Cocaine abuse, 1100–1101

Cocaine hydrochloride poisoning, acute, 1100
Coccidioidomycosis, 1101
Colitis, ulcerative, 1101
Colostomy, 1101–1102
Coma, 1102
  diabetic, 1102
Comfort diagnostic division
  in adult medical/surgical assessment tool, 1199
  discomfort, 229–237
  dry eye, risk for, 242–245
  dry mouth self-management, ineffective, 246–250
  end-of-life comfort syndrome, impaired, 297–300
  nursing diagnoses related to, 1206
  pain, acute, 684–692
  pain, chronic, and chronic pain syndrome, 692–702
  pain, labor, 702–708
  pain self-management, ineffective, 709–717
  in prototype plan of care, 1213–1214
Communication, impaired verbal, 151–160
Community/home (CH) specialty area, 1069
Compartment syndrome, extremity, 1102
Complex regional pain syndrome, 1103
Concept mapping, 1229–1230
Concussion, brain, 1103
Conduct disorder, 1103–1104
Confusion
  acute, 160–166
  chronic, 166–170
Congestive heart failure, 1104
Conn syndrome, 1104
Constipation, 1104
  chronic functional, 171–176
Contact dermatitis, 1111
Contamination exposure, 176–185
Continence, impaired fecal, 185–192
Coping
  difficulty, 192–199
  impaired community, 200–203
  impaired family, 203–208
Coronary artery bypass surgery, 1104
Coronary artery disease, 1104
Craniotomy, 1104–1105
Crohn disease, 1105
Croup, 1105
  membranous, 1105
Cubital tunnel syndrome, 1105–1106
Cues
  activity intolerance, 5–6
  acute substance withdrawal syndrome, 12
  airway clearance, impaired, 18–19
  allergy reaction, risk for, 24–25
  anxiety, 28–29
  aspiration, risk for, 35–36
  autonomic dysreflexia, risk for, 41
  bleeding, risk for excessive, 45
  blood glucose within normal limits, 51
  blood pressure, risk for imbalanced, 58–59
  body image, disturbed, 63–64
  body temperature, decreased, 70–71
  body temperature, decreased neonatal, 76–77
  body temperature, risk for decreased perioperative, 80–81

Index

Cues (*continued*)
- body weight problem, 83–84
- breastfeeding, difficulty performing, 90–91
- breastfeeding, interrupted, 98–99
- breathing pattern, ineffective, 105–106
- cardiac output, impaired, 111–112
- cardiovascular function, risk for impaired, 122
- caregiver child attachment, impaired, 127
- caregiving burden, excessive, 133–134
- childbearing process, ineffective, 141–142
- communication, impaired verbal, 152
- confusion, acute, 160–161
- confusion, chronic, 166
- constipation, chronic functional, 171–172
- contamination exposure, 176–177
- continence, impaired fecal, 186
- coping, difficulty, 192–193
- coping, impaired community, 200
- coping, impaired family, 204
- death anxiety, 209–210
- decision-making, impaired, 215
- development, delayed child, 220
- dignity, risk for compromised, 226
- discomfort, 230
- diversional activity engagement, decreased, 237–238
- dry eye, risk for, 242–243
- dry mouth self-management, ineffective, 246–247
- eating dynamics, ineffective adolescent, 251
- eating dynamics, ineffective child, 256–257
- elder frailty syndrome, 261–262
- elimination, impaired intestinal, 267–268
- elimination, impaired urinary, 276
- elopement, risk for, 283
- emancipated decision-making, impaired, 289
- emotion regulation, ineffective, 294
- end-of-life comfort syndrome, impaired, 297–298
- energy field, disrupted, 301
- exercise engagement, readiness for enhanced, 305–306
- fall, risk for, 309
- family identity syndrome, disrupted, 316–317
- family process, impaired, 322–323
- fatigue, 329
- fear, 336
- feeding behavior, impaired infant, 342–343
- female genital mutilation, risk for, 347
- fluid volume, excessive, 358–359
- fluid volume, inadequate, 365–366
- fluid volume balance, risk for impaired, 352
- gas exchange, impaired, 374–375
- gastrointestinal motility, impaired, 383
- grief, 391–392
- grief, dysfunctional, 396–397
- growth, delayed child, 403–404
- health knowledge, inadequate, 409–410
- health literacy, inadequate, 415–416
- health maintenance behaviors, ineffective, 420–421
- health management, ineffective community, 426
- health management, ineffective family, 430–431
- health self-management, ineffective, 434–435
- healthy aging, readiness for enhanced, 440
- home maintenance behaviors, ineffective, 443–444

hope, readiness for enhanced, 446–448
human milk production, inadequate, 451–452
hyperbilirubinemia, neonatal, 457
hyperthermia, 464
immigration transition, risk for disrupted, 472
immunologic impairment, 476–477
impulse control, ineffective, 483
incontinence, disability-associated urinary, 487–488
incontinence, mixed urinary, 494–495
incontinence, stress urinary, 503
incontinence, urge urinary, 510
infection, risk for, 517
injury, risk for burn, 525
injury, risk for cold, 531
injury, risk for corneal, 535
injury, risk for occupational physical, 538–539
injury, risk for perioperative positioning, 544–545
injury, risk for physical, 549
injury, risk for urinary tract, 555
interaction patterns, disrupted family, 559–560
latex allergy, risk for, 567
liver function, risk for impaired, 570
loneliness, excessive, 575–576
lymphedema self-management, ineffective, 581–582
maternal-fetal dyad, risk for impaired, 586
memory, impaired, 594
mobility, impaired bed, 598–599
mobility, impaired physical, 603–604
mobility, impaired wheelchair, 609
mood regulation, impaired, 613–614
moral distress, 617–618
motor development, delayed infant, 622
mucous membrane, impaired oral, 627–628
nausea, 634–635
neonatal abstinence syndrome, 640
neurodevelopmental organization, impaired infant, 646–647
neurovascular function, risk for impaired peripheral, 653
nipple-areolar complex integrity, impaired, 658–659
nutritional intake, inadequate, 664–665
occupational illness, risk for, 672
overweight self-management, ineffective, 675–676
pain, acute, 684
pain, chronic, and chronic pain syndrome, 692–693
pain, labor, 702–703
pain self-management, ineffective, 709–710
parenting, impaired, 718–719
personal identity, disturbed, 726
poisoning, risk for, 732
post-trauma syndrome, 738
pressure injury, adult, 751–752
pressure injury, child, 759–760
pressure injury, neonatal, 767
relationship, ineffective intimate partner, 773–774
relationship problem, 778
religiosity, impaired, 783
relocation stress, risk for, 789
resilience, lack of, 795
retention, risk for urinary, 802–803
role performance, impaired, 808–809
sedentary behaviors, excessive, 813
self-care deficit, 819–820

Index

Cues (*continued*)
- self-compassion, inadequate, 830–831
- self-concept, readiness for enhanced, 834
- self-esteem, chronic inadequate, 838–839
- self-esteem, situational inadequate, 845–846
- self-injurious behavior, non-suicidal, 851–853
- sensory deficit, 858–859
- sexual functioning, impaired, 865
- shock, risk for, 872
- sitting ability, impaired, 878
- skin integrity, impaired, 882–883
- sleep pattern, ineffective, 893–894
- social connectedness, inadequate, 897–898
- social identity, readiness for enhanced transgender, 904
- social support network, inadequate, 908–909
- spiritual well-being, impaired, 913–914
- standing ability, impaired, 920
- suck-swallow response, ineffective infant, 924–925
- sudden infant death, risk for, 928
- suffocation, risk for accidental, 933–934
- suicide, risk for, 938–939, 945–946
- surgical wound infection, risk for, 952
- swallowing, impaired, 956–958
- thermoregulation, ineffective, 964
- thought process, disrupted, 969
- thrombosis, risk for, 977–978
- tissue integrity, impaired, 981–982
- tissue perfusion, ineffective peripheral, 992–993
- tissue perfusion, risk for ineffective cerebral, 1000
- transferring ability, impaired, 1006–1007
- underweight self-management, ineffective, 1010–1012
- ventilation, impaired spontaneous, 1019–1020
- ventilatory weaning response, impaired adult, 1027–1028
- ventilatory weaning response, impaired child, 1034–1035
- violence, risk for other-directed, 1041–1042
- walking ability, impaired, 1051–1052
- water-electrolyte imbalance, risk for impaired, 1056
- weight self-management, readiness for enhanced, 1064

Cushing syndrome, 1106
Cystic fibrosis, 1106
Cystitis, 1106–1107
Cytomegalic inclusion disease, 1107
Cytomegalovirus (CMV) infection, 1107

D

Death anxiety, 209–214
Decision-making, impaired, 215–220
Deep vein thrombosis, 1107
Degenerative disc disease, 1107
Degenerative joint disease, 1107, 1158
Dehiscence, abdominal wound, 1107
Dehydration, 1107
Delirium tremens, 1107–1108
Delivery, precipitous/out of hospital, 1108
Delusional disorder, 1108–1109
Dementia
  AIDS, 1075
  HIV, 1109
  presenile/senile, 1109
Depressant abuse, 1109–1110

Depression
  major, 1110
  postpartum, 1110–1111
Dermatitis, contact, 1111
Development, delayed child, 220–225
Diabetes
  gestational, 1111
  juvenile, 1111–1112
Diabetes insipidus, 1111
Diabetes mellitus, 1112
  sample plan of care for client with, 1219–1228
Diabetic coma, 1102
Diabetic ketoacidosis, 1112
Diagnostic divisions (DDs), 1069, 1205–1210
Dialysis
  general, 1112–1113
  peritoneal, 1113
Diaper rash, 1113
Diarrhea, 1114
Digitalis toxicity, 1114
Dignity, risk for compromised, 225–229
Dilation and curettage, 1114
Dilation of cervix, premature, 1114
Discharge considerations, 1218
Discomfort, 229–237
Dislocation/subluxation of joint, 1114–1115
Disruptive behavior disorder, 1115
Disseminated intravascular coagulation (DIC), 1115
Dissociative disorders, 1115
Diversional activity engagement, decreased, 237–242
Diverticulitis, 1115–1116
Documentation focus
  activity intolerance, 11
  acute substance withdrawal syndrome, 17–18
  airway clearance, impaired, 24
  allergy reaction, risk for, 27
  anxiety, 35
  aspiration, risk for, 40
  autonomic dysreflexia, risk for, 44–45
  bleeding, risk for excessive, 50
  blood glucose within normal limits, 57–58
  blood pressure, risk for imbalanced, 62–63
  body image, disturbed, 69–70
  body temperature, decreased, 76
  body temperature, decreased neonatal, 80
  body temperature, risk for decreased perioperative, 83
  body weight problem, 89
  breastfeeding, difficulty performing, 97–98
  breastfeeding, interrupted, 104
  breathing pattern, ineffective, 110–111
  cardiac output, impaired, 121
  cardiovascular function, risk for impaired, 126
  caregiver child attachment, impaired, 132
  caregiving burden, excessive, 140
  childbearing process, ineffective, 151
  communication, impaired verbal, 159–160
  confusion, acute, 165
  confusion, chronic, 170
  constipation, chronic functional, 175–176
  contamination exposure, 185
  continence, impaired fecal, 191

Index

Documentation focus (*continued*)
- coping, difficulty, 199
- coping, impaired community, 203
- coping, impaired family, 208
- death anxiety, 214
- decision-making, impaired, 219–220
- development, delayed child, 225
- dignity, risk for compromised, 229
- discomfort, 237
- diversional activity engagement, decreased, 242
- dry eye, risk for, 245
- dry mouth self-management, ineffective, 250
- eating dynamics, ineffective adolescent, 255
- eating dynamics, ineffective child, 260
- elder frailty syndrome, 266–267
- elimination, impaired intestinal, 275
- elimination, impaired urinary, 282–283
- elopement, risk for, 288
- emancipated decision-making, impaired, 293
- emotion regulation, ineffective, 296–297
- end-of-life comfort syndrome, impaired, 300
- energy field, disrupted, 304–305
- exercise engagement, readiness for enhanced, 308
- fall, risk for, 315–316
- family identity syndrome, disrupted, 321
- family process, impaired, 328
- fatigue, 335
- fear, 341–342
- feeding behavior, impaired infant, 346–347
- female genital mutilation, risk for, 351
- fluid volume, excessive, 365
- fluid volume, inadequate, 373–374
- fluid volume balance, risk for impaired, 357–358
- gas exchange, impaired, 382
- gastrointestinal motility, impaired, 390–391
- grief, 395–396
- grief, dysfunctional, 402–403
- growth, delayed child, 408
- health knowledge, inadequate, 414–415
- health literacy, inadequate, 419–420
- health maintenance behaviors, ineffective, 425
- health management, ineffective community, 429–430
- health management, ineffective family, 433–434
- health self-management, ineffective, 439
- healthy aging, readiness for enhanced, 442–443
- home maintenance behaviors, ineffective, 447
- hope, readiness for enhanced, 450–451
- human milk production, inadequate, 456–457
- hyperbilirubinemia, neonatal, 463
- hyperthermia, 471
- immigration transition, risk for disrupted, 475–476
- immunologic impairment, 482
- impulse control, ineffective, 487
- incontinence, disability-associated urinary, 494
- incontinence, mixed urinary, 502
- incontinence, stress urinary, 509–510
- incontinence, urge urinary, 516
- infection, risk for, 524
- injury, risk for burn, 530–531
- injury, risk for cold, 534
- injury, risk for corneal, 538

injury, risk for occupational physical, 543
injury, risk for perioperative positioning, 548
injury, risk for physical, 554–555
injury, risk for urinary tract, 559
interaction patterns, disrupted family, 566
latex allergy, risk for, 569–570
liver function, risk for impaired, 574–575
loneliness, excessive, 580
lymphedema self-management, ineffective, 585–586
maternal-fetal dyad, risk for impaired, 593
memory, impaired, 597–598
mobility, impaired bed, 602
mobility, impaired physical, 608–609
mobility, impaired wheelchair, 612–613
mood regulation, impaired, 616–617
moral distress, 621
motor development, delayed infant, 626
mucous membrane, impaired oral, 633–634
nausea, 639–640
neonatal abstinence syndrome, 645
neurodevelopmental organization, impaired infant, 652–653
neurovascular function, risk for impaired peripheral, 657–658
nipple-areolar complex integrity, impaired, 663
nutritional intake, inadequate, 671
occupational illness, risk for, 674–675
overweight self-management, ineffective, 683
pain, acute, 691–692
pain, chronic, and chronic pain syndrome, 701–702
pain, labor, 708
pain self-management, ineffective, 717–718
parenting, impaired, 725
personal identity, disturbed, 731
poisoning, risk for, 737
post-trauma syndrome, 750–751
pressure injury, adult, 758
pressure injury, child, 766
pressure injury, neonatal, 772
relationship, ineffective intimate partner, 777
relationship problem, 782
religiosity, impaired, 788–789
relocation stress, risk for, 795
resilience, lack of, 802
retention, risk for urinary, 808
role performance, impaired, 812
sedentary behaviors, excessive, 817
self-care deficit, 829
self-compassion, inadequate, 833
self-concept, readiness for enhanced, 837
self-esteem, chronic inadequate, 845
self-esteem, situational inadequate, 851
self-injurious behavior, non-suicidal, 857–858
sensory deficit, 864
sexual functioning, impaired, 871–872
shock, risk for, 877
sitting ability, impaired, 881
skin integrity, impaired, 892–893
sleep pattern, ineffective, 896–897
social connectedness, inadequate, 903–904
social identity, readiness for enhanced transgender, 907–908
social support network, inadequate, 912–913
spiritual well-being, impaired, 919

Index

Documentation focus (*continued*)
    standing ability, impaired, 923–924
    suck-swallow response, ineffective infant, 927–928
    sudden infant death, risk for, 932
    suffocation, risk for accidental, 937–938
    suicide, risk for, 945, 951
    surgical wound infection, risk for, 956
    swallowing, impaired, 963
    thermoregulation, ineffective, 968
    thought process, disrupted, 977
    thrombosis, risk for, 980
    tissue integrity, impaired, 991–992
    tissue perfusion, ineffective peripheral, 999–1000
    tissue perfusion, risk for ineffective cerebral, 1005–1006
    transferring ability, impaired, 1009–1010
    underweight self-management, ineffective, 1018–1019
    ventilation, impaired spontaneous, 1026
    ventilatory weaning response, impaired adult, 1033
    ventilatory weaning response, impaired child, 1040–1041
    violence, risk for other-directed, 1050–1051
    walking ability, impaired, 1055
    water-electrolyte imbalance, risk for impaired, 1063–1064
    weight self-management, readiness for enhanced, 1067–1068
Down syndrome, 1116
Drug overdose, acute, 1116
Drug withdrawal, 1117
Dry eye, risk for, 242–245
Dry mouth self-management, ineffective, 246–250
Duchenne muscular dystrophy, 1117, 1152
Dysmenorrhea, 1117
Dysrhythmia, cardiac, 1117–1118

E

Eating dynamics, ineffective adolescent, 251–255
Eating dynamics, ineffective child, 256–260
Eclampsia, 1118
Ectopic pregnancy, 1118
Edema, pulmonary, 1119, 1172
Elder frailty syndrome, 261–267
Electrical injury, 1119
Electroconvulsive therapy (ECT), 1119
Elimination diagnostic division
    in adult medical/surgical assessment tool, 1199
    constipation, chronic functional, 171–176
    continence, impaired fecal, 185–192
    gastrointestinal motility, impaired, 383–391
    incontinence, disability-associated urinary, 487–494
    incontinence, mixed urinary, 494–503
    incontinence, stress urinary, 503–510
    incontinence, urge urinary, 510–517
    injury, risk for urinary tract, 555–559
    intestinal, impaired, 267–275
    nursing diagnoses related to, 1206
    in prototype plan of care, 1214
    retention, risk for urinary, 802–808
    urinary, impaired, 276–283
Elopement, risk for, 283–288
Emancipated decision-making, impaired, 289–293
Emotion regulation, ineffective, 293–297
Emphysema, 1119–1120

Encephalitis, 1120
Encopresis, 1120
Endocarditis, 1120
End-of-life comfort syndrome, impaired, 297–300
Endometriosis, 1121
Energy field, disrupted, 301–305
Enhanced exercise engagement, readiness for, 305–308
Enteral feeding, 1121
Enteritis, 1121
Enuresis, 1121
Epilepsy, 1121
Erectile dysfunction, 1121–1122
Esophageal varices, 1194

F

Failure to thrive
    adult, 1122
    infant/child, 1122
Fall, risk for, 309–316
Family identity syndrome, disrupted, 316–322
Family process, impaired, 322–328
Fatigue, 329–335
Fatigue syndrome, chronic, 1122
Fear, 336–342
Feeding
    enteral, 1121
    parenteral, 1161
Feeding behavior, impaired infant, 342–347
Female genital mutilation, risk for, 347–351
Femoral popliteal bypass, 1122–1123
Fetal alcohol syndrome, 1123
Fetal demise, 1123
Fibroids, 1193
Fibromyalgia syndrome, primary, 1123
Fluid volume
    balance, risk for impaired, 351–358
    excessive, 358–365
    inadequate, 365–374
Food/fluid diagnostic division
    in adult medical/surgical assessment tool, 1199
    blood glucose within normal limits, 51–58
    body weight problem, 83–89
    breastfeeding, difficulty performing, 90–98
    breastfeeding, interrupted, 98–105
    eating dynamics, ineffective adolescent, 251–255
    eating dynamics, ineffective child, 256–260
    feeding behavior, impaired infant, 342–347
    fluid volume, excessive, 358–365
    fluid volume, inadequate, 365–374
    fluid volume balance, risk for impaired, 351–358
    human milk production, inadequate, 451–457
    liver function, risk for impaired, 570–575
    mucous membrane, impaired oral, 627–634
    nausea, 634–640
    nipple-areolar complex integrity, impaired, 658–663
    nursing diagnoses related to, 1206–1207
    nutritional intake, inadequate, 663–671
    overweight self-management, ineffective, 675–683
    in prototype plan of care, 1214
    suck-swallow response, ineffective infant, 924–928

Food/fluid (*continued*)
 swallowing, impaired, 956–963
 underweight self-management, ineffective, 1010–1019
 water-electrolyte imbalance, risk for impaired, 1056–1064
 weight self-management, readiness for enhanced, 1064–1068
Foot sprain, 1183
Fractures, 1124
Frostbite, 1124

G

Gallstones, 1124
Gas, lung irritant, 1124
Gas exchange, impaired, 374–382
Gastritis
 acute, 1124
 chronic, 1125
Gastroenteritis, 1125
Gastroesophageal reflux disease (GERD), 1125
Gastrointestinal motility, impaired, 383–391
Gender dysphoria, 1125–1126
Genetic disorder, 1126
Gestational diabetes, 1111
Gestational hypertension, 1136–1137
Gigantism, 1126
Glaucoma, 1126
Glomerulonephritis, 1126
Goiter, 1126–1127
Gonorrhea, 1127
Gout, 1127
Grief, 391–396
 dysfunctional, 396–403
Growth, delayed child, 403–408
Guillain-Barré syndrome, 1127
Gulf War syndrome, 1127–1128
Gunshot wound, 1195–1196

H

Hallucinogen abuse, 1128
Hansen disease, 1128
Hantavirus pulmonary syndrome, 1128–1129
Hay fever, 1129
Health knowledge, inadequate, 409–415
Health literacy, inadequate, 415–420
Health maintenance behaviors, ineffective, 420–425
Health management diagnostic division
 in adult medical/surgical assessment tool, 1199–1200
 development, delayed child, 220–225
 elder frailty syndrome, 261–267
 emancipated decision-making, impaired, 289–293
 enhanced exercise engagement, readiness for, 305–308
 growth, delayed child, 403–408
 health knowledge, inadequate, 409–415
 health literacy, inadequate, 415–420
 health maintenance behaviors, ineffective, 420–425
 healthy aging, readiness for enhanced, 440–443
 ineffective community, 425–430
 ineffective family, 430–434
 nursing diagnoses related to, 1207
 in prototype plan of care, 1214–1215

self-management, ineffective, 434–440
surgical recovery, impaired, 945–951
Health promotion NDs, 2–3
Health self-management, ineffective, 434–440
Healthy aging, readiness for enhanced, 440–443
Heart failure, chronic, 1129
Heatstroke, 1129
Hematoma
  epidural, 1129–1130
  subdural-chronic, 1130
Hemodialysis, 1130
Hemophilia, 1130
Hemorrhage
  postpartum, 1130–1131
  prenatal, 1131
Hemorrhagic shock, 1181
Hemorrhoidectomy, 1131
Hemothorax, 1131
Hepatitis, acute viral, 1131–1132
Hernia, hiatal, 1132
Herniated nucleus pulposus, 1132
Heroin withdrawal, 1132–1133
Herpes simplex, 1133
Herpes zoster, 1133
High-altitude pulmonary edema (HAPE), 1133
High-altitude sickness, 1133
High-risk pregnancy, 1170
Hodgkin disease, 1134
Home maintenance behaviors, ineffective, 443–447
Hope, readiness for enhanced, 447–451
Hospice/end-of-life care, 1134–1135
Human immunodeficiency virus (HIV), 1133
  dementia, 1109
Human milk production, inadequate, 451–457
Hydrocephalus, 1135
Hyperactivity/attention-deficit disorder, 1135
Hyperbilirubinemia, 1135
  neonatal, 457–463
Hyperemesis gravidarum, 1136
Hypertension, 1136
  gestational, 1136–1137
  intrapartum, 1137
  pregnancy-induced, 1170
  pulmonary, 1137, 1172
Hyperthermia, 463–471
Hyperthyroidism, 1137
Hypoglycemia, 1137
Hypoparathyroidism, 1137–1138
Hypothermia, 1138
Hypothyroidism, 1138
Hypovolemic shock, 1181
Hysterectomy, 1138

I

Idiopathic thrombocytopenic purpura, 1172
Ileocolitis, 1138
Ileostomy, 1139
Ileus, 1139
Immigration transition, risk for disrupted, 472–476
Immunologic impairment, 476–482

Impetigo, 1139
Impulse control, ineffective, 483–487
Incontinence
    disability-associated urinary, 487–494
    mixed urinary, 494–503
    stress urinary, 503–510
    urge urinary, 510–517
Infant (at 4 weeks), 1139
Infection
    prenatal, 1139–1140
    puerperal, 1140
    risk for, 517–524
    wound, 1140
Infectious mononucleosis, 1151
Infertility, 1140
Inflammatory bowel disease, 1141
Influenza, 1141
Injury
    electrical, 1119
    pressure, 1171
    pressure, adult, 751–758
    pressure, child, 758–766
    pressure, neonatal, 767–772
    repetitive motion, 1176
    risk for burn, 525–531
    risk for cold, 531–534
    risk for corneal, 535–538
    risk for occupational physical, 538–544
    risk for perioperative positioning, 544–548
    risk for physical, 549–555
    risk for urinary tract, 555–559
    spinal cord, 1183
    sprain of ankle or foot, 1183
    traumatic brain, 1190–1191
Insulin shock, 1141
Interaction patterns, disrupted family, 559–566
International Classification for Nursing Practice (ICNP), 1, 4
Interventions
    activity intolerance, 6–11
    acute substance withdrawal syndrome, 12–17
    allergy reaction, risk for, 25–27
    anxiety, 29–35
    aspiration, risk for, 36–40
    autonomic dysreflexia, risk for, 42–44
    bleeding, risk for excessive, 46–50
    blood glucose within normal limits, 52–57
    blood pressure, risk for imbalanced, 59–62
    body image, disturbed, 65–69
    body temperature, decreased, 72–75
    body temperature, decreased neonatal, 78–79
    body temperature, risk for decreased perioperative, 81–83
    body weight problem, 84–89
    breastfeeding, difficulty performing, 91–97
    breastfeeding, interrupted, 99–104
    breathing pattern, ineffective, 106–110
    cardiac output, impaired, 113–121
    cardiovascular function, risk for impaired, 123–126
    caregiver child attachment, impaired, 128–132
    caregiving burden, excessive, 134–140
    childbearing process, ineffective, 142–151
    communication, impaired verbal, 153–159

confusion, acute, 161–165
confusion, chronic, 167–170
constipation, chronic functional, 172–175
contamination exposure, 177–185
continence, impaired fecal, 187–191
coping, difficulty, 193–199
coping, impaired community, 201–203
coping, impaired family, 205–208
death anxiety, 210–214
decision-making, impaired, 216–219
development, delayed child, 221–225
dignity, risk for compromised, 226–229
discomfort, 230–236
diversional activity engagement, decreased, 238–242
dry eye, risk for, 243–245
dry mouth self-management, ineffective, 247–250
eating dynamics, ineffective adolescent, 252–255
eating dynamics, ineffective child, 257–260
elder frailty syndrome, 262–266
elimination, impaired intestinal, 269–275
elimination, impaired urinary, 277–282
elopement, risk for, 284–288
emancipated decision-making, impaired, 290–293
emotion regulation, ineffective, 295–296
end-of-life comfort syndrome, impaired, 298–300
energy field, disrupted, 302–304
exercise engagement, readiness for enhanced, 306–308
fall, risk for, 310–315
family identity syndrome, disrupted, 317–321
family process, impaired, 323–328
fatigue, 330–335
fear, 337–341
feeding behavior, impaired infant, 343–346
female genital mutilation, risk for, 348–351
fluid volume, excessive, 359–365
fluid volume, inadequate, 366–373
fluid volume balance, risk for impaired, 352–357
gas exchange, impaired, 375–382
gastrointestinal motility, impaired, 384–390
grief, 392–395
grief, dysfunctional, 397–402
growth, delayed child, 404–408
health knowledge, inadequate, 410–414
health literacy, inadequate, 416–419
health maintenance behaviors, ineffective, 422–425
health management, ineffective community, 427–429
health management, ineffective family, 431–433
health self-management, ineffective, 435–439
healthy aging, readiness for enhanced, 441–442
home maintenance behaviors, ineffective, 444–446
hope, readiness for enhanced, 447–450
human milk production, inadequate, 453–456
hyperbilirubinemia, neonatal, 458–462
hyperthermia, 465–471
immigration transition, risk for disrupted, 472–475
immunologic impairment, 477–482
impulse control, ineffective, 484–486
incontinence, disability-associated urinary, 488–494
incontinence, mixed urinary, 495–502
incontinence, stress urinary, 504–509
incontinence, urge urinary, 511–516

Index

Interventions (*continued*)
  infection, risk for, 518–524
  injury, risk for burn, 525–530
  injury, risk for cold, 532–534
  injury, risk for corneal, 535–538
  injury, risk for occupational physical, 539–543
  injury, risk for perioperative positioning, 545–548
  injury, risk for physical, 550–554
  injury, risk for urinary tract, 556–558
  interaction patterns, disrupted family, 561–566
  latex allergy, risk for, 567–569
  liver function, risk for impaired, 571–574
  loneliness, excessive, 576–580
  lymphedema self-management, ineffective, 582–585
  maternal-fetal dyad, risk for impaired, 587–593
  memory, impaired, 595–597
  mobility, impaired bed, 599–602
  mobility, impaired physical, 604–608
  mobility, impaired wheelchair, 610–612
  mood regulation, impaired, 614–616
  moral distress, 618–621
  motor development, delayed infant, 623–626
  mucous membrane, impaired oral, 628–633
  nausea, 635–639
  neonatal abstinence syndrome, 641–645
  neurodevelopmental organization, impaired infant, 647–652
  neurovascular function, risk for impaired peripheral, 654–657
  nipple-areolar complex integrity, impaired, 659–663
  nutritional intake, inadequate, 665–671
  occupational illness, risk for, 673–674
  overweight self-management, ineffective, 677–683
  pain, acute, 685–691
  pain, chronic, and chronic pain syndrome, 694–701
  pain, labor, 704–708
  pain self-management, ineffective, 710–717
  parenting, impaired, 719–725
  personal identity, disturbed, 727–731
  poisoning, risk for, 733–737
  pressure injury, adult, 753–758
  pressure injury, child, 760–766
  pressure injury, neonatal, 768–772
  relationship, ineffective intimate partner, 774–777
  relationship problem, 779–782
  religiosity, impaired, 784–788
  relocation stress, risk for, 790–795
  resilience, lack of, 796–802
  retention, risk for urinary, 803–808
  role performance, impaired, 809–812
  in sample plan of care for diabetes mellitus, 1219–1228
  sedentary behaviors, excessive, 814–817
  self-care deficit, 820–829
  self-compassion, inadequate, 831–833
  self-concept, readiness for enhanced, 834–837
  self-esteem, chronic inadequate, 839–844
  self-esteem, situational inadequate, 846–850
  self-injurious behavior, non-suicidal, 853–857
  sensory deficit, 859–863
  sexual functioning, impaired, 866–871
  shock, risk for, 873–877
  sitting ability, impaired, 878–881
  skin integrity, impaired, 883–892

sleep pattern, ineffective, 894–896
social connectedness, inadequate, 898–903
social identity, readiness for enhanced transgender, 905–907
social support network, inadequate, 909–912
spiritual well-being, impaired, 915–919
standing ability, impaired, 921–923
suck-swallow response, ineffective infant, 925–927
sudden infant death, risk for, 929–932
suffocation, risk for accidental, 934–937
suicide, risk for, 939–944, 946–951
surgical wound infection, risk for, 952–955
swallowing, impaired, 958–963
thermoregulation, ineffective, 965–968
thought process, disrupted, 970–976
thrombosis, risk for, 978–980
tissue integrity, impaired, 983–991
tissue perfusion, ineffective peripheral, 993–999
tissue perfusion, risk for ineffective cerebral, 1001–1005
transferring ability, impaired, 1007–1009
underweight self-management, ineffective, 1012–1018
ventilation, impaired spontaneous, 1020–1026
ventilatory weaning response, impaired adult, 1028–1033
ventilatory weaning response, impaired child, 1036–1040
violence, risk for other-directed, 1042–1050
walking ability, impaired, 1052–1055
water-electrolyte imbalance, risk for impaired, 1056–1063
weight self-management, readiness for enhanced, 1065–1067
Intestinal obstruction, 1141
Iron-deficiency anemia, 1079
Irritable bowel syndrome, 1141

J

Juvenile diabetes, 1111–1112
Juvenile rheumatoid arthritis, 1084

K

Kawasaki disease, 1141
Kidney disease, polycystic, 1142
Kidney injury, acute, 1174
Kidney stone(s), 1142
Knowledge in sample plan of care for diabetes mellitus, 1223–1228

L

Labor
  induced/augmented, 1142
  precipitous, 1142
  preterm, 1142–1143
  stage I, 1143
  stage II, 1143
Laminectomy
  cervical, 1143
  lumbar, 1143–1144
Laryngectomy, 1144
Laryngitis, 1144
Latex allergy, 1144
  risk for, 567–570
Laxative abuse, 1144

Lead poisoning
  acute, 1145
  chronic, 1145
Leukemia
  acute, 1145–1146
  chronic, 1146
Liver function, risk for impaired, 570–575
Loneliness, excessive, 575–580
Long-term care, 1146–1147
Lumbar laminectomy, 1143–1144
Lung irritant gas, 1124
Lupus erythematosus, systemic (SLE), 1147
Lyme disease, 1147
Lymphedema self-management, ineffective, 581–586

M

Macular degeneration, 1147
Major depression, 1110
Malignant melanoma, 1149
Mallory-Weiss syndrome, 1147
Malnutrition, 1148
Mastectomy, 1148
Mastitis, 1148
Mastoidectomy, 1148–1149
Maternal-fetal dyad, risk for impaired, 586–593
Measles, 1149
Medical-surgical (MS) specialty area, 1069
Melanoma, malignant, 1149
Membranous croup, 1105
Memory, impaired, 594–598
Meningitis, acute meningococcal, 1149
Meniscectomy, 1149
Menopause, 1149–1150
Mental delay, 1150
Metabolic acidosis, 1072
Metabolic alkalosis, 1076
Metabolic syndrome, 1150
Mind mapping, 1229–1230
Miscarriage, 1151
Mitral stenosis, 1151
Mobility
  impaired bed, 598–603
  impaired physical, 603–609
  impaired wheelchair, 609–613
Mononucleosis, infectious, 1151
Mood disorders, 1151
Mood regulation, impaired, 613–617
Moral distress, 617–621
Motor development, delayed infant, 622–626
Mountain sickness, acute (AMS), 1151
Mucous membrane, impaired oral, 627–634
Multiple myeloma, 1153
Multiple personality, 1151
Multiple sclerosis, 1151–1152
Mumps, 1152
Muscular dystrophy (Duchenne), 1117, 1152
Myasthenia gravis, 1152–1153
Myeloma, multiple, 1153
Myocardial infarction, 1153–1154
Myocarditis, 1154

Myringotomy, 1154
Myxedema, 1154

N

NANDA-I, 1, 4
Narcolepsy, 1154
Nausea, 634–640
Necrotizing cellulitis/fasciitis, 1154
Necrotizing enterocolitis, 1155
Neglect/abuse, 1155
Neonatal abstinence syndrome, 640–645
Nephrectomy, 1155
Nephrolithiasis, 1155
Nephrotic syndrome, 1155
Neuritis, 1155
Neurodevelopmental organization, impaired infant, 646–653
Neurosensory diagnostic division
   in adult medical/surgical assessment tool, 1200
   confusion, acute, 160–166
   confusion, chronic, 166–170
   memory, impaired, 594–598
   neurodevelopmental organization, impaired infant, 646–653
   nursing diagnoses related to, 1207
   in prototype plan of care, 1215
   sensory deficit, 858–864
   thought process, disrupted, 968–977
Neurovascular function, risk for impaired peripheral, 653–658
Newborn
   at 1 week, 1156
   normal, 1155–1156
   premature, 1156–1157
Nicotine withdrawal, 1157
Nipple-areolar complex integrity, impaired, 658–663
Nonketotic hyperosmolar syndrome, 1157
Nursing diagnoses (NDs), 2–3, 1069, 1205–1210
   mind or concept mapping for, 1229–1230
Nursing outcomes & interventions classifications (NOC/NIC)
   activity intolerance, 11
   acute substance withdrawal syndrome, 18
   airway clearance, impaired, 24
   allergy reaction, risk for, 28
   anxiety, 35
   aspiration, risk for, 40
   autonomic dysreflexia, risk for, 45
   bleeding, risk for excessive, 50
   blood glucose within normal limits, 58
   blood pressure, risk for imbalanced, 63
   body image, disturbed, 70
   body temperature, decreased, 76
   body temperature, decreased neonatal, 80
   body temperature, risk for decreased perioperative, 83
   body weight problem, 89
   breastfeeding, difficulty performing, 98
   breastfeeding, interrupted, 105
   breathing pattern, ineffective, 111
   cardiac output, impaired, 121
   cardiovascular function, risk for impaired, 126
   caregiver child attachment, impaired, 132
   caregiving burden, excessive, 140

Nursing outcomes & interventions classifications (NOC/NIC) (*continued*)
- childbearing process, ineffective, 151
- communication, impaired verbal, 160
- confusion, acute, 166
- confusion, chronic, 170
- constipation, chronic functional, 176
- contamination exposure, 185
- continence, impaired fecal, 192
- coping, difficulty, 199
- coping, impaired community, 203
- coping, impaired family, 209
- death anxiety, 214
- decision-making, impaired, 220
- development, delayed child, 225
- dignity, risk for compromised, 229
- discomfort, 237
- diversional activity engagement, decreased, 242
- dry eye, risk for, 245
- dry mouth self-management, ineffective, 250
- eating dynamics, ineffective adolescent, 255
- eating dynamics, ineffective child, 260
- elder frailty syndrome, 267
- elimination, impaired intestinal, 275
- elimination, impaired urinary, 283
- elopement, risk for, 288
- emancipated decision-making, impaired, 293
- emotion regulation, ineffective, 297
- end-of-life comfort syndrome, impaired, 300
- energy field, disrupted, 305
- exercise engagement, readiness for enhanced, 308
- fall, risk for, 316
- family identity syndrome, disrupted, 322
- family process, impaired, 328
- fatigue, 335
- fear, 342
- feeding behavior, impaired infant, 347
- female genital mutilation, risk for, 351
- fluid volume, excessive, 365
- fluid volume, inadequate, 374
- fluid volume balance, risk for impaired, 358
- gas exchange, impaired, 382
- gastrointestinal motility, impaired, 391
- grief, 396
- grief, dysfunctional, 403
- growth, delayed child, 408
- health knowledge, inadequate, 415
- health literacy, inadequate, 420
- health maintenance behaviors, ineffective, 425
- health management, ineffective community, 430
- health management, ineffective family, 434
- health self-management, ineffective, 440
- healthy aging, readiness for enhanced, 443
- home maintenance behaviors, ineffective, 447
- hope, readiness for enhanced, 451
- human milk production, inadequate, 457
- hyperbilirubinemia, neonatal, 463
- hyperthermia, 471
- immigration transition, risk for disrupted, 476
- immunologic impairment, 482
- impulse control, ineffective, 487
- incontinence, disability-associated urinary, 494

incontinence, mixed urinary, 503
incontinence, stress urinary, 510
incontinence, urge urinary, 517
infection, risk for, 524
injury, risk for burn, 531
injury, risk for cold, 534
injury, risk for corneal, 538
injury, risk for occupational physical, 543
injury, risk for perioperative positioning, 548
injury, risk for physical, 555
injury, risk for urinary tract, 559
interaction patterns, disrupted family, 566
latex allergy, risk for, 570
liver function, risk for impaired, 575
loneliness, excessive, 580
lymphedema self-management, ineffective, 586
maternal-fetal dyad, risk for impaired, 593
memory, impaired, 598
mobility, impaired bed, 603
mobility, impaired physical, 609
mobility, impaired wheelchair, 613
mood regulation, impaired, 617
moral distress, 621
motor development, delayed infant, 627
mucous membrane, impaired oral, 634
nausea, 640
neonatal abstinence syndrome, 645
neurovascular function, risk for impaired peripheral, 658
nipple-areolar complex integrity, impaired, 663
nutritional intake, inadequate, 671
occupational illness, risk for, 675
overweight self-management, ineffective, 683
pain, acute, 692
pain, chronic, and chronic pain syndrome, 702
pain, labor, 708
pain self-management, ineffective, 718
parenting, impaired, 725
personal identity, disturbed, 731
poisoning, risk for, 737
post-trauma syndrome, 751
pressure injury, adult, 758
pressure injury, child, 766
pressure injury, neonatal, 772
relationship, ineffective intimate partner, 777
relationship problem, 782
religiosity, impaired, 789
relocation stress, risk for, 795
resilience, lack of, 802
retention, risk for urinary, 808
role performance, impaired, 812
sedentary behaviors, excessive, 817
self-care deficit, 829–830
self-compassion, inadequate, 834
self-concept, readiness for enhanced, 838
self-esteem, chronic inadequate, 845
self-esteem, situational inadequate, 851
self-injurious behavior, non-suicidal, 858
sensory deficit, 864
sexual functioning, impaired, 872
shock, risk for, 877
sitting ability, impaired, 882

Index

Nursing outcomes & interventions classifications (NOC/NIC) (*continued*)
    skin integrity, impaired, 893
    sleep pattern, ineffective, 897
    social connectedness, inadequate, 904
    social identity, readiness for enhanced transgender, 908
    social support network, inadequate, 913
    spiritual well-being, impaired, 920
    standing ability, impaired, 924
    suck-swallow response, ineffective infant, 928
    sudden infant death, risk for, 933
    suffocation, risk for accidental, 938
    suicide, risk for, 945, 951
    surgical wound infection, risk for, 956
    swallowing, impaired, 963
    thermoregulation, ineffective, 968
    thought process, disrupted, 977
    thrombosis, risk for, 980
    tissue integrity, impaired, 992
    tissue perfusion, ineffective peripheral, 1000
    tissue perfusion, risk for ineffective cerebral, 1006
    transferring ability, impaired, 1010
    underweight self-management, ineffective, 1019
    ventilation, impaired spontaneous, 1026
    ventilatory weaning response, impaired adult, 1034
    ventilatory weaning response, impaired child, 1041
    violence, risk for other-directed, 1051
    walking ability, impaired, 1055
    water-electrolyte imbalance, risk for impaired, 1064
    weight self-management, readiness for enhanced, 1068
Nursing process, 1–4
Nutritional intake, inadequate, 663–671

O

Obesity, 1157–1158
Obsessive-compulsive disorder, 1158
Obstetric/gynecological (OB/GYN) specialty area, 1069
Occupational illness, risk for, 672–675
Opioid abuse, 1158
Oppositional defiant disorder, 1158
Organic brain syndrome, 1158
Osteoarthritis, 1107, 1158
Osteomyelitis, 1158
Osteoporosis, 1159
Overweight self-management, ineffective, 675–683

P

Pain
    acute, 684–692
    chronic pain syndrome and chronic, 692–702
    labor, 702–708
    in sample plan of care for diabetes mellitus, 1222
    self-management, ineffective, 709–717
Palsy, cerebral, 1159
Pancreatitis, 1159
Panic disorder, 1159–1160
Paranoid personality disorder, 1160
Paraplegia, 1160
Parathyroidectomy, 1161

Parent-child relational problem, 1161
Parenteral feeding, 1161
Parenting, impaired, 718–725
Parkinson disease, 1161–1162
Pediatric (PED) specialty area, 1069
Pelvic inflammatory disease, 1162
Peptic ulcer, 1192
Periarteritis nodosa, 1162
Pericarditis, 1162
Perinatal loss/death of child, 1162–1163
Peripheral arterial occlusive disease, 1163
Peripheral vascular disease, 1163
Peritoneal dialysis, 1113
Peritonitis, 1163
Pernicious anemia, 1079
Personal identity, disturbed, 726–731
Pheochromocytoma, 1163–1164
Phlebitis, 1164
Phobia, 1164
Physical abuse, 1071
Placenta previa, 1164
Plan of care
    client situation and prototype, 1212–1218
    for client with diabetes mellitus, 1219–1228
    mind or concept mapping in, 1229–1230
Pleurisy, 1164
Pneumonia, 1164
Pneumothorax, 1164–1165
Poisoning
    lead, acute, 1145
    lead, chronic, 1145
    risk for, 732–737
Polyarteritis nodosa, 1165
Polycythemia vera, 1165
Polyradiculitis, acute inflammatory, 1165
Postoperative recovery period, 1165–1166
Postpartum depression, 1110–1111
Postpartum hemorrhage, 1130–1131
Postpartum period
    4 to 48 hours, 1166
    postdischarge to 4 weeks, 1166–1167
Postpartum psychosis, 1167
Postpolio syndrome, 1167
Post-trauma syndrome, 738–751
Post-traumatic stress disorder (PTSD), 1167–1168
Pregnancy
    1st trimester, 1168
    2nd trimester, 1169
    3rd trimester, 1169
    abortion, elective termination, 1070
    abortion, spontaneous termination, 1070
    abruptio placentae, 1070
    adolescent, 1169–1170
    cesarean birth, postpartal, 1097
    cesarean birth, unplanned, 1097–1098
    childbearing process, ineffective, 141–151
    delivery, precipitous/out of hospital, 1108
    dilation of cervix, premature, 1114
    eclampsia, 1118
    ectopic, 1118

Pregnancy (*continued*)
   gestational diabetes, 1111
   gestational hypertension, 1136–1137
   hemorrhage, prenatal, 1131
   high-risk, 1170
   hyperemesis gravidarum, 1136
   intrapartum hypertension, 1137
   placenta previa, 1164
   toxemia of, 1189
Pregnancy-induced hypertension, 1170
Premenstrual dysphoric disorder, 1170
Premenstrual tension syndrome, 1170
Prenatal infection, 1139–1140
Presenile/senile dementia, 1109
Pressure injury, 1171
   adult, 751–758
   child, 758–766
   neonatal, 767–772
Preterm labor, 1142–1143
Problem-focused NDs, 2
Prostatectomy, 1171
Pruritus, 1171
Psoriasis, 1171
Psychiatric/behavioral (PSY) specialty area, 1069
Psychological abuse, 1071
Puerperal infection, 1140
Puerperal sepsis, 1180
Pulmonary edema, 1119, 1172
Pulmonary embolus, 1172
Pulmonary hypertension, 1137, 1172
Purpura, idiopathic thrombocytopenic, 1172
Pyelonephritis, 1173

Q

Quadriplegia, 1173

R

Rape, 1173–1174
Raynaud disease, 1174
Reflex sympathetic dystrophy (RSD), 1174
Regional enteritis, 1174
Relationship, ineffective intimate partner, 773–777
Relationship problem, 778–782
   parent-child, 1161
Religiosity, impaired, 783–789
Relocation stress, risk for, 789–795
Renal disease, end-stage, 1174
Renal failure
   acute, 1174
   chronic, 1174–1175
Renal transplantation, 1175
Repetitive motion injury, 1176
Resilience, lack of, 795–802
Respiration diagnostic division
   in adult medical/surgical assessment tool, 1200–1201
   airway clearance, impaired, 18–24
   aspiration, risk for, 35–40
   breathing pattern, ineffective, 105–111
   gas exchange, impaired, 374–382

nursing diagnoses related to, 1207
in prototype plan of care, 1216
ventilation, impaired spontaneous, 1019–1026
ventilatory weaning response, impaired adult, 1027–1034
ventilatory weaning response, impaired child, 1034–1041

Respiratory acidosis, 1072
Respiratory alkalosis, 1076
Respiratory distress syndrome
  acute, 1176
  premature infant, 1176
Respiratory syncytial virus (RSV), 1176
Retention, risk for urinary, 802–808
Retinal detachment, 1177
Reye syndrome, 1177
Rheumatic fever, 1177
Rheumatoid arthritis, 1084
Rickets, 1177
Ringworm, tinea, 1177–1178
Risk NDs, 2
Role performance, impaired, 808–812
Roles/relationships diagnostic division
  in adult medical/surgical assessment tool, 1201
  caregiver child attachment, impaired, 126–132
  caregiving burden, excessive, 133–140
  communication, impaired verbal, 151–160
  coping, impaired community, 200–203
  coping, impaired family, 203–208
  family identity syndrome, disrupted, 316–322
  family process, impaired, 322–328
  interaction patterns, disrupted family, 559–566
  loneliness, excessive, 575–580
  nursing diagnoses related to, 1207–1208
  parenting, impaired, 718–725
  in prototype plan of care, 1216
  relationship, ineffective intimate partner, 773–777
  relationship problem, 778–782
  role performance, impaired, 808–812
  social connectedness, inadequate, 897–904
  social support network, inadequate, 908–913
Rubella, 1178
Ruptured intervertebral disc, 1132

S

Safety
  acute substance withdrawal syndrome, 11–18
  in adult medical/surgical assessment tool, 1201
  allergy reaction, risk for, 24–28
  body temperature, decreased, 70–76
  body temperature, decreased neonatal, 76–80
  body temperature, risk for decreased perioperative, 80–83
  contamination exposure, 176–185
  elopement, risk for, 283–288
  fall, risk for, 309–316
  hyperbilirubinemia, neonatal, 457–463
  hyperthermia, 463–471
  immunologic impairment, 476–482
  infection, risk for, 517–524
  injury, risk for burn, 525–531
  injury, risk for cold, 531–534

Safety (*continued*)
    injury, risk for corneal, 535–538
    injury, risk for occupational physical, 538–544
    injury, risk for perioperative positioning, 544–548
    injury, risk for physical, 549–555
    injury, risk for urinary tract, 555–559
    latex allergy, risk for, 567–570
    neonatal abstinence syndrome, 640–645
    nursing diagnoses related to, 1208
    occupational illness, risk for, 672–675
    poisoning, risk for, 732–737
    pressure injury, adult, 751–758
    pressure injury, child, 758–766
    pressure injury, neonatal, 767–772
    in prototype plan of care, 1216–1217
    sitting ability, impaired, 877–882
    skin integrity, impaired, 882–892
    sudden infant death, risk for, 928–933
    suffocation, risk for accidental, 933–938
    suicide, risk for, 938–945
    surgical wound infection, risk for, 952–956
    thermoregulation, ineffective, 964–968
    tissue integrity, impaired, 981–991
Scabies, 1178
Scarlet fever, 1178
Schizophrenia, 1178–1179
Sciatica, 1179
Scientific method, 1–2
Scleroderma, 1179
Scoliosis, 1179
Seasonal affective disorder, 1075
Sedentary behaviors, excessive, 813–818
Seizure disorder, 1180
Self-care diagnostic division
    in adult medical/surgical assessment tool, 1202
    deficit, 818–830
    home maintenance behaviors, ineffective, 443–447
    nursing diagnoses related to, 1209
    in prototype plan of care, 1217
Self-compassion, inadequate, 830–834
Self-concept, readiness for enhanced, 834–838
Self-esteem, chronic inadequate, 838–845
Self-esteem, situational inadequate, 845–851
Self-injurious behavior, non-suicidal, 851–858
Self-perception/concept diagnostic division
    in adult medical/surgical assessment tool, 1202–1203
    body image, disturbed, 63–70
    dignity, risk for compromised, 225–229
    hope, readiness for enhanced, 447–451
    impulse control, ineffective, 483–487
    mood regulation, impaired, 613–617
    nursing diagnoses related to, 1209
    personal identity, disturbed, 726–731
    in prototype plan of care, 1217
    resilience, lack of, 795–802
    self-compassion, inadequate, 830–834
    self-concept, readiness for enhanced, 834–838
    self-esteem, chronic inadequate, 838–845
    self-esteem, situational inadequate, 845–851
    social identity, readiness for enhanced transgender, 904–908
Sensory deficit, 858–864

Sepsis, 1180
  puerperal, 1180
Septic arthritis, 1084
Septic shock, 1181
Serum sickness, 1181
Sexual functioning, impaired, 865–872
Sexuality/reproduction diagnostic division
  in adult medical/surgical assessment tool, 1203
  childbearing process, ineffective, 141–151
  female genital mutilation, risk for, 347–351
  maternal-fetal dyad, risk for impaired, 586–593
  nursing diagnoses related to, 1209
  in prototype plan of care, 1217
  sexual functioning, impaired, 865–872
Sexually transmitted infection (STI), 1181
Shingles, 1133
Shock, 1181
  cardiogenic, 1094, 1181
  hypovolemic/hemorrhagic, 1181
  risk for, 872–877
  septic, 1181
Sickle cell anemia, 1079
Sick sinus syndrome, 1182
Sitting ability, impaired, 877–882
Skin integrity, impaired, 882–892
Skin/tissue abscess, 1071
Sleep apnea, 1182
Sleep pattern, ineffective, 893–897
Smallpox, 1182
Snow blindness, 1182–1183
Social connectedness, inadequate, 897–904
Social identity, readiness for enhanced transgender, 904–908
Social support network, inadequate, 908–913
Solutions
  activity intolerance, 6
  acute substance withdrawal syndrome, 12
  airway clearance, impaired, 19
  allergy reaction, risk for, 25
  anxiety, 29
  aspiration, risk for, 36
  autonomic dysreflexia, risk for, 42
  bleeding, risk for excessive, 46
  blood glucose within normal limits, 52
  blood pressure, risk for imbalanced, 59
  body image, disturbed, 64–65
  body temperature, decreased, 71
  body temperature, decreased neonatal, 77–78
  body temperature, risk for decreased perioperative, 81
  body weight problem, 84
  breastfeeding, difficulty performing, 91
  breastfeeding, interrupted, 99
  breathing pattern, ineffective, 106
  cardiac output, impaired, 112–113
  cardiovascular function, risk for impaired, 122
  caregiver child attachment, impaired, 127–128
  caregiving burden, excessive, 134
  childbearing process, ineffective, 142
  communication, impaired verbal, 153
  confusion, acute, 161
  confusion, chronic, 166–167

Solutions (*continued*)
  constipation, chronic functional, 172
  contamination exposure, 177
  continence, impaired fecal, 186
  coping, difficulty, 193
  coping, impaired community, 200
  coping, impaired family, 205
  death anxiety, 210
  decision-making, impaired, 216
  development, delayed child, 221
  dignity, risk for compromised, 226
  discomfort, 230
  diversional activity engagement, decreased, 238
  dry eye, risk for, 243
  dry mouth self-management, ineffective, 247
  eating dynamics, ineffective adolescent, 252
  eating dynamics, ineffective child, 257
  elder frailty syndrome, 262
  elimination, impaired intestinal, 268, 276–277
  elopement, risk for, 284
  emancipated decision-making, impaired, 289–290
  emotion regulation, ineffective, 294
  end-of-life comfort syndrome, impaired, 298
  energy field, disrupted, 301
  exercise engagement, readiness for enhanced, 306
  fall, risk for, 309–310
  family identity syndrome, disrupted, 317
  family process, impaired, 323
  fatigue, 329–330
  fear, 337
  feeding behavior, impaired infant, 343
  female genital mutilation, risk for, 347–348
  fluid volume, excessive, 359
  fluid volume, inadequate, 366
  fluid volume balance, risk for impaired, 352
  gas exchange, impaired, 375
  gastrointestinal motility, impaired, 383–384
  grief, 392
  grief, dysfunctional, 397
  growth, delayed child, 404
  health knowledge, inadequate, 410
  health literacy, inadequate, 416
  health maintenance behaviors, ineffective, 421–422
  health management, ineffective community, 426
  health management, ineffective family, 431
  health self-management, ineffective, 435
  healthy aging, readiness for enhanced, 440
  home maintenance behaviors, ineffective, 444
  hope, readiness for enhanced, 447
  human milk production, inadequate, 452
  hyperbilirubinemia, neonatal, 458
  hyperthermia, 465
  immigration transition, risk for disrupted, 472
  immunologic impairment, 477
  impulse control, ineffective, 483–484
  incontinence, disability-associated urinary, 488
  incontinence, mixed urinary, 495
  incontinence, stress urinary, 503
  incontinence, urge urinary, 511
  infection, risk for, 517–518
  injury, risk for burn, 525

injury, risk for cold, 531
injury, risk for corneal, 535
injury, risk for occupational physical, 539
injury, risk for perioperative positioning, 545
injury, risk for physical, 549
injury, risk for urinary tract, 555
interaction patterns, disrupted family, 560–561
latex allergy, risk for, 567
liver function, risk for impaired, 570–571
loneliness, excessive, 576
lymphedema self-management, ineffective, 582
maternal-fetal dyad, risk for impaired, 587
memory, impaired, 594–595
mobility, impaired bed, 599
mobility, impaired physical, 604
mobility, impaired wheelchair, 610
mood regulation, impaired, 614
moral distress, 618
motor development, delayed infant, 623
mucous membrane, impaired oral, 628
nausea, 635
neonatal abstinence syndrome, 641
neurodevelopmental organization, impaired infant, 647
neurovascular function, risk for impaired peripheral, 654
nipple-areolar complex integrity, impaired, 659
nutritional intake, inadequate, 665
occupational illness, risk for, 672–673
overweight self-management, ineffective, 677
pain, acute, 685
pain, chronic, and chronic pain syndrome, 693–694
pain, labor, 703
pain self-management, ineffective, 710
parenting, impaired, 719
personal identity, disturbed, 727
poisoning, risk for, 732
post-trauma syndrome, 739–750
pressure injury, adult, 752
pressure injury, child, 760
pressure injury, neonatal, 768
relationship, ineffective intimate partner, 774
relationship problem, 778–779
religiosity, impaired, 783–784
relocation stress, risk for, 790
resilience, lack of, 795
retention, risk for urinary, 803
role performance, impaired, 809
sedentary behaviors, excessive, 814
self-care deficit, 820
self-compassion, inadequate, 831
self-concept, readiness for enhanced, 834
self-esteem, chronic inadequate, 839
self-esteem, situational inadequate, 846
self-injurious behavior, non-suicidal, 853
sensory deficit, 859
sexual functioning, impaired, 866
shock, risk for, 872–873
sitting ability, impaired, 878
skin integrity, impaired, 883
sleep pattern, ineffective, 894
social connectedness, inadequate, 898
social identity, readiness for enhanced transgender, 905

Solutions (*continued*)
  social support network, inadequate, 909
  spiritual well-being, impaired, 914
  standing ability, impaired, 921
  suck-swallow response, ineffective infant, 925
  sudden infant death, risk for, 928
  suffocation, risk for accidental, 934
  suicide, risk for, 939, 946
  surgical wound infection, risk for, 952
  swallowing, impaired, 958
  thermoregulation, ineffective, 964
  thought process, disrupted, 970
  thrombosis, risk for, 978
  tissue integrity, impaired, 982
  tissue perfusion, ineffective peripheral, 993
  tissue perfusion, risk for ineffective cerebral, 1001
  transferring ability, impaired, 1007
  underweight self-management, ineffective, 1012
  ventilation, impaired spontaneous, 1020
  ventilatory weaning response, impaired adult, 1028
  ventilatory weaning response, impaired child, 1035–1036
  violence, risk for other-directed, 1042
  walking ability, impaired, 1052
  water-electrolyte imbalance, risk for impaired, 1056
  weight self-management, readiness for enhanced, 1065
Somatoform disorders, 1183
Spinal cord injury (SCI), 1183
Spiritual well-being, impaired, 913–920
Sprain of ankle or foot, 1183
Standing ability, impaired, 920–923
Stapedectomy, 1183
Stimulant abuse, 1184
Stress management diagnostic division
  in adult medical/surgical assessment tool, 1203
  anxiety, 28–35
  coping, difficulty, 192–199
  death anxiety, 209–214
  emotion regulation, ineffective, 293–297
  energy field, disrupted, 301–305
  fear, 336–342
  grief, 391–396
  grief, dysfunctional, 396–403
  immigration transition, risk for disrupted, 472–476
  nursing diagnoses related to, 1209
  post-trauma syndrome, 738–751
  in prototype plan of care, 1217–1218
  relocation stress, risk for, 789–795
  self-injurious behavior, non-suicidal, 851–858
  suicide, risk for, 935–945
  violence, risk for other-directed, 1041–1051
Substance dependence/abuse rehabilitation, 1184–1185
Suck-swallow response, ineffective infant, 924–928
Sudden infant death, 1185
  risk for, 928–933
Suffocation, risk for accidental, 933–938
Suicide, risk for, 938–945
Surgery, general, 1185
Surgical recovery, impaired, 945–951
Surgical wound infection, risk for, 952–956
Swallowing, impaired, 956–963
Syndrome NDs, 3

Synovitis (knee), 1185–1186
Syphilis, congenital, 1186
Syringomyelia, 1186
Systemic lupus erythematosus (SLE), 1147
Systems theory, 2

T

Tay-Sachs disease, 1186
Thermoregulation, ineffective, 964–968
Thought process, disrupted, 968–977
Thrombophlebitis, 1187
Thrombosis, risk for, 977–980
Thrush, 1187
Thyroidectomy, 1187
Thyrotoxicosis, 1188
Tic douloureux, 1188
Tissue integrity, impaired, 981–991
Tissue perfusion
 ineffective peripheral, 992–1000
 risk for ineffective cerebral, 1000–1006
Tonsillectomy, 1188
Tonsillitis, 1188
Total joint replacement, 1188–1189
Toxemia of pregnancy, 1189
Toxic shock syndrome, 1189
Traction, 1189
Transferring ability, impaired, 1006–1010
Transfusion reaction, blood, 1189
Transient ischemic attack (TIA), 1190
Transplantation, recipient, 1190
Traumatic brain injury (TBI), 1190–1191
Trichinosis, 1191
Tuberculosis, 1191–1192
Typhus, 1192

U

Ulcer
 peptic, 1192
 venous stasis, 1192
Unconsciousness, 1192
Underweight self-management, ineffective, 1010–1019
Urinary calculi, 1092
Urinary diversion, 1192–1193
Urolithiasis, 1193
Uterine bleeding, dysfunctional, 1193
Uterine myomas, 1193

V

Vaginitis, 1193
Values/beliefs diagnostic division
 in adult medical/surgical assessment tool, 1204
 decision-making, impaired, 215–220
 moral distress, 617–621
 nursing diagnoses related to, 1210
 in prototype plan of care, 1218
 religiosity, impaired, 783–789
 spiritual well-being, impaired, 913–920
Valvular heart disease, 1193–1194

Varices, esophageal, 1194
Varicose veins, 1194
Venereal disease, 1194
Venous stasis ulcer, 1192
Ventilation, impaired spontaneous, 1019–1026
Ventilator assist/dependence, 1194–1195
Ventilatory weaning response
  impaired adult, 1027–1034
  impaired child, 1034–1041
Ventricular aneurysm, 1080
Ventricular fibrillation, 1195
Ventricular tachycardia, 1195
Violence, risk for other-directed, 1041–1051

W

Walking ability, impaired, 1051–1055
Water-electrolyte imbalance, risk for impaired, 1056–1064
Weight self-management, readiness for enhanced, 1064–1068
West Nile fever, 1195
Wilms tumor, 1195
Wound, gunshot, 1195–1196
Wound infection, 1140
  in sample plan of care for diabetes mellitus, 1219–1220